Veterinary Neuroanatomy AND Clinical Neurology

THIRD EDITION

Veterinary Neuroanatomy
AND Clinical Neurology

Alexander de Lahunta
DVM, PhD, DACVIM, DACVP

James Law Professor of Anatomy-Emeritus
Rye, New Hampshire

Eric Glass
MS, DVM, DACVIM (Neurology)

Section Head, Neurology and Neurosurgery
Red Bank Veterinary Hospital
Tinton Falls, New Jersey

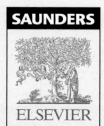

SAUNDERS

ELSEVIER

SAUNDERS

ELSEVIER

11830 Westline Industrial Drive
St. Louis, Missouri 63146

Library of Congress Cataloging-in-Publication Data

DeLahunta, Alexander, 1932-
 Veterinary neuroanatomy and clinical neurology / Alexander de Lahunta, Eric Glass.—
3rd ed.
      p.   ;   cm.
 Includes bibliographical references and index.
 ISBN 978-0-7216-6706-5 (hardcover : alk. paper) 1. Veterinary neurology. 2. Veterinary
anatomy. 3. Neuroanatomy. I. Glass, Eric. II. Title.
 [DNLM: 1. Anatomy, Veterinary. 2. Nervous System Diseases—veterinary. 3. Nervous
System—anatomy & histology. SF 895 D278v 2009]
 SF895. D44 2009
 636.089'18—dc22

978-0-7216-6706-5

Vice President and Publisher: Linda Duncan
Publisher: Penny Rudolph
Developmental Editor: Shelly Stringer
Publishing Services Manager: Julie Eddy
Project Manager: Laura Loveall
Designer: Teresa McBryan

Printed in China.

Last digit is the print number: 9   8   7   6   5   4   3   2

VIDEOS ONLINE

The disease portion of each chapter of this textbook is primarily presented in the form of individual patient case examples. Most of these case examples and clinical disorders are illustrated with videos. These online videos are hosted by Cornell University College of Veterinary Medicine. They are organized and identified by the chapters in this textbook where each video is described.

The videos can be accessed at **www.neurovideos.vet.cornell.edu.**

It is my profound privilege to write this foreword to the third edition of *Veterinary Neuroanatomy and Clinical Neurology*, a remarkable collaboration between Drs. Alexander de Lahunta and Eric Glass. This anxiously anticipated textbook recaptures and updates the multifaceted aspects of veterinary neurology, advanced neurodiagnostics, neuroanatomy, and neuropathology, many aspects of which Dr. de Lahunta himself defined during his distinguished career at Cornell University. The third edition undoubtedly will withstand the test of time as an invaluable contribution to the disciplines of veterinary internal medicine, neurology, and neurosurgery.

The emphasis of the third edition remains the *neuroanatomic diagnosis*, and this is accomplished elegantly in parallel with descriptions of key differential diagnoses and current diagnostic techniques. The textbook is referenced meticulously, providing the reader the opportunity to further explore individual neurologic disorders. Hundreds of color illustrations, case photographs, and web-based case videos are utilized to provide an invaluable resource for the student, general practitioner, or specialist wishing to develop or expand their understanding of neuroanatomy and clinical neurology.

Those who have been taught by or worked with Dr. de Lahunta invariably conclude that he is one of the greatest veterinary teachers of the past several generations. Dr. de Lahunta's innumerable college, national, and international teaching awards recognize his tremendous contributions to veterinary education. His inherent ability to teach such a complex topic is largely due to his steadfast commitment to a vertically integrated learning process whereby neuroembryology, neuroanatomy, clinical neurology, and neuropathology are taught as a continuum. For 42 years, Dr. de Lahunta preached that a basic understanding of neuroanatomy is indispensible for one to determine the anatomic localization and, in turn, to generate the correct differential diagnosis in neurological patients. Dr. de Lahunta recognized early in his career that neuroanatomy and clinical neurology are inseparable, and the third edition is a testament to this philosophy.

The inseparability of neuroanatomy and clinical neurology may be best epitomized by Dr. de Lahunta's ability to interpret MRIs of the brain and spinal cord, a technique that came to the forefront of the specialty during the last decade of his career. As his resident, I had the unique opportunity to observe Dr. de Lahunta develop an immediate and natural mastery of MR imaging, which undoubtedly evolved from his vast experience studying gross and histopathologic specimens from clinical cases. In the third edition, Dr. de Lahunta's unique appreciation for the complexities of the diseased nervous system, combined with Dr. Glass' clinical perspective derived from an immense caseload in specialty practice, seamlessly merge the disciplines of neuroanatomy and neuropathology together with clinical neurology and state of the art neurodiagnostics.

A foreword to this textbook would be remiss to ignore Dr. de Lahunta's warmth, selflessness, and humanistic qualities. Dr. de Lahunta has *always* found time to answer innumerable formal and informal consultation requests from all over the world, help students with their studies and projects, and mentor interns and residents, all the while making landmark contributions to the discipline of veterinary neurology. He has set the bar incredibly high for academic neurologists. We should all aspire to share of our time and experiences with others as Dr. de Lahunta has done so gracefully for over four decades.

In closing, the third edition of *Veterinary Neuroanatomy and Clinical Neurology* provides the critical building blocks necessary to gain competence in the discipline of veterinary neurology. On behalf of neurologists world wide, I would like to thank Drs. de Lahunta and Glass for collaborating on this new edition which promises to be the new *treatise* of neuroanatomic localization and clinical neurology.

Congratulations and please accept our sincere gratitude for all of the time, energy, and wisdom you have shared with all of us through the years.

S. J. Schatzberg

Scott J. Schatzberg, DVM, PhD, DACVIM (Neurology)
University of Georgia College of Veterinary Medicine

This third edition is a revision based on my 42 years of experience in teaching a vertically integrated course in veterinary neuroanatomy and clinical neurology to first year veterinary students at the Cornell University College of Veterinary Medicine. The clinical information evolved from my experience as a consultant to the Teaching Hospital that received patients with neurological disorders, consulting with veterinary practitioners, and my involvement with the neuropathological studies of hospital patients and specimens sent to me by veterinary practitioners and pathologists. My studies were greatly enhanced by my interaction with Drs. John Cummings and Brian Summers. I consider these two colleagues as close friends and brilliant veterinary scientists.

When I first organized a course in neuroanatomy for the veterinary curriculum at Cornell University in 1963, I was strongly influenced by two outstanding veterinary pathologists who in 1956 and 1965 published their experiences in correlating neurological signs with the location of lesions in the nervous system.[1,2] These were Dr. Jack McGrath at the University of Pennsylvania and Dr. Tony Palmer at Cambridge University. They set a standard that I wanted to pursue. I felt strongly that teaching neuroanatomy solely for the sake of the anatomical training was not a useful expenditure of the student's limited time or that of the busy teacher. It is the one system that needs to be closely correlated with the study of the clinical signs to be useful to the student as a veterinary practitioner. The teaching of clinical veterinary medicine is the primary objective of the curriculum at Cornell University. Drs. McGrath and Palmer set this standard that became the basis for my entire professional career and the correlated course that I taught to first year veterinary students for 42 years. This course provided all the useful neuroanatomy and clinical neurology simultaneously. This has been an exciting experience for me that has been rewarded by observing the success of my students in this clinical specialty and by observing the satisfaction expressed by the students who have mastered the ability to diagnose neurological disorders.

The emphasis of this third edition is the *anatomic diagnosis,* which is the basis for the successful practice of clinical neurology and is presented in the form of case examples. Disease descriptions are presented in the form of differential diagnoses of individual case examples. Although many neurological disorders will be described, this revision makes no attempt to present a complete synopsis of the veterinary neurological literature. This has been adequately covered in other textbooks of veterinary neurology. A unique feature of this text is the linking of the case descriptions to videos of these patients which are available on a website that is organized by the chapters of this text. There are 380 videotapes on this website that show most of the neurological disorders that are described in this text. This can be accessed at: www.neurovideos.vet.cornell.edu.

My coauthor, Dr. Eric Glass, is a former student of mine who graduated from the College of Veterinary Medicine at Cornell University in 1995. He is the senior neurologist at Red Bank Veterinary Hospital, a very active specialty practice in Tinton Falls, New Jersey, where he has ten years of practice experience. Eric brings a clinician's perspective to the understanding of neuroanatomy. I am honored to have his contributions to this textbook. Eric and I have agreed on most areas of controversy in clinical neurology and have presented our combined opinions in this text. We present these controversies as well as differences of opinion as challenges for the present and future veterinary neurologists to support or deny.

Alexander de Lahunta

1. McGrath, JT: *Neurologic examination of the dog with clinicopathologic observations*, 1956, Philadelphia, PA, Lea and Febiger.
2. Palmer, AC: *Introduction to animal neurology*, 1965, Philadelphia, PA, F.A. Davis.

CONTENTS

1 INTRODUCTION, *1*

2 NEUROANATOMY BY DISSECTION, *6*

3 DEVELOPMENT OF THE NERVOUS SYSTEM: MALFORMATION, *23*

4 CEREBROSPINAL FLUID AND HYDROCEPHALUS, *54*

5 LOWER MOTOR NEURON: SPINAL NERVE, GENERAL SOMATIC EFFERENT SYSTEM, *77*

6 LOWER MOTOR NEURON: GENERAL SOMATIC EFFERENT, CRANIAL NERVE, *134*

7 LOWER MOTOR NEURON: GENERAL VISCERAL EFFERENT SYSTEM, *168*

8 UPPER MOTOR NEURON, *192*

9 GENERAL SENSORY SYSTEMS: GENERAL PROPRIOCEPTION AND GENERAL SOMATIC AFFERENT, *221*

10 SMALL ANIMAL SPINAL CORD DISEASE, *243*

11 LARGE ANIMAL SPINAL CORD DISEASE, *285*

12 VESTIBULAR SYSTEM: SPECIAL PROPRIOCEPTION, *319*

13 CEREBELLUM, *348*

14 VISUAL SYSTEM, *389*

15 AUDITORY SYSTEM: SPECIAL SOMATIC AFFERENT SYSTEM, *433*

16 VISCERAL AFFERENT SYSTEMS, *441*

17 NONOLFACTORY RHINENCEPHALON: LIMBIC SYSTEM, *448*

18 SEIZURE DISORDERS: NARCOLEPSY, *454*

19 DIENCEPHALON, *476*

20 THE NEUROLOGIC EXAMINATION, *487*

21 CASE DESCRIPTIONS, *502*

1 INTRODUCTION

OBJECTIVE

ACCURATE DIAGNOSIS

Malformations
Inflammations
Injuries
Neoplasias
Degenerations

NEURON

FUNCTIONAL SYSTEMS

SENSORY (AFFERENT)

Somatic Afferent
    General Somatic Afferent
    Special Somatic Afferent
Visceral Afferent
    General Visceral Afferent
    Special Visceral Afferent

Proprioception
    General Proprioception
    Special Proprioception

MOTOR (EFFERENT)

General Somatic Efferent
General Visceral Efferent

FURTHER READING

OBJECTIVE

This book was written primarily for the veterinary student and secondarily for the veterinary practitioner. It is organized to provide the veterinary student with an anatomic basis and sufficient information about the development, organization, and function of the nervous system to be able to understand and diagnose the more common disorders of the nervous system of domestic animals. For the most part, these disorders are described in the chapter that discusses the functional system primarily affected by the disorder.

ACCURATE DIAGNOSIS

The major objective of this book is to teach enough of the morphologic and physiologic features of the nervous system to enable the student to make an accurate localization of the lesion in the nervous system. This is the *anatomic* diagnosis. The *differential* diagnosis is totally dependent on the anatomic diagnosis and that, in turn, determines the ancillary procedures that will be prioritized to arrive at the most accurate presumptive clinical diagnosis and the subsequent selection of treatment.

The diagnosis of clinical neurologic disorders starts with recognition of the problem—the clinical signs exhibited by the patient and your neurologic examination. This visual and hands-on experience is difficult to learn by reading text descriptions. Direct contact with the affected patient is the ideal teaching model but is impractical in a teaching environment. The most effective alternative is to visualize the clinical signs using video technology. This third edition includes linkage to a website consisting of 381 videos that provide the student with the classical appearance of the common disorders of the nervous system of domestic animals. The anatomic diagnosis is determined by the nature of the problem; that is, clinical signs that you have observed. You should first attempt to determine whether all the clinical signs can be explained by a lesion at one site in the nervous system, a focal lesion, because they are more common than multifocal or diffuse disorders. Based on this anatomic diagnosis, you will next establish a list of disorders that must be able to affect the anatomic location of the lesion. This is the differential diagnosis. You will learn various ways to remind yourself of the disorders to consider. One way is the MIIND system (malformation, injury, inflammation, neoplasia, and degeneration).

Malformations

Malformations are the disorders that result from abnormal development of the nervous system.

Inflammations

Inflammations involve a pathologic process and a reaction of blood vessels and tissues to physical, chemical, and biologic agents—the reaction of a tissue to an irritant. In the nervous system, this commonly refers to the tissues' reaction to a microorganism or an immune system abnormality. Suppurative inflammation is characterized by a neutrophilic response and the products of necrosis of tissue and inflammatory cells usually caused by a bacterium, protozoa, or fungus. Nonsuppurative inflammation is characterized by a lymphocytic or monocytic response and is usually caused by a viral agent or an immune system abnormality.

Injuries

Injuries occur when nervous tissue undergoes traumatic disturbance deriving from external or internal sources. These cause acute or chronic displacements and disruptions or vascular impairment of the nervous tissue, which may result in hemorrhage, edema, or parenchymal necrosis.

Neoplasias

Neoplasias are uncontrolled growth of cells. Primary central nervous system (CNS) neoplasias include the uncontrolled growth of nervous tissue cells—neurons, glia, and ependyma. Metastatic neoplasia of the nervous system is the spread of primary neoplasms in other body tissues to the nervous system.

Degenerations

Degenerations include the deterioration of cells due to lack of blood supply (ischemia), abnormal cellular metabolism caused by an inherited cellular defect, exposure to exogenous toxins, and abnormalities in other body systems (renal disorders with uremia, diffuse liver disorders with hyperammonemia, cardiorespiratory disorders with hypoxia). Abiotrophy is cell degeneration due to an intrinsic defect in the essential metabolism necessary for the survival and function of that cell, the neuron.

Do not forget to consider the breed of your patient and the possible inherited disorders that must be considered. You will prioritize these disorders in your differential on the basis of signalment, history, and course of the clinical signs and the characteristics of the various disorders being considered.

Based on this ranking of the differential diagnosis, the most useful ancillary procedures will be selected to further confirm or deny the diagnosis under consideration. This selection is especially critical now that neuroimaging by computed tomography and magnetic resonance are available to veterinarians. These procedures require general anesthesia and the costs to the owner of the patient are considerable. Therefore, it is crucial that the correct anatomic diagnosis be made prior to the selection of the ancillary procedures. Your knowledge of the characteristics of the disorders of the nervous system will then permit you to offer a therapy where it is appropriate and a prognosis.

▌ NEURON

The nervous system is composed of primary functional cells—the neurons and supporting cells, which include the glia and ependyma. In this book the neuron is defined as consisting of a dendritic zone, axon, cell body, and telodendron. The dendritic zone is the receptor portion, where a stimulus from the internal or external environment is converted into an impulse in the neuron. The axon is the cell process composed of neurofilaments that course from the dendritic zone to the telodendron. The telodendron is the termination of the neuron where the impulse leaves the neuron. It is often referred to as the synapse. This synapse may lie at an effector organ or at another neuron. The cell body consists of the nucleus and the major organelles necessary for the neuron to function and may be located anywhere along the axon.

For example, a sensory neuron in the peripheral nervous system for general proprioception may have its dendritic zone in a neuromuscular spindle in a skeletal muscle where it is stimulated by a stretching of the muscle. The axon courses toward the spinal cord through a specific peripheral nerve, then through the dorsal or ventral branch of one of the spinal nerves and into its dorsal root. It then enters the spinal cord and passes into the dorsal gray column of that spinal cord segment to synapse on a second neuron in a nucleus within that gray column. The telodendron is the nerve ending at the synapse on another neuron in that nucleus. The neuronal cell body is located in the spinal ganglion associated with the dorsal root that the axon coursed through to reach the spinal cord. It is actually intercalated in the axon at this point (Fig. 1-1).

The dendritic zone and cell body of a motor neuron in the peripheral nervous system that is innervating a skeletal muscle are closely associated and are located in the ventral gray column of a segment of the spinal cord. The axon leaves the cell body in that gray column and courses through the white matter of that segment to enter the ventral root of that segment. It continues into the spinal nerve of that segment and its dorsal or ventral branch and then travels in a specific peripheral nerve to reach the skeletal muscle cells being innervated. Here the axon ends in a telodendron at the neuromuscular ending in a motor end-plate.

Within the CNS, a neuron of the dorsal spinocerebellar tract is an example of a sensory or afferent neuron to the cerebellum. Its dendritic zone and cell body are closely associated in a nucleus in the dorsal gray column of the spinal cord. The impulse is initiated here by a synapse with the telodendron of a sensory general proprioceptive neuron of the peripheral nervous system. The axon courses through the gray matter into the white matter of the lateral funiculus to join other axons in a tract on the dorsal superficial surface of the lateral funiculus. This axon continues

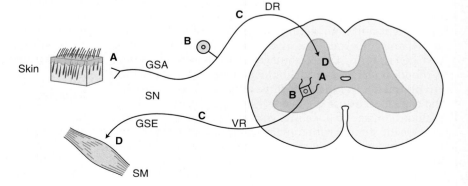

FIGURE 1-1 Diagram of a general somatic afferent *(GSA)* neuron and a general somatic efferent *(GSE)* neuron in a spinal nerve *(SN)*. **A,** Dendritic zone. **B,** Cell body. **C,** Axon. **D,** Telodendron. *DR,* Dorsal root; *SM,* skeletal muscle; *VR,* ventral root.

cranially in this dorsal spinocerebellar tract. It traverses the portion of the spinal cord cranial to the spinal cord segment where it originated, then continues into the medulla where it enters the cerebellum via the caudal cerebellar peduncle. It courses through the cerebellar medulla and into the white matter of a cerebellar folium. It enters the adjacent granular layer of the cerebellum and terminates in a telodendron that synapses with the dendritic zone of a granule cell neuron.

Within the CNS, the Purkinje neuron of the cerebellum is an example of an efferent neuron in the cerebellar cortex. Its dendritic zone consists of a branched structure located in the molecular layer of the cerebellar cortex on the surface of a folium. Here the telodendria of the granule cell neurons synapse at sites on these branches to initiate the impulse in the Purkinje neuron .The cell body is located in the Purkinje neuronal layer of the cerebellar cortex. The axon arises from this cell body and courses through the granular layer into and through the white matter of that cerebellar folium and enters the white matter of the cerebellar medulla. Here the axon ends in a telodendron on the dendritic zone of another efferent neuron located in a nucleus of the cerebellar medulla.

FUNCTIONAL SYSTEMS

This book is organized primarily by functional systems rather than by regions of the nervous system or by the chief clinical neurologic complaint. It is our opinion that for teaching purposes, this is the most effective way to learn the organization of the nervous system and provide the basis for understanding the disorders that affect the various components of the nervous system. Most of these functional systems are derived from a classification of the peripheral nervous system based on its functional components. The sensory portion has extensive components in the CNS. The classification is outlined in Table 1-1.

SENSORY (AFFERENT)

The sensory, or afferent, portion of the peripheral nervous system is classified on the basis of the location of the dendritic zone in the body. This is the site of the origin of the impulse.

Somatic Afferent

The somatic afferent system has its dendritic zone on or near the surface of the body derived from the somatopleura, where it receives the various stimuli from the external environment.

General Somatic Afferent

The general somatic afferent (GSA) system comprises the neurons distributed primarily by the fifth cranial nerve to the surface of the head and all the spinal nerves to the surface of body and limbs that are sensitive to touch, temperature, and noxious stimuli.

TABLE 1-1 Functional Classification of the Nervous System

System	Function and Anatomic Location
1. Afferent (A): Sensory	
Somatic (S)	
General (GSA)	Temperature, touch, noxious stimuli All spinal nerves, cranial nerve V
Special (SSA)	Vision: Cranial nerve II Hearing: Cranial nerve VIII
Visceral (V)	
General (GVA)	Organ content, distention, chemicals Spinal nerve splanchnic branches Cranial nerves VII, IX, X
Special (SVA)	Taste: Cranial nerves VII, IX, X Olfaction: Cranial nerve I
Proprioception	
General (GP)	Muscle and joint movement All spinal nerves, cranial nerve V
Special (SP)	Vestibular system: Cranial nerve VIII
2. Efferent (E): Motor	
Somatic (S)	
General (GSE)	Striated skeletal muscle All spinal nerves Cranial nerves III, IV, V, VI, VII, IX, X, XI, XII
Visceral (V)	
General (GVE)	Smooth and cardiac muscle and glands Sympathetic: All spinal nerves, splanchnic nerves Parasympathetic: Sacral spinal nerves Cranial nerves III, VII, IX, X, XI

Special Somatic Afferent

The special somatic afferent (SSA) system involves specialized dendritic zone receptor organs limited to one area deep to the body surface but stimulated by changes in the external environment. These include light to the eyeball (cranial nerve II) and air waves indirectly to the membranous labyrinth of the inner ear (cranial nerve VIII, cochlear division).

Visceral Afferent

The visceral afferent system has its dendritic zone in the wall of the various viscera of the body. This is tissue derived mostly from splanchnopleura and is stimulated by changes in the internal environment.

General Visceral Afferent

The general visceral afferent (GVA) system is composed of neurons distributed by the seventh, ninth, and tenth cranial nerves to visceral structures in the head and by the tenth cranial nerve and spinal nerves to the viscera of the body cavities and blood vessels throughout the neck, trunk, and limbs. This widely distributed system is stimulated primarily by the distention of visceral walls and chemical changes.

Special Visceral Afferent

The special visceral afferent (SVA) system contains the neurons in the seventh, ninth, and tenth cranial nerves, whose dendritic zones are limited to the specialized receptors for taste, and the first cranial nerve, whose dendritic zones are localized in the caudal nasal mucosa for olfaction.

Proprioception

The modality of general proprioception is sometimes included in the GSA system. In this book we consider it as a separate system because of its clinical significance. Disorders that affect this system express clinical signs different from those that affect the GSA system as we have classified it. Proprioception is the system responsible for detecting changes in the position of the head, neck, trunk, and limbs.

General Proprioception

The general proprioception (GP) system has its dendritic zones widely distributed in receptor organs located in muscles, tendons, and joints deep to the body surface. It is distributed widely throughout all the spinal nerves and the fifth cranial nerve. The receptors are sensitive to changes in the lengths and positions of the structures they innervate.

Special Proprioception

The special proprioception (SP) system's dendritic zones are limited to receptors specialized to respond to positions and movements of the head. They are located in a portion of the membranous labyrinth of the inner ear. These neurons concerned with the orientation of the head in space are in the vestibular division of the vestibulocochlear nerve (cranial nerve VIII).

MOTOR (EFFERENT)

The motor, or efferent, portion of the peripheral nervous system is classified on the basis of where the motor neuron terminates, which is the site of the telodendron. This peripheral motor system is also referred to as the lower motor neuron (LMN) because it is the final neuron to innervate the muscle cell. There are somatic and visceral components of the efferent system.

General Somatic Efferent

In the general somatic efferent (GSE) system, the telodendron is located in striated skeletal muscle throughout the entire body derived from somatic mesoderm, somites, and head somitomeres. The cell body and dendritic zone of these GSE neurons are in the spinal cord ventral gray column and in nuclei in the brainstem. Their axons are in the ventral root and spinal nerves or in cranial nerves, and they course through various named peripheral nerves to terminate in a muscle cell at the neuromuscular ending (junction). These GSE neurons are found in all the spinal nerves and in all the cranial nerves except cranial nerves I, II, and VIII.

General Visceral Efferent

The general visceral efferent (GVE) system has its telodendria in involuntary smooth muscle of viscera derived from splanchnic mesoderm as well as blood vessels, cardiac muscle, and glands. This system is the LMN of the autonomic nervous system, which has components in all segments of the brain and spinal cord. In some books, the GVE system is considered to be the entire autonomic system; we believe that to be an inappropriate concept that defies the true functional totality of this autonomic system, which includes peripheral afferent components and a plethora of nuclei and tracts at all levels of the CNS.

The GVE system, unlike the GSE system, is a two-neuron system in that there are two neurons between the CNS and the target organ. A synapse occurs in a peripheral ganglion between these two neurons. There are two divisions of this system: sympathetic and parasympathetic. They are further described in Chapter 7, which is devoted to the GVE system. These GVE neurons are distributed in the third, seventh, ninth, tenth, and eleventh cranial nerves and all the spinal nerves.

In previous editions of this book and in older books of developmental anatomy, a special visceral efferent system was described for the innervation of striated skeletal muscle in the head derived from branchial arch mesoderm. This classification has now been deleted because there is no difference between this head skeletal muscle and the muscles in the rest of the body. All this muscle is now considered to be innervated by the GSE system.

■ FURTHER READING

For further reading, the following list of textbooks is highly recommended. For all aspects of canine neuroanatomy, the most extensive and thorough descriptions are found in *Miller's Anatomy of the Dog* by Howard Evans. From our perspective, this should be considered the gold standard. The text by Tom Jenkins, *Functional Mammalian Neuroanatomy*, is an easy read, has many simplified line drawings of various neurologic concepts, and is based primarily on the dog. For the study of brain sections in all three planes, *The Brain of the Dog in Section* by Marcus Singer is unsurpassed. This is a superb text for correlation with MR images.

For further reading in veterinary clinical neurology, the six texts listed are all well written and provide thorough coverage of their areas of concern. Cheryl Chrisman's text is limited to small animals and is usefully organized by the patient's problem, the chief complaint. Kyle Braund's text is organized like a dictionary and is useful for looking up short, succinct reviews of any domestic animal's neurologic problem. All species are included in the handbook written by Mike Lorenz and Joe Kornegay, although their personal experience is mostly with small animals. The only text in veterinary neurology that is limited to large animals is that written by Joe Mayhew. This is a superb book that represents his extensive personal experience. The original textbook of veterinary neurology written by Ben Hoerlein, which included an extensive section on surgical and medical treatment, was revised by John Oliver and Joe Mayhew and was expanded to include some large-animal neurology. In our opinion the most current and most inclusive veterinary neurology text for small animals is the text published in 2003 and edited by Curtis Dewey. For spinal surgery, the textbook by Nick Sharp and Simon Wheeler details the contemporary aspects of spinal surgery for small animals. This text is supported by excellent diagrams and photos. The only textbook devoted to veterinary neuropathology is the one written by Brian Summers with the help of John Cummings and myself (Alexander de Lahunta). In addition to the descriptive neuropathology, this text includes considerable clinical correlations as well as descriptions of pathogenesis.

SUGGESTED READINGS

Domestic Animal Neuroanatomy

Jenkins TW: *Functional mammalian neuroanatomy*, ed 2, Philadelphia, 1978, Lea & Febiger.

Evans HE: *Miller's anatomy of the dog*, ed 3, Philadelphia, 1993, Saunders.

Singer M: *The brain of the dog in section*, Philadelphia, 1962, Saunders.

Veterinary Clinical Neurology

Braund KG: *Clinical syndromes in veterinary neurology*, ed 2, St Louis, 1994, Mosby.

Chrisman CL: *Problems in small animal neurology*, ed 2, Philadelphia, 1991, Lea & Febiger.

Chrisman CL, et al: *Neurology for the small animal practitioner*, Jackson, WY, 2003, Teton NewMedia.

Dewey CW: *A practical guide to canine and feline neurology*, Ames, IO, 2003, Iowa State Press.

Lorenz MD, Kornegay JN: *Handbook of veterinary neurology*, ed 4, Philadelphia, 2004, Saunders.

Mayhew IG: *Large animal neurology*, Philadelphia, 1989, Lea & Febiger.

Oliver JE, Hoerlein BF, Mayhew IG: *Veterinary neurology*, Philadelphia, 1987, Saunders.

Platt SR, Olby NJ: *BSAVA manual of canine and feline neurology*, ed 3, Gloucester, UK, 2004, British Small Animal Veterinary Association.

Sharp NJ, Wheeler SJ: *Small animal spinal disorders: diagnosis and surgery*, ed 2, Philadelphia, 2005, Elsevier.

Veterinary Neuropathology

Summers BA, Cummings JF, de Lahunta A: *Veterinary neuropathology*, New York, 1995, Mosby.

Other References

Crosby EC, Humphrey T, Lauer EW: *Correlative anatomy of the nervous system*, New York, 1962, Macmillan.

Fankhauser R, Luginbuhl H: *Pathologische Anatomie des zentralen und peripheren Nervensystem der Haustiere*, Berlin, Germany, 1968, Verlag Paul Perey.

Frauchiger E, Fankhauser R: *Neuropathologie des Menschen und der Tiere*, Berlin, Germany, 1957, Springer-Verlag.

Innes JRM, Saunders LZ: *Comparative neuropathology*, New York, 1962, Academic Press.

Nickle R, Schummer A: *Seiferle E: Lehrbuch der Anatomie der Haustiere, Band IV, Nervensystem, Sinnesorgane, Endokrine Drusen*, Berlin, Germany, 1975, Verlag Paul Perey.

Papez JW: *Comparative neurology*, New York, 1929, TY Crowell.

2 NEUROANATOMY BY DISSECTION

TRANSVERSE BRAIN SECTIONS

The neuroanatomic components of this textbook are based on and complement the dissection of the nervous system described in *Guide to the Dissection of the Dog* by H. E. Evans and A. de Lahunta (ed 6, Philadelphia, 2004, Elsevier). The peripheral nerves are described and dissected along with the regions of the body in which they are found. The dissection of the brain and spinal cord is found in the last section, titled "Nervous System." The split head of the embalmed dog used for the dissection of the entire dog is also used to demonstrate the blood vessels and meninges. A separate entire preserved dog brain is provided to each group of students for the dissection. The spinal cord can be dissected on the embalmed dogs or presented as prosections. On completion of the brain dissection, an additional preserved domestic animal brain is provided to each group for the study of the transverse sections.

In the Cornell curriculum this dissection is performed simultaneously with lectures and discussions of nervous system development, cerebrospinal fluid, and malformations, including hydrocephalus, which are the subjects of Chapters 3 and 4 of this book.

The nomenclature used in this third edition, as in *Guide to the Dissection of the Dog*, adheres to that published in the fifth edition of *Nomina Anatomica Veterinaria* in 2005, unless otherwise stated.

▎ TRANSVERSE BRAIN SECTIONS

The following transverse brain sections in Figs. 2-2 through 2-17 are arranged from rostral to caudal through the brain at irregular intervals, as indicated on the drawings in Fig. 2-1. In these sections the white matter has been stained and appears black, whereas the gray matter is relatively unstained.

Figs. 2-18 through 2-33 are transverse plane (axial) proton density MR images of a normal adult dog for comparison with Figs. 2-2 through 2-17. The images are 2 mm thick, but to select those that best demonstrate the anatomic features, the intervals between images vary.

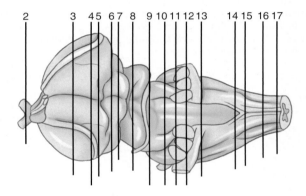

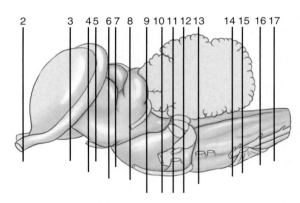

FIGURE 2-1 Dorsal and left lateral views of the brainstem, indicating the approximate levels of the following transverse sections.

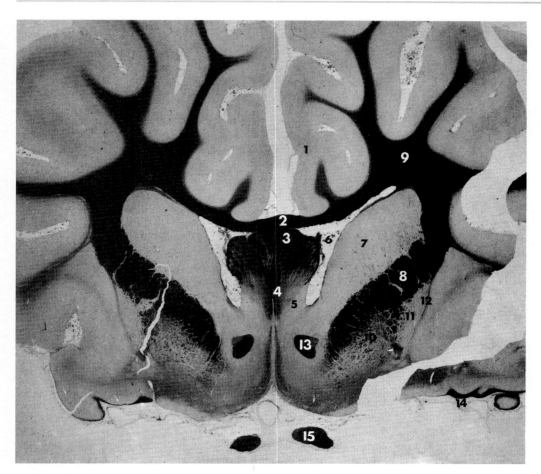

FIGURE 2-2
1. Cingulate gyrus
2. Corpus callosum
3. Body of fornix
4. Column of fornix
5. Septal nuclei
6. Lateral ventricle
7. Body of caudate nucleus
8. Internal capsule
9. Centrum semiovale
10. Globus pallidus
11. Putamen
12. External capsule
13. Rostral commissure
14. Lateral olfactory tract
15. Optic nerve

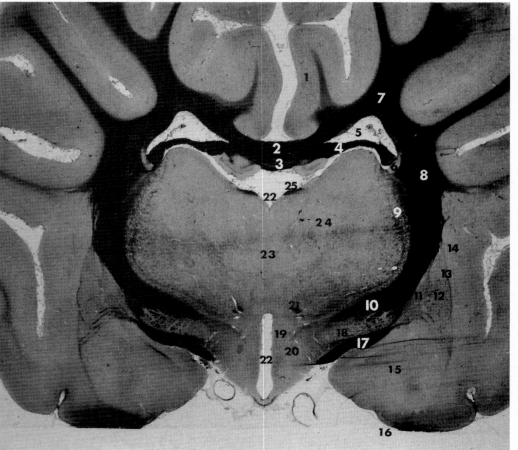

FIGURE 2-3
1. Cingulate gyrus
2. Corpus callosum
3. Body of fornix
4. Crus of fornix
5. Lateral ventricle
6. Caudal (tail) caudate nucleus
7. Centrum semiovale
8. Internal capsule
9. Thalamocortical projection fibers
10. Corticopontine, corticobulbar, and corticospinal projection fibers
11. Globus pallidus
12. Putamen
13. External capsule
14. Claustrum
15. Amygdaloid body
16. Pyriform lobe
17. Optic tract
18. Endopeduncular nucleus
19. Hypothalamic nuclei
20. Column of fornix
21. Mamilothalamic tract
22. Third ventricle
23. Interthalamic adhesion
24. Thalamic nuclei
25. Stria habenularis thalami

FIGURE 2-4
1. Cingulate gyrus
2. Corpus callosum
3. Hippocampus
4. Crus of fornix
5. Lateral ventricle
6. Parahippocampal gyrus
7. Lateral rhinal sulcus, caudal part
8. Internal capsule
9. Thalamocortical projection
10. Lateral geniculate nucleus
11. Thalamic nuclei
12. Habenular nucleus
13. Habenulointerpeduncular tract
14. Third ventricle
15. Interthalamic adhesion
16. Zona incerta
17. Crus cerebri
18. Optic tract
19. Subthalamic nucleus
20. Mammillary body
21. Mamillothalamic tract
22. Caudal hypothalamic region
23. Adenohypophysis
24. Neurohypophysis

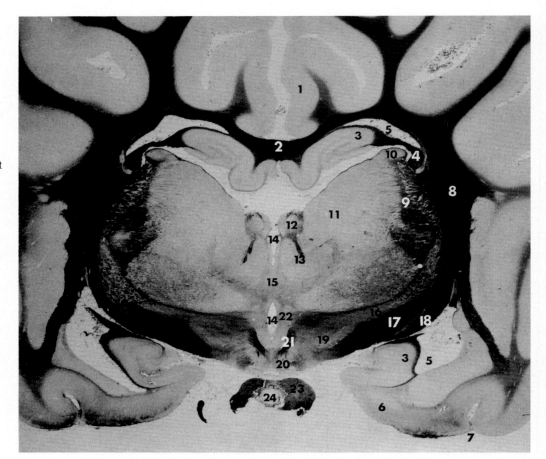

FIGURE 2-5
1. Cingulate gyrus
2. Splenium of corpus callosum
3. Hippocampus
4. Crus of fornix
5. Lateral ventricle
6. Parahippocampal gyrus
7. Lateral rhinal sulcus, caudal part
8. Optic tract
9. Lateral geniculate nucleus
10. Medial geniculate nucleus
11. Pretectal nuclei
12. Pineal body
13. Caudal commissure
14. Mesencephalic aqueduct
15. Parasympathetic nucleus of
    oculomotor nerve
16. Medial lemniscus
17. Substantia nigra
18. Crus cerebri

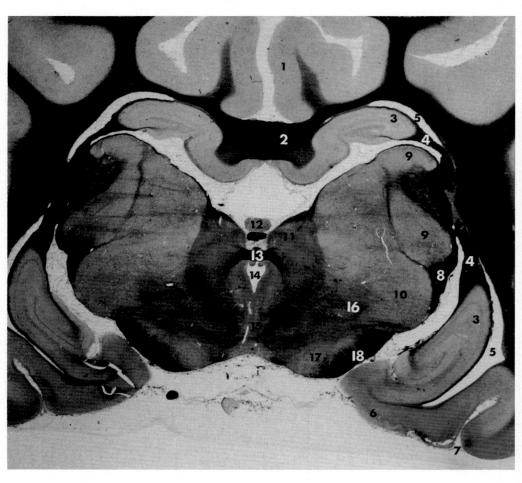

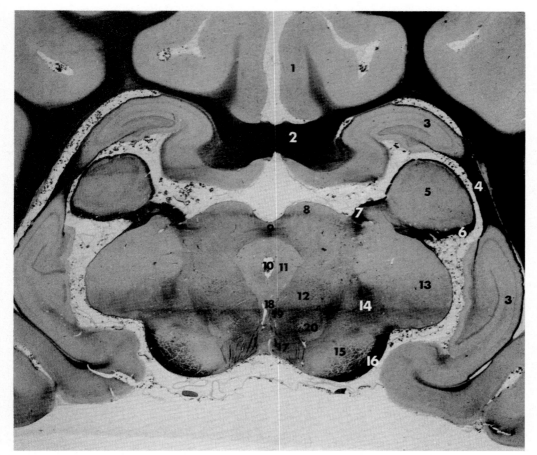

FIGURE 2-6
1. Cingulate gyrus
2. Splenium of corpus callosum
3. Hippocampus
4. Crus of fornix
5. Lateral geniculate nucleus
6. Optic tract
7. Brachium of rostral colliculus
8. Rostral colliculus
9. Commissure of rostral colliculus
10. Mesencephalic aqueduct
11. Central gray substance
12. Reticular formation
13. Medial geniculate nucleus
14. Medial lemniscus
15. Substantia nigra
16. Crus cerebri
17. Oculomotor nerve fibers
18. Parasympathetic nucleus of
    oculomotor nerve
19. Medial longitudinal fasciculus
20. Red nucleus

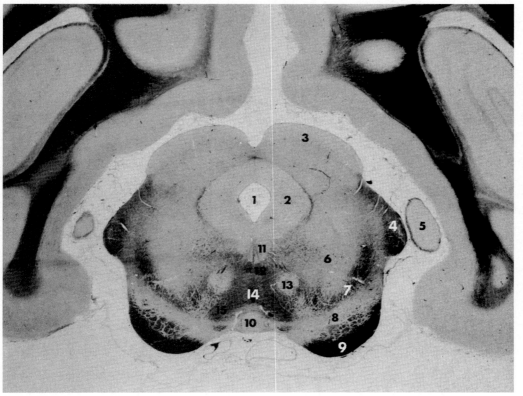

FIGURE 2-7
1. Mesencephalic aqueduct
2. Central gray substance
3. Rostral colliculus
4. Brachium of caudal colliculus
5. Medial geniculate nucleus
6. Reticular formation
7. Medial lemniscus
8. Substantia nigra
9. Crus cerebri
10. Interpeduncular nucleus
11. Oculomotor nucleus
12. Medial longitudinal fasciculus
13. Red nucleus
14. Ventral tegmental decussation
    (rubrospinal neurons)
15. Rubrospinal tract

FIGURE 2-8

1. Commissure of caudal colliculus
2. Mesencephalic aqueduct
3. Central gray substance
4. Caudal colliculus
5. Brachium of caudal colliculus
6. Lateral lemniscus
7. Reticular formation
8. Nucleus of trochlear nerve
9. Medial longitudinal fasciculus
10. Decussation of rostral cerebellar peduncle
11. Rubropsinal tract
12. Medial lemniscus
13. Interpeduncular nucleus
14. Crus cerebri
15. Pontine nuclei
16. Transverse fibers of pons

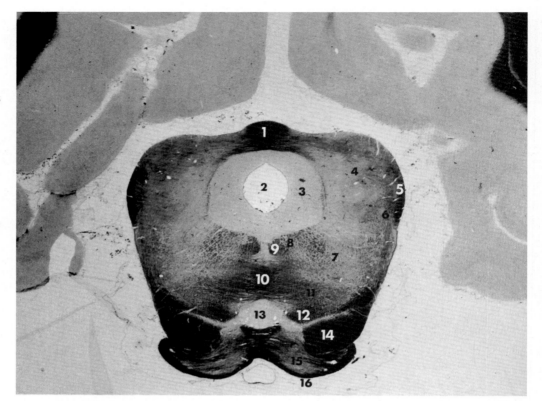

FIGURE 2-9

1. Medial longitudinal fasciculus
2. Fourth ventricle
3. Trochlear nerve
4. Caudal colliculus
5. Rostral cerebellar peduncle
6. Lateral lemniscus
7. Nucleus of lateral lemniscus
8. Middle cerebellar peduncle
9. Trigeminal nerve
10. Transverse fibers of pons
11. Pontine nuclei
12. Longitudinal fibers of pons
13. Medial lemniscus
14. Reticular formation
15. Locus ceruleus

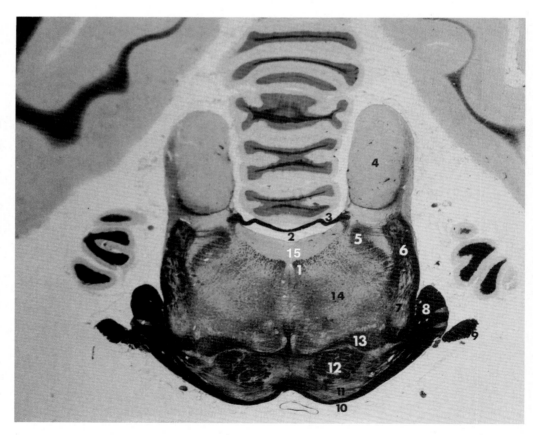

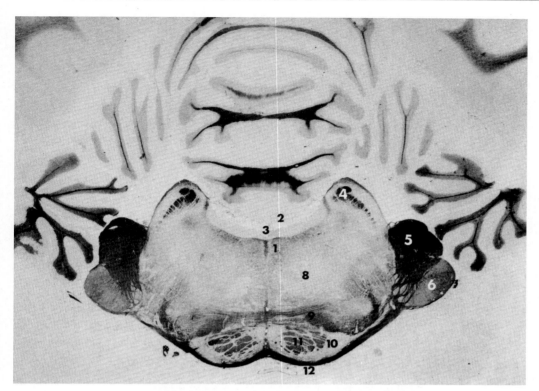

FIGURE 2-10
1. Medial longitudinal fasciculus
2. Rostral medullary velum
3. Fourth ventricle
4. Rostral cerebellar peduncle
5. Middle cerebellar peduncle
6. Trigeminal nerve
7. Lateral lemniscus
8. Reticular formation
9. Medial lemniscus
10. Pontine nuclei
11. Longitudinal fibers of pons
12. Transverse fibers of pons

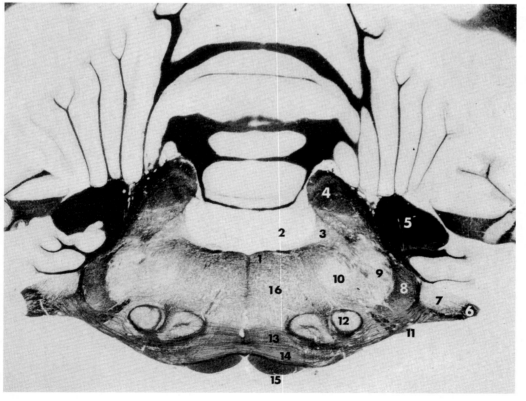

FIGURE 2-11
1. Medial longitudinal fasciculus
2. Rostral medullary velum
3. Rostral vestibular nucleus
4. Rostral cerebellar peduncle
5. Middle cerebellar peduncle
6. Vestibulocochlear nerve
7. Cochlear nucleus
8. Trigeminal nerve
9. Nucleus of spinal tract of trigeminal nerve, pontine sensory portion
10. Motor nucleus of trigeminal nerve
11. Facial nerve
12. Dorsal nucleus of trapezoid body
13. Medial lemniscus
14. Trapezoid body
15. Pyramid
16. Reticular formation

FIGURE 2-12

1. Medial longitudinal fasciculus
2. Abducent nerve fibers
3. Genu of facial nerve
4. Ventrolateral coursing facial nerve fibers
5. Medial vestibular nucleus
6. Vestibulocerebellar fibers
7. Lateral vestibular nucleus
8. Caudal cerebellar peduncle
9. Flocculus
10. Cochlear nuclei
11. Vestibulocochlear nerve
12. Spinal tract of trigeminal nerve
13. Nucleus of spinal tract of trigeminal nerve
14. Dorsal nucleus of trapezoid body
15. Trapezoid body
16. Pyramid
17. Medial lemniscus

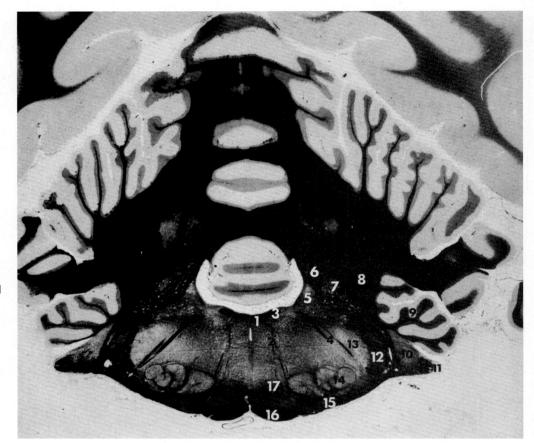

FIGURE 2-13

1. Fastigial cerebellar nucleus
2. Interposital cerebellar nucleus
3. Lateral cerebellar nucleus
4. Nodulus
5. Flocculus
6. Medial vestibular nucleus
7. Caudal vestibular nucleus
8. Acoustic stria
9. Caudal cerebellar peduncle
10. Spinal tract of trigeminal nerve
11. Nucleus of spinal tract of trigeminal nerve
12. Facial nucleus
13. Dorsomedial coursing facial nerve fibers
14. Reticular formation
15. Pyramidal tract
16. Medial lemniscus

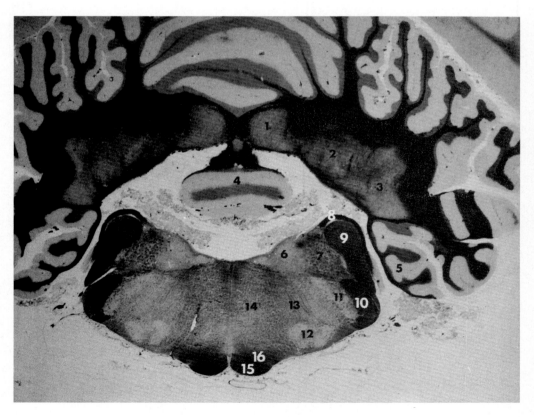

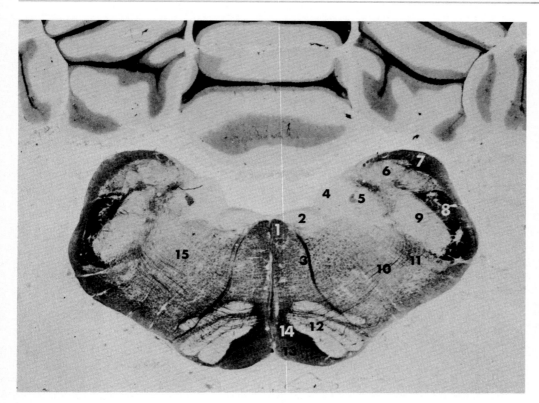

FIGURE 2-14

1. Medial longitudinal fasciculus
2. Hypoglossal nucleus
3. Radix of hypoglossal nerve
4. Parasympathetic nucleus of vagus nerve
5. Nucleus of solitary tract
6. Lateral cuneate nucleus
7. Caudal cerebellar peduncle
8. Spinal tract of trigeminal nerve
9. Nucleus of spinal tract of trigeminal nerve
10. Deep arcuate fibers
11. Nucleus ambiguus
12. Olivary nucleus
13. Pyramidal tract
14. Medial lemniscus
15. Reticular formation

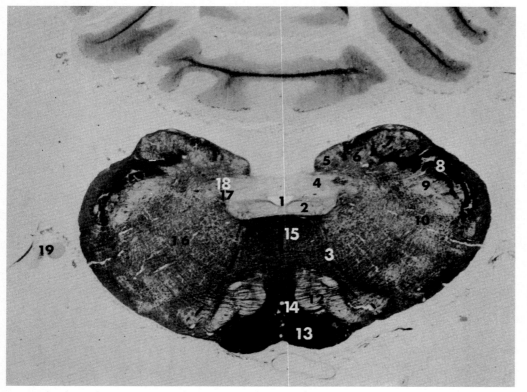

FIGURE 2-15

1. Central canal
2. Hypoglossal nucleus
3. Radix of hypoglossal nerve
4. Parasympathetic nucleus of vagus nerve
5. Nucleus gracilis
6. Medial cuneate nucleus
7. Lateral cuneate nucleus
8. Spinal tract of trigeminal nerve
9. Nucleus of spinal tract of trigeminal nerve
10. Nucleus ambiguus
11. Dorsal spinocerebellar tract
12. Olivary nucleus
13. Pyramidal tract
14. Medial lemniscus
15. Medial longitudinal fasciculus
16. Reticular formation
17. Nucleus of solitary tract
18. Solitary tract
19. Accessory nerve

FIGURE 2-16

1. Nucleus gracilis
2. Medial cuneate nucleus
3. Fasciculus gracilis
4. Spinal tract of trigeminal nerve
5. Nucleus of spinal tract of trigeminal nerve
6. Medial longitudinal fasciculus
7. Pyramidal decussation
8. Spinocerebellar tracts

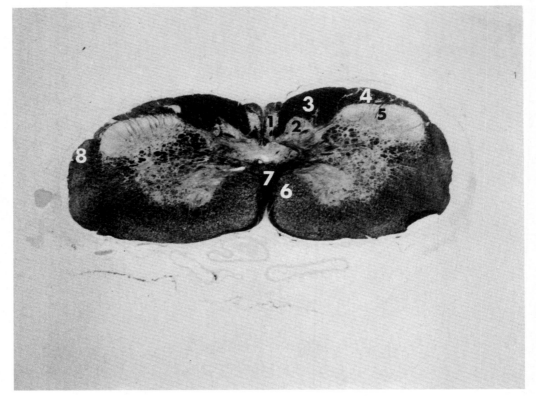

FIGURE 2-17

1. Fasciculus gracilis
2. Fasciculus cuneatus
3. Spinal tract of trigeminal nerve
4. Nucleus of spinal tract of trigeminal nerve: dorsal gray column, first cervical spinal cord segment
5. Rubrospinal tract
6. Lateral pyramidal (corticospinal) tract
7. Vestibulospinal tract
8. Ventral median fissure
9. Spinocerebellar tracts

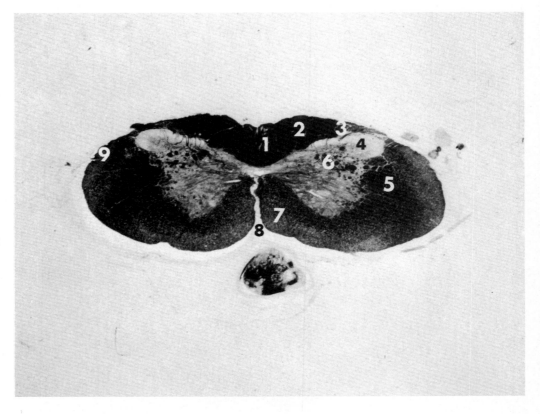

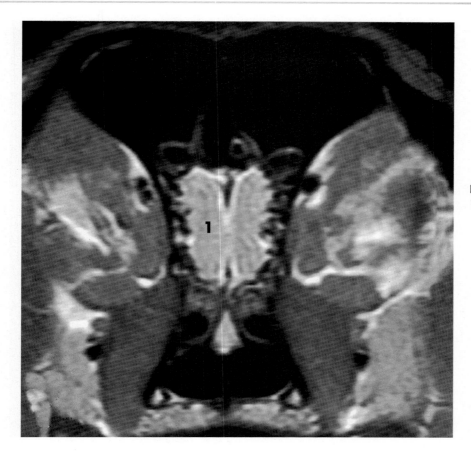

FIGURE 2-18
1. Olfactory bulb

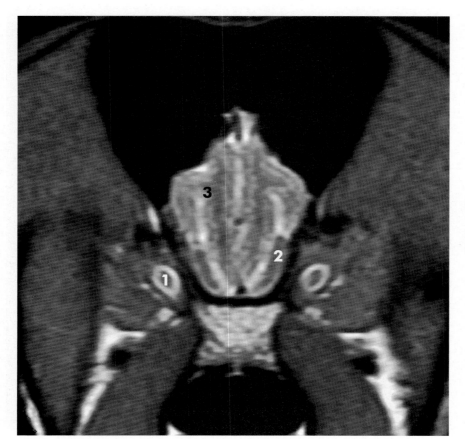

FIGURE 2-19
1. Optic nerve
2. Olfactory peduncle
3. Frontal lobe

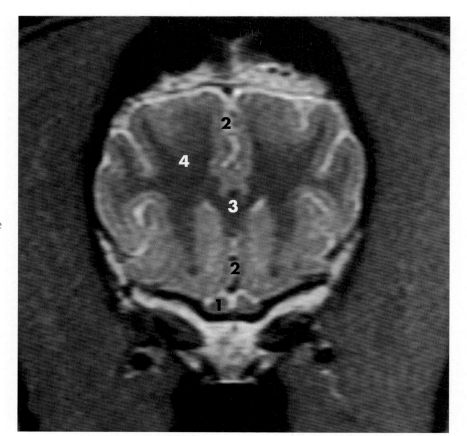

FIGURE 2-20
1. Optic nerve
2. Longitudinal cerebral fissure
3. Genu corpus callosum
4. Internal capsule

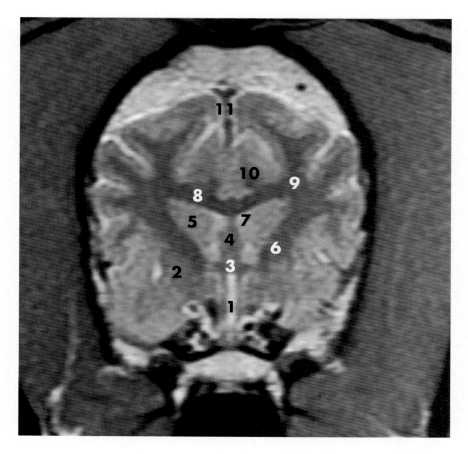

FIGURE 2-21
1. Third ventricle
2. Lentiform nucleus
3. Rostral commissure
4. Body of fornix at bend to columns of fornix
5. Caudate nucleus
6. Internal capsule
7. Lateral ventricle
8. Corpus callosum
9. Centrum semiovale
10. Cingulum in cingulate gyrus
11. Falx cerebri

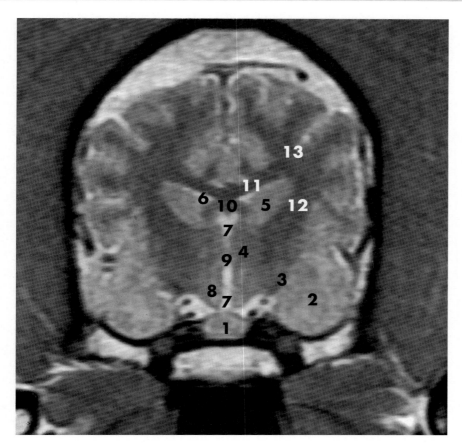

FIGURE 2-22
1. Pituitary gland
2. Amygdaloid body in piriform lobe
3. Optic tract
4. Thalamus
5. Caudate nucleus
6. Lateral ventricle
7. Third ventricle
8. Hypothalamus
9. Interthalamic adhesion
10. Body of fornix
11. Corpus callosum
12. Internal capsule
13. Centrum semiovale

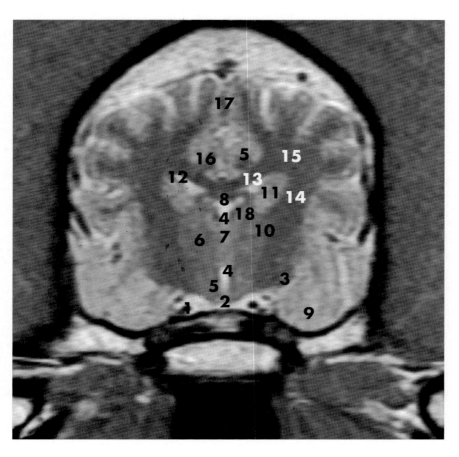

FIGURE 2-23
1. Cerebral arterial circle
2. Mamillary bodies
3. Optic tract
4. Third ventricle
5. Hypothalamus
6. Thalamus
7. Interthalamic adhesion
8. Body of fornix
9. Amygdaloid body in piriform lobe
10. Thalamocortical fibers
11. Caudate nucleus
12. Lateral ventricle
13. Corpus callosum
14. Internal capsule
15. Centrum semiovale
16. Cingulum in cingulate gyrus
17. Falx cerebri
18. Stria habenularis thalami

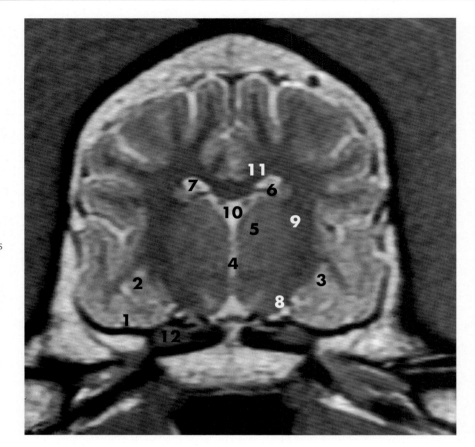

FIGURE 2-24
1. Parahippocampal gyrus
2. Hippocampus
3. Lateral ventricle
4. Third ventricle, caudal part
5. Thalamus
6. Crus of fornix
7. Choroid plexus in lateral ventricle
8. Internal capsule, just rostral to crus cerebri
9. Thalamocortical fibers
10. Subarachnoid space
11. Corpus callosum
12. Trigeminal nerve

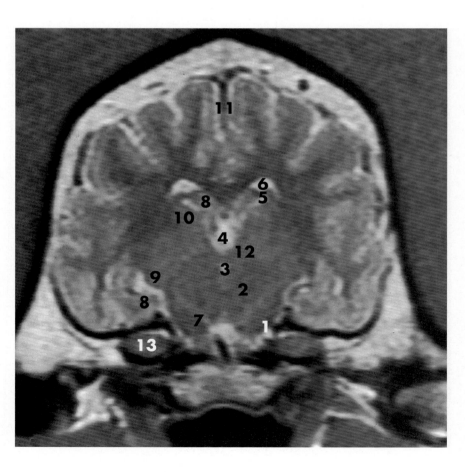

FIGURE 2-25
1. Crus cerebri
2. Mesencephalic tegmentum
3. Mesencephalic aqueduct
4. Subarachnoid space
5. Crus of fornix
6. Lateral ventricle
7. Substantia nigra
8. Hippocampus
9. Medial geniculate nucleus
10. Lateral geniculate nucleus
11. Falx cerebri
12. Pretectal nucleus
13. Trigeminal nerve

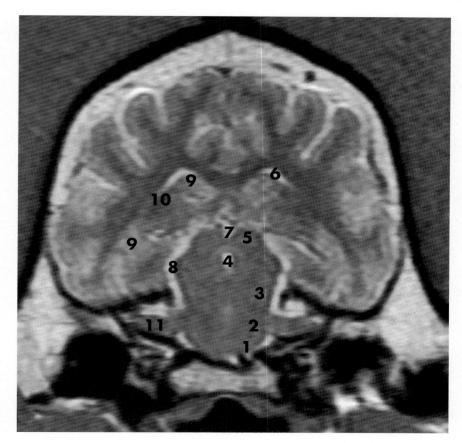

FIGURE 2-26

1. Transverse fibers of pons, rostral part
2. Crus cerebri at longitudinal fibers of pons
3. Mesencephalic tegmentum
4. Mesencephalic aqueduct
5. Rostral colliculus
6. Lateral ventricle
7. Subarachnoid space
8. Brachium of caudal colliculus
9. Hippocampus
10. Crus of fornix
11. Trigeminal nerve

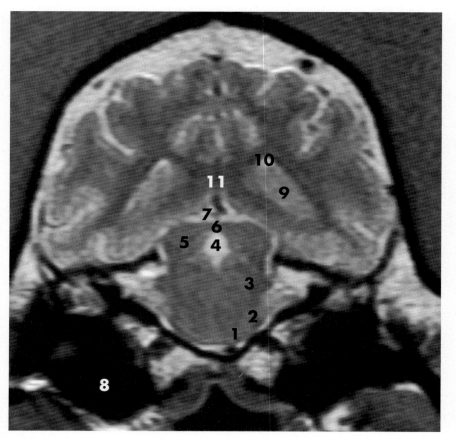

FIGURE 2-27

1. Transverse fibers of pons
2. Longitudinal fibers of pons
3. Mesencephalic tegmentum
4. Mesencephalic aqueduct
5. Caudal colliculus
6. Commissure of caudal colliculus
7. Subarachnoid space
8. Tympanic bulla
9. Hippocampus
10. Lateral ventricle
11. Splenium of corpus callosum

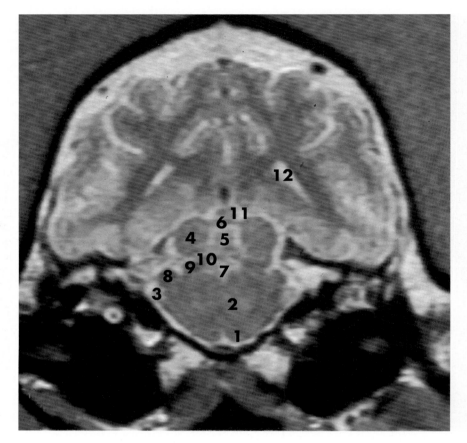

FIGURE 2-28
1. Pyramid
2. Pontine tegmentum
3. Trigeminal nerve
4. Caudal colliculus
5. Rostral cerebellar vermis and rostral medullary velum
6. Commissure of caudal colliculus
7. Fourth ventricle
8. Middle cerebellar peduncle
9. Rostral cerebellar peduncle
10. Trochlear nerve in rostral medullary velum
11. Subarachnoid space
12. Lateral ventricle

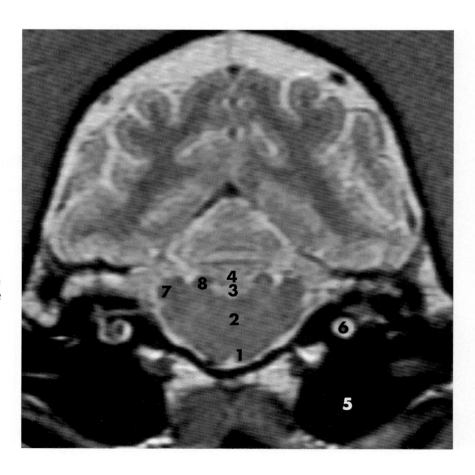

FIGURE 2-29
1. Pyramid
2. Rostral medulla
3. Fourth ventricle
4. Cerebellar vermis
5. Tympanic bulla
6. Cochlea in inner ear
7. Middle cerebellar peduncle
8. Rostral cerebellar peduncle

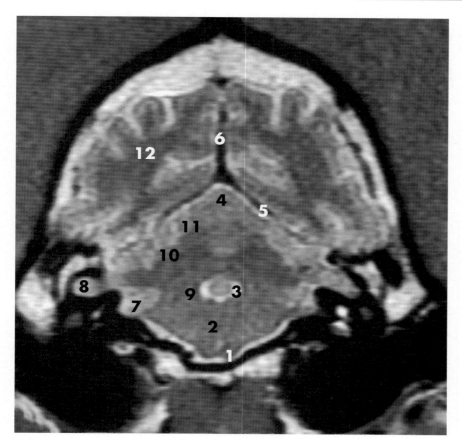

FIGURE 2-30
1. Pyramid
2. Medulla
3. Fourth ventricle
4. Cerebellar vermis
5. Tentorium cerebelli osseum
6. Falx cerebri
7. Vestibulocochlear nerve–cochlear nuclei
8. Paraflocculus of cerebellum
9. Confluence of cerebellar penducles
10. Cerebellar medulla
11. Cerebellar hemisphere
12. Occipital lobe

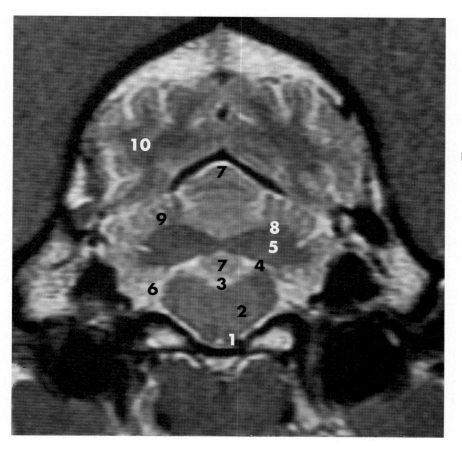

FIGURE 2-31
1. Pyramid
2. Medulla
3. Fourth ventricle
4. Caudal cerebellar peduncle
5. Interposital cerebellar nucleus
6. Subarachnoid space
7. Cerebellar vermis
8. Cerebellar medulla
9. Cerebellar hemisphere
10. Occipital lobe

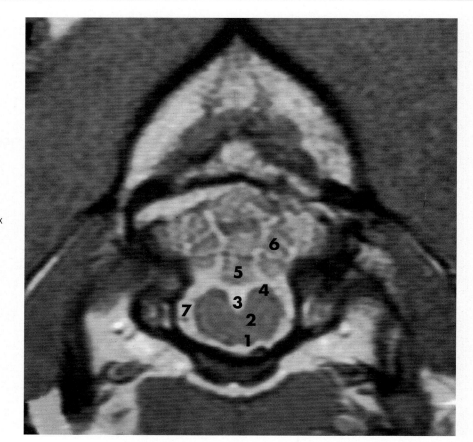

FIGURE 2-32
1. Pyramid
2. Medulla
3. Fourth ventricle near the obex
4. Caudal cerebellar peduncle
5. Cerebellar vermis
6. Paramedian lobule
7. Subarachnoid space

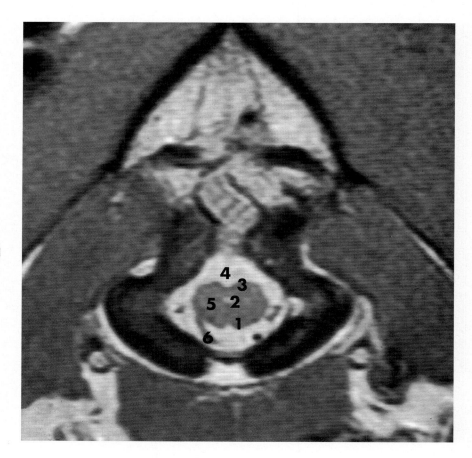

FIGURE 2-33
1. Pyramid at deccussation
2. Central canal
3. General proprioceptive nuclei
4. Subarachnoid space
5. Junction of medulla and first cervical spinal cord segment
6. Branch of basilar or vertebral artery

3 DEVELOPMENT OF THE NERVOUS SYSTEM: MALFORMATION

NEURAL TUBE

Cell Differentiation

MEDULLA SPINALIS: SPINAL CORD

Neural Crest

MYELENCEPHALON: MEDULLA OBLONGATA

METENCEPHALON: CEREBELLUM AND PONS

MESENCEPHALON: MIDBRAIN

DIENCEPHALON: INTERBRAIN

TELENCEPHALON: CEREBRUM

Cell Bodies

Axons

MALFORMATIONS

Brain Malformations
 Hydrocephalus
 Hypoplasia of the Prosencephalon:
  Cerebral (Telencephalic) Aplasia
  (Anencephaly)
 Meningocele: Meningoencephalocele
 Exencephaly
 Lipomeningocele

Duplication of the Prosencephalon
Holoprosencephaly-Arrhinencephaly
Hydranencephaly
Lissencephaly
Cerebellar Malformations
Complex Malformation of Calves
Occipital Bone Malformation and
 Syringohydromyelia
Calvarial Ossification
Spinal Cord Malformations
 Spina Bifida: Meningomyelocele
 Pathogenesis of Malformations
 CASE EXAMPLE 3-1

NEURAL TUBE

The central nervous system is a tubular structure originating from a proliferation of ectodermal epithelial cells referred to as the neurectoderm, which is located dorsal to the notochord along the axis of the embryo. This thickened ectoderm, known as the neural plate, invaginates along this axis, forming a groove until the lateral extremities of the original plate, the neural folds, meet centrally and fuse over the neural groove to form a neural tube and canal. As the neural tube forms, it separates from the nonneural ectoderm which grows over the dorsum of the tube to fuse along the midline. As this fusion and separation of ectodermal layers occurs, a longitudinal column of ectodermal epithelial cells arises from the junction of nonneural and neural ectoderm and separates from these two structures when the neural tube is formed. These two bilateral columns, situated dorsolateral to the neural tube throughout its length, are the columns of neural crest cells (Fig. 3-1).

Closure of the neural tube progresses rostrally and caudally from the level of the site of development of the rhombencephalon, the most caudal division of the brain. The caudal closure forms the majority of the spinal cord. Closure of the brain portion of the neural tube may initially occur at multiple sites and progress rostrally and caudally. The locations of these sites vary among species of animals. Prior to complete closure, the most rostral opening is the rostral neuropore (Fig. 3-2). The caudal portion of the spinal cord develops from the caudal end of the closed neural tube as an extension of a column of neuroepithelial cells that grows caudally on the midline between the notochord and skin ectoderm. A cavitation of this column of cells produces an extension of the neural tube and its neural canal. This portion of the neural tube will ultimately form the caudal,

the sacral, and a variable number of lumbar spinal cord segments. An opening may persist at the caudal end of the neural tube, allowing communication with the subarachnoid space of the leptomeninges at the conus medullaris.

The rostral end of the neural tube develops rapidly and produces three vesicles, from rostral to caudal: the prosencephalon, mesencephalon, and rhombencephalon (Fig. 3-3). Early in its development the prosencephalon has lateral enlargements, the optic vesicles, which grow laterally to contact the overlying skin ectoderm. The further development of this primordial eye is described in Chapter 14, Visual System. Two additional swellings emerge from the rostral prosencephalon and grow out of the neural tube on each side laterally and dorsally. These telencephalic vesicles completely overgrow the original vesicular system and form the cerebral hemispheres. The portion of the prosencephalon that remains at the rostral end of the neural tube is the diencephalon. The optic vesicles remain associated with the diencephalon. The neural canal within the diencephalon is the third ventricle. It communicates rostrolaterally with the neural canal of each telencephalon (cerebral hemisphere), which is the lateral ventricle (first and second ventricles). This small communication on each side is the interventricular foramen. The nuclei of the thalamus and hypothalamus develop in the diencephalon. The neurohypophysis is a ventral outgrowth of the diencephalon. The cerebral cortex and basal nuclei develop in the telencephalon.

The neural canal of the mesencephalon is reduced to a narrow tubular space called the mesencephalic aqueduct.

From the rostral rhombencephalon, the cerebellum or dorsal metencephalon develops dorsally. The remaining ventral metencephalon becomes the pons. The caudal rhombencephalon forms the myelencephalon or medulla oblongata. The fourth ventricle is the lumen of the neural

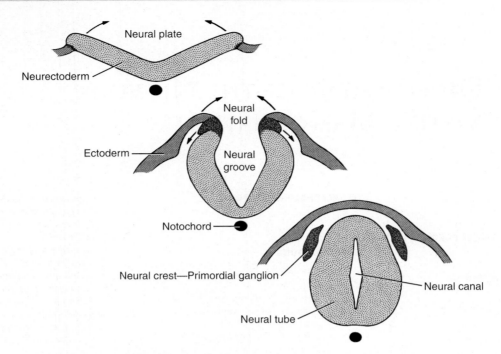

FIGURE 3-1 Development of the neural tube–transverse sections.

canal in the rhombencephalon. It communicates with the meningeal spaces that develop around the neural tube by way of openings that arise in the wall of the neural tube caudal to the developing cerebellum. These openings are called the lateral apertures (see Figs. 4-1 and 4-2). The neural canal continues caudally as the central canal of the spinal cord.

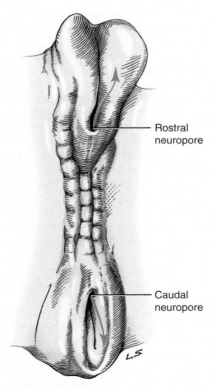

FIGURE 3-2 Dorsal view of neural tube closure.

Cell Differentiation

In the first stage of development within the wall of the neural tube, the cells, which are commonly referred to as neuroepthelial or neurectodermal cells, are organized in a pseudostratified arrangement; thus the neural tube is one cell in thickness. The cell membrane of each cell spans the full width of the neural tube but the nuclei are located at various levels within each cell. These cells are all mitotically active, increasing the thickness of the wall of the tube. The nuclei migrate within the cytoplasm of each cell, and their position is dependent on the cell's stage of mitosis.

During interphase, the nuclei are located on the external surface of the neural tube. Chromosomal DNA duplication occurs with the nucleus in that position. As the nucleus enters mitosis, it migrates through the cytoplasm to the neural canal's luminal surface. The peripheral portion of the cytoplasm and the cell membrane also retract to the luminal position where cell division is completed. The two new daughter cells extend their cytoplasm and cell membranes back to the external surface of the neural tube. The nucleus migrates back to the periphery again. In this position, this cell can undergo another mitosis or it can differentiate. Because the nucleus is at the external surface during interphase, differentiation occurs at the external surface of the neural tube. Thus, in a short time a new layer of differentiating cells appears on the external surface of the actively dividing layer. The mitotic layer of cells is the germinal layer. The cells undergoing differentiation form the mantle layer.

The cells that are differentiated are of two types: immature neurons and spongioblasts. Immature neurons are the primary parenchymal cells of the nervous system. They are often referred to as neuroblasts but this is a misnomer because once a neuron is formed it will not divide again as the term *neuroblast* implies. The differentiated immature neuron grows extensively, forming long processes in becoming a mature functioning cell, but it does not divide

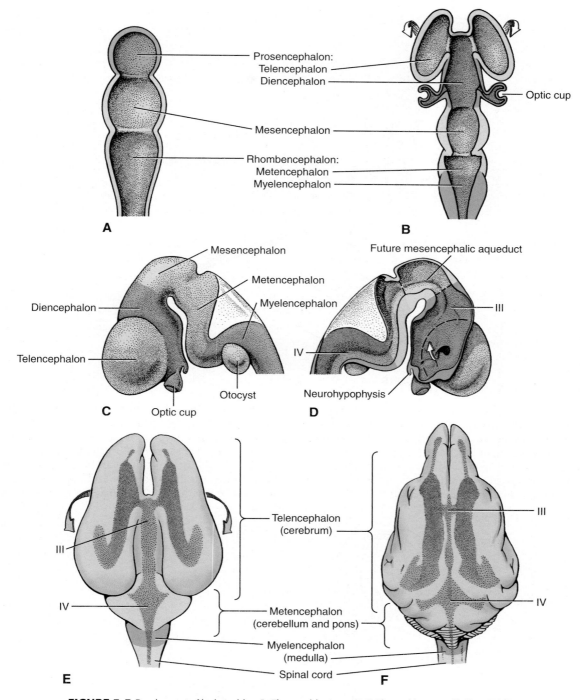

FIGURE 3-3 Development of brain vesicles. **A,** Three vesicle stages. **B-F,** Five vesicle stages, III, IV—ventricles.

again. Spongioblasts are the progenitors of the neurectodermal supporting cells of the nervous system, the neuroglia (glue). Two of the three forms of glial cells are derived from these spongioblasts: astrocytes and oligodendrocytes (Fig. 3-4). The third glial cell is the microglial cell, which is mesodermal in origin. It is a monocyte that enters the nervous system from its blood supply.

As the primitive neurons and spongioblasts are differentiated and grow and the neurons produce processes, the neural tube becomes arranged in three concentric layers (Fig. 3-5). Adjacent to the lumen of the neural tube is the germinal layer of proliferating neuroepithelial cells. This proliferative mitotic activity will ultimately be exhausted, reducing the germinal layer to a single layer of cells ranging from squamous to columnar and called ependymal cells. These ependymal cells line the entire lumen of the neural tube, which includes the ventricular system in the brain and the central canal of the spinal cord. Peripheral to this germinal layer in the embryonic neural tube is the thick layer of differentiated cells, the immature neurons, and spongioblasts. They form the mantle layer, which will ultimately become the gray matter of the definitive spinal cord, the

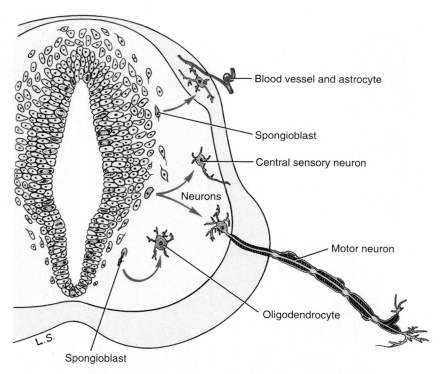

FIGURE 3-4 Mitosis and differentiation of neuroepithelial cells.

nuclei of the brainstem, the nuclei and cortex of the cerebellum, and the basal nuclei and cerebral cortex of the telencephalon. The latter requires a migration of these neurons from the mantle layer to the external surface of the neural tube. The external layer of the neural tube is the marginal layer; it is composed primarily of the growing axonal processes of the neuronal cell bodies in the mantle layer.

These axons will be myelinated by the oligodendroglial cells forming tracts in the white matter.

From the mesencephalon caudally, a longitudinal groove, the sulcus limitans, appears in the lateral wall of the neural canal. Thus the neural canal can be artificially divided into dorsal and ventral portions by an imaginary dorsal plane at the level of this sulcus. The dorsal portion is called the alar

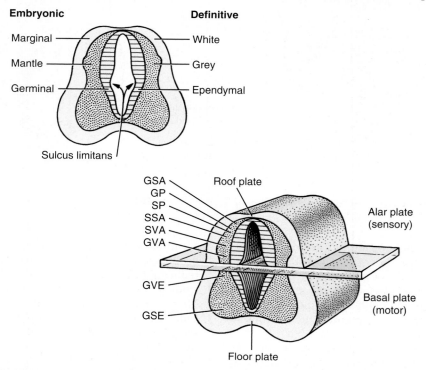

FIGURE 3-5 Functional organization of the neural tube. *GP,* General proprioception; *GSA,* general somatic afferent; *GSE,* general somatic efferent; *GVA,* general visceral afferent; *GVE,* general visceral efferent; *SP,* special proprioception; *SSA,* special somatic afferent; *SVA,* special visceral afferent.

plate and the ventral portion the basal plate. Functionally the alar plate mantle layer is concerned predominantly with sensory systems, and the basal plate mantle layer with motor systems (see Fig. 3-5).

MEDULLA SPINALIS: SPINAL CORD (See Fig. 2-17)

In this text, the term *spinal cord* is used rather than *medulla spinalis*, the nomenclature preferred by *Nomina Anatomica Veterinaria*. The spinal cord provides the best example of the symmetric development of the neural tube by layers. Ventral growth of the two basal layers and associated marginal layers beyond the level of the floor plate (Fig. 3-6) leaves a separation between the two sides, which is the ventral median fissure. The mantle and marginal layers of the alar plates grow dorsally. The dorsal marginal layers fuse on the median plane to form a dorsal median septum that may be poorly defined. The external margin of this septum forms the dorsal median sulcus. This midline growth displaces the roof plate region ventrally, resulting in a reduction of the neural canal to form the small central canal of the spinal cord lined by ependymal cells. The mantle layer of the alar plate becomes the dorsal gray column (also referred to as horn), and that of the basal plate becomes the ventral gray column. The mantle zone at the plane of the sulcus limitans becomes the intermediate gray column (see Fig. 3-6).

Not only is there a gross topographic differentiation of function of primitive neurons between the alar and basal plates, but within the mantle layer of each plate, neurons are further arranged in functional columns. The general visceral afferent and general visceral efferent neurons are located adjacent to each other in their respective gray columns on either side of the dorsal plane through the sulcus limitans. The general somatic afferent and general proprioceptive neuronal columns are located dorsally in the alar plate of the mantle layer,

and the general somatic efferent column is located ventrally in the basal plate of the mantle layer. Because the relative size of the components of each spinal cord segment depends on the volume of tissue being innervated, at the levels of the limbs the spinal cord segments responsible for their innervation are enlarged forming the cervical and lumbosacral intumescences. The ultimate growth to maturity of a neuron in the peripheral nervous system depends on its appropriate innervation of a muscle cell (general somatic efferent [GSE]) or formation of a peripheral receptor (general somatic afferent [GSA], general proprioception [GP]). The lack of such innervation results in the degeneration of that neuron. In the cervical and thoracolumbar regions where appendages are not innervated, the immature primitive neurons in the basal plate mantle layer and the adjacent spinal ganglion that fail to innervate structures will degenerate by a process of cell death referred to as apoptosis. The shape of the ventral gray column depicts this process.

In the basal plate mantle layer, the GSE neurons located medially innervate the axial skeletal muscles. Those located laterally innervate the appendicular skeletal muscles. Within these areas of the ventral gray column, the GSE neuronal cell bodies can be further grouped according to the specific peripheral nerve that contains their axon and by the specific muscles innervated.

The growth of axons of the basal plate neurons through the marginal layer and outside the neural tube forms the ventral root and part of the spinal nerve and further branching of the peripheral nerves. This includes the general somatic efferent neurons located in the ventral gray column and the general visceral efferent neurons located in the intermediate gray column adjacent to the sulcus limitans. These latter general visceral efferent (GVE) neurons are the preganglionic lower motor neurons of the autonomic nervous system. This intermediate gray column is only present in the thoracic, cranial lumbar and sacral spinal cord segments. In the other segments, it was present in the embryo but subsequently

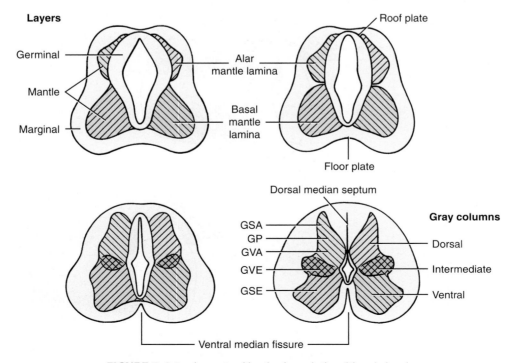

FIGURE 3-6 Development and functional organization of the spinal cord.

degenerated due to the absence of a target organ or biochemical attractant. These GVE neurons terminate in ganglia in the peripheral nervous system that contain cell bodies of the postganglionic neurons in this two-neuron lower motor neuron system (Figs. 3-7 and 3-8; see also Fig. 3-6).

Neural Crest

The neural crest cells are the cell bodies in the longitudinal column of cells that formed dorsolateral to the neural tube. Along the developing spinal cord segments, these cells provide the neurons that form the spinal ganglia at each segment. Adjacent to each somite a proliferation of neural crest cells forms the segmental spinal ganglion (see Figs. 3-1 and 3-7). One portion of the axon that emerges from each of these cell bodies grows centrally into the spinal cord segment to enter the alar plate dorsal gray column forming the dorsal root. The other portion of the axon grows distally to form a sensory component of the spinal nerve and further branches of the peripheral nerves. The point of penetration

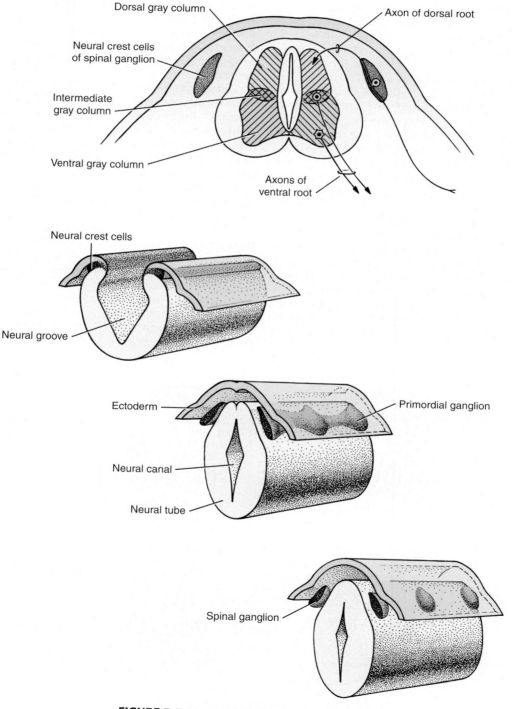

FIGURE 3-7 Spinal ganglia development from the neural crest.

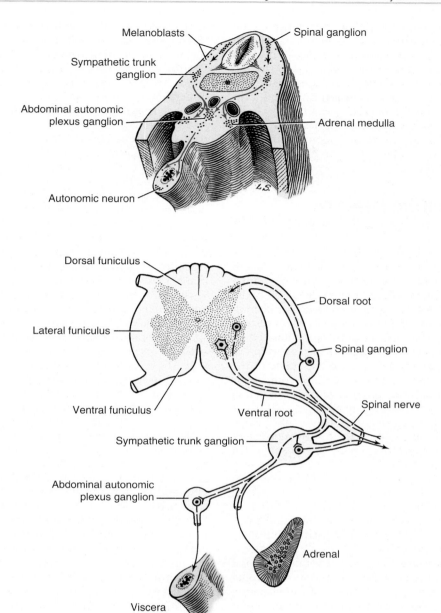

FIGURE 3-8 Neural crest contribution to the development of GVE neurons.

of the marginal white matter layer of the spinal cord segment by the axons in the dorsal and ventral roots divides the spinal cord white matter processes into three regions called funiculi. These are the dorsal, lateral, and ventral funiculi on each side of the spinal cord.

The formation of spinal ganglia is only one of many outcomes of neural crest differentiation. Prior to its segregation into spinal gangli, an early migration of cells from this neural crest column provides melanoblasts to the somitic dermatome and adjacent epidermis as well as to the cell bodies of postganglionic axons in the two-neuron GVE system.

These latter cell bodies form the ganglia of the sympathetic trunk and the abdominal plexus sympathetic ganglia as well as the medullary cells in the adrenal gland (see Fig. 3-8). These adrenal medullary cells do not grow any processes but synthesize and elaborate into the blood stream

the same endocrine substance, norepinephrine, that is the neurotransmitter released at the telodendron of the sympathetic postganglionic axon derived from the neural crest cells. Although the melanoblasts and GVE neurons seem unrelated, their common denominator is the unique metabolism of tyrosine, which provides melanin for the melanocytes and the norepinephrine for the neuron. In addition, there is extensive migration of the neural crest cells into the wall of the developing gastrointestinal tract. These will form the postganglionic neurons of the parasympathetic portion of the GVE lower motor neuron as well as interneurons; and they form the glial cells that develop in the wall of the bowel, creating what is referred to as the enteric nervous system. The latter is extremely extensive and complex and presumably is entirely derived from the neural crest cells. A similar migration forms the postganglionic parasympathetic neurons for the urogenital system.

In addition to these nervous system structures, the neural crest contributes to the formation of bone and cartilage in the skull and derivatives of the branchial arches; to the wall of the great vessels at the base of the heart; and to thyroid parafollicular (C) cells, odontoblasts, a portion of the leptomeninges and the lemmocytes, Schwann cells, that form the myelin of the peripheral nervous system. This is an amazing display of developmental capabilities in an initial column of cells. When a student is asked about the origin of a structure, if there is any doubt, relying on neural crest is a worthwhile consideration!

MYELENCEPHALON: MEDULLA OBLONGATA (See Figs. 2-11 through 2-16)

In this text, the term *medulla oblongata* is shortened to *medulla*. The medulla is the most caudal portion of the brainstem and is continuous caudally with the spinal cord. The basic formation of the medulla involves only a slight modification of the development described for the spinal cord. The narrow mid-dorsal roof plate of the initial neural tube (see Figs. 3-5 and 3-6) is stretched extensively instead of being obliterated by the proliferating alar plate and marginal tissue as it is in the spinal cord. Imagine grasping the midline roof plate of the neural tube with both hands and then pulling your hands apart sideways. This would stretch out a thin layer of neural tube (roof plate) and displace the entire alar and basal plates to a lateral and ventral position (Fig. 3-9). This would enlarge the lumen of the neural tube to form the fourth ventricle of the medulla, which is covered dorsally by only a single cell layer of neuroepithelial cells. At this site these cells will not enter mitosis but will remain as a single layer of ependymal cells. The sulcus limitans that is present on the ventrolateral wall of the fourth ventricle provides the plane of division of the medulla into a ventromedial basal plate and a dorsolateral alar plate, which have the same functional significance as in the spinal cord development.

Throughout the brainstem, the mantle layer of the neural tube is broken up into nuclei that are collections of neuronal cell bodies with a common purpose, and they are interspersed with neuronal processes. Some nuclei are more distinct than others. The functional columns described in the spinal cord have a similar location in the brainstem. In addition, there are neurons in the medulla that are organized into functional groups that are present only in cranial nerves (see Fig. 3-9).

In domestic animals, cranial nerves VI through XII and the trapezoid body are part of the medulla. The rostral border of the medulla is the caudal border of the pontine transverse fibers. In the primate and some nondomesticated species, the transverse fibers of the pons expand caudally to cover the trapezoid body, so cranial nerves VI through VIII are included with V in the pons. Cranial nerves VI, VII, IX, X, XI, and XII contain general somatic efferent neurons. The medullary nuclei of cranial nerves VI and XII are located in an interrupted column along the median plane adjacent to the fourth ventricle. The hypoglossal nucleus is very long. The GSE neuronal cell bodies of the facial nerve have migrated from their initial formation in the mantle layer to form the facial nucleus in a ventrolateral position, which is closer to their common source of sensory stimuli coursing into the medulla in the spinal tract of the trigeminal nerve. This phenomenon of migration is referred to as neurobiotaxis. As a result of this migration, the axons leaving this facial nucleus initially course dorsomedially to the floor of the fourth ventricle before turning to course ventrolaterally to leave the medulla and form the facial nerve. The GSE cell bodies of cranial nerves IX, X, and XI undergo a similar migration ventrolaterally and accumulate in nucleus ambiguus, which is well named because it is a poorly defined nucleus. The preganglionic neurons of the parasympathetic portion of the GVE system are located in an interrupted column just ventromedial to the sulcus limitans, similar to their location in the spinal cord. Their axons leave the medulla in cranial nerves VII, IX, X, and XI.

The sensory components of cranial nerves associated with the medulla arise primarily from primitive neurons that develop from the column of neural crest cells, with a few arising from ectodermal cells that proliferate from branchial arch ectoderm. The latter areas are referred to as cranial placodes. These two sources form the sensory ganglia of cranial nerves VII, IX, and X, which are concerned with general visceral afferent and special visceral afferent (taste) function. Ectodermal cells derived from the otic placode form the sensory ganglia of cranial nerve VIII, which is concerned with special proprioception for vestibular system function and with the special somatic afferent system for auditory function. These cranial nerve VIII ganglia are located in the inner ear within the petrosal portion of the temporal bone. Their axons course into the alar plate region of the medulla to synapse on cell bodies comparable to the dorsal gray column cell bodies in the spinal cord (see Fig. 3-9).

The leptomeninges that surround the entire developing central nervous system (CNS; neural tube) arise from neural crest cells and adjacent mesodermal cells. These meninges contain the bulk of the blood vessels that supply the CNS and the roots of the peripheral nerves. Dorsal to the stretched-out roof plate of the fourth ventricle, the capillary blood vessels proliferate to form the two longitudinal rows of a dense capillary bed. The adjacent ependymal cells enlarge into cuboidal cells, and the entire structure (cuboidal ependymal cells, pia mater, and capillary bed) hangs down into the lumen of the fourth ventricle (Fig. 3-10). This is called the choroid plexus of the fourth ventricle. By strict definition, only the proliferated capillary bed is the plexus. Thus the choroid plexus of the fourth ventricle comprises two sagittal lines parallel to and on either side of the median plane. These extend from the caudal part of the fourth ventricle rostrally to the level of the cerebellar peduncles where each plexus turns laterally. At this point there is an opening that develops in the medullary roof plate, called the lateral aperture. This aperture allows communication between the lumen of the fourth ventricle and the subarachnoid space that develops in the leptomeninges. At the level of this lateral aperture, the choroid plexus protrudes from the lumen of the fourth ventricle out through the aperture, where it is visible on each side at the cerebellomedullary angle (see Fig. 3-10). The aperture itself is invisible grossly because it is filled with this choroid plexus. The choroid plexus is a major site of formation of cerebrospinal fluid (see Chapter 4). In domestic animals, the lateral aperture is the only communication between the ventricular system of the brain and the subarachnoid space, which makes it critical for the maintenance of normal intracranial pressure. Primates have an additional aperture located caudally in the caudal medullary velum of the fourth ventricle.

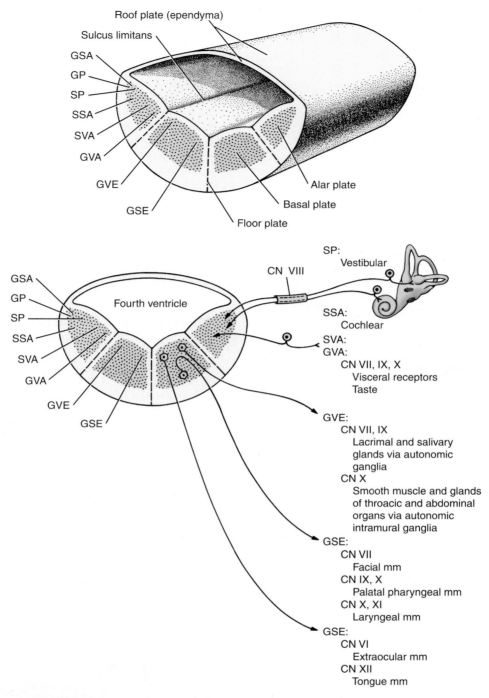

FIGURE 3-9 Functional organization of cranial nerves VI to XII in the myelencephalon. *CN VI,* Abducent; *CN VII,* facial; *CN VIII,* vestibulocochlear; *CN IX,* glossopharyngeal; *CN X,* vagus; *CN XI,* accessory; *CN XII,* hypoglossal; *GP,* general proprioception; *GSA,* general somatic afferent; *GSE,* general somatic efferent; *GVA,* general visceral afferent; *GVE,* general visceral efferent; *SP,* special proprioception; *SSA,* special somatic afferent; *SVA,* special visceral afferent.

METENCEPHALON: CEREBELLUM AND PONS (See Figs. 2-9 and 2-10)

The initial development of the metencephalon is comparable to that of the myelencephalon. Cranial nerve V, the trigeminal nerve, is associated with this segment of the brainstem (Fig. 3-11). Its motor neurons arise in the basal plate mantle layer, migrate a short way ventrolaterally into the parenchyma

of the pons, and form a small, well-defined motor nucleus. These neurons function in the general somatic efferent system and innervate the muscles of mastication derived from the somitomeres in branchial arch 1. The sensory neurons in cranial nerve V are derived primarily from neural crest cells and form the trigeminal ganglion. Most of these neurons are GSA and their dendritic zones are widely spread over the entire surface of the head and to the inner surface of the

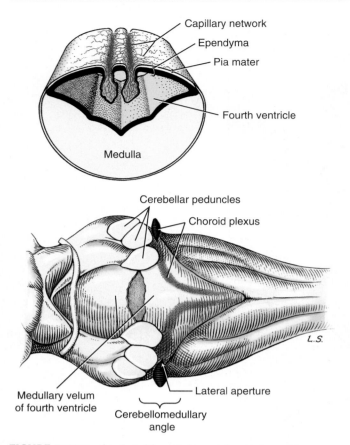

FIGURE 3-10 Development of the roof plate and choroid plexus of the fourth ventricle.

upper respiratory and digestive systems. A smaller component is composed of general proprioceptive neurons for the muscles and joints in the head region. These sensory neurons greatly outnumber the motor neurons. Therefore, when these sensory axons enter the alar plate region of the metencephalon, they spread out for a short distance rostrally and for a long distance caudally, forming the spinal tract of trigeminal nerve in the pons and medulla. These axons terminate in telodendria at synapses in the alar plate neurons, which form the sensory pontine nucleus of the trigeminal nerve in the pons and the nucleus of the spinal tract of the trigeminal nerve in the medulla. This spinal tract and nucleus extends the full length of the medulla, where caudally they meet the comparable functional neurons developing in the first cervical spinal nerves and spinal cord segment (see Fig. 3-11).

The cerebellum, or dorsal metencephalon, is formed primarily from the proliferation of the germinal epithelial cells of the alar plate, forming the rhombic lip (see Figs. 3-11 and 3-12). This growth dorsolaterally from each side overgrows the roof plate of the fourth ventricle so that the cerebellum forms part of the dorsal boundary of the fourth ventricle in the metencephalon. The development of the cerebellar cortex and nuclei are described in Chapter 13. The ventral metencephalon is the pons. A ventral migration of alar plate mantle layer neurons forms the pontine nucleus (see Fig. 3-12). The axons of these neurons cross the midline and course dorsally into the cerebellum. This forms the transverse fibers of the pons, which demarcate the ventral surface of the pons and the middle cerebellar peduncle.

MESENCEPHALON: MIDBRAIN
(See Figs. 2-5 through 2-9)

Symmetric proliferation of the walls of the neural tube in the mesencephalon reduces the size of the neural canal to a narrow tube, the mesencephalic aqueduct. This is smaller rostrally, where it joins the third ventricle of the diencephalon, and larger caudally, where it is continuous with the fourth ventricle beneath the rostral medullary velum.

Cranial nerves III (oculomotor) and IV (trochlear) are associated with the midbrain. These contain primarily GSE neurons that innervate extraocular muscles. The cell bodies are in nuclei derived from the basal plate mantle layer. They do not migrate but remain adjacent to the median plane ventral to the aqueduct, which is in the same topographic nuclear column as the abducent and hypoglossal GSE nuclei in the medulla (Fig. 3-13). The oculomotor nucleus also contains the neuronal cell bodies of the preganglionic parasympathetic innervation to the constrictor muscle of the iris. These are derived from the same basal plate mantle layer.

FIGURE 3-11 Development of the metencephalon: surface view and sagittal view of the afferent portion of cranial nerve V.

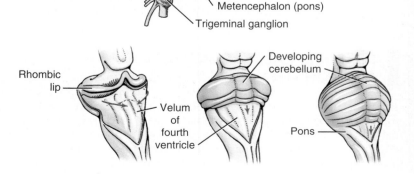

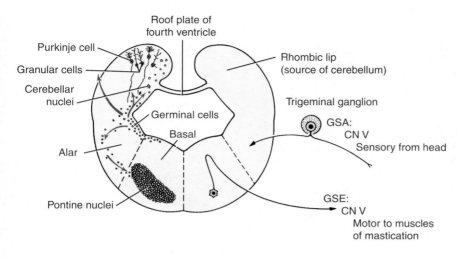

FIGURE 3-12 Development of the metencephalon: transverse section, pontine nucleus.

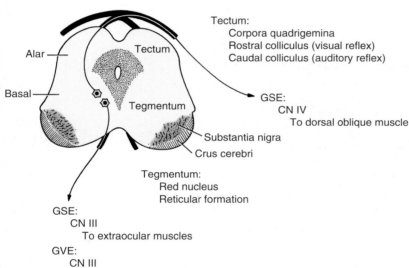

FIGURE 3-13 Development of the mesencephalon: transverse section.

The alar plate proliferates dorsally to form the tectum of the midbrain, which is divided into paired rostral and caudal colliculi, collectively known as the corpora quadrigemina. These are associated with visual and auditory reflex function, respectively. The crus cerebri on the ventral surface of the midbrain results from the caudal growth of descending axons from telencephalic projection neurons. These are continuous from the internal capsule in the diencephalon.

▌ DIENCEPHALON: INTERBRAIN
(See Figs. 2-3 through 2-6)

Rostral to the mesencephalon, the sulcus limitans is no longer evident in the neural tube and the diencephalon and telencephalon are considered to be developments of the alar plate. The symmetric development of the lateral walls of the neural tube in the diencephalon reduces the neural canal to a vertical slit on the median plane, the third ventricle. Adhesion of the developing thalamus in the center forms the interthalamic adhesion and separates the third ventricle into a small dorsal component and a larger ventral component. These two portions converge caudally at the mesencephalic aqueduct and rostrally at the level of the interventricular foramina, which connect to each telencephalic lateral ventricle (Fig. 3-14). On the dorsal median plane of the diencephalon, there is no proliferation of the neural tube epithelial cells, leaving a single-cell-thick roof plate, where a small choroid plexus develops in two parallel lines similar to those in the medulla. At the interventricular foramina each of these is continuous with the choroid plexus that develops in each lateral ventricle (Fig. 3-15).

In the diencephalon, a plethora of nuclei are formed from the mantle layer, which are dispersed diffusely through this brain segment forming a complex of nuclei and neuronal processes.

These nuclei form the thalamencephalon, hypothalamus, and subthalamus. The thalamencephalon consists of the thalamus, metathalamus, and epithalamus, which comprise those nuclei located dorsal to the ventral portion of the third ventricle. The hypothalamus includes the nuclei located on the sides and floor of the ventral portion of the third ventricle. The subthalamic nuclei are located ventrolaterally in the diencephalon. A ventral outgrowth of the hypothalamus, including an extension of the third ventricle, forms the neurohypophysis. The neurohypophysis

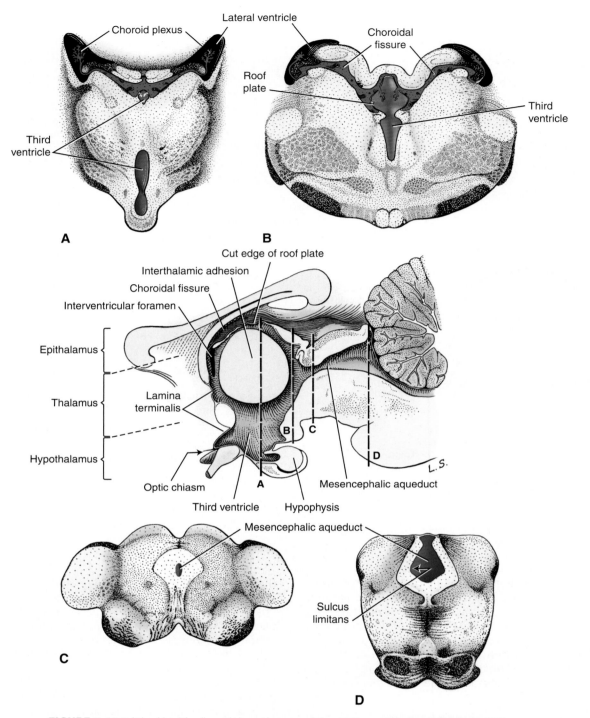

FIGURE 3-14 Relationship of the diencephalon and mesencephalon. **A,** Transverse section of mid-diencephalon. **B,** Transverse section of caudal diencephalon. **C,** Transverse section of rostral mesencephalon. **D,** Transverse section of caudal mesencephalon.

becomes associated with a dorsal extension of the adjacent oral ectoderm, the hypophyseal (Rathke's) pouch, to form the hypophysis (pituitary gland). The optic vesicles that initially grew out of the prosencephalon will form the neural layer of the eye and optic nerves, which become associated with the diencephalon (see Fig. 3-3). The axons that grow caudally from the retina in the optic nerve will form the optic tracts of the diencephalon, and many will terminate in a nuclear area of the thalamus. These optic nerves form cranial nerve II, the special somatic afferent neurons of the visual system. By definition, a nerve is a collection of axons outside the CNS that are myelinated by Schwann cells, which arise from the neural crest. Optic nerves are misnamed because they develop as extensions of the prosencephalon. They form in the optic stalk that extends from the diencephalon to the optic cup. Their axons are myelinated by CNS oligodendroglial cells. This is important to remember because the optic nerves are affected by diseases that are specific to the CNS.

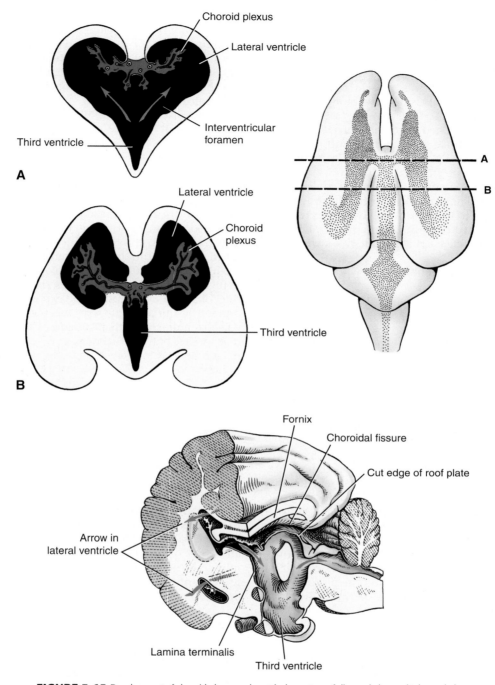

FIGURE 3-15 Development of choroid plexus and ventricular system of diencephalon and telencephalon.

Therefore, optic neuritis is a form of encephalitis. A polyneuritis does not affect the optic nerves.

 TELENCEPHALON: CEREBRUM
(See Figs. 2-2 through 2-7)

The rostral boundary of the brainstem is the lamina terminalis of the diencephalon. It is the rostral boundary of the third ventricle. The optic chiasm is located at the ventral portion of this lamina, and the rostral commissure develops in and remains in this lamina. It is at this level that the telencephalic vesicles grow out of the original prosencephalon to form the two cerebral hemispheres that comprise the cerebrum. The lamina terminalis is located on the median plane between these two outgrowths. The telencephalic vesicles grow out of the prosencephalon a short distance rostrally and then in a large curve caudally and ventrally. The neural canal in each telencephalon is the lateral ventricle, which communicates with the diencephalic third ventricle via the interventricular foramen on each side of the lamina terminalis (see Figs. 3-15 and 3-18).

At one aspect of the medial wall of the telencephalic vesicle, the neuroepithelial layer of the neural tube does not proliferate and remains a single layer of cells that become ependymal cells comparable to the roof plate of the myelencephalon over the fourth ventricle and the roof plate of the diencephalon over the third ventricle. As the rest of the telencephalon proliferates and differentiates, this telencephalic roof plate will be attached to the crus of the hippocampal fornix on one side and the stria terminalis on the other side. The choroid plexus of each lateral ventricle develops in this roof plate as was described for the choroid plexus in the medulla. This is a curved structure similar to the structures that it is attached to, and it protrudes into the lumen of the lateral ventricle. At each interventricular foramen, each lateral ventricular choroid plexus is continuous with the choroid plexus of the third ventricle.

An extensive development of projection axons occurs from diencephalic thalamic neurons to the cerebrum and telencephalic neurons to the brainstem. This gives rise to a thick layer of myelinated processes, white matter, between the diencephalon and telencephalon that is known as the internal capsule.

Telencephalic neuronal cell bodies and white matter can be organized as follows.

Cell Bodies

The telencephalic neuronal cell bodies are located in one of two general locations. One is on the external surface of the entire telencephalon, forming the various layers of the cerebral cortex. The other is deep to the surface in subcortical basal nuclei. These are often incorrectly called basal ganglia. Remember that ganglia are collections of neuronal cell bodies outside the CNS. Such collections inside the CNS are nuclei or cortices. Cortices are located superficially, and their neuronal cell bodies are in a continuous arrangement. Examples of basal nuclei are the caudate nucleus, globus pallidus, putamen, claustrum, and amygdaloid body. The cerebral cortex can be divided into three regions based on evolutionary and anatomic features. The archipallium (pallium is a synonym for cortex) is the hippocampus, which is an internal gyrus, an area of cerebral cortex that has been rolled into the lateral ventricle and is not visible on the surface of the cerebrum. The paleopallium is the olfactory system and is composed of the olfactory bulbs, the peduncles, and the piriform lobe cortex. In animal evolution, these are the most primitive

portions of the cerebrum. The neopallium is a more recent evolutionary brain development and makes up the surface of all the gyri of the cerebrum (Fig. 3-16).

Comparative evolutionary studies show the continual development of the neopallium in higher animals, relegating the archipallium and paleopallium to a lesser portion anatomically.

The surface of the amphibian cerebrum is smooth, lacking any gyri. It is composed of the archipallium dorsally, the paleopallium laterally, and the basal nuclei ventrally. In the advanced reptile, the basal nuclei have receded from the ventral surface and have been replaced by the paleopallium on the ventral surface. A small lateral area is neopallium and the dorsal area is archipallium. In mammals, the neopallium has overgrown the other divisions of the cerebral cortex so that the paleopallium is entirely on the ventral surface of the cerebrum, ventral to the rhinal sulcus, and the archipallium is rolled medially into the lateral ventricle as an internal gyrus, the hippocampus. Continual development of the neopallium in higher mammals has resulted in the characteristic gyri and sulci observed over most of the exposed surface of the cerebrum. The rhinal sulcus separates the neopallium from the paleopallium. This is characteristic of all of the domestic animal species, but most laboratory rodents and all birds have no gyri because in these animals the neopallium is unfolded, so the cerebrum has a smooth surface. Although at birth a few gyri and sulci are present in the puppy brain, they increase remarkably during the first 3 to 6 weeks of life.

Axons

The axons of telencephalic neurons form three groups of processes on the basis of their destinations. The association axons course between cortical areas within one cerebral hemisphere. They can be short and course between adjacent gyri or long and traverse the entire cerebral hemisphere, but they never leave that hemisphere. Projection axons leave the cerebral hemisphere where their cell bodies are located and enter the brainstem via the internal capsule. They terminate in nuclei in various parts of the brainstem, with a few reaching the spinal cord. Commissural axons cross from one cerebrum to the other (Fig. 3-17). All of these axons are

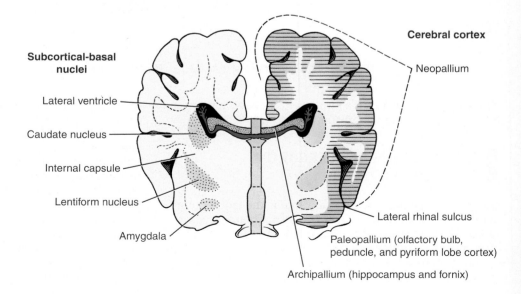

FIGURE 3-16 Development of the telencephalon.

Subcortical-basal nuclei

Lateral ventricle

Caudate nucleus

Internal capsule

Lentiform nucleus

Amygdala

Cerebral cortex

Neopallium

Lateral rhinal sulcus

Paleopallium (olfactory bulb, peduncle, and pyriform lobe cortex)

Archipallium (hippocampus and fornix)

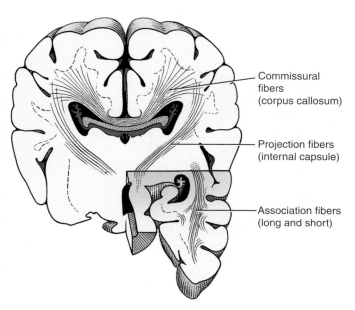

FIGURE 3-17 Development of the neuronal processes in the telencephalon, white matter.

their axons grow centrally, forming the white matter on the inside of the gray matter. Radial astrocytes participate in this migration by guiding the neurons to the surface of the neural tube. Ultimately, six layers of neurons will populate the cortex and are numbered from superficial (layer I) to deep (layer VI). The first neurons to migrate to the developing cerebral cortex will form layer VI. As more neurons arrive, they pass by those already there to form the rest of the layers in a reverse sequence. Thus the last to arrive form layer I. The basal nuclei are formed by neurons that migrate only a short distance from the mantle layer into the developing white matter so that they remain in a subcortical position. Remnants of the telencephalic germinal layer persist throughout the life of the animal, forming the subependymal layer, which consists of a variably sized population of small cells that are thought to be a continuous source of glia and neurons throughout the life of the animal. Postnatal neurogenesis is now a well-recognized event, especially in the olfactory system and the hippocampus. This subependymal-subventricular layer is thought to be the source of some of the glial neoplasms that arise in the brain.

The development of the choroid plexuses of the lateral, third, and fourth ventricles is similar, but the adult morphology varies. The choroid plexuses of the lateral and third ventricle are small and form a thin, undulating veil that projects into the ventricle. The fourth ventricle choroid plexus is more robust and lobulated, especially where it projects through the lateral apertures.

This is especially evident in horses and cattle. In addition, in older horses there often is an accumulation of cholesterol crystals resulting from chronic bleeding that enlarges the choroid plexus. The accumulation of these crystals may present a sparkling appearance in the choroid plexus. Occasionally, in the choroid plexus of the lateral ventricle, this chronic bleeding results in such a large accumulation of cholesterol crystals and associated chronic inflammation that the mass causes neurologic signs associated with increased intracranial pressure. This cholesterinic granuloma can be unilateral or bilateral (Figs. 3-19 and 3-20) and can be diagnosed by computed tomography (CT) or magnetic resonance (MR) imaging. They can be very large when neurologic signs occur. The choroid plexus can give rise to choroid plexus papillomas and carcinomas. The latter can spread to other sites by way of the cerebrospinal fluid (CSF) in the subarachnoid space. Meningiomas arise from arachnoid cells and expand in the subarachnoid space. Meningiomas that bulge into the ventricular system arise from the arachnoid cells associated with the choroid plexus.

intermixed in the white matter of each gyrus, which is the corona radiata, and in the centrum semiovale, which is the mass of white matter in the center of the cerebrum dorsal to the lateral ventricle. The semioval appearance of this structure can be appreciated only in a dorsal plane section of the cerebral hemisphere.

There are three groups of commissural axons, all of which initially develop in the lamina terminalis (Fig. 3-18). The rostral commissure is located ventrally in the lamina terminalis and courses primarily between paleopallial structures and basal nuclei (the amygdaloid body) on each side. This commissure remains at this site dorsal to the optic chiasm in the fully developed brain. Another small group of commissural axons courses between the archipallium (hippocampus) of each side. This commissure migrated caudodorsally as the telencephalon developed to reach a position dorsal to the caudal aspect of the diencephalon.

The largest group of commissural axons forms the corpus callosum, which also expands dorsally as the cerebrum develops so that it is positioned between the other two commissures. The corpus callosum serves primarily to connect the neopallial areas of each cerebral hemisphere. It begins in the lamina terminalis and as the telencephalic vesicle expands, the corpus callosum enlarges and extends caudally dorsal to the diencephalon. Near the median plane it is located between the neopallial cingulate gyrus dorsally and the archipallial hippocampus and body of the fornix ventrally. Laterally in each cerebral hemisphere, the corpus callosum forms the roof of the lateral ventricle. The septum pellucidum develops dorsally in the lamina terminalis between the genu of the corpus callosum and the rostral body of the fornix (see Fig. 3-18).

In the telencephalon, the neural tube germinal layer ultimately is replaced by the ependyma of the lateral ventricle. Except for the area of the basal nuclei, the mantle and marginal layers reverse their positions. This is the result of the migration of the newly formed primitive neurons to the surface of the neural tube to form the cerebral cortex, where

MALFORMATIONS

Brain Malformations

Hydrocephalus

Many circumstances can cause the ventricular system to enlarge. It is usually most evident in the lateral ventricles, and the most common cause is an interference with the flow of CSF from the ventricles into the subarachnoid space, which results in increased CSF pressure. This hypertensive hydrocephalus causes extensive degeneration of the telencephalon, especially the neopallium. The subject of hydrocephalus is considered in the discussion of CSF in Chapter 4.

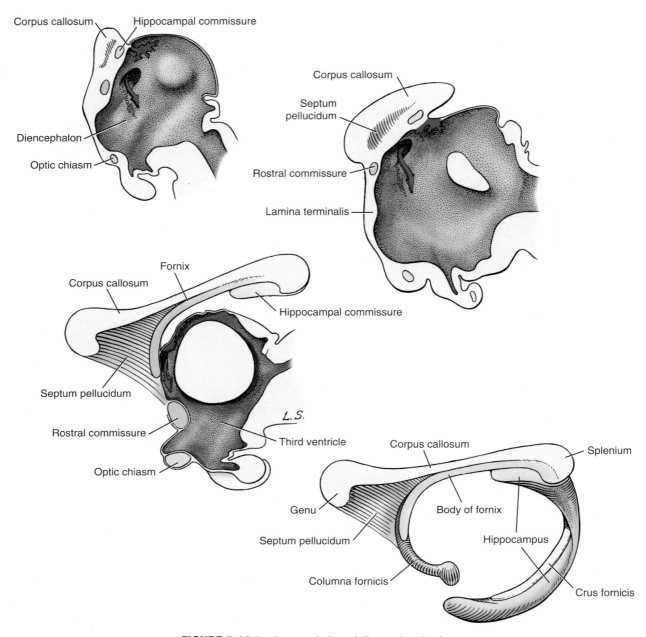

FIGURE 3-18 Development of telencephalic commissural pathways.

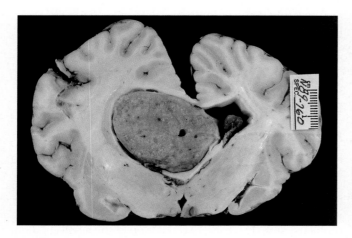

FIGURE 3-19 Transverse section of the brain of a 14-year-old Morgan horse with a unilateral cholesterinic granuloma of the choroid plexus in the left lateral ventricle.

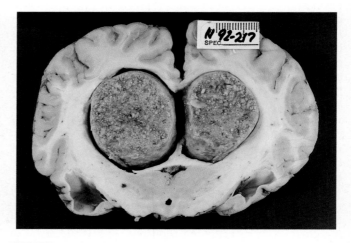

FIGURE 3-20 Transverse section of the brain of a 10-year-old Percheron horse with bilateral cholesterinic granulomas of the choroid plexuses of the lateral ventricles.

Hypoplasia of the Prosencephalon: Cerebral (Telencephalic) Aplasia (Anencephaly)

Calves have been observed at birth with a failure of the telencephalic vesicles to develop; this is associated with a small opening in the calvaria on the midline at the level of the orbits where fluid, presumably CSF, emerges (Fig. 3-21). The calvarial defect here is called a cranioschisis or cranium bifidum. The skin around this opening is continuous with a malformed diencephalon inside the small cranial cavity. There are no cerebral hemispheres. The brainstem and cerebellum are present but reduced in size and abnormally shaped. There are no recognizable thalamic geniculate nuclei or mesencephalic colliculi (Figs. 3-22 and 3-23). The eyes are well developed and all cranial nerves are present except for the first, the olfactory neurons. In human babies this is called anencephaly, an incorrect term because it implies that there is no brain development at all. No single term best describes this malformation.

Telencephalic (cerebral) aplasia accounts for the most extensive part of the malformation. One hypothesis about the mechanism involved in this brain malformation is as follows. If some factor caused the neurectoderm of the prosencephalon to fail to separate from the skin ectoderm at the level of the rostral neuropore, that could prevent the outgrowth of the telencephalic vesicles and create a defect in the closure of the calvaria, resulting in cerebral aplasia and cranioschisis, respectively. CSF could leak from the third ventricle of the diencephalon, which remains attached to the surface skin. The cause of this malformation in animals

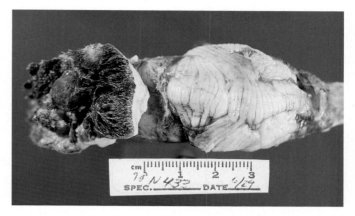

FIGURE 3-22 Dorsal view of the brain of a calf with prosencephalic hypoplasia. Note the complete absence of any cerebral hemispheres.

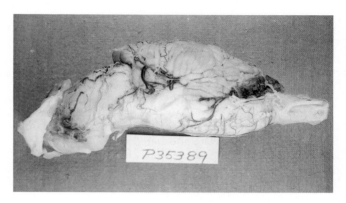

FIGURE 3-23 Lateral view of the brain of a calf with prosencephalic hypoplasia. Note the abnormally shaped brainstem and cerebellum.

is unknown but is one of the neural tube defects thought to result from a deficiency in folic acid in the diet of the human mother very early in development, before pregnancy may be diagnosed. Hyperthermia has also been implicated as a cause of this neural tube defect.

These calves are usually unable to get up at birth. **Video** **3-1** shows a newborn Guernsey calf with this malformation. When supported, these calves struggle to stand and exhibit considerable voluntary movement. They are blind because of the lack of any cerebral visual cortex for perception, but the cranial nerves function normally. Spinal reflexes are intact and surprisingly, there is some evidence of nociception (the perception of noxious stimuli), which supports the idea that some "conscious" perception can occur at the level of the diencephalon. The evidence for this is the occasional voluntary struggling that occurs when forceps pressure is applied to the digits as a noxious stimulus or when forceps are pressed against the nasal septum, and occasionally a loud noise elicits a voluntary response. We have not observed this malformation in other species of domestic animals.

Meningocele: Meningoencephalocele

A newborn animal with a large skin-covered, soft swelling outside the calvaria, usually on the midline, has a meningocele or meningoencephalocele. The latter has brain tissue in

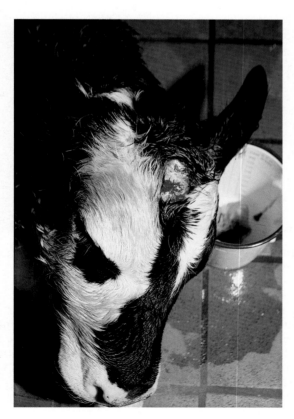

FIGURE 3-21 Calf with prosencephalic hypoplasia. Note the area in the center of the calvaria devoid of hair. The malformed diencephalon is fused to the skin here, and CSF leaked out of the third ventricle at this site.

the swelling along with the meninges and is by far the most common of these two malformations, but microscopic examination of the wall of the swelling is commonly required to appreciate the brain component (Figs. 3-24 and 3-25). The calvarial defect is called cranioschisis or cranium bifidum. This is usually on the midline and at any level of the length of the calvaria. This cranioschisis may be very large with both cerebral hemispheres bulging into the meningoencephalocele, or it can be small and involve an extension from the brainstem into the meningoencephalocele. In the large meningoencephalocele, the protruding cerebral hemispheres are usually very thin and fluid-filled due to dilation of their lateral ventricles, which results in the meningoencephalocele's being soft and fluctuant. Usually the cause is unknown. It is seen in all species of domestic animal but may be more common in pigs. In one kitten, a meningoencephalocele was associated with the queen's being treated orally with griseofulvin throughout the gestation period for a ringworm infection (Fig. 3-26).[26]

A very large meningoencephalocele occurs as part of an inherited craniofacial malformation in Burmese cats (Fig. 3-27).[31] Prior to its recognition as an inherited disorder, it was quite common in this breed in many different locations in the United States. It became apparent when a number of breeders attempted to breed for Burmese cats with shortened faces. In addition to the large meningoencephaloceles that often hung over their shortened faces, these kittens had significant facial malformations: the upper jaws and nasal areas were shortened and had no recognizable nares, planum nasale, or nasal cavities. There were no olfactory bulbs or peduncles in the malformed cerebrums. There was a philtrum on either side of the rostral midline of the face and vibrissae on both sides of the cleft (Fig. 3-28). Duplication was also evident in the two pairs of maxillary bones and two sets of maxillary canine teeth. There was no gross evidence of any eyes but one pair of orbits was present. No optic nerves or chiasm were associated with the diencephalon. The mandibles were prominent and the tongue was enlarged and protruded from the mouth. These facial deformities represent the result of abnormal cranial neural crest development. This is a prime example of what can happen when breeders select for a characteristic that in reality is a malformation, the shortened face; it is clear

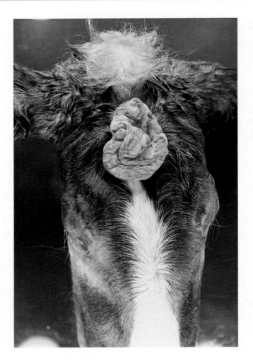

FIGURE 3-25 Head of a stillborn Belgian foal with a small meningoencephalocele. The hairless mass protruded through a small midline cranioschisis. On microscopic examination of the mass, brain tissue including choroid plexus was found adjacent to the dermis.

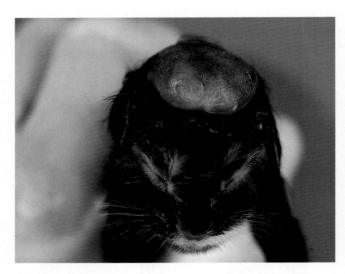

FIGURE 3-26 Newborn kitten with a meningoencephalocele. The queen had been treated with griseofulvin during gestation.

that more serious and life-threatening malformations can result. Selection for a longer cat skull shape will eliminate the problem. The malformation that occurs in Manx cats that are bred for the absence of a tail is a similar failure of judgment by misinformed breeders. This is described with the spinal cord malformations in this chapter.

Exencephaly

Exencephaly is now defined as brain tissue that protrudes out of the cranial cavity and is not covered by skin (Fig. 3-29).

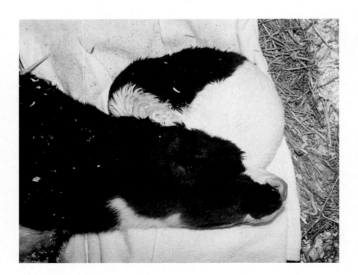

FIGURE 3-24 Newborn Holstein calf with a large meningoencephalocele.

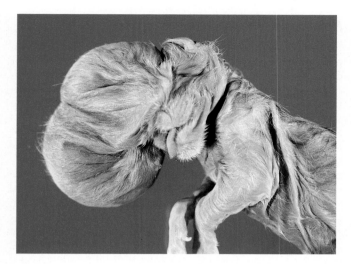

FIGURE 3-27 Newborn Burmese kitten with a large meningoencephalocele associated with facial duplication.

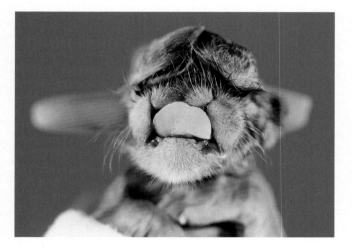

FIGURE 3-28 Another Burmese kitten with a smaller meningoencephalocele. Note the duplication of the philtrum and whisker pads.

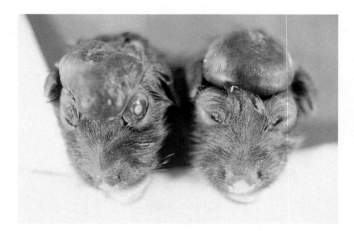

FIGURE 3-29 Two Pomeranian puppies with exencephaly.

There is no stratified squamous epithelium over the brain, only the connective tissue of the meninges. This can be determined only by microscopic study of the protruding tissue. When these malformations are studied microscopically, it is found that exencephaly is much less common than meningoceles or meningoencephaloceles. Both malformations require a cranioschisis, which is the opening in the calvaria where the bones have not fused.

Lipomeningocele

A lipomeningocele, as the term suggests, is a meningocele that has a large amount of fat associated with it. It can occur along the midline of the calvaria or the vertebral column through a cranioschisis or spina bifida, respectively. It consists of fat-filled meningeal tissue covered by skin that is continuous with the falx cerebri in the head and the dura of the spinal cord in the vertebral column (Fig. 3-30). With no associated neural tube malformation, there are no neurologic signs in these animals. These are rare malformations and the cause is unknown.

Duplication of the Prosencephalon

Prosencephalic duplication occurs most commonly in calves and is associated with varying degrees of duplication in the face that are called diprosopus or dicephalus (Fig. 3-31). The

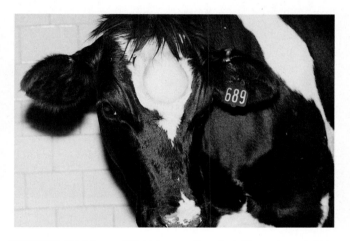

FIGURE 3-30 A 2-year-old Holstein cow with a calvarial lipomeningocele. This malformation was associated with the meninges of the falx cerebri with no cerebral involvement. This cow was clinically normal.

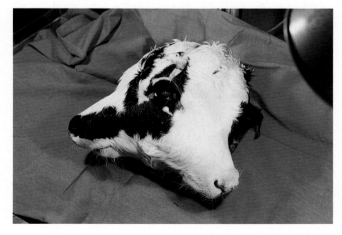

FIGURE 3-31 Dicephalic Holstein calf. Besides the enlarged midline orbit containing two fused eyes, there is an orbit and a complete eye on each side of the head.

diprosopus includes two separate nasal regions with four nares and nasal cavities, portions of two upper and lower jaws, and usually three orbits. The two complete orbits on the lateral sides of the head are normal. The central orbit is enlarged to accommodate two separate or fused eyeballs. The cranial region is broad but there are two normal ears and one normal atlantooccipital joint. In the widened cranial cavity there are four cerebral hemispheres (Fig. 3-32). There is one for each naris, formed from the embryonic olfactory placode that gave rise to the olfactory nerves. Each cerebral hemisphere has a normal olfactory bulb that resides in the cribriform plate of each of the two separate ethmoid bones. There are two diencephalons. Each diencephalon is associated with a pair of eyes, a pair of optic nerves, and an optic chiasm (Fig. 3-33). The brainstem usually becomes single somewhere in the mesencephalon. The pons, medulla, and cerebellum are all single structures. This is a partial dicephalus. These calves are usually born alive but are recumbent and unable to stand.

Holoprosencephaly-Arrhinencephaly

Holoprosencephaly-arrhinencephaly occurs with the cyclopian malformation. This is common in lambs when their dams are exposed through their diets to *Veratrum californicum* on their 14th or 15th day of gestation. This plant contains the alkaloid cyclopamine, which interferes with the sonic hedgehog signaling in the prechordal plate.[12] This results in a failure of the visual area on the ventral aspect of the prosencephalon to divide into two fields. One midline optic vesicle develops, producing a single eye. The interference with neural crest development results in the absence of any nasal portion of the respiratory system and olfactory system and the presence of a proboscis dorsal to the eye (Fig. 3-34). The interference with prosencephalic development results in only a single midline telencephalic vesicle (holoprosencephaly) that grows caudally on each side of the brainstem. Varying degrees of a longitudinal cerebral fissure develop caudally in the single cerebrum. This gives rise to three forms of holoprosencephaly: alobar, hemilobar, and lobar. In all three forms, the corpus callosum fails to develop. Arrhinencephaly is another term for this cerebral malformation because there is no development of the olfactory system. These lambs can be born alive and some survive for months. We have seen a semilobar holoprosencephaly as an isolated malformation with no ocular or facial abnormality in a 6-month-old Morgan with the clinical complaint of abnormal behavior and occasional seizures (Fig. 3-35).[14] The single cerebrum was partly divided caudally and had no olfactory system structures. The ethmoid bone had no cribriform plates. We have seen the cyclopian malformation on rare occasions in puppies, pigs, and kittens (Fig. 3-36). One case occurred in a kitten whose dam was treated throughout gestation with griseofulvin (Fig. 3-37).[26]

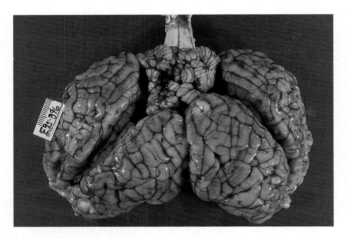

FIGURE 3-32 Dorsal view of the four cerebral hemispheres from a dicephalic calf.

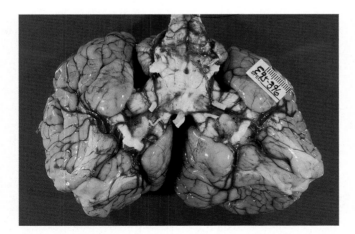

FIGURE 3-33 Ventral view of the four cerebral hemispheres and two diencephalons. Note the two prominent optic chiasms. Fusion occurs in the mesencephalon and there is no duplication of the pons, medulla, and cerebellum.

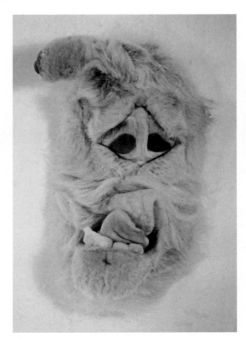

FIGURE 3-34 Newborn cyclopic lamb with a single median plane partially divided eyeball. Note the proboscis dorsal to the fused eye.

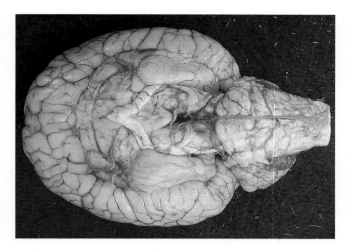

FIGURE 3-35 Ventral view of the brain of a 6-month-old Morgan with partial holoprosencephaly. Note the absence of any longitudinal cerebral fissure rostral to the optic chiasm and the absence of the olfactory bulbs and peduncles.

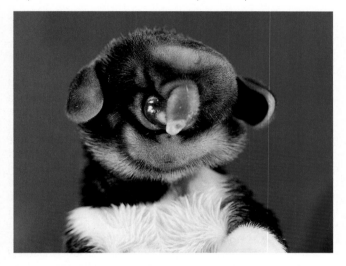

FIGURE 3-36 Beagle that is cyclopic, with unknown cause.

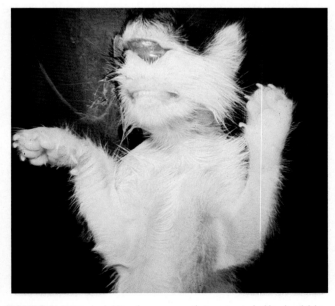

FIGURE 3-37 Cyclopic kitten from a queen that was treated with griseofulvin during gestation.

Hydranencephaly

Hydranencephaly is a model for a virus-induced cerebral malformation in animals. By definition hydranencephaly is the cerebral abnormality in which the neopallium is reduced to a thin, nearly transparent pial-glial membrane with no associated parenchyma other than a thin layer of ependyma lining the expanded lateral ventricle. The latter represents compensatory hydrocephalus because the increase in CSF volume and ventricular size are secondary to the absence of cerebral parenchyma. The loss of neopallial parenchyma represents both aplasia resulting from the viral destruction of germinal layer cells and atrophy resulting from the viral destruction of already differentiated neopallial neurons. Some of the destructive lesions may represent the effect of the viral agent on the developing vasculature and loss of adequate blood supply to the neopallium. Usually the olfactory paleopallium, the archipallium (hippocampus), and the basal nuclei are spared. The brainstem and cerebellum are also spared, but in some cases there are cerebellar lesions. The degree of lesion is dependent on the viral agent and the period during gestation when the infection occurs. There are no changes in the skull bones. The cranial cavity is normal in size and shape.

The bluetongue virus has been reported to produce this lesion in cattle and sheep in both clinical and experimental studies.[18-21] This virus causes systemic disease in sheep that is characterized by fever, lameness, and erosions and ulcerations of the oral and nasal mucosae. The live virus vaccine that was produced to establish immunity in sheep was found to cause brain malformations in lambs born of ewes immunized during gestation. These lambs were referred to as "dummy lambs" because of their depressed sensorium and lack of response to their environments. They were also blind. Experimental studies of direct inoculation of this vaccine into fetal sheep demonstrated that inoculation between 50 and 58 days of gestation consistently produced a severe necrotizing encephalitis that presented at term as hydranencephaly. Inoculation between 75 and 78 days of gestation caused a less severe multifocal encephalitis that presented at term as porencephaly. These are congenital cystic cavities in the cerebrum that commonly communicate with the lateral ventricle. Inoculation after 100 days of gestation caused a mild encephalitis with no resulting malformation. Thus the nature of the lesions at term depended on the gestational age at which infection of the fetus occurred.

The germinal cells of the telencephalon are especially susceptible to this infection and are most abundant at the end of the first trimester in the lamb fetus. Necrosis of the germinal cells in the first trimester prevents their contributing to the formation of the neopallium and, along with the necrosis of the initial neopallial cortical plate that is formed at that time, leads to the lesion referred to as hydranencephaly in lambs. At birth the inflammation has resolved, leaving the remaining neopallial membrane, which represents the "scar" resulting from the in utero infection. The lesion associated with this bluetongue virus infection represents a combination of abnormal development (hypoplasia-aplasia) and destruction (necrosis) of differentiated tissue, resulting in atrophy. A similar situation occurs primarily in the cerebellum as the result of a bovine viral diarrhea virus infection in cattle and the panleukopenia virus infection in cats.

Hydranencephaly occurs in calves that are exposed in utero to the same bluetongue virus (Fig. 3-38).[21] Like lambs, these calves are born lethargic, blind, and unable to suckle normally. The dams of these calves have no clinical illness but their serum contains antibodies to the bluetongue virus, and the presence of these same serum antibodies in the affected calves prior to the ingestion of colostrum indicates an in utero exposure to this virus. Hydranencephaly occurs in these calves when the infection occurs around 125 days of their in utero development.

The bovine viral diarrhea virus has been reported to cause hydranencephaly, but it has not been seen in the cattle in the northeast United States. The Cache Valley virus is another cause of hydranencephaly in ruminants in the United States.

In Australia, Japan, and Israel, hydranencephaly has been observed in ruminants in association with in utero infection with the Akabane virus in the first trimester (Fig. 3-39).[9,10] The same in utero viral infection has been associated with calves born with arthrogryposis. These calves have lesions in their spinal cords and loss of ventral gray column neurons. The denervation atrophy in muscles causes the arthrogryposis. In experimental studies in cattle, exposure to this virus between 74 and 104 days of gestation results in calves that have hydranencephaly. With exposure between 104 and 173 days, calves are born with arthrogryposis, and with exposure between 173 days and term, the calves have meningoencephalitis. Other viruses that are foreign to the United States and have been implicated in causing hydranencephaly in newborn ruminants include the Aino and Chuzan viruses.

Hydranencephaly was observed in a 3-month-old domestic shorthair kitten that had been blind and ataxic since birth.[8] The feline panleukopenia virus was implicated on the basis of direct immunofluorescence of the virus in the tissues. As a rule, the cerebellum is more severely affected by this virus, and there are few to no lesions in the cerebrum.

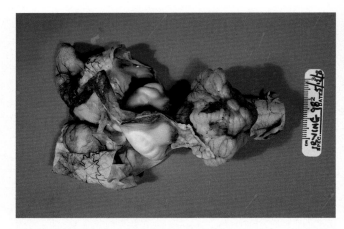

FIGURE 3-39 Brain of a calf with hydranencephaly caused by in utero infection with the Akabane virus. The white structures on the floor of the lateral ventricles are the hippocampi.

We have observed a bilateral hydranencephaly in related litters of Labrador retrievers. At necropsy they appeared to be caused by compromise of the blood flow in the cerebral arteries. Computed tomography and MR images were diagnostic.[1]

Unilateral hydranencephaly was found in an 8-month-old miniature poodle in which the only clinical sign was a contralateral visual deficit and sporadic seizures (Figs. 3-40 through 3-43). The primary lesion was limited to the right neopallium that was in the distribution of the right middle cerebral artery. The transparency of the remaining intact cerebral membrane allowed the observer to see the hippocampus on the floor of the lateral ventricle. The presence of polymicrogyria in the left cerebrum supported an in utero interference with the blood supply of the neopallium that was much worse on the right side. The cause of this vascular compromise was not established, and in dogs there has been no recognized in utero viral infection that causes congenital cerebral brain lesions. The early development of these lesions in this dog was supported by the secondary hypoplasia of the right side of the diencephalon and the much reduced size of the right cerebral projection pathways—that is, the crus cerebri, the longitudinal fibers of the pons, and the pyramid.

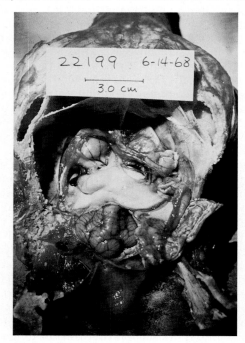

FIGURE 3-38 Hereford calf, 1 week old, with hydranencephaly. The calvaria has been removed. Note the normal cerebellum but the collapsed membranous neopallium bilaterally, exposing the hippocampi and caudate nuclei. This lesion was caused by an in utero infection by the bluetongue virus.

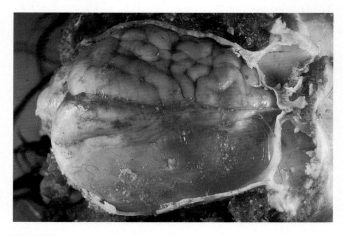

FIGURE 3-40 Unilateral hydranencephaly in an 8-month-old miniature poodle. The calvaria has been removed but the dura is still in place.

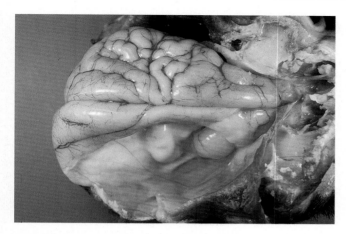

FIGURE 3-41 Same brain as in Fig. 3-40 except that the dura has been removed from the arachnoid. Note the thin red line of a blood vessel in the membranous neopallium.

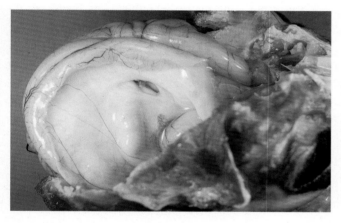

FIGURE 3-42 Lateral view of the same brain as in Figs. 3-40 and 3-41. Note the spared hippocampus and caudate nucleus in the floor of the lateral ventricle.

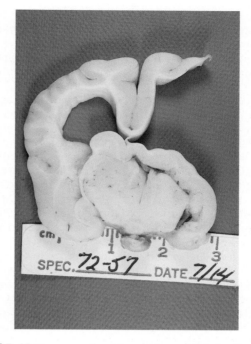

FIGURE 3-43 Transverse section of the miniature-poodle brain with unilateral hydranencephaly. Note the hypoplastic right half of the diencephalon and the polymicrogyria in the left cerebral hemisphere.

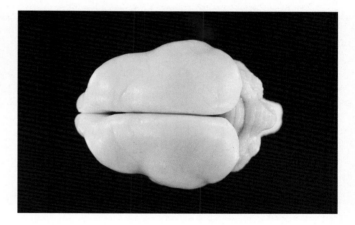

FIGURE 3-44 Lissencephaly in a 1-year-old Lhasa apso dog, dorsal view.

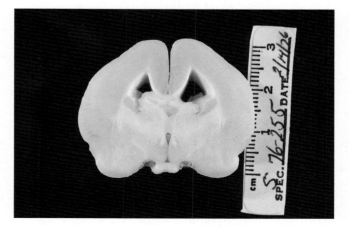

FIGURE 3-45 Transverse section of the brain in Fig. 3-44 at the level of the optic chiasm showing the thick pachygyrus with no folding into gyri.

Similar lesions have been produced experimentally with prenatal occlusion of the internal carotid artery in puppies. In humans, the pathogenesis of hydranencephaly includes infections, teratogens, genetic defects in cerebral vasculature, and genetic defects in neuronal migration.

Lissencephaly

Lissencephaly means a smooth brain without evidence of cerebrocortical folding to produce gyri and sulci. It is a congenital condition seen most commonly in the Lhasa apso breed of dogs (Figs. 3-44 and 3-45).[7,25,30] The cerebral cortex is thickened (pachygyria) owing to the abnormal distribution of neuronal cell bodies. The malformation presumably results from impaired neuronal migration, and an inherited genetic abnormality is presumed in this breed. In humans, intrauterine hypoxia or perfusion failure have also been suggested as possible causes of lissencephaly. Clinical signs seen in dogs with this malformation include difficulty in learning routine training programs, abnormal behavior, and occasionally slow postural reactions and poor menace responses. Generalized seizures may occur when the dogs are 10 to 12 months old.

We have seen lissencephaly in two related litters of Korat cats that exhibited abnormal behavior shortly after birth. This diagnosis can be made by MR imaging.[25]

Lissencephaly combined with a cerebellar hypoplasia and dysplasia occurs in children because of an autosomal recessive inheritance of a mutation in the gene known as the RELN gene. This gene normally encodes for reelin, which is a protein concerned with neuronal migration.[11] We have observed this same combination of dysplasias in a litter of wire fox terriers (Figs. 3-46 and 3-47) and a litter of Irish setters. These dogs exhibited a severe nonprogressive cerebellar quality ataxia from the time they began to walk. One wire fox terrier was provided with a cart to help with its ambulation and lived to be 4 years old. At 1 year of age this dog developed episodic generalized seizures that were presumed to be caused by the lissencephalic dysplasia. MR imaging confirmed this same diagnosis in a 4-year-old Samoyed. The cerebellar lesion similar to the cerebral lesion could be explained by an aberrant process of neuronal migration. Neuronal migration is a complex process involving astroglia and many extracellular factors, one of which is brain-derived neurotrophic factor. This factor has been shown to provide directional cues for the migration of the external germinal layer to the granule neuron layer of the cerebellum.

Cerebellar Malformations

Congenital cerebellar abnormalities include genetic disorders resulting in various forms of hypoplasia and dysplasia and in utero viral infections causing hypoplasia and atrophy. These are described in Chapter 13, which is devoted to the cerebellum.

Complex Malformation of Calves

A unique multifocal bone and neural tube malformation has been described in calves as the Arnold Chiari malformation, presumably because of an assumed similarity to a human malformation that has been given this eponym.[2] Although there are some similarities, the distinct differences in the bovine disorder make the use of this eponym incorrect. These calves are usually born alert and visual but recumbent and unable to coordinate their trunk and limb function to stand. They often exhibit opisthotonus and abnormal nystagmus. There is a sacrocaudal spina bifida with a meningiomyelocele, a malformed tail, and an associated loss of tone and reflexes in the anus and tail. At necropsy, the meningomyelocele consists of sacrocaudal nerves connecting from their spinal cord segments in the exposed vertebral canal into the skin-covered swelling over the spina bifida (Figs. 3-48 and 3-49). The ganglia of these spinal nerves are

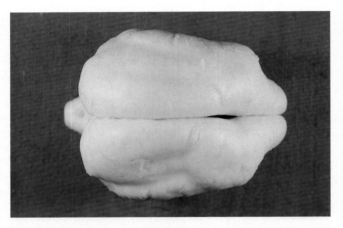

FIGURE 3-46 Lissencephaly and cerebellar hypoplasia in a 1-month-old wire fox terrier.

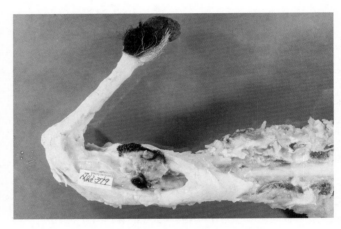

FIGURE 3-48 Holstein calf with malformed tail, spina bifida, and meningomyelocele.

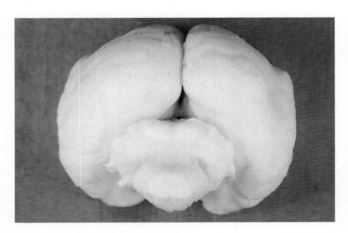

FIGURE 3-47 Lissencephaly and cerebellar hypoplasia in a 1-month-old wire fox terrier.

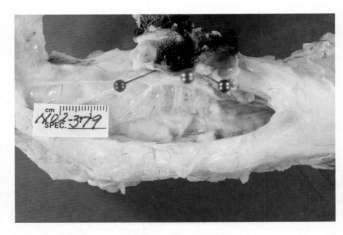

FIGURE 3-49 Same calf as in Fig. 3-48, showing the nerve roots extending into the patch of skin dorsal to the spina bifida.

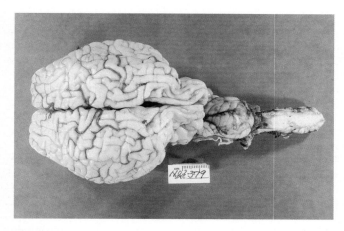

FIGURE 3-50 The same Holstein calf as in Figs. 3-48 and 3-49, showing the caudal extension of occipital lobes, which filled the caudal cranial fossa and the malformed cerebellum that was in the vertebral canal of C1 and C2.

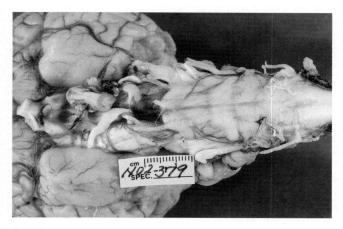

FIGURE 3-51 The same Holstein calf shown in Figs. 3-48 through 3-50. Ventral surface of the brain showing the rostral courses of the cranial nerves from their locations in the vertebral canal to enter the cranial cavity and access their respective foraminae.

located in the skin. Myelodysplasia is present in the sacrocaudal segments. In the brain, the cerebellum is flattened and elongated into a cone-shaped structure, and it is displaced caudally along with the caudal brainstem into the foramen of the atlas and axis. The associated cranial nerves are elongated to extend back into the cranial cavity to exit through their respective foramina. In addition, there is a bilateral abnormal extension of the occipital lobes into the caudal cranial fossa space vacated by the cerebellum. These abnormal extensions of the occipital lobes pass ventral to the tentorium, which results in a groove on the lateral side of each of these extensions. These are not herniations of the normal occipital lobes (Figs. 3-50 and 3-51). This malformation has been observed in calves since the early 1900s and is assumed to be an inherited defect.

Occipital Bone Malformation and Syringohydromyelia

A dilation of the central canal is hydromyelia; a cavitation of the spinal cord parenchyma is syringomyelia. They occur secondary to a herniation of the caudoventral cerebellar vermis through the foramen magnum. The cause of the herniation is presumed to be a caudal cranial fossa that develops to be too small for the volume of brain tissue that it contains.[5,6,22-24] Some veterinarians refer to this as an Arnold Chiari type 1 malformation, which is a human disorder that involves herniation of the cerebellar tonsils, which are not present in animals. Although the pathogenesis may be similar, we believe this eponym is inappropriate for the canine disorder. Until we better understand the skull malformation that leads to the small caudal cranial fossa, occipital bone malformation will be considered the primary defect in these dogs. Usually both hydromyelia and syringomyelia are present, and at some point there is a communication between these two fluid-filled spaces. Therefore, we refer to this spinal cord lesion as a syringohydromyelia.

Syringohydromyelia occurs most commonly in the cervical spinal cord segments as a multifocal or continuous lesion, but it is often present in the thoracolumbar segments as well. It is thought to result from the compromise of CSF flow at the foramen magnum caused by cerebellar herniation and the compression of the underlying medulla. The cranial cavity is a closed space and the movement of CSF is greatly influenced by the pulsation of arteries associated with the heartbeat. CSF pulsates in synchrony with the heartbeat and flows in both directions at the foramen magnum but primarily from the cranial cavity to the spinal cord subarachnoid space. When this normal pulsating flow is obstructed by cerebellar herniation, the smooth flow is converted into a higher-pressure pulsatile flow and turbulence results in the spinal cord subarchnoid space, forcing CSF, vascular fluid, or both into the parenchyma along the penetrating perivascular spaces. The area of least resistance in the spinal cord parenchyma is in the dorsal funiculi, where the syrinx is most commonly found. The pathogenesis of this spinal cord lesion in humans as well as animals is very complex and still under intense investigation. A new concept of the pathophysiology of the development of syringohydromyelia is based on research that showed a higher pressure of CSF in the spinal cord cavities than in the subarachnoid space.[24] In addition, it was determined that these cavities contained extracellular fluid and not just CSF. The driving force is still the intracranial systolic CSF pressure. This concept is based on obstruction of CSF flow and repeated pulsatile mechanical distention of the spinal cord. The latter results in the accumulation of extracellular fluid because of the high pressure in the spinal cord microcirculation. Edema in the less resistant dorsal funiculi would precede the development of the syrinx. The high-velocity jet of CSF created by the obstruction of CSF flow paradoxically decreases the hydrostatic pressure in the subarachnoid space (the Venturi effect). This augments the intramedullary distention of the spinal cord and causes the formation of edema, which leads to syringomyelia. It is well recognized now that surgical enlargement of the foramen magnum results in spontaneous resolution of the syringohydromyelia in many patients. Other lesions that cause excessive tissue mass in the brain, especially in the caudal cranial fossa, such as neoplasms and cysts, also cause the same interference with CSF flow dynamics and the same spinal cord lesions that resolve after surgical removal of the mass or enlargement of the foramen magnum. The occipital bone malformation is most common in the small breeds, especially the Cavalier King Charles spaniel, where there is evidence for a genetic basis.[23] Clinical signs vary in onset from a few months to the early adult years and most commonly relate to the cervical spinal cord.[22] The most common clinical sign is discomfort. Affected dogs may be hyperesthetic and act very sensitive to any touching of the head, neck, shoulder, or sternum. In addition, some dogs exhibit continual scratching anywhere from their ears to the thoracic limb shoulder region. This may relate to the tendency for the cervical syrinx to dissect laterally from the dorsal funiculus into the adjacent dorsal gray column and interfere with its role in sensory functions. Scoliosis can also result from this dorsal gray column lesion, with the neck bending away from the side of the dorsal gray column lesion. Some dogs exhibit a lower motor neuron paresis in one thoracic limb if the syrinx involves the ventral gray column of the cervical intumescence on that side. Others, with involvement of the lateral funiculus, may develop an upper motor neuron paresis and general proprioceptive ataxia. Occasionally, cerebellar-vestibular signs have been reported. Facial paresis and deafness have also been reported and rarely seizures may occur. The seizures probably relate to the alteration of pressure in the prosencephalic ventricular system. Once clinical signs are observed, they usually progress until surgery is performed to enlarge the foramen magnum. Diagnosis is made by MR imaging. The median plane T2-weighted MR images are the most successfully diagnostic of the herniation as well as the syringohydromyelia (Fig. 3-52). Veterinary surgeons have recognized that a thickening of the dura-arachnoid dorsal to the compressed medulla and first cervical spinal cord segment is associated with this chronic herniation. This fibrotic tissue is removed in the decompression procedure without apparent clinical complications resulting from surgical manipulation of the cerebellum and first cervical spinal cord segment or CSF leakage into the adjacent tissues, in our experience. Insertion of a titanium mesh may help to protect against the formation of scar tissue at the surgical site.

Calvarial Ossification

There are two variations of the ossification of the calvaria that are often mistakenly related to neurologic disorders. They are seen primarily in the small breeds. One involves the occipital bone at the foramen magnum and the other the frontoparietal suture. A dorsal notch or extension of the foramen magnum has been referred to as occipital dysplasia and has been mistakenly related to clinical signs of congenital or acquired neurologic disease. This anomaly

of the occipital bone occurs primarily in toy or medium-sized brachycephalic breeds, and there are no conclusive data to support that it is related to any clinical neurologic signs. This "keyhole" foramen is common in the Cavalier King Charles spaniel, with or without an associated occipital bone malformation and syringohydromyelia. A doctoral study of a large number of clinically normal dogs showed a considerable variation in the shapes and sizes of the foramen magnum.[28,29] A dorsal notch of the foramen magnum was commonly present in the skulls of the small dog breeds. This space in the occipital bone, where there was no bone, was filled by a membrane of connective tissue. This dorsal notch was considered to be an area of incomplete ossification of the ventromedial aspect of the supraoccipital bone. It is a variation in the normal morphology of the occipital bone that is most common in the small brachycephalic breeds and is not related to any disturbances of the nervous system.

Incomplete ossification at the frontoparietal suture is referred to as a molera or fontanelle. In many breeds, this is a normal feature at birth that rapidly closes in a few days to a few weeks. However, in the toy breeds, especially the Chihuahua, this molera may remain present in the adults. Unfortunately, some veterinarians have mistakenly related the presence of any persistent space here to a hydrocephalic condition in the brain. There is no basis for this. The breed standard accepts the presence of a small molera in the adult Chihuahua. The size of the acceptable space is difficult to define, but it varies in shape and usually is in the range of 5 mm in diameter, about the size of the end of one's little finger. If there is concern about hydrocephalus in a toy breed with a persistent molera, that diagnosis can be easily confirmed or denied by ultrasound evaluation of the lateral ventricles through the persistent molera.

Spinal Cord Malformations

A number of important features must be emphasized in regard to spinal cord malformations: The clinical signs will be present at birth or when the newborn animal first tries to walk, and they will not progress. Spinal cord malformations are most common in calves and most commonly occur in the thoracolumbar segments.[3] Vertebral column malformations often accompany the spinal cord malformations because of their close developmental relationship, and these vertebral malformations may be visible or palpable. Despite the many different forms of myelodysplasia that we have seen, there is no specific clinical sign that distinguishes one malformative spinal cord lesion from another. A very common lesion is a duplication of the spinal cord, with both components contained in one set of meninges, one dural sheath. This is called diplomyelia (Figs. 3-53 and 3-54). Less commonly there are two spinal cords, each with its own meningeal sheath and each in its own vertebral canal and separated by a bony partition. This malformation is called a diastematomyelia (Figs. 3-55 and 3-56). In less successful attempts at duplication, there may be a mass of excessive gray matter in the spinal cord and no demarcation into the respective columns, or there may be attempts at duplication of a dorsal or ventral gray column. The central canal is often absent or it may be dilated, which is known as hydromyelia. Cavities are commonly seen in the white matter and

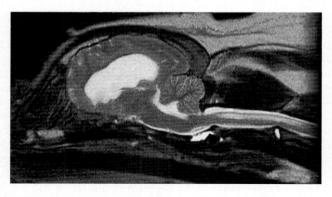

FIGURE 3-52 MR sagittal image of a dog, showing herniation of the caudal cerebellar vermis and a cervical spinal cord syringohydromyelia.

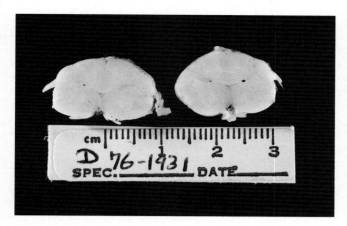

FIGURE 3-53 Diplomyelia in the lumbar spinal cord of a calf. Note the two central canals.

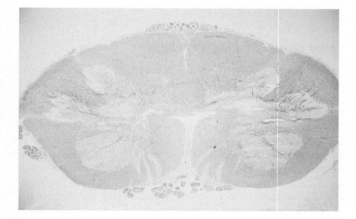

FIGURE 3-54 Microscopic section of diplomyelia in the lumbar spinal cord of a calf.

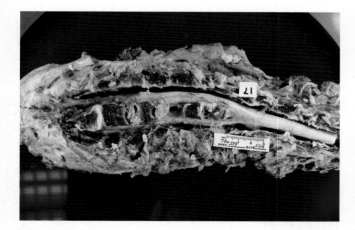

FIGURE 3-55 Diastematomyelia involving the lumbosacral spinal cord of a calf.

occasionally in the gray matter, which is known as syringomyelia. The ventral median fissure may be absent and neuronal cell bodies may be spread across the midline between the ventral gray columns. If a few spinal cord segments are smaller than normal, it is known as segmental hypoplasia. Sometimes these small segments contain only white matter tracts and no gray matter. No studies have been done on the inheritance of these bovine malformations.

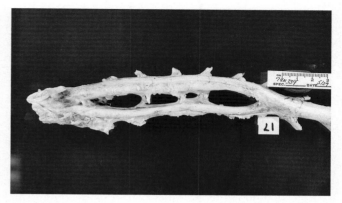

FIGURE 3-56 Duplicated spinal cord removed from the malformed vertebral column of the calf in Fig. 3-55. Each of the two separate portions of the lumbosacral segments had its own meninges.

Regardless of the nature of the thoracolumbar spinal cord malformation, if the animal is able to walk, it is common for the pelvic limbs to be used simultaneously in a "bunny-hopping" fashion. **Video 3-2** shows a 1-week-old Holstein that is able to walk unassisted with a mild lumbar scoliosis and associated myelodysplasia (Figs. 3-57 and 3-58). **Video 3-3** shows a 2-week-old Holstein that has been unable to stand

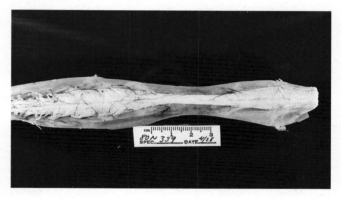

FIGURE 3-57 Lumbosacral spinal cord of the calf in Video 3-2, showing the segmental hypoplasia of the middle lumbar spinal cord segments.

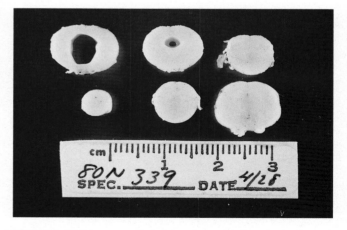

FIGURE 3-58 Transverse sections of the spinal cord in Fig. 3-57, showing a large syringohydromyelia, the absence of the central canal, and segmental hypoplasia.

since birth. Note the bunny-hopping movements when it is assisted to stand. Note the mild palpable lumbar (L2, L3) vertebral abnormality. The CT shows both the mild vertebral malformation and the segmental hypoplasia of the spinal cord. At necropsy there was a widespread thoracolumbar myelodysplasia and a sacral segment diplomyelia.

There is no specific gross or microscopic malformative lesion that relates to this unique bunny-hopping clinical sign. We assume that the disorder relates to an interference with the interneuronal connections between the ventral gray columns in the lumbosacral intumescence that are involved with the gait, so that usually the initial flexor muscle activation at the onset of protraction occurs alternatively. A submicroscopic alteration in these commissural interneurons may be the basis for the simultaneous bilateral flexor responses at the onset of protraction and when both limbs respond when the flexor reflex is stimulated in one limb. This bilateral response is not seen with the patellar reflex, which is a monosynaptic tendon reflex that does not involve interneuronal connections with the opposite side. We are comfortable stating that this bunny-hopping gait does not involve spinal cord tracts that project cranially or caudally in the spinal cord because we have seen it in a recumbent newborn Simmenthal calf with no cranial lumbar segments, an L1 to L3 segmental aplasia (Figs. 3-59 and

3-60). The isolated segments of the lumbosacral intumescence were entirely responsible for very brisk simultaneous bilateral pelvic limb protraction movements with any stimulus to the limbs. **Video 3-4** shows this 3-day-old Simmenthal calf. Note that this simultaneous pelvic limb protraction occurs whether the calf is recumbent or is supported by the tail in a position that allows walking. As soon as the hooves touch the floor, there is a brisk bilateral hip flexion to advance the limbs. This is a fabulous example of the spinal reflex walking present at birth and is a classic example of complete loss of the normal role of the upper motor neuron in the inhibition of extensor motor neurons. The pelvic limbs in this calf were in a constant state of hypertonicity due to an isolated intumescence that had no connections with any other part of the CNS. Do not be confused by the rapid bilateral flexor reflexes that respond to any noxious stimulus and think the calf is trying to avoid the stimulus. This calf is completely analgesic in the pelvic limbs and the pelvic and perineal areas.

Spina Bifida: Meningomyelocele

These are two separate malformations that are often confused. Spina bifida refers to the failure of the closure of the dorsal aspect of the vertebral foramen of one or a few vertebrae. If many adjacent vertebrae are involved, it is called a rachischisis. These are failures of the vertebral arches to develop. They are often associated with neural tube malformations. They include a meningocele or meningomyelocele with spina bifida and myeloschisis with a rachischisis. A meningocele is a protrusion of meninges and an accumulation of CSF outside the vertebral canal beneath the skin and therefore requires the presence of a spina bifida. A meningomyelocele is a protrusion of meninges and associated nervous tissue outside the vertebral canal. Usually the nervous tissue involved consists of spinal nerves and rarely of spinal cord segments. A myeloschisis is by definition a failure of the neural tube to close and usually involves a number of adjacent spinal cord segments. For this to occur, the skin ectoderm remains attached to the borders of the neural plate, which prevents any vertebral arches from forming and results in a rachischisis (Fig. 3-61). Prior to birth this open neural tube is exposed to amniotic fluid but after birth it is exposed to environmental air and

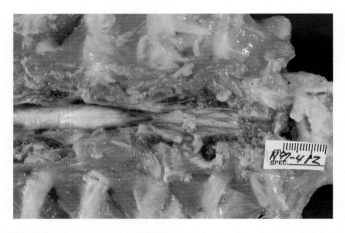

FIGURE 3-59 Simmenthal calf in Video 3-4, showing the end of the spinal cord at T10 and no vertebral arch in the first lumbar vertebrae.

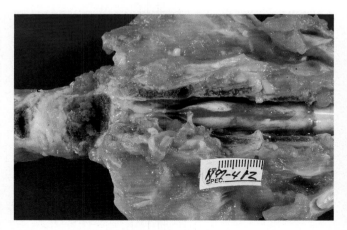

FIGURE 3-60 The same calf as in Fig. 3-59, showing the absent spinal cord and vertebral arches in the L3 and L4 vertebrae and the isolated dysplastic lumbosacral spinal cord segments caudal to them.

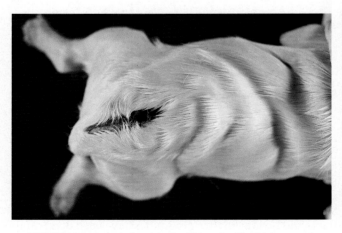

FIGURE 3-61 Lumbosacral myeloschisis and rachischisis in a puppy.

rapidly undergoes dessication, which is often associated with hemorrhage along the surface of the neural plate.

A sacrocaudal spina bifida and meningomyelocele are most common in the Manx breed of cat and in English bulldogs.[4,13] The Manx breed is known for the absence of its tail, which in fact is the trait that is selectively bred for by Manx owners. The caudal vertebral hypoplasia or aplasia is inherited as an autosomal dominant gene. In the homozygous state, this is a lethal factor. The clinically affected cats are heterozygotes with variable expression. This is unfortunate because in breeding for one malformation, the lack of a tail, these Manx cat owners are breeding for other associated malformations, especially in the adjacent vertebrae and the spinal cord. The various forms of spinal cord malformation, myelodysplasias, can result in excretory dysfunctions such as urinary and fecal incontinence sometimes associated with loss of tone, reflexes, and nociception in the anal and perineal area. In more severe myelodysplasias that involve the sacral and caudal lumbar spinal cord segments, there may be partial or complete interference with the ability to stand and walk with the pelvic limbs (Figs. 3-62 and 3-63).

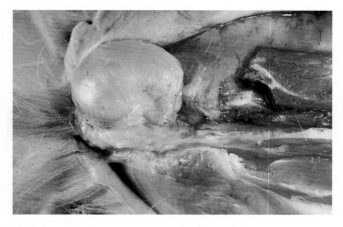

FIGURE 3-62 Necropsy of a Manx cat with the skin removed from the lumbosacral region, exposing a CSF-distended meningomyelocele.

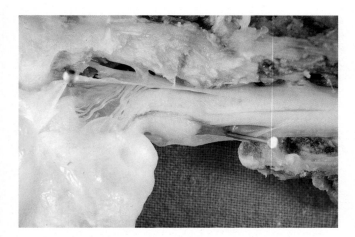

FIGURE 3-63 Further dissection of the Manx cat in Fig. 3-62, showing nerve roots extending into the meningomyelocele. Note the gray line at the site of the dorsal median septum of the lumbar segments. This is a thin membrane covering a syrinx. Note the white mass of hyperplastic spinal cord parenchyma on the right of the caudal end of the spinal cord.

Owners recognize these severe cases shortly after birth and euthanize the kittens. This prevents the profession from having any idea how widespread this malformation is in the breed. Affected cats that are able to stand and walk often use their pelvic limbs simultaneously in a bunny-hopping fashion, which is a common clinical sign of myelodysplasia in any species. If these cats with urinary and fecal incontinence are maintained by well-meaning breeders or owners, the cats may eventually develop urinary tract infections that lead to pyelonephritis. Most are euthanized between 4 and 8 months of age. The breeders should be urged to stop the program of breeding these cats for the absence of tails, and the veterinary profession should take the lead in providing this advice. The epitome of success in breeding for multiple system malformations in this breed was observed in an incontinent Manx cat that had a cloaca. In addition to the complete absence of the tail and the last two sacral vertebrae, there was only one external orifice in the perineum that served for the evacuation of both the feces and urine. Cloacas belong in birds, not cats! If you are not sure of the diagnosis, myelography or MR imaging will show the continuation of the subarachnoid space through the spina bifida into the subcutaneous area. **Video 3-5** shows a 6-month-old female Manx cat that was presented for incontinence and exhibits a bunny-hopping gait. Also note the simultaneous flexion of both pelvic limbs when only one pelvic limb receives a noxious stimulus.

In dogs the most renown and well-studied spinal cord malformation is the spinal dysraphism that is inherited in the weimaraner breed. Dr. Jack McGrath studied a colony of these dogs at the University of Pennsylvania and published his results in 1965.[15-17] This term actually is defined as an incomplete closure of a raphe or defective fusion of the neural tube, which is not what happens in these dogs. In Dr. McGrath's 1956 edition of his textbook he described this as syringomyelia in weimaraners because of the cavities that he observed in the dorsal funiculi.[14] In 1965, after further study, he described the primary malformative lesion to be microscopic and involving primarily midline structures: aberrations of the dorsal median septum, the absence of a ventral median fissure, hydromyelia or an absent central canal, and the presence of ventral gray column neuronal cell bodies scattered across the midline in the ventral funiculi as a result of their failure to migrate into the ventral gray columns.[16] These lesions occur in scattered thoracolumbar segments. In a few dogs it may be difficult to find any microscopic lesions at all. There is no term that is specific for these microscopic lesions, and we feel it is more accurate to refer to this as inherited myelodysplasia of weimaraners. Some of these weimaraners have other malformations, including scoliosis, abnormal hair patterns on the dorsal aspect of the neck, and a depression of the sternum known as koilosternia. The clinical signs are first observed as these dogs begin to walk, when they consistently exhibit a simultaneous gait with the pelvic limbs. A variable degree of paresis and ataxia may be present in some dogs that may limit their ability to be satisfactory pets. **Video 3-6** shows two 5-month-old weimaraners that have walked like this since birth. Whatever clinical signs are observed will not change with time. Many bunny-hopping weimaraners have found homes and have made delightful pets. These affected dogs and their parents should not be bred because this disorder is thought to be inherited as a codominant lethal gene where the homozygous condition is lethal and the clinically affected dogs are heterozygotes. It is important to remember that if you are presented with an adult weimaraner that has bunny-hopped since it was a pup and now has progressing spinal cord signs, it has a different disease! I (Alexander de Lahunta) have studied one litter of six weimaraners in which three of the dogs showed the bunny-hopping gait in all four limbs. Necropsy of one of these pups showed no gross or microscopic nervous system abnormality.

Myelodysplasias are occasionally seen in other breeds and in mixed breeds. I (AD) have studied three mixed-breed husky dogs from a litter of nine that had been exhibiting the bunny-hopping gait in the pelvic limbs since they were pups but had no other gait abnormality. Two others in the litter had undefined malformations of their appendicular skeleton. **Video 3-7** shows two 1-year-old chow shepherd mixed-breed dogs that were donated to Cornell University because since birth they showed the simultaneous use of both the pelvic and the thoracic limbs. You have to see this to believe it. They were normal in all other respects and made outstanding pets for the two veterinary students who adopted them. These two were really nice dogs who probably thought all dogs should walk like they did!

Pathogenesis of Malformations

The above examples show the variety of factors that can lead to abnormal development of the nervous system.

Only knowing the correct cause can permit prevention of further malformed newborn animals. Because inherited gene abnormalities are so common, breeders often jump to this conclusion without a scientific basis for the judgment. It is most important first to have a confirmation of the morphology of the malformation. This usually requires a necropsy diagnosis. If the disorder is inherited, a confirmed diagnosis is required before any judgments can be made about the parents of the affected offspring. For many inherited disorders, published data support the inherited basis of the malformation. When such data are lacking, breeders must carefully document all the confirmed cases of the disorder and determine from pedigree studies whether the disorder fits a pattern of inheritance. Planned repeat breedings may be necessary to establish inheritance, but that is expensive and very time consuming. With the rapid progress being made in understanding the gene codes of the various species of domestic animals, abnormalities are being understood at the gene level and this has led to the development of blood tests that can diagnose affected and carrier animals. Dedicated use of these genetic tests provides the opportunity to decrease significantly the incidence of and even to eliminate many of these malformations.

Consider the following Case Example of a Hereford calf brought into the Necropsy Service at the College of Veterinary Medicine at Cornell University from a small Hereford farm in upstate New York.

CASE EXAMPLE 3-1

Signalment: 1-day-old Hereford heifer calf

Chief Complaint: Recumbent since its unassisted birth and blind with "white" eyes

History: Following a normal parturition, this calf was unable to get up. The owner stated that the calf was representative of a herd problem of 3 years' duration. The herd consisted of one bull and seven Hereford cows. Six of these cows traced back to one female. Of the seven calves born 2 years earlier, two were similar to this calf, in the opinion of the owner, but no necropsy studies had been done. The year before this calf was born, five of the seven calves had been similarly affected. This calf was the second to be born in that year, and the first calf was normal.

Examination: The calf was obtunded, recumbent, and unable to get up. When stimulated, it demonstrated voluntary limb movements. Tone and spinal reflexes and nociception were normal. The calf was blind and had severe cataracts, which accounted for the owner's observation of white eyes. The pupils were unresponsive to light. There was bilateral ventral strabismus, and a positional abnormal nystagmus could be elicited.

Anatomic Diagnosis: Diffuse brain (prosencephalon and brainstem)

Necropsy: Both cerebral hemispheres were distended by dilated, CSF-filled lateral ventricles. The thinned neocortex suggested there had been increased CSF pressure. The dilated third ventricle supported that observation. The gyri were smaller and more numerous than normal (polymicrogyria). The optic nerves and chiasm were small and cystic. The brainstem was bent in a sharp dorsal deviation at the level of the mesencephalon. The colliculi were fused and stenotic. The mesencephalic aqueduct was malformed and stenotic. The cerebellum was misshapen and smaller than normal. On microscopic examination, there was cerebellar cortical dysplasia and areas of hypomyelination. There were bilateral cataracts, retinal dysplasia, and cone-shaped retinal detachments.

Pathogenesis: In 1964, H. K. Urman and O. D. Grace published a similar collection of lesions in newborn Hereford calves and described an inherited basis for it.[27] The unique collection of abnormalities in the calf described here was identical to that described by Urman and Grace, and it makes an inherited basis most presumptive; this is supported by the herd's history. In addition, the various viral disorders that affect bovine fetuses in utero have never been known to cause these kinds of lesions.

REFERENCES

1. Barone G, de Lahunta A, Sandler J: An unusual neurological disorder in the Labrador retriever, *J Vet Intern Med* 14: 315-318, 2000.
2. Cho DY, Leipold HW: Arnold-Chiari malformation and associated anomalies in calves, *Acta Neuropathol (Berl)* 39:129-133, 1977.
3. Cho DY, Leipold HW: Spina bifida and spinal dysraphism in calves, *Zentalbl Vetinarmed Med A* 24:680, 1977.
4. DeForest ME, Basrur PK: Malformations and the Manx syndrome in cats, *Can Vet J* 20:304, 1979.
5. Dewey CW, et al: Caudal occipital malformation syndrome in dogs, *Compend Contin Educ Pract Vet* 26: 886-896, 2004.

6. Dewey CW, et al: Foramen magnum decompression for treatment of caudal occipital malformation syndrome, *J Am Vet Med Assoc* 227:1270-1275, 2005.

7. Greene CE, Vandevelde M, Braund K: Lissencephaly in two Lhasa apso dogs, *J Am Vet Med Assoc* 169:405, 1976.

8. Greene CE, Gorgacz EJ, Martin CL: Hydranencephaly associated with feline panleukopenia, *J Am Vet Med Assoc* 180:767, 1982.

9. Hartley WJ, et al: Serological evidence for the association of the Akabane virus with epizootic bovine congenital arthrogryposis and hydranencephaly syndrome in New South Wales, *Aust Vet J* 51:103, 1975.

10. Hartley WJ, et al: Pathology of congenital bovine epizootic arthrogryposis and hydranencephaly and its association with the Akabane virus, *Aust Vet J* 53:319, 1977.

11. Hong SE, et al: Autosomal recessive lissencephaly with cerebellar hypoplasia is associated with human RELN mutations, *Nat Genet* 26:93-96, 2000.

12. Incardona JP, et al: The teratogenic Veratrum alkaloid cyclopamine inhibits sonic hedgehog signal transduction, *Development* 125:3553-3562, 1998.

13. James CCM, Lassman LP, Tomlinson BE: Congenital anomalies of the lower spine and spinal cord in Manx cats, *J Pathol* 97:269, 1969.

14. Koch T, et al: Semilobar holoprosencephaly in a Morgan horse, *J Vet Intern Med* 19:367-372, 2005.

15. McGrath JT: *Neurologic examination of the dog with clinicopathologic observations,* Philadelphia, 1956, Lea & Febiger.

16. McGrath JT: Spinal dysraphism in the dog, *Pathol Vet* 2(suppl 1): 1965.

17. McGrath JT: Spinal dysraphism. *Comp Path Bull* 8:2, 1976.

18. Osburn BI, et al: Experimental viral-induced congenital encephalopathies. I. Pathology of hydranencephaly and porencephaly caused by the bluetongue vaccine virus, *Lab Invest* 25:197, 1971.

19. Osburn BI, et al: I. Experimental viral-induced congenital encephalopathies. II. The pathogenesis of bluetongue vaccine virus infection in fetal lambs, *Lab Invest* 25:206, 1971.

20. Parsonson IM, et al: Congenital abnormalities in foetal lambs after inoculation of pregnant ewes with Akabane virus, *Aust Vet J* 51:585, 1975.

21. Richards WPC, Crenshaw GL, Bushnell RB: Hydranencephaly of calves associated with natural bluetongue virus infection, *Cornell Vet* 61:336, 1971.

22. Rusbridge C, et al: Syringomyelia in Cavalier King Charles spaniels, *J Am Anim Hosp Assoc* 36:34-41, 2000.

23. Rusbridge C, Knowler SP: Inheritance of occipital bone hypoplasia (Chiari type I malformation) in Cavalier King Charles spaniels, *J Vet Intern Med* 18:673-678, 2004.

24. Rusbridge C, Greitze D, Iskandar BJ: Syringomyelia: current concepts in pathogenesis, diagnosis, and treatment, *J Vet Intern Med* 20:469-479, 2006.

25. Saito M, et al: Magnetic resonance imaging features of lissencephaly in two Lhasa apsos, *Vet Radiol Ultrasound* 43:331-337, 2002.

26. Scott FW, et al: Teratogenesis in cats associated with griseofulvin therapy, *Teratology* 11:79, 1975.

27. Urman HK, Grace OD: Hereditary encephalopathy, a hydrocephalus syndrome in newborn calves, *Cornell Vet* 54:229, 1964.

28. Watson G: *The phylogeny and development of the occipito-atlas-axis complex in the dog,* Ph.D. dissertation, Cornell University, 1981.

29. Watson AG, de Lahunta A, Evans HE: Dorsal notch of foramen magnum due to incomplete ossification of supraoccipital bone in dogs, *J Small Anim Pract* 30:666-674, 1989.

30. Zaki F: Lissencephaly in Lhasa apso dogs, *J Am Vet Assoc* 169:1165, 1976.

31. Zook BC, Sostaric BR, Draper DJ: Encephalocele and other craniofacial anomalies in Burmese cats, *Vet Med Small Anim Clin* 78:695-701, 1983.

4

CEREBROSPINAL FLUID AND HYDROCEPHALUS

PRODUCTION

MENINGES: SUBARACHNOID SPACE

CIRCULATION

ABSORPTION

FLUID COMPARTMENTS

FUNCTION

CLINICAL APPLICATION OF CSF

CEREBELLOMEDULLARY CISTERN CSF COLLECTION

LUMBOSACRAL CSF COLLECTION IN LARGE ANIMALS

MYELOGRAPHY

HYDROCEPHALUS

    Compensatory Hydrocephalus
    Obstructive Hydrocephalus

Acquired Obstructive Hydrocephalus
Developmental Obstructive Hydrocephalus
Signalment, History, Clinical Signs
    Prosencephalic Signs
Differential Diagnosis
Diagnosis
Treatment

Cerebrospinal fluid (CSF) is a clear, colorless fluid that surrounds and permeates the entire central nervous system (CNS) and therefore protects, supports, and nourishes it. In general, the CSF is produced within the ventricles of the brain by the choroid plexuses, circulates to the subarachnoid space, and is absorbed into the venous sinuses.

PRODUCTION

The CSF originates from capillaries throughout the CNS and leptomeninges. A major site is the choroid plexus located in the lateral, third, and fourth ventricles. Small amounts enter the ventricles from the parenchyma through their ependymal lining and enter the subarachnoid space through the pial-glial membrane on the external surface of the parenchyma. Capillaries within the parenchyma are a small source via the microscopic interstitial spaces. Leptomeningeal capillaries in the subarachnoid space are an additional small source of CSF. One study of CSF production determined that 35% was derived from the third and lateral ventricles, 23% from the fourth ventricle, and 42% from the subarachnoid space.[3,4,8,15]

The choroid plexus consists of numerous fronds of villous processes that project into the CSF of the ventricular system. The simple cuboidal cells of the plexus are continuous with the ependymal cells that line the ventricular surface adjacent to the CNS parenchyma (Fig. 4-1).[19] At the choroid plexus, there are essentially two cell layers between the blood plasma and the ventricular CSF. The vascular endothelium is separated from the choroidal epithelial cells by a thin basement membrane and loosely arranged meningeal pial cells. The endothelial cells of the choroid plexus capillaries are considered to be fenestrated because they lack tight junctions. This is different from the capillary structure within the parenchyma. The epithelial cells of the choroid plexus are robust cuboidal cells with tight junctions at their ventricular surfaces. They have the characteristics of cells that function in the transcellular transport of materials. This includes microvilli on their luminal surface and infoldings of the basal portion of the cell membrane. This is a semipermeable barrier that selectively and actively transports some substances and inhibits others. The methods of CSF production are a selective ultrafiltrate from the blood plasma and active transport mechanisms that utilize energy.

Compared with blood plasma, CSF has less potassium and calcium and more chloride, sodium, and magnesium. It has slightly less glucose, about 80% of that in the blood, and much less protein. Plasma protein is measured in grams per deciliter (g/dl), whereas CSF protein is measured in milligrams per deciliter (mg/dl). In the dog, the normal total protein level does not exceed 25 to 30 mg/dl, and it is predominantly albumin. Bile salts, products of hemoglobin breakdown, and many pharmaceuticals, including penicillin, are prevented from entering the CSF from the blood.

The rate of production of CSF varies with the species and the method of determination but is remarkably rapid. The total volume of CSF is produced and absorbed about 3 to 5 times per day. The following rates have been determined: dog, 0.047 ml/min; cat, 0.017 ml/min. With this continuous turnover of CSF, there is evidence that it is produced at a constant flow rate, regardless of increases or decreases in CSF pressure in the ventricular system. In chronic obstructive hydrocephalus, atrophy of the choroid plexus decreases CSF production. The rate of CSF production is independent of the hydrostatic pressure of the blood but is influenced by the osmotic pressure of blood. Intravenous administration of hypertonic solutions reduces the rate of formation of CSF. This has clinical application in head injuries involving brain edema and in neurosurgery performed for space-occupying lesions. An osmotic diuretic is administered to decrease the rate of CSF formation and to decrease the vasogenic edema associated with the brain lesion. Brain volume will be reduced and intracranial pressure will be lowered. The most common osmotic agent used is mannitol, a hypertonic solution of a carbohydrate. It is administered intravenously at 0.25 to 2 g/kg

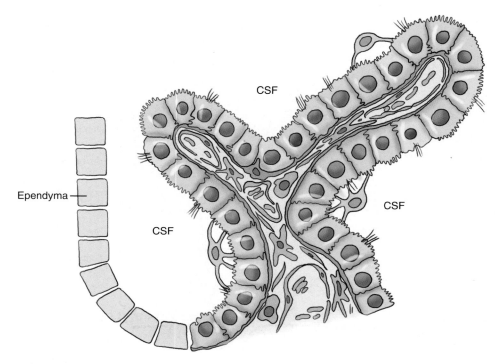

FIGURE 4-1 Transverse section of choroid plexus villi showing the main morphologic features of the choroidal tissue. *(From Strazille N, Ghersi-Egea S-F: Choroid plexus in the central nervous system: biology and physiopathology,* J Neuropathol Exp Neurol *59:561-574, 2000.)*

of a 20% solution. If mannitol is administered intraoperatively, the reduction in the size of the brain is grossly visible.

MENINGES: SUBARACHNOID SPACE

Before we consider the circulation of CSF, it is worthwhile to review the anatomy of the meninges, which is described with the dissection of the brain and spinal cord in *Guide to the Dissection of the Dog* (ed 6, by H. E. Evans and A. de Lahunta).

Recall that the entire CNS is covered by three layers of connective tissue (Fig. 4-2). These layers are derived predominantly from the neural crest with a small component of mesoderm. The most external layer is the thick, fibrous dura mater that, within the cranial cavity, closely adheres to the bones of the skull. Within the vertebral canal, the dura is separated from the vertebrae by the epidural space, which often contains fat. The arachnoid membrane is a thin layer of connective tissue that in life adheres to the dura by means of desmosomal attachments (Fig. 4-3).[10] There is *no* subdural space in

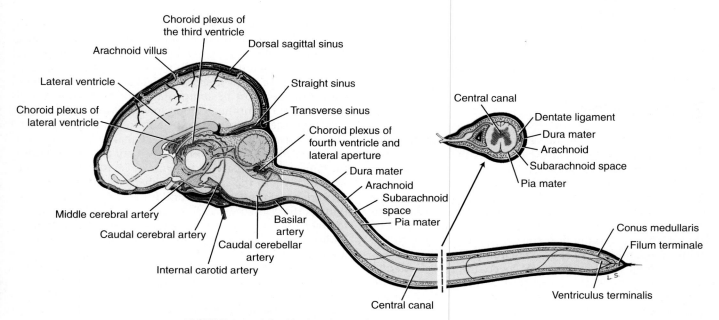

FIGURE 4-2 Relationship of meninges and subarachnoid space to ventricular system.

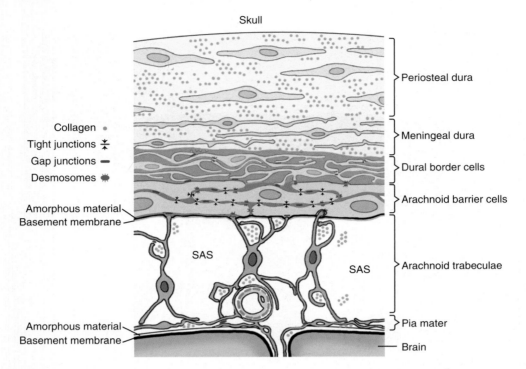

FIGURE 4-3 Ultrastructure of the meninges. *SAS,* Subarachnoid space. *(From Haines DE, Harkey HL, Al-Mefty O: The "subdural space": a new look at an outdated concept,* Neurosurgery *32:111-120, 1993.)*

the normal living animal, despite what you may read in the literature. These dura-arachnoid desmosomal attachments are easily disrupted by hemorrhage following an injury (subdural hematoma); by contrast agents inadvertently injected into the dura-arachnoid; and following death, when the CSF pressure is lost. It should be noted here that subdural hematomas are rare in veterinary medicine compared with their occurrence in humans. This arachnoid membrane is the external surface of the subarachnoid space, which contains CSF, blood vessels, spinal nerve roots, and arachnoid trabeculations. The latter are thin, collagenous extensions from the arachnoid membrane to the pia mater, which is the thin layer of connective tissue attached to the surface of the CNS parenchyma where it forms a pial-glial membrane. The thick dura mater is also called the pachymeninx, and the thin vascularized pia and arachnoid make up the leptomeninges.

CIRCULATION

The CSF circulates from the ventricular system to the subarachnoid space by way of the lateral apertures of the fourth ventricle (Fig. 4-4). In some animals there is a similar passage between the central canal and the subarachnoid space at the conus medullaris (see Fig. 4-2). Primates also have a median plane aperture (the foramen of Magendie) in the caudal part of the roof plate of the fourth ventricle. Much of the CSF passes dorsally over the cerebellum, ventral to the tentorium, and then over the cerebrum where it has access to the venous sinuses. The CSF covers the entire external surface of the brain and spinal cord, where it can penetrate the parenchyma along with the larger blood vessels in their perivascular spaces. These spaces are extensions of the subarachnoid space to the point where the pia mater blends

with the adventitia of the blood vessel. This is not a distinct point, and for some distance the cells of the leptomeninges and the adventitia of the blood vessel may be closely related and the perivascular space reduced to small clefts between cells. Ultimately the CSF has access to the very small extracellular interstitial spaces of the CNS parenchyma. Altered CSF flow patterns along the spinal cord subarachnoid space lead to syrinx formation when CSF enters the spinal cord parenchyma along these perivascular spaces. These flow pattern alterations may also contribute to the formation of a subarachnoid diverticulum. These diverticula are incorrectly referred to as subarachnoid cysts in the literature.

The flow of CSF in the ventricles is thought to be caused primarily by the pulsations of blood in the choroid plexuses. Remember that the cranial cavity is a closed space consisting of three components: the brain parenchyma, the blood, and the CSF (Fig. 4-5). Any increase in the volume of one of these compartments must be compensated for by a reduction in the volume of another compartment. With each arterial pulsation, the CSF pressure rises and surges toward the lateral apertures. The cilia on the ependymal cells may make a small contribution to this flow. Movement of the CSF within the subarachnoid space of the cranial cavity and from the cranial cavity to the spinal cord subarachnoid space is also dependent on cardiac systole and intracranial arterial pulsations in that closed space. Interference with this flow at the foramen magnum can lead to the development of a syringohydromyelia, as discussed in the section about brain malformations in Chapter 3. The effect of this arterial pulsation on CSF movement is remarkable when viewed using magnetic resonance (MR) imaging utilizing CSF flow analysis (see **Video 4-1**). In addition, during surgery that involves the ventricular system or subarachnoid space, the surgeon can directly view the arterial pulsatile effects on CSF flow.

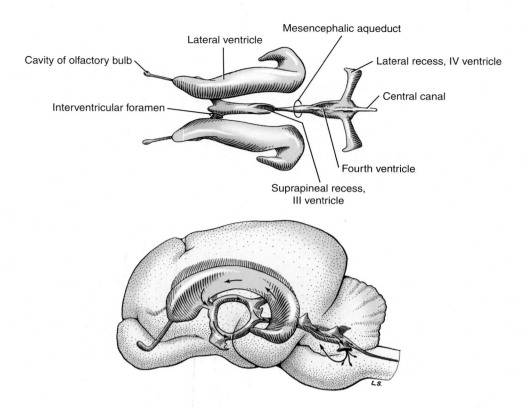

Cavity of olfactory bulb

Lateral ventricle

Mesencephalic aqueduct

Lateral recess, IV ventricle

Central canal

Interventricular foramen

Fourth ventricle

Suprapineal recess, III ventricle

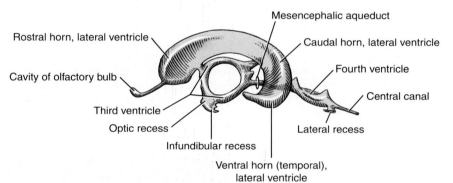

Rostral horn, lateral ventricle

Mesencephalic aqueduct

Caudal horn, lateral ventricle

Cavity of olfactory bulb

Fourth ventricle

Central canal

Third ventricle

Lateral recess

Optic recess

Infundibular recess

Ventral horn (temporal), lateral ventricle

FIGURE 4-4 The canine ventricular system.

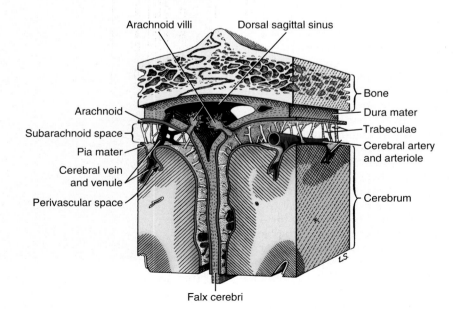

Arachnoid villi

Dorsal sagittal sinus

Arachnoid

Subarachnoid space

Pia mater

Cerebral vein and venule

Perivascular space

Bone

Dura mater

Trabeculae

Cerebral artery and arteriole

Cerebrum

Falx cerebri

FIGURE 4-5 Cerebral meninges and arachnoid villi at the attachment of the falx cerebri to the calvaria.

In relationship to cardiac systole and diastole, the CSF can move cranially and caudally, but the caudal flow predominates. Radioiodinated serum albumin injected into the lumbar cistern of humans can be followed by scanning radiographic procedures to the dorsum of the cerebrum in 12 to 24 hours. Similar injections into the lateral ventricle appear in the thoracolumbar subarachnoid space in 30 to 40 minutes, reflecting the predominant caudal flow of CSF.[6] Comparison of cerebellomedullary and lumbosacral CSF in animals with focal spinal cord disease supports the predominance of the caudal flow of CSF.

The sensitivity of the close relationship among the three compartments of the closed cranial cavity as well as a demonstration of the continuity of the intracranial and intravertebral subarachnoid spaces is seen when the CSF pressure is monitored at the cerebellomedullary cistern, and the external jugular veins are compressed. This extracranial venous compression causes an immediate increase in the intracranial blood volume, which requires more space. The CSF volume is compressed and displaced through the foramen magnum, causing an elevation in the pressure in the spinal cord subarachnoid space, which can be seen in the pressure-measuring manometer. For a similar reason, the CSF in the manometer will rise and fall in synchrony with respirations, reflecting the associated changes in thoracic venous pressure. If a pressure-measuring manometer is also placed in the lumbosacral subarachnoid space, the same observations will be made because of the continuity of this space for the full length of the spinal cord.

If the continuity of this CSF-filled space is compromised by a space-occupying lesion such as a neoplasm or abscess along the spinal cord, the CSF pressure measured at the lumbosacral subarachnoid space will not elevate when the external jugular veins are compressed. In humans this is called the Queckenstedt, or jugular compression, maneuver.

Other practical applications of the knowledge that the cranial cavity is a closed space relate to intracranial injury and neurosurgery. When an animal is positioned for intracranial or cervical spinal cord surgery, the head and neck should be elevated and suspended by a specialized holding device rather than placed on a padded surface so as to avoid compressing the external jugular veins. A practical test to ensure the avoidance of external jugular vein compression is that the surgeon can freely pass his or her hand between the surgical table and the ventral surface of the patient's neck. When an animal is presented following an intracranial injury, a cardinal rule in any emergency room is to be sure the patient has a patent airway. This not only ensures the proper oxygenation of the blood for the tissues but also prevents dilation of cerebral blood vessels, which would contribute to any increase in intracranial pressure. Hypercapnia causes cerebral arterial vasodilation and increases the volume of intracranial blood. If head injury has occurred, hypercapnia will augment any hemorrhage and vasogenic edema that is already present and compromising the space available in the cranial cavity. Hyperventilation will reduce this effect by increasing the oxygen and decreasing the carbon dioxide content of the blood vessels; this is a procedure that may be used during intracranial surgery. Some of the gas anesthetics may induce intracranial vasodilation, which makes the selection of anesthetics for intracranial surgery an important consideration.

When the intracranial space is compromised by developing lesions, the CNS is able to accommodate for it by physiologic mechanisms that are referred to as autoregulation. The purpose of this autoregulation is to attempt to maintain adequate cerebral perfusion in the presence of increased intracranial pressure caused by the lesions. This perfusion is independent of systemic blood pressure. Cerebral perfusion pressure is defined as the mean arterial blood pressure minus the intracranial pressure. It determines the oxygen and nutritional supply to the parenchyma. This autoregulation involves complex regulation of intracranial blood flow by chemical, neurogenic, and myogenic means. It is most effective with slow-growing lesions that occupy space. It is amazing how large neoplasms can be that develop within the prosencephalon or even in the extraparenchymal (extraaxial) space along the brainstem without producing neurologic signs as long as their growth is slow. Slowly growing extramedullary lesions can cause more than a 50% compression of the spinal cord before clinical signs are seen. CNS vascular autoregulation is the basis for the preservation of the parenchymal perfusion to these compromised tissues. Clinical signs occur when the tissue demands exceed the capability of this autoregulation. Vasogenic and cytotoxic edema follow. When this occurs within the cranial cavity, the uncontrolled increase in intracranial volume and pressure forces displacements of various components of the brain that are referred to as herniations. These represent attempts of the brain to squeeze out of the cranial cavity. Three of these herniations are regularly seen in domestic animals. The subfalcine herniation is a medial displacement of one cerebral hemisphere ventral to the falx cerebri. On computed tomography (CT) and MR imaging, a sign commonly seen is referred to as a midline shift; it represents an enlargement of one cerebrum (Figs. 4-6 and 4-7). When it is severe, a subfalcine herniation may occur. The portion of the enlarging cerebral hemisphere that is herniated is the cingulate gyrus. The transentorial

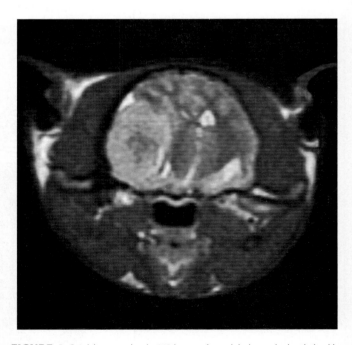

FIGURE 4-6 Axial proton density MR image of an adult domestic shorthair with a meningioma directly compressing the left cerebral hemisphere and displacing it to the right side of the midline. This is an example of a "midline shift" due to a mass lesion in one cerebral hemisphere that can lead to a subfalcine herniation.

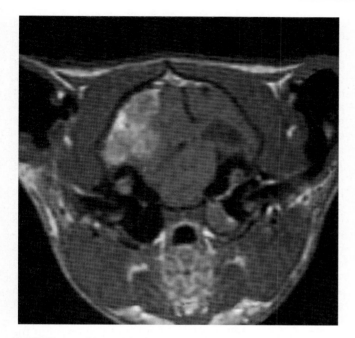

FIGURE 4-7 Axial T1-weighted, postcontrast MR image of an adult domestic shorthair with a meningioma compressing the left cerebral hemisphere and displacing it to the right side of the midline, a midline shift of the brain.

herniation is the displacement of the caudal aspect of one or both cerebral hemispheres ventral to the tentorium cerebelli. This directly compresses the mesencephalon and indirectly the rostral cerebellum. It can sometimes be seen on MR imaging but is recognized at necropsy by the marked oblique indentation in the caudomedial aspect of the occipital lobes and often includes the parahippocampal gyrus on the medial aspect of the cerebral hemisphere (Figs. 4-8 and 4-9). Herniation of the caudoventral aspect of the cerebellar vermis is commonly called cerebellar coning. This involves primarily the pyramis and uvula lobules, which compress the ventrally situated medulla. It can sometimes be seen on axial (transverse) MR images but is best seen on median-plane sagittal

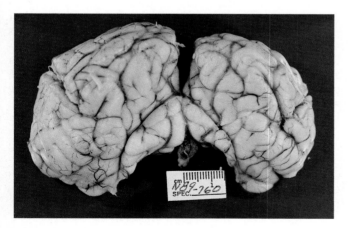

FIGURE 4-8 Gross lesion of the occipital lobes where a transtentorial herniation occurred. This is the cerebrum of the 14-year-old Morgan horse with the cholesterinic granuloma of the choroid plexus of the left lateral ventricle seen in Fig. 3-19. The herniation is worse on the left side. Herniation on the right side is due to the vasogenic edema crossing through the corpus callosum into the white matter of the right cerebral hemisphere.

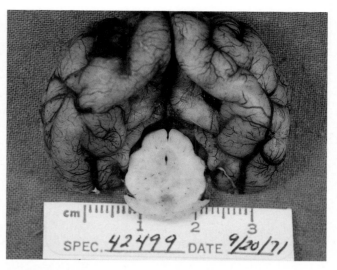

FIGURE 4-9 This is the brain of an adult dog that was struck by a car, causing a fracture of the right calvaria with contusion of the right cerebral hemisphere. Note the herniation of the occipital lobes (worse on the right side) the compressed mesencephalon, meningeal hemorrhage, and swelling of left cerebral hemisphere.

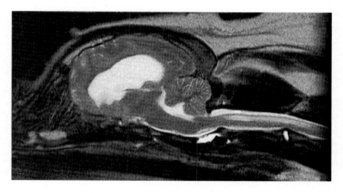

FIGURE 4-10 Sagittal T2-weighted MR image of a young Cavalier King Charles spaniel with occipital bone malformation syndrome and herniation of the caudoventral cerebellar vermis, or cerebellar coning. Note the hyperintensity in the dorsal portion of the cervical spinal cord where fluid is accumulating in the formation of a syrinx.

MR images (Figs. 4-10 and 4-11). It should not be referred to as "tonsillar" herniation because these paramedian lobules do not herniate in domestic animals, only in primates.

ABSORPTION

The major site of CSF absorption is at the arachnoid villi that are located in the venous sinuses or cerebral veins.[20] Collections of these arachnoid villi are known as arachnoid granulations. Occasionally they can be seen in some species on gross examination of the lumen of a large intracranial venous sinus.[8,9] The arachnoid villus is a prolongation of the arachnoid membrane and subarachnoid space into the lumen of the venous sinus covered by the endothelium of the vessel wall (see Fig. 4-5). Usually the portion of the villus within the lumen is reduced to a single endothelial cell between the CSF of the subarachnoid space and the lumen of the sinus. It is structured to act as a one-way valve that permits the CSF to flow into the lumen of the sinus when the CSF pressure exceeds venous pressure.

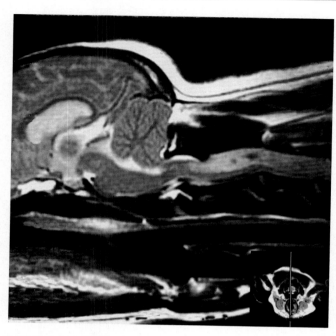

FIGURE 4-11 Sagittal proton density MR image of a young Cavalier King Charles spaniel with occipital bone malformation syndrome and herniation of the caudoventral cerebellar vermis. Note the extensive hyperintensity in the dorsal half of the spinal cord, where fluid is accumulating in the formation of a syrinx.

When the intravenous pressure exceeds the CSF pressure, these villi collapse, closing the "valves" so that no blood can pass into the subarachnoid space. Flow is one-way at these sinuses, only from the CSF into the blood.[17] Electron microscope studies of these endothelial cells that line the arachnoid villi have revealed transient transcellular channels that develop for the passage of materials from the CSF into the venous system.[1] These apparently develop in response to a pressure gradient between the CSF and venous blood.

Other sites of CSF absorption include the veins and lymphatics found around the spinal nerve roots and spinal nerves at the intervertebral foramina and associated with the first, second, and eighth cranial nerves where they pass through the skull bones. CSF passes through the cribriform lamina of the ethmoid bone, where it is absorbed or leaks into the nasal cavity, resulting in cerebrospinal rhinorrhea.[7] The small amount of CSF in the interstitial spaces of the parenchyma may be absorbed into the parenchymal blood vessels.

In reality, CSF is formed and absorbed throughout the ventricles and subarachnoid space. It is in constant motion and progresses over the surface of the brain and spinal cord. With its rate of production being independent of intracranial pressure, absorption is the primary homeostatic mechanism for the maintenance of the intracranial pressure by CSF. There are no lymphatics in the CNS, and the CSF provides for some of the lymphatic system functions that occur in other tissues.

▌ FLUID COMPARTMENTS

There are three extracellular fluid compartments in the cranial cavity that are associated with brain parenchyma: plasma, CSF, and extracellular fluid. Exchanges among them are critical to the normal maintenance of brain function. There are unique features to the morphologic and physiologic barriers among these compartments. The blood-brain barrier (BBB) exists between the plasma and the extracellular fluid of the interstitial spaces at the level of the capillaries. Morphologically, this BBB consists of a nonfenestrated, tightly joined layer of endothelial cells of the capillary wall surrounded by a thick basement membrane and a relatively complete layer of foot processes from astrocytes on the surface of the basement membrane. Much of the barrier is dependent on physiologic mechanisms within the endothelial cells. Numerous carrier-mediated transport systems have been defined for this barrier. They can function as bidirectional pathways or primarily for influx, such as for glucose and large neutral amino acids or just for efflux to rid the parenchyma of excessive glutamate or glycine and to maintain extracellular potassium at a level that will not interfere with neural transmission. When this barrier is normal it prevents therapeutic levels of the antibiotic penicillin from entering the parenchyma but allows ready passage of chloromycetin and sulfonamides to reach antibacterial levels in the extracellular fluid. In mammals the anthelmintic ivermectin is prevented from passage through the BBB by the presence of a p-glycoprotein. It is thought that the breeds of dogs that are susceptible to ivermectin toxicity lack this BBB structure. This is most common in the collie breeds but also occurs in Australian shepherds and Old English sheepdogs. This is important clinically because administration of this anthelmintic to susceptible dogs can result in severe neurologic signs and death.

The blood-CSF barrier exists between the plasma and the CSF at the choroid plexus and consists of two cell layers separated by a thin basement membrane. The vascular endothelial layer and its basement membrane have fenestrations, and the cells lack tight junctions. The choroidal epithelium consists of large cuboidal cells with tight junctions at their ventricular surfaces. Fragments of meningeal cells are interspersed among these endothelial and epithelial cells (see Fig. 4-1). They serve as a semipermeable membrane between the plasma and the CSF. In acid-base imbalances, CO_2 readily passes between the plasma and the CSF, whereas bicarbonate exchange is slow owing to the relative impermeability of this barrier to bicarbonate.

There is no significant barrier between the CSF in the ventricles or the subarachnoid space and very limited extracellular fluid in the minute interstitial spaces of the adjacent parenchyma. The ependymal cells that line the ventricles are mostly thin squamous cells with incomplete intercellular junctions and no basement membrane between them and the adjacent subependymal cells or neuroglial cells. CSF can move in either direction through this barrier. On the external surface of the CNS, the pia and astrocytic foot processes separated by a basement membrane form a permeable pial-glial membrane. There are no intercellular junctions in this membrane, which extends into the parenchyma along blood vessels for a short distance, where it defines a perivascular space. Thus, metabolites in the CSF have ready access to the extracellular fluid of the parenchyma that is important in maintaining normal brain function.

▌ FUNCTION

CSF serves to protect the CNS by its physical support, with the parenchyma suspended in this fluid medium. It protects the CNS by its role in modulating pressure changes that occur, especially in the closed cranial cavity. In conjunction with cerebral blood flow, the CSF helps to regulate the intracranial pressure. It protects the parenchyma by being a source of nourishment because it is a medium for the transport of metabolites and nutrients between the blood and the CNS parenchyma. It also serves to transport neuroendocrines and neurotransmitters within the parenchyma. CSF plays a role in maintaining the ionic balance necessary for neuronal function by acting as a chemical buffer for the parenchyma. By means of its close relationship to the extracellular fluid in the interstitial spaces, the CSF provides a more stable and closely controlled ionic environment than the blood plasma. At necropsy, when studying young animals with extensive leptomeningitis, it is surprising how profound their diffuse neurologic signs are with these lesions confined to the subarachnoid space in the absence of any microscopic parenchymal lesions. Cryptococcal meningitis in dogs and cats and bacterial meningitis in calves are examples of this observation, which reflects the importance of the CSF in providing vital nourishment to maintain parenchymal function.

CLINICAL APPLICATION OF CSF

CSF may be analyzed for its cellular and chemical constituents, antibodies, and infectious agents. CSF can be used in neuroradiographic procedures to demonstrate the shape of the CSF-containing ventricles or subarachnoid space and reveal changes caused by disease. Both of these require the anatomic knowledge and technical skill to access the subarachnoid space.

In the dog and cat, the most reliable source of CSF is at the cerebellomedullary cistern. The cistern at the conus medullaris is too small to be a reliable source. Lumbar myelograms are usually performed at the L5-L6 articulation in the dog and at the L6-L7 articulation in cats. Occasionally at these lumbar vertebral sites, enough CSF can be obtained prior to the injection of the contrast agent to allow its evaluation. In the horse, ox, sheep, goat, pig, and *Camelidae* species, both the atlantooccipital and lumbosacral sites are useful sources of CSF for clinical evaluation. The following are detailed descriptions for the dog and horse that are applicable to the other species.

CEREBELLOMEDULLARY CISTERN CSF COLLECTION

CSF collection at the cerebellomedullary cistern in all species requires general anesthesia to ensure restraint of the patient as well as to eliminate discomfort. The following description for small animals is the same for large animals except for the accommodations necessitated by the differences in their sizes. The skin over the occipital bone and first two cervical vertebrae must be surgically prepared. For right-handed individuals, the patient should be placed in left lateral recumbency, with its head and neck positioned level at the edge of the table. Have an assistant elevate the nose slightly so that it is parallel with the vertebral column and flex the atlantooccipital joint so that the median axis of the head is approximately at a right angle to the median axis of the neck. Excessive flexion can bend the endotracheal

tube and obstruct respiration. Right-handed persons should place the thumb of the left hand on the external occipital protuberance and the first finger of this hand on the cranial aspect of the right wing of the atlas. From these landmarks, an imaginary line is drawn caudally along the dorsal median plane from the external occipital protuberance, and another line is drawn transversely between the cranial edges of the wings of the atlas. Where these two lines cross is where the needle should be inserted, directed at the angle of the mandible. The needle should be approximately parallel with the ramus of the mandible. To avoid contamination, it is advisable to use sterile surgical gloves. In reality, you cannot palpate the space between the dorsal edge of the foramen magnum and the arch of the atlas, so there is no need to palpate the area where you performed a surgical preparation, and if you handle only the hub of the needle, there is no need for surgical gloving, although it is a worthy precaution.

For most dogs and cats, a spinal needle with a stylet that is 1.5 inches long and 20 or 22 gauge is adequate. A 3.5-inch, 20- or 22-gauge spinal needle may be necessary in some of the larger dog breeds. In the horse and ox, a 3.5-inch, 18- or 20-gauge spinal needle may be used (Fig. 4-12). With the bevel directed to one side, insert the needle through the skin and underlying fascia and muscle, directing it toward the angle of the mandible. To support the needle for removing the stylet, place the palm of your left hand on the head over the external occipital protuberance for support. Grasp the hub of the needle with the fingers of your left hand and do not move your left hand until the procedure is completed. Remove the stylet with your right hand and observe for fluid. You want to know how far to go! Well, we can not tell you because there is so much difference between a Chihuahua and a Great Dane. So use trial and error carefully. We recommend that you initially practice this on a few euthanized patients. Insert the needle progressively and observe for CSF at the hub at 1-mm intervals. Occasionally you will feel a slight loss of resistance when you penetrate the atlantooccipital membrane and dura together and enter the subarachnoid space, but do not count on that feeling. Because the cistern is small in all cats and the small breeds of dogs, holding the needle hub tightly, with the left hand braced on the head, will prevent you from dislodging the needle when you remove the stylet. If you strike bone, you may be able to judge which bone you are on and walk the needle either cranially off the atlas or caudally off the occipital bone before inserting the needle farther. Usually when you are in the cistern, the CSF will immediately appear in the needle hub. Do not advance the needle without the stylet so that tissue will not obstruct the needle. In small patients, such as cats and toy-breed dogs, use a 21-gauge butterfly needle because the capillary forces will contribute to the flow of CSF.

Usually the CSF pressure is not measured, but if that determination is desired, the manometer and its three-way valve should be attached to the needle hub as soon as the CSF appears. The opening pressure can be recorded, a sample of CSF obtained, and the closing pressure recorded by redirecting the valve. Recording CSF pressures from the cerebellomedullary cistern was more common before MR and CT imaging were so readily available. Elevated pressures were considered to be consistent with CNS disease. A sterile syringe may be attached to the needle hub and 1 to 2 ml of CSF obtained. If

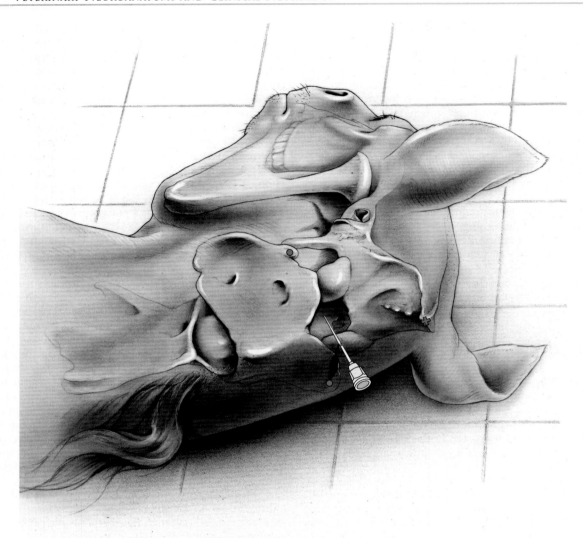

FIGURE 4-12 Atlantooccipital cisternal CSF collection from a recumbent horse. The spinal needle is in position, with the stylet removed. Palpable landmarks are the cranial borders of the transverse processes of the atlas (●-●) and the median eminence of the nuchal crest (⊕).

you have difficulty accessing the cistern, especially in cats or very small dogs where the space is small, you may prefer to let the CSF drip into a sterile test tube to avoid attaching a syringe and possibly dislodging the needle from the cistern. About 15 drops of CSF equals 1 ml. Applying pressure to both external jugular veins may assist the flow of CSF.

There are many large veins at the atlantooccipital site, most of which are extradural. It is common to have whole blood appear in the hub of your needle because you have penetrated one of these veins. If this is an extradural vein, the CSF has not been contaminated and you should remove the needle, obtain a new needle, and repeat the procedure. On one occasion, after describing this procedure to a class of 80 students, I (Alexander de Lahunta) performed a demonstration on an anesthetized beagle dog. After using six needles and obtaining whole blood each time, assuring the students that the CSF was still there and not contaminated by blood, the clear CSF showed up in the seventh needle! If there is blood in the CSF, it may result from injury by the needle to a blood vessel in the subarachnoid space of the cistern or it may be part of the disease process. If it is caused by

the procedure, the amount of blood should decrease as more CSF is withdrawn, and the first aliquots with the most blood should be discarded so that the least contaminated CSF is evaluated. If hemorrhage is part of the disease process, the amount will not change in the CSF as it is withdrawn. If you are uncertain about the reason for the blood, centrifugation will remove all the blood from the sample, leaving a clear, colorless fluid if the hemorrhage has been caused by the procedure. If the hemorrhage is part of the disease process, centrifugation will remove the erythrocytes that are present, but the supernatant will have a yellow color (xanthochromia) because of the hemoglobin breakdown products of the erythrocytes in the hemorrhage. Small amounts of iatrogenic hemorrhage are common and will not interfere significantly with the interpretation of the CSF evaluation.

Warning! When you have had some experience performing this procedure and you have a patient in which you are having difficulty obtaining the CSF, *do not become aggressive*. Stop and make your clinical assessment without the CSF evaluation. If you persist in your attempts to obtain the fluid, there is a good chance that you will injure the medulla or first cervical spinal cord segment. The needle should never be allowed to penetrate the CNS at this site. This is called pithing and is a technique used to kill an animal. It is common in these patients that the disease process has obliterated the cistern, preventing you from obtaining any CSF. I (Eric Glass) have a three-strikes rule. There should be no more than three attempts to obtain CSF by one individual. Increased frustration will result only in a misplaced needle. If a second clinician also fails on three attempts, abandon the procedure. A common reason for failure is that the disease process has obliterated the cistern.

Warning! If you suspect there may be an increase in intracranial pressure such as an increase secondary to a space-occupying lesion, either do not proceed with the procedure or be very cautious, when you remove the stylet, to attach the syringe so that there is no sudden release of CSF under high pressure; this could lead to cerebellar vermal herniation and an exacerbation of the neurologic signs. As a rule, it is best to delay your collection of CSF until after the neuroimaging. This will allow you to know whether there is an anatomic reason to avoid this procedure.

LUMBOSACRAL CSF COLLECTION IN LARGE ANIMALS

The collection of CSF from the subarachnoid space at the lumbosacral articulation is described for the horse but is applicable to all farm animal species.[14] It is important to know which spinal cord segments are present in the vertebral canal at this level because they vary significantly among species. Table 4-1 addresses this subject and includes the small animals for the clinical importance of this anatomy. CSF collection here in small animals is not reliable.

The disparity between the location of the spinal cord segments and the vertebrae occurs when the vertebral column outgrows the spinal cord. The two develop in direct relationship to each other, with the paired spinal nerves growing laterally through the respective intervertebral or lateral vertebral foramina. With growth, as the spinal cord is displaced cranially in the vertebral canal, the spinal nerves grow in length to accommodate this displacement. This growth takes time. Therefore, Table 4-1 refers to adult animals. All of these spinal cord segments are farther caudal in the vertebral canal in young animals. Because of the remarkable variation in size of the various dog breeds, some adjustment is necessary in adult animals. As a rule of thumb, in the large breeds, adjust the spinal cord segments one vertebra cranially so that the three sacral segments are

in the foramen of L4. In the small breeds, adjust the spinal cord segments one vertebra caudally so that the three sacral segments are in the foramen of L6.

Lumbosacral CSF collection in the horse is best done when the horse is standing and is under light restraint.[14] Only in overtly excited animals is a tranquilizer advised because it tends to cause the horse to stand with most of its weight supported by one pelvic limb, which results in a displacement of the landmarks used for the procedure. For the same reason, this procedure is more difficult in the laterally recumbent horse. The landmarks used to locate the site for needle insertion are often difficult to palpate, and there is some variation between the sexes and among individual animals. The site of skin penetration is within the depression bordered laterally by the medial surface of the rim of the tuber sacrale, cranially by the caudal edge of the spine of the sixth lumbar vertebra, and caudally by the cranial edge of the second sacral vertebra (Fig. 4-13). The spine of the first sacral vertebra is short and too deep to palpate. When you palpate the lumbar spines, be aware that the spine of L6 is shorter than the spine of L5, and do not mistake this depression dorsal to L6 as the site for skin penetration. Usually you can palpate the tuber sacrale. Estimate a transverse line between the cranial edge of these two protuberances. Palpate the caudal ventral portion of the tuber coxae on each side, and estimate a line between these two protuberances. Where the two lines cross, the dorsal median plane should demarcate the area for skin penetration. Prepare this area surgically. Use local anesthesia of the skin at the needle insertion site and incise the skin before insertion of the needle. Use a 6-inch, 18-gauge, thin-walled needle with stylet for adult horses up to about 17 hands tall. Very tall horses may require a special 8- or 9-inch spinal needle. A 3.5-inch, 18- or 20-gauge spinal needle with stylet can be used in ponies and foals up to about 12 hands tall. A right-handed person should stand on the right side of the horse and rest the right wrist on the dorsal median plane of the horse, cranial to the needle insertion site. Holding the needle hub firmly, advance the needle into the axial tissues. Be sure the needle is perpendicular to the dorsum of the horse in both directions. You may need an assistant to stand an appropriate distance behind the horse to help you with the needle position. The depth of penetration to reach the subarachnoid space varies with the size of the horse. It is about 5 inches in a 450 kg horse. Fig. 4-14 shows the thickness of tissue that must be penetrated to reach this space. The space between the arches of S1 and L6 is about 1 inch in diameter. If you strike either of these arches, the needle must be removed and the procedure repeated

TABLE 4-1 Relationship of Lumbosacral Spinal Cord Segments to the Vertebrae in Adult Animals

Species	Number of Lumbar Vertebrae	Number of Sacral Segments	Location of Sacral Segments	End of Conus Medullaris	Segments at Lumbosacral Site
Dog	7	3	L5	L6, L7	None
Cat	7	3	L6	L7	None
Ox	6	5	L6	S1	Caudal
Horse	6	5	S1-3 = L6 S4, 5 = S1	S2	Sacral
Llama	6	5	S1, 2	S2	Sacral

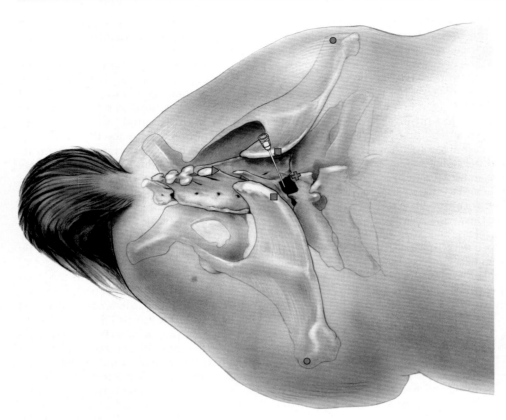

FIGURE 4-13 Lumbosacral CSF collection from a standing horse. The spinal needle is in position, with the stylet removed. Palpable landmarks are the caudal borders of each tuber coxae (●-●), the caudal edge of the spine of L6 (✦), the cranial edge of the spine of S2 (▶), and the cranial edge of each tuber sacral (■-■).

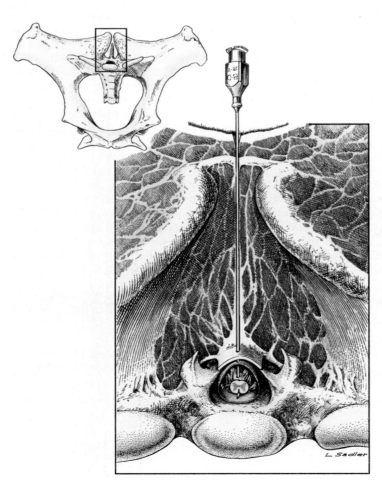

FIGURE 4-14 Lumbosacral CSF collection from a horse. Cranial view of a transverse section at the level of the lumbosacral articulation. The spinal needle passes through the skin, thoracolumbar fascia, interspinous ligament, yellow ligament, dorsal dura mater and arachnoid, dorsal subarachnoid space, and conus medullaris. The needle point is in the ventral subarachnoid space. The drawing insert is a cranial view of the pelvis and sacrum at the level of the transverse section.

L. Sadler

because the site is too deep to allow you to "walk" the end of the needle any distance. There may be a slight loss of resistance when the needle penetrates the yellow ligament and enters the epidural space. When the dura-arachnoid is penetrated, there may be a slight reaction by the horse, with a tail movement, slight pelvic limb flexion, or axial muscle contraction. A light application of a restraining twitch may be useful at this time. At this level, advance the needle slowly, remove the stylet, and look for CSF flow at 1-mm intervals. Ideally, you want to remove the CSF from the subarachnoid space that is dorsal to the spinal cord. Often you cannot get the CSF to flow here and it is necessary to carefully pass the needle through the caudal sacral segments and meninges to the floor of the vertebral canal and slowly back the needle up dorsally into the ventral subarachnoid space (see Fig. 4-14). In adult horses, the fourth and fifth sacral spinal cord segments are here, and it is expected that the needle will pass through these segments to reach the ventral subarachnoid space. Therefore, the needle insertion should be done carefully. Clinical signs of injury to these segments resulting from this procedure are rare. Compression of the external jugular veins may aid in the flow of CSF in difficult patients. Rotating the needle may also help to free the needle tip from obstruction by meninges or spinal nerve roots. Gentle aspiration using a syringe is also an option.

In the ox, it is usually not difficult to palpate the depression between the spines of L6 and S1. This site is generally where the dorsal median plane intersects a transverse line between the palpable tuber coxae on each side. A 3.5-inch, 20-gauge spinal needle with stylet is adequate for most adult cattle. There are only a few caudal segments at this site in adults.

In this text, we do not describe the methods of evaluating the contents of the CSF or the results of these evaluations. That subject is aptly covered in textbooks of clinical pathology and other textbooks of neurology.

A few of our observations follow. Be cautious in your interpretation of the results of CSF examination. They often do not reflect the nervous system disorder that exists. We have studied brains with extensive neoplastic or inflammatory lesions in which the CSF was normal. Likewise, we have studied brains that have had minimal evidence of parenchymal inflammation and no obvious meningeal inflammation but in which the CSF has been profoundly inflammatory. Where did the excessive cells and protein come from? Did we miss the lesion? We cannot answer these questions but they support our advice to be cautious. Despite massive neoplasia with neoplastic cells in the subarachnoid space, the presence of these neoplastic cells in CSF is rare, or we lack the ability to recognize them. Except for *Cryptococcus neoformans,* it is rare to find infectious agents in the CSF. In granulomatous meningoencephalitis in dogs, the CSF can vary from being normal to being profoundly abnormal. The presence of a few neutrophils is rare but does not rule out the diagnosis. Eosinophils may not be present in the CSF of cats with CNS *Cuterebra* larval myiasis or in small ruminants or *Camelidae* species with CNS infection by *Parelaphostrongylus tenuis.* Remember that lumbosacral CSF normally may have more cells and protein than cerebellomedullary cistern CSF. This is especially true for the protein level at the lumbosacral site. Be careful of overinterpreting abnormalities in CSF that is contaminated by blood during the procedure to obtain the CSF. An excellent example of this is the evaluation of lumbosacral CSF in horses for antibodies to *Sarcocystis neurona.* An experimental study showed that blood contamination that included just eight red blood cells could be the source of a positive antibody level in the CSF. It is common to get a small amount of blood when the lumbosacral site is used. Be aware that there are differences in the normal levels reported for the various species of domestic animals, especially the protein levels. Normal CSF protein rarely exceeds 20 mg/dl in cats, 25 to 30 mg/dl in dogs, 40 mg/dl in cattle, and 80 mg/dl in horses. Now that MR imaging has nearly replaced the use of myelograms in many small-animal neurology practices, there is no need to place a needle in the subarachnoid space, so many neurologists do not obtain CSF for evaluation as a routine procedure. The CSF is evaluated only in patients in which the MR imaging suggests inflammation—with the exception of a cat with possible feline infectious peritonitis (FIP), when the cerebellomedullary cistern may be obliterated by the inflammation or herniated cerebellum.

■ MYELOGRAPHY

Myelograms may be performed by injecting contrast at the cerebellomedullary cistern or at a subarachnoid site between two lumbar vertebrae. The choice depends on the location of the anatomic diagnosis or the preference of the neurologist or radiologist. At present, iohexol (Omnipaque, 240 mg of iodine/ml) is the contrast agent used most commonly at either site. A small amount of CSF is removed and replaced by the recommended dose and concentration of the contrast agent for the size of the patient. When injected at the cerebellomedullary cistern, there is no epidural space and the contrast will enter the subarachnoid space, which will appear as two straight, thin parallel lines on either side of the spinal cord, whether the patient is in lateral or ventral recumbency. The contrast surrounds the spinal cord but the lines appear where it is most concentrated due to the thickness of the subarachnoid space in that position. On rare occasions, if the end of the needle is partly in the dura, the contrast will be injected into the subarachnoid space, but a portion will enter the dura where it will separate the fragile desmosomal attachments of the arachnoid membrane to the dura, creating a subdural space (see Fig. 4-3). This is recognized by the irregularity of the contrast lines. It may extend for the entire length of the cervical spinal cord.

Lumbar myelograms are performed in the average-sized dog between the L5 and L6 vertebrae, where the conus medullaris is located. This site is chosen to provide an adequately sized subarachnoid space with a minimal amount of spinal cord parenchyma, usually only the caudal segments. Remember the variation in the locations of the spinal cord segments in dogs of different sizes. It is preferable to use the site between L6 and L7 in small dogs and between L4 and L5 in larger dogs. The lumbosacral site is not used because the subarachnoid space there is so small, if it is present at all. After surgical preparation of the injection site, the needle is inserted on the median plane between the palpable lumbar vertebral spines. A 1.5- to 3.5-inch, 20- or 22-gauge spinal needle with stylet is used. If CSF is not obtained when the needle first enters the vertebral canal at this site, the needle is advanced to the floor of the vertebral canal and slowly withdrawn to enter the subarachnoid space. You must be cautious because the needle may penetrate the small amount of parenchyma located here to enter the subarachnoid space. It is difficult to keep the end of the needle solely in the subarachnoid space here, and some contrast often enters the epidural space as well as the subarachnoid space. This can be recognized by the irregularity of the radiopaque lines that course along the spinal cord, especially the wavy line that is seen ventral to the spinal cord on the lateral views, the "seagull" appearance. At the level of the middle of the vertebral body you may see a small ventral extension of this wavy line where the epidural space extends into the foramen for the basivertebral vein. Pooling of contrast will also occur where the spinal nerves pass through the intervertebral foramina. When this epidural contrast is extensive, it may be necessary to repeat the myelogram at another time for better interpretation of the lesion. Alternatively, fluoroscopy can be used or a test radiograph can be made to ensure that the contrast is located primarily in the subarachnoid space. Occasionally, a seizure will occur in the immediate postanesthetic period. This is more common in the large dogs in which a cisternal myelogram is performed. Although a chemically induced meningitis will occur briefly, this should not be a deterrent to utilizing myelography. In T2-weighted MR images, CSF is hyperintense relative to the spinal cord parenchyma, which mimics what is seen on a myelogram. The major deterrent to MR imaging is the cost, and occasionally the lesion can be better defined by myelography than by MR imaging, especially in cases of dynamic lesions.

Lesions are classified into three locations (Fig. 4-15).[18]

1. Extradural: This means that the lesion is in the epidural space where, if it occupies space, it will displace and compress the spinal cord and its subarachnoid space. Either the contrast will not pass by the lesion at all and may be deflected centrally, or the contrast will be displaced centrally away from the lesion and thin out as it passes by the lesion. Examples of extradural lesions are intervertebral disk protrusions or extrusions, discospondylitis, primary or metastatic neoplasms of the vertebrae, and epidural hemorrhages or abscesses (Figs. 4-16 and 4-17).

2. Intradural-extramedullary: This means that the lesion is in the subarachnoid space. It may block the flow of contrast in the CSF completely, causing the contrast to form a cuplike shape as it attempts to get around and past the lesion. This cup appearance is referred to as a golf tee sign. The contrast may be able to get past the lesion in the subarachnoid space but will narrow and usually will still show this cup shape. The most common intradural-extramedullary lesions are neoplasms, such as a nerve sheath neoplasm, meningioma, or nephroblastoma (Figs. 4-18 and 4-19).

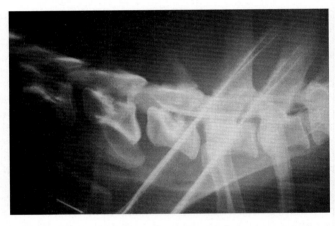

FIGURE 4-16 Lumbar myelogram of a 5-year-old Doberman pinscher with an extradural mass lesion causing a ventral compression of the spinal cord at the C6-C7 articulation. The mass lesion is a protrusion of the annulus fibrosis of the intervertebral disk.

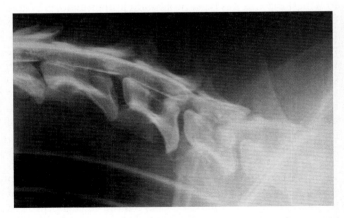

FIGURE 4-17 Cisternal myelogram of a 7-year-old Doberman pinscher with an extradural mass lesion causing a dorsal and ventral compression of the spinal cord at the C5-C6 articulation. The lesion is a protrusion of the annulus fibrosis of the intervertebral disk and a proliferation of the articular processes and joint capsules of the synovial joints.

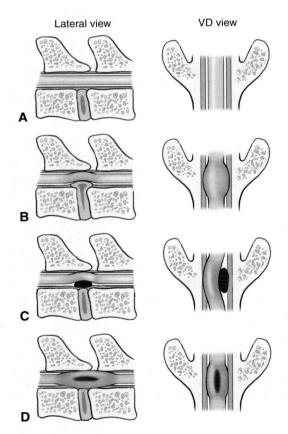

Lateral view   VD view

A

B

C

D

FIGURE 4-15 Three myelographic patterns. **A,** Normal myelographic pattern. **B,** Pattern of an extradural lesion. **C,** Pattern of an intradural-extramedullary lesion. **D,** Pattern of an intramedullary lesion. *(From Roberts RE, Selcer BA: Myelography and epidurography, Vet Clin North Am Small Anim Pract 23:307-329, 1993.)*

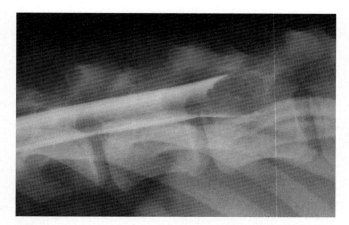

FIGURE 4-18 Cisternal myelogram of a 5-month-old Labrador retriever with an intradural-extramedullary mass lesion compressing the spinal cord at the level of the T12 vertebra. The lesion is a nephroblastoma growing in the subarachnoid space. Note the cupping shape of the contrast as it attempts to pass by the neoplasm that obstructs the subarachnoid space.

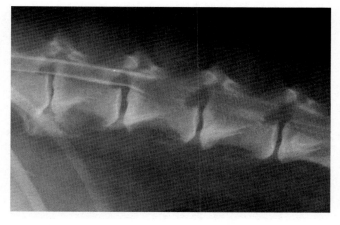

FIGURE 4-20 Cisternal myelogram of a 7-year-old basset hound with an intramedullary mass lesion at the level of the L3 vertebra. The contrast lines deviate to the sides of the vertebral foramen in both this lateral view and the dorsal view. The mass lesion is in the spinal cord parenchyma and at necropsy was a hemangioendothelioma.

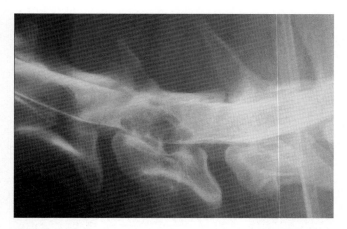

FIGURE 4-19 Cisternal myelogram of a 6-year-old Labrador retriever with an intradural-extramedullary mass lesion compressing and displacing the spinal cord at the level of the C6 vertebra. The mass lesion is a nerve sheath neoplasm involving the C7 spinal roots and nerve on one side. Note the numerous cup shapes made by the contrast as it surrounds the neoplasm that is growing in the subarachnoid space.

3. Intramedullary: This means that the lesion is developing within the parenchyma of the spinal cord. As the segment enlarges, the contrast lines will narrow and be displaced to the periphery of the vertebral canal. The contrast may be completely prevented from continuing past the area of the lesion and will be deflected to the periphery before it stops. Examples of intramedullary lesions are primary neuroectodermal neoplasms such as gliomas and metastatic neoplasms and granulomatous inflammations (Fig. 4-20). Intramedullary lesions are sometimes difficult to distinguish from intradural-extramedullary lesions on MR imaging.

▌ HYDROCEPHALUS

Hydrocephalus is described here because it involves the accumulation of excessive amounts of CSF in the brain or cranial cavity. In fact, the correct definition of hydrocephalus is any increase in the volume of CSF, which means that it is not always related to the cause of any neurologic signs. A number of terms have been used over the years in reference to hydrocephalus, with varying usefulness:

- Internal hydrocephalus is ventricular dilation with CSF accumulation.
- External hydrocephalus is subarachnoid space dilation with CSF accumulation. This is also referred to as hydrocephalus ex vacuo.
- Noncommunicating hydrocephalus is ventricular dilation due to an intraventricular obstruction of CSF flow preventing communication between the ventricular system and the subarachnoid space.
- Communicating hydrocephalus is ventricular dilation secondary to an extraventricular obstruction of CSF flow.
- Normotensive hydrocephalus is associated with normal CSF pressure.
- Hypertensive hydrocephalus is associated with an increase in CSF pressure.
- The two major categories of hydrocephalus are compensatory and obstructive.

Compensatory Hydrocephalus

In compensatory hydrocephalus, a disease process has caused the loss of parenchyma, and the CSF volume has increased (hydrocephalus) to take up the space previously occupied by that portion of the parenchyma. The CSF is increasing in volume to compensate for the loss of parenchyma. The clinical signs relate to the primary disease process that has resulted in the loss of parenchyma. Some examples include in utero viral infections that cause hypoplasia and atrophy of portions of the parenchyma, such as the cerebellum with bovine virus diarrhea (BVD) viral infections in calves and the cerebrum with Akabane viral infection in calves, which result in hydranencephaly (Figs. 4-21 and 4-22). With the former, the CSF accumulation is in the subarachnoid space where the cerebellar

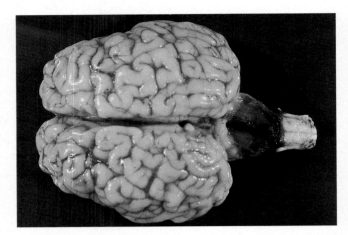

FIGURE 4-21 Brain of a 3-week-old calf with cerebellar hypoplasia and atrophy due to an in utero infection by the bovine virus diarrhea virus. CSF fills up the space where the cerebellar tissue is absent.

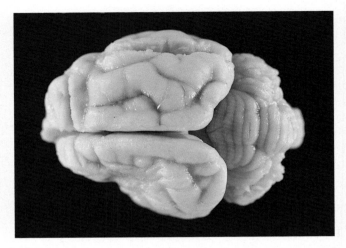

FIGURE 4-23 Brain of a 2-year-old cat necropsied 3 months after an intracranial migration of a *Cuterebra* species larva caused a compromise of the left middle cerebral artery that resulted in a cerebral infarct. CSF filled the space where the cerebral tissue atrophied.

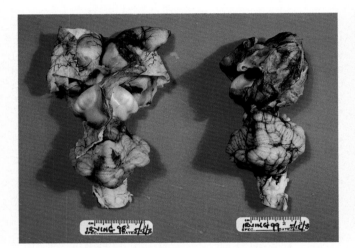

FIGURE 4-22 Two 1-week-old calf brains with severe hydranencephaly due to an in utero infection by the Akabane virus. At necropsy, the thin pial-glial membrane of the neocortical portion of the cerebral hemispheres collapsed when the CSF in the dilated lateral ventricles was released. The CSF replaced the absent cerebral tissue.

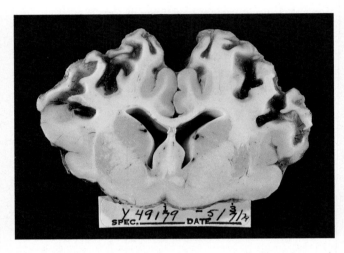

FIGURE 4-24 Transverse section of the brain of a 10-month-old steer just rostral to the rostral commissure and diencephalon. This steer was necropsied 4 months after an acute metabolic encephalopathy due to thiamin deficiency from which it recovered the ability to stand and walk but remained lethargic and blind. CSF filled the cerebral sulci where the polioencephalomalacia occurred with complete loss of the neocortex.

tissue is absent. In hydranencephaly, the CSF accumulation is usually in the lateral ventricles and is normotensive and communicating because there is no obstruction to its flow to and through the lateral apertures. In feline ischemic encephalopathy related to a *Cuterebra* species larval migration, thrombosis or vasospasm of the middle cerebral artery will, in time, result in a significant loss of the parenchyma in its area of distribution on the lateral side of the cerebral hemisphere. CSF will accumulate in the enlarged subarachnoid space at this site (Fig. 4-23). In thiamin-deficient cattle, the resulting cerebrocortical necrosis (polioencephalomalacia) may result in a complete loss of the affected neocortex if the animal survives. CSF will accumulate in the widened subarachnoid spaces between the shrunken gyri (Figs. 4-24 and 4-25). These are all examples of normotensive communicating compensatory hydrocephalus.

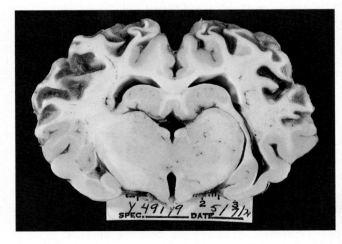

FIGURE 4-25 Transverse section of the brain of the steer in Fig. 4-24 at the level of the mid-diencephalon.

Obstructive Hydrocephalus

Obstruction to the flow or the absorption of CSF causes the CSF pressure to increase and the ventricular system to expand. As a rule, the lateral ventricles are most susceptible to this expansion, which results in more loss of the adjacent cerebral white matter than the gray matter. The cerebral cortex is relatively spared. A number of different conditions can cause the obstruction of CSF flow, and the CSF pressure varies with the disease process and when it is measured. Obstructive hydrocephalus can be subdivided into acquired forms and developmental forms.

Acquired Obstructive Hydrocephalus

Neoplasia may interfere with CSF flow through the interventricular foramen, third ventricle, mesencephalic aqueduct, or lateral apertures. This will produce a noncommunicating hypertensive hydrocephalus in the ventricular compartments rostral to the obstruction (Figs. 4-26 through 4-28). Most of the clinical signs relate to

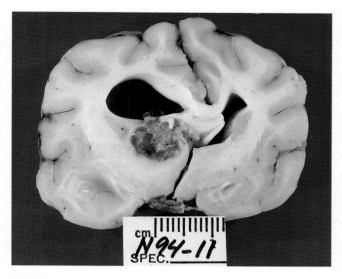

FIGURE 4-28 Transverse section of the same brain as in Figs. 4-26 and 4-27 at the level of the rostral diencephalon.

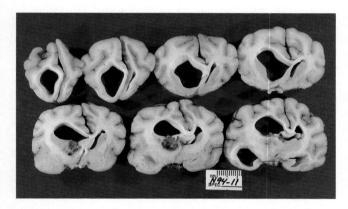

FIGURE 4-26 Transverse sections of the brain of a 5-year-old golden retriever, showing a dilated left lateral ventricle due to a choroid plexus papilloma obstructing the left interventricular foramen.

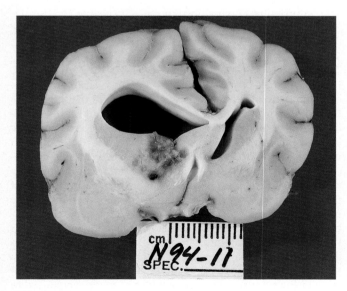

FIGURE 4-27 Transverse section of the same brain as in Fig. 4-26 at the level of the columns of the fornix.

the effect of the growth of the neoplasm in the involved parenchyma, but the hypertensive hydrocephalus may contribute to these signs. Neoplasia may interfere indirectly with CSF absorption through the arachnoid villi because of its compression of the venous sinuses. The CSF volume may not be obviously increased, but its pressure will be increased at the cerebellomedullary cistern. Caudal cranial fossa neoplasms, which interfere with the flow of CSF through the foramen magnum, may cause an expansion of the entire ventricular system, including the fourth ventricle. In addition, a syringohydromyelia may occur in the spinal cord.

Inflammations that involve the ependyma at the narrow components of the CSF flow pathway in the brain may cause obstruction and a hypertensive noncommunicating hydrocephalus.[12] The best example of this is the feline infectious peritonitis (FIP) viral infection in cats. This is the most common inflammation in the CNS of cats, and the virus has a predilection for the ependymal lining of the entire ventricular system, including the choroid plexuses and the central canal in the spinal cord. Mesencephalic aqueductal obstruction is common in this infection and results in expanded third and lateral ventricles (Figs. 4-29 and 4-30). When a pathologist examines the transverse sections of a cat brain and cannot see the normal small opening of the aqueduct, infection with the FIP virus is strongly suspected. Bacterial meningoencephalitis in young farm animals may also obstruct the mesencephalic aqueduct, resulting in expanded lateral ventricles (Figs. 4-31 and 4-32). CSF flow may be obstructed at the lateral apertures by the choroid plexitis because of these same viral and bacterial agents. A periventricular, choroidal, and meningeal suppurative inflammation has been associated with hydrocephalus in 6- to 8-week-old dogs; it was assumed to be of bacterial origin.[11] Some of these lesions may be confused with a traumatic or ischemic lesion that commonly occurs in the white matter adjacent to markedly expanded lateral ventricles in young dogs with developmental obstructive hydrocephalus. This is described later.

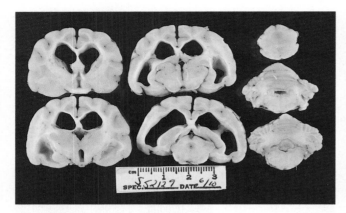

FIGURE 4-29 Transverse sections of the brain of an 8-month-old Siamese cat with the gross lesions of meningoencephalitis caused by a FIP viral infection (see Case Example 12-11). Note the obstructive hydrocephalus and the lack of patency of the mesencephalic aqueduct.

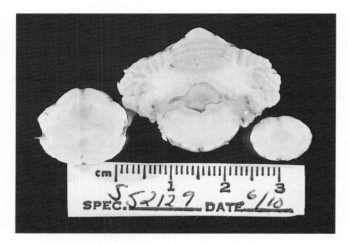

FIGURE 4-30 The same animal as in Fig. 4-29; close-up view of the mesencephalic aqueductal obstruction by inflammation. Note the inflammation of the choroid plexus of the fourth ventricle, which could obstruct the lateral apertures, and note the inflammation filling the central canal in the first cervical spinal cord segment.

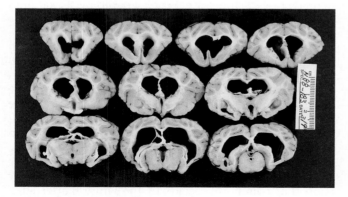

FIGURE 4-31 Transverse sections of the brain of a 3-week-old lamb with a bacterial suppurative meningoencephalitis with severe suppurative ependymitis. Note the obstructive hydrocephalus.

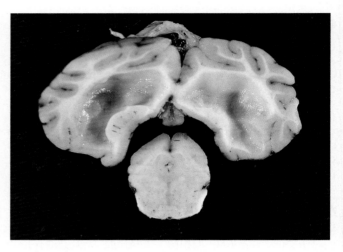

FIGURE 4-32 The same animal as in Fig. 4-31; close-up view of the suppurative inflammation obstructing the mesencephalic aqueduct.

Vitamin A deficiency in calves causes a dural fibrosis that affects the arachnoid villi and interferes with the absorption of CSF, resulting in CSF hypertension. The degree of CSF hypertension directly correlates with the degree of vitamin A deficiency.[16] Minimal hydrocephalus is associated with this deficiency. It occurs most commonly in western North American ranges in 6- to 8-month-old beef cattle kept on dry, vitamin A–deficient pastures with no green feed for a number of months. We have also seen an older German shepherd that had late onset of seizures and dementia with hydrocephalus that was thought to be due to degeneration of the arachnoid villi, similar to that seen in some older humans. Resolution of the clinical signs occurred after placement of a ventriculoperitoneal shunt.

Occipital bone hypoplasia that results in a small caudal cranial fossa and a herniation of the caudal cerebellar vermis into the foramen magnum often backs the CSF up through the entire ventricular system, which expands to include the fourth ventricle in addition to generating a syringohydromyelia. This can be seen on Video 4-1, which shows MR imaging of CSF circulation in a dog with this abnormality. This ventricular expansion may be responsible for the seizures that occasionally occur in these dogs.

Developmental Obstructive Hydrocephalus

Developmental obstructive hydrocephalus, also known as congenital hydrocephalus, is associated with malformations that interfere with the flow or absorption of CSF. The inheritance of these malformations is poorly understood in domestic animals but has been reported for cattle.[2] The most common malformation involves a stenosis of the mesencephalic aqueduct, which produces a hypertensive noncommunicating hydrocephalus. This is often associated with a malformation of the mesencephalon that consists of the development of a single mound of parenchyma for a rostral colliculus and, rarely, partially fused or incompletely divided caudal colliculi (Figs. 4-33 through 4-35). In laboratory rodents this has been described as being inherited as a recessive gene. These dogs are born with markedly expanded lateral ventricles and a third ventricle that is wider than normal. The cerebral hemispheres are reduced to 1 to 2 mm in thickness with occasional foci in the temporal or occipital lobes of only a pial-glial membrane. These dogs often

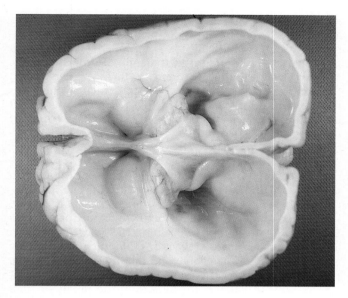

FIGURE 4-33 The brain of a 4-month-old beagle with developmental obstructive hydrocephalus. The dorsal half of the cerebrum has been removed to expose the markedly dilated lateral ventricles and the thinned, stretched-out body of the fornix.

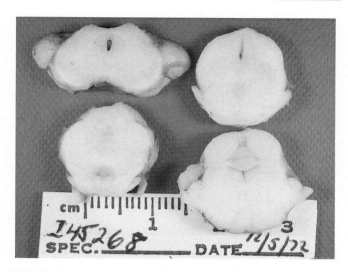

FIGURE 4-35 Transverse sections of the brainstem in Fig. 4-34. Note the lack of a recognizable mesencephalic aqueduct at the level of the rostral mesencephalon where the single rostral colliculus is present. This rostral mesencephalic malformation is a reliable marker for the deficient aqueductal development at this level, which results in a developmental obstructive hydrocephalus.

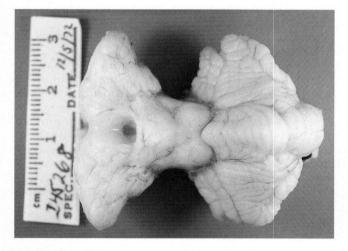

FIGURE 4-34 The brainstem and cerebellum of the brain in Fig. 4-33, after removal of the cerebrum. Note the single mound on the dorsal aspect of the rostral mesencephalon, which is a fused or undivided rostral colliculus.

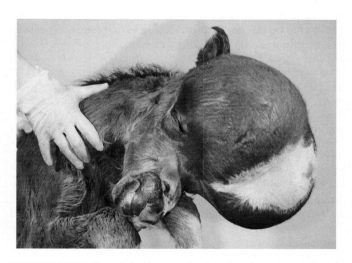

FIGURE 4-36 Stillborn foal with a severely enlarged cranium. Large portions of the calvaria were not ossified and consisted only of a palpable membrane.

have a prominent dome-shaped skull with a prominent molera at the frontoparietal suture and sometimes one or more small molerae in the thinned occipital bone. Occasionally in a newborn foal or farm animal with this same mesencephalic aqueductal stenosis, the cranial cavity is huge, and large areas of nonossified membrane make up the calvaria. Lining the inner surface of this calvaria is a thin layer of cerebral mantle covering a huge volume of CSF in the expanded lateral ventricle (Figs. 4-36 and 4-37). These animals rarely survive.

The same degree of severe expansion of the lateral ventricles and similar prosencephalic clinical signs occur in dogs that have no morphologic abnormalities in the brain at necropsy to explain an obstruction. In addition, these dogs demonstrate normal CSF circulation when a contrast ventriculogram is performed antemortem. We hypothesize two possibilities to explain the severe congenital hydrocephalus in these dogs.

1. At a critical time in the fetal development of the mesencephalic aqueduct, the aqueduct was inadequate to accommodate the flow of CSF produced in the third and lateral ventricles. A partial obstruction occurred and the lateral ventricles expanded at the expense of the extremely delicate fetal cerebrum. With growth, the aqueduct developed to its normal size and CSF pressures normalized but the compromised atrophied cerebrum persisted.
2. A malformation of the arachnoid villi with a deficiency in the number produced or an abnormality in their structure could prevent normal CSF absorption. A communicating obstructive hydrocephalus would result with expansion of the lateral ventricles. There would be no evidence of any obstructive lesions at necropsy. These arachnoid villi are very difficult to locate and study microscopically, which makes this hypothesis difficult to evaluate.

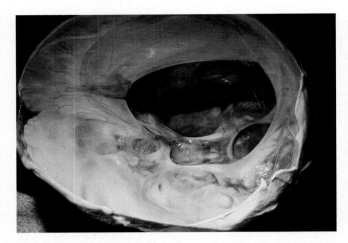

FIGURE 4-37 The same foal as in Fig. 4-36, after removal of the brain. Rostral is to the left of the photo, and the left side of the enlarged cranial cavity is exposed. The dorsal sheet of tissue is the falx cerebri. The rostral mesencephalon had only one midline rostral colliculus, and there was no recognizable mesencephalic aqueduct at this level.

Signalment, History, Clinical Signs

Although developmental obstructive hydrocephalus occurs sporadically in all breeds of dogs, there is a much higher incidence in the toy and brachycephalic breeds, especially the Chihuahua, Pekingese, pug, Boston terrier, Yorkshire terrier, Pomeranian, and English bulldog. This disorder is uncommon in cats. Despite the presumed fetal genesis of the obstruction, clinical signs may not be evident at birth. Most will be observed by 3 months of age, some between 3 and 12 months, and rarely beyond 12 months. Some dogs exhibit no clinical signs despite markedly enlarged lateral ventricles with significant cerebral atrophy. This suggests that the clinical signs may be related to the level of CSF pressure, which can be quite variable in these dogs.

The most common clinical signs observed are prosencephalic in origin because of the severe expansion of the lateral ventricles, with compromise of the cerebral tissue and compression of the diencephalon. The following description of prosencephalic signs is introduced here but applies to any prosencephalic disorder.

Prosencephalic Signs

Seizures and abnormal behavior will have been observed by the owner but commonly are not observed by you during your examination. Mild changes in the animal's behavior may be appreciated only by the owner, who can recognize such changes. They include loss of trained habits, abnormal behavior, lack of recognition by the animal of its environment, and changes in attitude toward the owner. Some of these dogs cannot be housebroken, unlike their littermates. Progressive loss of the animal's sensorium or its level of consciousness or response to the owner or you is described by the following terms: depression, lethargy, obtundation, semicoma (stupor), and coma. The last two usually implicate involvement of the ascending reticular activating system in the diencephalon. The anatomy of this system is described in Chapter 19. The owner is better able to recognize a mild change in attitude to more docile or more aggressive behavior. The latter may include hysterical or

maniacal behavior, which also will be obvious to you. Head and neck turning to one side (pleurothotonus) and propulsive pacing and circling are commonly associated with frontoparietal lobe or rostral thalamic disorders. Usually, but not always, the patient tends to turn or circle toward the side on which the lesion exists, which is the basis for the term *adversive* ("to turn to") *syndrome*. Seizures or behavioral changes may be the only clinical signs present in a prosencephalic disorder, and your neurologic examination may be normal.

In your neurologic examination of the patient, there are only three responses you can test that may be abnormal in the presence of prosencephalic disorders. The specific anatomy of these tests is described in later chapters. If the lesion is confined to the prosencephalon, without any pressure on the caudal brainstem or cerebellum, the gait is normal on a flat surface but postural reactions, of which the hopping response is the most reliable, are mildly abnormal. Visual perception tested by the menace response is depressed or absent, with no change in the size of the pupils or their reaction to a bright light. Nociception tested on the surface of the body is depressed, especially when evaluated on the mucosa of the nasal septum because of its reliable sensitivity. With unilateral prosencephalic lesions, all three of these responses (hopping, menace, nasal septum nociception) are abnormal on the side of the body contralateral to the prosencephalic disorder.

Dogs with developmental obstructive hydrocephalus most commonly exhibit a change in behavior or a loss of sensorium. Loss of vision is common due to the compromise of the optic radiation in the centrum semiovale and the occipital cortex. The gait is usually unaffected on a flat surface. Postural reactions and nociception may or may not be depressed. If intracranial pressure is significantly elevated, pressure may be exerted on the brainstem, which will cause a spastic paresis and general proprioceptive ataxia in the gait. The ataxia may also have a cerebellar or vestibular quality, especially if the fourth ventricle has been expanded by the increase in CSF volume. Syringohydromyelia may also occur in these dogs and contribute to the gait abnormality, and it may also cause excessive neck scratching and a cervical vertebral scoliosis. The frequency of syringohydromyelia with obstructive hydrocephalus is unknown because it has not been consistently looked for at necropsy or during imaging procedures. In all dogs in which MR imaging reveals an obstructive form of hydrocephalus, the cervical spinal cord should be imaged for this lesion.

In addition to these neurologic signs, the cranial cavities may be enlarged enough that the skulls of these dogs may have a dome shape and there may be a palpable molera. Remember that many toy breeds, especially the Chihuahua, normally have small molerae as adults. Some dogs with enlarged cranial cavities have orbits with abnormal shapes, causing the eyes in some head positions to deviate ventrally and slightly laterally ("sunset eyes"). We believe that this strabismus is not due to compression of the oculomotor nerves on the floor of the cranial cavity because the strabismus is not always apparent, and on moving the head repeatedly from one side to the other to test for normal physiological nystagmus, each eye adducts well, indicating normal oculomotor nerve innervation of the medial rectus muscles. In addition, the pupillary size and response to light is normal.

The following four videos of dogs demonstrate the clinical signs of developmental obstructive hydrocephalus:

1. **Video 4-2** shows a 7-week-old keeshond that was lethargic and blind. Note the enlarged cranium, the strabismus, and the retained ability to walk.

2. **Video 4-3** shows a 7-week-old beagle in which blindness was the only complaint. Note the enlarged cranium and the strabismus. At necropsy, this beagle and the keeshond in Video 4-2 both had mesencephalic aqueductal stenosis, with extremely enlarged lateral ventricles and cerebral atrophy. Despite the severe prosencephalic compromise, note that these two dogs have normal gaits.

3. **Video 4-4** shows a 9-week-old Labrador retriever that is lethargic and blind and has mild vestibular ataxia and a tendency to circle to its right side. Postural reactions are slow bilaterally. The vestibular ataxia was presumed to be due to the pressure of the enlarged cerebrum on the caudal brainstem. The cranium is not noticeably enlarged.

4. **Video 4-5** shows a 4-month-old pug dog with propulsive circling to the right and a normal gait, but poor postural reactions in the left limbs and a poor left-side menace response. These clinical signs suggest that the lesion was worse in the right cerebral hemisphere. The cranium is enlarged and has a large frontoparietal molera. The CT shows these extensive cerebral lesions and the small diencephalon. Note the loss of parenchyma ventrally on the right side in the rostral sections at the level of the head and body of the caudate nucleus. The bone window CT at the end shows the large molera. At necropsy no obstruction was found but, associated with the extremely dilated lateral ventricles, there were tears in the cerebral white matter, especially in the right cerebrum. The presumed diagnosis was obstructive hydrocephalus due to an arachnoid villi abnormality. Figures 4-38 through 4-42 show the features of this dog's calvaria and brain at necropsy.

Occasionally, sudden exacerbations of clinical signs occur in these dogs and are sometimes associated with an expression of considerable discomfort by the patient. We believe

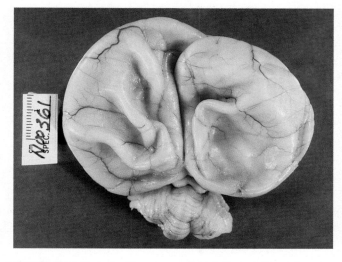

FIGURE 4-39 The brain of the same pug that is in Fig. 4-38. The cerebrum is collapsed due to the postmortem release of CSF from the excessively dilated lateral ventricles.

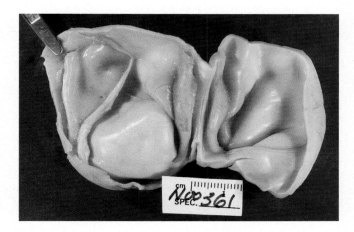

FIGURE 4-40 Inner surface of the dorsal aspect of the cerebrum after its removal from the brain seen in Fig. 4-39. Note the separation of a sheet of thinned white matter in the right cerebral hemisphere.

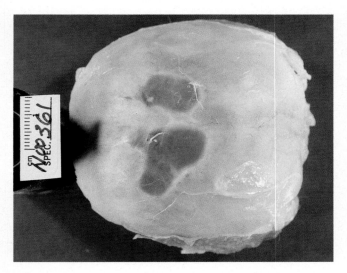

FIGURE 4-38 Calvaria of the 4-month-old pug seen in Video 4-5. Note the large molerae, which were palpable antemortem.

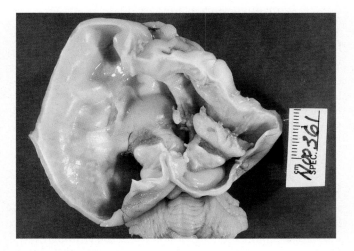

FIGURE 4-41 Dorsal view of the brain seen in Fig. 4-39 after removal of the dorsal portion of the cerebrum. In the left cerebrum, note the thinned but intact cerebral tissue and the smooth tan mound toward the midline, which is the normal left caudate nucleus. In the right cerebrum, this nucleus is obscured by a tear in the tissue where the caudate nucleus lies adjacent to the internal capsule.

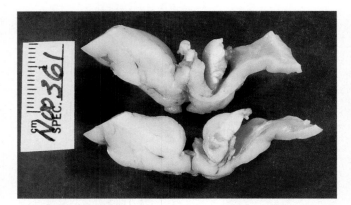

FIGURE 4-42 Two transverse sections of the brain in Fig. 4-41, showing the caudal surfaces and the torn tissue on the right side.

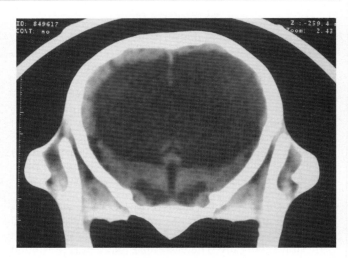

FIGURE 4-43 CT image of a 1-week-old miniature horse with developmental obstructive hydrocephalus. Note the very small diencephalon ventrally.

this may be a result of episodes of bleeding into the expanded ventricle. The discomfort may occur because this blood gets access to the subarachnoid space. It is common at necropsy to see a mild yellow discoloration of either side of the atrophic cerebrum and occasionally to see blood clots on the wall or in the lumen of the lateral ventricle. These findings are associated with tears in the thin layer of white matter in the atrophic cerebral hemisphere.[21] The most common sites of these tears extend from the lateral surface of the distended lateral ventricle ventrally, lateral to the caudate nucleus. This tear is primarily in the internal capsule but may extend medially into the caudate nucleus or laterally into the lentiform nucleus. On microscopic examination of these areas of tissue disruptions, there are foci of ischemic necrosis and scattered inflammation that include macrophages and neutrophils. We believe that the latter reflect recent acute tissue injury, not an infectious process as indicated in some of the literature.[11] The constant stretching of the thinned wall of the cerebrum may lead to ischemia and susceptibility to tearing as the result of mild trauma. MR imaging may reveal this lesion in the ventral internal capsule where it separates the lentiform nucleus from the caudate nucleus. Another possible cause of episodic discomfort is the development of a cervical syringohydromyelia in these dogs.

Differential Diagnosis

The disorder that is most common at this age and that causes similar prosencephalic signs is the hepatic encephalopathy associated with portosystemic shunts. A major difference is that the dogs with the liver disorder usually have episodic signs related to the quality of the diet and the feeding times. Infectious diseases and inherited storage diseases are other considerations.

Diagnosis

Numerous ancillary procedures may be used to confirm the diagnosis of enlarged lateral ventricles. Both CT and MR imaging readily demonstrate such lesions (Figs. 4-43 through 4-47). MR imaging is the most accurate means of defining all components of the intracranial CSF compartments, and it also allows the clinician to evaluate the spinal cord for a syringohydromyelia. Ultrasound can be used by probing through a molera or even the calvaria, if it is thin enough, as in a puppy.

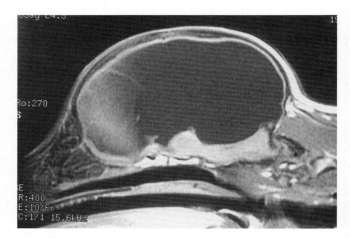

FIGURE 4-44 Sagittal T1-weighted MR image of a 14-week-old Labrador retriever with developmental obstructive hydrocephalus due to a mesencephalic aqueductal stenosis.

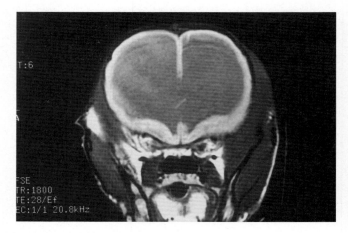

FIGURE 4-45 Axial T1-weighted MR image of the dog in Fig. 4-44 at a level just rostral to the diencephalon.

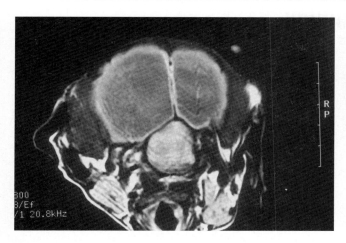

FIGURE 4-46 Axial T1-weighted MR image of the dog in Figs. 4-44 and 4-45 at the level of the occipital lobes and rostral mesencephalon. Note the single median mound of the mesencephalic tectum that represents a single rostral colliculus and no evidence of any mesencephalic aqueduct.

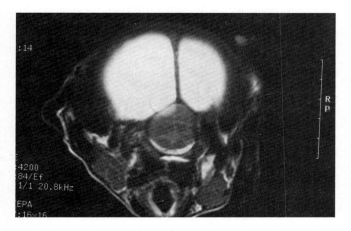

FIGURE 4-47 Axial T2-weighted MR image at the same level as the image in Fig. 4-46, showing the hyperintense CSF in the dilated lateral ventricles in the occipital lobes but none where the mesencephalic aqueduct should be located.

A lateral radiograph may show loss of the cerebral gyral pattern, a diffuse homogenous "ground-glass" appearance where the lateral ventricle is enlarged and filled with CSF, and a flattened appearance of the cribriform lamina. Before CT and MR imaging were available, this diagnosis was confirmed by injecting air or contrast into the lateral ventricle. The site of injection is on the dorsal aspect of the calvaria, 3 to 5 mm to one side of the median plane and at a transverse level that is one half the distance from the lateral angle of the eye to the external occipital protuberance. A hole is made in the calvaria there by rotating the spinal needle if the bone is thin or rotating an intramedullary pin held in an orthopedic handle. A spinal needle with stylet is slowly inserted through this opening in the bone and into the parenchyma until CSF appears in the needle hub. With severe enlargement of the lateral ventricle, this will occur within 2 to 3 mm from the bone opening. It is often difficult to place the end of the needle in the thin slit of a normal lateral ventricle. To be safe, do not pass the needle into the brain more than one half the height of the cranial cavity, as measured on the lateral radiograph.

For diagnosis, remove a few milliliters of CSF and replace it with a similar volume of air. In this pneumoventriculogram, the radiolucency of the air dorsal to the more radiopaque CSF is obvious in a lateral radiograph (Fig. 4-48). If progressive radiographs are made with the head rotated in different positions, the entire lateral ventricle can be defined by the position of the air. To diagnose the location of the obstruction that caused the ventricular expansion, a radiopaque contrast agent can be injected to replace the CSF that was removed. Within a short time, a lateral radiograph of a normal animal will show the contrast in all of the brain ventricles and in the subarachnoid space intracranially and around the spinal cord. The presence of a myelogram confirms that the CSF can circulate through the ventricles and exit through the lateral apertures. If the mesencephalic aqueduct is stenotic, there will be no contrast in the fourth ventricle or subarachnoid space (Figs. 4-49 and 4-50). If the lateral apertures are inadequate, contrast fills the expanded fourth ventricle and is not present in the subarachnoid space. If the obstruction is at the level of the arachnoid villi, the distribution of contrast is similar to that of a normal animal except for the expanded lateral ventricles. Warning! Be careful in cases of severe hydrocephalus that you remove only a very small amount of CSF before you inject air or contrast so as to avoid a collapse of the thin atrophied cerebrum. Electroencephalograms of dogs with expanded lateral ventricles and atrophic cerebral mantles typically show slow wave patterns with markedly increased amplitude in all leads.[5,13]

Treatment

If severe developmental obstructive hydrocephalus is diagnosed in a recently purchased puppy that has debilitating neurologic signs, we believe that euthanasia is advisable because of the poor quality of life expectancy for the puppy, even with an attempt at treatment. This advice should be given before the owners and their children become bonded

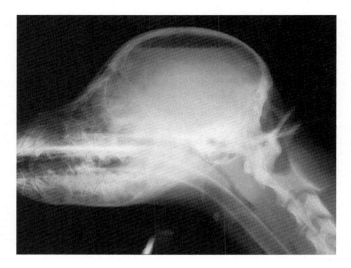

FIGURE 4-48 Skull radiograph of a 4-month-old mixed-breed dog with developmental obstructive hydrocephalus. Note the homogenous appearance of the CSF-filled lateral ventricles and the small volume of air dorsally that was injected into one lateral ventricle to produce a pneumoventriculogram. Note the flattened cribriform lamina, which is a feature of the moderate enlargement of the cranial cavity in this dog.

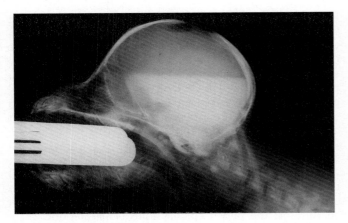

FIGURE 4-49 Skull radiograph of a 3-month-old beagle with developmental obstructive hydrocephalus. A small amount of air can be seen dorsally after it had been injected into one of the dilated lateral ventricles, indicating that the remaining cerebral tissue was extremely thin. Contrast has also been injected into one lateral ventricle. Note that no contrast is evident in the fourth ventricle or in the subarachnoid space in the cranial cavity or around the spinal cord. This indicates that there is a mesencephalic aqueductal stenosis that has blocked the circulation of CSF.

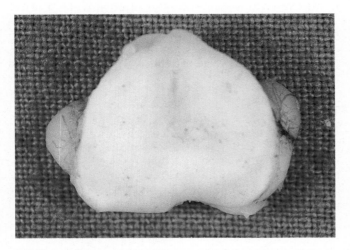

FIGURE 4-50 Transverse section of the rostral mesencephalon of the dog in Fig. 4-49, confirming the severe aqueductal stenosis associated with a single median rostral colliculus.

with the puppy. Although low levels of corticosteroids may decrease the rate of production of CSF, the most effective treatment is surgical. A shunt may readily be placed in the lateral ventricle and tunneled subcutaneously to the abdomen, where it is inserted into the peritoneal cavity. The surgical outcome is usually good but is not a cure for all cases, and it requires life-long maintenance of the shunt. Returning the affected puppy to the breeder is highly recommended.

REFERENCES

1. Andres KH: Zur Feinstruktur der Arachnoidalzotten bei Mammalia, *Z Zellforsch Mikrosk Anat* 82:92, 1967.
2. Baker ML, Payne CA, Baker GN: The inheritance of hydrocephalus in cattle, *J Hered* 52:135, 1961.
3. Cserr HF: Physiology of the choroid plexus, *Physiol Rev* 51:273, 1971.
4. Davson H: *Physiology of cerebrospinal fluid*, London, 1971, JA Churchill.
5. de Lahunta A, Cummings JF: The clinical and electroencephalographic features of hydrocephalus in three dogs, *J Am Vet Med Assoc* 146:954, 1995.
6. DiChiro G, Hammock MK, Bleyer WA: Spinal descent of cerebrospinal fluid in man, *Neurology* 26:1, 1976.
7. DiChiro G, Stein SC, Harrington T: Spontaneous cerebrospinal fluid rhinorrhea in normal dogs: radiographic studies of an alternate pathway of CSF drainage, *J Neuropathol Exp Neurol* 31:447, 1972.
8. Gomez DG, Potts DG: The choroid plexus of the dog, *Anat Rec* 181:363, 1975.
9. Gomez DG, Potts DG: Deonarine V: Arachnoid granulations of the sheep, *Arch Neurol* 30:169, 1974.
10. Haines DE, Harkey HL, Al-Mefty O: The "subdural space": a new look at an outdated concept, *Neurosurgery* 32: 111-120, 1993.
11. Higgins RG, Vandevelde M, Braund FG: Internal hydrocephalus and associated periventricular encephalitis in young dogs, *Vet Pathol* 14:236, 1977.
12. Johnson RT: Hydrocephalus and viral infections, *Dev Med Child Neurol* 17:807, 1975 (review).
13. Klemm WR, Hall CL: Electroencephalograms on anesthetized dogs with hydrocephalus, *Am J Vet Res* 32:1859, 1971.
14. Mayhew IG: Collection of cerebrospinal fluid from the horse, *Cornell Vet* 56:500, 1975.
15. Milhorat TH, et al: Cerebrospinal fluid production by the choroid plexus and the brain, *Science* 173:330, 1971.
16. Mills JH, et al: Experimental pathology of dairy calves ingesting one-third the daily requirement of carotene, *Acta Vet Scand* 8:324, 1967.
17. Pollay M, Welch K: The function and structure of the canine arachnoid villi, *J Surg Res* 2:307, 1962.
18. Roberts RE, Selcer BA: Myelography and epidurography, *Vet Clin No Am Small Anim Pract* 23:307-329, 1993.
19. Strazille N, Ghersi-Egea S-F: Choroid plexus in the central nervous system: biology and physiopathology, *J Neuropathol Exp Neurol* 59:561-574, 2000.
20. Tripathi RC: The functional morphology of the outflow systems of ocular and cerebrospinal fluid, *Exp Eye Res* (suppl): 65, 1977.
21. Wunschmann A, Oglesbee M: Periventricular changes associated with spontaneous canine hydrocephalus, *Vet Pathol* 38:67-73, 2001.

5 LOWER MOTOR NEURON: SPINAL NERVE, GENERAL SOMATIC EFFERENT SYSTEM

LOWER MOTOR NEURON

SPINAL NERVE: GSE-LMN

SPINAL CORD SEGMENTS: VERTEBRAL COLUMN

FUNCTION

PELVIC LIMB AND PERINEAL REFLEXES

THORACIC LIMB REFLEXES

LOWER MOTOR NEURON DISEASE: NEUROMUSCULAR DISEASE

Clinical Signs
Wallerian Degeneration
Electrodiagnostic Techniques in Neuromuscular
  Disease

NEUROMUSCULAR DISEASES: DISEASES OF THE GSE-LMN

CASE EXAMPLE 5-1: NMD TETRAPLEGIA—DOG
  Polyradiculoneuritis
  Botulism
  Myasthenia Gravis
  Tick Paralysis
  Polymyositis
  Other Differential Diagnoses
CASE EXAMPLE 5-2: NMD TETRAPARESIS—DOG
  Polyradiculoneuritis
  Botulism
  Myasthenia Gravis
  Tick Paralysis
  Polymyositis
  Hypokalemic Myopathy
CASE EXAMPLE 5-3: NMD TETRAPARESIS—DOG
  Type II Deficiency Autosomal Recessive
    Polymyopathy in Labrador Retrievers
CASE EXAMPLE 5-4: NMD TETRAPARESIS—DOG
  Dystrophinopathy, a Sex-Linked Recessive
    Muscular Dystrophy

Exercise-Induced Collapse in Labrador Retrievers
Exercise-Induced Fatigue
Motor Neuron Disease: Congenital
Equine Motor Neuron Disease: Acquired
CASE EXAMPLE 5-5: NMD MONOPARESIS—
  THORACIC LIMB—DOG
  Malignant Nerve Sheath Neoplasm
  Brachial Plexus Neuritis
  Chronic Neuritis
  Brachial Plexus Root Avulsion
CASE EXAMPLE 5-6: NMD MONOPARESIS—
  THORACIC LIMB—HORSE
  Lymphoma
  Equine Protozoal Myelitis
  Injury
CASE EXAMPLE 5-7: INFRASPINATUS
  CONTRACTURE—DOG
CASE EXAMPLE 5-8: LMN PARAPLEGIA—DOG
  Fibrocartilaginous Embolic Myelopathy
CASE EXAMPLE 5-9: SACROCAUDAL
  DYSFUNCTION—HORSE
  Polyneuritis Equi, or Neuritis of the Cauda
    Equina
CASE EXAMPLE 5-10: SACROCAUDAL
  DYSFUNCTION—DOG
  Lumbosacral Syndrome, or Cauda Equina
    Syndrome
  Intervertebral Disk Protrusion
  Diskospondylitis
  Neoplasm
  L7 Fracture
  Limber Tail Syndrome, or Acute Caudal Myopathy
CASE EXAMPLE 5-11: NMD PARAPARESIS—DOG
  Neosporosis
  Swimmer Puppies
CASE EXAMPLE 5-12: NMD PARAPLEGIA—CAT
  Aortic Thromboembolism
CASE EXAMPLE 5-13: NMD PARAPLEGIA—CAT
  Ischemic Poliomyelomalacia

Postoperative Poliomyelomalacia: Horse
  and Calf
Poliomyelomalacia in Pigs
Poliomyelomalacia in Ayshire Calves
CASE EXAMPLE 5-14: LMN TETRAPLEGIA—DOG
  Diffuse Myelomalacia
CASE EXAMPLE 5-15: PELVIC LIMB
  MONOPLEGIA—DOG
  Sciatic Nerve Injury
CASE EXAMPLE 5-16: LMN PARAPARESIS—COW
  Injury
  Lymphoma
  Diskospondylitis
CASE EXAMPLE 5-17: LMN PARAPARESIS—DOG
  Leonberger Inherited Neuropathy
  Metabolic Neuropathy
  Inherited Neuromyopathy–Dancing
    Doberman
  Inherited Hypertrophic Neuropathy
  Inherited Giant Axonal Neuropathy
CASE EXAMPLE 5-18: LMN
  PARAPARESIS—HORSE
CASE EXAMPLE 5-19: LMN PARAPARESIS—COW
  Dystocia Injury: Femoral Nerve
CASE EXAMPLE 5-20: LMN PARAPARESIS—DOG
  Intervertebral Disk Extrusion
CASE EXAMPLE 5-21: PELVIC LIMB
  DYSFUNCTION—DOG
  Fibrosis: Caudomedial Thigh Muscles
  Plantigrade Posture
CASE EXAMPLE 5-22: STIFFNESS IN A KID
  Vitamin E Deficiency Myopathy

LOWER MOTOR NEURON

The lower motor neuron (LMN) is the efferent neuron of the peripheral nervous system (PNS) that connects the central nervous system (CNS) with the muscle to be innervated. The entire function of the CNS is manifested through the lower motor neuron. The LMN includes two components: the general somatic efferent system (GSE) and general visceral efferent system (GVE).

The general somatic efferent system of the lower motor neuron includes the neurons that innervate striated voluntary skeletal muscle that is derived from somites and somatic mesoderm in the body wall's limb buds and from somitomeres in the head. These neurons are located in all of the spinal nerves and all of the cranial nerves except I, II, and VIII. This chapter describes the spinal nerve GSE-LMN. Chapter 6 describes the GSE-LMN present in cranial nerves.

SPINAL NERVE: GSE-LMN

The neuronal cell bodies of this system are located in the ventral gray columns throughout the entire spinal cord. The shape and size of the ventral gray column reflect the number of neurons present, which is determined by the volume of striated muscle that is innervated. The GSE neurons innervating the axial muscles populate the medial portion of the column. Those innervating the appendicular muscles are located laterally and cause the lateral bulge of the ventral gray column that is evident at the cervical and lumbosacral intumescences (Fig. 5-1). These lateral portions of the ventral gray column can be subdivided further into motonuclear columns representative of muscle groups and peripheral nerves present in the limbs. GSE neurons that innervate proximal limb muscles are located in the ventral portion of the lateral part of the ventral gray column. Those innervating the more distal limb muscles are in the dorsal portion. These motonuclear columns have been identified by transecting peripheral nerves or ablating specific muscles and then observing in the spinal cord ventral gray column the retrograde chromatolysis of the neuronal cell bodies whose axons were destroyed in the experimental procedure.

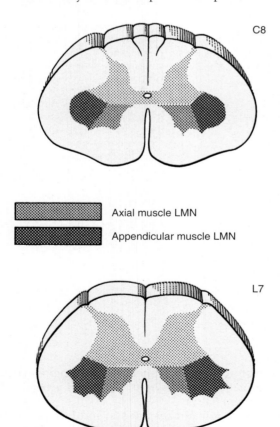

Axial muscle LMN

Appendicular muscle LMN

FIGURE 5-1 Spinal cord topography depicted at the cervical *(C8)* and lumbar *(L7)* intumescences.

The dendritic zone of the multipolar GSE neuron is confined to the gray matter of the spinal cord adjacent to the cell body of that neuron. The axon courses through the white matter between the lateral and ventral funiculi to leave the spinal cord as part of a ventral rootlet. It continues in a ventral root and then into the spinal nerve, which that root forms. Then it travels into the limbs as part of a specific peripheral nerve that is distributed to a specific group of striated skeletal muscles (Fig. 5-2). The part of the axon that is located within the spinal cord (intramedullary) is myelinated by oligodendroglial cells, whereas the part of the axon located within the PNS is myelinated by Schwann cells.

At the level of the striated skeletal muscle, each axon of a GSE neuron divides into several branches. Each of these axonal branches ends on a muscle cell at a motor end-plate. Each adult muscle cell is innervated only by the axon of one motor neuron. In the fetus and newborn, more than one neuron may innervate a striated muscle cell, but during early postnatal development this polyneuronal innervation is reduced to a single neuron.[82] The number of muscle cells innervated by one GSE neuron is called the motor unit. It varies from 100 to 150 muscle cells in the proximal limb muscles to 3 to 4 in extraocular muscles. Muscles involved in functions that require a large degree of coordination are innervated by motor neurons with small motor units (only a few muscle cells per neuron).

The strength of a muscle contraction depends on the number of motor units activated in a muscle. At the motor end-plate the myelin sheath is absent, and the axon terminates in several small branches that form a cluster in a localized area near the longitudinal center of the muscle cell. Each of these small branches terminates on specialized modification of the sarcolemma. This terminal is called the neuromuscular ending, junction, or synapse (Fig. 5-3).

The neuromuscular junction consists of a distended axonal terminal covered by a Schwann cell that has not formed myelin up to the point where the axon extends into a sarcoplasmic trough on the surface of the muscle cell. The endoneurium of the nerve and the endomysium of the muscle cell are continuous outside this trough. Inside the trough the axolemma and sarcolemma are juxtaposed. The axon terminal contains numerous mitochondria and synaptic vesicles. The latter are the source of the neurotransmitter substance acetylcholine. The sarcoplasmic trough is located on an area of the muscle cell membrane at which the sarcoplasm has accumulated. This is called the sole plate and abounds with muscle cell nuclei and mitochondria. The sarcoplasmic trough is extended farther by invaginations of the sarcoplasm to form postsynaptic membrane folds (subneural clefts). The synaptic cleft is the space between the presynaptic membrane (axolemma) and the postsynaptic membrane (sarcolemma) and is about 200 angstroms (A). The postsynaptic membrane abounds with acetylcholine receptors. These receptors consist of five subunits formed from the integral proteins of the cell membrane and arranged in a circular shape that forms a channel for sodium ions.

When the action potential traveling along the axon arrives at the neuronal presynaptic membrane, calcium channels on the axolemmal surface open. The increase in axoplasmal calcium triggers the release of acetylcholine from the synaptic vesicles into the synaptic cleft where the acetylcholine molecules bind to the receptors in the sarcolemma of the sole plate. This binding opens these sodium

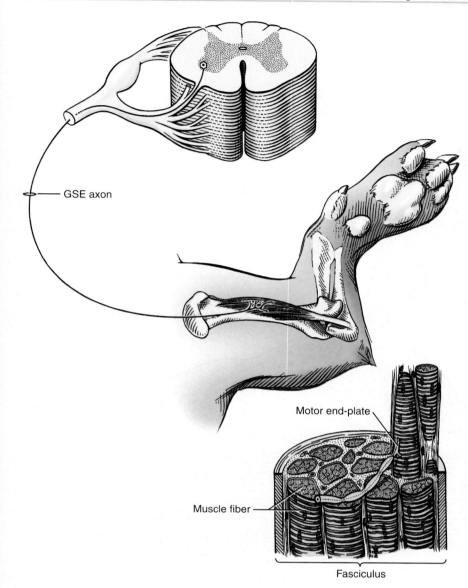

GSE axon

Motor end-plate

Muscle fiber

Fasciculus

FIGURE 5-2 GSE-LMN innervation of the medial head of the triceps brachii.

channels and the influx of sodium results in depolarization of the sole plate region; if enough channels are opened, the depolarization spreads, resulting in muscle cell contraction. The acetylcholine released into the synaptic cleft is rapidly eliminated by diffusion away from the cleft site and by hydrolysis by acetylcholinesterase that is released into the cleft through the muscle cell membrane.

SPINAL CORD SEGMENTS: VERTEBRAL COLUMN

For clinical purposes, it is important to know in which spinal cord segments the neuronal cell bodies of the GSE motor neurons are located, whose axons are in specific peripheral nerves, and to know the specific vertebrae (vertebral foramen) in which these segments are found. For example, if your neurologic examination of a medium-sized dog determines that your patient has a deficiency localized to the sciatic nerve innervation of the pelvic limb, the anatomic diagnosis includes all components of that nerve as well as the neuronal cell bodies in the L6, L7, and S1 spinal cord

segments. These spinal cord segments are located in the L4 and L5 vertebral foramina and their spinal nerves course caudally in the vertebral canal to leave through the intervertebral foramina between vertebrae L6 and L7, L7 and S1, and S1 and S2.[57] In the dog, the spinal cord is composed of about 36 segments: 8 cervical, 13 thoracic, 7 lumbar, 3 sacral, and usually 5 caudal. Each segment has a number of dorsal and ventral rootlets that attach respectively to the dorsolateral and ventrolateral aspects of each side. The segmental spinal ganglion is found in the dorsal root just prior to its union with the ventral root at the level of the intervertebral foramen. The spinal nerve emerges from the intervertebral foramen and immediately branches into a dorsal and a ventral branch. Thus each spinal cord segment is connected to the tissues of the body by a spinal nerve on each side. The dorsal branch innervates epaxial tissues and the ventral branch innervates hypaxial tissues, which include the limbs.

The development in the embryo of the spinal cord segments and that of the vertebral column are closely related, which accounts for the manner in which the roots and spinal nerves of each segment are distributed among the

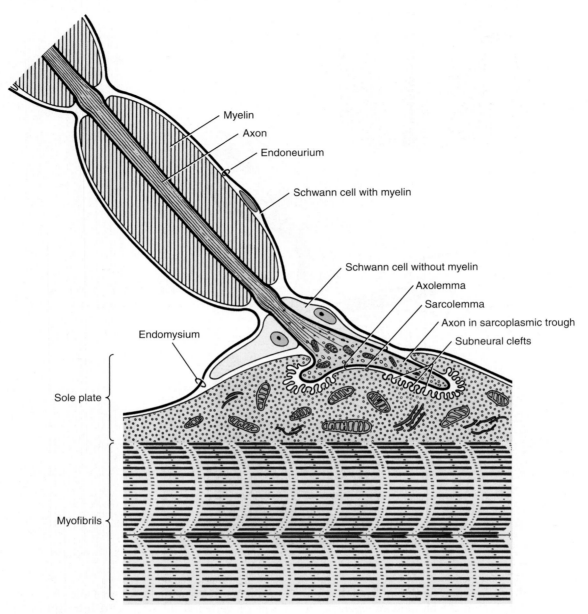

FIGURE 5-3 Neuromuscular junction of a motor end-plate.

vertebrae. The first cervical spinal nerves leave the vertebral canal through the lateral vertebral foramina in the arch of the atlas (Fig. 5-4). All the remaining spinal nerves leave this canal between vertebrae via intervertebral foramina or though the sacral foramina. This is also true for the cat. Other species have a variable number of vertebrae with lateral vertebral foramina. The spinal nerves of the second through the seventh cervical spinal cord segments leave the canal through the intervertebral foramina cranial to the vertebra of the same number. Therefore, the seventh cervical spinal nerves leave the vertebral canal cranial to the C7 vertebrae (see Fig. 5-4). Because there are always only seven cervical vertebrae and there are eight cervical spinal cord segments, the spinal nerves of the eighth cervical spinal cord segment leave the vertebral canal cranial to the first thoracic vertebra. All the remaining spinal nerves leave the vertebral canal through the intervertebral foramina that are caudal to the vertebrae of the same number. This segmental relationship

of the spinal cord and vertebral column is established in the embryo.

After birth, as the animal grows, there is more growth in the vertebral column than in the spinal cord, and this alters the relationship of the spinal cord segments to the vertebrae by means of a cranial displacement of most of the spinal cord segments. In the dog, only the first and second cervical spinal cord segments and the last two thoracic and first two or three lumbar segments lie in the vertebral canal within the vertebra of the same numbers. All the remaining segments reside in the canal cranial to the vertebrae of the same number. To accommodate for this cranial displacement, the spinal nerves must grow in length because the place where they exit the vertebral canal can not be altered. This is especially evident in the caudal lumbar and sacral vertebrae, where the arrangement of the long spinal roots and nerves adjacent and caudal to the conus medullaris is called the cauda equina for its resemblance to the tail of a horse. (See the table and discussion in Chapter 4, where the positions of the sacral segments within the vertebral canal are described.) This cranial displacement of the caudal lumbar, sacral, and caudal segments is most apparent in the large dog breeds in which the three sacral segments are located in the fourth lumbar vertebra. In all dogs and cats, the only nervous system tissue in the vertebral foramen of L7 is the collection of spinal nerves passing caudally to their respective intervertebral foramina to leave the vertebral canal (Fig. 5-5).

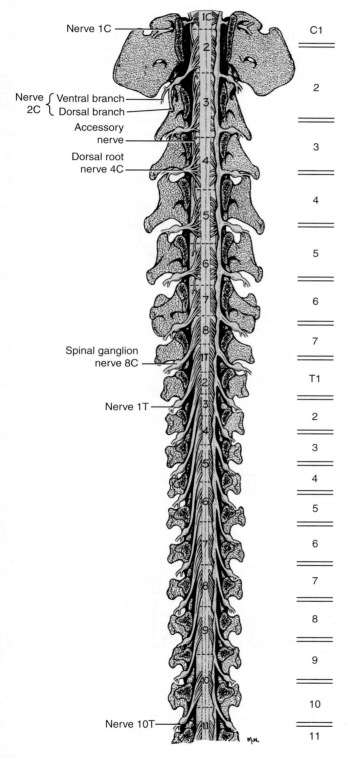

FIGURE 5-4 Spinal cord segmental relationship to vertebral bodies. From C1 to T11 the spinal cord, roots, ganglia, and nerves have been exposed by removal of the vertebral arches. The dura mater has been removed except on the right side. The numbers on the right represent the levels of the vertebral bodies. *(From Evans HE: Anatomy of the dog, ed 3, Philadelphia, 1993, Saunders. Drawn by M. Newsom)*

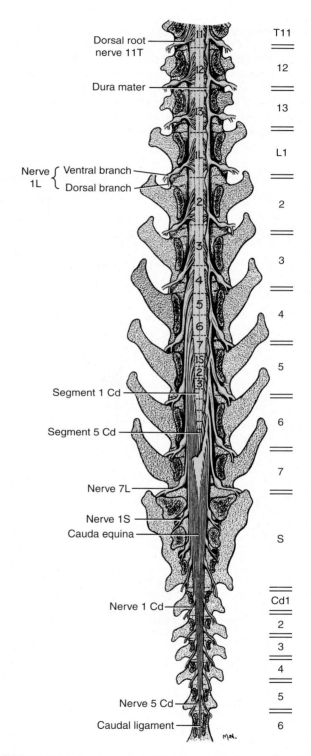

FIGURE 5-5 Spinal cord segmental relationship to vertebral bodies. From T11 through the caudal segments, the spinal cord, roots, ganglia, and nerves have been exposed by removal of the vertebral arches. The dura mater has been removed except on the right side. The numbers on the right represent the levels of the vertebral bodies. *(From Evans HE: Anatomy of the dog, ed 3, Philadelphia, 1993, Saunders. Drawn by M. Newson)*

FUNCTION

The GSE portion of the LMN provides the final motor innervation of the muscles whose contractions are necessary to maintain posture, support weight, and provide the gait. They are also the motor component of the spinal reflexes that are tested in the neurologic examination. Knowledge of the anatomy of these reflexes is critical to localizing lesions to portions of the PNS or the spinal cord.

The sensory components of these reflexes are neurons of the general somatic afferent (GSA) and general proprioceptive (GP) systems. These systems are described in Chapter 9. These sensory neurons consist of a dendritic zone (receptor) in the skin or neuromuscular spindle and an axon that courses through a specific peripheral nerve, spinal nerve, and dorsal root and enters the spinal cord dorsal gray column of the corresponding spinal cord segment. Here it usually terminates in a telodendron on a dendritic zone of a second neuron, whose cell body is located in the dorsal gray column (Fig. 5-6). The cell body of the GSA or GP neuron initially stimulated is located in the spinal ganglion at the lateral aspect of the dorsal root.

The patellar reflex (see Fig. 5-6) is a tendon reflex that is composed of only two neurons. The sensory neuron terminates directly on the GSE neuron in the ventral gray column without involving a synapse on a second neuron in the gray column. The peripheral sensory neuron of the flexor, or withdrawal spinal reflex, has its telodendron on

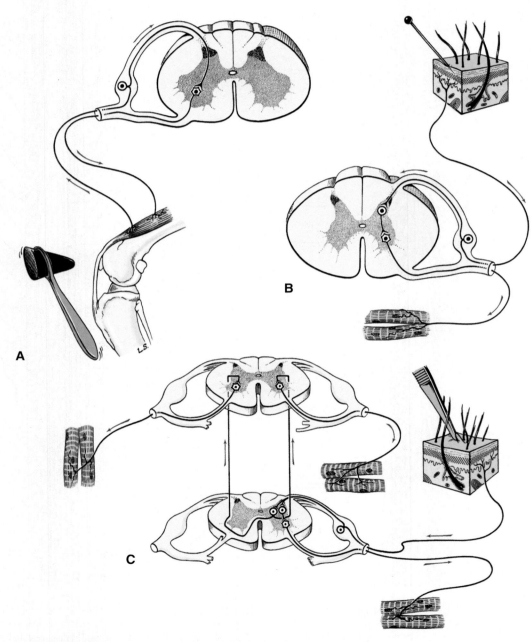

FIGURE 5-6 Spinal nerve reflexes. **A,** Monosynaptic myotatic-patellar reflex. **B,** Polysynaptic flexor reflex to a noxious stimulus. **C,** Polysynaptic reflex with intersegmental transmission of impulses.

an interneuron in the gray matter that in turn terminates on a GSE neuron in the ventral gray column.

For these spinal reflexes to function, they need only the peripheral nerve components and their associated spinal cord segments. They will still function when these segments have been cut off and isolated from the rest of the CNS. For example, if you examined a dog 2 days after it had been hit by a car, which fractured the thirteenth thoracic vertebra and transected the thirteenth spinal cord segment, the spinal reflexes in the pelvic limbs and perineal region would still function because there was no direct disturbance to the spinal cord segments and peripheral nerves involved with these reflexes. In order to interpret these spinal reflexes properly it is vital to understand their anatomic components (Table 5-1). This is critical to making an accurate anatomic diagnosis of peripheral nerve and spinal cord disorders.

■ PELVIC LIMB AND PERINEAL REFLEXES

The lumbosacral plexus innervates the muscles that are involved with pelvic limb movement and the cutaneous region of the pelvic limb. The sacral plexus innervates the muscles and skin of the perineal region. The lumbosacral plexus is widespread, with most of it located in the hypaxial muscles associated with the lumbar and sacral vertebrae. In most animals it includes ventral branches of all the lumbar and sacral nerves. Most of the named peripheral nerves are formed in the hypaxial muscles or close to them. The pelvic limb spinal reflexes test the femoral nerve and the sciatic nerve with its peroneal and tibial nerve branches.

The patellar tendon reflex is the only reliable tendon reflex and the only one that I (Alexander de Lahunta) test in my examinations. Both the sensory and motor components are in the femoral nerve. The femoral nerve is formed from the spinal nerves of the L4, L5, and L6 spinal cord segments (Fig. 5-7). The L5 segment makes the largest contribution to this nerve.[141] The L6 segment may not contribute to this nerve in some dogs. The patient should be held in lateral recumbency and must be relaxed. This reflex cannot be tested in a struggling patient. Lightly strike the patellar tendon with a blunt instrument. A pediatric patellar hammer or pleximeter is the most satisfactory instrument for veterinarians, but the handle of a pair of scissors will work as

well. In my experience (Eric Glass) the pediatric pleximeter is especially useful in cats and small dogs, but a larger pleximeter or heavy bandage scissors may be more reliable in large dogs such as German shepherds. This will elicit a brief extension of the stifle if all components of the femoral nerve are functioning. We usually grade the response as normal (+2), depressed (+1), or brisk (+3). The response is called clonus if, with one stimulation, repetitive stifle extensions occur. The paw will appear to tremor. There are degrees of clonus but we do not find them to be of much help in prognosis. Occasionally, this patellar reflex will not be present in the nonrecumbent limb but will be present when the dog is rolled over and you test the reflex when that limb is on the recumbent side. We do not know the reason for this but have learned never to record that the reflex is absent until it has been tested in both positions. Be aware that this reflex may be depressed or even absent in some old dogs that have no other recognizable neurologic abnormality.[87]

The flexor or withdrawal reflex in the pelvic limb is a test primarily for the sciatic nerve and its spinal cord segments L6, L7, and S1. Within the sciatic nerve, the neurons that will be associated with the peroneal nerve tend to be components of the L6 and L7 spinal cord segments, and those associated with the tibial nerve are components of the L7 and S1 segments. The S2 components innervate primarily muscles in the pelvis that do not participate in this test or in the animal's posture or gait. The sensory component of the reflex depends on the area of skin that is stimulated. In a routine exam, the skin at the base of the claw of the fifth digit is compressed using a pair of forceps. Finger pressure can be used but is not always sufficient, in our experience. This area of skin is innervated by cutaneous branches of the peroneal nerve dorsally and by the tibial nerve on the plantar surface. The motor response is a flexion of all the joints in the limb to withdraw the limb from the stimulus. Except for the hip, flexion of the pelvic limb is a function of the GSE components of the sciatic nerve. The major flexor muscle of the hip is the iliopsoas, which is innervated by all the lumbar spinal nerve ventral branches, with a contribution caudally from the femoral nerve. The latter also innervates the rectus femoris, which is the one component of the quadriceps muscle that flexes the hip. Because of this anatomy, a patient with complete sciatic nerve dysfunction will have no reflex if the fifth digit is stimulated, but if the first digit is

TABLE 5-1 Topographic Anatomy of Spinal Nerve Reflex Testing in Dogs

Limb	Reflex	Peripheral Nerve	Spinal Cord Segments	Level in Vertebral Canal
Thoracic	Flexor	All thoracic limb peripheral nerves	C6-T2	C5-T1
	Biceps*	Musculcutaneous	C6-C8	C5-C7
	Triceps*	Radial	C7-T2	C6-T1
	Extensor carpi radialis*	Radial	C7-T2	C6-T1
Pelvic	Flexor	Sciatic	L6-S1	L4-L5
	Patellar	Femoral	L4-L6	L3-L4
	Cranial crural*	Peroneal	L6-L7	L4
	Gastrocnemius*	Tibial	L7-S1	L4-L5

*Not always present in normal dogs.

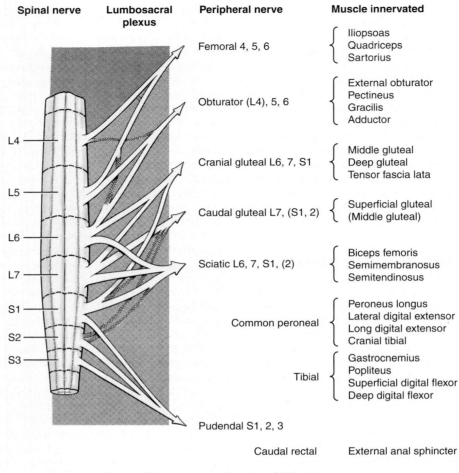

Spinal nerve	Lumbosacral plexus	Peripheral nerve	Muscle innervated

Femoral 4, 5, 6
- Iliopsoas
- Quadriceps
- Sartorius

Obturator (L4), 5, 6
- External obturator
- Pectineus
- Gracilis
- Adductor

Cranial gluteal L6, 7, S1
- Middle gluteal
- Deep gluteal
- Tensor fascia lata

Caudal gluteal L7, (S1, 2)
- Superficial gluteal
- (Middle gluteal)

Sciatic L6, 7, S1, (2)
- Biceps femoris
- Semimembranosus
- Semitendinosus

Common peroneal
- Peroneus longus
- Lateral digital extensor
- Long digital extensor
- Cranial tibial

Tibial
- Gastrocnemius
- Popliteus
- Superficial digital flexor
- Deep digital flexor

Pudendal S1, 2, 3

Caudal rectal   External anal sphincter

Flexor reflex: sensory and motor: sciatic nerve
Patellar reflex: sensory and motor: femoral nerve
Perineal reflex: sensory and motor: pudendal

FIGURE 5-7 Segmental innervation from lumbosacral intumescence of pelvic limb muscles in the dog. The shaded nerve roots represent contributions in some but not all dogs.

stimulated, the hip will flex to pull the limb away from the stimulus but the rest of the joints will not flex. The first digit usually receives its cutaneous innervation from the saphenous nerve branch of the femoral nerve. Be sure to look for this disparity. The same strong hip flexion in the absence of any flexion in the other joints will occur with severe but not complete sciatic nerve dysfunction when the fifth digit is stimulated. As a rule, there is more clinical evidence of loss of the motor function with some preservation of the sensory function in a partially compromised peripheral nerve.

The flexor reflex is not only a test of the reflex arc that utilizes the sciatic nerve; it is also a test for nociception, which requires the sensory portion of the peripheral nerves involved with the reflex plus a pathway through the spinal cord and brainstem to the neocortex. This is described with the GSA system in Chapter 9. Because of this nociceptive pathway, you must be gentle with the degree of compression of the digit that you use or you may rightfully be abused by your patient.

Other muscle and tendon reflexes that are used by some neurologists (EG) include the gastrocnemius reflex in which, with the tarsus slightly flexed, the common calcanean tendon is lightly tapped with a pleximeter or blunt instrument. In the normal animal this will elicit a slight extension of the tarsus. This is a test for the tibial nerve branch of the sciatic

nerve. When you perform this tendon reflex, you may also observe a brief twitch of the caudal thigh muscles, which suggests that this monosynaptic reflex has spread in the spinal cord to involve other branches of the sciatic nerve. The cranial crural muscle reflex is elicited by lightly tapping on these muscles, with the tarsus held in slight extension, and observing a slight flexion of the tarsus. This is a test of the peroneal nerve branch of the sciatic nerve. My (AD) concern is that I am not convinced that these muscle tendon reflexes can be elicited in all normal animals, so I rely on the features of the animal's posture and gait to differentiate between a tibial and peroneal nerve disorder. In general, these reflexes are more significant when they are present than when absent.

The perineal reflex is a test of the branches from the sacral plexus that is located in the pelvic canal. These branches supply the external sphincter muscle of the anus; the striated muscles of the penis, vulva, and vestibule; the urethralis muscle; and the skin of the anus, perineum, and caudal thigh. It is not necessary to learn the names of the specific nerve branches or their individual areas of innervation. Mild compression of the skin of the perineum or anus with forceps will elicit an immediate contraction of the anal sphincter and flexion of the tail. The latter response requires that the caudal spinal cord segments and nerves be intact.

THORACIC LIMB REFLEXES

As a rule, we rely only on the flexor-withdrawal reflex in the thoracic limb. In reality, it is a crude test of many anatomic components. The peripheral sensory component depends on the area of skin that is stimulated by compression. These areas are more accurately defined in Chapter 9, the GSA system. Compression of the lateral digit stimulates primarily the cutaneous endings of branches from the ulnar nerve dorsally and from the ulnar and median nerves on the palmar surface. The muscles that contract to flex the joints and withdraw the limb are innervated by the GSE-LMN systems present in many nerves: for shoulder flexion, it is the axillary, radial, and thoracodorsal nerves; for elbow flexion, it is the musculocutaneous nerve; for carpal and digital flexion, it is the median and ulnar nerves.

These nerves have their central components in the cervical intumescence, which includes the spinal cord segments (C5), C6, C7, C8, T1, and T2. The ventral branches of the spinal nerves from these segments intertwine medial to the shoulder to form the brachial plexus from which the specific named peripheral nerves emerge (Fig. 5-8). For example, the radial nerve contains primarily branches from spinal nerves and segments C7, C8, and T1. All of these components must be intact for the withdrawal reflex to be normal. Remember that, as in the pelvic limb, the stimulus used is a noxious stimulus that tests the nociceptive pathway as well as the flexor reflex. Always start with a gentle compression.

There are three tendon-muscle reflexes that are used by some neurologists, but the reliability of these reflexes may be questioned. For the biceps reflex, hold the elbow in partial extension with your first finger on the distal bellies of the biceps brachii and brachialis muscles. Lightly tap your finger with your patellar hammer or some other blunt instrument and observe a slight flexion of the elbow or feel the muscles contract beneath your finger. This is a test for the musculocutaneous nerve and the C6 and C7 spinal cord segments. For the triceps reflex, hold the elbow relaxed in slight flexion and lightly tap the triceps tendon just proximal to the olecranon tuber and observe for a slight elbow extension. This tests for the radial nerve and spinal cord segments C7, C8, and T1. For the extensor carpi radialis reflex, hold the thoracic limb so that the carpus is relaxed. Lightly tap the proximal belly of this muscle and observe for carpal extension. This tests the extension of the radial nerve into

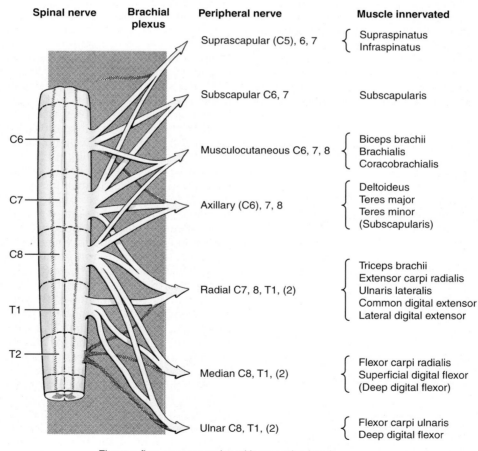

FIGURE 5-8 Segmental innervation from cervical intumescence of thoracic limb muscles in the dog. The shaded nerve roots represent contributions in some but not all dogs.

the antebrachium by its deep branch. The presence of these tendon-muscle reflexes indicates that the nervous system components involved are able to function. Their absence may be of no consequence because these reflexes are not always present in all normal animals.

The cutaneous trunci reflex involves a larger portion of the spinal cord (Fig. 5-9). It is useful for locating C8 and T1 spinal cord lesions and their contributions to the lateral thoracic nerve, and it is also useful for locating the level of a transverse thoracolumbar spinal cord lesion. The sensory stimulus is a mild compression of the skin of the trunk using forceps, and the motor response is a brief contraction of the cutaneous trunci muscle, which causes the skin of the trunk to twitch. This reflex is usually performed using progressive stimuli starting in the caudal lumbar region and progressing cranially along the dorsal midline of the trunk. The cutaneous nerves that are stimulated are from the dorsal branches of the lumbar and thoracic spinal nerves (see Fig. 5-9). The sensory impulse courses through the dorsal roots and enters the dorsal gray column of each respective spinal cord segment. Here the axons of the GSA neurons synapse on long interneurons whose axons enter the fasciculus proprius on both sides of the spinal cord but predominantly the contralateral side. The fasciculus proprius is the white matter of the lateral funiculus that is adjacent to the gray matter. These axons course cranially to the T1 and C8 spinal cord segments where they terminate in the ventral gray column by synapsing on GSE neurons whose axons emerge from the brachial plexus as a component of the lateral thoracic nerve that innervates the cutaneous trunci muscle. Any disorder that interrupts this pathway will interfere with this reflex. On rare occasions this reflex cannot be elicited in a normal dog. Sometimes it takes rigorous stimulation to elicit it. Normal dogs vary in how far caudally in the lumbar region the reflex can be stimulated. Most will show the reflex by the middle of the lumbar region. Its use in locating the level of a transverse spinal cord lesion is described with spinal cord disorders.

LOWER MOTOR NEURON DISEASE: NEUROMUSCULAR DISEASE

Clinical Signs

The terms *LMN disease* and *neuromuscular disease (NMD)* are used interchangeably. The latter term includes the muscle as well as the LMN because the clinical signs are very similar. Disorders of any part of the GSE-LMN system will cause muscle paresis or paralysis, along with hyporeflexia or areflexia, hypotonia or atonia, and neurogenic atrophy. Normal muscle tone is dependent on a closely regulated, constant stimulation of the LMN that innervates the striated muscles. The LMN forms the motor component of the spinal reflexes.

The dictionary definition of *paresis* is weakness. The student tends to interpret this to mean loss of muscle strength with loss of tone and difficulty supporting weight, which characterizes the paresis caused by LMN disease. However, in medicine there are two qualities of paresis. When severe, both forms can result in complete paralysis and inability to move, but the quality of the paralysis is very different in the two forms. These two forms are LMN and upper motor neuron (UMN) paresis or paralysis. The word *paralysis* should be used only when there is complete absence of any voluntary movement. LMN paresis is described in this chapter. UMN paresis is described with the anatomy of that system in Chapter 8. The two forms are compared in that chapter.

Neurologists define paresis as a deficiency in the generation of the gait or in the ability to support weight. The lack of ability to support weight characterizes LMN paresis. If the patient is ambulatory, the gait will be short-strided and will appear as a lameness. The gait in LMN disease is identical to that of an animal that has discomfort when the diseased limb attempts to support weight. The inability to support weight looks the same as when an animal expresses pain whenever weight is supported. This animal walks as you would with a stone in your shoe. The stride is shortened. It is important to rule out any orthopedic disorder in your evaluation of an animal with LMN disease by doing a complete orthopedic examination. When you see a shortened stride in the gait, always ask yourself if it is because the patient is unable to support its weight or is unwilling to support its weight. If multiple limbs are affected with LMN disease, the animal will tend to collapse and have difficulty standing up from a recumbent position. When both pelvic limbs are affected, the animal may walk by simultaneously flexing both hips to advance the limbs. This is referred to as bunny-hopping. Be aware that animals that have pelvic or pelvic limb noxious stimuli may also bunny-hop as an expression of pain. When standing, the affected limbs may exhibit a tremor in the muscles, and the affected animal may continually shift its weight from one limb to another and look for an opportunity to lie down. This is especially evident in horses with diffuse LMN disease. An animal with diffuse LMN disease that is still ambulatory may stumble on uneven surfaces. This state is often confused with ataxia, which implies a sensory system abnormality—a general

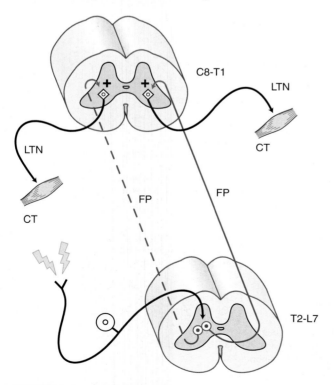

FIGURE 5-9 Cutaneous trunci reflex. *CT,* Cutaneous trunci; *FP,* fasciculus proprius; *LTN,* lateral thoracic nerve.

proprioceptive, vestibular, or cerebellar disorder. LMN disease does not cause ataxia, only paresis!

An animal with only a LMN disorder knows exactly where its paws or hooves are located because the sensory systems that convey cutaneous and proprioceptive information to the CNS are unaffected. The major problem is support and degree of limb advancement, which result in the short stride. When evaluating an abnormal gait, also ask yourself the following question: does this animal know where its limbs are located? The patient with LMN disease knows their locations and therefore moves the paw or hoof very rapidly when it attempts to move the limb. When the GP system is affected, this knowledge is lost and there is a delay in the limb movement. Loss of UMN function also causes a delay in the initiation of limb movement.

Postural reactions are complex, and they require that multiple components of the central and PNS, including the LMN, be intact. Many postural reactions are described, but the most useful is the animal's ability to hop on each limb. To evaluate these reactions correctly you need to practice eliciting them. If you are falling all over the patient as you elicit them, you will not know who is ataxic—you or the patient!

Your patient must be reasonably cooperative. So what do we do about a fractious dog or cat that fights any restraint? The answer is simply that we do not try to perform them and rely instead on whatever manipulations the patient will allow. First, make friends with your patient. Use the animal's name. Tell the patient what you are going to do. This may sound foolish, but you have to gain the trust of the animal. It is much better to do this examination without the presence of the owner, who tends to distract the attention of the patient. Also, many owners do not understand what you are doing and are liable to get upset. You also should perform this examination on a surface that provides some grip for the patient. A carpet is the best surface (AD). This is critical for the interpretation of mild abnormalities. Buy one that can be hosed off because we can guarantee that your patient will excrete on it.

To test the hopping responses, stand over the patient facing in the same direction as the patient and keep scratching those ears! Place one of your forearms beneath the patient's abdomen and lift the pelvic limbs just free of the ground surface. If you rest your elbow on your thigh, you can avoid stress to your back. With your other forearm, pick up the patient's thoracic limb on that side and move the patient in the direction of the supporting limb. As you look down that limb and slowly move the patient toward it, as soon as the paw disappears beneath the shoulder, the animal should hop. Get three or four hops and then shift your hands, pick up the limb that just hopped, and move the patient toward the supporting limb until you get three or four hops on that limb. Keep repeating this until you are comfortable that these are normal hopping responses or that there is an abnormality. Always evaluate the limb as you make it hop laterally. You should not have to move at all during this test.

For the pelvic limbs, stand beside your patient. Place your forelimb that is nearest the patient's head beneath its neck and between its thoracic limbs. Lift the patient's thorax and thoracic limbs off the ground. With your other forelimb, pick up the patient's pelvic limb that is on your side and push the patient away from you so that it has to hop on the opposite pelvic limb. Change sides and repeat this in the opposite limb. The pelvic limbs normally do not hop as fast as the thoracic limbs. In very large dogs that are too heavy to lift, these hopping actions can be performed by hemiwalking your patient. Stand beside the patient, pick up both of its limbs on one side, slowly push the dog away from you, and watch the hopping responses in the limbs on the opposite side. Remember to compare one thoracic limb with the other and then one pelvic limb with the other.

In patients that have LMN disease and are still able to stand and walk, the hopping responses will be as fast as normal if you help them support their weight. With all their weight supported on one limb without your assistance, the patient will collapse or have difficulty trying to hop without collapsing. The attempts are brisk because their proprioception is unaffected.

For the paw/hoof replacement reaction, stand over or beside the patient, turn the paw/hoof over, and place it on the ground surface. Usually the normal patient will immediately replace the paw/hoof onto its palmar or plantar surface. As long as the patient with LMN disease has enough strength to move its joints, this response will be normal. The patient with severe paralysis that is unable to move its limbs will obviously be unable to replace its paws from this abnormal position. Like other postural reactions, this paw/hoof replacement reaction requires that multiple CNS and PNS pathways be intact: the GP, GSA, UMN, and LMN systems. It is inappropriate to refer to this paw/hoof replacement test as a test for conscious proprioception (CP) because of the involvement of the other neuroanatomic systems in the response. This anatomically incorrect and misleading term is deeply embedded in the vocabulary of the veterinarian but should be expunged!

Severe diffuse LMN disease produces the same degree of paralysis as a severe focal midcervical spinal cord lesion. Recumbent immobile patients appear to be the same as each other. The first clue that they are very different will be when you attempt to pick the patient off the ground surface. The patient with diffuse LMN disease will be atonic and just hang limply over your forearms. When you lift the patient up and down, the limbs will flop uselessly like wet dish rags. This is a flaccid (originally pronounced flack-sid) paralysis. When all four limbs are affected, it is referred to as a tetraplegia or quadriplegia. Thus a patient with severe diffuse LMN disease has flaccid tetraplegia. A patient with a severe focal cervical spinal cord lesion will be paralyzed in recumbency because of the loss of function in its UMN pathways, resulting in the inability to generate any LMN function and releasing the reflex arcs from inhibition. The latter results in hypertonia that is referred to as spasticity. This will be obvious when you attempt to pick up the recumbent animal. All the muscles will feel taut, giving the trunk and limbs a remarkably stiff feeling. This will be especially obvious as you lift the patient up and down or try to flex any of the limbs. This is spastic paralysis of all four limbs, or spastic tetraplegia. Video 10-24 shows two dogs (described in Chapter 10) that make it easy to appreciate the comparison.

The patient with the severe diffuse LMN disease described earlier will have no tone in the limbs when they are manipulated—atonia—and no patellar tendon or flexor reflexes—areflexia. The latter reflex requires a noxious stimulus, and many diffuse LMN diseases do not affect the GSA pathways; therefore, nociception may be intact. The only evidence of nociception will be jaw and facial movements and an increase in the rate of respirations because any voice sounds may be absent or muffled. Animals that are recumbent because of LMN disease but still have some voluntary movements may exhibit hypotonia and depressed spinal reflexes. In the diffuse LMN disease known as myasthenia gravis, the recumbent animal may still have normal tone and normal spinal reflexes. The patient that has diffuse LMN disease and is still able to ambulate may have reduced muscle tone and reflexes or they may be normal. Remember to examine the muscle tone and reflexes in the anus, perineum, and tail because they will be affected with sacrocaudal LMN disorders.

Denervation of muscles occurs when the LMN of that muscle is unable to function. The loss of axonal impulses results in a rapid degeneration of the denervated muscle that is referred to as denervation or neurogenic atrophy. It is rapid and severe. It can be first observed in a muscle group about 7 days after the denervation. The health of the muscle cell is dependent on its constant innervation. Without that innervation, the muscle cell rapidly loses protein and after many weeks the cell will die and be replaced by fat and fibrous tissue. The rate and degree of denervation atrophy varies with the species and the specific muscle that is denervated. Denervated muscles can be severely atrophic for weeks and still return to normal size when reinnervated. This is especially evident in dogs with severe acute polyradiculoneuritis (coonhound paralysis), an immune-mediated disease that affects primarily the LMN. Disuse atrophy is usually much slower to develop and less severe than denervation atrophy. This occurs in limbs that are immobile when placed in a cast or in a limb with a chronic joint disorder that causes discomfort when the limb is used and therefore results in a decrease in the use of the limb. An example of this occurs in rapidly growing, very active retrievers that develop a painful osteochondrosis lesion in the shoulder, resulting in significant disuse atrophy of the lateral scapular muscles. These muscles are especially prone to disuse atrophy that is severe enough to mimic a suprascapular nerve disorder.

Remember that when you make the anatomic diagnosis of an LMN disorder, whether it is a focal or a diffuse abnormality, you must consider all components of that LMN for the lesion site because the same LMN signs will occur whether the lesion is in the spinal cord and is affecting the neuronal cell bodies of that LMN or the lesion is in the axons in the ventral roots, spinal nerves, ventral branches of the spinal nerves, the plexus these form, or the named specific peripheral nerve that terminates at the affected muscle. And do not forget that the lesion may be in the muscle itself.

As a general rule, the dysfunction caused by the loss of function of a peripheral nerve exceeds that caused by the loss of function of an entire ventral root or spinal nerve. This is because the peripheral nerve supplies the entire innervation to the muscle it innervates, whereas a single ventral root or spinal nerve contributes the axons of a few neurons to many peripheral nerves and their muscles but not to the entire innervation of a muscle. For example, the C7 spinal nerve contributes LMNs to the suprascapular, subscapular, musculocutaneous, axillary, and radial nerves but it is not the only source of LMNs to any of these nerves. Therefore, a radial nerve lesion causes a much more severe clinical deficit than a C7 spinal nerve lesion.

Wallerian Degeneration

Wallerian degeneration is an important concept that is useful in mapping the anatomic components of peripheral nerves and spinal cord segments, in recognizing peripheral or central nervous system disorders microscopically, and in understanding and predicting reinnervation by peripheral nerves. When a peripheral nerve axon is destroyed at some point in its course away from the cell body, it will completely degenerate from the point of destruction to the structure innervated. This is because the axon requires the axoplasmic flow of cytoplasmic materials from the cell body for its survival.

Dr. Augustus Waller (1816-1870) described this degeneration of peripheral nerves; hence its designation as wallerian degeneration. The same process occurs in neurons within the CNS, where it is useful for the recognition and location of lesions.

Wallerian degeneration is a trophic degeneration that occurs in the neuron at the site of the lesion and travels in a distal direction from the cell body as follows (Fig. 5-10). The axon degenerates through a process of swelling and subsequent granulation that takes about 3 to 4 days. The myelin degenerates simultaneously with the axons. There is a close interaction between the axon and its myelin, and myelin cannot survive if the axon degenerates. In this process of wallerian degeneration, there is a secondary demyelination that includes the formation of swellings along the internodes, called ellipsoids, and the fragmentation of myelin into droplets. *Digestion chamber* is a term used for a myelin ellipsoid containing axonal granules. The telodendron and motor end-plate disintegrate. The Schwann cells that are now reduced to their nuclei and cytoplasmic organelles rapidly proliferate to form a column of cells known as a Büngner band. The adjacent endoneurial cells also proliferate. These columns of Schwann cells provide pathways for regenerating axons to follow to the target that was denervated. They also provide growth factors that induce the outgrowth of axonal buds from the proximal portion of the neuron where the axon is still intact. This regeneration begins in about 7 days. Each axon puts out a number of processes called axonal buds that grow into the existing cords of proliferating Schwann cells. The rate of growth is about 1 to 4 mm per day. This process is dependent on close proximity of the axonal buds and the Büngner bands. With this knowledge, you can estimate for the owner of a patient that has a peripheral nerve injury how long it will take for some evidence of regeneration to occur by measuring the distance from the site of the lesion to the middle of the denervated muscles. Using the slowest rate (1 mm/day), the distance in millimeters is the same as the number of days.

When a nerve has been completely severed, it is important to suture the cut ends to provide the least impediment to this effort to regenerate. If an impediment such as hemorrhage or fibrosis prevents the axonal buds from reaching the nearest bands of Schwann cells, the axonal buds will continue to grow in a haphazard manner and form an observable swelling known as a neuroma. These neuromas can be a source of considerable discomfort. They are often a sequel to the neurectomies that are performed in the distal extremities of the horse to eliminate a source of discomfort such as a degeneration of the distal sesamoid bone, referred to as navicular disease. The resultant neuroma may then be an additional source of irritation to the patient.

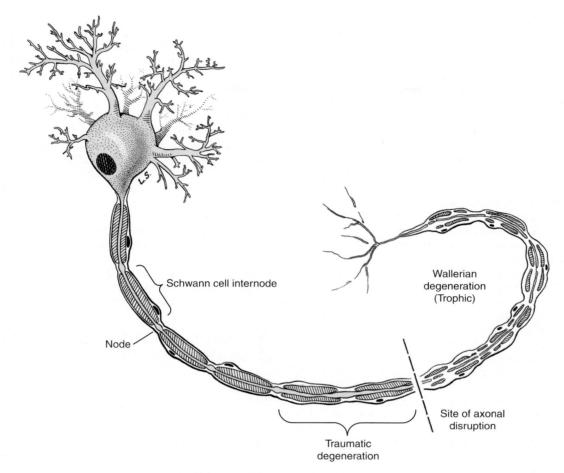

FIGURE 5-10 Wallerian degeneration of a LMN.

Along with the changes that occur in the neuron distal to the lesion, other changes occur proximal to the lesion. If the lesion is an injury, the trauma will produce degeneration of a few internodes proximal to the lesion in a manner similar to the trophic degeneration that occurs distal to the lesion. A reaction occurs in the cell body in the spinal cord, called the axonal reaction, in which there is a slight swelling of the cell body, a displacement of the nucleus to one side of the cytoplasm (an eccentric nucleus), and a disbursement of the granular endoplasmic reticulum of the Nissl substance within the cytoplasm. The last event is referred to as central chromatolysis and represents the efforts of the cell body to produce more products for the axoplasmic flow necessary for the regeneration to progress. This central chromatolysis has been used in the anatomic mapping of the components of the ventral gray columns in the spinal cord and the LMN nuclei in the brainstem.

Electrodiagnostic Techniques in Neuromuscular Disease

The most common electrodiagnostic techniques[9,13,64,77] used in veterinary medicine are electromyography (EMG) and the determination of conduction times. EMG is the study of the electric activity of muscle by inserting a recording electrode into the muscle and observing the electric activity with the aid of an amplifier on an oscilloscope. An audible signal accompanies this recording. It is used clinically to determine whether the LMN, its myelin, or the muscle fibers themselves is the site of the lesion. Like any ancillary procedure, it is used to confirm and more precisely locate a clinical observation of a neuromuscular disorder, and it may contribute to the prognosis.

Normal resting muscle shows no or very limited electric activity on EMG once the electrode placement has been stabilized and there is no audible signal. This is the resting potential of the muscle being studied. In LMN disease muscle cells become denervated. About 5 days after denervation in the patient, continuous spontaneous potentials called fibrillations develop; they have amplitudes of less than 200 μV. They are biphasic, last 1 to 2 ms (fewer than 7 ms), and produce a sound like eggs frying. They may occur as often as 2 to 30 times per second. They represent the spontaneous action potential or contraction of an individual denervated muscle cell that can not be seen through the skin surface of the patient. Denervation disturbs the metabolism of the muscle cell and makes it sensitive to circulating acetylcholine, which makes it contract spontaneously. The prevalence of fibrillations in denervated muscle may decrease after 3 weeks. Positive sharp waves (potentials) may also accompany the fibrillations recorded in denervated muscle. They are characterized by an initial low-voltage, sharp positive deflection and a slow return to the baseline. Voltage is variable, ranging from 50 to 1000 μV. The sharp waves usually last several times longer than the fibrillations and they have a dull sound. Spontaneous contraction of an entire motor unit, called a muscle fasciculation, may be visible on the surface of the patient. It varies from 300 to 2000 µV in amplitude and lasts 4 to 10 ms. Fasciculations occur in LMN disease and occasionally are seen in normal muscle. As a general rule, the fibrillations and positive sharp waves that occur with denervation imply a dysfunction of the axon, whereas a severe myelin disorder is more likely to be reflected in impairment in the rate of impulse transmission, and motor nerve conduction will be slowed.

Motor nerve conduction can be determined using much the same equipment that was used for the EMG study. In this study a motor nerve will be stimulated and the evoked muscle potential will be observed on the oscilloscope. In the thoracic limb, this is usually performed using the ulnar nerve, which can be stimulated at the elbow and in the carpal canal while recording the evoked response from the interosseous muscles. By measuring the distance between the two stimulating electrodes, the conduction time can be measured in meters per second. In the pelvic limb, the tibial nerve is stimulated at the stifle and proximal to the tarsus, and the responses are recorded from the interosseous muscles. Other motor nerves and the muscles they innervate can be used. Normal conduction times are dependent on age and temperature; they vary from 50 to 60 meters per second. Nerves that have been injured and avulsed and have undergone wallerian degeneration for 4 to 5 days will not conduct impulses. Decreased conduction velocities usually occur in nerves after severe loss of their myelin sheaths. The evoked potential resulting from motor nerve stimulation is the summated motor unit potential recorded on the oscilloscope. Normally it is a smooth bi- or triphasic wave that lasts 5 to 10 ms and varies in amplitude but is often greater than 3000 µV. In LMN disease, the evoked potential may be polyphasic and prolonged if some nerve fibers are conducting slowly. Loss of some motor units prevents the smooth summation of response. In myositis, if the inflammation involves the neuromuscular junctions, denervation potentials may occur in an EMG study. Polyphasic potentials of decreased amplitude may be observed in motor nerve conduction studies in patients with myositis. These electrodiagnostic studies are useful for confirming a neuromuscular anatomic diagnosis but may be less useful for distinguishing between an LMN and a muscle cell disorder.

Another use of an EMG study is to elicit a form of myotonia that implicates a disorder of the muscle cell membrane. Myotonia is defined as the continuous contraction of muscle cells that persists after the stimulation or voluntary effort has stopped. In the EMG study, it is stimulated by the needle insertion and appears as a repetitive high-frequency discharge that initially increases in amplitude and frequency and then decreases over 4 to 5 seconds. This produces an audible and distinct sound that waxes and wanes and is described as the sound of a dive bomber or a dirt bike. This is referred to as true myotonia. Another form, called pseudomyotonia or complex repetitive discharges, has an abrupt onset when the muscle first contracts; after a few seconds, it abruptly stops. Both forms result from a hyperexcitable muscle cell membrane. Although myotonic bursts can occur in many muscle cell disorders, the most common diffuse myotonias are inherited and are seen in young animals or accompany hyperadrenocorticoidism in older dogs. Myotonia is described further in Chapter 8 and is illustrated by videos.

Sensory nerve conduction velocity may also be recorded by stimulating a sensory nerve distally and recording the response at some proximal point in the same nerve. As a rule, the superficial branches of the radial nerve in the antebrachium are used in the thoracic limb and the superficial peroneal nerve is used in the pelvic limb. For more details on these studies, other textbooks should be consulted.

NEUROMUSCULAR DISEASE: DISEASES OF THE GSE-LMN

NMD is defined as a disorder of the entire GSE-LMN and the muscle cells that it innervates. These diseases include those that affect any part of the entire motor unit: the cell bodies in the CNS; the axons and their myelin sheaths in the spinal and cranial nerve roots; the spinal and cranial nerves and their entire peripheral distribution; the neuromuscular junctions; the striated skeletal muscle; and the striated visceral muscles of the larynx, pharynx, and esophagus that are innervated by GSE-LMNs.

In the first two editions of this text, these neuromuscular diseases were organized anatomically, starting with the neuromuscular junction and progressing proximally to the neuronal cell bodies in the CNS, with consideration of focal and diffuse disorders at each anatomic level. We believe it is more useful to the student and practitioner to describe these disorders as they would be considered in a differential diagnosis for a patient, in which a specific anatomic diagnosis has been made involving its LMN. In this text, only the most salient features of these disorders are described, and rare considerations are excluded. More detailed information can be found in other veterinary neurology texts.

CASE EXAMPLE 5-1

NMD Tetraplegia—Dog

Signalment: 3-year-old spayed female red bone coonhound, Kulman

Chief Complaint: Recumbent, with no voluntary movement

 Examination: Video 5-1 shows the total flaccid paralysis of the entire neck, trunk, limbs, and tail that spares anal tone and the cranial nerves, except for a slight facial paresis. Despite the diffuse atonia and areflexia, nociception was intact. The only evidence of this was the movement of the jaw and eyes. No voice was audible due to the lack of expiratory effort.

Anatomic Diagnosis: Diffuse neuromuscular

Differential Diagnosis: Acute polyradiculoneuritis, botulism, acute fulminating myasthenia gravis, tick paralysis, polymyositis, snake envenomation, organophosphate toxicity

POLYRADICULONEURITIS

Acute polyradiculoneuritis (PRN) is an immune-mediated disorder of myelin or axons or both that usually presents as an acute or peracute onset of diffuse LMN paresis that usually progresses rapidly to tetraplegia.*

*References 23, 26, 34, 69, 70, 98.

There is often a history of possible exposure to a raccoon bite, but that is not a requirement for this diagnosis. Paresis often begins in the pelvic limbs, but not always. Owners often recognize a voice change because there is considerable loss of its usual volume. Tetraplegic dogs may have no audible voice. Cranial nerves are spared except for a few dogs that have a mild facial paresis. Megaesophagus is not seen in this disease. Chronic forms exist, some of which may wax and wane in the severity of the clinical signs, but tetraplegia does not usually occur. There is no evidence of any sensory loss because the major site of the lesion is in the ventral roots, which is the basis for the term *radix* in the name of the inflammation (Figs. 5-11 and 5-12). However, some dogs may appear to be hyperesthetic for which there are hypotheses but no reliable explanation. Muscle atrophy is observed by 7 to 10 days and rapidly becomes very severe.

In the human literature, this polyradiculoneuritis is referred to as inflammatory polyneuropathy, which seems superfluous when an inflammation of nerves is a neuritis. It is also known as the Landry-Guillain-Barré disease, the most common cause of total paralysis in humans today. Some forms cause predominantly a primary demyelination with axonal sparing. Others affect primarily axons, and the demyelination is secondary. There is good evidence that molecular mimicry is involved in the pathogenesis.[113] In this mechanism, the patient's immune system is exposed to an exogenous antigen such as the bacterium *Campylobacter jejuni,* in which the lipopolysaccharide capsule of the bacterium has components that act as antigens that are similar to the gangliosides found in the myelin of the patient's PNS. The antibodies formed by the immune system attack and destroy the peripheral nerve, recognizing it as being similar to the bacterium's lipopolysaccharide capsule. Other exogenous antigens have components that mimic molecules found in axons. The degree and rate of recovery is dependent on whether the immune system

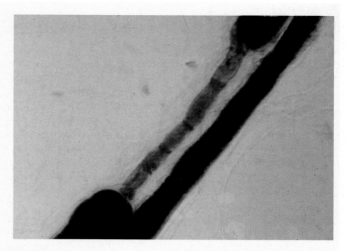

FIGURE 5-12 A teased nerve specimen from the dog in Fig. 5-11 with an osmic acid stain of its myelin. Note the unstained portion of axon where segmental primary demyelination has occurred.

is directed primarily at the myelin sheaths or the axons. The former recover faster and more completely because of the remarkable ability of the Schwann cells to proliferate and remyelinate the intact axons. Electrodiagnostic testing may help contribute to the prognosis by determining which portion of the peripheral nerve is more affected. Recovery can take a few weeks to many months; it is assumed to be a reflection of the degree of axonal involvement. Occasionally recovery does not occur.

The antigenic stimulus in dogs is unknown. Because of the high incidence of this disease in the dogs used to hunt raccoons, the saliva of the raccoon is thought to be a source of the antigen involved in this molecular mimicry. This is the reason the disorder is often called coonhound paralysis. There may also be a genetic predisposition for this PRN in breeds of coonhounds. In our attempts to reproduce the disease using raccoon saliva, it was successful only in coonhounds that had previously had the disease and had recovered. However, it is important to know that exposure to raccoon saliva is not required for this disease to occur. This supports the theory that there are other sources of antigen that have not yet been discovered. We believe that to acquire PRN, two conditions must be satisfied. One is the exposure to a specific antigen, which can have a variety of sources. The other is that there has to be some alteration in the immune system of the patient. In humans, this PRN occasionally follows a vaccination, yet only a very small portion of individuals who receive this vaccine develop PRN.

The high rate of recovery from PRN suggests that the immune system disorder is short-lived. This is supported by the fact that immunosuppressive drugs do not appear to enhance the recovery, and repeat exposures to raccoon saliva can induce another episode of PRN. Dr. John Cummings and I (AD) studied one red bone hound that had the disorder five times, with complete recovery from each episode. In large kennels of working coonhounds, repeat episodes are common.

Diagnosis is based primarily on the characteristic clinical appearance of a rapidly progressive LMN tetraparesis to tetraplegia. No ancillary procedures will confirm this diagnosis of PRN. CSF evaluation that shows a significant elevation of protein, with or without a pleocytosis, is strongly supportive of this diagnosis but requires general anesthesia.

(Continued)

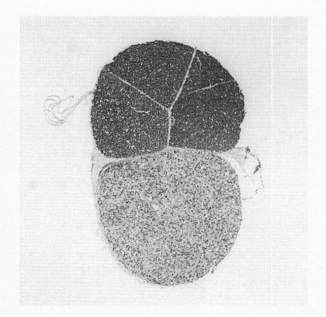

FIGURE 5-11 Transverse section of a dorsal and a ventral root in a dog that died of severe polyradiculoneuritis. These roots were stained with luxol-fast-blue for myelin. Note the severe primary demyelination of the ventral root with sparing of the dorsal root, which correlates well with the clinical signs of LMN disease.

CASE EXAMPLE 5-1—cont'd

These CSF changes occur because the nerve roots, where the lesion is most pronounced, are bathed in CSF. Most of the ancillary procedures that are used help to rule down the other disorders in the differential diagnosis, including intravenous edrophonium (Tensilon), serum antibody levels for acetylcholine, receptor antibodies for myasthenia gravis, and serum enzyme levels for polymyositis. Nerve biopsies are nonspecific because the primary nonsuppurative inflammation is most prevalent in the ventral roots.

Treatment involves rigorous, persistent nursing care. Placing the patient on a waterbed is the best way to prevent pressure-induced skin ulcerations. In a rural environment, bed the patient in a stall with many feet of straw, and change the straw daily. These dogs should be turned over hourly. They usually are able to excrete if they are supported and helped by abdominal pressure. The cranial nerves involved with prehension and swallowing are unaffected, but the patient will have to be supported to eat and drink. A regular daily schedule of physical manipulation and muscle massage is recommended. With the recent interest in physical therapy in veterinary medicine, facilities are now available to aid in the treatment of these patients. Be patient. It may take many weeks for recovery to evolve. I (AD) have personally observed patients that required 6 months before they could stand and walk. In humans with severe signs of PRN, intravenous gamma globulin and plasmapheresis have been effective treatments, but there are no reliable data on their use in animals.

PRN is occasionally seen in cats but is rare in other domestic animals.[85]

Based on the examination of this red bone coonhound, Kulman, and prior to any ancillary procedures, PRN is the most presumptive clinical diagnosis of the disorders listed in the differential diagnosis.

BOTULISM

Botulism is a LMN disorder caused by the toxin produced by the bacterium *Clostridium botulinum*.[2,3,8] There are at least eight recognized neurotoxins. The organisms that produce these toxins vary in their geographic location. The type B–producing organisms are common in the mid-Atlantic states where foals are abundant and are commonly exposed. There are species differences in susceptibility to botulism as well as to the specific types of neurotoxins. Dogs, cats, and pigs are the most resistant to botulism. In affected dogs, the type C neurotoxin is most commonly involved. Ruminants and horses are highly susceptible and deaths are common. Cattle are most commonly affected by the type C and D neurotoxins and horses by types B and C.[138,139]

There are three methods by which intoxication can occur. The most common is by the ingestion of a preformed neurotoxin in a feed source. Hay and silage are often implicated, but the identification of the feed source is often very difficult. Infected dead animals are a source for carnivorous animals. A second and common method of intoxication in young animals, especially foals, is by the absorption of a neurotoxin that is produced within the gastrointestinal tract from spores that have been ingested from the environmental soil. This method is referred to as toxicoinfectious botulism. A third but rare method is the circulation of toxin produced by organisms growing in the anaerobic environment of an infected wound. This is wound botulism.

Ingestion of toxin from a feedstuff available to a herd of animals can cause a significant loss of animals. This occurs most commonly in cattle. More often, individual horses are affected but herd outbreaks can occur. Foals are especially at risk when they ingest the bacterial spores from their environment and the toxin produced in their digestive system is able to be absorbed. These have been referred to as shaker foals because of the diffuse muscle tremors that occur when they are standing and walking.[125,140] Without antitoxin therapy, the mortality rate is very high because of paralysis of the respiratory muscles. There may be circumstances in which an excessive growth of this bacterium in the intestine of adult horses may be the source of intoxication. Dogs and cats are relatively resistant to botulism and if removed from the source of the toxin, they usually recover in a few weeks. Kennels of hunting dogs can be exposed to the toxin in a feed source. An individual dog may be exposed to the neurotoxin present in a dead animal that it consumes. Beware of dead birds in public parks, where dogs often run free.

The mechanism of action of the neurotoxin is at the neuromuscular junction where the neurotoxin binds to receptors on the axon terminal. It translocates into the axon and interferes with the release of acetylcholine. Because this affects only neuromuscular junctions, all the clinical signs are limited to an LMN deficiency. There are no sensory system signs.

In cattle and horses, affected animals can be found dead at pasture when no prior clinical signs have been observed.[92,138] Be aware of the horse that suddenly becomes less active and constantly wants to lie down.[91,122,124,139,140] When you urge the animal to stand, it trembles all over, walks with short strides, and immediately starts to lie down again. If it lies in sternal posture, it will rest its chin on the ground to support its head. You may mistake this tendency to lie down for an onset of colic and the more you make this horse stand the more it will be stressed, and severe diffuse sweating and an elevated pulse rate will follow. Cattle with diffuse NMD such as botulism may lie in sternal recumbency with their necks flexed to one side and their heads resting on their thoraxes. This is the classic posture of milk fever, which is a metabolic muscular disorder caused by hypocalcemia. Cattle with acute signs of hypokalemic myopathy will assume the same posture (see the Case Example 5-2 discussion that follows in this chapter). It is presumed that they assume this posture because of the weight of the head and neck, which they cannot support in a normal extended position. The GSE components of cranial nerves are usually affected in botulism, resulting in paresis of the facial muscles and the muscles of prehension and swallowing. Affected foals that try to nurse typically dribble milk from their noses. Eyelid and tongue paresis and dysphagia are common. There is also a loss of tail tone in large animals. Dogs usually remain ambulatory but lose tone and spinal reflexes and often exhibit dysphagia. It is important to recognize that when these animals are able to walk with this diffuse LMN disorder, they are short-strided but are not ataxic.

Video 5-2 shows a 5-year-old castrated male thoroughbred with the presumptive clinical diagnosis of botulism. Clinical signs of inactivity, a shortened stride, and frequent periods of lying down in the stall were first observed 3 days before this video was made. Note the slightly lowered neck, the shifting of its weight between its limbs, the trembling, the difficult prehension with dropping of its feed, the paretic tongue, the hypotonic anus, and the shortened strides with no indication of ataxia. Note that when he was placed in a stall, he immediately lay down. This horse received specific type B antitoxin on the second day of clinical signs, but by the fifth day was unable to stand and died the next day. We thank Dr. Caroline Hahn and Dr. Ian Mayhew of the University of Edinburgh for sharing this video with us.

In this case example, the red bone coonhound, it would be unusual to have such an acute diffuse LMN tetraplegia due to botulism without greater evidence of cranial nerve involvement.

MYASTHENIA GRAVIS

Myasthenia gravis (grave muscle weakness) is a disorder at the neuromuscular junction. There are two forms: congenital and acquired. Congenital forms are observed primarily in puppies, and most represent a developmental disorder of the acetylcholine receptor that may be inherited. The acquired form is more common; it occurs in adults (although cases have been diagnosed as early as 3 months of age), and it is an autoimmune disease.[38-40,51,59,118]

The basis for the autoimmune disorder is unknown. It is hypothesized that a spontaneous disorder occurs in the immune system that results in the production of antibodies against the nicotinic acetylcholine receptor. The trigger for this is unknown. A genetic predisposition may be involved, but its nature remains undefined. Although the disease is diagnosed more commonly in the larger breeds, especially the golden retriever, German shepherd, Akita, and German short hair pointer, any breed and mixed breeds can be affected. A familial basis has been proposed for the Newfoundland and Great Dane breeds. These antibodies bind to the acetylcholine receptor and prevent the attachment of the acetylcholine released from the axonal terminal in response to the neuronal impulse. Once the antibody is bound to the acetylcholine receptor, the entire unit is internalized into the muscle and is no longer available; it must be replaced by the forming of a new receptor. The large abundance of receptors provides a safety factor because many are spared from this antibody binding. This is the basis for the classical signs of exercise-induced fatigue, which is an episodic paresis associated with exertion. Signs of paresis are present only when there are inadequate numbers of acetylcholine receptors to bind with the acetylcholine that is released from the axonal terminal. Three clinical syndromes are observed in dogs: generalized, focal, and fulminating.

In the generalized syndrome, if a patient is presented to you after a period of rest and relaxation, your examination will be normal. If you vigorously exercise this animal for a variable period of time, usually less than 10 minutes, the paresis will first be seen in the pelvic limbs, with the development of a short stride and a crouched posture. Thoracic limb paresis usually follows, accompanied by a flexed neck posture, and collapse may occur. Even when collapsed, the spinal reflexes are usually preserved. This is often accompanied by some dyspnea, drooling, and eyelid and lip paresis. If the patient is placed in a cage to rest for 30 to 60 minutes, the signs of paresis disappear, and the patient comes out of the cage normal; but after walking briskly for just a few minutes, the paresis usually recurs. Be aware that this episodic feature is not a requirement for the diagnosis. Occasionally the antibodies are able to bind nearly all of the receptors, causing a fulminating form of myasthenia gravis, and the clinical signs will be similar to those of the red bone coonhound presented at the beginning of this discussion.

An owner commonly observes that the dog is unable to keep its food down. From the description of this event, you usually can determine that this is regurgitation, not vomiting. It is the result of a megaesophagus that is commonly present in dogs that have diffuse paresis due to myasthenia gravis. Remember that most of the esophageal muscle in dogs is striated voluntary muscle innervated by GSE neurons, and these muscle cells have acetylcholine receptors identical to those in skeletal muscle. It is paramount that the clinician distinguish regurgitation from vomiting in these patients by obtaining appropriate history at the time the patient is presented. Aspiration pneumonia commonly accompanies this regurgitation and may be life-threatening.

Focal forms of myasthenia gravis occur in muscles innervated by cranial nerves. They can occur in combination or as isolated events. The most common focal form is limited to the esophagus and causes a megaesophagus and regurgitation, especially in older dogs. Myasthenia gravis can be limited to the laryngeal muscles, causing dyspnea; to the pharyngeal muscles, causing dysphagia; and to the facial muscles, causing weak eyelids and lips. In humans, myasthenia gravis can be limited to the extraocular muscles, causing a diplopia, a diagnosis that is difficult to make in our patients.

Acquired myasthenia gravis is much less common in cats than in dogs.[51] The Abyssinian and Somali breeds have a high incidence. Myasthenic cats tend to exhibit the episodic characteristic much less commonly. Cats are usually difficult to exercise in a hospital environment. Sometimes their refusal to walk provides a huge problem in your desire to evaluate their gait in the case of a neurologic disorder. Unfortunately, most cats are not leash trained. A cat commonly carries its head and neck in a flexed position when it has a neuromuscular disorder such as myasthenia gravis. Megaesophagus is less common in cats with acquired myasthenia gravis and the focal forms are less commonly diagnosed.

In the congenital form of myasthenia gravis, clinical signs are usually seen by 3 to 8 weeks of age in multiple puppies in a litter, and they commonly progress as the puppies grow and may result in their inability to walk.[42,73,74,105] This form usually involves an abnormality in the development of the acetylcholine receptor, when its abnormal structure prevents the binding with acetylcholine, or when insufficient numbers of receptors have developed. There is strong evidence that this disease is inherited as an autosomal recessive gene in the smooth fox terrier, the Parson (Jack) Russell terrier, and the Gammel Dansk honsehund. It has been reported in the springer spaniel and the miniature smooth dachshund, and I (AD) have seen it in the Samoyed breed. The inherited disorder in the Gammel Dansk honsehond is presynaptic and involves an abnormality in the release of sufficient acetylcholine from the axonal terminal. Megaesophagus has been reported only in the smooth fox terrier. Congenital myasthenia gravis is rare in cats.

A congenital form of myasthenia gravis has been recognized in Brahman calves that exhibit a muscle paresis at birth or within the first month of life.[127] This is inherited as an autosomal recessive gene that codes for one of the subunits of the acetylcholine receptor. A polymerase chain reaction (PCR)-based DNA test performed on blood or semen will confirm the diagnosis in affected calves and detect the clinically normal carrier animals.

Be aware that a neonatal myasthenia gravis occurs in children born to mothers who have acquired myasthenia gravis, presumably from the passage of antibodies across the placenta. The same could occur in puppies after ingestion of colostral antibodies. We are not aware of any published report of this in domestic animals.

Diagnosis

The most common ancillary procedure used to diagnose myasthenia gravis is an intravenous injection of an ultra-short-acting anticholinesterase, edrophonium chloride (Tensilon). By blocking the degradating enzyme, it allows more opportunity for the acetylcholine to be available to those receptors that are not bound to antibody. Exercise your patient first so that the LMN paresis is obvious. Inject the edrophonium intravenously at 0.1 to 0.2 mg/kg (in a cat, use 0.25 to 0.5 mg). You should expect any response to occur in just a few seconds, but it will be short-lived and last only 2 to 3 minutes because the drug is rapidly metabolized. This test is reliable for most cases, but a few dogs with the episodic form will not respond, and a few dogs with other LMN disorders will show

(Continued)

CASE EXAMPLE 5-1—cont'd

some response. Most dogs with the fulminating form of myasthenia gravis will not respond because most of their acetylcholine receptors are bound with antibody. Some congenital forms will not respond. Toxicity to this drug is uncommon but may occur in the normal dog or in an overdosed patient because of the overstimulation of the acetylcholine receptor, which causes a depolarizing blockade. You should have atropine available to treat this possibility of toxicity. I (EG) often pretreat patients with atropine prior to the injection of edrophonium.

In the acquired forms of myasthenia gravis, there are usually circulating antibodies against the acetylcholine receptor; they can be determined by laboratory analysis. These antibody levels are generally lowest in the patients with focal signs and highest in the fulminating cases, in our experience. However, no definitive evidence exists in scientific studies to support this relationship. Indeed, some mild focal forms of this disease have the highest antibody levels. False negatives can occur with no clear explanation. This ancillary procedure is of no use in the congenital forms. However, the total volume of acetylcholine receptor can be assayed in the laboratory from a sample of an external intercostal muscle. This can help confirm the diagnosis of congenital myasthenia gravis when it involves a deficiency of acetylcholine receptor formation.

All patients should undergo radiographs of the thorax to determine whether megaesophagus is present; to look for the presence of aspiration pneumonia, which is common with a megaesophagus and is life-threatening; and to look for a thymic mass. The latter is seen in less than 5% of dogs and in about 25% of cats with acquired myasthenia gravis. It is thought that thymic hyperplasia or neoplasia may play a role in the production of the antibodies against the acetylcholine receptor. In humans, the recovery from myasthenia gravis is enhanced by the removal of this thymic mass. It is believed that the antibodies produced against the thymic mass cells are similar to those produced for the acetylcholine receptor.

There is a significant incidence of hypothyroidism in dogs with acquired myasthenia gravis that justifies evaluating the thyroid function in these patients.

If electrodiagnostic equipment is available, the diagnosis can be supported by repetitive stimulation of a peripheral nerve and observation of the immediate decrement in the response of the muscle. This decrement will be reduced or will resolve after the intravenous administration of edrophonium (Tensilon). Single-fiber electromyography is a more specific determination but requires specialized needles and operator expertise. These tests require generalized anesthesia, which may be contraindicated in certain patients.

The following videos show examples of myasthenia gravis:

- **Video 5-3** shows Bright, a 5-year-old spayed female Labrador retriever with a history of 10 weeks of occasional episodes of paresis associated with exercise. The frequency had increased in the past week, along with occasional regurgitation. This dog had been resting in her cage for a few hours before the video was made. She walked through the hospital and continued outdoors with a normal gait but then became paretic, as seen on the video. Note the progression of the paresis as she is walked, her response to intravenous edrophonium, and the recurrence of the paresis at the end of the video. Radiographs showed a megaesophagus.
- **Video 5-4** shows Sailor, a 7-year-old castrated male standard poodle with a 1-week history of episodes of pelvic limb paresis. Note the response to intravenous edrophonium.

- **Video 5-5** shows Ruddy, an 8-year-old male Abyssinian with 1 month of progressive inactivity, inability to climb stairs or jump up onto the bed, and less vocalizing than usual. Note the flexed neck posture, the reluctance to walk, the slight facial paresis, and the response to intravenous edrophonium.
- **Video 5-6** shows Maya, a 5-week-old female English springer spaniel. She was one in a litter of six that appeared to be less active when the others began to walk, and she had difficulty walking. She would tremor when she tried to interact with her littermates. Note the crouched posture, flexed neck, and short strides. She showed some response to intravenous edrophonium and was diagnosed as a presumptive congenital myasthenic. She improved on oral treatment with pyridostigmine, which is a long-term anticholinesterase drug. This can be seen at the end of the video, which was made about 1 week after the start of therapy. By 16 weeks she was normal and was weaned off the drug. Presumably, this is an example of an insufficient development of acetylcholine receptors.
- **Video 5-7** shows a 2-week-old Brahman calf that had exhibited diffuse signs of NMD since birth. The calf spent most if its time lying down, was slow to get up, and walked short-strided. Note the response to intravenous edrophonium. This is a calf with an inherited acetylcholine receptor abnormality, and it will not recover. We thank Dr. Peter Thompson at the University of Pretoria for providing us with this video.[127]
- **Video 5-8** shows a 1-week-old female Holstein that since birth had been inactive and short-strided and spent most of her time lying down. Note her response to intravenous edrophonium. She was normal by 6 weeks of age, which suggests that there was a delay in her formation of acetylcholine receptors.

Treatment

Treatment of acquired myasthenia gravis can be palliative by providing a constant source of anticholinesterase by oral administration, or treatment can be directed at the antibody production itself by the use of immunosuppressant drugs. Pyridostigmine bromide (Mestinon) is the most common oral anticholinesterase that is used. In dogs, use 0.5 to 3.0 mg/kg every 8 to 12 hours. Start with a low dose and slowly increase the amount used until satisfactory improvement in the clinical signs occurs without signs of toxicity. In cats, use 0.25 mg/kg every 8 to 12 hours. If regurgitation interferes with this oral administration, either administer it by a gastrostomy tube or use an intramuscular injection of neostigmine (Prostigmine) until the oral route is accepted.

Be aware that an overdose of anticholinesterase will cause paralysis due to excessive depolarization of the muscle. This is the nicotinic effect of the overdose. It will sometimes be accompanied by the muscarinic effect, which includes excessive salivation, vomiting, diarrhea, miosis, and bradycardia. This cholinergic crisis should be treated with atropine. To distinguish an overdose from an inadequate dose of the medication, an edrophonium test can be done carefully.

Corticosteroids and azathioprine have been used successfully as immunosuppressants.[41] In dogs, prednisone should be started at a low dose of 0.5 mg/kg every 12 hours to prevent the initial exacerbation of the neuromuscular signs. Gradually increase the dose to immunosuppressive levels over 1 to 2 weeks. Try to attain an alternate-day schedule that will control the disorder. Cats are treated with 1 to 4 mg/kg every 12 hours. The dose of azathioprine in dogs is

1 mg/kg every 12 hours. Recently, cyclosporine has been used for the treatment of myasthenia gravis.

The goal of the treatment is essentially to buy time for the spontaneous resolution of the immune disorder and the replacement of the internalized receptors. After a few months of successful therapy, the drug used should be slowly withdrawn. When the serum level of acetylcholine antibodies decreases to an undetectable level, treatment can be stopped. Occasionally, a recurrence will occur and require more treatment. This spontaneous recovery suggests that the immune system disorder is short-lived. The megaesophagus may persist despite the therapy and postprandial regurgitation will be a constant threat for aspiration pneumonia. The latter must be treated aggressively. It is important to feed these dogs when their strength is at its best following the treatment. It may help to feed a moist food or slurry in small portions more frequently and from an elevated position.

Be aware that the successful long-term treatment of myasthenia gravis can be frustrating and unsuccessful. Many patients will develop aspiration pneumonia and require multiple hospitalizations. Therefore, owners must be warned about this possibility and the associated costs.

Some congenital forms of myasthenia gravis will be improved by anticholinesterase therapy. Occasionally puppies will outgrow the clinical signs that were presumed to be due to an insufficient development of acetylcholine receptors.

For Kulman, the recumbent red bone coonhound in the case discussion, only the fulminating form of myasthenia gravis would be a concern. This degree of severe atonia and areflexia would be less likely in most cases of myasthenia gravis. A negative response to edrophonium would not eliminate this diagnosis. Determination of serum antibodies to acetylcholine receptor would be necessary to support this diagnosis. This red bone coonhound had no response to intravenous edrophonium and had no serum antibodies for acetylcholine receptors.

TICK PARALYSIS

For tick paralysis to occur, it is essential that the animal be exposed to a species of tick that has in its saliva a neurotoxin that is injected into the animal when the tick bites to extract blood from the animal.[16] We are all taught to obtain a travel history for our patients because it may be important in diagnosing disorders that are not indigenous to our practice area. Tick paralysis is an excellent example of this because a dog can acquire a tick attachment on the mid-Atlantic coast and travel to a state that has no toxin-carrying ticks before that dog shows any signs of paralysis. The only diagnosis that I (AD) ever made of tick paralysis in a patient at the College of Veterinary Medicine at Cornell University was in a dog from Ithaca, New York, that had spent the previous week on the shores of North Carolina. The few species of ticks that inhabit the Ithaca area do not carry the necessary neurotoxin. I (EG) made this diagnosis in a young Labrador retriever that had traveled over one weekend from southern Virginia to New York City and developed the clinical signs of tick paralysis a few days later.

In North America, tick paralysis is most common in dogs and children, but all species of domestic animals and some species of birds are also susceptible to this neurotoxin. In the United States, the common wood tick, *Dermacentor variabilis*, and *Dermacentor andersoni* are incriminated most often. Clinical signs can occur after feeding by a single female tick. The neurotoxin enters the circulation and gains access to the neuromuscular junctions where the toxin interferes with the function of calcium in the release of acetylcholine from the axonal terminal. Clinical signs occur 5 to 9 days after the tick

infestation, with a rapid onset of LMN paresis starting in the pelvic limbs and spreading to the thoracic limbs. Dogs may become recumbent in 24 to 72 hours. Spinal reflexes are depressed or absent. Nociception is normal and there is no hyperesthesia. Cranial nerve LMN signs are uncommon except for severe cases. Megaesophagus is uncommon. Death may occur as the result of respiratory paralysis in 1 to 5 days.

Diagnosis is based on a history of possible exposure to toxin-bearing ticks and a careful search of the affected animal for a tick. If the history and signs are compatible with this diagnosis and the offending tick cannot be found, it is worth giving the patient an insecticide dip to kill any hidden ticks. Removal of the tick will be followed by recovery in 24 to 72 hours.

In eastern Australia, the neurotoxin secreted by the species of tick *Ixodes holocyclus* produces an extremely severe, rapidly progressive paralysis that is commonly lethal.[16] Death can occur rapidly in all species, including humans, sometimes even after removal of the offending tick.

Video 5-9 shows Lola, a 6-month-old female Maltese with sudden onset of a stumbling gait that progressed to recumbency in 24 hours. Note the hypotonia and areflexia but intact nociception based on the head movements. The voice was not audible. There was facial paresis and jaw hypotonia. A veterinary student found a tick and removed it. The last part of the video shows Lola 24 hours after removal of the tick. (We thank Dr. Marc Kent of the University of Georgia for sharing this case with us.)

The red bone coonhound under discussion was from upstate New York where there are no ticks that secrete a neurotoxin, and this dog had no history of travel from the farm where he was housed. No ticks were found on this dog, and no insecticide dip was considered necessary.

POLYMYOSITIS

A generalized polymyositis is most commonly the result of an autoimmune disorder associated with antibodies circulating against striated skeletal muscle.[53,81] There are a number of infectious agents that cause a myositis: *Toxoplasma gondii*, *Neospora caninum*, and *Leptospira icterohaemorrhagiae*. They usually affect body systems other than the muscle and are less often generalized. Autoimmune myositis can be focal and limited to the muscles of mastication, the extraocular muscles, or the muscles of the pharynx and esophagus or can be generalized.

Masticatory myositis is the focal form most commonly diagnosed. Any breed is susceptible, but there is a high incidence in the German shepherd. There are acute and chronic forms. In the acute form, the masticatory muscles are swollen and very painful. Do not try to open the animal's mouth because this hurts the patient! The reluctance to open the mouth prevents the dog from eating. The swelling is so severe that the eyes may protrude from the orbits. Fever and swollen palatine tonsils and mandibular lymph nodes may be present. Biopsy of these swollen muscles will reveal a diffuse necrotizing inflammation with hemorrhage and edema. Inflammatory cells include macrophages, plasma cells, lymphocytes, occasionally neutrophils, and sometimes eosinophils. Serum muscle enzymes usually are remarkably elevated and there will be circulating antibodies to the type II M muscle fibers that predominate in these muscles.

Treatment with immunosuppressant drugs will alleviate the acute clinical signs but recurrences may occur. In the chronic phase, muscle atrophy can be severe, and the fibrosis that occurs in the muscle can in time mechanically prevent the mouth from opening. Some dogs only have a chronic myositis only of the masticatory muscles, but it results in the same severe atrophy and inability to open the mouth.

(Continued)

CASE EXAMPLE 5-1—cont'd

Do not try to force the jaw to open under anesthesia—you will fracture the mandible. If immunosuppressant drug therapy is ineffective, consider surgically cutting the attachments of the temporal and masseter muscles to the ramus of the mandible. There is no neurologic disorder other than tetanus that causes the inability to open the jaw. Only a fibrosing muscle disorder will do this. The term *trismus* refers to the excessive uncontrolled contraction of the masticatory muscles that is present in tetanus. It is not an appropriate term for the fibrosing stage of chronic myositis, which is a mechanical resistance. I (EG) have used corticosteroids, azathioprine, and oral cyclosporine to treat these patients and have seen varying responses.

Other focal forms of presumptive autoimmune myositis have been reported in young adult dogs: it may involve the extraocular muscles, causing a prominent exophthalmos; the laryngeal muscles, causing dyspnea; or the pharyngeal muscles, causing dysphagia.

Generalized autoimmune polymyositis can mimic the LMN signs seen in a dog that has polyradiculoneuritis but is ambulatory. It is rare for this muscle disorder to cause recumbency and tetraplegia. In the acute phase, the affected muscles may be swollen and when palpated, discomfort will be evident. Usually the spinal nerve reflexes will be preserved. In the chronic phase, muscle atrophy will be significant. Be aware that the clinical signs of paresis in these dogs may worsen with exercise and sometimes they will show a moderate response to an intravenous injection of edrophonium. Involvement of the esophagus will result in megaesophagus and regurgitation. As a rule, the diagnosis can be supported by a marked elevation of the serum enzymes. A biopsy of an affected muscle that reveals necrosis of muscle cells, with macrophages and prominent lymphoplasmacytic interstitial inflammation, confirms the diagnosis. Serum assay often detects circulating antibodies against skeletal muscle antigens. EMG studies are nonspecific in that the abnormalities seen do not clearly distinguish a neuronal disorder from a muscle disorder. Observing normal nerve conduction studies may be helpful. Magnetic resonance (MR) imaging has been used to help diagnose focal forms of myositis, including the form that affects the extraocular muscles. Occasionally dogs with immune-mediated polymyositis also have hypothyroidism caused by the same kind of inflammation that is affecting their thyroid glands. Maybe this suggests that there is a common factor triggering these two autoimmune disorders. It is to be hoped that this may be determined as our ability to study the canine genome progresses.

Generalized polymyositis is uncommon in cats. A dermatomyositis occurs primarily in collies and Shetland sheepdogs. Treatment of polymyositis with immunosuppressant drugs should be initiated and continued until serum enzyme levels return to normal. Recurrences may occur, and alternate-day therapy may be necessary for prolonged therapy.

 Video 5-10 shows a 4-year-old male Labrador retriever that had had a slowly progressing gait disorder for 3 to 4 weeks. It became worse with exercise, and he never had normal periods. Note the crouched posture, the short strides without any ataxia, the decreased range of jaw movement, and the diffuse moderate muscle atrophy. All of his serum muscle enzymes were elevated: CK-3033 U/l (normal <241); AST-252 U/l (normal <52); ALT-256 U/l (normal <99). The muscle biopsy showed an extensive nonsuppurative inflammation associated with muscle necrosis.

Our tetraplegic red bone coonhound is an unlikely candidate for acute polymyositis because of the severity of his flaccid paralysis with atonia and areflexia. His serum enzyme levels were only moderately elevated, which would be expected in a recumbent patient.

OTHER DIFFERENTIAL DIAGNOSES

Other considerations for this recumbent red bone coonhound with the LMN tetraplegia include snake envenomation and possibly organophosphate toxicity. Snake envenomation obviously requires exposure of the patient to the bite of a snake whose venom is toxic. The two most common species of snake whose venom causes a postsynaptic blockade of the neuromuscular junction are the coral snakes found in the southeastern states and the North American rattlesnake in the southern and southwestern states. The onset of clinical signs of a rapidly progressive LMN tetraparesis vary from 30 minutes to a few hours but less than 24 hours, so there is little time for travel to a state that is free of the offending snake. When recumbent, there will be loss of spinal nerve reflexes and significant paresis of cranial nerve GSE neurons. Death results from respiratory muscle paralysis. This can often be prevented with the immediate administration of specific antivenom. Less severely affected animals may recover spontaneously in 7 to 10 days. The observation of hemolysis and hemoglobinuria will help support this diagnosis when the snake bite is not observed.

Organophosphate toxicity can occur in different forms.[97] The form that is a possible consideration in this tetraplegic dog is one in which the toxin causes a blockade of the acetylcholine receptor. Chlorpyrifos and fenthion are acetylcholineesterase inhibitors. The resultant accumulation of acetylcholine will eventually cause a blockade at the receptor and produce LMN paralysis. Clinical signs are usually observed within minutes to hours of the exposure. Diagnosis is supported by a history of exposure and detection of decreased levels of cholinesterase in the blood. Treatment should include atropine for the muscarinic signs and 2-PAM (pralidoxime chloride) for the nicotinic signs; in some toxicities diphenhydramine (Benadryl) may help block the action of the toxin.

Kulman, the red bone coonhound in this case example, had no possibility of exposure to a snake toxin and no history of exposure to any organophosphate. The severe degree of flaccid paralysis would be extreme for the latter diagnosis, especially with the absence of any muscarinic signs. It was concluded that the most presumptive clinical diagnosis for Kulman was polyradiculoneuritis. Only supportive therapy was provided. Despite being bedded on a thick layer of blankets, skin ulcerations occurred, as can be seen at the end of the video when he had regained the ability to walk after 3 weeks of recumbency. These ulcerations rarely occur when a dog like this is kept on a waterbed. By 5 weeks, Kulman's gait was normal. Given the relatively rapid rate of recovery, it was presumed that the major lesions in Kulman involved the myelin rather than the axons in his peripheral nerves.

The following videos show three additional examples of polyradiculoneuritis-coonhound paralysis in dogs used for hunting raccoons.

 Video 5-11 shows Swampfox, a 6-year-old male red bone coonhound crossbreed that was presented for examination 24 hours after the owner recognized that the dog was lame and his voice was altered. One week before this, Swampfox had been bitten in the ear by a raccoon. Note the severely lame gait affecting all four limbs that is due to a rapidly progressing diffuse neuromuscular disorder, not a joint disease. Note his preference for sitting, which is very abnormal for an active working coonhound. The second portion of the video, which shows the dog inside the hospital, was made 24 hours after the outdoor portion of the video. Now the dog is recumbent due to flaccid tetraplegia. Spinal nerve reflexes are absent but nociception is intact and exaggerated. Note the howling attempts caused just

by palpation of his thigh muscles. Normally these coonhounds are minimally affected by mild noxious stimuli. Note the flaccid paralysis of the trunk and neck as well as the limbs but the preservation of function in the head muscles innervated by cranial nerves. Swampfox was able to eat and drink well but had to be held up to do so. The portion of the video with Swampfox in the cage under a blanket was made 24 hours after the second video. He died the next day because of the severity of his polyradiculoneuritis, which was confirmed at necropsy.

 Video 5-12 is another case of polyradiculoneuritis that caused a less severe recumbency. This is Blackjack, a 1.5-year-old male mixed-breed retriever from a farm in New York State where he is exposed to raccoons. Blackjack had experienced a 2-week history of progressive difficulty in walking that began in the pelvic limbs and progressed to the thoracic limbs by the start of the second week; he had been recumbent for 2 days. Note the presence of more strength in the trunk and neck than in the limbs. When encouraged to come out of his cage, he cannot stand and squirms toward the door using his axial muscles but has only feeble movement in his appendicular muscles. The second time he is shown coming out of his cage, 3 weeks had passed since the first portion of the video was taken; the portion taken outdoors was recorded 1 week later. Blackjack made a full recovery. All of his muscle mass returned and, with no further contact with raccoons, the polyradiculoneuritis has not recurred. At present, Blackjack is a healthy, robust 8-year-old dog.

Video 5-13 is a delightful and instructive video made by the owner of his affected dog, Woody, on his farm near Buffalo, New York, and sent to us for our use in teaching. Woody is a 6-year-old male mixed-breed dog that had been clinically affected for about 2 months at the time the video was made. The first indication of a problem was when Woody was slow to return to the owner while hunting. It was followed by his inability to jump into the owner's truck. The pelvic limbs were initially the most seriously affected, and Woody became recumbent after about 3 days of rapidly progressive paresis. His flaccid tetraplegia involved all of the muscles of his limbs, trunk, and neck but spared the head muscles innervated by cranial nerves. About 2 weeks before this video was made, the owner noticed some movement in Woody's head, neck, and tail. Woody had experienced a similar clinical disorder when he was 3 years old. It was 3 months before he had completely recovered.

One addendum is needed here because this discussion of LMN tetraplegia involves only adult dogs. John Cummings and I (AD) studied four puppies in a litter of eight Labrador retrievers that at 6 weeks of age developed LMN paraparesis. In a few days it had progressed to LMN tetraplegia, with prehension difficulties and dysphagia, followed by death. These puppies all had a severe diffuse polyradiculoneuritis caused by *N. caninum*.[31] The young age is critical here because this organism usually affects only spinal nerve roots in puppies under 12 weeks of age and usually is limited to the lumbosacral roots (see Case Example 5-11). This study emphasizes the importance of a necropsy. The diagnosis was not suspected during our clinical study of these puppies, and it is critical knowledge for breeders so that they can prevent future occurrences.

CASE EXAMPLE 5-2

NMD Tetraparesis—Dog

Signalment: 2-year-old male German shepherd, Cosmos
Chief Complaint: Gait abnormality
History: Two days of rapidly progressive difficulty in walking, especially with the pelvic limbs
Examination: Video 5-14 shows the rapid, short-strided gait in the pelvic limbs when he was assisted. Mild support loss in the thoracic limbs was more evident when he was hopped. Muscle tone was normal. Spinal nerve reflexes were mildly depressed. Nociception was normal. Cranial nerves were normal.
Anatomic Diagnosis: Diffuse neuromuscular disease
Differential Diagnosis: The same as for the dog in Case Example 5-1

POLYRADICULONEURITIS

The dog had experienced no known exposure to raccoons but such exposure could not be totally denied. The cerebrospinal fluid (CSF) contained 4 leucocytes per cmm and 40 mg protein per dl (normal <30). This albuminocytologic dissociation is supportive of the diagnosis.

BOTULISM

There was no known exposure. The clinical signs were mild and there were no cranial nerve signs. The CSF should be normal in botulism patients.

MYASTHENIA GRAVIS

There was no history of improvement with rest and worsening with exercise. There was no response to intravenous edrophonium. The CSF should be normal.

TICK PARALYSIS

This dog could have been exposed to ticks while on a camping trip in Virginia 1 week prior to the development of the neurologic signs. No ticks were found on the dog, and no improvement followed an insecticide bath. The CSF should be normal.

POLYMYOSITIS

Serum enzymes were normal. The CSF should be normal.

HYPOKALEMIC MYOPATHY

This is a rare cause of tetraparesis in the dog but is more commonly seen in cats and occasionally in cattle. It usually occurs in older cats that often have a chronic renal disorder with excessive renal loss of potassium. Decreased dietary intake can contribute to this disorder. Be sure that the potassium content of the cat's diet is adequate. The onset of paresis is usually acute, with a stiff, short-strided gait, reluctance to walk, and ventroflexion of the head

(Continued)

and neck. Spinal nerve reflexes and postural reactions are normal. Serum potassium levels are low and serum muscle enzymes are elevated. Be aware that a presumably inherited hypokalemic myopathy occurs in 2- to 6-month-old Burmese kittens.[75] Signs of paresis are episodic and are associated with intermittent hypokalemia and elevation of creatine kinase (CK). The episodes are commonly transient and usually can be avoided by means of dietary supplementation.

Hypokalemic myopathy in cattle is an iatrogenic disorder associated with the use of the mineralocorticoid drug isoflupredone (9-fluoro-prednisolone acetate) for the treatment of ketosis or clostridial mastitis.[119] With the sudden loss of potassium through the urine, these cattle are usually found recumbent, with no muscle tone, with their necks flexed laterally, and with their heads resting on their thoraxes, similar to the posture of a cow with "milk fever," which is associated with her hypocalcemic myopathy (Fig. 5-13). These cattle may be found dead. Recumbent cattle treated for hypokalemia have a guarded prognosis. To make the correct diagnosis, it is important to recognize that in cattle the recumbent posture, with the head and neck resting on the side of the thorax, is a clinical sign of a neuromuscular disorder as is the ventroflexion of the head and neck in a standing animal, especially a cat.

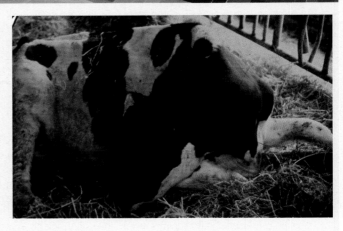

FIGURE 5-13 Recumbent 5-year-old Holstein with diffuse neuromuscular paresis due to treatment with isoflupredone for clostridial mastitis.

The most presumptive clinical diagnosis for this German shepherd was polyradiculoneuritis. Only supportive care was provided, and the dog began to improve in about 2 weeks. The last portion of the video shows the improved walking at that time.

CASE EXAMPLE 5-3

NMD Tetraparesis—Dog

Signalment: 5-month-old male Labrador retriever, Nemo
Chief Complaint: Poor growth, progressive paresis, exercise-induced collapse
History: When this dog was purchased at 3 months of age, he was smaller than his littermates and was less playful. He has progressively become less active, and he becomes fatigued with exercise, which recently resulted in his collapse and the necessity of his being carried home from a long hike. His growth has been slow and his muscle development poor.
 Examination: Video 5-15 shows the short strides, the arched back, the lowered head and neck, the diffuse muscle atrophy, and the lack of patellar reflexes in this Labrador retriever.
Anatomic Diagnosis: Diffuse neuromuscular disease
Differential Diagnosis: The differential diagnosis would include the seven major disorders described in the first two case examples. However, the age of onset and the very slow and insidious progression of the clinical signs would be unusual for any of these seven disorders.

In any consideration of a differential diagnosis, always be sure to ask yourself whether there is any disorder that could produce these signs that is unique to this breed. In this case, two inherited muscle disorders should be considered. The most common is a polymyopathy that is inherited as an autosomal recessive gene disorder. The less common is a muscular dystrophy associated with a deficiency of a cytoskeletal glycoprotein, dystrophin, which is inherited as a sex-linked recessive gene. This is described in Case Example 5-4.

TYPE II DEFICIENCY AUTOSOMAL RECESSIVE POLYMYOPATHY IN LABRADOR RETRIEVERS

Nemo's clinical signs are typical of the polymyopathy inherited as an autosomal recessive gene. It was originally studied and published by Jack Kramer of Washington State University in 1976 as an autosomal recessive inherited deficiency of type II muscle fibers.[83,84] The disorder has now been recognized in Labrador retrievers in many countries throughout the world.[78,95,100] More recently it has been described as an autosomal recessive muscular dystrophy. This name is inappropriate because the muscle lesion is not a muscular dystrophy in which the histologic examination of affected muscle should show both degeneration and regeneration of muscle cells. It has also been called a centronuclear-like myopathy, but this is a nonspecific muscle cell abnormality seen in many myopathic disorders. Immunocytochemical studies of the dystrophin-glycoprotein complex in the muscle cell membrane cytoskeleton have not yet defined any specific abnormality. Until we have a better understanding of the nature of the muscle cell disorder, it is best to refer to this as type II deficiency Labrador retriever polymyopathy.

The video of Nemo, the dog presented in this case example, shows the classical clinical signs of this type II deficiency polymyopathy. The depressed or absent patellar reflex is a common clinical sign and may reflect involvement of the small striated intrafusal muscle cells in neuromuscular spindles.

The ancillary studies supported this diagnosis: There was no response to an intravenous injection of edrophonium. Serum muscle enzyme levels were normal (occasionally they are slightly elevated in this muscle disorder). The CSF was normal. An EMG revealed a few denervation potentials and a few bursts of complex repetitive discharges. Nerve conduction times were normal. Such an electrodiagnostic study is quite typical of this disorder. The nerve biopsy was normal. The muscle biopsy showed a variation in muscle fiber size, a depletion of type II muscle fibers, and a few cells with centrally positioned nuclei but no necrosis of muscle cells.

This type II deficiency Labrador retriever polymyopathy has a good prognosis for life because it is self-limited. It rarely progresses for more than 9 or 10 months and rarely causes recumbency. Owners learn to limit the amount of exercise to avoid having to carry the dog home. Obviously, such a dog and its parents should not be used for breeding. Nemo's clinical signs had remained essentially unchanged when he was last examined at 10 years of age.

CASE EXAMPLE 5-4

NMD Tetraparesis—Dog

Signalment: 7-month-old male Labrador retriever, Jake
Chief Complaint: Abnormal gait and abnormal prehension
History: This dog was the smallest of the litter and did not grow well. By 9 to 10 weeks of age, he was less active than the others, lay down much of the time, rapidly fatigued with exercise, drooled constantly, and was a very sloppy eater. These clinical signs have slowly progressed over the subsequent few months.
Examination: Video 5-16 shows Jake's examination.
Anatomic Diagnosis: Diffuse neuromuscular disease
Differential Diagnosis: It is the same as that described in Case Example 5-3.

The major difference between Nemo (Case Example 5-3) and Jake is the constant drooling exhibited by Jake and the decreased range of motion on trying to open the mouth. The diffuse muscle atrophy, the short gait in all four limbs, the arched back, and the lowered head and neck position are similar. However, Jake had normal patellar reflexes; they were absent in Nemo.

DYSTROPHINOPATHY, A SEX-LINKED RECESSIVE MUSCULAR DYSTROPHY

These clinical signs exhibited by Jake are typical of the sex-linked inherited muscular dystrophy caused by a deficiency of dystrophin.[6] In addition, a very early clinical sign is the decrease in range of mouth opening associated with prehension difficulties and sialosis. As the disease progresses, the tongue and pharyngeal muscles begin to feel enlarged between the mandibles. Although there is diffuse atrophy of most axial and appendicular muscles, some of the caudal thigh muscles will hypertrophy along with the diaphragm.

To support the clinical diagnosis of muscular dystrophy with dystrophinopathy, an ancillary test that is extremely reliable is the determination of a marked elevation of serum muscle enzyme levels. In dystrophinopathy, muscle fiber necrosis is usually severe, which results in the marked elevation of the serum enzymes CK, aspartate aminotransferase (AST), and alanine aminotransferase (ALT). In Jake's serum the CK was 59,200 U/l (normal <359); the AST was 725 U/l (normal <56); and the ALT was 431 U/l (normal <92). Muscle biopsy shows the extensive muscle cell necrosis that is responsible for the high levels of circulating serum muscle enzymes. This necrosis is associated with large accumulations of macrophages, with fibrosis, and with lipid accumulation in the presence of rows of proliferating satellite cells in regenerating muscle cells. Immunocytochemistry clearly shows the lack of dystrophin in the muscle cell membrane.

This muscular dystrophy is inherited as a sex-linked recessive gene. Therefore, as a rule, only male dogs are clinically affected. This is a spontaneous mutation of a very large gene associated with the X chromosome that was first recognized in male golden retrievers.* These golden retrievers have served as a reliable model for the similar human disorder referred to as Duchenne muscular dystrophy. Since its original recognition in golden retrievers, this dystrophinopathy has been found in many different breeds of dogs. The clinical signs vary considerably among affected dog breeds according to the nature of the spontaneous mutation in this very large gene. It is a rare disease in cats, in which there is a diffuse hypertrophy of muscles that severely limits their rate and range of motion. The clinical signs vary with the nature of the gene mutation. It can be lethal in young puppies. Severely affected dogs have limited life spans and often develop complications associated with their cardiomyopathy.

Video 5-17 shows the first two affected golden retrievers, Shadow and Goldie, that I (AD) studied in 1972. They came from a litter raised in Ithaca, New York. **Video 5-18** shows the third dog, which came from northwest Pennsylvania and was studied in 1982. Note the stiff, rolling movements of the limbs, this reflects both muscle fibrosis and a degree of myotonia in the affected muscles. Note the posture of the tarsus, the arch of the back, and the reduced range of motion of the temporomandibular joint. Compare Jake and these two golden retrievers with **Video 5-19** of Stubby, a 10-month-old rat terrier that was presented at 7 months old because of a stiff gait and dysphagia. Note the remarkably enlarged neck muscles at 10 and 14 months of age. This video was made during the clinical study of this dog by Dr. Ken Harkin at Kansas State University.[137] Stubby had a CK level of 66,420 U/l and he had no dystrophin in his skeletal muscle cell membranes. These videos show some of the remarkable range of clinical signs that can occur with the various mutations of this dystrophin gene. As we are able to define these various mutations, we should be able to associate them with their respective phenotypes.

Carrier females often have mildly elevated serum enzymes but rarely develop clinical signs. This relates to the volume of skeletal muscle cells that have the X chromosome with the mutated dystrophin gene. At the time these young male golden retrievers were studied in 1972, a similar clinical muscular dystrophy was being studied in young male Irish terriers in the Netherlands.[136]

Be aware of young dogs that are presented to you because of fatigue on exercising, inactivity, and slow growth. Any one or more of these clinical signs may reflect a muscular dystrophy related to a mutation in the genes responsible for the multiple components of the

---

*References 14, 80, 112, 130-132, 134, 136, 137.

(Continued)

CASE EXAMPLE 5-4—cont'd

dystrophin-glycoprotein complex. This cytoskeletal complex resides in the skeletal muscle cell membrane and is responsible for anchoring the actin myofilaments to the cell membrane and the adjacent basement membrane to support the cell during muscle contraction. A loss of any one of these components can result in muscle cell necrosis, a muscular dystrophy.[99,100] Be persistent in your clinical study of these often quite subtle clinical signs. Muscle specimens can be submitted to Dr. Diane Shelton at the Comparative Neuromuscular Laboratory at the University of California at San Diego for immunocytochemistry to determine whether there is any abnormality in this dystrophin-glycoprotein complex.

EXERCISE-INDUCED COLLAPSE IN LABRADOR RETRIEVERS

The previous two case examples of polymyopathy in Labrador retrievers are very different from a unique, presumably inherited disorder in Labrador retrievers that clinically affects adult dogs and causes collapse after vigorous exercise.[126] **Video 5-20** shows a 1-year-old male Labrador retriever in Oregon that had been exhibiting episodes of collapse for the past 2 months when exercised vigorously. He had been chasing the ball for about 10 minutes when the video was recorded. The owner stated that the same degree of exercise in the ocean surf never caused any fatigue in this dog. **Video 5-21** shows a 4-year-old male Labrador retriever in Ohio being exercised and exhibiting a collapsing episode. This had been occurring for at least 1 year. Both of these dogs recovered completely after about 15 minutes of rest. Exercise-induced collapse occurs in juvenile and young adult (7 months to 2 years), heavily muscled Labrador retrievers that are hyperexcitable and aggressively pursue their physical activities. Many of these cases are recognized when the dogs commence their training as field trial dogs. After a brief period of vigorous exercise (5 to 15 minutes) the affected dog starts to collapse in the pelvic limbs. The dog vigorously struggles to continue but rapidly loses its ability to stand, and collapses, usually in sternal recumbency. At the time of its collapse, the dog pants excessively and develops a fever of 107° to 108° F. Be aware that this hyperthermia occurs also in normal Labrador retrievers after vigorous exercise.[93] As these affected dogs struggle to stand, they exhibit some loss of balance and fall to one side. They never exhibit the typical quick, short strides of a dog with diffuse NMD. When the dog has collapsed, the patellar reflexes are usually absent, but the withdrawal reflexes and nociception are normal. These dogs always remain very alert and exhibit what we would interpret as frustration as they continually struggle to stand. They never show any loss of cranial nerve function. After a period of 10 to 20 minutes of rest, these dogs recover completely.

The anatomic diagnosis is not clear in these dogs. A diffuse NMD has been suspected, but the character of the collapse and the loss of balance suggest a possible central disorder with a vestibular system component. Possibly this is a striated muscle cell disorder and in addition to involving the extrafusal muscle fibers, it also affects the intrafusal muscle cells in the neuromuscular spindles. The loss of function in these spindles in the axial muscles, especially where they are so abundant in the cervical muscles, might account for the appearance of a loss of balance as these dogs struggle to keep from falling and as they attempt to get up. All ancillary studies performed in animals during collapse have been normal. They include blood chemistries, metabolic studies, MR imaging, edrophonium testing, and muscle biopsies. Necropsy has revealed no abnormalities.

Because of our lack of knowledge of the pathogenesis of this disorder, there is no specific treatment. The disorder is not progressive. Therefore, these dogs should lead healthy lives, as long as their exercise is limited so as to prevent episodes of collapsing. Death has occurred in dogs that have been excessively exercised. It has been observed that affected dogs do not collapse when they are exercised in water. Tests for malignant hyperthermia have all been negative for that disorder. Littermates and related dogs have been affected. Therefore, this should be considered to be an inherited disorder. The nature of the genetic defect has not yet been established. This exercise-induced collapse has been under intense investigation by a team of veterinarians led by Dr. Susan Meric Taylor at the University of Saskatchewan in Canada. We look forward to future achievements by this group.

EXERCISE-INDUCED FATIGUE

This is an appropriate point in the text to consider the differential diagnosis for the clinical complaint of exercise-induced fatigue in a dog.[56,89] Based on the presentation of this dog and the results of your examination, exercise-induced fatigue can be organized into two groups: dogs that are normal on your examination and those that are abnormal. For those that are normal and in which the paresis cannot be induced with exercise, it is useful to have the owner provide a video of the disorder so that you can determine whether this so-called exercise-induced fatigue is related to a diffuse NMD or another disorder, such as cataplexy, syncope, partial seizure, or a movement disorder.

When a dog is normal on your examination but the owner's description or the video clearly indicates diffuse NMD, the following disorders should be considered: myasthenia gravis, hypoglycemia, hyperkalemia, hypokalemia, muscular dystrophy, and, in Labrador retrievers, exercise-induced collapse.

Appropriate ancillary tests can help to differentiate these disorders. If the studies are unrewarding, be sure to include a thorough cardiovascular examination because the episodic paresis may be the only clinical sign of cardiac disease. Any decrease in cardiac output may result in peripheral hypoxia and paresis.

In dogs that show evidence of NMD on your examination but are worsened by exercise, you should consider study of the following disorders: myasthenia gravis, polymyopathy, muscular dystrophy, polymyositis, hypoglycemia, hyperkalemia, and hypokalemia.

MOTOR NEURON DISEASE: CONGENITAL

Return to Case Examples 5-3 and 5-4, where it was emphasized that you should be sure to consider disorders related to the breed of the animal you are examining. Another group of disorders that must be considered for the anatomic diagnosis of diffuse NMD in the young animal is a motor neuron disease (MND) that is also referred to as spinal muscular atrophy.* The primary lesion is an abiotrophy of GSE neurons in the spinal cord ventral gray column and brainstem nuclei.

By definition, an abiotrophy is the lack of a biologic substance in the cell that is necessary for the maintenance of the cell. This is an intrinsic cellular abnormality that is an inherited developmental defect. It results in the premature degeneration of that cell. In the nervous system, the parenchymal neurons normally live for the life of the animal and cannot be replaced. In an abiotrophy, these cells degenerate prematurely at various times after their initial formation in the embryo. Usually this degeneration does not occur until after birth, or at least, the clinical signs caused by this abiotrophy are often not recognized until a few weeks postnatally. It depends on the population

---

*References 19, 33, 55, 76, 90, 111, 114-116, 124.

of neurons that are affected and the rate of the progression of the abiotrophy. Neuronal abiotrophy most commonly affects Purkinje neurons in the cerebellum and GSE neurons in the spinal cord and brainstem. Often, multiple neuronal systems are affected. Clinical signs usually reflect the loss of those neurons most important for the animal's ability to support weight and to generate a coordinated gait.

Congenital MND is caused by an abiotrophy that affects GSE neurons, especially in the spinal cord. It occurs in young dogs and is commonly recognized as soon as the puppy begins to walk. It progresses at variable rates depending on the nature of the genetic abnormality. These are breed-related disorders. There is no published description of a congenital MND in the Labrador retriever. However, I (AD) have seen these lesions in the spinal cord and brainstem of a young Labrador retriever that was euthanized because of a progressive LMN gait disorder.

The most thoroughly studied canine congenital MND occurs in Brittany spaniels; it has been published as hereditary spinal muscular atrophy.[19,90] This is inherited as an autosomal dominant gene and presents as three phenotypes. The puppies that are homozygous for the dominant gene have an accelerated form that results in clinical signs by 6 to 8 weeks of age with tetraparesis, difficult prehension, and dysphagia. By 3 to 4 months of age the tetraparesis may progress to tetraplegia, along with severe neurogenic atrophy and associated limb deformities. Two phenotypes are seen in the heterozygote dogs. The intermediate form shows clinical signs of LMN tetraparesis at 6 to 12 months of age, and it slowly progresses to the inability to walk by 2 to 3 years of age. The chronic form consists of a subtle paresis that is not observed until a few years of age and is accompanied by mild neurogenic atrophy.

An example of a multisystem neuronal abiotrophy occurs as an autosomal recessive inherited disorder in Swedish Lapland dogs.[111] Clinical signs of LMN paresis are seen as the puppies start to walk at 5 to 7 weeks of age. Tetraparesis progresses to recumbency by a few months of age and is associated with severe neurogenic atrophy and deformity of the limbs, which is referred to as arthrogryposis. The latter contractures are the result of the shortening of the denervated skeletal muscles in the rapidly growing dog relative to the normally growing bones. The disparity in growth between the bones and the muscles results in the fixation of joints in a flexed (carpus) or extended (stifle, tarsus) position. These dogs have an extensive abiotrophy of GSE neurons in the spinal cord ventral gray columns but also of neurons in the spinal cord dorsal gray columns, spinal ganglia, and Purkinje neurons in the cerebellar cortex. The clinical signs all relate to the loss of the GSE neurons. You cannot expect to appreciate cerebellar ataxia in an animal with diffuse LMN disease. This disease was studied in the 1970s and was successfully eradicated by careful selection of dogs for breeding. We studied a similar multisystem abiotrophy in two Doberman pinscher puppies (in a litter of eight) that began to walk at about 4 to 5 weeks of age and then rapidly developed LMN tetraparesis and became recumbent, with severe muscle atrophy and rigid limbs due to the shortening muscles and the growing bones.

An inherited congenital MND limited to the spinal cord GSE neurons has been described in rottweiler puppies in which the signs include regurgitation due to the associated megaesophagus.[114,115] This is inherited as an autosomal recessive gene. A similar diffuse spinal cord GSE abiotrophy is inherited as an autosomal recessive gene in brown Swiss calves.[55] These calves usually show clinical signs of progressive LMN tetraparesis before 1 month of age.

Focal forms of neuronal abiotrophy have been reported but are rare. In 1936 Dr. C. R. Stockard was studying the musculoskeletal system of large-breed dogs by mating Great Danes with bloodhounds and Saint Bernards.[124] In a few litters, there were puppies that developed a rapidly progressive LMN paraparesis and priapism at 11 to 14 weeks of age. This was determined to be an inherited abiotrophy of lumbar GSE and GVE sympathetic preganglionic neurons. To our knowledge, this has never been diagnosed outside this laboratory experimental setting. In 1989, Dr. John Cummings published our observations of a focal abiotrophy of GSE neurons limited to the cervical intumescence in two littermate German shepherd puppies with progressive thoracic limb LMN paresis.[33] We have also studied two littermate Doberman pinscher puppies with a similar abiotrophy of GSE motor neurons in the intumescences, which resulted in their recumbency with thoracic limb contractures by the age of 6 weeks. A similar diagnosis was made in a 9-week-old saluki that had generalized LMN paresis and deformed thoracic limbs.[76]

EQUINE MOTOR NEURON DISEASE: ACQUIRED

Equine motor neuron disease (EMND) is an acquired disorder of adult horses that is strongly associated with an inadequate amount of vitamin E in the diet.* As a rule, it occurs in older adult horses, especially those that have been kept for a long period in a riding stable and fed hay and little grain, with no access to pasture. The most common chief complaints are generalized weakness, fatigue, and weight loss. The loss can be as much as 200 to 300 pounds, even though these horses have good appetites, because the weight loss is secondary to the denervation atrophy associated with the MND. The owner often observes the weight loss 3 to 6 weeks before recognizing the other clinical signs. Paresis is usually subacute in onset and progresses and does not usually occur until about 30% of the GSE neurons are lost from the spinal cord ventral gray columns (Figs. 5-14 and 5-15). Owners recognize that the affected horse is less active, does not perform as expected, trembles, and spends much more time lying down when in its stall. When you examine this horse, you will note that the horse acts uncomfortable when

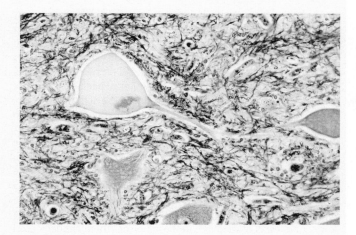

FIGURE 5-14 GSE neuron in the ventral gray column of a 12-year-old Quarter horse with EMND; it shows the swelling and chromatolysis of the cell body in the intitial stages of degeneration. Note the three normal neuronal cell bodies.

*References 25, 28, 29, 43-46, 72, 96, 110, 134.

(Continued)

CASE EXAMPLE 5-4—cont'd

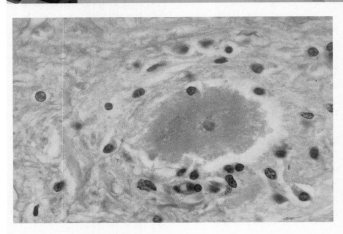

FIGURE 5-15 Same horse as in Fig. 5-14, showing neuronal cell body atrophy. Note the accumulating astrocytes and macrophages.

just standing. It keeps all of its limbs placed inappropriately under its trunk camped under rather than the usual stance; it continually shifts its weight from one limb to another, trembles in the muscles in all four limbs, sweats excessively, and holds its head and neck in a lowered position. You will observe that this horse will be unable to "lock its stifles" to help support its weight. In more chronic cases the tail may be carried in a slightly elevated position and occasionally a bizarre "stringhalt-like" movement may be seen as the limbs are protracted. These two clinical signs may be the result of denervation atrophy and fibrosis of affected muscles. There is no question that these horses prefer to walk rather than stand, which relates to the predilection of the MND for the GSE neurons that have the most active oxidative metabolism and that innervate the type 1 antigravity postural muscles. The observation that affected horses "walk better than they stand" is a very reliable guideline for separating EMND from virtually all other spinal cord diseases. The horses walk with short strides and circle with no delay in the onset of protraction. There is no evidence of any ataxia. When returned to their stalls, they usually immediately start circling to lie down. Once they are down, they act much more comfortable and will eat as soon as feed is offered to them. When not eating, they often rest the chin on the ground to support the weight of the head and neck. All of these clinical signs relate to the increased effort of supporting weight because of the loss of neurons to the postural muscles. **Video 5-22** shows Forget-Me-Not, a 9-year-old male thoroughbred with the history and many of the clinical signs that were just described.

It is believed that the GSE motor neurons that innervate the type 1 postural muscles have the most active oxidative metabolism, and their degeneration is the result of the oxidative stress that is created by an imbalance between pro- and antioxidants in the CNS tissues. The most significant of these is the dietary deficiency of the antioxidant vitamin E, which can be documented by determining low serum levels of vitamin E in these horses. There are decreased levels of superoxide dismutase in the CNS and blood. This enzyme normally converts the highly toxic superoxide radicle into hydrogen peroxide. There is no recognized genetic abnormality in the equine genome to explain these low levels; therefore, they may reflect an

overwhelming of this system by the patient's need for antioxidant activity. There are increased levels of copper in the nervous system and of iron in the liver and in the visible dental tartar on the incisors. Both of these are prooxidant catalysts for the production of highly toxic hydroxyl ion radicles that initiate lipid peroxidation and may contribute to the neuronal oxidative stress. There may be other components of the pathogenesis of this disorder, but all studies strongly support the deficiency of vitamin E as the most significant cause. In support of this, clinically normal adult horses that have low vitamin E levels when purchased will develop the identical clinical signs and lesions of EMND when maintained on a diet deficient in vitamin E for about 2 years. **Video 5-23** shows Teka, a 12-year-old saddle horse with the clinical signs of EMND that resulted from being fed a vitamin E–deficient diet for about 2 years. At necropsy, the microscopic lesions were identical to those in natural cases of this disorder.

In subacute to chronic cases with the anatomic diagnosis of diffuse NMD, the only significant disorder that explains the clinical signs is EMND. The occasional case of a horse with very acute onset may be confused with cases of botulism or acute diffuse exercise-induced rhabdomyolysis. For botulism, look for some evidence of a paretic tongue, paretic facial muscles, dysphagia, and anal and tail hypotonia. For rhabdomyolysis, look for elevated serum muscle enzyme levels. There are a number of ancillary procedures that help support the diagnosis of EMND:

1. The serum levels of vitamin E are usually extremely low.
2. In most affected horses, biopsy of the sacrocaudal dorsomedial muscle at the base of the tail, using a sacrocaudal epidural local anesthesia, reveals denervation atrophy in this muscle, which normally consists of a large component of type 1 muscle fibers.
3. In most affected horses, biopsy of the branch of the spinal accessory nerve to the sternocephalicus muscle where it enters the muscle at the origin of its tendon near its termination on the mandible reveals wallerian degeneration in the neuronal processes.[72] This degeneration follows the loss of the cell bodies of these neuronal processes in the cervical spinal cord ventral gray column. However, general anesthesia is usually necessary for this procedure.
4. Fundic examination reveals a yellowish discoloration in the retina in about 30% of affected horses; it results from the accumulation of retinal lipopigment that occurs in this disease.[110] The associated retinal degeneration is enough to be determined on electroretinography, but clinical evidence of any visual deficit has not been observed.[28]

Treatment with vitamin E supplements and access to good-quality pasture will stop the progress of the disorder, and some improvement may be seen, but a return to the athletic activity of the horse prior to clinical signs should not be expected because some degree of paresis and atrophy will persist. The disorder is readily prevented by providing a good source of vitamin E in the diet. Now that EMND is well known in the equine industry, vitamin E supplementation is a normal husbandry practice, and the incidence of clinical cases has decreased significantly.

EMND is an important animal model for a similar sporadic acquired MND in humans, which is known as amyotrophic lateral sclerosis (ALS), or Lou Gehrig disease.

CASE EXAMPLE 5-5

NMD Monoparesis—Thoracic Limb—Dog

Signalment: 10-year-old male Labrador retriever, Moose

Chief Complaint: Lame in the left thoracic limb

History: For the past 6 months this dog has exhibited a lame gait in the left thoracic limb, and it has slowly progressed. Numerous orthopedic examinations, including radiography, have been normal.

Examination: Video 5-24 shows Moose walking normally in all limbs except the left thoracic limb, which he carried flexed at the elbow (musculocutaneous nerves C6, C7) with the carpus bouncing on the floor, usually on its dorsal surface because of the inability to extend the carpus (radial nerves C7, C8, T1). He hopped well on the three normal limbs but collapsed if any weight was placed on the left thoracic limb (radial nerve). When the limb was manipulated, there was no tone in the carpus (radial nerve, median and ulnar nerves C7, C8, T1, T2). On elbow extension, resistance was felt in the elbow flexors (musculocutaneous nerve). On muscle palpation, only mild atrophy was perceived in the lateral scapular muscles (suprascapular nerves C6, C7), and it may be the result of disuse. There was significant atrophy in the triceps muscle (radial nerve) and in all the antebrachial muscles (radial nerve cranially, median and ulnar nerves caudally). The superficial pectoral muscle was normal (cranial pectoral nerves C6, C7), whereas the deep pectoral muscle was atrophied (caudal pectoral nerves C8, T1). There was no cutaneous trunci reflex on the left side (lateral thoracic nerves C8, T1), but Moose perceived the forceps stimulus. Sensory testing of the skin of the left thoracic limb did not reveal any areas of analgesia. Hypalgesia was difficult to determine with any degree of confidence. Palpation of the axilla and the ventral branches of C7 and C8 where they cross the cranial surface of the first rib was normal. Pupil size was normal.

Anatomic Diagnosis: Left (C7), C8, T1, and T2 spinal cord segments; spinal roots; spinal nerves and their ventral branches; the brachial plexus; the radial, median, ulnar, caudal pectoral, and lateral thoracic nerves

Differential Diagnosis: Malignant nerve sheath neoplasm, intervertebral disk protrusion, lymphoma, brachial plexus neuritis, chronic neuritis

MALIGNANT NERVE SHEATH NEOPLASM

Malignant nerve sheath neoplasm is the most common peripheral nerve neoplasm in the dog. It is usually located in spinal nerves, their roots, or both, where it occasionally can compress the spinal cord.[12] Involvement of the cervical spinal nerves is the most common site. This has to be the first consideration in Moose, the dog in this case example. Occasionally, the mass extends into the brachial plexus and is palpable in the axilla. It was not palpated in Moose. Sometimes these neoplasms cause considerable discomfort and it is difficult to determine how much of the lameness is caused by the discomfort and how much by the inability to support weight. EMG will confirm denervation when it is difficult to differentiate a neurologic disorder from an orthopedic disorder, but it will not indicate the cause of the denervation. Although significant atrophy commonly follows the denervation associated with a nerve sheath neoplasm, be aware that disuse atrophy can be surprisingly severe.

It is common to find that a portion of the neoplasm is located in the vertebral canal or is growing into it along the course of the spinal nerve through the intervertebral foramen. In time, this will result in compression of the spinal cord, and additional clinical signs will be observed (Figs. 5-16 through 5-18). The compression can

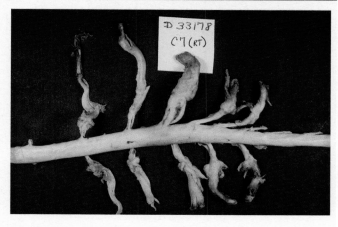

FIGURE 5-16 A 10-year-old male beagle. Dorsal view of the cervical intumescence with the associated spinal cord roots and spinal nerves (C5 to T2). It shows a malignant nerve sheath neoplasm of the right C7 spinal nerve dorsal and ventral roots and the spinal nerve.

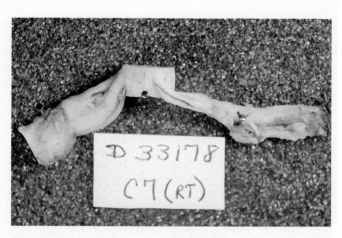

FIGURE 5-17 Ventral surface of the same specimen as in Fig. 5-16; it shows the C7 spinal cord segment with its associated spinal nerves and their roots and the nerve sheath neoplasm on the right side.

be extradural or, if the nerve roots are involved, it can be intradural and extramedullary. Occasionally both forms of compression occur. A myelogram will support this diagnosis when there is significant involvement of the vertebral canal. MR imaging is the ancillary procedure of choice because it can diagnose a neoplasm that lies anywhere between the axilla and the vertebral canal.

Surgery is the treatment of choice, but this neoplasm is so prolific that it extends into many nerve branches, making it very difficult to remove all of the neoplasm. Recurrences are common in a few months. In a dog like Moose, where there are no clinical signs to support the growth of a neoplasm in the vertebral canal, you should always evaluate the latter by imaging to help determine the prognosis and how extensive your surgery should be. If, as far as you can determine, the neoplasm involves primarily the brachial plexus, then amputation is the only surgical alternative. However, be aware that the neoplastic cells most likely are growing proximally in the ventral branches of the spinal nerves that contribute to the brachial plexus and in the spinal

(Continued)

CASE EXAMPLE 5-5—cont'd

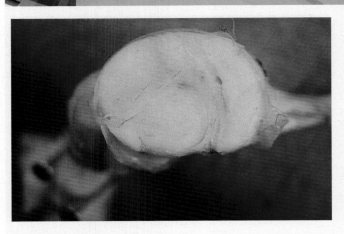

FIGURE 5-18 Same specimen as in Fig. 5-16; it shows the cranial surface of the C7 segment with the nerve sheath neoplasm on its right side. Note the marked compression and displacement of the spinal cord to its left side. At this stage, this dog would have exhibited a right side hemiparesis and ataxia: LMN paresis in the right thoracic limb, UMN paresis, and general proprioceptive ataxia in the right pelvic limb.

nerves themselves, where they are difficult to remove with the limb (Fig. 5-19). The prognosis for long-term recovery is guarded. Always remember carefully to evaluate the patient's ipsilateral pelvic limb for any paresis and ataxia that would suggest growth of the neoplasm within the vertebral canal and resulting spinal cord compression.

A degenerate intervertebral disk that protrudes laterally into an intervertebral foramen and compresses the spinal nerve located there is a common cause of lameness in one thoracic limb. However, this lameness is more the result of the discomfort caused by the compression of the meninges associated with that spinal nerve than

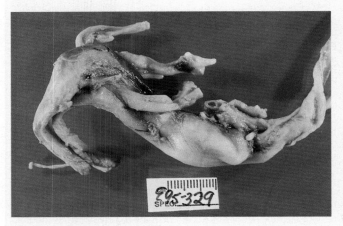

FIGURE 5-19 Brachial plexus removed from the amputated limb of a 12-year-old spayed female Labrador retriever; it shows a malignant nerve sheath neoplasm. The two nerves on the left of the photograph are the ventral branches of the C5 and C6 spinal nerves that also contained neoplastic cells in locations where they can grow into the vertebral canal.

the loss of motor neurons to extensor muscles. In Moose, there was much more evidence of inability to support weight than of discomfort, and the distribution of the neurogenic atrophy could not be explained by compression of a single spinal nerve. Radiography and MR imaging can help to support this diagnosis of intervertebral disk protrusion. Surgical removal of the protrusion is recommended.

BRACHIAL PLEXUS NEURITIS

Brachial plexus neuritis is a rare cause of LMN signs in one or both thoracic limbs.[27] This usually is a very acute disorder and would not be a consideration in Moose, the dog in this case example. The pathogenesis is poorly understood, but an allergic response that causes swelling of the spinal nerves at their intervertebral foramina has been proposed. We studied one Great Dane dog with an acute onset of brachial plexus neuritis in both thoracic limbs that was associated with eating horse meat.

CHRONIC NEURITIS

A chronic neuritis affecting the brachial plexus or its branches is more compatible with the prolonged history of slow progression of clinical signs in Moose. This is a nonsuppurative neuritis that probably is an autoimmune disorder.[11,23,24] The involvement of one limb would be unusual. We observed a chronic hypertrophic neuritis in a 6-year-old golden retriever that was most developed in the C7 and C8 spinal nerves on one side and caused clinical signs very similar to those seen in Moose. The involvement of the spinal nerve roots was seen on a computed tomography (CT) myelogram. The diagnosis was made on the basis of the histologic examination of the enlarged C7 nerve roots that were removed surgically. A nerve sheath neoplasm is more likely to result in greater nerve enlargement than is a chronic hypertrophic neuritis. MR imaging is necessary to determine the degree of extravertebral nerve enlargement and to diagnose involvement of the nerves in the vertebral canal when there is no displacement of the subarachnoid space. Myelography requires the latter to be diagnostic. Definitive diagnosis requires biopsy of an involved nerve. Bilateral hypertrophic neuritis of the brachial plexus has been diagnosed in a cat by means of MR imaging.[58]

BRACHIAL PLEXUS ROOT AVULSION

Avulsion of all or a portion of the roots of the brachial plexus is a peracute severe neurologic disorder caused by the patient's being struck by a car or motorcycle; it would not be considered in explaining the clinical signs in Moose, the dog in this case example. However, the character of the neurologic signs causing the lameness in this dog is similar to that which follows an injury that tears some of the spinal nerve roots or the spinal nerves, or both, that contribute to the brachial plexus.[61,62] This is considered to be a partial avulsion.

Video 5-25 shows Kaiser, a 6-month-old German shepherd, 2 days after being struck by a car. The inability to support weight is due to the loss of function of the radial nerve (C7, C8, T1). In this dog, the injury spared the C6 and possibly some of the C7 roots, enabling the dog to advance the limb by extending the shoulder (suprascapular nerve—C6, C7; nerve to brachiocephalicus muscle—C6) and to lift the limb off the floor by flexing the elbow (musculocutaneous nerve—C6, C7). The area of analgesia is in the autonomous zone of the radial nerve. A miosis was observed in the right eye; this places the lesion at the level of the spinal nerve roots or spinal nerves before they branch. Always carefully examine the eyes of these dogs. Avulsion of the ventral roots of T1 or of the T1 spinal nerve will cause a miosis because of the interruption of the preganglionic neuronal fibers located there. An elevated third eyelid and ptosis require interruption of the ventral roots of the T2 and T3 spinal cord segments. Only at this level can the GSE neurons to the thoracic limb and the GVE neurons to the head be simultaneously affected. The same GSE-LMN paralysis observed in the thoracic limb would occur if the injury were located within the brachial plexus, but this lesion could not affect the GVE innervation of the head because those preganglionic neurons leave the GSE neurons just lateral to the intervertebral foramen, where the ramus communicans leaves the spinal nerve to join the cranial portion of the thoracic sympathetic trunk. MR images obtained in Kaiser suggested a lesion at the nerve root level without an avulsion. This dog was much improved after 1 month (see video) and was normal by 6 weeks, which supports the resolution of hemorrhage and edema, and not a tearing-avulsion of the roots.

The majority of these injuries cause a nerve root or spinal nerve avulsion of most of the spinal nerves that contribute to the brachial plexus (Figs. 5-20 and 5-21). This causes complete flaccid LMN paralysis of the affected limb. **Video 5-26** shows Luke, an 8-year-old Labrador retriever mixed breed that was struck by a car as he was being used in a narcotic search. This occurred 2 weeks before he was videoed, and no change had occurred in his clinical signs in that time. The limb hangs dropped beside the body and is dragged, limp and useless, as the dog walks or runs normally on the other three limbs. The paralyzed limb is atonic, areflexic, and entirely analgesic distal to the elbow and in patches proximal to it that represent autonomous zones supplied by the C6 to T1 spinal

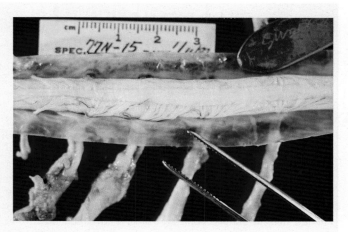

FIGURE 5-21 Same dog as in Fig. 5-20, with the dura reflected to show the avulsion of the left C7 to T1 dorsal roots.

nerve roots. This analgesia represents the loss of the GSA neurons as a result of the avulsion of the dorsal roots from C6 to T1. Note the analgesic patch just caudal to the neck of the scapular, which is the autonomous zone of the cranial lateral cutaneous brachial nerve (axillary—C7, C8), but the immediate nociceptive response just caudal to it, which is innervated by lateral cutaneous branches of the second or third thoracic spinal nerve. The cutaneous trunci reflex contraction was present on the right but not the left when the skin on the dorsal midline was pinched with forceps at any thoracic level (lateral thoracic nerve—C8, T1). There was miosis in the left eye (T1—preganglionic sympathetics).

Surgical reattachment of the torn ventral roots to the surface of the spinal cord to provide a guide for neuronal reinnervation has shown some success experimentally.[65]

Because your clinical examination can define only the degree of functional neurologic deficit and not the actual structural disorder responsible for it (i.e., hemorrhage and edema or an avulsion), it is important to provide supportive care for a few weeks to allow for recovery of the occasional dog that does not have an avulsion. If there is no indication of recovery after at least a 6-week period, the paralyzed limb should be amputated because it will impede the dog's efforts to move freely and can easily become abraded and infected.

The latter may result in osteomyelitis, sepsis, and even death. If, during the waiting period, the dog begins to chew on the limb or abrades it extensively, it should be amputated then. Dogs with only one thoracic limb do very well in most activities except swimming. Owners are often hesitant to elect amputation because of the aesthetics involved. It can be very helpful for them to see how well a dog actually does after an amputation. We recommend that you make a video of one of these dogs with an amputated thoracic limb to show reluctant owners so they can appreciate the extent to which these dogs can enjoy a good quality of life.

We have made this diagnosis of a brachial plexus root avulsion in cats and in many species of birds.[37]

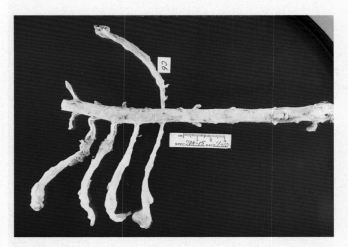

FIGURE 5-20 Dorsal view of the cervical and cranial thoracic spinal cord of a 3-year-old mixed-breed dog, showing avulsion of the left C7, C8, and T1 spinal nerves.

CASE EXAMPLE 5-6

NMD Monoparesis—Thoracic Limb—Horse

Signalment: 16-year-old male Clydesdale horse, Starlane

Chief Complaint: Right thoracic limb lameness

History: This lameness has progressed for 4 weeks. No abnormality has been found on orthopedic examination.

Examination: Video 5-27 shows Starlane's right thoracic limb lameness. In the absence of any discomfort on weight bearing and with a normal orthopedic examination, including nerve blocks, the lameness must be considered an inability to support weight and must therefore involve some component of the radial nerve. The degree of atrophy could be caused by disuse or could be neurogenic. There was no loss of nociception in the right thoracic limb, but remember that the horse is the only domestic animal in which the radial nerve has no autonomous zone for the branches that provide cutaneous innervation. On the cranial nerve examination, the only abnormality was the deviation of the nose and lip to the left side.

Anatomic Diagnosis: C7, C8, and T1 spinal cord segments, spinal nerve roots, spinal nerves, the brachial plexus, the radial nerve, and the buccal branches of the right facial nerve

Differential Diagnosis: Equine protozoal myelitis, malignant nerve sheath neoplasm, lymphoma, polyneuritis equi, other neoplasms

Equine protozoal myelitis caused by *Sarcocystis neurona* is the most common cause of inflammatory spinal cord lesions in the horse and is more completely described in Chapter 11, which discusses spinal cord diseases in large animals.[10,48,94] This form of myelitis involves both the gray and the white matter and occasionally is nearly limited to one area of gray matter and therefore must be a strong consideration in diagnosing this horse. Usually the gray matter lesion involves the adjacent white matter which, at the level of this anatomic diagnosis, could affect the UMN and GP systems running to and from the right pelvic limb. No pelvic limb signs were seen in Starlane. The normal lumbar CSF analysis in this horse would not rule out this diagnosis. The horse received antiprotozoal treatment based on this diagnosis for 2 weeks but showed no improvement.

Malignant nerve sheath neoplasm would be the most presumptive clinical diagnosis in a dog of this age and with these clinical signs and progressive history, but to our knowledge, this diagnosis involving spinal nerves has not been reported in the horse. In addition, it would not explain the facial nerve involvement.

LYMPHOMA

Lymphoma would be the most presumptive diagnosis in a cat of this age and with these clinical signs and history. In cats and cattle, extradural lymphoma is a common cause of progressive spinal cord compression. Occasionally in cats, the lymphoma develops and grows within peripheral nerves. Involvement of a spinal nerve and its roots may cause an intradural-extramedullary spinal cord compression.[68] Malignant nerve sheath tumor is rare at this level in cats.

Polyneuritis equi typically involves the nerves of the cauda equina and occasionally cranial nerves. It would be an unlikely cause of the anatomic diagnosis in this horse. See Case Example 5-9 for an example and description of this equine disease.

Spinal cord neoplasms are rare in horses of any age.

When this horse did not respond to antiprotozoal therapy, the owners requested euthanasia. The necropsy diagnosis in this horse was peripheral nerve lymphoma that involved primarily the C8 spinal nerve roots (without spinal cord compression), the C8 spinal nerve and its ventral branch, and a portion of the brachial plexus (Figs. 5-22 through 5-25). The clinical signs reflected the major contribution of

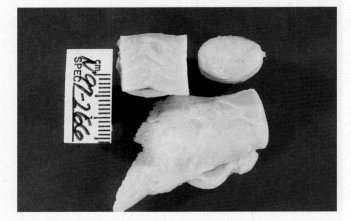

FIGURE 5-22 The 16-year-old male Clydesdale of this case example, showing gross enlargement of the ventral branch of the right C8 spinal nerve caused by an infiltrating lymphoma.

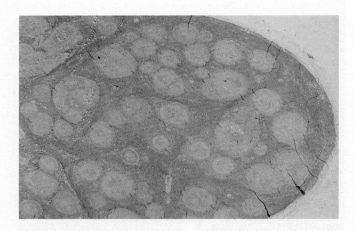

FIGURE 5-23 Microscopic view of the transverse section seen in Fig. 5-22. Note the infiltration of neoplastic lymphocytes within and surrounding the nerve fascicles bounded externally by the epineurium.

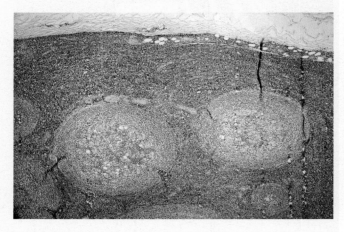

FIGURE 5-24 A high-power magnification of the tissue section in Fig. 5-23, showing the neoplastic lymphocytes in all components of the ventral branch of the C8 spinal nerve.

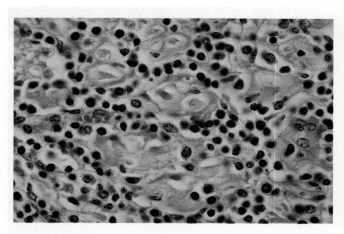

FIGURE 5-25 High-power magnification of the section in Figs. 5-23 and 5-24, showing the neoplastic lymphocytes infiltrating the endoneurium around individual myelinated axons.

this C8 spinal nerve to the radial nerve. The same lesion was present in the buccal branches of the right facial nerve. Figures 5-26 through 5-28 show an 18-month-old domestic shorthair with a similar infiltrating lymphoma affecting the left C7 and C8 spinal nerves and their roots.

EQUINE PROTOZOAL MYELITIS

Video 5-28 shows a 4-year-old thoroughbred gelding that had raced 10 days before he fell in the crossties and exhibited a reluctance to walk and lameness in both thoracic limbs. Note the normal pelvic limb gait and the hesitant short strides in the thoracic limbs. The right thoracic limb is slightly worse and has mild atrophy of the lateral scapular muscles. The anatomic diagnosis is C6 to T2 spinal cord ventral gray columns, spinal nerve roots, and spinal nerves. The differential diagnosis is the same as in this case example. The serum was positive for antibodies to *S. neurona*. The CSF was normal. This horse was treated with antiprotozoal drugs but became recumbent

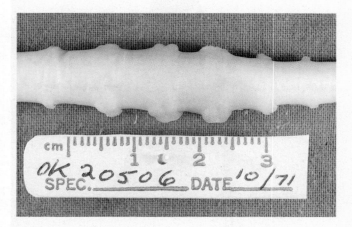

FIGURE 5-26 Cervical intumescence of an 18-month-old domestic shorthair with a history of LMN paresis of its left thoracic limb that over months progressed to left hemiparesis and ataxia, followed by tetraparesis and ataxia of all four limbs. Note the discoloration and swelling of the left C7 and C8 spinal nerve roots caused by an infiltrating lymphoma. This was incorrectly published as a lesion caused by an intervertebral disk extrusion.[53] At the time the report was published, no microscopic examination had been performed.

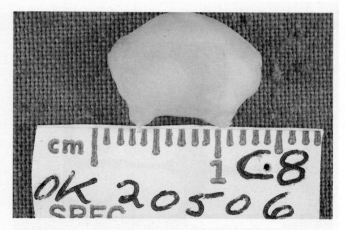

FIGURE 5-27 Transverse section of the C8 spinal cord segment of the specimen in Fig. 5-26. Note the marked displacement and compression of the spinal cord by the lymphoma.

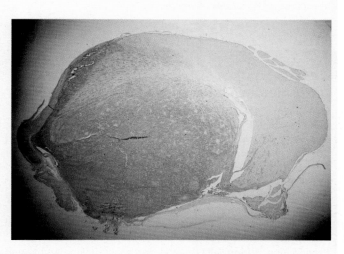

FIGURE 5-28 Microscopic view of the tissue section seen in Fig. 5-27, with the lymphoma growing in the nerve roots and compressing the spinal cord.

2 days later and was euthanized. Necropsy revealed an extensive hemorrhagic myelitis centered in the ventral gray columns of the cervical intumescence bilaterally. Protozoal organisms were found in the lesion (Fig. 5-29).

INJURY

Video 5-29 shows a 6-month-old male thoroughbred that was found at pasture with a severe non–weight-bearing left thoracic limb lameness. Note the dropped position of the elbow and the complete inability to support weight. Palpation and manipulation of this limb caused no discomfort and showed hypotonia. This is a complete radial paralysis presumed to be due to an injury of the radial nerve at the level of the brachial plexus as the result of some form of trauma that occurred while at pasture. About 50% of young horses with these signs, including this one, recover spontaneously in a few weeks. Necropsies of these cases show lesions compatible with an injury of the brachial plexus where it lies between the scapula and the first rib. A spinal nerve root avulsion has not been diagnosed in the horse.

(Continued)

CASE EXAMPLE 5-6—cont'd

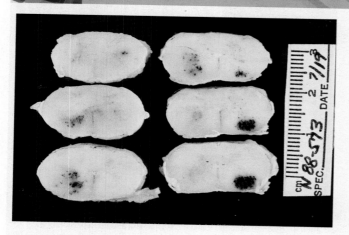

FIGURE 5-29 Transverse section of the cervical intumescence of the horse seen in Video 5-28. The discoloration of the spinal cord gray matter is due to a hemorrhagic myelitis caused by *S. neurona*.

Compare Video 5-29 of this 6-month-old thoroughbred with **Video 5-30** of a 15-month-old Belgian that had been lame in the right thoracic limb since being kicked in the region of the elbow a few days before. The swelling had disappeared but not the lameness. Note the ability of this Belgian to support weight but the hesitation in the extension of the carpus and digit due to the injury of the distal portion of the radial nerve. After innervating the extensors of the elbow, the radial nerve courses distally on the lateral surface of the brachialis muscle, where it terminates in muscular branches to the extensors of the carpus and digit and in cutaneous branches to the cranial and lateral surfaces of the antebrachium. The cutaneous distribution overlaps with the cutaneous branches from other peripheral nerves, so there is no autonomous zone for the radial nerve in the horse. This Belgian was kicked at the level of the elbow, where the radial nerve is subcutaneous on the surface of the brachialis muscle. The same signs are seen in dogs that are injured at this site by moving vehicles.

CASE EXAMPLE 5-7

Infraspinatus Contracture—Dog

Signalment: 2-year-old female Brittany spaniel, Seafuss
Chief Complaint: Left thoracic limb lameness
History: While bird hunting with her owner, this dog disappeared from the owner's sight, and when she reappeared shortly later she would not bear weight on the left thoracic limb. There was no evidence of any swelling or obvious fracture. The owner rested her in the kennel and Seafuss began to use the limb cautiously after a few days. Over the next 3 to 4 weeks, the presumptive discomfort disappeared and she readily used the limb, but the owner has noticed that it is still not normal.

Examination: Video 5-31 shows how the thoracic limb is protracted with the medial rotation of the elbow and lateral course of the paw. Use slow motion to fully appreciate this movement. The elbow appears mildly deviated medially when the limb is supporting weight but is exacerbated as soon as the limb is lifted off the floor for protraction. When the examiner stands over this dog to assess the degree of rotation of the shoulders by rotating the brachium medially and laterally, note the decreased range of motion when the left brachium is rotated medially. This is due to restriction caused by a shortening of the lateral rotator muscles of the shoulder (infraspinatus and teres minor). Normally the potentially very mobile shoulder joint is kept in its straight craniocaudal course during protraction by the balance between the medial rotators (subscapularis and teres major muscles) and the lateral rotators (infraspinatus and teres minor muscles). This dog has experienced a shortening of the left infraspinatus muscle, which she most likely injured while hunting. If she stepped into a hole while running and overextended her left shoulder, the distal edge of the spine of the scapular would be suddenly forced into the distal belly of the infraspinatus muscle, causing it to tear. As this injury healed and fibrosis occurred in the muscle, it could shorten and create a mechanical tension that would force lateral rotation and limit medial rotation. Note that when you force excess lateral rotation at the shoulder, the elbow rotates medially. This is not a problem at the elbow. The abnormal position of the elbow reflects the primary

shoulder disorder (Fig. 5-30). Treatment requires removing the fibrous portion of the affected infraspinatus muscle. The last portion of the video of Seafuss shows her normal gait after this surgery.

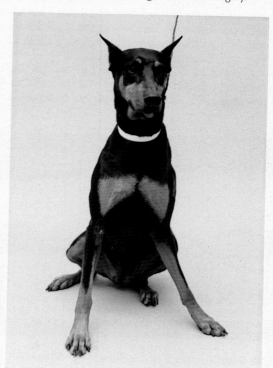

FIGURE 5-30 A 2-year-old Doberman pinscher that was struck by a vehicle and 1 month later was presented for a persistent abnormality in the use of the left thoracic limb. Its gait was similar to that seen in Videos 5-31 through 5-33, and this dog sits with the characteristic posture of a dog with excessive lateral rotation of the shoulder, which results in medial displacement of the elbow. This is an example of the infraspinatus contracture that follows an injury to the muscle and the healing by fibrosis.

The next three videos show two dogs with this same infraspinatus contraction[5,120] and histories similar to that of the dog in this case example. **Video 5-32** shows a 4-year-old pointer crossbreed and **Video 5-33A** shows an 8-year-old male Labrador retriever. **Video 5-33B** shows the same Labrador retriever viewed in slow motion. (We thank Dr. Marc Kent of the University of Georgia for the use of this video.)

This disorder is presented here because it is often confused with a peripheral nerve disorder, but that cannot explain what is happening here. Experimental sectioning of the suprascapular nerve will denervate the supraspinatus and infraspinatus muscles, but this will not cause any gait abnormality in the dog or cat, only atrophy of these muscles.[116] Horses that run into a doorway or fence post with the cranial aspect of the scapula may injure this nerve where it crosses the scapular notch on the cranial surface of the neck of the scapula. This may cause a slight lateral deviation, abduction, or lateral buckling of the shoulder when weight is borne on that limb. The collar used with the draft horse may chronically compress this nerve at this site if the collar is too tight. Usually the denervation atrophy of these muscles is the most obvious clinical sign; the lateral deviation of the shoulder during walking is very mild. The disorder is often referred to as sweeney, which was the name of a type of collar made for working draft horses. This equine occupational hazard is similar to the carpal tunnel syndrome in humans.

Lesions that involve the other thoracic limb peripheral nerves do not produce any significant clinical signs. Experimental sectioning of both the median and ulnar nerves causes only a slight carpal overextension-drop of the carpus. More important, when you observe a significant carpal overextension that produces a palmigrade posture, it is a reflection of loss of the integrity of the palmar carpal ligaments. If you remove all the nerves and muscles from a thoracic limb specimen, you cannot manually force the carpus into a palmigrade position as long as the palmar carpal ligaments are intact. These ligaments become stretched when the thoracic limb has to bear more weight than usual, such as when a young dog has a fracture in one thoracic limb and bears all its weight on the normal limb for a period of weeks. That normal limb will slowly assume a more palmigrade posture. Older dogs that are overweight often assume this carpal posture. Chronic neuromyopathies cause dogs that have lost the normal muscle strength necessary to support weight to assume a palmigrade posture. This clinical sign reflects the secondary loss of integrity of the palmar carpal ligaments and is not a sign of a specific neuromuscular disorder. A plantigrade posture in a pelvic limb has a very different pathogenesis; it will be described in Case Examples 5-17 and 5-21 in this chapter with the pelvic limb disorders.

CASE EXAMPLE 5-8

LMN Paraplegia—Dog

Signalment: 5-year-old male Great Dane, Figliaro

Chief Complaint: Unable to walk with the pelvic limbs

History: Two days before our examination of this dog, he was outdoors walking on a leash with his owner. On the way back into their home, he stumbled going up the stairs and collapsed in the house. The next morning he was seen by a veterinarian who diagnosed paraplegia and who then made arrangements to get specialty studies for this dog.

Examination: Video 5-34 shows that this dog could get up only on his thoracic limbs. When supported by his tail, he walked well with the thoracic limbs but the pelvic limbs were dragging on the ground, and there was only an occasional slight hip flexion to try to advance the limbs. The pelvic limbs were hypotonic, with normal patellar reflexes but no flexor reflexes when digits 3 through 5 were stimulated. Noxious stimulation of the medial side of the limb or the cranial aspect of the thigh elicited a slight flexion of the hip. This dog was very stoic and displayed only minimal displeasure in response to this method of stimulation. The tail and anus were atonic, areflexic, and analgesic. There was analgesia of the perineum, the caudal thigh, and all of the crus and paw except for the medial surface. There was a line of analgesia at about the L7 vertebral level. This could be reliably determined only by using an electric cattle prod. The bladder was enlarged and urine was constantly dribbling from the penis. No discomfort was elicited when the lumbar and sacral vertebrae were palpated.

Anatomic Diagnosis: L6, L7, all the sacral and caudal spinal cord segments, the spinal nerve roots, the spinal nerves. Possibly, there is some mild involvement of a few more cranial lumbar segments.

The basis for this anatomic diagnosis is as follows. The examination showed complete lack of LMN and GSA function to the tail (caudal nerves); anus; perineum (pudendal nerve branches from the sacral plexus); caudal thigh (caudal cutaneous femoral nerve from the sacral plexus); caudal thigh muscles and all the crural muscles and the skin of the crus and paw except for the medial surface (sciatic nerve—L6, L7, S1). Function was normal in the distribution of the femoral nerve (L4, L5) to the quadriceps femoris and the medial side of the distal thigh, crus, and paw (saphenous branch of the femoral nerve); in the distribution of the lateral cutaneous femoral nerve (L3, L4) to the cranial and craniolateral side of the proximal thigh; and in the distribution of the genitofemoral nerve (L3, L4) to the skin of the proximal medial thigh. When these intact nerves were stimulated, the dog's response was a mild flexion of the hip using his iliopsoas muscle, which is innervated by almost all of the ventral branches of the lumbar spinal nerves. The line of analgesia along the dorsal lumbar area is usually about two vertebrae caudal to the cranial aspect of the lesion because the dorsal branches of the lumbar spinal nerves that are stimulated course caudally from their intervertebral foramen for the distance of about two vertebrae. The response to the electric prod at about the L7 level occurred because of impulses passing through the intact dorsal branches of the L5 spinal nerves. The lack of much hip flexion when the dog was supported to walk suggested that there was perhaps more involvement of the white matter cranial to the L6 level. Not shown on the video is the analgesia of the skin of the penis (dorsal nerve of the penis, a branch of the pudendal nerve from the sacral plexus) and the normal nociception in the skin of the prepuce (genitofemoral nerve from the ventral branches of the L3, L4 spinal nerves).

(Continued)

CASE EXAMPLE 5-8—cont'd

Differential Diagnosis: External injury, fibrocartilaginous embolic myelopathy (FCEM), intervertebral disk extrusion, neoplasia, myelitis, and lumbosacral syndrome

When a history supports a peracute onset and no obvious progression of clinical signs after 24 hours, two major disorders should be considered: external or internal trauma and vascular compromise. When the clinical signs involve the spinal cord or cauda equina, the possibility of an acute intervertebral disk extrusion must be included; it would be considered a form of internal trauma. The history of Figliaro in this case example denies any external trauma. This dog is a breed in which intervertebral disk extrusions usually do not occur until middle age or older, so because the dog is 5 years of age, this diagnosis must be considered. The absence of any indication of discomfort when the lumbosacral vertebrae were palpated would be more likely with a vascular compromise than with an intervertebral disk extrusion, but there are many exceptions to this clinical observation. The most common vascular compromise is a sudden hemorrhagic or ischemic infarction of the spinal cord secondary to a shower of fibrocartilaginous emboli that blocks the arterial supply.*

Such a peracute onset would be unusual for a neoplasm, especially one that was intramedullary (within the spinal cord parenchyma). However, extramedullary neoplasms, either intradural or extradural, that grow and compress the spinal cord slowly may suddenly produce clinical signs when the autoregulatory system that maintains the vascular perfusion of the spinal cord fails or a hemorrhage occurs in the neoplasm. Myelitis in these spinal cord segments would produce a progressive clinical disorder. The same chronic clinical course would be expected for a lumbosacral syndrome, and it would not produce the severe degree of neurologic deficit that has occurred in this dog.

FIBROCARTILAGINOUS EMBOLIC MYELOPATHY

Radiographs were normal in this dog, and a cisternal myelogram showed a mild intramedullary swelling at the level of the lumbosacral intumescence. This study supported the diagnosis of FCEM, which could cause this swelling from hemorrhage and edema. Treatment for this disorder is mostly supportive. The use of corticosteroids has not been shown to be of any significant value in spinal cord injury and may have serious side effects. When FCEM causes such severe gray matter damage as has occurred in this case, the prognosis for spontaneous recovery is poor. However, when it occurs at other levels of the spinal cord, and when the signs are caused by dysfunction of the white matter and are less severe, spontaneous recovery is common. Our rule of thumb is that if there is no indication of any improvement of clinical signs in 14 days, it is very unlikely that any recovery will occur.

This dog was euthanized after 2 weeks of supportive care, and necropsy showed an extensive hemorrhagic and ischemic infarction of most of the components of the spinal cord, from the L6 segment caudally (Figs. 5-31 through 5-33). These lesions were associated with numerous emboli of fibrocartilage in arteries and a few veins on the surface of the spinal cord as well as in the parenchyma. This disease is described in Chapter 10, along with diseases of the spinal cord in small animals.

*References 36, 67, 79, 109, 128, 146, 147.

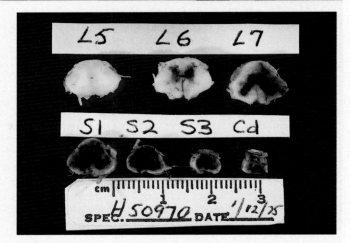

FIGURE 5-31 Transverse sections of the lumbosacral intumescence of the dog in this case example, showing the gross lesions of hemorrhagic necrosis due to fibrocartilaginous emboli.

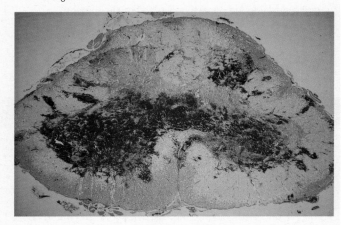

FIGURE 5-32 Microscopic view of the L7 spinal cord segment seen in Fig. 5-31, showing diffuse hemorrhagic and ischemic necrosis.

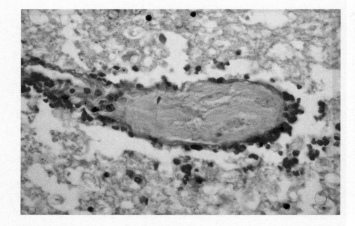

FIGURE 5-33 High-power magnification of the section of L7 in Fig. 5-32, showing a fibrocartilaginous embolus in a blood vessel in the right ventral funiculus.

CASE EXAMPLE 5-9

Sacrocaudal Dysfunction—Horse

Signalment: 8-year-old male warm blood horse

Chief Complaint: Abnormal facial expression and rectal impaction

History: About 10 days prior to examination, the owner noticed that the right ear drooped and the nose was deviated to the left side. For 1 week, there was no movement of the tail, feces occluded the anus and rectum and had to be removed manually, and the penis often protruded from its sheath.

Examination: Video 5-35 shows that a slow, plodding gait and circling were normal for this horse. Note the prominent palpable buccal branches of the right facial nerve. The skin of the penis, which is innervated by branches of the dorsal nerve of the penis from the sacral plexus, was analgesic. However, the skin of the prepuce, which is innervated by branches of the genitofemoral nerve from the ventral branches of spinal nerves L3 and L4, had normal nociception. Note the atonia, areflexia, and analgesia of the tail, anus, and perineum. The area of cutaneous analgesia was in the autonomous zones of the caudal and caudal sacral spinal nerves.

Anatomic Diagnosis: Right facial nerve, bilateral sacral 3 to 5 and caudal spinal cord segments, spinal nerve roots and spinal nerves

Differential Diagnosis: Polyneuritis equi (neuritis of the cauda equina), equine protozoal myelitis, diskospondylitis-abscess, cryptococcal leptomeningitis and radiculitis, neoplasm

POLYNEURITIS EQUI, OR NEURITIS OF THE CAUDA EQUINA

Polyneuritis equi, which is also known as neuritis of the cauda equina because of the location of the major lesions,[32,35,104] is the most presumptive diagnosis in this horse. The cause of this disease is unknown but an autoimmune disorder is most suspect. The intradural spinal nerve root lymphoplasmacytic inflammatory lesions are very similar to those seen in polyradiculoneuritis in dogs, but in the horse there is an additional extradural granulomatous lesion that enlarges and causes the extradural portion of the spinal nerves to adhere, forming a mass lesion within the vertebral canal (Figs. 5-34 through 5-36). The reason for the formation of this extradural lesion is unknown. Lumbar CSF often has an elevated protein content and

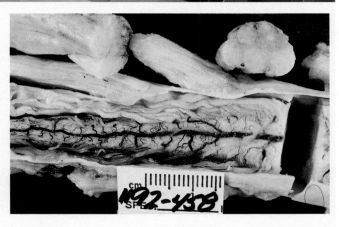

FIGURE 5-35 Closer view of the enlarged inflammed extradural spinal nerves compared with the intradural nerve roots. Note the shrunken, discolored right intradural dorsal roots.

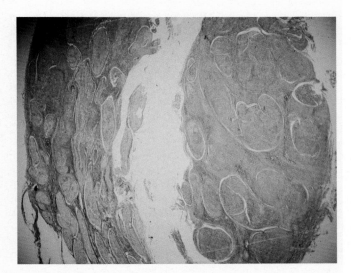

FIGURE 5-36 Microscopic section of a transverse section of one of the enlarged extradural spinal nerves in the horse in Fig. 5-34. The inflammation proliferates around and within the nerve fascicles.

a pleocytosis with nonsuppurative leucocytes. The prognosis for recovery is poor. Continual care is necessary to assure elimination of feces and urine. Occasionally there is a mild pelvic limb gait deficit if the lesions become extensive enough in the caudal lumbar and cranial sacral spinal nerve roots. This will appear as a partial sciatic nerve dysfunction. There may be histologic evidence of lesions in many of the spinal nerve roots but only occasionally are clinical signs seen in the limbs. However, involvement of cranial nerves VII, VIII and, less often, V is seen in some horses; it relates to the facial paralysis in this horse. It is unusual for the cranial nerve deficits to occur before those that involve the sacrocaudal nerve roots, as happened in this horse.

Equine protozoal myelitis limited to these spinal cord segments is the most likely other cause of these clinical signs. To affect the

(Continued)

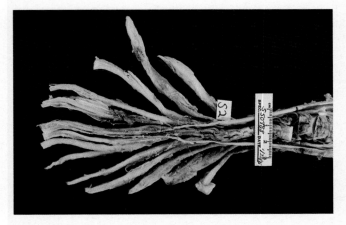

FIGURE 5-34 Dorsal view of the cauda equina of an 8-year-old warm blood gelding with polyneuritis equi after the adhered extradural spinal nerves were torn apart at necropsy.

CASE EXAMPLE 5-9—cont'd

facial nucleus in the brainstem and no other system located there is possible for this protozoal agent, but it is unusual. If there are no serum antibodies to *S. neurona*, this diagnosis can be considered unlikely.

Diskospondylitis at the L6-S1 articulation or an abscess at this site would be much more likely in a foal than in a horse of this age.

Neoplasms of the spinal cord, nerve roots, and extradural space are rare in horses.

I (AD) have seen one case of cryptococcal leptomeningitis and radiculitis that involved this anatomic site in an adult horse with identical sacrocaudal clinical signs. This fungal agent should be observed in the lumbar CSF.[1]

CASE EXAMPLE 5-10

Sacrocaudal Dysfunction—Dog

Signalment: 10-year-old male German shepherd, Max
Chief Complaint: Loss of control of excretions and expresses discomfort when he stands up
History: For the past few weeks, when he stands up after a nap, a puddle of urine or occasionally a small clump of feces has been left on the floor, and his tail has often been soiled with feces. Max gets up slowly and occasionally cries out, and he resents any petting over his pelvic region.
Examination: Max had a normal gait except for a slight overflexion of each tarsus. He had no patellar reflex in the left pelvic limb and it was depressed in the right pelvic limb. The flexor reflexes and postural reactions were normal. Tail and anal tone were poor. The perineal reflex seemed depressed. Max strongly resented firm palpation at the level of the lumbosacral articulation, especially if it was done while his pelvic limbs were raised off the floor.
Anatomic Diagnosis: L7, sacral and caudal spinal cord segments, spinal nerve roots or spinal nerves. This anatomic diagnosis explains the paretic tail, the incontinence, and the overflexed tarsus. Be aware that a mild overflexion of the tarsus is normal in this breed and often difficult to differentiate from the posture of a mild tibial nerve deficit. The neuronal cell bodies of the tibial nerve portion of the sciatic nerve are located in the L7 and S1 spinal cord segments. A lesion at the L4, L5 spinal cord segments, their roots or spinal nerves, or the femoral nerves would be needed to explain the abnormal patellar reflexes. However, this abnormality may have nothing to do with the chief complaint or the other clinical signs in this dog; a small percentage of old dogs lose one or both of their patellar reflexes with no other indication of any femoral nerve dysfunction. It is age related and probably represents some disturbance to the sensory portion of the reflex arc because there is no evidence of any inability to support weight or any atrophy of the quadriceps muscle.[87]

Two anatomic features that relate to this anatomic diagnosis are important to appreciate. The involvement of the caudal nerves leading to the tail strongly supports the theory that the lesion is within the vertebral canal because these nerves only course through this canal, then leave it through the intervertebral foramina to innervate the axial muscles of the tail directly. They never have any course through the pelvic cavity. If you destroyed all the neural components that are located in the vertebral canal at the lumbosacral articulation in the adult dog, it would include all the caudal and sacral nerves and possibly the L7 spinal nerves. Note how such a partial destruction agrees with the anatomic diagnosis in this case. Note also that the only gait abnormality that a lesion at this site can explain is a partial sciatic-tibial nerve deficit. Some dogs that have severe discomfort localized

to this articulation have an entrapment of one or both of the L7 spinal nerves caused by the degenerative joint disease at this articulation.
Differential Diagnosis: Lumbosacral-cauda equina syndrome, intervertebral disk protrusion, diskospondylitis, neoplasm, external injury (*Note:* Some authors include all of the disorders listed here except for external injury as part of the lumbosacral syndrome. We have joined the majority and limited the use of the term *syndrome* to those disorders that are a form of degenerative joint disease [DJD].)

LUMBOSACRAL SYNDROME, OR CAUDA EQUINA SYNDROME

Lumbosacral syndrome, or cauda equina syndrome,[86,101,107,108] is the most presumptive clinical diagnosis for Max. These are the two names most commonly used for this DJD that occurs at the L7-S1 articulation in older dogs, especially the larger breeds. Do not confuse this cauda equina syndrome with the equine disease that was just described; that one is a neuritis of the cauda equina. There is no precise anatomic definition of the cauda equina, which is the name applied to the collection of nerves that courses along the surface of the conus medullaris. Most authors include the caudal, sacral, and L7 spinal nerves in this term. Other names for this degenerative joint disease include lumbosacral malformation-malarticulation, lumbosacral instability or spondylolisthesis, and lumbosacral spondylopathy. The term *lumbosacral stenosis* fits the compression here but has been more commonly used for a malformative vertebral disorder at this articulation that occurs in young adults of small breeds.

The lumbosacral syndrome represents a plethora of lesions that classify as chronic DJD. It can involve the fibrous articulation, with proliferation of the annulus fibrosis of the intervertebral disk dorsally into the vertebral canal. Spondylosis with excessive bony proliferation on the caudoventral and lateral aspects of the body of L7 and on the cranioventral and lateral aspects of the body of S1, often with fusion, is common at this articulation and can be found in many dogs with no clinical signs of any nerve compression. DJD of the articular processes results in a marked thickening of the processes and the joint capsules. Proliferation of the associated yellow and dorsal longitudinal ligaments can contribute to the narrowing of the vertebral canal at this site. The cause of the DJD at this articulation is unknown but may reflect a chronic malarticulation with or without some instability. Prior to MR and CT imaging, many radiographic contrast procedures were used to try to confirm this lesion but were hampered by the termination of the subarachnoid space cranial to this articulation in many of the large-breed dogs, or else the space was as narrow as a thread at this site. Fat in the epidural space sometimes interfered with epidurography.

The use of intraosseous vertebral venography to show compromise of the internal ventral vertebral venous plexus at this articulation was only sporadically reliable. Most neurologists now prefer MR imaging. Decompressive surgery is the treatment of choice but has variable results. Paramount for successful surgery is early detection of the disorder, prior to permanent fecal or urinary incontinence.

INTERVERTEBRAL DISK PROTRUSION

Intervertebral disk protrusions can occur at any of the intervertebral fibrous articulations; they are more completely described along with spinal cord disease in Chapter 10. Such a protrusion could occur at the L7-S1 articulation without other evidence of any DJD and cause the clinical signs observed in this dog. Diagnosis and treatment are the same as for the lumbosacral syndrome.

DISKOSPONDYLITIS

Diskospondylitis resulting from bacterial or fungal causes is common at this site but can occur at any fibrous intervertebral articulation. This lesion is often associated with severe discomfort and sometimes causes the systemic effects of an infection, with fever and leucocytosis. In some dogs the same infectious agent may cause cystitis. This diagnosis can often be made by plain radiographs, but remember that the radiographic changes take a few weeks to become evident and you should not rule out this diagnosis just because there are no radiographic changes. MR and CT imaging may be useful in subtle cases. The ideal antibiotic treatment is based on culture of the blood or lesion aspirate with identification of the organism and antibiotic-sensitivity testing. Occasionally, surgical decompression is necessary in these cases.

NEOPLASM

All of the clinical signs exhibited by Max in Case Example 5-8 could relate to a neoplasm that is growing at this site. The tumor could be extradural, such as lymphoma, sarcoma, or a metastatic vertebral tumor such as hemangiosarcoma. A malignant nerve sheath tumor could occur here but not a glioma because there is no spinal cord at this level. Diagnosis requires imaging first and then histologic examination of a specimen obtained surgically or by aspiration. Treatment is dependent on this diagnosis.

L7 FRACTURE

External injury is included here because L7 fractures are fairly common after an animal has been struck by a car, and if the nervous tissue damage is limited to this site, the clinical signs are similar to those seen in this case. However, the onset of clinical signs will, of course, be sudden and they will not progress. As a rule, traumatic lesions here usually cause more severe clinical signs: complete LMN paralysis and analgesia of the tail and anus, analgesia of the perineum, continual urinary incontinence resulting from overflow and lack of urethralis muscle function, and more significant signs of sciatic nerve dysfunction. **Video 5-36** shows a 2-year-old male miniature poodle 10 days after a fracture of L7, with ventral displacement of the caudal portion of the L7 body that compromised the vertebral canal by more than 50% (Fig. 5-37). Note the ability of this dog to support weight (normal femoral nerves) and the ability to flex the hips to advance the limbs (normal lumbar spinal nerve ventral branch innervation of the psoas major muscle); but note also the loss of stifle flexion, tarsal

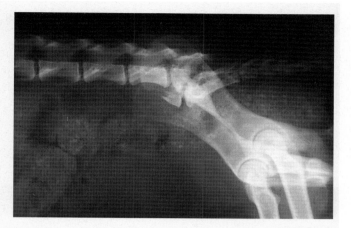

FIGURE 5-37 Radiograph of the L7 fracture in the miniature poodle seen in Video 5-36.

flexion or extension, and digital extension (abnormal sciatic nerve function bilaterally). The L6-S1 spinal nerve lesions at the site of the fracture are not complete because nociception is intact on the lateral digits. Note the dilated areflexic, analgesic anus that, along with the analgesic perineum and tail, indicates complete dysfunction of the sacral and caudal nerves. This dog shows how a dog can ambulate despite a bilateral sciatic nerve dysfunction.

The diagnosis of the lumbosacral syndrome was made in Max, the dog in this case example, by MR imaging and was treated by means of a dorsal laminectomy, including removal of the protruding portions of the articular processes and their joint capsule and of the protruding annulus fibrosis.

LIMBER TAIL SYNDROME, OR ACUTE CAUDAL MYOPATHY

Limber tail syndrome, or acute caudal muscle injury, is a disorder of the muscles in the tail that has been described in hunting dogs, especially pointers and Labrador retrievers.[123] Other terms for the syndrome include cold tail, swimmer's tail, frozen tail, and sprain tail. Until the precise pathogenesis is determined, we will refer to this disorder as acute caudal myopathy. The term *caudal* has replaced *coccygeal* for the tail vertebrae, muscles, blood vessels, and nerves. Dogs with this syndrome often present with a completely flaccid tail or a tail that is held in a dorsal plane (horizontally) for several inches from the tail base and then hangs ventrally with no tone. The clinical signs of tail paresis and discomfort most commonly develop after vigorous exercise, which includes hunting or swimming. I (EG) most commonly see Labrador retrievers with this syndrome 1 to 2 days after spending a day swimming at the beach. Other predisposing factors include prolonged cage transportation and exposure to cold, wet weather. Despite the marked degree of flaccidity in the tail, nociception is intact. Ancillary studies show a mild elevation in the level of serum creatine kinase and spontaneous electric activity on EMG that is restricted to the caudal muscles. Thermography and scintigraphy also show abnormalities restricted to these caudal muscles. Histologic study of the affected caudal muscles shows muscle fiber lesions compatible with ischemia. These lesions are similar to those seen in human muscles affected by an acute compartmental syndrome. This syndrome occurs in muscles that are enclosed by a relatively thick layer of fascia and are adjacent to

(Continued)

CASE EXAMPLE 5-10—cont'd

bone. Stressful events that affect these muscles lead to edema and subsequent ischemia due to the noncompliant fascial sheath. This disorder must be differentiated from other causes of tail trauma and lesions that affect the caudal spinal cord segments or caudal spinal nerves, such as intervertebral disk protusion-extrusion, neoplasia, the lumbosacral syndrome, and radiculitis. Most dogs with this myopathy recover spontaneously with a few days of rest. The use of nonsteroidal antiinflammatory therapy may enhance recovery, and drugs to decrease the patient's discomfort are recommended when that is a complaint.

CASE EXAMPLE 5-11

NMD Paraparesis—Dog

Signalment: 3-month-old male English springer spaniel

Chief Complaint: Unable to use pelvic limbs normally

History: All four puppies in the litter began to walk at 4 to 5 weeks of age. By 7 weeks, three of the four exhibited difficulty walking with the pelvic limbs. In two puppies, this progressed to paraplegia, with the pelvic limbs fixed in an extended position, and they were euthanized. The third puppy, this patient, was still able to move one pelvic limb, and his clinical signs stabilized at about 10 weeks of age.

Examination: Video 5-37 shows this dog at 4 months of age. Note the occasional acquired bunny-hopping the dog used to get around. Note the better use of the left pelvic limb, which flexed well at the hip to advance the limb, but the tarsus was overflexed because of his lack of ability to extend it (tibial nerve). Occasionally he stood on the dorsum of the paw (peroneal nerve). The left stifle was overextended to accommodate for the overflexed tarsus, but no patellar reflex could be elicited (femoral nerve). This left pelvic limb was hypotonic and only flexed well at the hip when the flexor reflex was tested (sciatic). The right pelvic limb moved only by hip flexion (intact lumbar spinal nerve ventral branches to the psoas major muscle). The rest of the joints were nearly immobile because of the severe denervation atrophy of all the muscles and the forced overextension of the stifle and tarsus, both of which were angled in the wrong direction. These joint abnormalities are the result of denervation atrophy in a young dog whose bones are growing in length. These limb contractures (arthrogryposis) result from the disparity in the normal growth of bones in the limbs and the abnormal shortening of the associated muscles. Denervation atrophy does not do this in the adult dog. The tail, anus, and perineum were normal in this patient. The thoracic limbs were normal, as were the cranial nerves.

Anatomic Diagnosis: L4-S1 spinal cord segments, spinal nerve roots, spinal nerves, femoral and sciatic nerves, the muscle these nerves innervate

Differential Diagnosis: Protozoal radiculitis, motor neuron disease, myelitis (canine distemper, fungal, granulomatous), diskospondylitis, neoplasm, intervertebral disk extrusion-protrusion

NEOSPOROSIS

Protozoal radiculitis, most commonly caused by *N. caninum* and rarely *T. gondii,* is the most presumptive diagnosis in these dogs, based on their ages and the character of the clinical signs. Neosporosis[21,31,47,50] can affect the nervous system at any age but for reasons that are not known, this protozoan has a predilection for the lumbosacral spinal nerve roots of young dogs. Lesions also are present in these spinal cord segments (myelitis) and in the pelvic limb muscles (myositis), but the spinal nerve lesions are the most extensive (Figs. 5-38 and 5-39). Serum antibodies for *N. caninum* will confirm infection. Confirmation of this agent as the cause of the disease requires necropsy with immunocytochemical staining to demonstrate the organism in the lesions. CSF will show a protein elevation and a pleocytosis of a mixed population of leucocytes. Serum muscle enzymes will be elevated when there is an associated myositis. In adult dogs, the lesions are

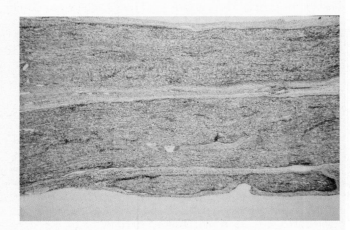

FIGURE 5-38 Longitudinal section of the dorsal and ventral roots of the L7 spinal nerve of a dog with severe radiculitis caused by *N. caninum.*

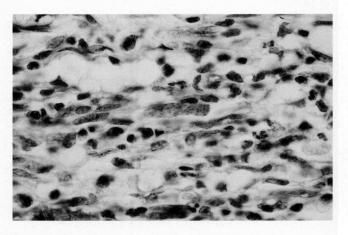

FIGURE 5-39 High-power magnification of the ventral root in Fig. 5-38, showing the extensive nonsuppurative inflammation with a cluster of protozoal organisms in the center.

usually confined to the CNS, and although the lesions can occur at any level, there is a predilection for the cerebellum. Be aware that this organism can be acquired by vertical transmission from the bitch to the puppies in utero and may occur in subsequent litters. It has been recognized that if you start antiprotozoal treatment as soon as there is any evidence of neurologic clinical signs in the puppies, the disease can be prevented from progressing. Adult dogs most likely acquire the protozoal agent from the infected feces in their environment as well as by ingesting tissue cysts in the muscles of intermediate hosts. Infected dogs serve as a source of this agent to pregnant cattle, where it is a common cause of abortion.

Video 5-38 shows Phoebe, a 3-month-old female mixed-breed puppy that was taken to the Teaching Hospital at Cornell University by the Society for the Prevention of Cruelty to Animals (SPCA) because she had been abandoned. Note the bilateral pelvic limb abnormality, which is similar to that in the right pelvic limb of this case example. These rigid limbs have severe muscle atrophy, and the stifle and tarsus cannot be moved. The presumptive diagnosis of an L4 to S1 radiculitis caused by *N. caninum* was supported by the presence of serum antibodies for this agent. Based on the assumption that the disease had run its course in Phoebe and would not progress, and with the understanding that she would never recover from these clinical signs, a veterinary student adopted this puppy and provided it with boots to prevent abrasions of the digits and a harness or a carriage for longer walks, and Phoebe has lived a high-quality life well into her teens as she has followed the professional accomplishments of her adopted owner. It should be noted that historically, prior to the discovery of *N. caninum* in the late 1980s and the development of immunocytochemical procedures, many cases of neosporosis were incorrectly diagnosed as toxoplasmosis.

MND in this springer spaniel and his littermates in this case example would explain the LMN clinical signs at that age, but the asymmetry, the limitation to the pelvic limbs, and the lack of continued progression would be unexpected.

Granulomatous meningomyelitis would be unusual at this young age. Canine distemper virus and fungal agents would be unlikely to cause a focal lesion limited to the L4-S1 spinal cord segments; they usually cause multifocal disease and clinical signs that continue to progress. A neoplasm at this level or intervertebral disk extrusion-protrusion would not be expected at this age.

The young springer spaniel in this case example had serum antibodies for *N. caninum* but none for *T. gondii* and was euthanized because of the poor quality of life expected for this dog. The diagnosis of a radiculitis, myelitis, and myositis caused by *N. caninum* was confirmed at necropsy.

SWIMMER PUPPIES

Swimmer syndrome in puppies is a developmental abnormality that occurs at a critical period of growth when a normal puppy is just starting to be able to stand and walk. These are usually large puppies that lack the strength to stand. As they struggle to stand, their limbs progressively become abducted. This places excess weight on their sternums, and that causes an excessive curvature or bowing of the ribs, resulting in a flattened thorax. In their attempts to stand in this abducted position, the flailing limbs make the puppy appear as if it were swimming—hence the name of the syndrome. In time, secondary joint deformities and ankylosis may occur. Breeders who are aware of this condition have learned to prevent the problem by hobbling the puppies by loosely tying their limbs together to prevent the abduction and by providing nonskid surfaces during this critical growth period. Providing a bed of deep, soft material such as blankets can be helpful. This is not a neurologic problem or a primary muscle disorder. It is the result of a disparity in growth between the muscles and the bones and soft tissues. One or more of a litter can be affected.

CASE EXAMPLE 5-12

NMD Paraplegia—Cat

Signalment: 2-year-old castrated male domestic shorthair, Simba
Chief Complaint: Inability to use his pelvic limbs
History: About 2 weeks before the examination shown on the video, this cat had been missing for 4 days and when found, he was unable to use his pelvic limbs. Initially he was reluctant to move at all. After a few days, whenever he tried to move, the hips would flex to advance the limbs but there was no function of the joints distal to the hips. This pelvic limb dysfunction has not changed since that time.

Examination: Video 5-39 shows the characteristic gait that was described in the history: all the pelvic limb function was limited to hip flexion. Note the normal tone that was elicited when the tail and the hips were manually extended but the lack of any tone distal to the hips, especially in the tarsus, each of which is flaccid. Note the atrophy of the crural muscles, the areflexia and analgesia distal to the stifle, the absent left patellar reflex, and the depressed right patellar reflex. Cutaneous nociception was absent bilaterally in all the digits and the crus but was normal on all surfaces of both thighs. In an examination of this cat, it is important to recognize that the tail, anus, perineum, and excretory functions are all normal. At the time of this examination, the temperature of the paws was normal. Femoral pulses were present but difficult to feel.

Anatomic Diagnosis: Sciatic and femoral nerves and the crural muscles: the pattern of the analgesia can be explained only by the loss of function in these peripheral nerves in their course through the limbs distal to the distal thigh level. This also explains the loss of function in the muscles distal to this level A primary muscle disorder and would not explain the analgesia. This unique pattern can be explained only by an ischemic neuromyopathy secondary to a compromise of the blood supply at the level of the caudal aorta or external iliac arteries. The veterinarian that first examined this cat could not feel any femoral artery pulses; the caudal crural muscles were swollen, and palpation elicited discomfort. The pelvic limb paws felt cool.

AORTIC THROMBOEMBOLISM

Once you recognize this anatomic diagnosis, there is no clinical disorder to consider other than a thromboembolism of the caudal aorta or the external iliac arteries.[63,71] The spinal cord is unaffected because the aortic lumbar spinal arteries provide adequate blood flow.

(Continued)

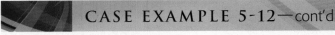

CASE EXAMPLE 5-12—cont'd

In most cats, this disorder is associated with hypertrophic cardiomyopathy, which in itself can be life-threatening and the source of repeat thromboembolism. No reliable treatment protocol has proven to be effective in these cats. Most treatments include the use of aspirin. Many cats will make partial improvement by walling off the clot and reestablishing an endothelial-lined channel through the obstruction. These clinical signs can be limited to one limb if only one external iliac artery is occluded.

Euthanasia should be recommended to the owners of these cats because the thromboembolic event is very likely to recur and initially causes the patient to express pain.

Simba, the cat in this case example, would not be expected to make much more improvement in his pelvic limb gait. The owners elected to keep him as a pet and accommodate him for his abnormal ambulation.

CASE EXAMPLE 5-13

NMD Paraplegia—Cat

Signalment: Adult spayed female domestic shorthair, French
Chief Complaint: No use of the pelvic limbs
History: This pet house cat had been missing for 10 days. When the owner found the cat, she had no use of her pelvic limbs and dragged herself around using her thoracic limbs.
Examination: Video 5-40 shows the severe bilateral flaccid paraplegia with atonia and areflexia of the pelvic limbs, tail, and anus. These same areas were also analgesic except for an occasional mild response from the right pelvic limb digits. The abdomen was also atonic. There was no palpable abnormality in the alignment of the lumbar vertebral spines.
Anatomic Diagnosis: About L1-L7, sacral and caudal spinal cord segments, spinal nerve roots, and spinal nerves
Differential Diagnosis: External injury, fibrocartilaginous embolic myelopathy, diffuse myelomalacia secondary to an acute intervertebral disk extrusion, abscess-suppurative leptomeningitis and myelitis

ISCHEMIC POLIOMYELOMALACIA

External injury could produce this anatomic diagnosis in two ways: (1) multiple lumbar vertebral fractures and spinal cord contusion. They were not palpated, and subsequent radiographs were normal; (2) severe abdominal compression such as would occur if an automobile tire ran over the cat and caused a prolonged vasospasm of the lumbar arteries and ischemic poliomyelomalacia. This spinal cord lesion can be produced experimentally in dogs, cats, and laboratory animals by ligating the aorta at or cranial to the level of the renal arteries. The severity of the lumbosacrocaudal spinal cord gray matter lesion is dependent on the duration of the vascular compromise. As a rule, about 30 minutes are required for the permanent destruction of this gray matter. I (AD) have now studied the nervous system at necropsy of three cats with the same history of being missing for a few days and found paraplegic with these identical signs, including this patient. None of these cats had any radiographic evidence of fractures. Two had radiographic evidence of soft tissue lesions of possible retroperitoneal hemorrhage. At necropsy there was gross evidence of this retroperitoneal hemorrhage in all three cats, one of which had an avulsed kidney. There were no gross lesions in the vertebral canal or the spinal cord until it was preserved and sectioned, and a softening was felt in the central portion of the spinal cord segments that extended from L2 through all the spinal cord segments caudal to it. On microscopic examination there was complete ischemic-type necrosis of the gray matter and the adjacent white matter of the fasciculus proprius (Figs. 5-40 through 5-42). The gray matter is the most sensitive to hypoxia, and the white matter lesion here is in the terminal watershed zone of the branches of the ventral spinal artery via the gray matter and the arteries to the white matter that branch from the

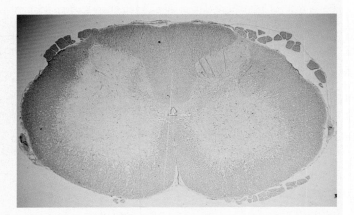

FIGURE 5-40 This figure and Figs. 5-41 and 5-42 show three domestic shorthair cats with necropsy diagnoses of poliomyelomalacia of the lumbosacrocaudal spinal cord segments, related to presumptive abdominal injury by compression by the tire of a vehicle. Fig. 5-40 is the L5 spinal cord segment approximately 5 to 7 days after the injury.

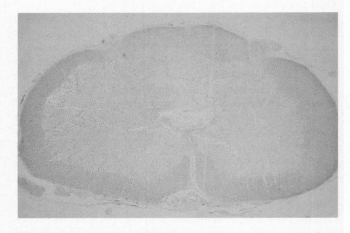

FIGURE 5-41 This is the L6 spinal cord segment in a cat about 2 weeks after the injury.

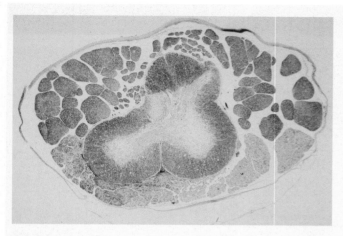

FIGURE 5-42 The S3 spinal cord segment about 2 months after the injury. This is a luxol-fast-blue stain for myelin. Note the loss of myelin in the transverse sections of the ventral roots due to wallerian degeneration caused by the loss of the neuronal cell bodies in the ventral gray column necrosis.

plexus of arteries on the external surface of the spinal cord (see Fig. 10-4). These lesions are identical to those described earlier following experimental occlusion of the midportion of the aorta.[56] In these three cats, no blood vessel lesions were found, but the lumbar arteries were not examined. Our hypothesis is that all three of these cats were run over by cars and that the tire compressed the abdomens, causing varying degrees of hemorrhage and prolonged spasm of the lumbar arteries. In support of this hypothesis, EG examined a cat with identical clinical signs and no radiographic evidence of fractures but with the history of having been run over; the owner knew that she had run over her cat with her car. No necropsy was allowed to prove the similarity of the lesion.

Video 5-41 shows Winky, a 2-year-old spayed female domestic shorthair. An ovariohysterectomy was performed at a hospital with no complications. She was discharged a few hours after the surgery and was normal at that time, but within a few hours, she lost the ability to use her pelvic limbs. The video was made about 48 hours after the surgery. The clinical signs are identical to those in this case example. The cat was euthanized and no gross lesions were seen in the abdomen, including the aorta. However, the spinal cord had the same gross and microscopic lesions as the three cats described earlier. The cause of the presumptive lumbar artery vasospasm remains an enigma in this cat.

Fibrocartilaginous embolic myelopathy (FCEM) occurs in cats but is much more common in dogs. The extent of the vascular compromise rarely is more than a few spinal cord segments, which may mean that the emboli arise from one degenerate intervertebral disk. The lesion is often asymmetric and often has a significant hemorrhagic component. Usually the fibrocartilaginous emboli can be found on microscopic examination. This disorder is described more completely in the Chapter 10, which discusses small-animal spinal cord diseases.

An acute intervertebral disk extrusion with subsequent progressive diffuse myelomalacia could produce these clinical signs in a dog, but we have never seen this spinal cord lesion in cats. This necrotizing lesion affects all components of the spinal cord and is described in Case Example 5-14.

Extensive development of an abscess that spread as a suppurative leptomeningitis through the subarachnoid space in the area of this anatomic diagnosis presumably could cause the clinical signs mentioned, but that would be a progressive disorder and would occur rarely.

POSTOPERATIVE POLIOMYELOMALACIA: HORSE AND CALF

This same ischemic poliomyelomalacia of the lumbosacrocaudal spinal cord segments occasionally occurs during surgery in young horses[7] that have general anesthesia for surgery that requires dorsal recumbency (cryptorchidism, colic, stifle arthroscopic surgery). They recover well from the anesthesia but are unable to get up on their pelvic limbs, which exhibit flaccid paralysis. The extent of the lesion, when seen microscopically, depends on the time interval between the surgery and euthanasia (Fig. 5-43). It is hypothesized that during the period of dorsal recumbency, the heavy bowel causes enough compression of the aorta or its lumbar branches to result in these lesions. Fortunately, this is not a common occurrence, but once is enough to make a surgeon wary and consider shifting the position of the patient periodically during the anesthesia. I (AD) have seen these same clinical signs and these same lesions in a young calf that was anesthetized and placed in dorsal recumbency for evacuation of its abomasum as a treatment for its digestive disorder.

POLIOMYELOMALACIA IN PIGS

A unique poliomyelomalacia occurs in pigs[142-144] that ingest excessive amounts of selenium in their diets. Selenium is used as a feed additive, and occasionally an excessive amount is mistakenly added to the feed mixture. As a result, multiple pigs fed this diet are at risk for developing neurologic signs. They are usually young pigs, 1 to 5 months old, that exhibit a sudden onset of a LMN tetraparesis. The toxic effect of the excessive selenium causes a bilateral symmetric degeneration of the center of the ventral gray columns, primarily in the cervical and lumbosacral intumescences and in a few brainstem GSE nuclei. Neuronal cell bodies are spared on the borders of the lesion, which consists of an abundance of macrophages and has numerous small blood vessels coursing through it (Figs. 5-44 through 5-47). Identical lesions occur when pigs are fed 6-amino-nicotinamide, an antagonist to the nicotinic acid that functions as a coenzyme.[102,103] It is suspected that this metabolic disorder is initially toxic to the astrocytes and that the neuronal degeneration follows their loss. There is no treatment. Recognizing and removing the source of the

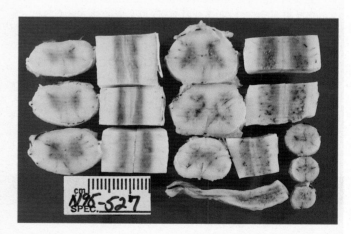

FIGURE 5-43 Transverse sections of the spinal cord from T17 through the caudal segments of a 2-year-old thoroughbred, showing the bilateral symmetric discoloration of the gray matter by a poliomyelomalacia associated with recumbency for cryptorchid surgery.

(Continued)

CASE EXAMPLE 5-13—cont'd

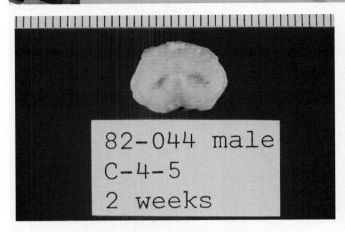

FIGURE 5-44 Transverse section of the C5 spinal cord segment from a 4-month-old mixed-breed pig with poliomyelomalacia due to selenium toxicity.

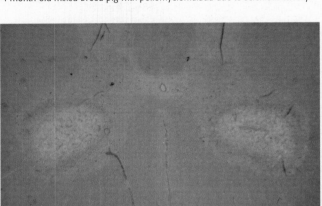

FIGURE 5-45 Microscopic view of a section of cervical intumescence from a pig with selenium toxicity. Note the bilateral symmetry of the central lesion in each ventral gray column.

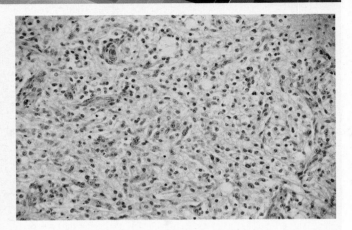

FIGURE 5-46 High-power magnification of the central portion of the lesion in Fig. 5-45, where most of the cells are macrophages.

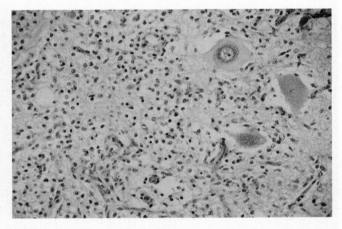

FIGURE 5-47 High-power magnification of the periphery of the lesion seen in Figs. 5-45 and 5-46, showing intact and degenerating neuronal cell bodies.

excess selenium prevents additional cases. Similar lesions have been reported in sheep in Africa and goats in California, but no causes have been identified.

POLIOMYELOMALACIA IN AYSHIRE CALVES

A poliomyelomalacia was reported in three Ayshire calves in one herd in the United Kingdom, and I (AD) studied a similar Ayshire calf in

Ontario, Canada, in the 1970s.[106] These calves were all normal at birth but at about 10 days of age, three calves developed a rapidly progressive LMN paresis of the pelvic limbs, and one calf developed it in all four limbs. The bilaterally symmetric ventral gray column lesions in the respective spinal cord intumescences were identical to those described in pigs with selenium toxicity. No toxin was identified in the environment of these calves. A metabolic disorder was proposed but not identified.

CASE EXAMPLE 5-14

LMN Tetraplegia—Dog

Signalment: 5-year-old female dachshund, Chloe
Chief Complaint: Unable to move
History: Three days before this examination, Chloe suddenly had difficulty using her pelvic limbs. Rapidly, in a few hours, she became

unable to move them at all and dragged herself around with her thoracic limbs. The local veterinarian diagnosed a thoracolumbar spinal cord lesion and suspected an intervertebral disk extrusion. On the following day, while Chloe was hospitalized, the veterinarian reported that Chloe could not get into a sternal position and had begun to lose reflexes in her pelvic limbs. By the third day she was recumbent but still alert and responsive.

Examination: Video 5-42 was made on the fourth day. Note the flaccid paralysis of all four limbs and the atonia of the entire body except for the neck. This was especially evident in the abdomen. Note the atonia, areflexia, and analgesia of the tail, anus, perineum, pelvic limbs, abdomen, and thorax. The analgesia extended as far cranial as the caudal borders of the scapulae. The thoracic limbs were hypotonic and nearly areflexic, but nociception was still intact. When the noxious stimulus was perceived, Chloe looked anxious, moved her head and her jaws slightly, and tried to bark but had no voice due to the LMN paralysis of her thorax and abdomen. Her respirations were entirely dependent on the function of her diaphragm. Note the abdominal movements that relate to this form of respiration.

Anatomic Diagnosis: C6 through the last caudal spinal cord segments, spinal nerve roots or spinal nerves; from C6 to T2 this lesion is severe but incomplete; from T3 caudally there is no clinical evidence of any spinal cord function.

Differential Diagnosis: Only diffuse myelomalacia can explain this diffuse anatomic diagnosis with such an extensive loss of the GSE-LMN and GSA pathways as well.

DIFFUSE MYELOMALACIA

Diffuse myelomalacia[60] most commonly follows an acute intervertebral disk extrusion that initially causes a severe transverse spinal cord hemorrhage and necrosis (Figs. 5-48 through 5-50). Most of these extrusions occur between the T10 and L3 vertebrae and initially cause spastic paraplegia. Usually within 1 to 3 days, progressive ischemic-type necrosis spreads through the spinal cord cranially and caudally from the initial lesion. However, I (EG) have seen one dog develop this progressive myelomalacia 12 days after the initial onset of the acute paraplegia. Varying degrees of hemorrhage are associated with this necrosis. The lesion appears to reflect primarily a vascular compromise and may be the result of a sudden vasospasm of all the parenchymal arterioles. The spinal cord nerve roots in the subarachnoid space are spared, whereas all structures within the pial-glial membrane degenerate. The vasospasm or the necrosis may be the result of the sudden release into the parenchyma of biologic amines, such as glutamate, norepinephrine, dopamine, histamine, and serotonin. These amines are thought to be involved with the extension of the spinal cord necrosis that occurs with focal spinal cord injury but usually is limited to the adjacent spinal cord segments. This is called secondary spinal cord injury; it occurs within the first 1 to 3

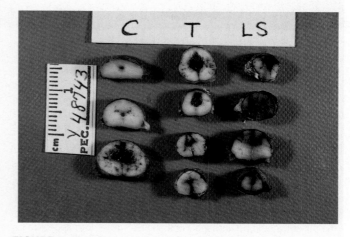

FIGURE 5-49 Transverse sections of the spinal cord shown in Fig. 5-48, showing the extensive hemorrhagic necrosis associated with this diffuse myelomalacia.

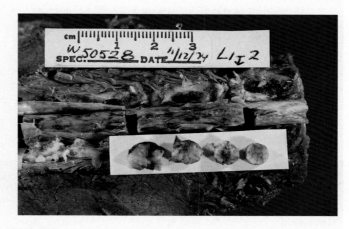

FIGURE 5-50 Dorsal view and transverse sections of the spinal cord of a 5-year-old dachshund with clinical signs of diffuse myelomalacia. When making these transverse sections, it felt like cutting toothpaste because they were so soft (malacia). These show the discoloration of necrosis resulting more from ischemia than hemorrhage.

days after the initial injury. Extensive research efforts are being directed toward determining ways to prevent this secondary necrosis.

This diffuse myelomalacia has never followed a cervical intervertebral disk extrusion and appears to be limited to those that occur between the T10 and L3 vertebrae. A possible explanation may be based on the blood supply, which appears to be severely compromised within the affected spinal cord segments. The normal blood supply to the thoracolumbar spinal cord comes from the spinal branches of the intercostal and lumbar arteries. This is a bilaterally symmetric system that can provide a spinal artery at every intervertebral foramen. However, anatomic studies show that there is a marked variation in the numbers and sizes of these spinal arteries and even the occasional absence of a spinal branch on one or both sides. In humans, one of the spinal arteries between T10 and T12 is exceptionally large and is called the arteria radicularis magna, the artery of Adamkiewicz. It supplies many spinal cord segments both cranial and caudal to the level where the artery enters the vertebral canal. Surgeons are very careful to avoid compromising this vessel. Studies in the dog show that

(Continued)

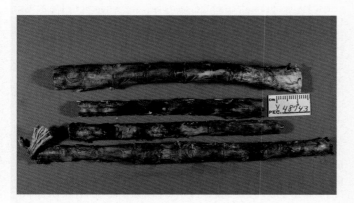

FIGURE 5-48 Dorsal view of the entire spinal cord of a 4-year-old dachshund with diffuse myelomalacia.

a similar large spinal artery exists usually at the L5 or L6 level. Possibly, the small percentage of dogs that develop progressive myelomalacia are exceptions in which this large artery appears at a more cranial level, where the disk extrusion that is related to the development of this progressive myelomalacia occurs. Sacrifice of this large artery has the potential to compromise a large segment of the spinal cord, and the secondary effects of the spinal cord injury could extend the necrosis into the less well-vascularized segments, the watershed zones, both cranially and caudally.

When this progressive necrosis reaches the cervical spinal cord, death occurs as the result of respiratory paralysis. Occasionally the spread of the necrosis stops before the thoracic limbs are affected. As soon as you recognize the clinical signs of a diffuse myelomalacia, the patient should be humanely euthanized. These dogs appear to be in considerable discomfort, which may be due to the subarachnoid hemorrhage at the cranial aspect of the lesion. No ancillary procedures should be performed to diagnose this lesion because no treatment can alter the disorder.

As described in Chloe in this case example, this diffuse myelomalacia most commonly follows an explosive intervertebral disk extrusion. I (AD) have seen this disorder associated with an extensive diffuse epidural hemorrhage without any intervertebral disk extrusion, in one dog with an extradural neoplasm and in two dogs where was no evidence of any

vertebral canal lesion at necropsy. We have not seen this associated with external trauma and have seen it only in dogs, not in cats.

To appreciate the incidence of this disorder, you must be aware that thoracolumbar intervertebral disk protrusions and extrusions in dogs are very common (see Chapter 10). The majority of these protrusions and extrusions cause only discomfort. Many cause a mild to moderate degree of spastic paraparesis and ataxia in the pelvic limbs. Only a small percentage cause the clinical signs of a transverse spinal cord lesion that results in a spastic paraplegia and analgesia of the portion of the body and limbs caudal to the lesion. Of this latter group, no more than about 5% will develop progressive diffuse myelomalacia, but no way has been found to prevent its occurrence in these few dogs. It can occur in the face of the most appropriate and aggressive medical and surgical treatment for acute spinal cord injury. This disorder can occur even if decompressive surgery is performed prior to the development of any recognizable signs of progression of a myelomalacia. If you wait 3 days to see whether progressive myelomalacia is going to occur, you will lose the critical time advantage in your surgical treatment of the much larger percentage of this group of spastic paraplegics that only have focal lesions. MR imaging may be useful in the early detection of the disorder in these patients, when the mixed signal on T2-weighted images begins to spread into the spinal cord segments adjacent to the initial site of injury from the intervertebral disk extrusion.

CASE EXAMPLE 5-15

Pelvic Limb Monoplegia—Dog

Signalment: 18-month-old castrated male shepherd-mixed breed, Leo

Chief Complaint: Unable to use the right pelvic limb

History: Leo had been struck by a car 5 days prior to the video, and there had been no change since that time.

 Examination: Video 5-43. Note that Leo walked well with three limbs, but the right pelvic limb was dragged along the floor, unable to protract or support weight. It was atonic and areflexic. There was analgesia of the entire limb distal to the stifle and the caudal thigh and right side of the perineum and tail. Nociception was normal in the proximal medial thigh (genitofemoral—L3, L4) and in the cranial and craniolateral thigh (lateral cutaneous femoral—L3, L4). At the end of the video, the dog is facing away from you and I am straddling the dog and facing toward you. Tail tone was normal but it was held deviated to the left side. When I stimulated the normal left side of the tail, his nose suddenly appeared. This was followed by my palpation of the iliac crests to show the marked ventral displacement of the right ilium. There also was a palpable deviation of the tail that I indicated.

Anatomic Diagnosis: Right L4 through caudal spinal cord segments, spinal nerve roots, spinal nerves, femoral and sciatic nerves, and sacral plexus

The asymmetry of the clinical signs strongly suggests that the lesion is in the peripheral nerves, not in the spinal cord, especially given the history of external trauma and the palpable displacement of the ilium. We have not seen a nerve root avulsion in the pelvic limb without a fracture and bony displacement.

The history of an observed external trauma eliminates any need to discuss a differential diagnosis. Radiographs showed fractures of the right pubis and ischium and a right sacroiliac luxation with severe ventral and lateral displacement of the ilium (Figs. 5-51 and 5-52). The latter was probably associated with a tearing of the termination of the iliopsoas muscle, which would account for the lack of hip flexion. It also would account for an injury to the femoral nerve, which emerges from the iliopsoas muscle to enter the quadriceps femoris. The sciatic nerve is commonly injured in pelvic trauma because it is formed by the L6 and L7 spinal nerve ventral branches that pass across the ventral surface of the sacroiliac joint, where they are at risk for injury by luxations.[4,145] These two branches are joined by the ventral branch of S1 to form the sciatic nerve, which then courses across the dorsal surface of the body of the ilium where fractures are common. Surgeons must be aware of this nerve and not injure it when repairing fractures of the body of the ilium. The obturator nerve courses on the medial surface of the ilium and is at risk for injury by these fractures, but we probably do not recognize the slight sliding-out of the limb during weight bearing when the dog is walking on a slippery surface. This would not be seen when the dog walked on a rug or on dirt or a grassy surface. The femoral nerve is rarely affected by these pelvic fractures because it is never directly associated with bones of the pelvis in its course from the psoas major muscle, where it is formed primarily by the ventral branches of the L4 and L5 spinal nerves and enters the quadriceps femoris. In Leo, the dog in this case example, the degree of iliac displacement ventrally from the sacrum was unusual and therefore injured the femoral nerve. The right sacral plexus may

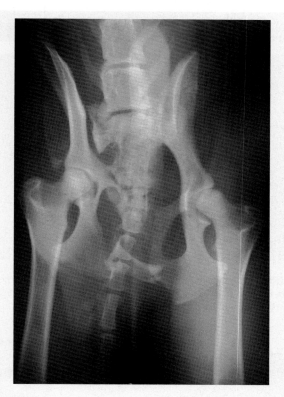

FIGURE 5-51 Ventrodorsal pelvic radiograph of Leo, the dog in this case example, showing the right sacroiliac luxation and the fractures of the right pubis and ischium.

also have been torn by this marked displacement. There was a fracture of the first two caudal vertebrae that caused the analgesia of the right side of the tail.

The prognosis for recovery from such severe neurologic signs was poor but the owners elected to have the sacroiliac luxation repaired. This repair was successful, but after waiting for 6 weeks, the neurologic signs did not change, so the limb was amputated. Leo was certainly given the benefit of the doubt and was fortunate to have such dedicated owners.

Video 5-44 shows Keane, a 1-year-old collie that had been struck by a car 1 week earlier and had suffered a fracture of the left pubis, ischium, and body of the ilium (Fig. 5-53). The fracture and displacement of the ilium injured the sciatic and obturator nerves. Note how readily the limb is protracted by hip flexion and the ability to support weight, but the paw is often placed on its dorsal surface. The stifle flexors and the tarsal flexors and extensors are hypotonic. These signs indicate a sciatic and peroneal nerve paresis.[144] Nociception is intact when the lateral digit is compressed, which indicates that the sciatic nerve is still anatomically intact. Note that the left hind paw occasionally slides laterally on the slippery floor. This is due to the obturator nerve injury. Figs. 5-54 and 5-55 show a domestic shorthair with a similar pelvic fracture and injury to the sciatic nerve.

Video 5-45 shows Hershey, a 10-year-old male Gordon setter that experienced 1 month of progressive gait abnormality in the right pelvic limb. Note the skipping-type gait, which is characteristic of a sciatic nerve dysfunction and is caused by the brisk, unopposed flexion of the hip. Weight support is normal but during this support, the tarsus

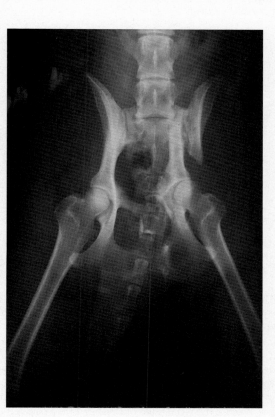

FIGURE 5-52 Lateral pelvic radiograph of Leo, showing the marked displacement of the right ilium, which caused the injury of the right femoral nerve and the ventral branches of the L6, L7, and S1 spinal nerves. Note the sacrocaudal fracture.

FIGURE 5-53 Ventrodorsal pelvic radiograph of Kean, the dog in Video 5-44. The fracture and displacement of the left ilium is located where the ventral branches of the L6, L7, and S1 spinal nerves form the sciatic nerve.

(Continued)

CASE EXAMPLE 5-15—cont'd

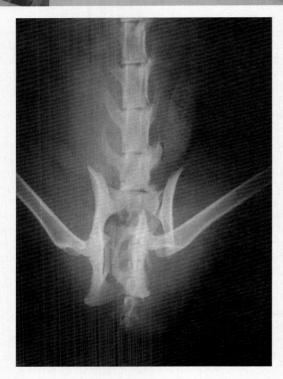

FIGURE 5-54 Ventrodorsal radiograph of a 2-year-old domestic shorthair that was struck by a vehicle.

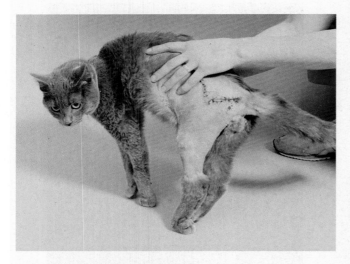

FIGURE 5-55 This is the cat that was radiographed in Fig. 5-54 after its surgery to repair the fractured ilium. Note the posture of the left pelvic limb paw, showing the peroneal portion of the sciatic nerve injury.

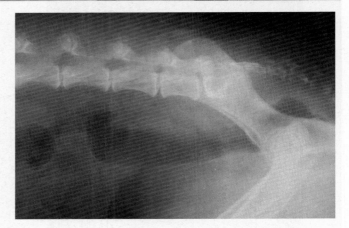

FIGURE 5-56 Lateral radiograph of Hershey, the 10-year-old Gordon setter in Video 5-45. Note the soft tissue mass ventral to the L6, L7, and sacral vertebrae and the displacement of the descending colon.

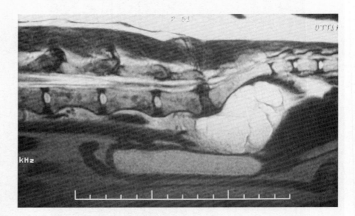

FIGURE 5-57 Sagittal T2-weighted MR image of the dog in Fig. 5-56, showing the same view as the radiograph and the hyperintensity of the soft tissue mass lesion.

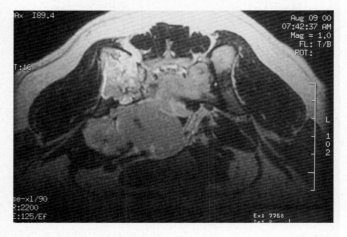

FIGURE 5-58 Axial T2-weighted MR image of the dog in Figs. 5-56 and 5-57, showing the hyperintense mass involving the right ilium where the sciatic nerve was involved and lost its function.

is overflexed and the hind paw is occasionally placed on its dorsal surface. Remember the course of the nerves that form the sciatic nerve along the medial side of the ilium to cross the body at the greater ischiatic notch. On a rectal exam of Hershey, I (EG) palpated a mass. This was confirmed by radiographic and MR imaging, which showed involvement of the ilium by the neoplasm (Figs. 5-56 through 5-58). Microscopic examination of the mass diagnosed a sarcoma.

Video 5-46 shows an adult parakeet with a right pelvic limb that could not be used to perch on its stand. This had been a slowly progressive problem that had progressed to complete inability to move the right pelvic limb. Note the normal brisk flexion of the left limb after being manually extended and especially the flexion of the digits (sciatic nerve), which the bird needs to be able to perch. The right limb was analgesic and areflexic, and the muscles were atrophied. This was diagnosed as a sciatic and femoral nerve disorder. One recognized cause of this neuropathy in a parakeet is a compression of these nerves by a renal adenocarcinoma because they course adjacent to the dorsal surface of the kidney. The avian kidney is an elongated structure that is embedded on the ventral surface of the synsacrum, where these nerves are formed by the spinal nerves that emerge at this level. This diagnosis was confirmed at neuropsy.

SCIATIC NERVE INJURY

Be very aware of the course of the sciatic nerve when you are performing intramuscular injections in the gluteal or caudal thigh muscles, when you are placing a needle into the trochanteric fossa to obtain a bone marrow sample, and when you are placing an intramedullary pin through that same fossa for fracture repair. If you are going to use the caudal thigh muscles for the injection, grasp the stifle from the caudal side with your hand. With your fingers wrapped around the cranial aspect of the extended stifle, your thumb will fit into a depression between the biceps femoris laterally and semitendinosis medially. The sciatic nerve is directly cranial to your thumb at this level. Intramuscular injections in young animals should be placed in the neck muscles to avoid this possible nerve injury.

CASE EXAMPLE 5-16

LMN Paraparesis—Cow

Signalment: 4-year-old Holstein cow
Chief Complaint: Abnormal pelvic limb gait
History: The owner noticed abnormal posture in the left pelvic limb 2 months prior to the examination. Over the next 2 to 3 weeks the same abnormal posture occurred in the right pelvic limb, and the cow spent most of her time lying down.
Examination: Video 5-47 shows her ability to advance her pelvic limbs and support weight but with overflexion of each tarsus ("dropped tarsus") and with dorsal buckling of the metatarsophalangeal (fetlock) joints. Nociception was normal on all surfaces of the digits, metatarsus, and crus. Tail and anal function were normal, and she was not incontinent.
Anatomic Diagnosis: S1, S2 spinal cord segments, spinal nerve roots, spinal nerves, sciatic or tibial nerves

This posture of the tarsus and digits is typical of a tibial nerve dysfunction in cattle. The overflexed tarsus is the result of loss of the innervation to the tarsal extensors (gastrocnemius and superficial digital flexor muscles). The basis for the dorsal buckling of the metatarsophalangeal joints is not clearly understood but presumably represents the loss of the function of the digital flexors. It is a very reliable sign of tibial nerve dysfunction in cattle. This dorsal buckling of the metatarsophalangeal joints does not occur with peroneal nerve paralysis. A ruminant with peroneal nerve paralysis stands on the dorsal aspect of the digits because of loss of the function of the digital extensor muscles, but the posture of the metatarsophalangeal joints is normal.
Differential Diagnosis: Injury, lymphoma, diskospondylitis

INJURY

The most common injury in this area in adult cattle is fracture of the sacrum or the caudal vertebrae as the result of being mounted by a bull or another cow. Most of these injuries damage the caudal nerves to the tail and the sacral nerves to the anus and perineum. If the injury affects the first two sacral nerves, a tibial nerve dysfunction will be observed. In this cow the tail, anus, and perineum were normal, and the tibial nerve signs were progressive.

LYMPHOMA

Lymphoma is a common extradural tumor in adult cattle that are 4 or 5 years old or older. If this lymphoma had been located in the craniosacral vertebral canal, it could readily explain the progressive clinical signs observed in this cow.

DISKOSPONDYLITIS

Diskospondylitis at the L6-S1 articulation, with abscess development in the craniosacral vertebral canal, could also explain these progressive signs. **Video 5-48** shows one of two 2-year-old Holstein cows with this lesion, which was thought to be secondary to tail-docking surgery performed a few weeks prior to the onset of clinical signs. In addition to the clinical signs of tibial nerve paresis, there was hypotonia and hypalgesia in the tail and anus and hypalgesia in the perineum due to the involvement of the sacrocaudal segments, spinal nerve roots, or spinal nerves.

A rectal examination of the cow in this case example diagnosed a bony protrusion on the ventral aspect of the sacrum; it was thought to be a healed displaced fracture. This cow was euthanized and at necropsy the bony mass was a large callus associated with a healed displaced fracture of S2. Both the S1 and S2 spinal nerve ventral branches were enclosed in fibrous tissue bilaterally, causing a compressive neuropathy and explaining the progressive bilateral tibial nerve paresis in this cow.

Be aware that a common cause of unilateral sciatic nerve paralysis in calves is iatrogenic in origin, resulting from the intramuscular injection of drugs into the gluteal or caudal thigh muscles (Fig. 5-59). These muscles are poorly developed at that age, making the sciatic nerve more easily accessed by these injections than they are in older animals. However, the gluteal muscles of adult dairy cattle are also thin and should not be used for intramuscular injections. These affected animals may not recover if the drug that is injected causes disruption of the neuronal axons. To avoid such injury, place intramuscular injections into the neck muscles. When this happens in a pen of young pigs, the denervated analgesic digits may be mutilated by the carnivorous activity of the penmate pigs. Figures 5-59 and 5-60 show a 2-month-old calf and a 5-year-old cow demonstrating the results of injury to portions of the sciatic nerve by intramuscular injection of drugs into the pelvic limb.

(Continued)

CASE EXAMPLE 5-16—cont'd

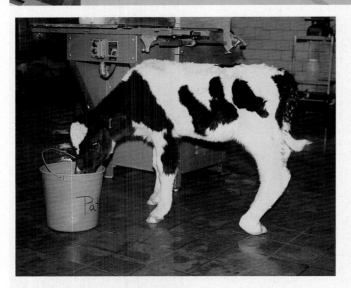

FIGURE 5-59 A 2-month-old Holstein calf with left sciatic nerve paralysis due to an intramuscular injection of a drug in the caudal thigh muscles.

Be aware that if a cow is bitten in the pelvic limb by a rabid fox or another rabid animal, the first signs of rabies virus encephalomyelitis may reflect the involvement of the gray matter in the lumbosacral intumescence. The clinical signs change rapidly because this disease progresses very fast and usually causes recumbency in a few days and death in 7 to 10 days.

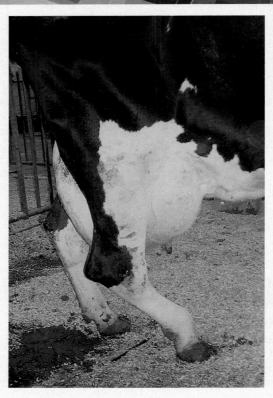

FIGURE 5-60 A 5-year-old Holstein cow with right tibial nerve paralysis due to a large abscess related to an intramuscular injection of a drug into the caudal thigh muscles. Note the swelling caudal to the stifle.

CASE EXAMPLE 5-17

LMN Paraparesis—Dog

Signalment: 4-year-old castrated male Leonberger, Beau

Chief Complaint: Abnormal pelvic limb gait

History: The abnormal gait in both pelvic limbs had been slowly progressing for 4 to 6 weeks. At 3 years of age, laryngeal paralysis was diagnosed as the cause of an inspiratory dyspnea, and "tie-back" surgery was performed on the larynx.

 Examination: Video 5-49 shows the skipping-type gait in the pelvic limbs, which is related to the brisk overflexion of the hips. This has sometimes been confused with a cerebellar hypermetria. It may represent the loss of tone in the antagonistic caudal thigh hip extensor muscles that are innervated by the sciatic nerve. Note the mild overflexion of the tarsus and the occasional placement of the hind paw on its dorsal surface during the hopping test. The flexor response to a noxious stimulus of the digits occurred mostly at the hip and was depressed at the stifle and tarsus. Nociception was intact throughout both pelvic limbs. The tarsus was hypotonic bilaterally, and crural muscle atrophy was extensive.

Anatomic Diagnosis: Bilateral L6, L7, S1 spinal cord segments, spinal nerve roots, spinal nerves, sciatic nerves

Differential Diagnosis: Inherited distal polyneuropathy, metabolic neuropathy, neoplasm

LEONBERGER INHERITED NEUROPATHY

An inherited distal polyneuropathy is the most presumptive diagnosis in Beau, based on the breed, the bilateral signs, and the history of previous laryngeal paralysis.[117] This has been described as a dying-back neuropathy affecting the distal portions of long peripheral neurons; the onset of clinical signs varies from 1 to 3 years. The recurrent laryngeal nerves and the sciatic nerves contain the longest peripheral neurons in domestic animals, and their degeneration is responsible for the clinical signs seen in this disorder. Electrodiagnostic studies show abnormalities in all the distal appendicular muscles. This is presumed to be inherited as a sex-linked recessive gene because it has been observed only in male Leonbergers. This canine disorder has been compared to the Charcot-Marie-Tooth polyneuropathy in humans. (The Leonberger breed was derived from the crossing of the Newfoundland, Saint Bernard, and Great Pyrenees breeds.)

METABOLIC NEUROPATHY

Diabetes and hypothyroidism are metabolic disorders that may cause a neuropathy.[54] Tibial nerve paresis is the most common diabetes-related neuropathy and is most common in cats. The resultant tarsal overflexion causes a plantigrade posture that is quite remarkable in these cats. It often resolves when the diabetes is well controlled. **Video 5-50** shows an 11-year-old domestic shorthair, Snowball, with diabetic neuropathy. We have also seen diffuse neuromuscular paresis associated with diabetes in cats and resulting in tetraparesis. Hypothyroid neuropathy is a canine disorder with a more varied clinical expression. It can affect the tibial nerves, the recurrent laryngeal nerves, the facial or vestibular nerves, and possibly the vagal nerves to the esophagus. Only a very small portion of dogs with chronic hypothyroidism develop a neuropathy and exhibit clinical signs. Old dogs commonly have a moderate degree of atrophy of the muscles of mastication and of the lateral scapular muscles; such atrophy may have a metabolic basis.

INHERITED NEUROMYOPATHY–DANCING DOBERMAN

Video 5-51 shows a 6-year-old spayed female Doberman pinscher that has exhibited a progressive pelvic limb gait abnormality for about 1 year. Note the flexed posture of the tarsus and the severe atrophy of the caudal crural muscles, suggesting a chronic tibial nerve disorder. Note the frequent elevation of each limb as the dog shifts its weight from one pelvic limb to the other and often sits down. Dogs in this situation act as if they are in some discomfort, but palpation does not elicit discomfort. This shifting type of lameness has led to this disorder's being called dancing Doberman disease.[15] There is some discrepancy in the understanding of the underlying lesions responsible for this disorder. Some dogs have severe chronic neuropathy and denervation atrophy. Others have no neuropathy but severe primary myopathy of the caudal crural muscles. Until this dilemma is resolved, we consider this to be a neuromyopathy that is presumably inherited in the Doberman pinscher. The clinical signs can commence at anywhere from 6 months to 7 years, and they slowly progress, but the clinical signs remain in the distribution of the tibial nerve and the muscles that it innervates. I (EG) followed one dog with this syndrome for 6 years, and the clinical signs slowly progressed but the dog remained able to walk.

INHERITED HYPERTROPHIC NEUROPATHY

Two other inherited disorders that involve the PNS are rare but worth mentioning. One is an autosomal recessive inherited hypertrophic neuropathy that occurs in Tibetan mastiffs (there are a small number of this breed in the United States).[17,18,22,121] Clinical signs usually begin between 7 and 12 weeks of age and progress rapidly. Paresis starts in the pelvic limbs with a symmetrically decreased ability to support weight, the development of plantigrade posture, hypotonia, loss of the patellar reflexes, and decreased flexor reflexes but intact nociception (Fig. 5-61). In most dogs, the clinical signs progress to the thoracic limbs in a few days, with decreased ability to support weight. Severely affected dogs become recumbent within about 3 weeks but retain voluntary limb movements (nonambulatory tetraparesis). Limb contractures may occur in the recumbent dogs. A few recumbent dogs improve after 6 to 7 weeks and regain the ability to stand and to walk with a shuffling plantigrade gait. Muscle atrophy is mild. On EMG

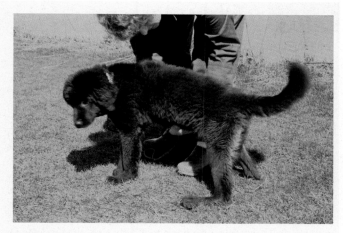

FIGURE 5-61 A 3-month-old Tibetan mastiff with overflexed tarsi due to an inherited hypertrophic neuropathy affecting the tibial nerves.

studies, there are rare denervation potentials, but nerve conduction rates are markedly prolonged, suggesting a myelin disorder. This is supported by the light and electron microscopic studies of peripheral nerves that show a widespread primary demyelination with Schwann cell hyperplasia and onion-bulb formation with minimal axonal degeneration. The Schwann cell hyperplasia and onion-bulb formation are the basis for the gross finding of nerve hypertrophy. This inherited defect appears to involve the Schwann cells and their ability to form and maintain stable myelin sheaths. The role of the axon signaling in this process is unknown. This inherited disorder first occurred in a kennel in which 15 affected puppies were diagnosed with this neuropathy out of a total of 62 puppies from 10 litters.

INHERITED GIANT AXONAL NEUROPATHY

The second inherited disorder is an autosomal recessive inherited giant axonal neuropathy that occurs in the German shepherd breed.[52] Clinical signs begin around 15 months of age with a symmetric paraparesis and ataxia of the pelvic limbs that slowly progresses. After many months, these dogs become unable to stand with the pelvic limbs and exhibit patellar reflex loss, distal muscle atrophy, and hypalgesia in the pelvic limbs. By 16 to 20 months, the bark may be reduced, and fecal incontinence and regurgitation may occur. EMG studies early in the course of the disorder show decreased amplitude of evoked muscle and sensory neuron action potentials. Denervation potentials occur later in the disease process. Lesions of focal axonal swelling (spheroids) that contain dense whorls of 10-nm neurofilaments occur in the distal portions of the longest peripheral nerves as well as in the distal portions of long neurons in the CNS. The clinical signs are thought to represent primarily the peripheral nerve lesion. This axonal disorder may involve an inherited metabolic defect that causes a disorder of the 10-nm neurofilaments and results in impaired axonal transport.

CASE EXAMPLE 5-18

LMN Paraparesis—Horse

Signalment: 12-year-old Quarter horse gelding, Tommy

Chief Complaint: About 3 weeks before examination, this horse suddenly was observed to be severely lame in the left pelvic limb. No injury was found, but the lameness got worse despite changing the shoes and providing a chiropractic adjustment.

Examination: An extensive orthopedic examination, including nerve blocks and local anesthesia of joints, did not diagnose any abnormality. **Video 5-52** shows the examination.

Note the severe weight-bearing lameness with no indication of any reluctance to use the limb. This lameness in the presence of a normal orthopedic examination must be considered an inability to support weight. Note that the right pelvic limb is also mildly paretic, based on how easy it is to push the horse to its right side. Note the normal response to a noxious stimulus on the medial side of the left crus.

Anatomic Diagnosis: L4, L5 spinal cord segments, spinal nerve roots, spinal nerves, femoral nerves worse on the left side. For weight support in the pelvic limb, the femoral nerve and the quadriceps femoris muscle must be intact. Because of the reciprocal apparatus in the horse, when the stifle flexes on collapsing, the tarsus also flexes, which exacerbates the limb collapse. Some femoral nerve GSA neurons are still functional, according to the normal nociception observed when the medial surface of the left crus was pinched with forceps. This cutaneous area is in the autonomous zone of the saphenous nerve, which is the cutaneous branch of the femoral nerve.

Differential Diagnosis: Equine protozoal myelitis, lymphoma, other neoplasm, neuritis

Equine protozoal myelitis is the most presumptive clinical diagnosis, based on the progression of signs, the asymmetry of the signs, the gray matter involvement, and the common occurrence of this disease in adult horses.[10,48,94] The clinical onset can vary from being remarkably acute and rapidly progressive to having a slow onset and chronic progression. This disease is described in Chapter 11 with Case Example 11-2.

Lymphoma is an uncommon disease of the nervous system of horses. However, infiltration of the L4 and L5 spinal nerve roots, spinal nerves, or femoral nerve could cause these signs, but the lesion would have to be bilateral.

Other neoplasms are quite rare in the spinal cord or peripheral nerves of horses.

The only recognized neuritis in the horse is polyneuritis equi (neuritis of the cauda equina), and the anatomic diagnosis of Tommy would be very unusual for this disorder.

Be aware that the first clinical signs of rabies virus encephalomyelitis may involve the gray matter of the lumbosacral intumescense and cause LMN signs in the pelvic limbs. This will change rapidly because the disease progresses fast, and most horses will be down in 4 days and dead by 7 to 10 days. The West Nile virus also causes a poliomyelitis, and the early signs of this disease may reflect this gray matter lesion.

Lumbar CSF obtained from Tommy contained a slight elevation of mononuclear cells (9 white blood cells per cmm), 2 red blood cells per cmm, and 43 mg protein/dl). Serum was positive for antibodies against *S. neurona*. He was treated with antiprotozoal drugs for 2 weeks, but there was continued progression of clinical signs in the right pelvic limb. He was euthanized, and the necropsy diagnosed an extensive nonsuppurative myelitis, primarily within the caudal lumbar spinal cord segments. The lesion was typical of that caused by *S. neurona* but no organisms were found in the lesion. This is typical in a horse that has received treatment for this organism.

CASE EXAMPLE 5-19

LMN Paraparesis—Cow

Signalment: 3-day-old Holstein cow

Chief Complaint: Lame in the left pelvic limb

History: Since its birth, this calf has exhibited pelvic limb lameness. The birth was difficult and required manual assistance. The calf's head and thoracic limbs presented but to free the calf's pelvic region from the cow's pelvic canal required the extraction efforts of two people. Initially the calf needed help to stand, and the lameness had not changed since birth.

Examination: Video 5-53 shows the marked inability to support weight with the left pelvic limb but no reluctance to try. A similar but much milder lameness was present in the right pelvic limb. There was no patellar reflex in the left pelvic limb. Nociception was normal on all surfaces of both pelvic limbs.

Anatomic Diagnosis: L4, L5 spinal cord segments, spinal nerve roots, spinal nerves, or femoral nerves

Differential Diagnosis: Injury, malformation, myelitis

DYSTOCIA INJURY: FEMORAL NERVE

The presence of these clinical signs at birth, with no change over the period of 3 days, strongly supports an injury to the femoral nerves that is worse on the left side. It is well recognized that the femoral nerves are at risk for being injured when a dystocia due to a "hip lock" leads to vigorous overextension of the hips when the extraction of the calf requires manual assistance.[20,129,135] This overextension puts traction on the femoral nerve or its roots. Most publications describe hemorrhages or disruption of the femoral nerve where it emerges from the iliopsoas muscle to enter the quadriceps femoris. If the injury is mild, spontaneous recovery may occur in a 2- to 4-week period, as it did in this calf.

Malformation of the spinal cord must be considered when the signs are present at birth and are nonprogressive. However, we have never seen a myelodysplasia cause a neurologic deficit that is asymmetric and is limited to the femoral nerves. Recall that most calves with myelodysplasia that are ambulatory will show a bunny-hopping simultaneous protraction of the pelvic limbs.

The only myelitis present at birth that would concern us in calves would be that caused by an in utero infection by *N. caninum,* which is a common cause of abortion in cattle.[49] Occasionally, calves that are infected late in gestation are born with signs of spinal cord dysfunction due to the myelitis portion of a diffuse encephalomyelitis. It would be very unusual for these signs to involve only the gray matter of the L4 and L5 spinal cord segments.

Video 5-54 shows a 1-week-old female Holstein calf that since birth had walked lame on its left pelvic limb. The initial diagnosis was a congenital patellar luxation. Note the lack of discomfort in using the limb, the inability to support weight, the atonic cranial thigh muscles, the laxity of the patella, the lack of a patellar reflex, and the analgesia of the medial aspect of the left crus. Compare the response of the calf to a noxious stimulus at the medial crus of the left pelvic limb with response at the same area of the right pelvic limb and the plantar aspect of the left metatarsus. Your anatomic diagnosis should be complete dysfunction of the left femoral nerve. What does this tell you about which pelvic limb nerve the calf needs to kick you? The analgesia in the distribution of the saphenous nerve branch of the left femoral nerve makes the prognosis for spontaneous recovery guarded. The owners raised this calf and at a follow–up, when she was 18 months old, her gait was unchanged.

Video 5-55 shows a 3-month-old Hereford calf with a similar history of a dystocia that required manual assistance and a diagnosis of right femoral nerve paralysis since birth that had not changed. This calf was euthanized, and a necropsy revealed an avulsion of the L4 and L5 spinal nerve roots on the right side. This is the only spinal nerve root avulsion we have seen involving the pelvic limbs that was not associated with a fracture. Small animals that are struck by moving vehicles and suffer sacrocaudal fracture with significant displacement are at risk for avulsion of the sacrocaudal nerves.

Femoral nerve injury may also occur in adult cattle that are recumbent due to a metabolic disorder such as hypocalcemia. This occurs when a cow is on a concrete surface and struggles to stand up. If the pelvic limbs slide out caudally, the femoral nerves may be stretched and torn, and the quadriceps femoris muscle may be injured. This can be avoided by keeping the cattle in stalls that have sand surfaces when they calve or have an illness that may cause recumbency resulting from paresis.

A cow is also at risk for a peripheral nerve injury during a dystocia. The obturator nerve can be compressed where it lies on the medial surface of the body of the ilium. The loss of the abductor muscles that this nerve innervates will not be seen if the cow freshens at pasture or in a box stall with a dirt floor. If she is on a concrete surface, she will severely abduct the limb when she tries to stand up, and this may tear the adductor muscles on the medial side of the thigh. Similarly, dystocia may cause compression of the ventral branch of the L6 spinal nerve, which lies against the prominent ventral surface of the cranial aspect of the sacrum as it courses caudally to join the ventral branches of S1 and S2 spinal nerves to form the sciatic nerve. Most of these L6 nerve fibers are destined to form the peroneal nerve. Their compression causes the cow to have difficulty extending her digits, and she will stand on their dorsal surfaces. The same clinical signs of peroneal nerve paralysis can occur in a cow that is recumbent in a stanchion and her recumbent pelvic limb lies across the edge of the gutter. Pressure can be placed on this nerve where it is subcutaneous as it crosses the lateral head of the gastrocnemius muscle to enter the cranial crural muscles.

CASE EXAMPLE 5-20

LMN Paraparesis—Dog

Signalment: 9-year-old castrated male Doberman pinscher, Zappa
Chief Complaint: Unable to stand in the pelvic limbs
History: Just 6 days prior to our examination, the owner noticed that Zappa was having difficulty with his pelvic limbs when he went up or down stairs, and he tripped when crossing thresholds. He was treated with corticosteroids and a muscle relaxant. The owner thought he was better the next day but the following day he was worse and became unable to get up using his pelvic limbs.

Examination: Video 5-56 shows that this dog cannot stand by himself. When assisted, note how he exerts himself to try to stand and walk and how fast he moves his pelvic limbs. He takes very rapid short strides, always in a crouched position because he cannot support his weight. Hip flexion is normal for protraction but stifle extension is inadequate. There was a mild decrease in tone distal to the hips, especially in the left pelvic limb, and the left patellar reflex was more depressed than the right. Flexor reflexes and nociception were normal. Anal tone was normal but the tail was too short to evaluate well. During the examination, there was constant dribbling of a small amount of urine. Occasionally, Zappa resented firm palpation of his lumbar vertebrae.

Anatomic Diagnosis: Bilateral L4, L5 spinal cord segments, spinal nerve roots, spinal nerves, and femoral nerves; slight involvement of the same sacral components

This anatomic diagnosis is uncommon. More often dogs with spinal cord disease cannot stand because of a UMN dysfunction. If some UMN is still intact and the dog is assisted to stand, there will be a delay in protraction of the limbs and the movements will be slow. This is in contrast to the rapid protraction efforts by Zappa, where the dysfunction was due primarily to the lack of sufficient support because of loss of femoral nerve activity.

Differential Diagnosis: Intervertebral disk extrusion, FCEM, neoplasm

INTERVERTEBRAL DISK EXTRUSION

An acute intervertebral disk extrusion was the most presumptive diagnosis in Zappa, based on the rapid onset of clinical signs, the brief improvement followed by rapid progression of clinical signs, and the suggestion of some discomfort on palpation of his lumbar vertebrae.

FCEM is a strong possibilty, but the history of a brief improvement and then progression of clinical signs would be unusual in that disorder. The occasional discomfort is more common with intervertebral disk extrusions but can occur occasionally with FCEM.

Extramedullary neoplasms can slowly compress the spinal cord without causing clinical signs until the vascular autoregulation is suddenly overwhelmed and clinical signs occur rapidly. Thus, neoplasm must be a consideration here.

The video shows the radiographs, the myelogram, and the CT myelogram that were performed on Zappa. They showed a large accumulation of intervertebral disk material over the body of L5. The CT sections start at the cranial aspect of L4 and continue to the caudal aspect of L5. Zappa was euthanized, and this diagnosis was confirmed at necropsy.

CASE EXAMPLE 5-21

Pelvic Limb Dysfunction—Dog

Signalment: 6-year-old male German shepherd, Jerry
Chief Complaint: Right pelvic limb lameness
History: For the past 2 months this dog had had an abnormal gait in the right pelvic limb; after 3 to 4 weeks of progression, it had been static. It did not interfere with his level of activity.

Examination: Video 5-57 shows that Jerry exhibited no discomfort when chasing the dummy. There was no impairment in his ability to advance the right pelvic limb and support weight, and the positions of the tarsus and digits were normal. Note that at the end of protraction (swing phase), the right hind paw was suddenly slightly elevated and quickly placed on the ground. At the same time there was a slight medial deviation of the stifle and lateral deviation of the tarsus.

FIBROSIS: CAUDOMEDIAL THIGH MUSCLES

There is no neurologic disorder that causes this abnormality. It is the result of the development of a fibrous band associated with the muscles on the caudomedial aspect of the thigh that arise from the pelvis and terminate on the proximomedial surface of the tibia. These are the semitendinosus, semimembranosus, and gracilis muscles. Most commonly this fibrous band is associated with the semitendinosus muscle. Full extension of the protracting limb depends on smooth relaxation of these antagonistic muscles. The fibrous band prevents this and mechanically terminates the protraction prematurely, resulting in the brief elevation of the paw and its sudden return to the ground. At the same time, the medial termination of this taut band on the proximal tibia forces a medial rotation of the stifle. When the stifle rotates medially, the tarsus always rotates laterally. In most dogs this fibrous band can be palpated on the caudomedial aspect of the thigh.

In the literature, this has been referred to as fibrotic myopathy of the caudomedial thigh muscles.[88] It is most common in the German shepherd breed. It has been proposed that an injury that tears a muscle in this group will result in fibrosis associated with the healing of the tear, and this will shorten the length of that muscle and result in the clinical signs seen here. This is a concept similar to that of the infraspinatus fibrosis that occurs in the thoracic limb. I (AD) have studied three surgical specimens of semitendinosus muscles with this fibrous band that were removed from Jerry and dogs similar to Jerry. In all of them, there was a dense fibrous band on one surface of the muscle, but the adjacent muscle was normal. There was no indication of any myopathy, no fibrosis associated with the healing of an injured portion of muscle. The band consisted of well-organized bundles of collagen (Fig. 5-62). The cause of this fibrous band is unknown but it must be removed to return the gait to normal. However, recurrence of this fibrous band is likely and therefore surgery should be considered with caution. There is no indication that this fibrous band causes the dog any discomfort. They readily run, jump and play with vigor like Jerry in this tape. Occasionally this disorder occurs bilaterally. I (EG) have now examined or observed videotapes of numerous working police dogs, mostly German Shepherds, and in all cases the trainers report that the dog's performance is not impeded by this disorder.

Video 5-58 shows another example of this muscle disorder in a 7-year-old male German shepherd with his trainer. This was a working police dog.

Video 5-59 shows a 17-year-old female standardbred. At 7 years of age she fell and fractured her pelvis and left greater

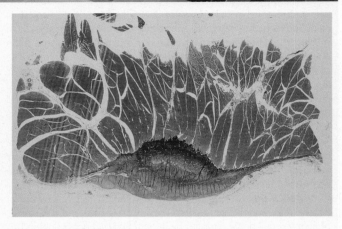

FIGURE 5-62 Microscopic transverse section of a surgical specimen of a semitendinosus muscle with a fibrous band in its epimysium and deep fascia. The muscle is normal.

trochanter. She had been used as a brood mare since then. It is not known when her lameness first developed, but it had been present for a number of years. Note the same abrupt termination of the protraction phase of the gait in the left pelvic limb as was seen in Jerry, but there is no medial rotation of the stifle. Note the taut band that is palpated on the caudomedial side of the left thigh. This mare was euthanized, and at necropsy there was extensive fibrosis of the proximal medial thigh muscles as well as considerable denervation atrophy to the branches of the sciatic nerve to these thigh muscles, all resulting from the injury. This gait disorder has been reported in horses that injure these muscles when they rest their caudal thighs on the chains that hold them in trailers for transportation or when these muscle are injured by repeated intramuscular injections of large quantities of drugs. Injury to the intramuscular branches of the sciatic nerve may play a role in the chronic shortening of these muscles in the horse.

PLANTIGRADE POSTURE

Whereas a significant palmigrade posture is the result only of loss of the integrity of the palmar carpal ligaments, a plantigrade posture has at least four different anatomic causes:

1. A tibial nerve dysfunction with denervation of the tarsal extensor muscles, the gastrocnemius, and the superficial digital flexors
2. A rupture of part or all of the common calcanean tendon
3. A fracture of the calcaneus
4. A disruption of the long plantar ligament.

Video 5-60 shows Chet, an 11-year-old castrated male domestic shorthair with a bilateral rupture of the gastrocnemius tendon, but the superficial digital flexor tendon has been spared. He is reluctant to move due to the discomfort of the lesion. Note that when the tarsus overflexes, the digits flex because of the stress put on the intact superficial digital flexor tendon that attaches to the calcaneus. Ultrasound examination showed changes suggestive of degeneration within the ruptured gastrocnemius tendon. In Figs. 5-63 through 5-65, note the same posture of a Doberman pinscher with a similar gastrocnemius tendon rupture at the level of the left pelvic limb

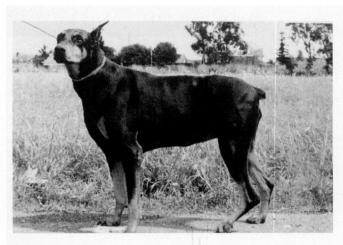

FIGURE 5-63 An 8-year-old Doberman pinscher with an overflexed left tarsus due to rupture of the tendon of insertion of the gastrocnemius muscle at the calcaneus. Note the flexion of the digits due to the stress placed on the intact superficial digital flexor muscle.

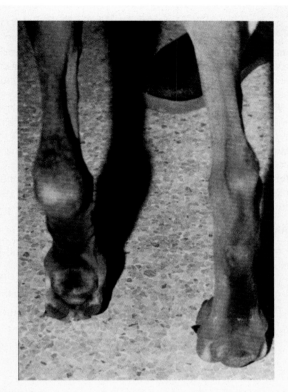

FIGURE 5-65 Caudal view of the dog seen in Figs. 5-63 and 5-64. Note the swelling at the calcaneus.

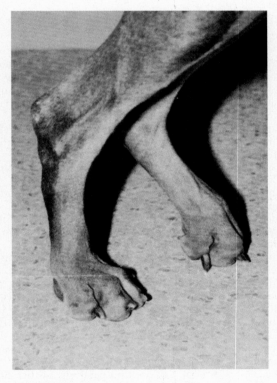

FIGURE 5-64 Lateral view of the dog seen in Fig. 5-63.

calcaneus, with sparing of the superficial digital flexor. The cause of these tendon ruptures was unknown.

Video 5-61 shows two 8-month-old German shepherd littermates that developed both a palmigrade and a plantigrade posture bilaterally. It was a slowly progressive disorder that started when they were about 3 months of age. Their neurologic examinations were normal. Only a collagen disorder affecting the palmar carpal ligaments and the common calcanean tendon would explain how both of these postures could result from a single cause. At necropsy, these dogs had no recognizable microscopic lesions in any of the samples of CNS or PNS tissue that were studied or in the numerous specimens of connective tissue that were studied. This is a poorly understood sporadic connective tissue disorder that is seen in this breed. A similar clinical presentation has been reported in rottweilers; it is caused by a form of muscular dystrophy.[66]

CASE EXAMPLE 5-22

Stiffness in a Kid

Signalment: 1-month-old female mixed-breed kid goat, Gimp

Chief Complaint: Unable to stand

History: The day before examination, this kid could not stand up without assistance. There was no obvious change during the short

period before the examination. This goat farm had a history of listeriosis in kids that appeared to be related to the time when they were losing their deciduous teeth. Gimp was taken to Cornell for a necropsy to confirm the diagnosis of listeriosis, but a clinical examination was requested by the pathologist prior to euthanasia.

(Continued)

CASE EXAMPLE 5-22—cont'd

Examination: Video 5-62 shows severe hypertonia, especially in the pelvic limbs, related to any stimulation. Note the absence of any obvious ataxia and the normal postural reactions by the thoracic limbs as well as attempts to overcome the hypertonia and perform the actions using the pelvic limbs. The hypertonia was too severe to permit the testing of the spinal nerve reflexes in the pelvic limbs. The muscles were prominent and firm on palpation.

Anatomic Diagnosis: Diffuse muscle disorder or diffuse spinal cord ventral gray column loss of inhibition

Differential Diagnosis: Vitamin E deficiency myopathy, inherited myotonia, myositis, dystrophinopathic (Duchenne) muscular dystrophy, tetanus

VITAMIN E DEFICIENCY MYOPATHY

The most common muscle disorder in young ruminants and foals is the myopathy-rhabdomyolysis associated with vitamin E and selenium deficiency. This is known as stiff lamb disease in sheep, and certainly the primary clinical sign in this goat was stiffness. The most likely cause is myotonia or pseudomyotonia as a result of disturbance of the muscle cell membranes. We are not aware of any EMG studies in these cases that would support or deny this hypothesis. In contrast, inherited myotonia is an episodic disorder in goats, evidenced by short periods of stiffness between long periods of normal muscle function (see Videos 8-2 and 8-3 in Chapter 8). Protozoal myositis caused by infection by *T. gondii* is uncommon, especially when accompanied by such diffuse severe hypertonia. A dystrophinopathic type of muscular dystrophy has not been reported in farm animals or horses. A moderate form of tetanus has to be considered in this kid. Only the lack of head muscle involvement makes it less likely.

Severe muscle necrosis was confirmed by the remarkable elevation of serum muscle enzymes: CK was 110,435 IU (normal is less than 446 IU). AST was 1393 IU (normal is less than 158 IU). Based on this information, the presumptive diagnosis was vitamin E deficiency myopathy. The necropsy was cancelled, and Gimp was treated with vitamin E and selenium and given a guarded prognosis because of the severity of her clinical signs. She was adopted and lost to follow-up evaluation.

REFERENCES

1. Barclay WP, de Lahunta A: Cryptococcal meningitis in a horse, *J Am Vet Med Assoc* 174:1236-1238, 1979.
2. Bargi V, Cohen A, Benado A: An outbreak of botulism in a dairy herd, *Refuah Vet* 30:135, 1973.
3. Barsanti JA, et al: Type C botulism in American foxhounds, *J Am Vet Med Assoc* 172:809, 1978.
4. Bennett D: Anatomical and histological study of the sciatic nerve relating to peripheral nerve injuries in the dog and cat, *J Small Anim Pract* 17:379, 1976.
5. Bennett RA: Contraction of the infraspinatus muscle in dogs: a review of 12 cases, *J Am Anim Hosp Assoc* 22:481-487, 1996.
6. Bergman RL, et al: Dystrophin-deficient muscular dystrophy in a Labrador retriever, *J Am Anim Hosp Assoc* 38:255-261, 2002.
7. Blakemore WF, et al: Spinal cord malacia following general anesthesia in the horse, *Vet Rec* 114:569-570, 1984.
8. Blakemore WF, Rees-Evans ET, Wheeler PEG: Botulism in foxhounds, *Vet Rec* 100:57, 1977.
9. Bowen JM: Electromyography. In Oliver JE, Hoerlein BF, Mayhew IG, editors: *Veterinary neurology*, Philadelphia, 1987, Saunders.
10. Boy MG, Galligan DT, Divers TJ: Protozoal encephalomyelitis in horses, 82 cases (1972-1986), *J Am Vet Med Assoc* 196:623-634, 1990.
11. Braund KG, Vallat JM, Steiss JE: Chronic inflammatory demyelinating polyneuropathy in dogs and cats, *J Periph Nerv Syst* 1:149-155, 1996.
12. Brehm DM, et al: A retrospective evaluation of 51 cases of peripheral nerve sheath tumors in the dog, *J Am Anim Hosp Assoc* 31:349-359, 1995.
13. Brown MO, Zaki FA: Electrodiagnostic testing for evaluation of neuromuscular disorders in dogs and cats, *J Am Vet Med Assoc* 174:86, 1979.
14. Cardinet GH, Holliday TA: Neuromuscular diseases of domestic animals: a summary of muscle biopsies from 159 cases, *Ann N Y Acad Sci* 317:290, 1979.
15. Chrisman CL: Dancing Doberman disease: clinical findings and prognosis, *Prog Vet Neurol* 1:83-90, 1990.
16. Cooper BJ: *Studies on the pathogenesis of tick paralysis*, Thesis, Sydney, Australia, 1976, University of Sydney.
17. Cooper BJ, et al: Canine inherited hypertrophic neuropathy: clinical and electrodiagnostic studies, *Am J Vet Res* 45:1172-1177, 1984.
18. Cooper BJ, et al: Defective Schwann cell function in canine inherited hypertrophic neuropathy, *Acta Neuropathol* 63:51-58, 1984.
19. Cork LC, et al: Hereditary canine spinal muscular atrophy, *J Neuropathol Exp Neurol* 38:209, 1979.
20. Cox VS, Breazile JE, Hoover TR: Surgical and anatomic study of calving paralysis, *Am J Vet Res* 36:427, 1975.
21. Cuddon P, et al: Neospora caninum infection in English springer spaniel littermates: diagnostic evaluation and organism isolation, *J Vet Intern Med* 6:325-332, 1992.
22. Cummings JF, et al: Canine inherited hypertrophic neuropathy, *Acta Neuropathol* 53:137, 1981.
23. Cummings JF, de Lahunta A: Chronic relapsing polyradiculoneuritis in a dog: a clinical, light and electron-microscopic study, *Acta Neuropathol* 28:191-204, 1974.
24. Cummings JF, de Lahunta A: Hypertrophic neuropathy in a dog, *Acta Neuropathol* 29:325-336, 1974.
25. Cummings JF, et al: Equine motor neuron disease: a preliminary report, *Cornell Vet* 80:357-379, 1990.
26. Cummings JF, et al: Coonhound paralysis: further clinical studies and electron microscopic observations, *Acta Neuropathol* 56:167-178, 1982.
27. Cummings JF, et al: Canine brachial plexus neuritis: a syndrome resembling serum neuritis in man, *Cornell Vet* 63:590, 1973.
28. Cummings JF, et al: Endothelial lipopigment as an indicator of alpha tocopherol deficiency in two equine neurodegenerative diseases, *Acta Neuropathol* 90:266-272, 1995.
29. Cummings JF, et al: Equine motor neuron disease: a new neurologic disorder, *Eq Pract* 13:15-18, 1991.
30. Cummings JF, et al: Reduced subtance P-like immuno-reactivity in hereditary sensory neuropathy of Pointer dogs, *Acta Neuropathol* 63:33-40, 1984.
31. Cummings JF, et al: Canine protozoan polyradiculoneuritis, *Acta Neuropathol* 76:46-54, 1988.

32. Cummings JF, de Lahunta A, Timoney JF: Neuritis of the cauda equina, a chronic idiopathic polyradiculoneuritis in the horse, *Acta Neuropathol* 46:17, 1979.

33. Cummings JF, et al: Focal spinal muscular atrophy in two German shepherd pups, *Acta Neuropathol* 79:113-116, 1989.

34. Cummings JF, Haas DC: Coonhound paralysis: an acute idiopathic polyradiculoneuritis in dogs resembling the Landry-Gullain-Barre syndrome, *J Neurol Sci* 4:51, 1967.

35. Dahme E, Deutschlander N: Die Neuritis der Cauda Equina beim Pferd in Elektronenmikroskopischen Bild, *Zentrallblat Vet Med* 23:502, 1976.

36. de Lahunta A, Alexander JM: Ischemic myelopathy secondary to presumed fibrocartilaginous embolism in nine dogs, *J Am Anim Hosp Assoc* 12:37, 1976.

37. de Lahunta A, et al: Avulsion of the roots of the brachial plexus in five birds, *Comp Anim Pract* 2:38-40, 1988.

38. Dewey CW: Acquired myasthenia gravis in dogs, Part I, *Compend Cont Ed* 19:1340-1353, 1997.

39. Dewey CW: Acquired myasthenia gravis in dogs, Part II, *Compend Cont Ed* 20:47-57, 1998.

40. Dewey CW, et al: Clinical forms of acquired myasthenia gravis in dogs: 25 cases (1988-1995), *J Vet Intern Med* 11: 50-57, 1997.

41. Dewey CW, et al: Azathioprine therapy for acquired myasthenia gravis in five dogs, *J Am Anim Hosp Assoc* 35:396-402, 1999.

42. Dickinson PJ, et al: Congenital myasthenia gravis in smooth-haired Dachshund dogs, *J Vet Intern Med* 19: 920-923, 2005.

43. Divers TJ, et al: Equine motor neuron disease, *Am Coll Vet Intern Med Proc* 13:918-921, 1995.

44. Divers TJ, et al: Equine motor neuron disease-update, *Am Coll Vet Intern Med Proc* 20:1442, 2002.

45. Divers TJ, et al: Equine motor neuron disease: a new cause of weakness, trembling and weight loss, *Compend Cont Ed* 14:1222-1226, 1992.

46. Divers TJ, et al: Equine motor neuron disease: findings in 28 horses and proposal of a pathophysiological mechanism for the disease, *Eq Vet J* 26:409-415, 1994.

47. Dubey JP, Carpenter JL, Speer CA: Newly recognized fatal protozoan disease of dogs, *J Am Vet Med Assoc* 192: 1269-1285, 1988.

48. Dubey JP, Davis SW, Speer CA: Sarcocystis neurona N. sp. (Protozoa: Apicomplexa), the etiologic agent of equine protozoal myeloencephalitis, *J Parasitol* 77:212-218, 1991.

49. Dubey JP, de Lahunta A: Neosporosis associated congenital limb deformities in a calf, *Appl Parasitol* 34:229-233, 1993.

50. Dubey JP, Hattel AL, Lindsay DS: Neonatal *Neospora caninum* infection in dogs: isolation of the causative agent and experimental transmission, *J Am Vet Med Assoc* 193: 1259-1263, 1988.

51. Ducote M, Dewey CW, Coates JR: Clinical forms of myasthenia gravis in cats, *Am Coll Vet Intern Med Proc* 16:238, 1998.

52. Duncan ID, Griffiths IR: Canine giant axonal neuropathy, *Vet Rec* 101:438, 1977.

53. Duncan ID, Griffiths IR: Inflammatory muscle disease in the dog. In Kirk RW, editor: *Current veterinary therapy VII: small animal practice*, Philadelphia, 1980, Saunders.

54. Dyck PJ, Lambert EH: Polyneuropathy associated with hypothyroidism, *J Neuropathol Expt Neurol* 29:631, 1970.

55. el-Hamidi M, et al: Spinal muscular atrophy in brown Swiss calves, *Zentralbl Veterinarmed A* 36:731-738, 1998.

56. Farrow BRH: Episodic weakness. In Kirk RW, editor: *Current veterinary therapy VII: small animal practice*, Philadelphia, 1980, Saunders.

57. Fletcher TF: Lumbosacral plexus and pelvic limb myotomes of the dog, *Am J Vet Res* 31:35, 1970.

58. Garosi L, et al: Bilateral hypertrophic neuritis of the brachial plexus in a cat: magnetic resonance imaging and pathological findings, *J Fel Med Surg* 8:63-68, 2006.

59. Gaschen F, Jaggy A, Jones B: Congenital diseases of feline muscle and neuromuscular junction, *J Fel Med Surg* 6: 355-366, 2004.

60. Griffiths IR: The extensive myelopathy of intervertebral disk protrusions in dogs (the ascending syndrome), *J Sm Anim Pract* 13:425, 1972.

61. Griffiths IR: Avulsion of the brachial plexus. 1. Neuro-pathology of the spinal cord and peripheral nerves, *J Small Anim Pract* 15:165, 1974.

62. Griffiths IR: Avulsion of the brachial plexus. 2. Clinical aspects, *J Small Anim Pract* 15:177, 1974.

63. Griffiths IR: Ischemic neuromyopathy in cats, *Vet Rec* 104:518, 1979.

64. Griffiths IR, Duncan ID: The use of electromyography and nerve conduction studies in the evaluation of lower motor neuron disease or injury, *J Small Anim Pract* 19:329, 1978.

65. Hallin RG, et al: Spinal cord implantation of avulsed ventral roots in primates: correlation between restored motor function and morphology, *Exp Brain Res* 124: 304-310, 1999.

66. Hanson SM, et al: Juvenile-onset distal myopathy in rottweiler dogs, *J Vet Intern Med* 12:103-108, 1998.

67. Hayes MA, et al: Acute necrotizing myelopathy from nucleus pulposus embolism of arteries and veins in large dogs with early disk degeneration, *J Am Vet Med Assoc* 173:289, 1978.

68. Heavner J: Intervertebral disk syndrome in the cat, *J Am Vet Med Assoc* 159:425-427, 1971.

69. Holmes DF, de Lahunta A: Experimental allergic neuritis in the dog and its comparison with the naturally occurring disease: coonhound paralysis, *Acta Neuropathol* 30:329-337, 1974.

70. Holmes DF, et al: Experimental coonhound paralysis, an unusual model for Guillain-Barré syndrome, *Neurology* 29:1186-1187, 1979.

71. Imhoff RK: Production of aortic occlusion resembling embolism syndrome in cats, *Nature* 192:979-980, 1961.

72. Jackson CA, et al: Spinal accessory nerve biopsy as an ante mortem diagnostic test for equine motor neuron disease, *Equine Vet J* 28:215-219, 1996.

73. Jenkins WL, Van Dyke E, McDonald CB: Myasthenia gravis in a fox terrier litter, *J S Afr Vet Assoc* 47:59, 1976.

74. Johnson RP, et al: Myasthenia in springer spaniel littermates, *J Small Anim Pract* 16:641, 1975.

75. Jones BR, Swinney GW, Alley MR: Hypokalemic myopathy in Burmese kittens, *N Z, Vet J* 36:150-151, 1988.

76. Kent MK, et al: Motor neuron abiotrophy in a Saluki, *J Am Anim Hosp Assoc* 35:436-439, 1999.

77. Kimura J: *Electrodiagnostics in diseases of nerve and muscle: principles and practice*, ed 3, New York, 2001, Oxford University Press.

78. Klopp LS, Smith BF: Autosomal recessive muscular dystrophy in Labrador retrievers, *Compend Cont Ed* 22: 121-130, 2000.

79. Kornegay JM: Ischemic myelopathy due to fibrocarti-ginous embolism, *Compend Cont Ed* 11:402, 1980.

80. Kornegay JN: Golden retriever muscular dystrophy: a model of Duchenne muscular dystrophy, *Discuss Neurosci* 5:118-123, 1988.

81. Kornegay JN, et al: Polymyositis in dogs, *J Am Vet Med Assoc* 176:431, 1976.

82. Korneliussen H, Jansen JKS: Morphological aspects of the elimination of polyneuronal innervation of skeletal muscle fibers in newborn rats, *J Neurocytol* 5:591, 1976.

83. Kramer JW, et al: A muscle disorder of Labrador retrievers characterized by deficiency of type II muscle fibers, *J Am Vet Med Assoc* 169:817, 1976.

84. Kramer JW, Hegreberg GA, Hamilton MJ: Inheritance of a neuromuscular disorder of Labrador retrievers, *J Am Vet Med Assoc* 179:380, 1981.

85. Lane JR, de Lahunta A: Polyneuritis in a cat, *J Am Anim Hosp Assoc*, 20:1006-1008, 1984.

86. Lenehan TM: Canine cauda equina syndrome, *Compend Cont Ed Pract Vet* 5:941-951, 1983.

87. Levine JM, et al: The influence of age on patellar reflex response in the dog, *J Vet Intern Med* 16:244-246, 2002.

88. Lewis DD, Shelton GD, Piras A: Gracilis or semitendinosus myopathy in 18 dogs, *J Am Anim Hosp Assoc* 33:177-188, 1997.

89. Lorenz MD: Episodic weakness in the dog. In Kirk RW, editor: *Current veterinary therapy, V: Small Animal Practice*, Philadelphia, 1974, Saunders.

90. Lorenz MD, et al: Hereditary spinal muscular atrophy in Brittaney spaniels: clinical manifestations, *J Am Vet Med Assoc* 175:833, 1979.

91. MacKay RD, Berkoff GA: Type C toxicoinfectious botulism in a foal, *J Am Vet Med Assoc* 180:163, 1982.

92. Martin S: *Clostridium botulinum* type D intoxication in a dairy herd in Ontario Canada, *Vet J* 44:493-495, 2003.

93. Matwichuk CL, et al: Changes in rectal temperature and hematologic, biochemical, blood gas, and acid-base values in healthy Labrador retrievers before and after strenuous exercise, *Am J Vet Res* 60:88, 1999.

94. Mayhew IG, de Lahunta A, Whitlock RH: Spinal cord disease in the horse, *Cornell Vet* 68(suppl 6):1-207, 1978.

95. McKerrell RE, Braund KG: Hereditary myopathy in Labrador retrievers: clinical variations, *J Small Anim Pract* 28:479-489, 1986.

96. Mohammed HO, et al: Epidemiology of equine motor neuron disease, *Vet Res* 25:275-278, 1994.

97. Nicholson SS: Bovine posterior paralysis due to organophosphate poisoning, *J Am Vet Med Assoc* 165:280, 1974.

98. Northington JW, et al: Acute idiopathic polyneuropathy in the dog, *J Am Vet Med Assoc* 179:375, 1981.

99. O'Brien DP, et al: Laminin alpha 2 (merosin)-deficient muscular dystrophy and demyelinating neuropathy in two cats, *J Neurol Sci* 189:37-43, 2001.

100. Olby NJ, et al: Evaluation of the dystrophin-glycoprotein complex, alpha actinin, dysferlin and calpain 3 in an autosomal recessive muscular dystrophy in Labrador retrievers, *Neuromusc Disord* 11:41-49, 2001.

101. Oliver JE, Selcer RR, Simpson S: Cauda equina compression from lumbosarcal malarticulation and malformation in the dog, *J Am Vet Med Assoc* 173:207-214, 1978.

102. O'Sullivan BM, Blakemore WF: Acute nicotinamide deficiency in pigs, *Vet Rec* 103:543, 1978.

103. O'Sullivan BM, Blakemore WF: Acute nicotinamide deficiency in the pig induced by 6-aminonicotinamide, *Vet Pathol* 17:748, 1980.

104. Pallaske G: Pathologie der chronischen Neuritis der Cauda Equina, *Dtsch Tierarztl Wochenschr* 73:415, 1966.

105. Palmer AC, Goodyear JV: Congenital myasthenia in the Jack Russell terrier, *Vet Rec* 103:433, 1978.

106. Palmer AC, Lamont MH, Wallace WE: Focal symmetrical poliomalacia of the spinal cord in Ayshire calves, *Vet Pathol* 23:506-509, 1986.

107. Palmer RH, Chambers JN: Canine lumbosacral diseases. Part I. Anatomy, pathophysiology and clinical presentation, *Compend Cont Ed Pract Vet* 13:61-69, 1991.

108. Palmer RH, Chambers JN: Canine lumbosacral disease. Part II. Definitive diagnosis, treatment and prognosis, *Compend Cont Ed Pract Vet* 13:213-222, 1991.

109. Pass DA: Posterior paralysis in a sow due to cartilaginous emboli in the spinal cord, *Aust Vet J* 54:100, 1978.

110. Riis RC, et al: Ocular manifestations of equine motor neuron disease, *Equine Vet J* 31:99-110, 1999.

111. Sandefelt E, et al: Hereditary neuronal abiotrophy in the Swedish Lapland dog, *Cornell Vet* 63(suppl 3):1, 1973.

112. Schatzberg S, Olby N, Breen M: Molecular analysis of a spontaneous dystrophin "knockout" dog, *Neuromusc Disord* 9:289-295, 1999.

113. Schwerer B: Antibodies against gangliosides: a link between preceding infection and the immunopathogenesis of Guillain-Barré syndrome, *Microbes Infect* 4:373-384, 2002.

114. Shell LG, Jortner BS, Leid MS: Spinal muscular atrophy in two rottweiler littermates, *J Am Vet Med Assoc* 190: 878-880, 1987.

115. Shell LG, Jortner BS, Leid MS: Familial motor neuron disease in rottweiler dogs: neuropathological studies, *Vet Pathol* 24:135-139, 1987.

116. Shelton GD, et al: Adult-onset motor neuron disease in three cats, *J Am Vet Med Assoc* 212:1271-1275, 1998.

117. Shelton GD, et al: Inherited polyneuropathy in Leonberger dogs: a mixed or intermediate form of Charcot-Marie-Tooth disease? *Muscle Nerve* 27:471-477, 2003.

118. Shelton GD, Schule A, Kass PH: Risk factors for acquired myasthenia gravis in dogs: 1,154 cases (1991-1995), *J Am Vet Med Assoc* 210:240-243, 1997.

119. Sielman ES, et al: Hypokalemia syndrome in dairy cows: 10 cases (1992-1996), *Am Coll Vet Intern Med Proc* 14:491-492, 1997.

120. Siems JJ, Breur GE, Blevins WE: Use of two-dimensional real-time ultrasound for diagnosing contracture and strain of the infraspinatus muscle in a dog, *J Am Vet Med Assoc* 212:77-80, 1998.

121. Sponenberg DP, de Lahunta A: Hereditary hypertrophic neuropathy in Tibetan mastiff dogs, *J Hered* 72:287, 1981.

122. Sprayberry KA, Carlson GP: Review of equine botulism, *Am Assoc Eq Pract Proc* 43:379-381, 1997.

123. Steiss J, et al: Coccygeal muscle injury in English pointers (limber tail), *J Vet Intern Med* 13:540-548, 1999.

124. Stockard CR: A hereditary lethal for localized motor and preganglionic neurons with a resulting paralysis in the dog, *Am J Anat* 59:1, 1936.

125. Swerczek TW: Toxicoinfectious botulism in foals and adult horses, *J Am Vet Med Assoc* 176:217, 1980.

126. Taylor SM: *Exercise induced collapse in Labrador retrievers* (website): www.thelabradorclub.com/library/eicstudy.html. Accessed April 16, 2003.

127. Thompson PN, et al: Congenital myasthenic syndrome of Brahman cattle in South Africa, *Vet Rec* 27:779, 2003.

128. Tosi L, Rigoli G, Beltramelo A: Fibrocartilaginous embolism of the spinal cord: a clinical and pathogenetic consideration, *J Neurol Neurosurg Psychiatry* 60:55-60, 1996.

129. Tryphonas L, Hamilton GF, Rhodes CS: Perinatal femoral nerve degeneration and neurogenic atrophy of quadriceps femoris muscle in calves, *J Am Vet Med Assoc* 154:801, 1974.

130. Valentine BA, et al: Progressive muscular dystrophy in a golden retriever dog: light microscopic and ultrastructural features at 4 and 8 months, *Acta Neuropathol* 71:301-310, 1986.

131. Valentine BA, et al: Canine X-linked muscular dystrophy: morphologic lesions, *J Neurol Sci* 97:1-23, 1990.

132. Valentine BA, Cooper B, de Lahunta A: Canine X-linked muscular dystrophy: an animal model of Duchenne muscular dystrophy: clinical studies, *J Neurol Sci* 88:69-81, 1988.

133. Valentine BA, et al: Acquired motor neuron disease, *Vet Pathol* 31:130-138, 1994.

134. Valentine BA, et al: Canine X-linked muscular dystrophy as an animal model of Duchenne muscular dystrophy: a review, *Am J Med Genet* 42:615-621, 1992.

135. Vaughan LC: Peripheral nerve injuries: an experimental study in cattle, *Vet Rec* 76:1293, 1964.

136. Wentink GH, et al: Myopathy with a possible recessive X-linked inheritance in a litter of Irish terriers, *Vet Pathol* 9:328, 1972.

137. Wetterman CA, et al: Hypertrophic muscular dystrophy in a young dog, *J Am Vet Med Assoc* 216:878-881, 2000.

138. Whitlock RH: Botulism in large animals, *Am Coll Vet Intern Med Proc* 8:681-684, 1990.

139. Whitlock RH: Botulism type C: experimental and field cases in horses, *Am Coll Vet Intern Med* 13:720-723, 1995.

140. Wilkins PA, Palmer JE: Botulism in foals less than 6 months of age: 30 cases (1989-2002), *J Vet Intern Med* 127:702-707, 2003.

141. Wilson JW: Relationship of the patellar tendon reflex to the ventral branch of the fifth lumbar spinal nerve in the dog, *Am J Vet Res* 39:1174, 1978.

142. Wilson TM, et al: Porcine focal symmetrical poliomyelomalacia: experimental reproduction with oral doses of encapsulated sodium selenite, *Can J Vet Res* 52:83-88, 1988.

143. Wilson TM, Scholz RW, Drake TR: Selenium toxicity and porcine focal symmetrical poliomyelomalacia: description of a field outbreak and experimental reproduction, *Can J Comp Med* 47:412-421, 1983.

144. Wilson TM, Sprake TR: Porcine focal symmetrical poliomyelomalacia, *Can J Comp Med* 46:218, 1982.

145. Worthman RP: Demonstration of specific nerve paralysis in the dog, *J Am Vet Med Assoc* 131:174, 1957.

146. Zaki F, Prata RG: Necrotizing myelopathy secondary to embolization of herniated intervertebral disk material in the dog, *J Am Vet Med Assoc* 169:222, 1976.

147. Zaki F, Prata RG, Kay WJ: Necrotizing myelopathy in five Great Danes, *J Am Vet Med Assoc* 165:1080, 1974.

6 LOWER MOTOR NEURON: GENERAL SOMATIC EFFERENT, CRANIAL NERVE

CRANIAL NERVE III: OCULOMOTOR NEURONS

Anatomy

CRANIAL NERVE IV: TROCHLEAR NEURONS

Anatomy

CRANIAL NERVE VI: ABDUCENT NEURONS

Anatomy

FUNCTION OF CRANIAL NERVES III, IV, AND VI

Function
Clinical Signs
Diseases

CRANIAL NERVE V: TRIGEMINAL NEURONS

Anatomy
Clinical Signs
Diseases
  Malignant Nerve Sheath Neoplasm
  Lymphoma

  Trigeminal Neuritis
  Myositis

CRANIAL NERVE VII: FACIAL NEURONS

Anatomy
Clinical Signs
Diseases
  Otitis Media
  Facial Nerve Tetanus (Hemifacial Spasm)
  Idiopathic Facial Neuropathy-Neuritis

CRANIAL NERVES IX, X, AND XI: GLOSSOPHARYNGEAL, VAGAL, ACCESSORY NEURONS

Anatomy
  Glossopharyngeal Nerve
  Vagus Nerve
  Accessory Nerve
Clinical Signs
Diseases
  Megaesophagus
  Guttural Pouch Mycosis

  Equine Laryngeal Hemiparesis-Hemiplegia
  Toxicity
  Cranial Mediastinal Lesions
  Canine Laryngeal Paralysis

CRANIAL NERVE XII: HYPOGLOSSAL NEURONS

Anatomy
Clinical Signs
Diseases
  Diffuse Lower Motor Neuron Diseases
  Encephalitis
  Prosencephalon
  CASE EXAMPLE 6-1
    Listeriosis
    Abscess
    Rabies
    Thrombotic Meningoencephalitis
    Malignant Catarrhal Fever
  CASE EXAMPLE 6-2
    Equine Protozoal Encephalomyelitis
    Polyneuritis Equi
    Equine Herpesvirus 1

The general somatic efferent (GSE) lower motor neurons (LMN) in cranial nerves innervate the voluntary striated skeletal muscle derived from occipital somites (i.e., tongue: cranial nerve XII) and from the head somitomeres that migrate into the branchial arches (i.e., extraocular muscles: cranial nerves III, IV, and VI; muscles of mastication: cranial nerve V; facial muscles: cranial nerve VII; larynx: cranial nerve X; and pharynx and esophagus: cranial nerves IX and X). Like spinal nerves, these cranial nerves contain neurons relating to other functional systems. Cranial nerves III, VII, IX, and X contain general visceral efferent (GVE) preganglionic neurons, and most contain some form of sensory neurons. The cell bodies of these GSE neurons are found in nuclei in the brainstem from the mesencephalon through the caudal medulla (Fig. 6-1).

CRANIAL NERVE III: OCULOMOTOR NEURONS

Anatomy

The GSE neuronal cell bodies of oculomotor neurons are located in the oculomotor nucleus in the rostral mesencephalon at the level of the rostral colliculi (Fig. 6-2; see also Figs. 2-6, 2-7, and 6-1). The nucleus is adjacent to the midline within the ventral portion of the central gray substance that surrounds the mesencephalic aqueduct. This nucleus is rostral to the trochlear nucleus and caudal to the pretectal nucleus. The GSE neuronal cell bodies are in the more caudal portion of the oculomotor nucleus, and the GVE parasympathetic preganglionic neuronal cell bodies are in the more rostral portion of this nucleus. These GVE neurons are described in Chapter 7. The oculomotor nucleus is dorsal and medial to the red nucleus. The medial longitudinal fasciculus is located just medial and ventral to this oculomotor nucleus. One function of this fasciculus is to interconnect the oculomotor, trochlear, and abducent neurons that innervate the extraocular muscles to permit coordinated conjugate movements of the eyes.

The axons of the GSE oculomotor neuronal cell bodies pass ventrally through the reticular formation of the mesencephalic tegmentum medial to the red nucleus, substantia nigra, and crus cerebri. They emerge on the lateral side of the interpeduncular fossa to form the oculomotor nerve on the medial side of the crus cerebri. This nerve courses rostrally in the middle cranial fossa beside the pituitary gland,

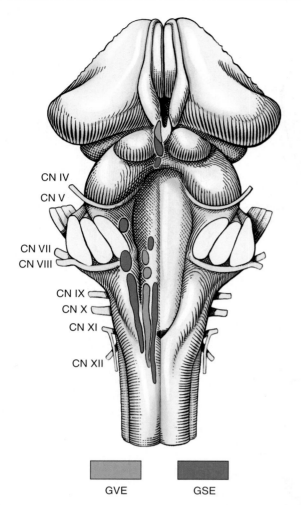

CN IV
CN V
CN VII
CN VIII
CN IX
CN X
CN XI
CN XII

GVE   GSE

FIGURE 6-1 Functional organization of cranial nerve nuclei in the brainstem: general somatic efferent *(GSE)* and general visceral efferent *(GVE)*.

adjacent to but *not in* the cavernous sinus. The oculomotor nerve leaves the cranial cavity through the orbital fissure and within the periorbita; the oculomotor nerve branches to supply the medial, dorsal, and ventral recti muscles, the ventral oblique muscle, and the levator palpebrae superioris muscle.

The clinical signs caused by lesions in these oculomotor neurons are described after the description of the anatomy of all three cranial nerves that innervate the extraocular muscles.

CRANIAL NERVE IV: TROCHLEAR NEURONS

Anatomy

The GSE neuronal cell bodies are located in a very small nucleus in the caudal mesencephalon at the level of the caudal colliculi (see Fig. 2-8 and Figs. 6-1 and 6-2). This trochlear nucleus is adjacent to the midline in the ventral portion of the central gray substance that surrounds the mesencephalic aqueduct. It is caudal to the larger oculomotor nucleus. The medial longitudinal fasciculus, which

connects the vestibular nuclei with these nuclei that innervate the extraocular muscles, lies just medial and ventral to the trochlear nucleus.

The axons of the GSE neuronal cell bodies in these trochlear nuclei course progressively in lateral, dorsal, and caudal directions to enter the rostral medullary velum, where they continue across this velum to the opposite side and emerge just caudal to the caudal colliculus (see Fig. 2-9). These axons continue rostrally and ventrally on the side of the mesencephalon to reach the floor of the middle cranial fossa. They continue rostrally beside the pituitary gland adjacent to but *not in* the cavernous sinus and leave the cranial cavity through the orbital fissure. Within the periorbita, the trochlear neurons innervate the dorsal oblique muscle. This is the only cranial nerve with GSE neurons that innervates a muscle solely on the side opposite from its nucleus (see the discussion of the clinical signs caused by lesions that affect these trochlear neurons; it follows the description of the anatomy of the abducent neurons).

CRANIAL NERVE VI: ABDUCENT NEURONS

Anatomy

The GSE neurons of the abducent nerve are located in the abducent nucleus in the rostral medulla (see Fig. 2-12). This is a small nucleus at the level of the medulla where the caudal cerebellar peduncle merges with the cerebellum. It is adjacent to the midline and floor of the fourth ventricle. The GSE axons of the genu of the facial nerve pass over this nucleus (Fig. 6-3; see also Fig. 6-1 and 6-24). The axons of the abducent neuronal cell bodies in the nucleus pass directly ventrally through the reticular formation of the medulla medial to the distinct dorsal nucleus of the trapezoid body. They pass through the trapezoid body and emerge just lateral to the pyramid. The abducent nerve courses rostrally on the floor of the middle fossa beside the pituitary gland, adjacent to but *not in* the cavernous sinus, and leaves the cranial cavity through the orbital fissure. It branches within the periorbita to innervate the lateral rectus and retractor bulbi muscles.

FUNCTION OF CRANIAL NERVES III, IV, AND VI

Function

To understand the clinical signs resulting from lesions that interfere with the function of one or more of these three cranial nerves that innervate the extraocular muscles, the normal action of these muscles on the eyeball must be understood. If the eyeball is assumed to have three axes for rotation, the muscles can be grouped into three opposing pairs. If you assume a horizontal axis through the center of the eyeball, the dorsal rectus will elevate the eyeball, and the ventral rectus will depress the eyeball. If you assume a vertical axis through the center of the eyeball, the medial rectus will adduct the eyeball and the lateral rectus will abduct it. If you assume an anterior-to-posterior axis through the center of the eyeball, the dorsal oblique will intort the

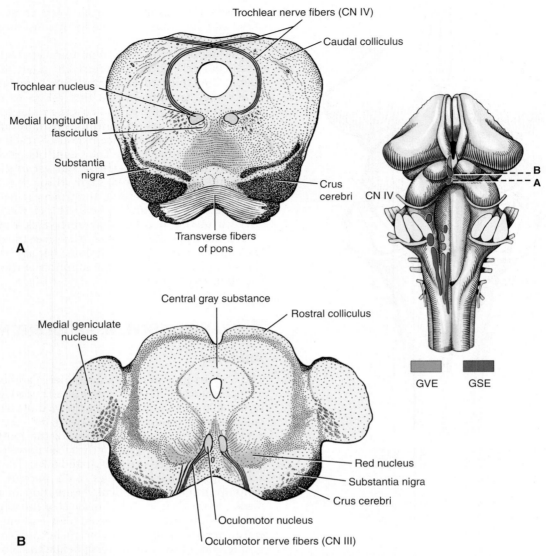

FIGURE 6-2 Transverse sections through the mesencephalon. **A,** At the level of the trochlear. **B,** At the level of the oculomotor nuclei.

eyeball, or rotate the dorsal portion medioventrally toward the nose, and the ventral oblique will extort the eyeball, or rotate the dorsal portion lateroventrally away from the nose. These muscles do not function alone but continuously act together in a synergistic or antagonistic manner to provide for conjugate movements of both eyeballs in the same direction at the same time. This is easiest to appreciate by considering the action of the medial and lateral recti muscles in horizontal conjugate movements. To test the action of these muscles as part of your cranial nerve examination, you obviously cannot depend on your patient to respond to your command to look in different directions. However, the function of the oculomotor nerve to the medial rectus and the abducent nerve to the lateral rectus is readily assessed by testing for normal or physiologic nystagmus, a vestibuloocular test.

Nystagmus is defined as involuntary movements of the eyes, and there are normal and abnormal forms of nystagmus. The normal nystagmus that occurs with this test is a jerk nystagmus, meaning that there is a fast and a slow phase of the eye movement. The direction of the fast phase defines the direction of the nystagmus. Stand over your small animal patient so that you both are headed in the same direction; with large animals, stand so that you face them and can observe both eyes. Move the head at a moderate rate from one side to the other and keep repeating this as you watch the movements of the eyes. It may help in small animals to hold the eyelids open as you do this test so that you can observe the limbus. Moving the head stimulates the sensory receptors in the inner ear that are innervated by the vestibular portion of cranial nerve VIII. Impulses are relayed into the vestibular nuclei in the medulla and then passed rostrally via the medial longitudinal fasciculus to the abducent, trochlear, and oculomotor nuclei. As you move the head to the right, both eyes will exhibit a rapid movement, a jerk, toward the right. This is a normal right nystagmus. As you move the head back to the left, both eyes will jerk to the left, a normal left nystagmus. In neuroanatomic terms, when the head is moved to the right, the right eye will jerk to the right via

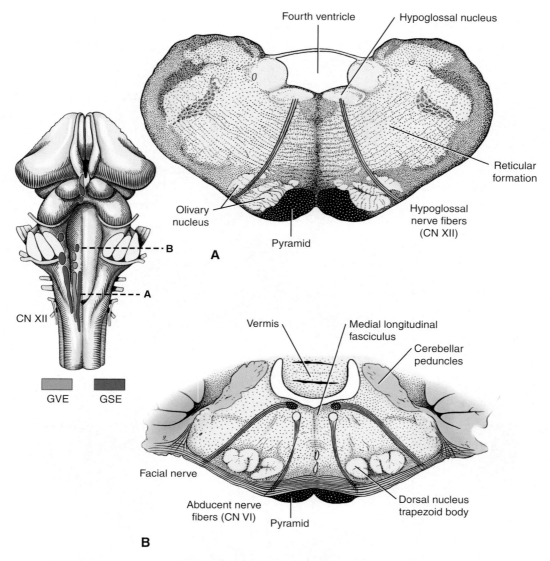

Fourth ventricle   Hypoglossal nucleus

Reticular formation

Olivary nucleus

Pyramid

Hypoglossal nerve fibers (CN XII)

A

CN XII

GVE   GSE

Vermis   Medial longitudinal fasciculus

Cerebellar peduncles

Facial nerve

Abducent nerve fibers (CN VI)   Pyramid   Dorsal nucleus trapezoid body

B

FIGURE 6-3 Transverse sections through the medulla. **A,** At the level of the hypoglossal. **B,** At the level of the abducent nuclei.

contraction of the lateral rectus innervated by the abducent nerve, and at the same time the left eye will jerk to the right via the contraction of the medial rectus innervated by the oculomotor nerve. When you swing the head back to the left, the opposite innervations and muscles will be activated. This action tests the function of cranial nerves III and VI as well as the vestibular nerve (VIII) and the pathway of the medial longitudinal fasciculus through the brainstem. These are conjugate eye movements related to the movement of the head and have nothing to do with vision. This test can be performed in blind animals.

This test is very reliable in most dogs, horses, and farm animals but may be difficult to elicit in some cats. Often in cats, the nystagmus (the eyeball jerk) will not occur until the very end of the head movement, and you must look carefully if you are to see it occur. Occasionally, you will not be able to elicit this eye movement in a normal cat. Serious brainstem lesions that interrupt this pathway will prevent any movement of the eyes when this normal physiologic nystagmus is tested. This is discussed further with the vestibular system.

Clinical Signs

Neuromuscular strabismus is an abnormal position of the eyeball due to a loss of innervation of extraocular muscles or due to a primary extraocular muscle disorder. In dogs with developmental obstructive hydrocephalus, it may result from a malformation of the orbit. The direction of the strabismus is determined by the muscles that have been denervated. Neuromuscular strabismus is present in most positions of the head.

Lesions of the abducent neurons cause paralysis of the lateral rectus and retractor bulbi muscles. Loss of the lateral rectus innervation results in a medial strabismus (Fig. 6-4) due to the unopposed contraction of the medial rectus muscle. When you test for normal nystagmus by moving the head from one side to the other in a horizontal plane, the affected eye will not abduct when the head is moved toward that eye. Carefully compare the degree of abduction of the two eyes to appreciate this clinical sign. There is no reliable test for eyeball retraction by the retractor bulbi muscle because all the rectus muscles also have this retractor function.

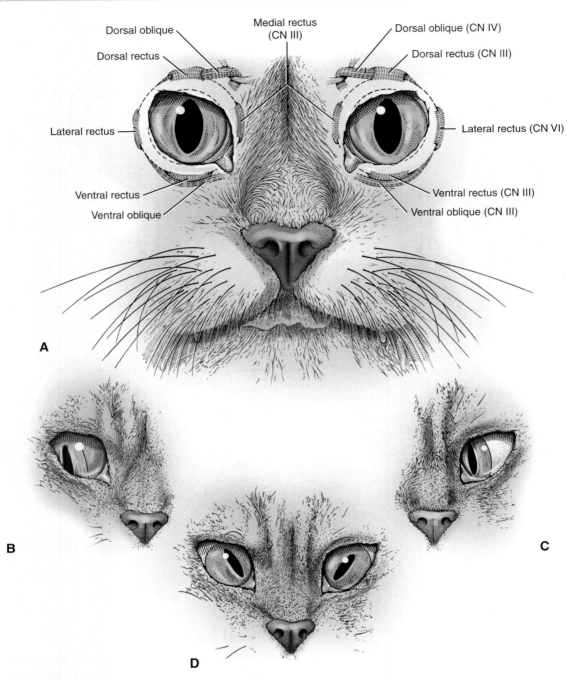

FIGURE 6-4 A, Functional anatomy of the extraocular muscles. Directions of strabismus following **B,** paralysis of the oculomotor neurons; **C,** paralysis of the abducent neurons; and **D,** paralysis of the trochlear neurons. *CN III,* Oculomotor nerve; *CN IV,* trochlear nerve; *CN VI,* abducent nerve.

Lesions of the trochlear neurons cause paralysis of the dorsal oblique muscle, and you will observe a strabismus caused by the unopposed contraction of the ventral oblique muscle. This strabismus will be contralateral to a nuclear lesion in the mesencephalon and ipsilateral to a trochlear nerve lesion after it emerges from the rostral medullary velum. In cats, which have vertical pupils, the dorsal, 12-o'clock position of the pupil will be extorted, deviated laterally. In horses and ruminants, which have horizontal pupils, the medial aspect of the pupil will be extorted dorsally. This is often referred to as a dorsomedial strabismus.

In ruminants, this is a clinical sign that commonly occurs in severe cases of a metabolic disorder caused by thiamin deficiency and is referred to as polioencephalomalacia. This is thought to represent dysfunction of the trochlear nucleus. In dogs, with their round pupils, extorsion cannot be appreciated unless you do a fundic examination and look for the position of the superior retinal vein that normally courses in a superior direction from the optic disk. It will be deviated laterally in a trochlear nerve paralysis. Trochlear nerve strabismus is rarely observed except in the ruminant disorder just described.

Lesions of the GSE oculomotor neurons cause paralysis of the dorsal and ventral rectus, the ventral oblique, and the medial rectus muscles as well as the levator palpebrae superioris. Loss of the function of the levator muscle causes a smaller palpebral fissure due to ptosis resulting from the inability to elevate the upper eyelid. Paralysis of the extraocular muscles causes a ventrolateral strabismus (see Fig. 6-4). The lateral deviation is explained by the unopposed contraction of the lateral rectus muscle. The mild ventral deviation has no obvious explanation other than the collective result of the loss of function of the other extraocular muscles innervated by the oculomotor nerve. The loss of the ability to adduct the eye can be readily observed when you test the patient for normal nystagmus by moving the head in a horizontal plane. The affected eye will not adduct fully when the head is moved in the direction of the normal eye. In small animals, when the head and neck are extended, the eyes normally move dorsally to stay in the center of the palpebral fissure. Paralysis of the dorsal rectus muscle prevents this in the affected eye, and you will observe the dorsal aspect of the sclera when you perform this movement. In the horse and ruminants, especially cattle, the eyes normally do not move dorsally as the head and neck are extended, and you normally observe the dorsal aspect of the sclera in both eyes.

Lesions that involve all components of the oculomotor nerve also cause dilated pupils that are unresponsive to light due to the loss of the GVE parasympathetic preganglionic neurons that innervate the iris constrictor muscle.[36] This is described in Chapter 7 when we discuss the GVE system.

A vestibular strabismus is a ventrolateral strabismus that is observed in some positions of the head when the vestibular system is affected by a lesion. The strabismus is ipsilateral to the vestibular system lesion. It can be differentiated from an oculomotor nerve strabismus because it is not present in all positions of the head, and when you test for normal (physiologic) nystagmus, the affected eye will adduct as well as the opposite eye. A GSE neuronal strabismus will be present in all positions of the head.

Strabismus may also occur with some congenital anomalies in the architecture of the central projections of the visual system. A mild bilateral medial strabismus is observed in Siamese cats. This breed has a higher portion of retinal ganglion cell neurons whose axons cross at the optic chiasm and project to the contralateral lateral geniculate nucleus.[33]

Diseases

The most common lesion to involve one or more of these cranial nerves that innervate the extraocular muscles is a neoplasm that is retrobulbar or extraparenchymal (extraaxial or extramedullary) in the middle cranial fossa. Meningiomas and germ cell neoplasms are the most common in the middle cranial fossa to affect these cranial nerves.[35] In the literature, the clinical signs of neoplasms located here that affect cranial nerves III, IV, and VI and the ophthalmic and maxillary nerves from V have been referred to as the cavernous sinus syndrome. This term should be discarded, because these nerves have nothing to do with the cavernous sinus other than to course by it to leave the cranial cavity. Pituitary macroadenomas rarely affect these nerves.

CRANIAL NERVE V: TRIGEMINAL NEURONS

Anatomy

The GSE neuronal cell bodies are located in the motor nucleus of the trigeminal nerve, which is a small, well-defined nucleus in the pons (see Fig. 2-11). This nucleus is found at the level of the middle and rostral cerebellar peduncles just rostral to where all three cerebellar peduncles merge with the cerebellum. It is medial to the pontine sensory nucleus of the trigeminal nerve and dorsal to the dorsal nucleus of the trapezoid body (Fig. 6-5; see also Fig. 6-1).

The axons pass ventrolaterally through the middle cerebellar peduncle to join the sensory neurons of the trigeminal nerve that are entering the pons. As these motor neurons emerge from the pons, they may be seen as a small separate motor nerve root on the medial aspect of the sensory portion of the trigeminal nerve before the nerve disappears into the canal for the trigeminal nerve in the petrosal portion of the temporal bone. Within this canal, these motor neurons pass through the large trigeminal ganglion to join the mandibular nerve that passes through the oval foramen, where the motor neurons are distributed to the muscles of mastication: masseter, temporal, pterygoid, rostral digastricus, and mylohyoideus.

Clinical Signs

Unilateral loss of function of the trigeminal motor neurons will be recognized only when atrophy occurs in the muscles of mastication (Figs. 6-6 and 6-7). This will be observed more readily in the shorthaired breeds. In your neurologic examination, be sure to palpate these muscles or you will miss this important clinical sign, especially in longhaired breeds such as the old English sheepdog. In the horse, there may be a slight deviation of the lower jaw toward the normal side, but this may be difficult to recognize. There must be bilateral loss of function in these trigeminal motor neurons to result in failure to prehend food because the mouth cannot be closed. An open mouth due to a dropped jaw that the patient cannot close but that you can close manually requires the anatomic diagnosis of bilateral motor cranial nerve V.

Diseases

Malignant Nerve Sheath Neoplasm

The most common lesion that causes a unilateral loss of the GSE-LMN in the trigeminal nerve is a malignant nerve sheath neoplasm. This is a neoplasm of Schwann cells that occurs in older dogs. The first indication of the neoplasm is usually recognition of atrophy in the muscles of mastication (see Figs. 6-6 and 6-7). There is no recognizable loss of jaw function. Be aware that the loss of general somatic afferent (GSA) neurons in the ophthalmic nerve from of the trigeminal nerve may cause a neurotrophic keratitis, which may be the first clinical sign observed. Often, there is no detectable loss of sensory function with this neoplasm, but it commonly expands into the cranial cavity and slowly compresses the brainstem, with its mass centered at the pons (Figs. 6-8 and 6-9). This will lead to other cranial nerve signs (facial and vestibulocochlear) on the same side and abnormal postural reactions and gait in the ipsilateral limbs.

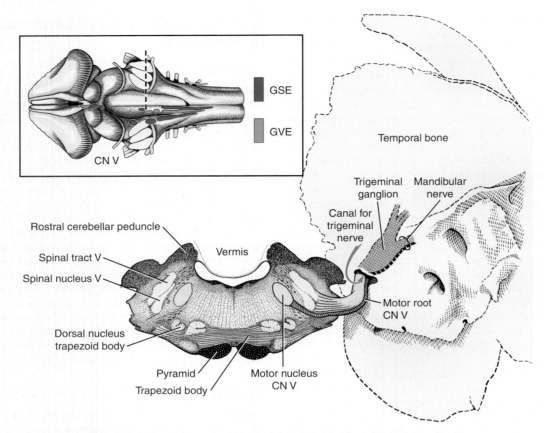

FIGURE 6-5 Transverse section of the medulla at the level of the facial and abducent nuclei.

Computed tomography (CT) and magnetic resonance (MR) imaging will diagnose this mass lesion and determine the extent of its growth (Figs. 6-10 through 6-14). Surgical removal is difficult because of the location of the mass, but it has been described. Usually this neoplasm is treated by radiation, and corticosteroids are used to control perilesional edema. The trigeminal nerve is the most common cranial nerve to develop this nerve sheath neoplasm in animals.

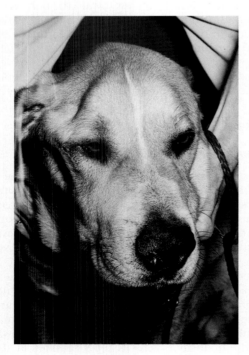

FIGURE 6-6 A 10-year-old beagle with severe denervation atrophy of the muscles of mastication on its right side due to a nerve sheath neoplasm in the trigeminal nerve, affecting the mandibular branch.

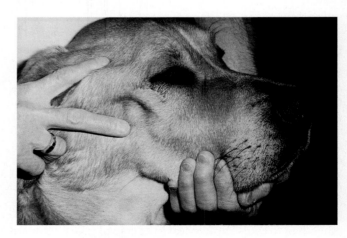

FIGURE 6-7 Lateral view of the dog in Fig. 6-6.

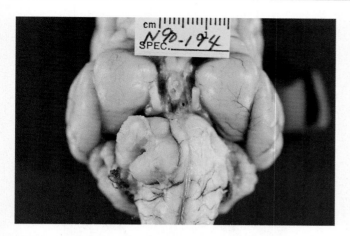

FIGURE 6-8 Ventral view of the brain of an 8-year-old West Highland white terrier with a nerve sheath neoplasm in the right trigeminal nerve. Note the severe compression of the pons.

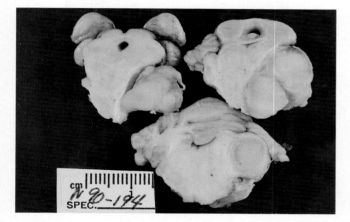

FIGURE 6-9 Transverse sections of the brain of the dog in Fig. 6-8, showing the severe compression of the mesencephalon and ventral metencephalon (pons). In addition to the atrophy of the right muscles of mastication, this dog exhibited right spastic hemiparesis and ataxia. However, the quality of the ataxia reflected predominantly dysfunction of the vestibular system rather than of the general proprioceptive system.

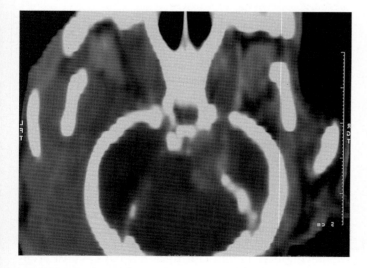

FIGURE 6-10 Dorsal plane CT image of the head of a 10-year-old West Highland white terrier with contrast enhancement of a nerve sheath neoplasm in the right trigeminal nerve intracranially that extends through the round and rostral alar foramina with the maxillary nerve.

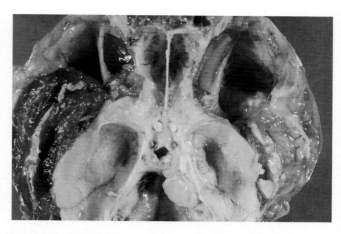

FIGURE 6-11 Dorsal view of the floor of the cranial cavity in the dog shown in Fig. 6-10. Note the large mass at the level of the canal for the trigeminal nerve in the right petrosal portion of the temporal bone, where it was cut away from the portion of the neoplasm that compressed the brainstem. Note the normal maxillary nerve on the dorsal surface of the left medial pterygoid muscle on the floor of the left orbit. Compare this with the floor of the right orbit, where the denervated muscle is severely atrophied and the maxillary nerve is enlarged by the nerve sheath neoplasm.

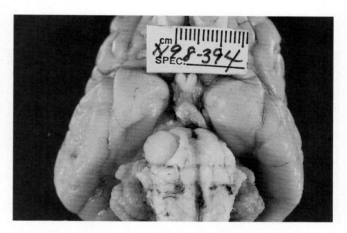

FIGURE 6-12 Ventral view of the brain of the dog in Figs. 6-10 and 6-11. Note the continuation of the nerve sheath neoplasm in the right trigeminal nerve at its attachment to the pons.

Lymphoma

Lymphoma can also develop within this cranial nerve, especially in cats.[25] **Video 6-1** shows Smokey, a 10-year-old spayed female domestic shorthair cat, who had been unable to close her mouth for 10 days during which time she was fed and watered by hand. In addition to the dropped lower jaw that she could not move, there was bilateral facial analgesia due to the loss of function of the GSA neurons in all three branches of the trigeminal nerves. Note the spontaneous blinking of the eyelids but no palpebral reflex because of the loss of the trigeminal sensory neurons. Also note the normal menace response and the ear movement, which supports normal functioning of the facial neurons. There is normal nociception in the ear because it has numerous sources of sensory innervation in addition to the small area supplied by the trigeminal nerve. Figures 6-15 through 6-17 show the brain of this cat and the bilaterally enlarged trigeminal nerves caused by an infiltrating lymphoma.

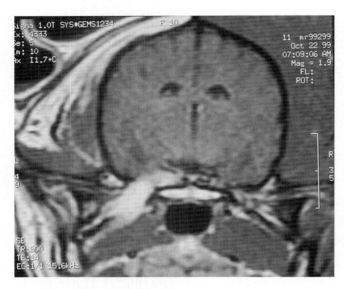

FIGURE 6-13 Axial T1-weighted MR image with contrast of the head of a 10.5-year-old castrated male American Eskimo dog, showing contrast enhancement of a nerve sheath neoplasm in the left trigeminal nerve (left side of figure) and its extension through the oval foramen in the mandibular nerve to the surface of the atrophied medial pterygoid muscle. Note the severe atrophy of the left temporalis muscle.

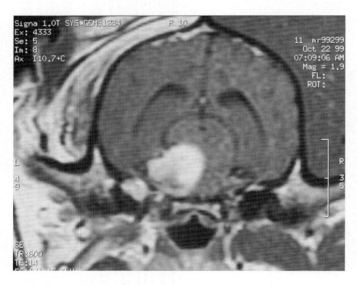

FIGURE 6-14 Axial T1-weighted MR image with contrast caudal to the level of the MR image in Fig. 6-13, showing contrast enhancement of the nerve sheath neoplasm where it compresses the caudal mesencephalon.

Trigeminal Neuritis

The most common cause of sudden inability to close the mouth in dogs is a bilateral nonsuppurative trigeminal neuritis.[23] This is also referred to as trigeminal neuropathy, but it is an inflammatory disease that is thought to be an autoimmune disorder. In my (Alexander de Lahunta) necropsy study of one affected dog, this inflammatory lesion was in all components of the trigeminal nerve bilaterally, including the ganglia. Demyelination was prominent and axonal degeneration was rare, indicating that this was predominantly a primary demyelination. There were numerous lymphoplasmatic perivascular cuffs and many macrophages engulfing the degenerate myelin.

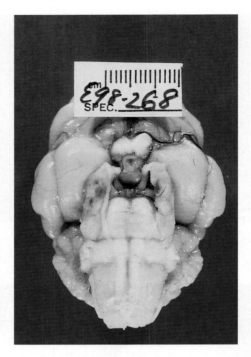

FIGURE 6-15 Ventral view of the brain of the 10-year-old domestic shorthair seen in Video 6-1. It shows the marked enlargement of both trigeminal nerves, which was caused by an infiltrating lymphoma.

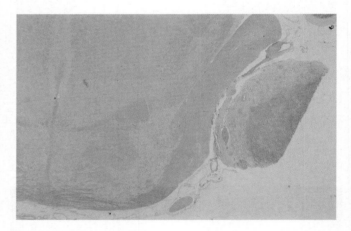

FIGURE 6-16 Low-power magnification of a microscopic section of one enlarged trigeminal nerve at its attachment to the pons. Note the lymphoid infiltration in the nerve.

This lesion is similar to that found in the ventral roots of dogs with polyradiculoneuritis. When you examine dogs with trigeminal neuritis, you find that the lower jaw has dropped and just hangs loose. You can manually close the mouth by elevating the lower jaw, but when you release it, the lower jaw drops back to its initial position. Usually, these dogs have normal use of their tongues and can swallow when food or water is placed in the caudal portion of the oral cavity and oral pharynx. Occasionally, swallowing may be difficult for a few days. Saliva accumulates around the lips and nose (Fig. 6-18). About one third of these dogs also has loss of facial sensation due to the involvement of the GSA neurons that are abundant in all three major branches of this nerve. A few dogs exhibit

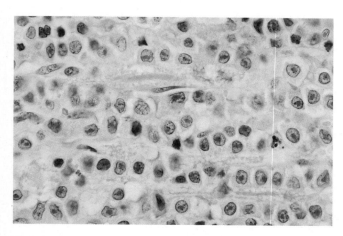

FIGURE 6-17 Higher magnification of the trigeminal nerve lymphoma seen in Figs. 6-15 and 6-16.

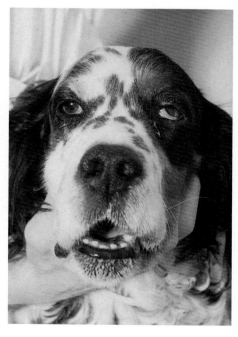

FIGURE 6-19 A 7-year-old English setter with a dropped jaw due to trigeminal neuritis that also exhibits a left Horner syndrome.

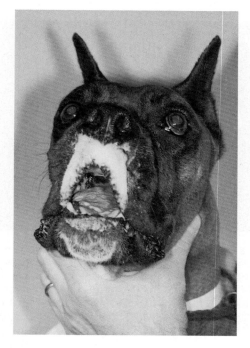

FIGURE 6-18 A 5-year-old boxer exhibiting sialosis due to the inability to close its mouth as a result of trigeminal neuritis, which was presumed to have been caused by an autoimmune disorder.

sympathetic paralysis of the head, which is referred to as Horner syndrome. This is presumed to be due to the involvement of the postganglionic sympathetic neurons that join the ophthalmic nerve from the trigeminal nerve to reach the smooth muscle of the eye, eyelids, and periorbita (Fig. 6-19). Rarely there is mild facial neuritis and paresis. Most of these dogs spontaneously recover in about 3 weeks, with or without significant atrophy of the masticatory muscles. The degree of atrophy reflects the degree of axonal involvement. Unilateral cases may be overlooked because they will be recognized only by this atrophy. MR imaging shows diffuse enlargement of the affected nerves, with hyperintensity on T2-weighted

images and contrast enhancement of T1-weighted images.[31] Bilaterally affected dogs must be fed and supplied with water by hand for the first 7 to 10 days. We do not treat these dogs with immunosuppressive drugs such as corticosteroids because there is no evidence that they have any influence on the rate of recovery. That probably reflects the degree of axonal injury. Recovery is short if the axons have been spared and only remyelination is necessary. Recurrences of this disorder are uncommon. We have made this clinical diagnosis in cats, but it is much less common in that species (Fig. 6-20). Despite what has been written, you cannot injure the mandibular nerve branches of the trigeminal nerve that innervate these muscles by opening the mouth too wide. The following two videos are examples of this disorder.

Video 6-2 shows a 5-year-old spayed female English springer spaniel, Jazz, 2 days after a sudden onset of inability to close the mouth to prehend food. Note that there is no loss of facial sensation.

Video 6-3 shows a 4-year-old spayed female schnauzer, Haley, 1 day after a sudden onset of inability to close its mouth to prehend food. Note the marked bilateral facial hypalgesia. There is no palpebral reflex, but note the spontaneous blinking of the eyelids, which indicates normal facial nerve function. Stimulating the skin of the external ear canal tests multiple cranial and cervical spinal nerves and is not reliable for cranial nerve V. The ear movement supports normal facial nerve function.

Encephalitis that involves the motor nuclei of the trigeminal nerve bilaterally causes paresis or paralysis of the muscles of mastication that results in a paretic or paralyzed dropped jaw and an open mouth that cannot be closed to prehend food. Infections by *Listeria monocytogenes* in ruminants and by *Sarcocystis neurona* in horses are examples of this (Figs. 6-21 through 6-23).

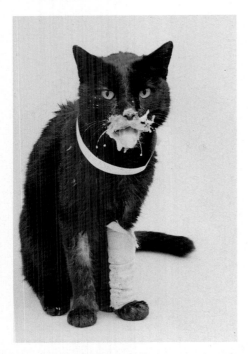

FIGURE 6-20 A 12-year-old domestic shorthair with food and saliva around its mouth because it cannot close its mouth as a result of a presumed trigeminal neuritis.

Myositis

Myositis of the muscles of mastication is described in Chapter 5. It is not a cause of dropped lower jaw and the inability to close the mouth and has no relationship to any dysfunction of the trigeminal nerve. In the acute stage, when the muscles are swollen, any movement of the jaw causes extreme discomfort. In the chronic stage, when the muscles are severely atrophied, the fibrosis that has developed in the muscles may mechanically prevent the jaw from being opened. This myositis is treated by long-term corticosteroids and more recently by oral cyclosporine.

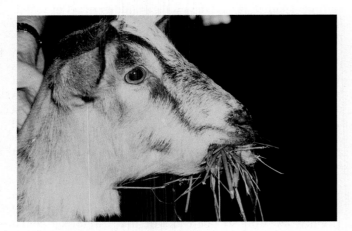

FIGURE 6-21 A 5-month-old mixed-breed goat unable to close its mouth and prehend food due to listeriosis, which caused necrosis of both motor nuclei of the trigeminal nerves in the pons.

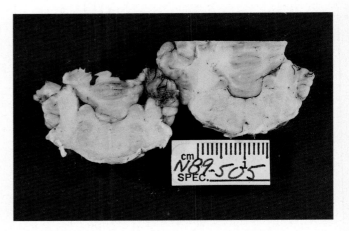

FIGURE 6-22 Transverse section of the pons and rostral medulla of the goat in Fig. 6-21. Note the slight bilateral discoloration in the pons, where the necrosis affected both of the motor nuclei of the trigeminal nerves.

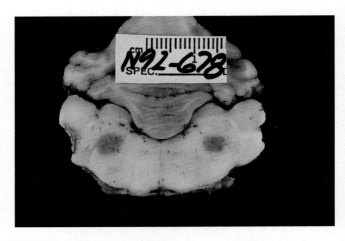

FIGURE 6-23 The caudal surface of a transverse section of the pons of a 4-year-old standardbred gelding with a dropped atonic jaw and inability to close the mouth. The bilateral symmetric discolorations reflect a chronic astrocytosis that has replaced all of the neuronal cell bodies in the nuclei of the motor component of the trigeminal nerves. There were areas of active nonsuppurative inflammation and necrosis in the pons and medulla that were presumed to be caused by infection by *S. neurona* organisms.

▌ CRANIAL NERVE VII: FACIAL NEURONS

Anatomy

The cell bodies of the GSE neurons in the facial nerve are located in the facial nucleus in the rostral medulla. This well-defined nucleus is ventrolateral in the medulla, midway between the pyramid medially and the spinal nucleus of the trigeminal nerve laterally, caudal to the trapezoid body and the level of attachment of the caudal cerebellar peduncle to the cerebellum (see Fig. 2-13). It is caudal to the dorsal nucleus of the trapezoid body and rostral to the olivary nucleus (see Fig. 6-24; see also Figs. 6-1 and 6-3).

The axons of these cell bodies initially pass dorsomedially to the midline of the floor of the fourth ventricle. Here they course rostrally for 1 to 2 mm, dorsal to

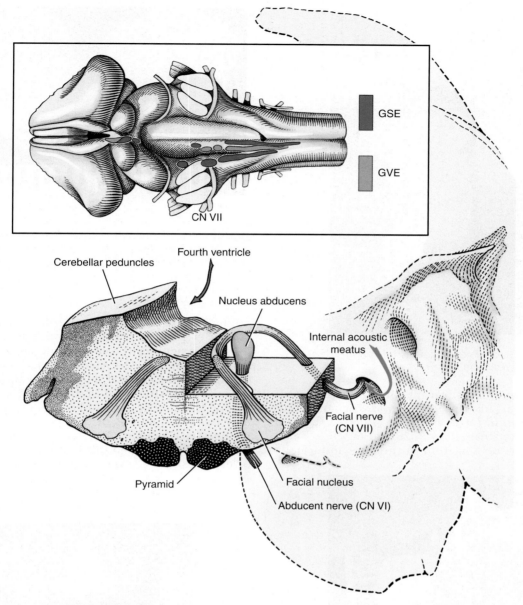

FIGURE 6-24 Transverse section of the pons at the level of the motor nucleus of the trigeminal nerve.

the abducent nucleus in the genu of the facial nerve. Then they course ventrolaterally through the medulla, medial to the spinal nucleus and tract of the trigeminal nerve and lateral to the dorsal nucleus of the trapezoid body. They emerge through the lateral aspect of the trapezoid body ventral to the vestibulocochlear nerve (see Fig. 2-12). The facial nerve accompanies the vestibulocochlear nerve into the internal acoustic meatus of the petrosal portion of the temporal bone.[1] The facial nerve is more dorsal; it enters the facial canal within the temporal bone and emerges through the stylomastoid foramen. Branches of the facial nerve are distributed to the muscles of facial expression. These are the relatively thin muscles of the ear, eyelids, nose, cheeks, and lips. The facial nerve also innervates the caudal portion of the digastricus muscle, which belongs to the muscles of mastication.

Clinical Signs

Lesions of the facial nucleus or the facial nerve to the point where it emerges from the stylomastoid foramen result in complete facial paresis or paralysis and inability to move these facial muscles normally. Paralysis may be recognized by asymmetry of the face, but that depends on the species. The most obvious asymmetry occurs in the horse (Fig. 6-25); on the paralyzed side the ear droops, the palpebral fissure is decreased in size, the lower lip droops, and the nose and upper lip are markedly deviated toward the normal side because of the unopposed contractions of the muscles of the lip and nose on that side. Even the angle of the upper eyelid lashes are decreased on the affected side when the two sides are carefully compared. The ear droop, small palpebral fissure, deviated nose, and lip droop are usually

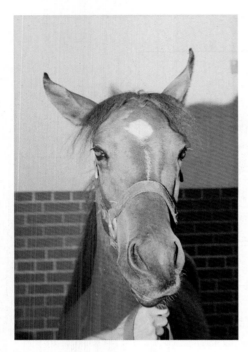

FIGURE 6-25 A 6-year-old standardbred gelding with complete right facial paralysis associated with otitis media.

seen in small ruminants, except for the ear in breeds with pendular ears like the Nubian goat. The same clinical signs are seen in cattle, but there is no deviation of the planum nasolabiale (Figs. 6-26 and 6-27). In small animals, there is no deviation of the nose and usually

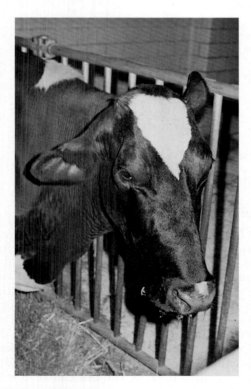

FIGURE 6-26 Right facial paralysis in a 4-year-old Holstein cow that is depressed and exhibits mild spastic tetraparesis and ataxia in all four limbs when she walks. The cause was encephalitis in the caudal brainstem resulting from infection by *L. monocytogenes*.

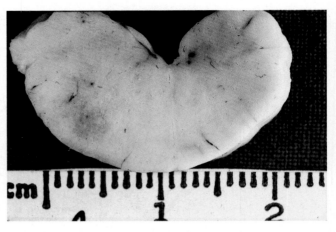

FIGURE 6-27 The rostral surface of a transverse section of the medulla of the cow in Fig. 6-26. Note the discoloration caused by the inflammation and necrosis at the site of the right facial nucleus (left side of photo).

no decrease in size of the palpebral fissure (Fig. 6-28). The latter suggests that the levator anguli oculi medialis plays a significant role in eyelid elevation in horses and farm animals. Occasionally, this fissure is slightly enlarged on the affected side in small animals. Be aware that the sympathetic and facial nerves can be affected by middle ear disorders, and a smaller palpebral fissure may be caused by loss of the sympathetic innervation to the eye. However, this is accompanied by pupillary miosis and an elevated third eyelid. With facial paresis or paralysis, there is no ear droop in cats and in many

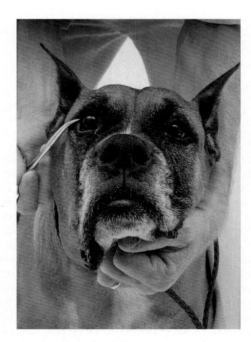

FIGURE 6-28 A 5-year-old spayed female boxer with complete right facial paralysis secondary to otitis media. Note the normal erect ear position and the normal size of the palpebral fissure despite the paralysis of the ear and the eyelid muscles. Note the droop of the atonic right lips.

dogs with erect ears because the ear cartilage is taut enough to keep the ear erect despite the paralysis of the ear muscles (see Figs. 6-28 and 6-35).

If you elevate the head of a small animal and examine the corners of the lips, you are likely to find that more mucosa is exposed on the paralyzed side, and more saliva may be lost on this side. Loss of tone in the lips is more difficult to feel in small animals than in the horse and farm animals. There will be no spontaneous eyelid blinking on the affected side, and you may observe that there is no movement of the naris on that side during inspiration. The most reliable test for facial nerve function is the palpebral reflex, which can be elicited by touching the corners of the eyelids or blowing into the eye (see Fig. 6-34). The sensory neurons stimulated are in the branches of the trigeminal nerve. They enter the pons with the trigeminal nerve and course through the medulla in the spinal tract of the trigeminal nerve. Synapse occurs on neuronal cell bodies in the adjacent spinal nucleus of the trigeminal nerve; they in turn synapse on the GSE neurons in the facial nucleus in the rostral medulla to complete the reflex arc. This results in a brisk closure of the eyelids. We usually avoid doing the corneal reflex, which is stimulated by touching the cornea, so as not to injure the cornea, which in animals is much less sensitive than in humans. In patients with facial paresis, you may be able to determine the paresis by trying to elevate the upper eyelid with your fingers. In normal horses and cattle, this may be difficult to do. In breeds with erect ears that do not droop with facial paralysis, you may be able to determine the inability to move the ear by blowing into the ear or mildly stimulating the skin of the external ear canal with a blunt instrument and comparing the ear movement responses on each side. On the affected side, the ear will not move but the patient may move its head away from you or might bite or scratch you!

When lesions affect the individual branches of the facial nerve, along their course to the muscles they innervate, the lesions produce paresis or paralysis that is restricted to those muscle groups. In horses, the buccal branches of the facial nerve are close together where they course laterally across the caudal border of the ramus of the mandible to reach the surface of the masseter muscle where they separate and continue on to innervate the muscles of the nose and lips. Where these branches cross this ramus, they are subject to compression injury when the horse is tabled for surgery and this area is not protected by padding, especially if the halter is not removed. The clinical signs are limited to a drooped lower lip and a deviated nose and upper lip. Eyelid and ear position and movement are normal (Fig. 6-29). Cattle that struggle to pull their heads out of stanchions may injure one or both of the palpebral branches of the auriculopalpebral nerve as it courses across the zygomatic arch, which is the widest portion of the skull. Usually, only eyelid paresis or paralysis results. This nerve can be blocked by a local anesthetic at this same point to permit examination of the eye in animals that will not allow you to open the eyelids, especially horses. Occasionally, cattle that struggle vigorously may also injure the auricular branches of the auriculopalpebral nerves and cause ipsilateral ear droop and loss of ear motion. This injury is referred to as stanchion paralysis.

Be aware that the facial and vestibulocochlear nerves are very closely associated from the medulla into the petrosal portion of the temporal bone.[1] As a result, the same lesion

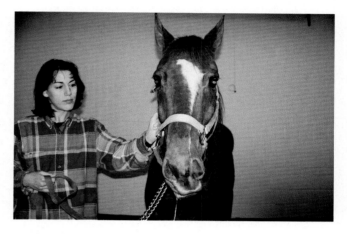

FIGURE 6-29 A 6-year-old thoroughbred gelding with paralysis limited to the right nose and lip muscles due to compression of the buccal branches of the facial nerve at the ramus of the mandible following prolonged lateral recumbency for surgery.

often causes dysfunction of both of these cranial nerves. A neoplasm compressing the medulla or otitis media-interna may cause dysfunction in these two cranial nerves. It is important to recognize clinical signs of involvement of other functional systems when the medulla is the site of the lesion because they will greatly influence the differential diagnosis, the selection of ancillary procedures, the therapy, and the prognosis. These other functional systems in the medulla include the upper motor neuron (UMN), causing a hemiparesis or tetraparesis; general proprioception, producing ataxia; the ascending reticular activating system, causing depression or lethargy; and the nuclei of other cranial nerves. Remember that any animal with complete facial paralysis can have a lesion anywhere between the level of the facial nucleus in the medulla and the level of the stylomastoid foramen. The recognition of the presence or absence of other clinical signs is critical to making the correct anatomic diagnosis (see Figs. 6-26 and 6-27).

Diseases

Otitis Media

By far, the most common cause of facial paralysis in all species is otitis media; the inflammation in the middle ear involves the facial nerve as it courses through the facial canal in the petrosal portion of the temporal bone. A portion of this canal that is adjacent to the tympanic (middle ear) cavity lacks a bony wall, and the nerve is separated from the cavity by only a few micra of loose connective tissue (Fig. 6-30). A lesion at this level causes complete facial paresis or paralysis (Figs. 6-31 and 6-32). It may be accompanied by peripheral vestibular system dysfunction due to involvement of the receptors in the inner ear.[12] Unilateral deafness caused by loss of the receptors for hearing on one side cannot be determined by your physical neurologic examination. This diagnosis requires a brainstem auditory-evoked response test, which is an electrophysiologic evaluation. In small animals, middle ear inflammation may involve the GVE postganglionic sympathetic neurons in their course from the cranial cervical ganglion to the ophthalmic nerve from the trigeminal nerve to innervate the smooth muscle of the eyelid, periorbita, and iris dilator muscle. (See Chapter 7 for a

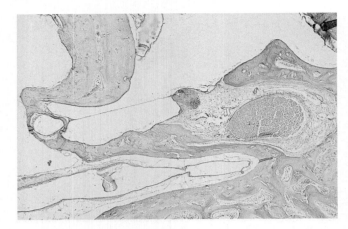

FIGURE 6-30 Dorsal plane microscopic section of a dog's temporal bone that includes portions of the petrosal and tympanic parts. The tubular structures at the bottom are a semicircular canal and its associated semicircular duct. The transverse section of the nerve adjacent to the right end of the semicircular canal is the facial nerve. The empty space above these structures is the tympanic cavity. This portion of the facial nerve is at risk for being involved with inflammatory lesions in the middle ear tympanic cavity.

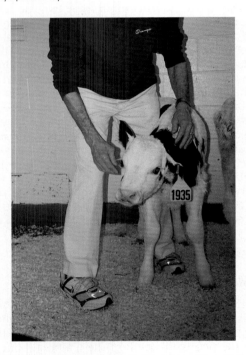

FIGURE 6-31 A 3-week-old Holstein calf with a left head tilt and facial paralysis resulting from a left-side otitis media-interna.

discussion of this pathway.) The loss of function of these sympathetic neurons causes Horner syndrome. Figures 6-33 through 6-35 show a young domestic shorthair with facial paralysis, peripheral vestibular signs, and Horner syndrome caused by unilateral otitis media-interna.

The diagnosis of otitis media can often be supported by head radiographs or MR or CT imaging. CT imaging may provide the best detail for both the osseous and soft tissue changes that occur in this disorder (Figs. 6-36 through 6-38).

Otitis media-interna should be treated aggressively to prevent extension of the infection from the inner ear into the cranial cavity. Caudal brainstem and cerebellar abscesses

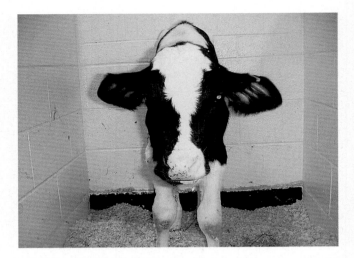

FIGURE 6-32 A 1-month-old Holstein calf with bilateral facial paralysis caused by bilateral otitis media.

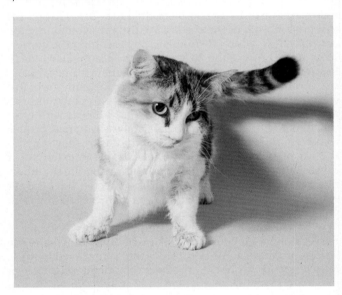

FIGURE 6-33 This figure and Figs. 6-34 and 6-35 show the same 10-week-old domestic shorthair kitten with peripheral vestibular system dysfunction, facial paralysis, and Horner syndrome caused by a left-side otitis media-interna. Here, the left head tilt reflects the involvement of the left vestibular nerve or its receptors in the inner ear.

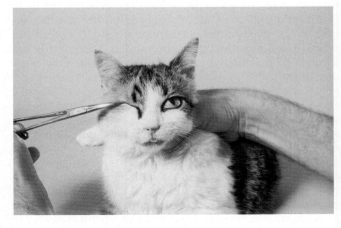

FIGURE 6-34 Note the left-side Horner syndrome and the normal right palpebral reflex.

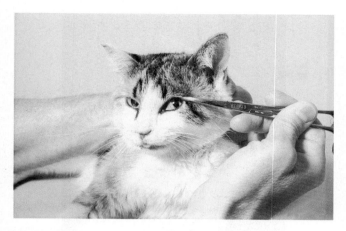

FIGURE 6-35 Note the absent left palpebral reflex and the erect left ear, which was immobile. Facial sensation was normal bilaterally.

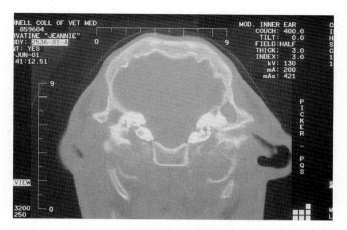

FIGURE 6-38 Axial CT of a 1-month-old Holstein calf with severe bilateral otitis media.

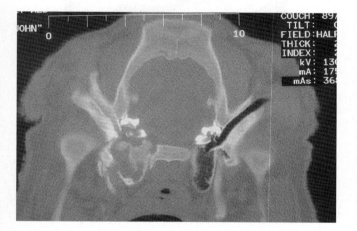

FIGURE 6-36 Axial CT image of a 1-month-old pig with right-side (left side of photo) otitis externa, media, and interna. Note the normal long osseous external acoustic meatus in a pig.

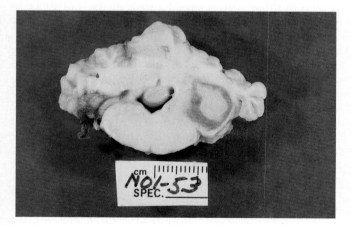

FIGURE 6-37 Caudal surface of a transverse section of the medulla and cerebellum of the pig in Fig. 6-36. It shows an abscess secondary to the intracranial extension of the right otitis media-interna.

commonly occur secondary to otitis in young farm animals, especially calves, lambs, and pigs (see Fig. 6-37). It occasionally occurs in cats, in which otitis media is very common and often subclinical. A significant percentage of cats that come to necropsy for other reasons also have incidental otitis media. Be aware that long-term therapy with corticosteroids

for undiagnosed facial or vestibular nerve dysfunction in an animal that has otitis media can lead to petrosal bone osteomyelitis and brainstem compression or infection.

Video 6-4 shows two Holstein calves with otitis media-interna. The smaller calf is 2 months old and exhibits a right-side facial paralysis and clinical signs of a right-side peripheral vestibular system dysfunction. Diagnosis was made by radiography. The larger calf is 4 months old and has left facial paralysis caused by otitis media but also shows involvement of the medulla: depression, need of assistance to stand, and an extended neck. The latter clinical signs were caused by the abscess that had formed in the medulla and pons due to invasion by the ear infection into the cranial cavity.

Video 6-5 shows a 1-month-old Holstein calf with bilateral ear droop resulting from facial paralysis secondary to bilateral otitis media. The video includes the CT images that led to this diagnosis.

In horses, otitis media has been associated with a proliferative bone lesion involving the articulations of the stylohyoid, tympanohyoid, and the temporal bone.[2,3,26,40] The cause of these bone lesions is unknown. Both inflammatory and mechanical hypotheses have been invoked. The bony proliferation causes ankylosis of these articulations, fusing the stylohyoid bone to the temporal bone. This prevents any movement of the hyoid apparatus associated with swallowing and vocalization and may lead to fracture of the temporal bone. Facial paralysis, with or without clinical signs of dysfunction of the peripheral vestibular system, can precede the fracture due to the otitis or follow the fracture due to injury of the facial nerve. If you suspect the possibility of this joint fusion, palpate the mobility of the hyoid apparatus by placing your fingers on the basihyoid bone or its lingual process and lifting up on it. Experiment with normal horses to learn how much mobility there is in the normal hyoid apparatus when it is manipulated this way. You will find that when this temporohyoid joint is fused, there is considerable resistance when you lift up on the basihyoid bone. In most cases, this stylohyoid osteopathy can be confirmed by endoscopic examination of the guttural pouch. **Video 6-6** shows guttural pouch endoscopy of an 8-year-old horse with a sudden onset of left facial paralysis. The left compartment of the guttural pouch is shown first.

Note the enlargement of the stylohyoid bone at the tympanohyoid articulation and the lack of any motion here due to the fusion that has occurred. Compare this with the view of the right compartment that follows and shows the normal stylohyoid bone and the movement at this joint. Head radiographs may reveal this bone lesion but CT imaging is the most reliable procedure for confirming this diagnosis (Figs. 6-39 through 6-41). The otitis is treated by antibiotics; surgical removal of the keratohyoid bone prevents further trauma to the temporal bone. If the diagnosis of this stylohyoid osteopathy is made before any neurologic signs are present, this surgery may be done as a prophylactic measure.

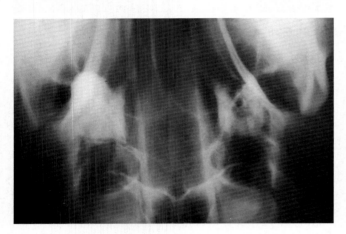

FIGURE 6-39 Ventrodorsal radiograph of the head of an anesthetized adult horse with stylohyoidosteopathy. Note the general thickening of the right (left side of figure) stylohyoid bone and its marked enlargement where it is fused to the temporal bone at its articulation.

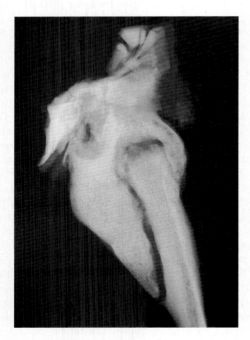

FIGURE 6-40 Radiograph of the necropsy specimen of the bone in Fig. 6-41 at its articulation. Note the marked thickening of both the stylohyoid and temporal bones.

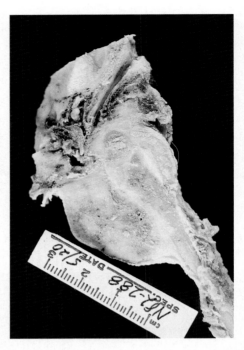

FIGURE 6-41 The necropsy specimen that was radiographed in Fig. 6-40. Note the inflammatory material in the tympanic cavity (middle ear) but no evidence of the osteopathy extending into this cavity.

Videos 12-22 through 12-24 in Chapter 12, the vestibular system, show horses with this disorder.

Facial Nerve Tetanus (Hemifacial Spasm)

Facial nerve tetanus is a unique disorder of the facial nerve in dogs that has been related to otitis media, but this correlation is poorly documented and inconsistent.[24,27] The clinical signs show continual contraction of the muscles innervated by the facial nerve on one side. The facial nerve function on the opposite side is usually normal. These dogs present with a slight elevation of the ear, a narrowed palpebral fissure, taut lips with the angle drawn caudally, and a nose slightly deviated toward the affected side (Figs. 6-42 and 6-43). Some of these dogs exhibit slight movement of the eyelids, lips, and ear when those areas are stimulated. This syndrome has been called hemifacial spasm, but that is a misnomer because it is not a spasm of the muscles in the true sense. The neuromuscular activity is constant. Some clinicians have described it to be the result of complete facial paralysis with denervation atrophy that causes shortening (contracture) of the facial muscles. We disagree with this hypothesis for the following reason. If general anesthesia is administered to one of these dogs or if the affected buccal branches are blocked by a local anesthetic, the clinical signs immediately disappear; they return when the anesthetic has resolved. This supports the idea that a neurogenic stimulus is the basis for these clinical signs rather than a denervation atrophy or other myopathic disorder. A more accurate name for this disorder is facial tetanus. As a clinical sign, tetanus is defined as the sustained contraction of muscles without relaxation; it

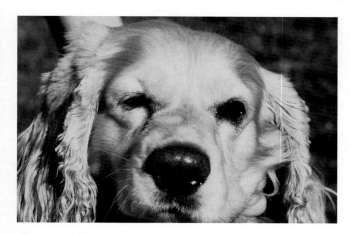

FIGURE 6-42 Right facial tetanus (hemifacial spasm) of a 6-year-old cocker spaniel with right otitis media.

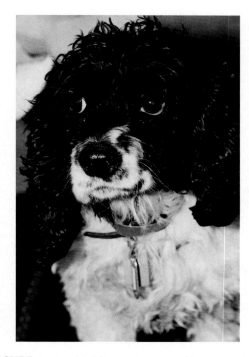

FIGURE 6-43 Left facial tetanus in a 3-year-old mixed-breed dog.

is caused by high-frequency repetitive stimulation of the motor neurons innervating the muscles involved. Some of these dogs have otitis media on the affected side, with or without any signs of dysfunction in the vestibular system or in the sympathetic innervation of the head. However, a significant number have no clinical signs of otitis media, and MR and CT images are normal. I (Eric Glass) recently performed extensive MR imaging on an affected dog in which the combined facial and vestibulocochlear nerves were visible on both sides of the medulla and no lesions were recognized, nor was there any evidence of otitis media. These tetanic signs may be the first indication of a disorder of the facial nerve or may follow a facial paralysis. The tetanic signs do not respond well to antibiotic

therapy for otitis media when it is present. It appears that facial tetanus is permanent in most patients. The neurophysiologic mechanism of facial tetanus is unknown. If it were a central functional disinhibition at the level of the facial nucleus, we would expect it to be bilateral. Until we have a better explanation, we assume facial tetanus is the result of an irritative lesion such as a neuritis affecting the LMN within the extramedullary facial nerve. In humans, there exists a hemifacial spasm that is a true spasmodic disorder and is related to abnormal contact between the facial nerve and an aberrant blood vessel that may be a branch of the labyrinthine artery because they both enter the internal acoustic meatus. The facial nerve excitation is related to the compressive neuropathy caused by the anomalous blood vessel. Decompression often relieves the clinical signs. We have never observed this facial tetanus preceding a progressive central nervous system (CNS) disorder, and we have not seen it in any other species of domestic animal.

Video 6-7 shows Baron, a 5-year-old male golden retriever with a 1-month history of right otitis externa, a right head tilt 2 weeks later, and a few days of drooling from the left lips. Note the normal gait and normal postural reactions. There was no head tilt at the time of this examination. Note the signs of facial tetanus on the dog's right side and the paralysis on his left side. The absent palpebral reflex on the left could be caused by loss of sensory nerve V or motor nerve VII. If a dog reacts to the placing of a blunt instrument on the nasal septal mucosa, sensory V innervation is intact. In this dog, when the conjunctiva was touched with forceps, the eye was retracted, indicating normal sensory V innervation. Similarly, the absent menace response could result from loss of vision or motor VII. To determine that he can still see with that eye, watch carefully for the eye to retract (and thus for the third eyelid to elevate) when you menace the eye. *Be careful* not to touch the dog or create an air current when you menace the eye or you will change the sensory stimulus to cranial nerve V. Radiographic studies confirmed bilateral otitis media in Baron. We assumed that neuritis occurred in the facial nerves, causing paralysis on the left and facial tetanus on the right.

Idiopathic Facial Neuropathy-Neuritis

Idiopathic facial paralysis occurs in older dogs; the cocker spaniel and beagle are at some risk for this disorder, but we have seen it in many breeds. Occasionally, an affected dog has hypothyroidism, but its relationship to the facial nerve disorder is still speculative. Clinical laboratory studies should support a primary hypothyroidism and severe hyperlipidemia. An ischemic neuropathy may be the result of hypothyroid-induced atherosclerosis or increased blood viscosity. In some dogs, the facial paralysis is accompanied by clinical signs of involvement of the vestibular portion of cranial nerve VIII.[39] Response of these dogs to thyroid supplementation is usually satisfactory. Ultimately, this idiopathic disorder is a diagnosis of exclusion that is based on your inability to diagnose any causative abnormality using routine MR or CT imaging, evaluation of the cerebrospinal fluid (CSF), and metabolic studies. A recent MR imaging study of the intratemporal course of the facial nerve in patients with this clinical diagnosis showed contrast enhancement in at least one segment of the facial nerve in three of the five dogs that were studied.[35] Further studies are needed to correlate this information with morphologic change in the affected facial nerve segment. It is not known whether any neuritis is involved. Bell palsy in humans is a similar facial paralysis and is thought to be related to infection by the herpes simplex virus. One study of biopsies of the buccal branches of the facial nerves in dogs with this diagnosis showed degeneration of the neuronal processes, a neuropathy, but that could be a result of neuritis in the nerve prior to its emergence from the stylomastoid foramen. No other cranial nerves are clinically affected by this facial nerve disorder. The prognosis should be guarded. Spontaneous recovery may occur in weeks to months or might not occur at all. No effective treatment is recognized. Be aware that corneal lesions may occur because of exposure due to the lack of eyelid closure or to the absence of tears if the parasympathetic preganglionic neurons that innervate the lacrimal gland and the gland of the third eyelid are affected in the proximal part of the facial nerve. Occasionally, this disorder progresses to affect both facial nerves.

CRANIAL NERVES IX, X, AND XI: GLOSSOPHARYNGEAL, VAGAL, ACCESSORY NEURONS

Anatomy

Cranial nerves IX, X, and XI are considered together because their medullary GSE neuronal cell bodies are all located in one nucleus, the nucleus ambiguus. The accessory nerve also has a spinal cord component. These medullary cell bodies are topographically organized in the nucleus ambiguus, with the most rostral portion contributing to the glossopharyngeal nerve and the most caudal to the accessory nerve. Nucleus ambiguus is an ill-defined column of neuronal cell bodies located ventrolaterally in the medulla, medial to the spinal tract and nucleus of the trigeminal nerve (see Figs. 2-14 and 2-15). It extends from the facial nucleus rostrally through the caudal medulla to a level slightly caudal to the obex. It is continued by the motor nucleus of the accessory nerve through the gray matter of all the cervical spinal cord segments (Fig. 6-44).

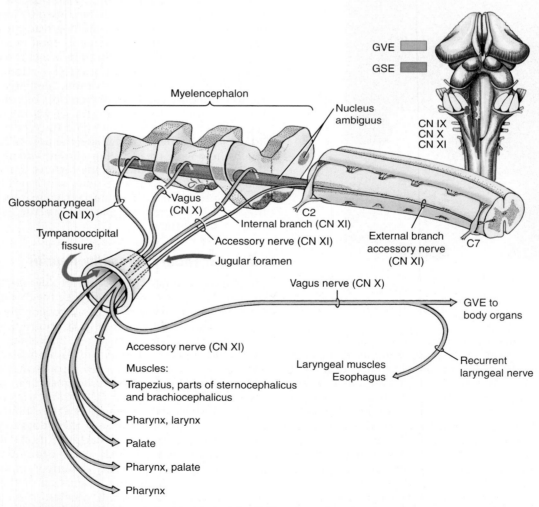

FIGURE 6-44 Schematic drawing of the medulla with the nucleus ambiguus and its efferent neurons and the cervical spinal cord with the external branch of the accessory nerve.

Glossopharyngeal Nerve

The GSE neuronal cell bodies are located in the rostral portion of the nucleus ambiguus. Their axons arch slightly dorsally and then ventrolaterally to emerge along the lateral aspect of the medulla along with the GVE preganglionic neurons from cell bodies in the parasympathetic nucleus of the glossopharyngeal nerve. These two sets of axons form the motor portion of the glossopharyngeal nerve just caudal to the vestibulocochlear nerve. The glossopharyngeal nerve courses through the jugular foramen and emerges from the tympanooccipital fissure, where it contributes pharyngeal branches to innervate the styloglossus muscle and other pharyngeal muscles via the pharyngoesophageal plexus, which includes a contribution from the vagus nerve.

Vagus Nerve

The axons of the GSE cell bodies in the middle portion of the nucleus ambiguus take a similar intramedullary course and emerge on the lateral side of the medulla rostral to the internal branch of the accessory nerve. They are joined by the GVE preganglionic neurons from the parasympathetic nucleus of the vagus to form the motor portion of the vagus nerve. The vagus nerve leaves the cranial cavity through the jugular foramen and emerges from the skull via the tympanooccipital fissure. Here on the dorsal surface of the pharynx, it provides pharyngeal branches that form a plexus with pharyngeal branches of the glossopharyngeal nerve. This pharyngoesophageal plexus innervates the striated muscles of the palate, pharynx and cervical esophagus. A cranial laryngeal branch innervates the cricothyroid muscle. The recurrent laryngeal nerves are branches of the vagus nerves in the cranial mediastinum. They contain the GSE neurons of the internal branch of the accessory nerve that innervate all the other intrinsic muscles of the larynx via the caudal laryngeal nerve as well as the cervical and cranial thoracic esophagus. As the vagus nerve courses caudally in the thorax on the surface of the esophagus, small branches supply its striated muscle with GSE innervation.[17,41]

Accessory Nerve

The axons of the neuronal cell bodies in the caudal portion of the nucleus ambiguus arch slightly dorsally and course ventrolaterally to emerge from the lateral aspect of the medulla as the cranial roots of the accessory nerve. Here they are joined by GVE neurons from the caudal portion of the parasympathetic nucleus of cranial nerve X to form the internal branch of the accessory nerve. The external branch of the accessory nerve is formed by the spinal roots of this nerve, whose cell bodies are located in the lateral portion of the ventral gray column of the eight cervical spinal cord segments. The axons of these cell bodies pass laterally to emerge from the lateral side of the cervical spinal cord as the spinal roots of the accessory nerve. These join to form a common bundle, the external branch of the accessory nerve, which courses cranially just dorsal to the denticulate ligament and between the segmental dorsal and ventral rootlets of the cervical spinal nerves (see Fig. 6-44). More GSE neurons are added to this external branch at each successive cervical segment. The external branch passes cranially through the foramen magnum into the caudal cranial fossa of the cra-

nial cavity. Here it is joined by the internal branch but for only a few millimeters. The two branches that comprise the accessory nerve pass through the jugular foramen. Within the short passageway between the jugular foramen and the tympanooccipital fissure, the internal branch of the accessory nerve joins the vagus nerve. Therefore, the accessory nerve that emerges from the tympanooccipital fissure contains only the GSE neurons from the external branch, and these neurons innervate the trapezius, sternocephalicus, and cleidocephalicus muscles. The GSE neurons in the internal branch of the accessory nerve that join the vagus nerve innervate the intrinsic muscles of the larynx and cervical and cranial thoracic esophagus by way of the recurrent laryngeal nerve that branches from the vagus nerve in the cranial thorax.

Clinical Signs

Lesions in the caudal portion of the nucleus ambiguus, in the GSE axous of the internal branch of the accessory nerve, in the cervical portion of the vagus nerve or its recurrent laryngeal branch, or in the caudal laryngeal nerve or the muscles of the larynx result in laryngeal paralysis. This causes an inspiratory dyspnea. When this is recognized in most small animals, there is bilateral paralysis. In racehorses, unilateral laryngeal paralysis is a common cause of poor performance; the inspiratory dyspnea may be severe enough to be audible in the exercised horse and is referred to as roaring. The inspiratory dyspnea is due to the failure of the cricoarytenoideus dorsalis muscles to completely abduct the vocal folds, which interferes with the air flow on inspiration.

Lesions in the rostral two thirds of nucleus ambiguus, in the GSE axons in the vagus and glossopharyngeal nerves, or in the muscles of the pharynx or esophagus result in varying degrees of difficulty in swallowing, which is referred to as dysphagia. In unilateral pharyngeal paresis, there is partial ability to swallow, but choking, gagging, and loss of food through the nares occur. With bilateral lesions, swallowing cannot be accomplished, choking and gagging are worse, and food commonly appears at the nares. There is no gag reflex in small animals, but with partial lesions this is a very difficult reflex to assess because of the marked variation in normal animals. In some dog breeds, especially the Labrador and golden retrievers, this reflex is very difficult to assess reliably. The most reliable indication of a problem with swallowing is the owner's description of the patient's attempts to eat and drink.

We have not observed in any domestic animal reliable clinical signs of lesions involving portions of the GSE neurons in the accessory nerve that innervate the cervical muscles.

Diseases

Oropharyngeal dysphagia as the only clinical sign is uncommon in small animals.[34] It occasionally occurs with extracranial neoplasms that involve the pharyngoesophageal plexus.

Megaesophagus

Regurgitation, associated with megaesophagus as the only clinical sign occurs in two forms, congenital and acquired.

A congenital idiopathic megaesophagus causes regurgitation that is first observed as the puppy is weaned from a liquid to a solid-food diet. A late-onset acquired form of megaesophagus occurs in older dogs and in many dogs is thought to be a form of focal myasthenia gravis. (This is described with the spinal nerve LMN diseases in Chapter 5.) Congenital idiopathic megaesophagus has been reported in most breeds of dogs but there is a high incidence in the German shepherd, Great Dane, Irish setter, Labrador retriever, Chinese shar pei, and Newfoundland. An inherited pathogenesis has been reported in the wire fox terrier and miniature schnauzer breeds.[8] The most salient clinical sign is postprandial regurgitation. A secondary aspiration pneumonia is a major risk. Thoracic radiographs confirm the presence of a diffuse megaesophagus that differentiates this cause of regurgitation from the megaesophagus associated with vascular ring malformations, which obstruct the esophagus at the base of the heart. These vascular ring malformations also cause regurgitation in the puppy at the time it is weaned. For many years this congenital idiopathic diffuse megaesophagus was thought to be a neuromuscular disorder based on being able to reproduce it by experimental vagotomies or the bilateral electrolytic destruction of the nucleus ambiguus.[5,28] However, no microscopic or physiologic studies could confirm this in affected dogs. Although the esophageal hypomotility is associated with the failure of the gastroesophageal junction to open, there is no evidence of any increased muscle tone at this junction. More recently, there has been physiologic evidence of dysfunction in the general visceral afferent (GVA) system involved in reflex esophageal function.[16] The cause of the dysfunction has not been defined. Fig. 6-45 shows a schematic diagram of the GSE and GVA innervation of the esophagus. There is no definitive treatment for this megaesophagus, but the movement of food from the esophagus into the stomach can be improved by feeding a soft semisolid diet to the patient that has been trained to eat while standing erect on its pelvic limbs, with its forepaws elevated on a stool or table, and to maintain that position for 15 to 20 minutes after consuming the food. This is one situation when feeding the dog at the table is appropriate, as long as the correct quality of food is offered! This esophageal disorder is uncommon in cats.

Guttural Pouch Mycosis

In adult horses, dysphagia is one of the two most common clinical signs of a fungal infection of the guttural pouch. The other clinical sign is epistaxis.[6,7,13,14,18] The guttural pouch is a saclike ventral diverticulum of the auditory tube that is situated dorsal to the pharynx on each side and ventral to the cranium and atlas (Fig. 6-46 through 6-48). A species of *Aspergillus* that normally may inhabit the guttural pouch is the most common cause of this infection. The infection causes inflammation of the mucosa of the guttural pouch that extends deep to the mucosa to invade the structures it covers, which include a number of cranial nerve branches and blood vessels (Fig. 6-49). The most common site for this inflammation is the dorsocaudal aspect of the medial compartment. The pharyngeal branches of cranial nerves IX and X course ventrally adjacent to this medial

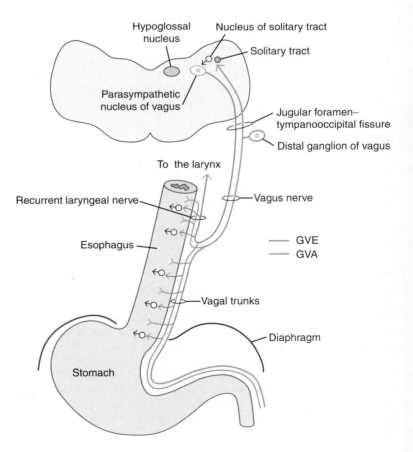

FIGURE 6-45 Schematic drawing of the general visceral efferent *(GVE)* and general visceral afferent *(GVA)* innervation of the esophagus.

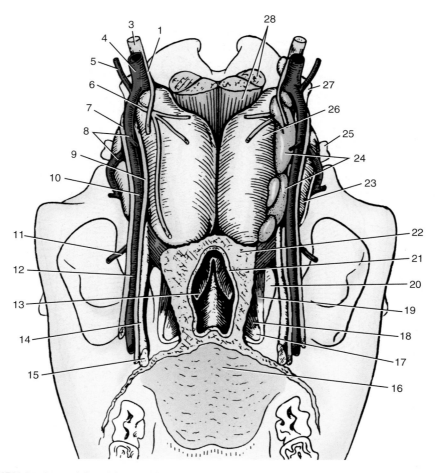

FIGURE 6-46 Ventral view of the guttural pouches after removal of the lower jaw, tongue, larynx, and oral and laryngeal parts of the pharynx. The upper border of the drawing is caudal.

1. Cranial laryngeal nerve
3. Vagosympathetic trunk
4. Common carotid artery
5. Occipital artery
6. Pharyngeal branch of vagus nerve
7. Hypoglossal nerve
8. External carotid artery
9. Glossopharyngeal nerve
10. Linguofacial nerve
11. Facial artery
12. Lingual artery
13. Ridge (torus tubarius) formed by the medial lamina of the cartilage of the auditory tube (the pharyngeal orifice of the tube is at the rostral end of the ridge below the leader line in the drawing and is foreshortened in this view)
14. Stylohyoid bone

15. Cut surface where the keratohyoid was severed from the stylohyoid in removing the tongue (the epihyoid is rudimentary)
16. Soft palate
17. Hamulus of pterygoid bone
18. Musculus pterygopharyngeus
19. Musculus tensor veli palatini
20. Pyramidal (pterygoid) process of palatine bone
21. Cut edge of pharyngeal mucosa
22. Cut surface of pharyngeal muscles
23. Right guttural pouch, lateral compartment
24. Right medial retropharyngeal lymph nodes
25. External acoustic meatus
26. Right guttural pouch, medial compartment
27. Paracondylar process of occipital bone
28. Musculus rectus capitis ventralis (above) and musculus longus capitis

(From de Lahunta A, Habel RE: Applied veterinary anatomy, *Philadelphia, 1986, Saunders.)*

compartment to reach the pharyngeal muscles that are ventral to the guttural pouch. When the inflammation involves these nerve branches, a partial dysphagia results and food is observed at the nares of these horses. The epistaxis is most commonly associated with the inflammation eroding into the internal carotid artery or occasionally into the maxillary artery. Bleeding occurs into the guttural pouch and from there, the blood drains through the pharyngeal orifice into the nasopharynx, then into the nasal cavities and out

the nares. Other neurologic signs associated with guttural pouch mycosis include laryngeal hemiparesis caused by involvement of the vagus nerve: Horner syndrome, resulting from lesions in the cranial cervical ganglion or its postganglionic branches in the internal carotid nerve that is associated with the internal carotid artery: less commonly, facial nerve paresis and hypoglossal nerve paresis; and, rarely, clinical signs of vestibular nerve dysfunction resulting from the inflammation eroding into the tympanic cavity and causing

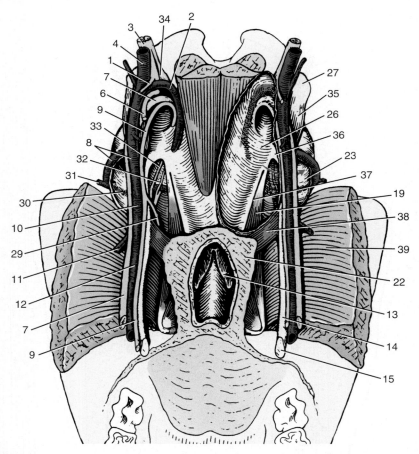

FIGURE 6-47 Same specimen as in Fig. 6-46 after removal of the medial compartment of the left guttural pouch and the ventral wall of the right pouch.

1. Cranial laryngeal nerve
2. Internal carotid artery
3. Vagosympathetic trunk
4. Common carotid artery
6. Pharyngeal branch of vagus nerve
7. Hypoglossal nerve
8. External carotid artery
9. Glossopharyngeal nerve, also shown on the right side, enclosed with the hypoglossal nerve in a fold of the pouch
10. Linguofacial artery
11. Facial artery
12. Lingual artery
13. Ridge (torus tubarius) formed by the medial lamina of the cartilage of the auditory tube (the pharyngeal orifice of the tube is at the rostral end of the ridge below the leader line in the drawing and is foreshortened in this view)
14. Stylohyoid bone
15. Cut surface where the keratohyoid was severed from the stylohyoid in removing the tongue (the epihyoid is rudimentary)
19. Musculus tensor veli palatine
22. Cut surface of pharyngeal muscles

23. Right guttural pouch, lateral compartment
26. Medial compartment (the pointer is on the bulla tympanica)
27. Paracondylar process of occipital bone
28. Musculus rectus capitis ventralis (above) and musculus longus capitis (below)
29. Pharyngeal branch of glossopharyngeal nerve
30. Maxillary artery
31. Masseteric artery
32. Nerve of musculus tensor tympani, a recurrent branch of the pterygoid nerve, the latter originating from the mandibular branch of the trigeminal nerve, dorsal to the maxillary artery
33. Chorda tympani
34. Cranial cervical ganglion
35. Musculus occipitohyoideus
36. Temporohyoid joint
37. Slit in the ventral wall of the auditory tube through which it communicates with the guttural pouch
38. Musculus stylopharyngeus caudalis
39. Musculus pterygoideus medialis

(From de Lahunta A, Habel RE: Applied veterinary anatomy, *Philadelphia, 1986, Saunders.)*

otitis media-interna. Treatment of this mycosis is difficult. Surgical procedures to prevent epistaxis by occluding the blood flow in the internal carotid artery or the maxillary artery are commonly followed by resolution of the inflammatory lesion.

Equine Laryngeal Hemiparesis-Hemiplegia

The most common laryngeal disorder that is recognized clinically occurs in racehorses. This is primarily a left hemiparesis that causes an inspiratory dyspnea, which interferes

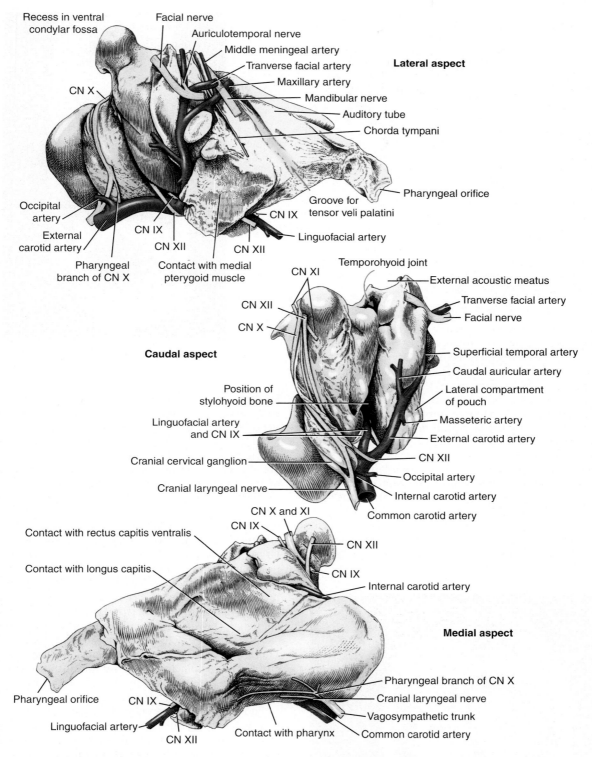

Recess in ventral condylar fossa
Facial nerve
Auriculotemporal nerve
Middle meningeal artery
Tranverse facial artery
Maxillary artery
Mandibular nerve
Auditory tube
Chorda tympani

Lateral aspect

CN X

Pharyngeal orifice

Occipital artery
External carotid artery
Pharyngeal branch of CN X
CN IX
CN XII
CN IX
CN XII
Contact with medial pterygoid muscle
Groove for tensor veli palatini
Linguofacial artery

CN XI
Temporohyoid joint
External acoustic meatus
CN XII
Tranverse facial artery
CN X
Facial nerve

Caudal aspect

Superficial temporal artery
Caudal auricular artery
Lateral compartment of pouch
Masseteric artery
External carotid artery
CN XII
Occipital artery
Internal carotid artery
Common carotid artery

Position of stylohyoid bone
Linguofacial artery and CN IX
Cranial cervical ganglion
Cranial laryngeal nerve

Contact with rectus capitis ventralis
Contact with longus capitis
CN X and XI
CN IX
CN XII
CN IX
Internal carotid artery

Medial aspect

Pharyngeal orifice
CN IX
Linguofacial artery
CN XII
Contact with pharynx
Pharyngeal branch of CN X
Cranial laryngeal nerve
Vagosympathetic trunk
Common carotid artery

FIGURE 6-48 Dissection of the right guttural pouch of a horse with its associated cranial nerves and vessels. *(From de Lahunta A, Habel RE: Applied veterinary anatomy, Philadelphia, 1986, Saunders.)*

with the athletic performance of the patient.[9-11,18,21,22] Most of the horses at risk for this disorder are 15 hands tall or taller and have long necks. It is not seen in ponies. Many of the pathogenetic mechanisms that have been proposed for this disorder relate to the asymmetric origin of the recurrent laryngeal nerves from the vagus nerves in the cranial mediastinum. The left recurrent laryngeal nerve has a longer course, having to pass around the ligamentum arteriosum and aortic arch before continuing cranially along the trachea to the larynx. The right recurrent laryngeal nerve has to pass

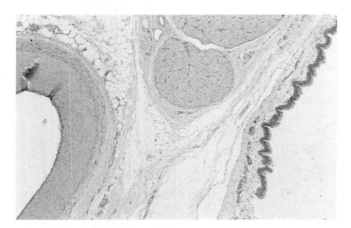

FIGURE 6-49 High-power magnification of the normal guttural pouch mucosa on the right, the internal carotid artery on the left, and the pharyngeal branches of the glossopharyngeal and vagal nerves in the middle. Mycotic lesions in the guttural pouch mucosa have ready access to the internal carotid artery to cause epistaxis and to the pharyngeal branches to cause a partial dysphagia.

only around the right subclavian artery to reach the trachea. In the first two editions of this text, I (AD) supported the hypothesis that the longer left recurrent laryngeal nerve was at risk for injury where it coursed around the aorta and could be stretched there by movements of the long neck. We now know that this hypothesis is incorrect, but the long length of these recurrent laryngeal nerves is important. There is denervation atrophy of only the laryngeal muscles innervated by the recurrent laryngeal nerves, which is much more extensive on the left side (Figs. 6-50 and 6-51). Microscopic study of the recurrent laryngeal nerves shows an axonal degeneration and demyelination that is most pronounced at the larynx and decreases as you progress retrograde along the more proximal components of these nerves. The current hypothesis is that this disorder is a dying-back neuropathy caused by the inability of the cell bodies in the nucleus ambiguus to maintain the integrity of such long motor neurons. In

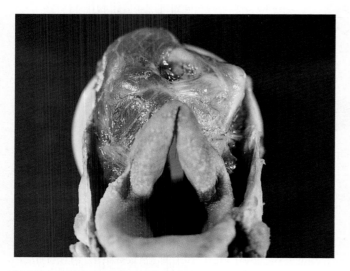

FIGURE 6-50 Craniocaudal view of the larynx of a horse with a left-side paralysis that resulted in severe denervation atrophy of all the intrinsic muscles of the larynx except for the cricothyroid. This is especially evident here in the cricoarytenoideus dorsalis muscle.

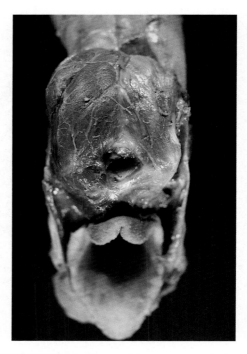

FIGURE 6-51 Dorsal surface of the same larynx as in Fig. 6-50.

affected horses, lesions can be found in both recurrent laryngeal nerves, but they are much more extensive in the left nerve, which further supports a dying-back neuropathy. Similar lesions can be found in the distal branches of the sciatic nerve where they innervate the crural muscles. These are also very long neurons, but no clinical signs of the loss of these neurons have been recognized. This hypothesis is supported by the absence of any lesions in the cranial laryngeal nerve, which is a short branch of the vagus nerve that innervates the cricothyroid muscle. Although the recurrent laryngeal nerve innervates all the intrinsic muscles of the larynx except the cricothyroid, the muscle most essentially necessary to open the glottis and increase the size of the airway is the cricoarytenoideus dorsalis muscle. As these lesions progress, varying degrees of paresis occur in the function of dilating the glottis. When the vocal folds cannot be fully abducted, they interfere with the flow of air on inspiration, causing the characteristic inspiratory dyspnea (Fig. 6-52). This is exacerbated by the air entering the laryngeal ventricle and further displacing the vocal fold into the airway. When the paresis is severe, a noise is audible, and that has led to calling this equine syndrome roaring.

Equine practitioners define four grades of laryngeal hemiparesis based on the endoscopic examination of the larynx at rest and during treadmill exercise **(Video 6-8)**. Treatments and prognosis depend on the grade of hemiparesis that is determined. Surgery is recommended for the more severely affected horses with the goal of maintaining the left vocal fold in a permanently abducted position. A suture is placed in the position of the cricoarytenoideus dorsalis muscle between the muscular process of the arytenoid cartilage and the caudal aspect of the cricoid cartilage.[21] Tension on this suture mechanically abducts the vocal fold. An inherited basis of this laryngeal disorder is suspected but has not been defined other than the risk involved in selection for taller long-necked horses.

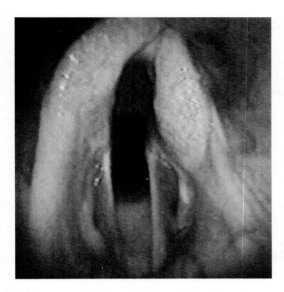

FIGURE 6-52 Endoscopic view of the larynx of a thoroughbred with left laryngeal paralysis.

Toxicity

Laryngeal paralysis has been reported in Arabian foals in association with the administration of the organophosphate anthelmintic haloxone starting at 2 days of age.[29] Chronic lead poisoning in horses causes a polyneuropathy that includes the recurrent laryngeal nerves and results in laryngeal paresis.

Cranial Mediastinal Lesions

The recurrent laryngeal nerves are at risk for being involved with lesions that develop in the cranial mediastinum. In horses, they include lymph node abscesses caused by *Streptococcus equi.* In cats and dogs, lymphoma is a concern at this location.

Canine Laryngeal Paralysis

Canine laryngeal paralysis occurs as an inherited disorder or an acquired disease.

Inherited. Laryngeal paralysis in dogs is most commonly an inherited degenerative disorder of the neurons in the recurrent laryngeal nerves. The neuropathy may affect only the recurrent laryngeal nerves, or their dysfunction may be part of a more diffuse polyneuropathy or may be a combination of neuropathy and encephalomyelopathy. It is critical to discuss with owners the possibility of a generalized neuromuscular disorder or encephalomyelopathy prior to any surgical correction of the larynx.

In our opinion, the most thorough study of inherited laryngeal paralysis was performed at the University of Utrecht in young Bouvier des Flandres dogs.[37,38] These young dogs were presented at 4 to 6 months of age for not growing well, exhibiting fatigue to the point of collapse and even cyanosis when exercised, and noisy breathing due to the marked inspiratory dyspnea. These severe clinical signs of laryngeal paralysis required that laryngeal surgery be performed if the patients were to survive.

Studies determined that this progressive laryngeal paresis was caused by bilateral abiotrophy of neurons in the caudal part of the nucleus ambiguus that innervated the larynx, and this abiotrophy was inherited as an autosomal dominant genetic disorder. Responsible dedicated breeders in the Netherlands were able to eliminate this disorder from the breed in a few years of careful control of their selection of dogs for breeding. North American dog breeders could take some lessons from these responsible individuals. A similar progressive laryngeal paresis-to-paralysis is inherited in young Siberian and husky cross-bred racing dogs, bull terriers, and dalmatians. The dalmatians may also have other signs of polyneuropathy. The patterns of inheritance and the pathologies of these disorders are less well defined than are those of the Bouviers. In Chapter 5, we describe laryngeal paralysis in 1- to 3-year-old male Leonbergers that is followed in a few weeks by the clinical signs of progressive sciatic-tibial nerve deficit.[32] It is inherited as a sex-linked recessive genetic disorder.

Be aware of the 8- to 10-week-old rottweiler pup that is presented to you with the clinical signs of progressive laryngeal paresis. Inspiratory dyspnea may be the only clinical sign that you recognize, and you perform surgery to establish a more adequate airway. At 12 to 14 weeks of age, the owner returns this dog to you because of a progressive gait abnormality that you recognize as a dysfunction of the UMN and general proprioceptive tracts in the spinal cord. This is an inherited autosomal genetic disorder that affects the CNS, especially the spinal cord tracts and the peripheral nervous system, and especially the recurrent laryngeal nerves. The initial clinical signs may involve the pelvic limb gait, the larynx, or both. If the clinical signs of laryngeal paresis occur first, you might perform surgery on a dog that will, in a few weeks to months, exhibit the signs of a progressive gait disorder that will ultimately cause recumbency and warrant euthanasia. This inherited disease of rottweiler dogs was published in 1997 as a neuronal vacuolation and spinocerebellar degeneration, but in reality this is a diffuse encephalomyelopathy and polyneuropathy.[19] This disorder is described in Chapter 10, in the discussion of small-animal cervical spinal cord diseases, Case Example 10-7. Progressive laryngeal paresis has also been reported in rottweiler dogs as part of a diffuse polyneuropathy that causes LMN tetraparesis.[20] We are not aware of a progressive laryngeal paresis in the rottweiler breed that is not associated with other neurologic signs and lesions, so great care should be taken before performing laryngeal surgical intervention.

Acquired: Idiopathic. An acquired idiopathic laryngeal paralysis occurs in older large-breed dogs without other significant signs of neuromuscular disease. It is common in Labrador retrievers, Saint Bernards, Newfoundlands, and Chesapeake Bay retrievers. Many of these dogs suffer from chronic hypothyroidism and some may improve when treated for their hypothyroidism. Most require laryngeal surgery to improve their inspiration and ability to exercise. The relationship between the chronic hypothyroidism and the laryngeal paralysis is not well understood. Both myopathy and neuropathy occur with this endocrine disorder in humans. Other cranial nerve and even brainstem signs have been associated with hypothyroidism solely on the basis of some response to therapy. No adequate pathologic studies have been performed in these dogs (see previous discussion with idiopathic facial neuropathy-neuritis). Occasionally, the dogs with this laryngeal paralysis also have megaesophagus. Until we understand this disorder better, these dogs should be evaluated for their thyroid status and the possibility of focal myasthenia gravis by evaluating their serum for antibodies against acetylcholine receptors.

Feline Laryngeal Paralysis. Laryngeal paralysis in cats is uncommon.[30] Unilateral paresis may follow injury to the carotid sheath during venipuncture, dog bites, or thyroid surgery. An infiltrative lymphoma can cause unilateral or bilateral laryngeal paresis. It is likely that a unilateral paralysis will not be recognized clinically because of the relative inactivity of this species.

Injury. Be aware that laryngeal hemiparesis or hemiplegia can follow an injury to the recurrent laryngeal nerve where it is still a component of the vagus nerve in the carotid sheath in the neck.

At this site, it is at risk for injury by aggressive attempts at external jugular venipuncture in any species, dog bites in small animals, ventral surgical approaches to the cervical intervertebral disks in dogs, and thyroid surgery. I (EG) have caused laryngeal paralysis in a middle-aged springer spaniel by the surgical approach to a ventral slot procedure in the cervical vertebrae. The carotid sheath is only a few millimeters deep to the external jugular vein and they are separated only by soft tissues. Serious injury to the contents of this sheath causes laryngeal hemiparesis or hemiplegia due to injury to the recurrent laryngeal nerve and Horner syndrome due to injury to the preganglionic sympathetic neurons in the cervical sympathetic trunk coursing to the head. I (AD) have seen a small pony with a heavily muscled neck collapse as the result of bilateral laryngeal paralysis following unsuccessful attempts to access the external jugular vein on both sides of the neck. Injury to the general visceral efferent and afferent neurons of one vagus nerve will not be recognized clinically.

CRANIAL NERVE XII: HYPOGLOSSAL NEURONS

Anatomy

The GSE neuronal cell bodies are located in the hypoglossal nucleus in the medulla (see Figs. 2-14 and 2-15).[4] This nucleus is adjacent to the median plane and to the floor of the fourth ventricle. It is a long nucleus (3 to 5 mm), extending from the obex caudally nearly to the level of the acoustic stria rostrally (see Figs. 6-1 and 6-3). The axons pass directly ventrally and slightly laterally through the reticular formation and across the lateral portion of the olivary nucleus. They emerge lateral to the pyramid as a longitudinal series of small roots. This row of hypoglossal roots merges at the small hypoglossal canal to form the hypoglossal nerve. The neurons course to innervate the extrinsic tongue muscles (styloglossus, hyoglossus, and genioglossus), the intrinsic tongue muscles, and the geniohyoideus. The hypoglossal nerve is much smaller inside the cranial cavity than outside the skull. This is the result of the increase in myelination and connective tissue that occurs after the nerve emerges from the hypoglossal canal.

Clinical Signs

Lesions in any parts of these hypoglossal neurons result in impairment of the function of the tongue in prehension, deglutition, mastication, and speech. The most reliable clinical sign of a unilateral lesion is atrophy of the tongue. Be sure to look at the tongue carefully in your cranial nerve exam because it is easy to miss mild unilateral atrophy. If the patient protrudes its tongue, it may deviate toward the denervated side because of contraction of the normal contralateral genioglossus and intrinsic tongue muscles. The animal may be observed to lick its lips only on the paralyzed side. An early sign of a unilateral hypoglossal nerve lesion may be the presence of fasciculations of the denervated half of the tongue.

Diseases

In the dog, unilateral tongue atrophy is most commonly due to an extramedullary lesion involving the hypoglossal nerve roots (Fig. 6-53). In the horse, unilateral tongue atrophy is almost pathognomonic for an *S. neurona* infection of the hypoglossal nucleus in the medulla (see Case Example 6-2). This can occur with or without other signs of medullary disease. In some horses the lesion is limited to this nucleus and at necropsy the cell bodies have been replaced by astrocytes. In cattle, the most common cause of tongue paresis is encephalitis in the medulla caused by *L. monocytogenes* (Fig. 6-54). Be sure to pull the tongue out of the mouth in horses and cattle to assess tongue strength as well as look for atrophy. This is much more difficult to do in normal cattle than in horses. Be careful not to be too aggressive because it is possible to injure the hypoglossal innervation and have the tongue fail to be retracted into the mouth. A hyoid bone

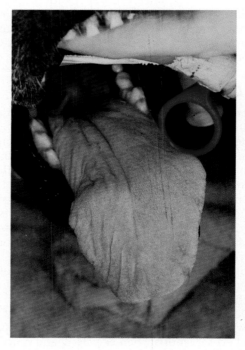

FIGURE 6-53 Atrophy of the right side of the tongue in a 14-year-old golden retriever due to a meningioma that involved the right hypoglossal nerve roots in the caudal cranial fossa.

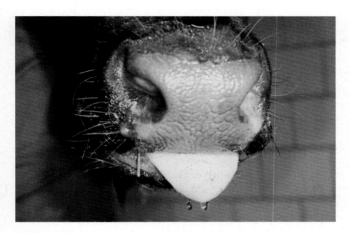

FIGURE 6-54 Tongue paresis in a 4-year-old Holstein cow with listeriosis; extensive inflammation and necrosis affected the hypoglossal nuclei and their intramedullary nerve roots bilaterally.

fracture or careless stylohyoid bone surgery in horses can also injure the hypoglossal nerve on one side. Clinical signs of vestibular nerve dysfunction associated with otitis media-interna are common in domestic animals. To avoid overlooking a central cause of these clinical signs, it is important to look carefully for involvement of other closely associated cranial nerves such as the hypoglossal nerve.

Diffuse Lower Motor Neuron Diseases

Many of the diseases described in Chapter 5 that diffusely affect spinal nerve GSE-LMN also affect cranial nerve GSE-LMN or the muscle innervated. Botulism is a good example of this because it commonly causes dysphagia, facial paresis, and jaw and tongue paresis. An acute onset of diffuse spinal nerve LMN signs that are accompanied by these cranial nerve LMN signs makes botulism a strong consideration for the clinical diagnosis. Myasthenia gravis may cause facial and laryngeal paresis and commonly causes regurgitation due to esophageal muscle paresis. North American tick paralysis and polyradiculoneuritis in dogs usually cause only mild facial paresis. Polyneuritis equi may cause facial paresis. Diffuse autoimmune polymyositis may include masticatory and pharyngeal muscles and cause dysphagia or the esophagus and cause regurgitation.

Encephalitis

Encephalitis involving the brainstem may produce clinical signs that include dysfunction of one or more of the cranial nerves that contain GSE-LMN. This is common in listeriosis in ruminants and when *S. neurona* affects the brainstem in horses. The type C retrovirus that causes caprine arthritis encephalitis (CAE) in goats and rabies in all species are other examples.

Prosencephalon

Be aware that acute prosencephalic disorders may cause mild cranial nerve signs as a result of a sudden interference with the UMN corticonuclear pathways that are involved in voluntary efforts that require cranial nerve GSE-LMN activity.[15] This is observed more commonly in horses and farm animals and is usually exhibited as dysphagia. Less commonly, facial paresis may be observed. For example, in horses, dysphagia may follow the sudden destruction of cerebral white matter, a leukoencephalomalacia caused by "moldy corn poisoning." This results from the ingestion of fumonisin B1, the mycotoxin produced by the fungus *Fusarium moniliformis* that grows on forages. In cattle, dysphagia may occur with severe acute prosencephalic hemorrhagic necrosis caused by *Histophilus somnus* vasculitis.

CASE EXAMPLE 6-1

Signalment: 2-year-old Holstein cow

Chief Complaint: Walking in circles and difficulty eating

History: For the past 6 days this cow has been walking in circles, usually to her right side. For 3 days, she was noticed to have difficulty in swallowing, and she developed a left ear droop.

Examination: Video 6-9 shows the bilateral ear droop and lack of closure of the eyelids to a menace or a direct stimulus with forceps. She was visual and would move away from the menacing gestures. Facial sensation was normal as is seen when the nasal septal mucosa was stimulated. Note the constant tongue protrusion and the lack of response when the tongue was handled. Note the lack of tone in the jaw and inability to close the mouth. There was poor abduction and adduction of the eyes when the head was moved in a horizontal plane to test normal physiologic nystagmus. Pupil size and light response were normal. Note her tendency to circle to the right when free in the pen, and watch her scuff the digits of her left limbs.

Anatomic Diagnosis: The brainstem nuclei or nerves of cranial nerves III, V, VI, VII, IX, X, and XII bilaterally; caudal brainstem UMN; and general proprioceptive pathways on the left side

It was impossible to tell how much of the dysphagia was due to the dysfunction of V and XII, the pharyngeal neurons of IX and X, or both. Involvement of the ascending reticular activating system in the more rostral brainstem could account for her mild depression. Circling may occur with asymmetric vestibular disorders and may be related to the loss of balance, or it may be propulsive and be related to an asymmetric frontoparietal basal nuclear lesion. The latter correlation is not well defined, and propulsive circling may occur with diencephalic or even mesencephalic lesions when the latter involves the substantia nigra. Most of the time propulsive circling is directed to the side of the lesion, but not always. The extensive bilateral cranial nerve dysfunction with minimal gait disorder suggests that this lesion may be extraparenchymal—perhaps an abscess that has spread along the floor of the cranial cavity. However, the left-side gait deficit requires involvement of neurons in the pons and medulla, and the circling does not appear to be related to a balance problem. Therefore, the indication is that the lesion involves central motor systems, not cranial nerve VIII.

Differential Diagnosis: Listeriosis, abscess, rabies, thrombotic meningoencephalitis, malignant catarrhal fever

LISTERIOSIS

Listeriosis is the most common inflammation in the brain of dairy cattle and is characterized by the involvement of cranial nerve neurons in the medulla and pons. The infectious agent is the bacterium

(Continued)

CASE EXAMPLE 6-1—cont'd

L. monocytogenes, which is thought to gain access to the brain by invading the sensory nerve endings in the oral mucosa and migrating over these nerves to the pons, where the trigeminal nerve enters the brainstem. This accounts for the predominance of lesions at this site. Prosencephalic lesions are very uncommon, which is why central blindness is not seen in this encephalitis. Various combinations of facial paralysis and vestibular ataxia with a head tilt are the most common cranial nerve signs observed in listeriosis. These clinical signs are also seen in otitis media-interna. However, in cattle with listeriosis, the recognition of other cranial nerve signs or gait abnormalities caused by UMN and general proprioceptive pathway dysfunction make otitis an untenable clinical diagnosis. The extent of cranial nerve involvement in this cow is unusual for listeriosis, which is why an extraparenchymal suppurative leptomeningeal infection was given strong consideration. (See the earlier discussion concerning the anatomic diagnosis.)

ABSCESS

A suppurative leptomeningitis resulting from a pituitary abscess or an extension from an otitis media-interna could spread on the floor of the cranial cavity and readily explain the severe bilateral involvement of the cranial nerves in this cow. If the lesion were more severe on the left side and compressed the caudal brainstem, this lesion could account for the mild left-side gait deficit. A lesion at this site would be less likely to cause the circling that was observed.

RABIES

In the opinion of Dr. Francis Fox at Cornell University, a large-animal veterinarian with more than 50 years of experience, the most typical clinical signs related to a rabies virus infection are their atypical appearance. This is a neurotrophic virus that includes infection of GSE neurons. The only reason for listing this diagnosis of rabies after the other two is that usually after 6 days of neurologic signs caused by the rabies virus, this cow would be unable to stand.

THROMBOTIC MENINGOENCEPHALITIS

Thrombotic meningoencephalitis caused by the bacterium *H. somni* is an acute brain disorder in cattle that would not be expected to affect the cranial nerves in such an extensive and bilateral manner. This disease is more common in the feed lots of the Midwest than in a New York State dairy farm, which was the location of this cow.

MALIGNANT CATARRHAL FEVER

Malignant catarrhal fever causing neurologic signs is uncommon in upstate New York. It is caused by a herpesvirus that infects cattle that reside on the same premises as sheep. It is usually an acute fulminating systemic disease that affects only the nervous system in the chronic stages, and cranial nerve signs are uncommon.

Polioencephalomalacia due to thiamin deficiency, sulfur intoxication, or lead poisoning is not included in this discussion because it is primarily a disorder of the prosencephalon and therefore would not be correlated with the anatomic diagnosis of this cow.

Lumbosacral CSF in the cow in this case example contained 17 white blood cells per cmm (normal <5), with 71% macrophages, 19% lymphocytes, and 19% neutrophils and with 66 mg/dl of protein (normal <40). This is most compatible with listeriosis or possibly rabies and is less likely to be suppurative leptomeningitis. Listeriosis

is treated with large doses of penicillin and has a fair prognosis if the cow is still standing, but the severity of the cranial nerve involvement in this cow suggested a guarded prognosis. This cow was treated but went down on the second day of treatment and was euthanized. At necropsy, an extensive inflammation was present in the brainstem, and the *L. monocytogenes* organism was identified in the lesion by using an immunocytochemical procedure. Be aware that this organism can be zoonotic and cause infection in the brain of humans, and you should protect yourself when examining a patient like this.

Video 6-10 shows a 6-month-old Holstein heifer with a 4-day history of depression, lying down excessively, having a protruding tongue, producing excessive salivation, and having difficulty eating. Note the ability to walk but with a slight vestibular ataxia (cranial nerve VIII deficit). Note the frequent bumping of her head into the wall and the lack of any response to a menace. Not seen are the dilated pupils that would not respond to light (cranial nerve II and/or III deficit). Note the dropped atonic jaw that she cannot move (bilateral motor cranial nerve V deficit); the protruded hypotonic tongue (bilateral cranial nerve XII deficit); the mild facial hypalgesia that is worse on the right side (sensory cranial nerve V deficit); the moderately weak eyelids (cranial nerve VII deficit); and the lack of normal physiologic nystagmus (bilateral cranial nerve III and VI deficit).

Anatomic Diagnosis: Bilateral cranial nerve II, III, V, VI, (VII, VIII, IX, X), XII

This anatomic diagnosis is similar to that made in this case example of a 2-year-old cow, and it should engender the same discussion concerning the differential diagnosis. However, this 6-month-old heifer had no clinical signs that could occur only in the brainstem, such as propulsive circling or a gait disorder involving the UMN and general proprioceptive systems; therefore, an extraparenchymal lesion would be more likely than a brainstem lesion. This observation and the knowledge that cattle with listeriosis are usually 1 year old or older and are not blind supports the presumptive clinical diagnosis of a suppurative leptomeningitis spread on the floor of the cranial cavity from the optic canals to the hypoglossal canals.

Because of the poor prognosis, this heifer was euthanized, and at necropsy a large, firm mass of highly organized suppurative meningitis was found to extend from the optic nerves to the caudal medulla (Figs. 6-55 through 6-57). This mass could be peeled off the ventral

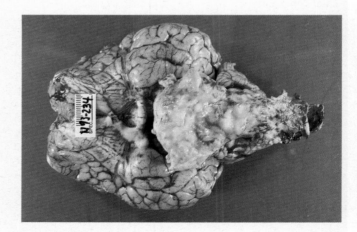

FIGURE 6-55 Ventral surface of the brain of the heifer in Video 6-10. Note the mass of thick tissue that covers and obscures the ventral surface of the entire brainstem, with its rostral border at the level of the optic chiasm. This mass consisted of a chronic fibrotic suppurative inflammation that may have resulted from a rupture of a pituitary abscess.

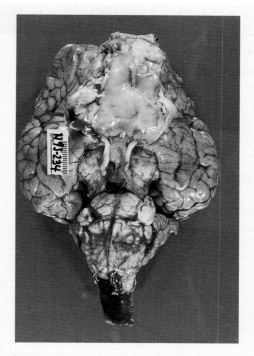

FIGURE 6-56 Same brain as in Fig. 6-55, with the mass of organized suppurative inflammation reflected rostrally to expose the ventral surface of the brainstem. The clinical signs that were observed were caused by the involvement of the cranial nerves as they passed through this inflammatory tissue ventral to the brainstem.

surface of the brainstem with tearing of the cranial nerves that were entrapped in it. It was suspected that this large mass of suppuration may have come from a pituitary abscess that had ruptured.

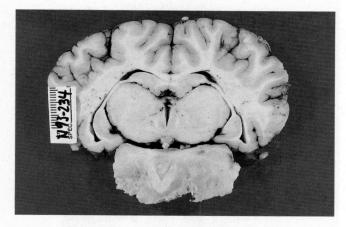

FIGURE 6-57 Transverse section of the preserved brain seen in Figs. 6-55 and 6-56 at the level of the caudal diencephalon. Note the thick mass of chronic inflammatory tissue ventral to the diencephalon.

CASE EXAMPLE 6-2

Signalment: 5-year-old thoroughbred gelding, Case

Chief Complaint: Head and pelvic muscle atrophy, inability to rise

History: The clinical signs observed in this horse were progressive over about a 3-month period. The initial clinical sign observed was atrophy of the left muscles of mastication (Fig. 6-58). This occurred while the gelding was still racing. A few weeks later atrophy was observed in the right gluteal muscles (Fig. 6-59), and the gait was altered in the right pelvic limb. Case was taken out of racing and stall-rested. In the week before the video was made, his pelvic limb gait problems progressed rapidly and he went down. When assisted, he could stand only on his thoracic limbs, like a sitting dog.

Examination: Video 6-11 shows the atrophy of the left masseter and temporal muscles and the right side of the tongue (Fig. 6-60). When assisted to stand with the help of Professors Robert Whitlock (University of Pennsylvania) and Ian Mayhew (Massey University) when they were on the faculty at Cornell University, Case could still move his pelvic limbs, but with difficulty. The quality of the paresis was difficult to evaluate. There was a mild loss of tone in the tail and anus and a mild atrophy of the right caudal thigh muscles. Thoracic limbs were normal.

Anatomic Diagnosis: Left motor V nucleus or the mandibular nerve from cranial nerve V; right hypoglossal nucleus or the hypoglossal nerve; L5, L6, sacral and caudal spinal cord segments; spinal nerve roots; spinal nerves: right sciatic and cranial gluteal nerves

Differential Diagnosis: Equine protozoal encephalomyelitis, polyneuritis equi, equine herpesvirus 1 vasculitis, and encephalomyelopathy

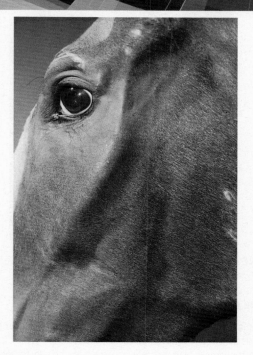

FIGURE 6-58 Left side of the head of the thoroughbred described in this case example, showing severe denervation atrophy of the left masseter muscle. The left temporal muscle was similarly affected.

(Continued)

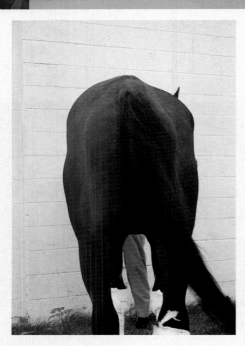

FIGURE 6-59 Atrophy of the gluteal muscles on the right side of the 5-year-old thoroughbred gelding shown in Fig.6-58 and described in this case example.

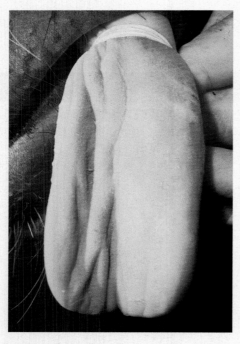

FIGURE 6-60 Atrophy of the right side of the tongue in the horse shown in Figs. 6-58 and 6-59 and described in this case example.

EQUINE PROTOZOAL ENCEPHALOMYELITIS

A chronic form of infection by *S. neurona* is the most presumptive diagnosis for this horse based on the multifocal asymmetric clinical signs of predominantly gray matter lesions, especially the very focal brainstem nuclear lesions without other clinical signs of brainstem disease. We have never seen such a localized nuclear lesion in any other equine disease. (See Case Example 11-2 for a complete description of this disease.)

POLYNEURITIS EQUI

Most horses with polyneuritis equi have a more severe and bilateral lesion in the sacrocaudal spinal nerves but not enough lumbar spinal nerve involvement to cause the patient to go down. If cranial nerves are affected, it is less severe than in this case, and we are not aware of any involvement of the hypoglossal nerves in polyneuritis equi. (This disease is described in Case Example 5-9.)

EQUINE HERPESVIRUS 1

Equine herpesvirus 1 causes vasculitis of small blood vessels in the CNS, which results in thrombosis and a myelopathy with ischemic or hemorrhagic infarction of the CNS parenchyma. The clinical signs are always acute in onset and nonprogressive after about 72 hours. In mild cases the lesions are mostly in the thoracolumbar spinal cord white matter, causing a UMN paresis and general proprioceptive ataxia limited to the pelvic limbs. In addition, there is usually a mild loss of tone in the tail and anus and difficulty in emptying the bladder. We have not seen cranial nerve signs in this disorder. (See Case Example 11-3 for a complete description of this disease.)

In this case example, the lumbosacral CSF was xanthochromic and contained 31 white blood cells per cmm (normal <5) and 106 mg/dl of protein (normal <80). At the time that this horse was studied, there were no antibody assays for the protozoal agent, which had yet to be identified. This horse was euthanized and at necropsy, there were grossly visible discolorations at the sites of the anatomic diagnosis. Figures 6-61 through 6-71 show these lesions and provide descriptions of their relationships to the clinical signs. Protozoal organisms were present in the lumbosacral lesion.

It is assumed that the *S. neurona* protozoal agent gains access to the CNS from the blood, but the focal GSE motor neuronal lesions observed in this horse suggest that a possible route of entry may be from the muscles, with the organism passing retrograde through the motor innervation to the GSE cell bodies in the brainstem nuclei or spinal cord ventral gray column. No organisms have been described in the muscles of any of these horses, but these studies have been few. The volume of horse muscle that should be studied is awesome!.

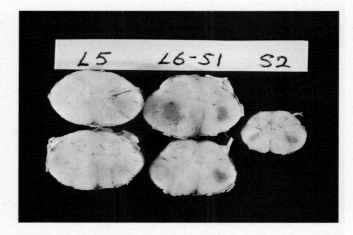

FIGURE 6-61 Caudal surface of transverse sections of the preserved L5 to S2 spinal cord segments of the horse in Figs. 6-58 through 6-60 and described in this case example. Discolorations centered in the ventral gray columns represent an acute necrotizing inflammation on the left side that includes the adjacent white matter and a chronic astrogliosis on the right side that is limited to the ventral gray column.

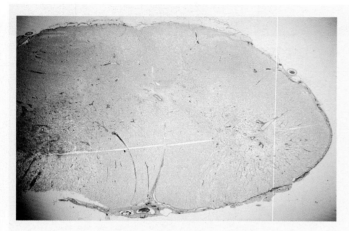

FIGURE 6-62 Low-power magnification of a microscopic section of the L6 spinal cord segment, showing the bilateral lesions in Fig. 6-61.

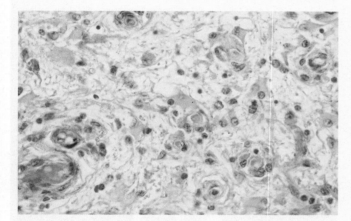

FIGURE 6-63 High-power magnification of the lesion in the right ventral gray column in the L6 spinal cord segment seen in Figs. 6-61 and 6-62, showing the replacement of the neuronal cell bodies with reactive astrocytes. This lesion correlates with the location of the neuronal cell bodies of the cranial gluteal nerve and the denervation atrophy of the right middle gluteal, deep gluteal, and tensor fascia lata muscles.

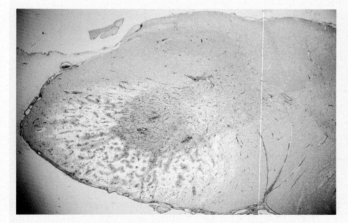

FIGURE 6-64 Low-power magnification of a microscopic section of the L6 spinal cord segment, showing the left side where there is active inflammation with extensive necrosis and hemorrhage.

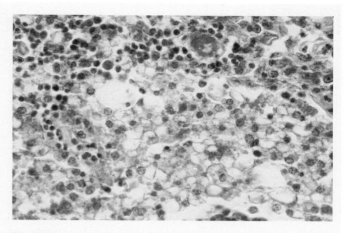

FIGURE 6-65 High-power magnification of the microscopic section seen in Fig. 6-64. Note the necrosis and nonsuppurative inflammation.

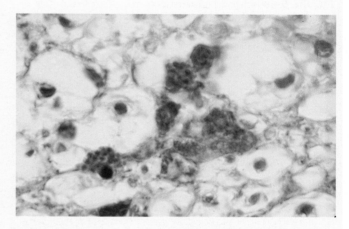

FIGURE 6-66 High-power magnification of the microscopic section seen in Figs. 6-64 and 6-65, showing clusters of basophilic organisms presumed to be *S. neurona.*

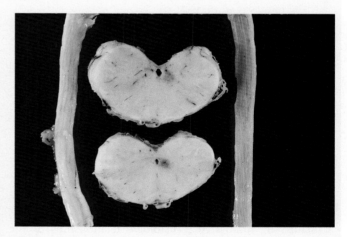

FIGURE 6-67 Caudal surface of transverse sections of the preserved caudal medulla and the left and right hypoglossal nerves of the horse in this case example. Note the small focal discoloration adjacent to the right side of the central canal. This represents a chronic lesion in the right hypoglossal nucleus. The discoloration of the right hypoglossal nerve reflects the diffuse wallerian degeneration of its neuronal processes.

(Continued)

CASE EXAMPLE 6-2—cont'd

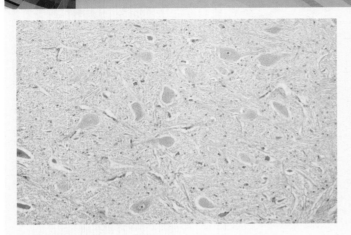

FIGURE 6-68 High-power magnification of a microscopic section of the normal left hypoglossal nucleus seen in Fig. 6-67, showing the normal neuronal cell bodies located at this level.

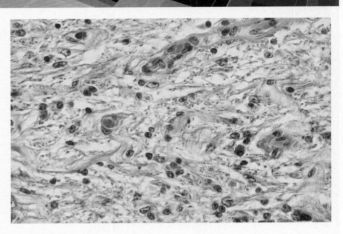

FIGURE 6-70 High-power magnification of the right hypoglossal nucleus seen in Fig. 6-69, where the neuronal cell bodies have been replaced by reactive astrocytes similar to the lesion seen in the right ventral gray column in the L6 spinal cord segment shown in Figs. 6-62 and 6-63. This lesion correlates with the wallerian degeneration in the right hypoglossal nerve and the atrophy in the right side of the tongue.

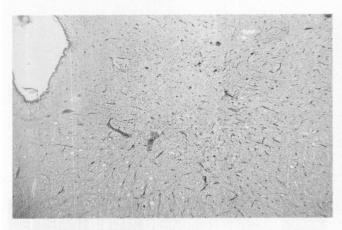

FIGURE 6-69 Low-power magnification of a microscopic section of the right hypoglossal nucleus seen in Fig. 6-67, where there is no evidence of any neuronal cell bodies.

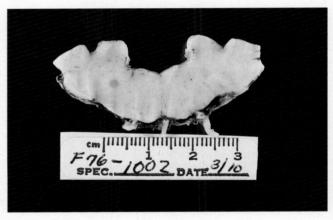

FIGURE 6-71 Caudal surface of a transverse section of the pons of the horse in this case example. The oval discoloration on the left side represents the left motor nucleus of the trigeminal nerve in which the neuronal cell bodies have been replaced by reactive astrocytes as seen in Figs. 6-63 and 6-70. This lesion correlates with the atrophy of the left masseter and temporal muscles.

REFERENCES

1. Blauch B, Strafuss AC: Histologic relationships of the facial (7th) and vestibulocochlear (8th) nerves within the petrous temporal bone in the dog, *Am J Vet Res* 35:481, 1974.
2. Blythe LL, et al: Otitis media/interna in the horse: a cause of head shaking and skull fractures, *Proc Am Assoc Eq Pract* 37:517-528, 1991.
3. Blythe LL, et al: Prophylactic partial stylohyoidostectomy for horses with osetoarthropathy of the temporohyoid joint, *J Eq Vet Sci* 14:32-37, 1994.
4. Chibuzo GA, Cummings JF: An enzyme tracer study of the organization of the somatic motor center for the innervation of different muscles of the tongue: evidence for two sources, *J Comp Neurol* 205:273, 1982.
5. Clifford DH, et al: Comparison of motor nuclei of the vagus nerve in dogs with and without esophageal achalasia, *Proc Soc Exp Biol Med* 142:878, 1973.
6. Cook WR: The clinical features of guttural pouch mycosis in the horse, *Vet Rec* 83:336, 1968.
7. Cook WR, Campbell RS, Dawson C: The pathology and etiology of guttural pouch mycosis in the horse, *Vet Rec* 83:422, 1968.

8. Cox VS, et al: Hereditary esophageal dysfunction in the miniature schnauzer dog, *Am J Vet Res* 41:326, 1980.
9. Duncan ID, Griffiths IR: Pathological changes in equine laryngeal muscles and nerves, *Proc Am Assoc Equine Pract* 19:97, 1973.
10. Duncan ID, Griffiths IR, Madrid RE: A light and electron microscopic study of the neuropathy of equine idiopathic laryngeal hemiplegia, *Neuropathol Appl Neurobiol* 4:483, 1978.
11. Duncan ID, et al: The pathology of equine laryngeal hemiplegia, *Acta Neuropathol* 27:337, 1974.
12. Firth EC: Vestibular disease and its relationship to facial paralysis in the horse: a clinical study of 7 cases, *Aust Vet J* 53:560, 1977.
13. Freeman DE: Diagnosis and treatment of diseases of the guttural pouch, part I, *Compend Cont Ed* 2:S3-S11, 1980.
14. Freeman DE: Diagnosis and treatment of diseases of the guttural pouch, part II, *Compend Cont Ed* 2:S25-S30, 1980.
15. Hockman CH, Bieger D, Weerasuriya SA: Supranuclear pathways of swallowing, *Prog Neurobiol* 12:15, 1979.
16. Holland CT, Satchell PM, Farrow BRH: Selective vagal afferent dysfunction in dogs with congenital idiopathic megaesophagus, *Auton Neurosci* 99:18-23, 2002.
17. Hudson LC: *The origins of innervation of the esophagus and the caudal pharyngeal muscles with histochemical and ultrastructural observations on the esophagus of the dog,* PhD dissertation, Ithaca, NY, 1982, Cornell University.
18. Koch C: Diseases of the larynx and pharynx of the horse, *Compend Cont Ed* 2:73, 1980.
19. Kortz GD, et al: Neuronal vacuolation and spinocerebellar degeneration in young rottweiler dogs, *Vet Pathol* 34:296-302, 1997.
20. Mahony OM, et al: Laryngeal paralysis-polyneuropathy complex in young rottweilers, *J Vet Intern Med* 12:330-337, 1998.
21. Marks D, et al: Etiology and diagnosis of laryngeal hemiplegia in horses, *J Vet Intern Med* 157:429, 1970.
22. Marks D, et al: Observations on laryngeal hemiplegia in the horse and treatment by abductor muscle prosthesis, *Equine Vet J* 2:159, 1978.
23. Mayhew PD, Bush WW, Glass EN: Trigeminal neuropathy in dogs: a retrospective study of 29 cases (1991-2000), *J Am Anim Hosp Assoc* 38:262-270, 2002.
24. Parker AJ, et al: Hemifacial spasm in a dog, *Vet Rec* 93:514, 1973.
25. Pfaff A-M D, March PA, Fishman C: Acute bilateral trigeminal neuropathy associated with nervous system lymphosarcoma in a dog, *J Am Anim Hosp Assoc* 36:57-61, 2000.
26. Power HT, Watrous BJ, de Lahunta A: Facial and vestibulocochlear nerve disease in six horses, *J Am Vet Med Assoc* 183:1076-1080, 1983.
27. Roberts SA, Vainisi SJ: Hemifacial spasm in dogs, *J Am Vet Med Assoc* 150:381-385, 1967.
28. Rogers WA, Fenner WR, Sherding RG: Electromyographic and esophagomanometric findings in clinically normal and dogs with idiopathic megaesophagus, *J Am Vet Med Assoc* 174:181, 1979.
29. Rose RJ, Hartley WJ, Baker W: Laryngeal paralysis in Arabian foals associated with oral haloxone administration, *Equine Vet J* 13:171, 1981.
30. Schachter S, Norris CR: Laryngeal paralysis in cats: 16 cases (1990-1999), *J Am Vet Med Assoc* 216:1100-1103, 2000.
31. Schultz RM, et al: Magnetic resonance imaging of acquired trigeminal nerve disorders in six dogs, *Vet Radiol Ultrasound* 48:101-104, 2007.
32. Shelton GD, et al: Inherited polyneuropathy in Leonberger dogs: a mixed or intermediate form of Charcot-Marie-Tooth disease? *Muscle Nerve* 27:471-477, 2003.
33. Stone J, Campion JE, Leicester J: The nasotemporal division of retina in the Siamese cat, *J Comp Neurol* 180:783, 1978.
34. Suter PF, Watrous BJ: Oropharyngeal dysphagias in the dog: a cinefluorographic analysis of experimentally induced and spontaneously occurring swallowing disorders, *Vet Radiol* 21:24, 1980.
35. Varejao AS, Munoz A, Lorenzo V: Magnetic resonance imaging of the infratemporal facial nerve in idiopathic facial paralysis in the dog, *Vet Radiol Ultrasound* 47:328-333, 2006.
36. Valentine BA, et al: Suprasellar germ cell tumors in the dog: a report of five cases and review of the literature, *Acta Neuropathol* 76:94-100, 1988.
37. Venker-van Hagen AJ: *Investigations on the pathogenesis of hereditary laryngeal paralysis in the Bouvier,* Thesis, Utrecht, the Netherlands, 1981, University of Utrecht.
38. Venker-van Hagen AJ, Bouw J, Hartman W: Hereditary transmission of laryngeal paralysis in young Bouviers, *J Am Anim Hosp Assoc* 17:75, 1981.
39. Vitale CL, Olby NJ: Neurologic dysfunction in hypothyroid, hyperlipidemic labrador retrievers, *J Vet Intern Med* 21:1316-1322, 2007.
40. Walker AM, et al: Temporohyoid osteoarthropathy in 33 horses (1993-2000), *J Vet Intern Med* 16:697-703, 2002.
41. Watson AG: *Some aspects of vagal innervation of the canine esophagus: an anatomical study,* Thesis, Massey, NZ, 1974, Massey University.

7 Lower Motor Neuron: General Visceral Efferent System

GENERAL ANATOMY

CONTROL OF THE PUPILS

Parasympathetic Innervation
  of the Eye
    Anatomy
    Clinical Signs
Sympathetic Innervation
  of the Eye
    Anatomy
    Clinical Signs
    CASE EXAMPLE 7-1
Anisocoria
Pupils in Acute Brain Disease

Protrusion of the Third Eyelid

CONTROL OF MICTURITION

Sacral Parasympathetic GVE-LMN
Caudal Lumbar Sympathetic GVE-LMN
Sacral GSE-LMN
General Visceral Afferent Neurons
Brainstem Centers
Continence and Storage of Urine
Micturition, Urination
Urinary Incontinence
  Lower Motor Neuron Bladder
  Upper Motor Neuron Bladder

CONTROL OF DEFECATION

**PARASYMPATHETIC GVE-LMN OF THE
MEDULLA: FACIAL, GLOSSOPHARYNGEAL,
VAGUS, AND ACCESSORY NEURONS**

DYSAUTONOMIA

**COMPLEX REGIONAL PAIN
SYNDROME, REFLEX SYMPATHETIC
DYSTROPHY**

GENERAL ANATOMY

General visceral efferent (GVE) neurons innervate the smooth muscle associated with blood vessels and visceral structures, glands, and cardiac muscle. This is an involuntary system that represents the lower motor neuron (LMN) for the autonomic nervous system. The autonomic nervous system is an anatomic and physiologic system with central and peripheral components. It includes higher centers located in the hypothalamus, midbrain, pons, and medulla. The hypothalamus is the primary integrating center of the autonomic nervous system. Nuclei in its rostral portion subserve the parasympathetic division of the GVE-LMN. Nuclei in its caudal portion subserve the sympathetic division of the GVE-LMN. These hypothalamic nuclei receive afferents from the cerebrum by way of numerous pathways, from thalamic nuclei, and from ascending general visceral afferent (GVA) pathways. The hypothalamus influences the activity of the metabolic centers in the reticular formation of the midbrain, pons, and medulla. These centers control the activity of visceral smooth muscle, glands, and cardiac muscle by means of the GVE-LMN, which is located in specific cranial nerves and all spinal nerves.

Some texts consider that the autonomic nervous system is only the GVE-LMN, but this is too simplistic and not realistic. The autonomic nervous system is concerned with activating emergency mechanisms and with the repair and preservation of the internal environment of the body. It maintains a steady state in the internal environment for the continuous efficient function of the body, which is called homeostasis. In order to carry out these functions, the autonomic nervous system must receive information from the body via sensory neurons in the GVA system, then process this information in centers in the brain and send responses back to the body by brainstem and spinal cord pathways that activate LMNs in the GVE system.

The GVE system is grouped physiologically and anatomically into two components: the sympathetic and parasympathetic systems. This LMN is a two-neuron system between the central nervous system (CNS) and the effector organ innervated. These two neurons are referred to as the preganglionic and postganglionic neurons. The cell body of the preganglionic neuron is in the gray matter of the CNS, and the cell body of the postganglionic neuron is in a ganglion in the peripheral nervous system. The telodendron of the preganglionic neuron synapses on the dendritic zone of the postganglionic neuron in this ganglion. To be accurate, only the axon of the second neuron is actually postganglionic. The sympathetic system is referred to as the thoracolumbar system based on the location of the cell body of the first neuron, the preganglionic neuron, that is in the lateral gray column from spinal cord segments T1 to about L4 or L5. As a general rule, the sympathetic ganglia are located fairly close to the CNS, and the postganglionic axons are fairly long. With a few exceptions, the neurotransmitter released at the telodendron of the sympathetic postganglionic neuron is norepinephrine. Thus the sympathetic system is referred to as the adrenergic system. The parasympathetic system is referred to as the craniosacral system because the cell bodies of the preganglionic neurons are located either in the brainstem nuclei of cranial nerves III, VII, IX, X, and XI or in the sacral spinal cord segments. As a general rule, the ganglia of this parasympathetic system are located in or fairly close to the effector organ, and the postganglionic axons are short. Acetylcholine is the neurotransmitter released at the telodendron of the postganglionic axon. Thus, this system is known as the cholinergic system. The anatomic components of this GVE-LMN should have been learned in your dissection course on the anatomy of the dog. (Refer to *Guide to the Dissection of the Dog* by H. E. Evans and A. de Lahunta, ed 6, Philadelphia, 2004, Elsevier). For clinical purposes, the GVE-LMN can be divided into four components, and the veterinary student must understand the functional anatomy of all four: control of the pupils, of micturition and defecation, of the enteric system, and of the cardiorespiratory system.

CONTROL OF THE PUPILS

For the purposes of clinical neurology, you can think of the size of the pupils as representing a constant balance between the amount of light in the environment and the emotional status of the patient. The parasympathetic GVE system regulates the response of the eye to environmental light. The sympathetic GVE system regulates the response of the pupil to environmental factors that elicit stress, such as excitement, fear, and anger.

Parasympathetic Innervation of the Eye

As part of the cranial nerve evaluation in your neurologic examination of any patient, you will always evaluate the size of the pupils and their response to a strong source of light. Always evaluate the size of the resting pupils first, and do it from a distance, with just enough light to allow you to see the pupils. In some animals, the pupils are difficult to see in ambient light. The examination can be facilitated by holding a light source on the median plane at about the level of the end of the patient's nose or a few inches beyond in cats and brachycephalic dog breeds—just far enough away so that you do not elicit significant pupil constriction. Appreciate the size of the resting pupils and look for any asymmetry, called anisocoria. Remember that an overly excited patient may have equally dilated pupils as the result of circulating epinephrine. Place your light source up close to the eye without touching it. Record the response, and swing the light quickly to the other eye. Record that response, and swing the light back to the first eye. Repeat this a number of times to be sure of your evaluation. This requires patience, both yours and that of the animal being evaluated. Usually, a normal, excited patient with dilated pupils will respond to a bright light source. To appreciate the pupillary responses or lack thereof, you must know all the anatomic components involved by the test that you just performed and all the factors that control the size of the pupils. These follow.

Anatomy

The sensory anatomic pathway stimulated by the light is described in detail in Chapter 14, the visual system. In brief (Fig. 7-1), the light must initially stimulate receptors in the retina. The area centralis of the retina is the most sensitive to light and in carnivores is just lateral to the optic disk.

The impulses generated in the retina travel through the optic nerve of that eye and continue in both optic tracts to the most dorsal caudal and lateral aspects of the thalamus, where they pass over the lateral geniculate nuclei and enter the pretectal nuclei in the most rostral part of the midbrain (see Fig. 2-5). Synapse occurs there, and the majority of the axons of the pretectal neurons cross through the caudal commissure to synapse on the GVE parasympathetic LMNs in the most rostral part of the contralateral oculomotor nucleus in the midbrain (see Fig. 2-6). A smaller number of pretectal neurons project directly to the rostral part of the ipsilateral oculomotor nucleus. Thus, light directed into one eye stimulates a series of neurons that terminate in both parasympathetic nuclei of the oculomotor nerve, resulting in a response in both eyes.

For this GVE-LMN pathway, the cell bodies of the preganglionic neurons are located in the parasympathetic nucleus of the oculomotor nerve in the rostral part of the mesencephalon. In humans, this nucleus is known as the nucleus of Edinger-Westphal. It is located in the ventral part of the central gray substance next to the median plane, where it is continuous caudally with the general somatic efferent (GSE) motor nucleus of the oculomotor nerve that is described in Chapter 6. The GVE axons course ventrally and emerge with the GSE axons in the lateral aspect of the interpeduncular fossa on the medial side of the crus cerebri. The GVE axons in the canine oculomotor nerve are located superficially on the medial side of this cranial nerve, where they are at risk for being compressed by extraparenchymal neoplasms and by disorders that cause the mesencephalon to swell or be displaced. The oculomotor nerve, with the GVE preganglionic axons, passes through the orbital fissure into the orbit within the periorbita, where it is adjacent to the lateral side of the optic nerve for a few millimeters. The oculomotor nerve then abruptly branches to the extraocular muscles. Located at this point of branching is a small ganglion, the ciliary ganglion. In this ganglion, the telodendrons of the GVE preganglionic neurons synapse on the dendritic zones of the cell bodies of the postganglionic neurons. The postganglionic axons pass by way of short ciliary nerves along the surface of the optic nerve to the eyeball to innervate the smooth muscle of the ciliary muscle and the sphincter of the pupil.[13] The more light that enters the eyes and stimulates the retina, the more impulses will reach this parasympathetic pathway and cause the sphincter muscles to contract and the pupils to constrict. In diminished light there is less stimulus to these sphincter muscles, so the pupils passively dilate. Turn off the lights in the room and watch this happen.

When you direct the light into one eye, you evaluate the direct response in that eye and the indirect or consensual response in the opposite eye. You appreciate this consensual response when you swing the light to the opposite eye. This terminology can be very confusing and it is much better to record what happens in each eye when you direct the light into one eye and repeat it for the other eye. Sometimes, the degree of constriction seen in the eye in which the light is directed (the direct response) is slightly greater than the degree of constriction seen in the opposite eye (indirect, consensual response). This is normal. It occurs because the majority of the axons cross in the optic nerve at the optic chiasm. A similar crossing back of the

Pathway for pupillary control

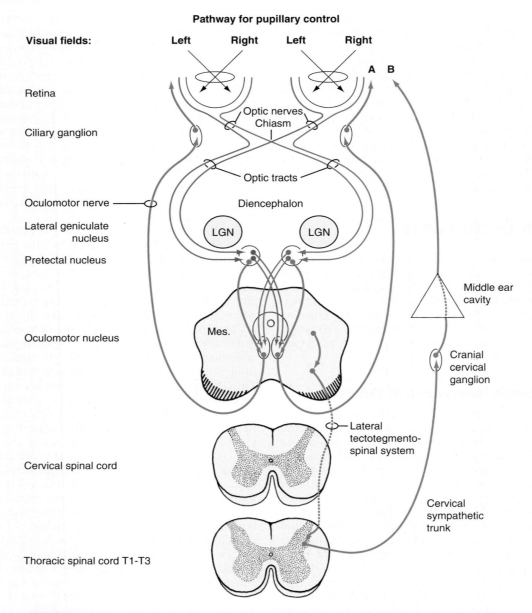

FIGURE 7-1 Neuroanatomic pathway for pupillary control. **A,** Constrictor. **B,** Dilator of pupil. *LGN,* Lateral geniculate nucleus; *Mes.,* mesencephalon.

majority of the axons of the neurons occurs in the pretectal nucleus in the midbrain via the caudal commissure. As a result, the parasympathetic nucleus of the oculomotor nerve on the side ipsilateral to the eye being stimulated receives the greater stimulus. This difference is more obvious in horses and farm animals than in small animals; this correlates with the larger number of axons that cross in the optic chiasm in the former. Be aware that the rate of pupillary constriction varies among species and among individuals of the same species. The rate of constriction is slowest in horses and cattle.

Clinical Signs

Lesions restricted to the visual pathways in the cerebrum can cause blindness but the pupillary light responses are normal. Note that in Fig. 7-1, no cerebral structures are present. Compare this with Fig. 14-5, which depicts the entire

pathway of vision. For the examples presented in Table 7-1, imagine the site of the lesion in Fig. 7-1 and consider the clinical signs that would result. For these examples, consider that each lesion causes complete dysfunction of the structure indicated. These clinical signs are summarized in Table 7-1 and the description follows. Remember that the normal menace response requires the entire visual system pathway from the eye to the cerebral cortex to be intact as well as a pathway to the facial nuclei in the medulla. The term *oculus sinister* (OS) refers to the left eye. The term *oculus dextra* (OD) refers to the right eye. *Oculi uterque* (OU) refers to both eyes.

1. A lesion in the right optic nerve causes an absent menace response in that eye only. The resting size of the pupils may be the same, or the right pupil may be slightly dilated. The room light entering the left eye stimulates both parasympathetic oculomotor nuclei, so both pupils respond the same to room light; or, because of the unequal

TABLE 7-1 Clinical Signs of Visual Deficit

Lesion	OS Menace	OS Pupil	OD Menace	OD Pupil
1. Right optic nerve	Present	Normal size Light in OS; both constrict	Absent	Normal size to partial dilation Light in OD; neither constricts
2. Right cranial nerve III	Present	Normal size Light in OS; only OS constricts	Present	Complete dilation Light in OD; only OS constricts
3. Right retrobulbar	Present	Normal size Light in OS; only OS constricts	Absent	Complete dilation Light in OD; neither pupil constricts
4. Right optic tract	Mostly absent	Normal size Light in OS; both pupils constrict	Mostly present	Normal size Light in OD; both pupils constrict
5. Right visual cortex	Mostly absent	Normal size Light in OS; both pupils constrict	Mostly present	Normal size Light in OD; both pupils constrict

OD, Oculus dexter (right eye); OS, oculus sinister (left eye).

double crossing, the response of the left pupil may be slightly greater than that of the right pupil. To prove this further, cover the normal left eye with your hand and watch the right pupil immediately dilate. Light directed into the right eye will elicit no response in either eye. Light directed into the left eye will cause both pupils to constrict. This is easier to write then to actually observe. Watch carefully when you swing the light from the abnormal right eye, where no light could get through the retina or optic nerve lesion, to the normal left eye. The pupil immediately constricts because it had not done so when the light was directed into the right eye. Now swing the light back to the right eye and watch the right pupil dilate because it had constricted when the light was directed into the left eye and reached both parasympathetic oculomotor nuclei. Look at Fig. 7-1 and imagine these responses or the absence thereof.

2. A lesion in the right oculomotor nerve GVE neurons does not interfere with the menace response in either eye. In room light, the right pupil will be widely dilated (mydriatic). Light directed into either eye causes constriction of the left pupil only.

3. A right retrobulbar lesion within the periorbita that affects both the optic nerve and the GVE oculomotor neurons causes an absent menace response in the right eye only. At rest in room light, the right pupil will be widely dilated. Light directed into the left eye will cause constriction of the left pupil only. Light directed into the right eye will cause no pupillary constriction in either eye.

4. Unilateral optic tract lesions usually do not interfere with the pupillary light responses enough to be observed. This is because a large number of the optic nerve axons cross at the optic chiasm and enter the opposite optic tract. However, a significant number of the optic nerve axons do not cross, and they enter the ipsilateral optic tract. As a result, optic nerve axons from both eyes are present in both optic tracts. If there is any difference in the pupillary light responses in a patient with a lesion in one optic tract, there will be slightly less response when the eye opposite the optic tract lesion is stimulated by light. This subject is addressed further in Chapter 14, which concerns the visual system.

Be aware that it takes a severe retinal or optic nerve lesion to interfere with the pupillary response to light. Clinical blindness and absent menace responses may occur in the presence of retinal and optic nerve lesions before the pupil response to light is lost. Usually animals with bilateral retinal or optic nerve lesions have pupils that are more dilated than normal in room light because of the loss of some of the pupillary light neurons bilaterally. This is commonly seen in acute optic neuritis or sudden acquired retinal degeneration syndrome.[2]

Remember that a complete oculomotor nerve lesion causes not only a dilated pupil unresponsive to light; that eye also exhibits ptosis and ventrolateral strabismus and will not adduct well on testing normal nystagmus. These three clinical signs are caused by the loss of function of the GSE-LMNs in the oculomotor nerve, as described in Chapter 6.

Fig. 7-2 shows a 9-year-old male malamute that was presented for asymmetry of the pupils, the only clinical complaint. The neurologic examination was normal except for the eyes. Menace responses were normal in both eyes. There was a persistent anisocoria in room light, with the left pupil always being more dilated than the right pupil. Light directed into the patient's left eye caused the right pupil to constrict but not the left pupil. Light directed into the right

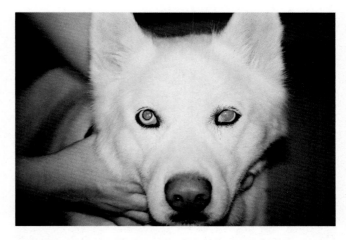

FIGURE 7-2 A 9-year-old male malamute with a dilated, unresponsive left pupil but normal menace responses bilaterally. Note the slight ptosis in the left eye. There was poor adduction of the left eye when tested for normal nystagmus. The anatomic diagnosis is left oculomotor nerve dysfunction with complete GVE neuronal deficit and partial GSE neuronal deficit. About 6 months later generalized seizures occurred, and computed tomography imaging was performed (see Fig. 7-3).

eye caused only the right pupil to constrict, not the left pupil. There is a slight ptosis in the left eye but no strabismus. On testing for normal nystagmus, when the head was moved to the dog's right, the left eye would not adduct as far as the right eye would when the head was moved to the dog's left side. Your anatomic diagnosis should be as follows: left cranial nerve III, with complete dysfunction of the GVE-LMNs and some loss of the GSE neurons to the medial rectus and levator palpebrae superioris. You must consider a lesion from the origin of this nerve on the ventral aspect of the midbrain to its terminal branching within the periorbita. Remember the superficial location of the GVE preganglionic neuronal axons and their susceptibility to compressive lesions in the cranial cavity. This could be direct compression resulting from an extraparenchymal neoplasm adjacent to this nerve, or it could be indirect compression resulting from a prosencephalic neoplasm that is causing a shift in the position of the midbrain. In the presence of either of these lesions, you would expect to see other neurologic signs, especially with indirect compression. Be aware that what this dog exhibits may be the first indication of an expanding neoplasm in the middle cranial fossa. We have seen this with germ cell neoplasms and meningiomas but not with pituitary neoplasms. The middle cranial fossa is a common site for a germ cell neoplasm, which is also more common in young dogs from 6 months to 3 years of age.[47] About 6 months later, this malamute had generalized seizures, and computed tomography (CT) imaging was performed (Fig. 7-3). Figs. 7-4 through 7-6 show magnetic resonance (MR) images and the gross lesions of canine germ cell neoplasms.

There is a pharmacologic testing procedure that can be used to try to determine whether the GVE-LMN dysfunction is in the preganglionic or postganglionic neuron.[4] It involves the denervation hypersensitivity that would be present only if the postganglionic neuron was affected. This hypersensitivity concept is similar to that which is the basis for the denervation potentials (fibrillations and positive sharp waves) seen in electromyograms that occur in skeletal muscle when that muscle has lost its GSE innervation. This pharmacologic testing involves exposing the eye

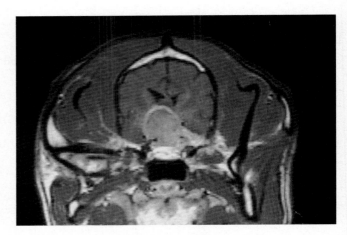

FIGURE 7-4 Axial MR T1 weighted image with contrast of a 3-year-old Doberman pinscher at the level of the mid-diencephalon. The image shows a germ cell neoplasm in the middle cranial fossa. The initial clinical sign was a dilated, unresponsive left pupil. The MR imaging was done 1 month later, when the dog was obtunded and reluctant but still able to walk. The right side of the image seen here is the left side of the dog. At necropsy this mass lesion was diagnosed as a germ cell neoplasm. Refer to Case Example 14-1 concerning abnormal pupils.

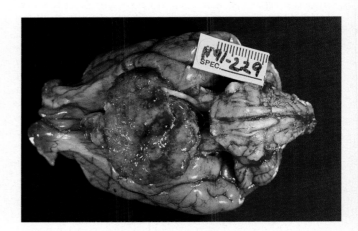

FIGURE 7-5 Gross appearance of a germ cell neoplasm in a 4-year-old golden retriever with clinical signs similar to those in the dog in Fig. 7-4.

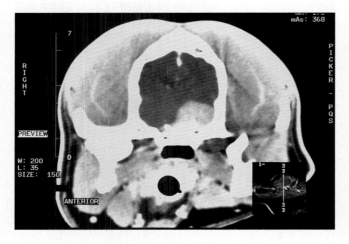

FIGURE 7-3 Contrast-enhanced CT image of the dog in Fig. 7-2 at the level of the mid-diencephalon and middle cranial fossa. It shows a large contrast-enhancing mass on the left (right side of figure), which is presumed to be a meningioma on the basis of its degree of contrast enhancement and its broad association with the bone of the cranium.

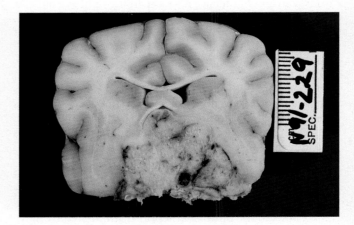

FIGURE 7-6 Transverse section of the preserved brain of the dog in Fig. 7-5 at the level of the diencephalon. The mass has obliterated the optic chiasm. The white structures in the center that form the shape of an inverted V are the columns of the fornix.

to direct- and indirect-acting parasympathomimetic drugs. The direct-acting drugs elicit a more rapid and more complete response in the hypersensitive denervated muscle (postganglionic lesion), whereas the indirect-acting drugs require the postganglionic neurons to be intact and able to release their endogenous neurotransmitter at the sphincter muscle in the iris. This is a timed response and, in our opinion, is not reliable. Imaging procedures are available, and we strongly recommend their use in locating lesions in this pupillary light reflex pathway.

Watch out for iatrogenic pupillary dilation if you are a consultant on a case in a large specialty practice or in a teaching hospital. In these environments, the most common cause of dilated pupils is the mydriatic drug used to dilate the pupils for the ophthalmologic examination of the fundus of the eyes!

Sympathetic Innervation of the Eye

Anatomy

The preganglionic neuronal cell bodies are located in the lateral gray column of the first three or four thoracic spinal cord segments (see Fig. 7-1). The axons pass through the ventral gray column and adjacent white matter to join the ventral roots of these segments and the proximal portion of the segmental spinal nerve. Just beyond where the spinal nerve emerges from the intervertebral foramen and before it branches, these preganglionic neuronal axons leave the spinal nerve in the segmental ramus communicans, which joins the thoracic sympathetic trunk. The latter courses longitudinally inside the thorax along the vertebral bodies. The preganglionic neuronal axons destined for the head usually do not synapse in a trunk ganglion but continue cranially in the trunk, pass through the cervicothoracic and middle cervical ganglia, and course cranially in the neck in the cervical sympathetic trunk. This trunk is associated with the vagus nerve forming the vagosympathetic trunk, which is located in the carotid sheath (see Fig. 7-25).

At the head, medial to the origin of the digastricus muscle and ventromedial to the tympanic bulla, the cervical sympathetic trunk separates from the vagus nerve and terminates in the cranial cervical ganglion. Here the preganglionic neuronal telodendria synapse on the dendritic zones of the neuronal cell bodies of the postganglionic neuronal axons. The pathway from this ganglion to the ocular structures is not well defined.[1,3,41,46] As a rule, these postganglionic sympathetic neuronal axons follow the blood vessels to the effector organs. A 1932 description of this pathway in the cat showed these axons to pass through the tympanic bulla on the ventral surface of the petrous portion of the temporal bone, but it is not clear whether these are sympathetic postganglionic axons or the parasympathetic preganglionic axons of the glossopharyngeal nerve that form the tympanic plexus known to course in this position.[41] It is also possible that the sympathetic postganglionic axons may join this plexus. From this location in the tympanic cavity, these axons enter the cranial cavity ventral to the trigeminal ganglion and join the ophthalmic nerve from the trigeminal nerve, which enters the orbit within the periorbita. Here, these sympathetic axons innervate the orbitalis muscle, which is the smooth muscle in the periorbita and the eyelids, including the third eyelid, the smooth ciliaris muscle, and the smooth dilator muscle of the pupil in the iris (Fig. 7-7). This pathway correlates well with our clinical experience of recognizing a paralysis of these muscles (Horner syndrome) in the presence of otitis media in small animals and trigeminal neuritis in dogs.

Another route from the cranial cervical ganglion to the ophthalmic nerve from of the trigeminal nerve is in the internal carotid nerve, which leaves the cranial cervical ganglion and follows the internal carotid artery. This artery lies adjacent to this ganglion, where these postganglionic neuronal axons can join it. The artery then passes through the tympanooccipital fissure and enters the carotid canal. At the rostral end of this canal, the artery and these axons gain access to the cranial cavity through the foramen lacerum, which is located just ventral to where the trigeminal nerve emerges from the rostral aspect of the canal of the trigeminal nerve in the petrous portion of the temporal bone. At this point, these axons can join the ophthalmic nerve from the trigeminal nerve. Some axons may continue along the internal carotid artery to the cerebral arterial circle and leave the circle with the internal ophthalmic artery, which courses along the optic nerves through the optic canals to enter the orbit within the periorbita. This last pathway has recently been described in humans. I (Alexander de Lahunta) have seen microscopically numerous unmyelinated axons coursing with the internal carotid artery in the carotid canal. The exact route of the axons from this cranial cervical ganglion to the smooth muscle of the ocular structures remains to be better defined, but however it turns out, there is an anatomic site where infections in the tympanic cavity (middle ear) of small animals can readily involve these axons. Otitis media in horses and farm animals does not affect these sympathetic neurons. Other postganglionic axons leave the cranial cervical ganglion and course with the blood vessels and cranial and spinal nerves to innervate the smooth muscles of blood vessels and the sweat glands of the skin in the head and cranial cervical area.

In addition to this GVE-LMN, note in Fig. 7-1 the CNS tract that is labeled *lateral tectotegmentospinal system*. This is an upper motor neuron (UMN) system that is part of the CNS portion of the autonomic nervous system. It actually

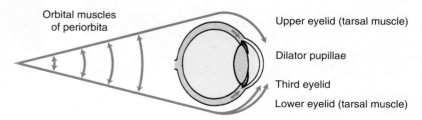

FIGURE 7-7 Smooth orbitalis muscles and the dilator pupillae that are innervated by the sympathetic GVE neurons.

begins in the hypothalamus and has components that continue caudally in the brainstem; it then continues in the lateral funiculus of the spinal cord. It terminates in the lateral gray column from the T1 to L4, L5 spinal cord segments, where the UMNs synapse on the preganglionic cell bodies of the sympathetic GVE-LMN system. The activity of this UMN system is necessary for the GVE-LMN to function. Noxious stimuli or emotional responses may cause dilation of the pupils. Noxious stimuli to the trunk and limbs utilize spinothalamic and spinotectal pathways to reach the sympathetic centers in the hypothalamus and activate the UMN that projects to the appropriate preganglionic sympathetic neurons in the cranial thoracic spinal cord to cause pupillary dilation. Emotional responses utilize corticohypothalamic pathways to activate this sympathetic pathway. Some texts refer to this sympathetic innervation as a three-order neuron system, with the first-order neuron being the UMN pathway that we just described. The second-order neuron is the preganglionic neuron; the third-order neuron is the postganglionic neuron. This is a confusing concept that is unnecessary for understanding the anatomic diagnosis, so it will not be utilized in this text.

Clinical Signs

The smooth muscle of the eye that is innervated by the sympathetic postganglionic axons includes the orbitalis muscle and the dilator pupillae (see Fig. 7-7). The orbitalis muscle consists of three sheets. A sheet of circular fibers in the periorbita makes the eyeball protrude. A ventral sheet of longitudinal fibers extends from the sheath of the ventral rectus muscle to the lower eyelid and the third eyelid. A medial sheet of longitudinal fibers extends from the sheath of the medial rectus muscle and the trochlea into the upper eyelid and the third eyelid. The ventral and medial sheets retract the eyelids. Loss of this innervation causes the signs that are often referred to as Horner syndrome, including a smaller pupil (miosis), a smaller palpebral fissure (ptosis is the droop of the upper eyelid), a protruded third eyelid, and enophthalmos that is mild and difficult to appreciate (Figs. 7-8 through 7-11). Be aware that a marked enophthalmos is most commonly associated with atrophy of the muscles of mastication that form a

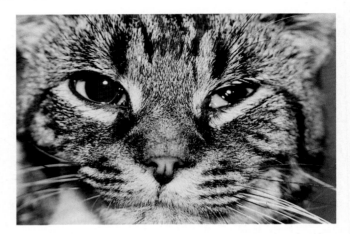

FIGURE 7-9 Horner syndrome in an adult domestic shorthair following aggressive attempts to obtain blood from the left external jugular vein.

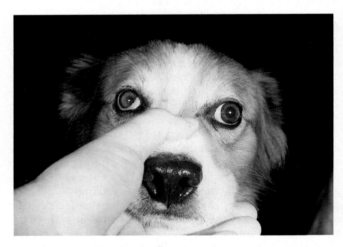

FIGURE 7-10 Horner syndrome in a young adult mixed-breed dog that was struck by a vehicle and had clinical signs of avulsion of the roots of its right brachial plexus.

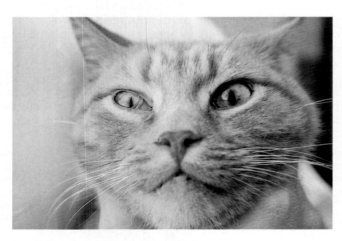

FIGURE 7-8 Horner syndrome in an adult domestic shorthair with a palpable right thyroid adenocarcinoma.

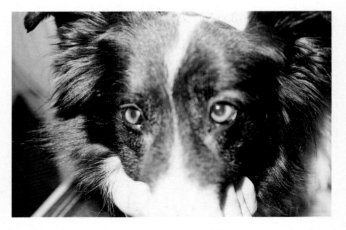

FIGURE 7-11 Horner syndrome in a 3-year-old border collie with an acute onset of right hemiplegia, with LMN paralysis of the right thoracic limb and UMN paralysis of the right pelvic limb due to fibrocartilaginous embolic myelopathy. Refer to Video 10-43 and Case Example 10-11.

significant portion of the border of the periorbita. With this atrophy, the eyeball sinks into the orbit and as a result, the palpebral fissure is smaller and the third eyelid passively protrudes. These clinical signs can be mistaken for sympathetic paralysis, except that there is no miosis. In some dogs with Horner syndrome, there may be congestion in the bulbar conjunctiva due to lack of vasoconstriction—a "red eye"—and a fundic exam may show congested retinal blood vessels. The miotic pupil, despite loss of sympathetic innervation to the dilator of the iris, can still dilate slightly when the room light is reduced and the iris constrictor muscle relaxes. The anisocoria may be more pronounced if you examine your patient in reduced light. In addition to these clinical signs related to the eyeball and extraocular structures, the sympathetic paralysis in the head causes peripheral vasodilation that may be detected by noting increased warmth of the skin on the affected side as well as pinkness where the skin is not pigmented, in the oral mucosa and external ear canal. Nasal mucosal vasocongestion will decrease the volume of airflow in the ipsilateral nasal cavity. In all domestic animals except the horse, there is decreased sweating on the affected side. This hypohydrosis, or anhydrosis, is difficult to appreciate except in the planum nasolabiale of the ox (see Fig. 7-13).[42]

In cattle, sheep, and goats, the most consistent and reliable clinical signs of loss of the GVE-LMN sympathetic innervation to the head are the smaller palpebral fissure and the palpable hyperthermia of the ear. The miosis and protrusion of the third eyelid are often very subtle. In cattle there is less sweating in the planum nasolabiale on the affected side (Figs. 7-12 and 7-13).[42] If you warm the muzzle with a heat lamp, this anhydrosis will be more pronounced. The vasodilation in the nasal mucosa may narrow the airway enough on the affected side to be felt on expiration by placing your hand in front of the naris or recognizing the lack

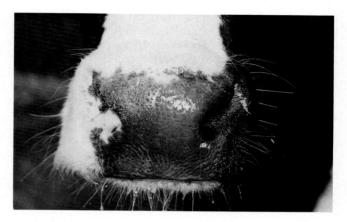

FIGURE 7-13 The planum nasolabiale of the cow in Fig. 7-12, showing the anhydrosis of the right side.

of mist on a cold morning (Fig. 7-14). The cow in this photo can be seen in **Video 7-1.** She is a 12-year-old Holstein cow from a farm in upstate New York. The farmer called for assistance because he astutely noticed that on cold mornings, there was less mist coming from her right nostril, and she also had developed a large swelling on the right side of her neck. About 2 months previously, he had treated this cow for what he assumed to be milk fever by administering calcium gluconate into the external jugular vein. The swelling had been slowly enlarging over the past few weeks. Note the clinical signs of Horner syndrome exhibited by this cow. It was assumed that the swelling in the neck was an infection associated with the treatment the farmer had administered—that at least some of the calcium gluconate had been

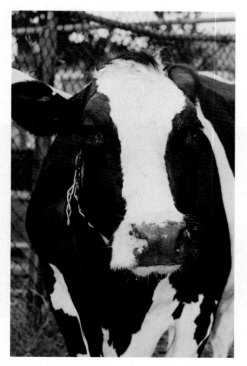

FIGURE 7-12 Right-sided Horner syndrome in an adult cow following venipuncture injury to the right carotid sheath. Note the dry right planum nasolabiale.

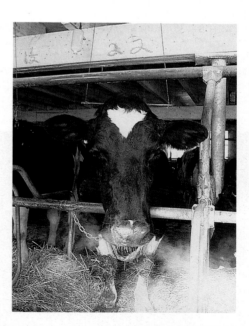

FIGURE 7-14 This is the 12-year-old Holstein cow seen in Video 7-1 on a cold winter morning, Note the lack of mist exiting from her right naris as she expires air. This is caused by right sympathetic paralysis in the head and the vasodilation of the right nasal mucosa due to loss of the sympathetic innervation of vasoconstrictor smooth muscle.

injected into the perivascular tissues. The infection involved the cervical sympathetic trunk in the carotid sheath, causing the Horner syndrome. This cow also probably had a right laryngeal hemiplegia, which was not detected. It would have been caused by the involvement of the recurrent laryngeal nerve GSE axons contained in the right vagus nerve.

The horse is unique among the domestic animals in that a sympathetic paralysis causes excessive sweating in the area of skin that is denervated.[16,25,38,42] This is often the first clinical sign that is observed, especially if the disorder is acute. An example that most equine practitioners have experienced at some point in their careers and is common in the veterinary college teaching environment relates to the intended intravenous administration of drugs into the external jugular vein. If in this process, some hemorrhage occurs in the adjacent carotid sheath, or if the drug is injected into the sheath, the sudden interference with the sympathetic trunk neurons causes sympathetic paralysis of the head and cranial neck, and almost as soon as the needle is removed from the tissues, the horse starts to sweat from the end of its nose to about the most cranial 15 cm of the neck.

If the paralysis persists, the sweating may decrease with time. In chronic cases it may be present only at the base of the ear. As in ruminants, the smaller palpebral fissure will be obvious, the miosis will be mild, and the protrusion of the third eyelid may be very subtle or not visible (Figs. 7-15 through 7-17). An additional indication of loss of sympathetic innervation to the head is the decrease in the angle of the eyelashes of the upper eyelids, which is associated with the loss of upper eyelid elevation and the loss of innervation to the arrector ciliorum muscles. This difference between the eyelashes of the two eyes can be seen if you elevate the head slightly and observe the eyelashes from the median plane of the head. The loss of sympathetic innervation can be an early sign of equine grass sickness in the countries where that disorder occurs. However, that disease typically affects the eyelash angle bilaterally. To confirm the loss of sympathetic innervation, you can apply a few drops of 0.5% phenylephrine to one eye.[19] This is an alpha-1 adrenergic agonist that will rapidly correct the eyelash angle associated with this disorder (Fig. 7-18). Presumably, this eyelash response occurs because of denervation hypersensitivity.

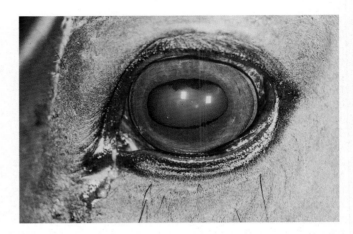

FIGURE 7-16 The normal left eye of the horse in Fig. 7-15. Compare this with Fig. 7-17.

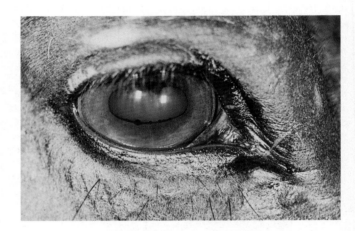

FIGURE 7-17 The right eye of the horse in Figs. 7-15 and 7-16. Note the slight miosis and smaller palpebral fissure.

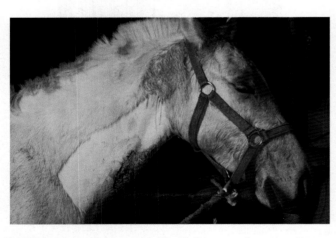

FIGURE 7-15 An adult horse with right-sided Horner syndrome caused by a needle puncture injury to its right carotid sheath. Note the sweating, from its nose to about 15 cm of the right cranial cervical region.

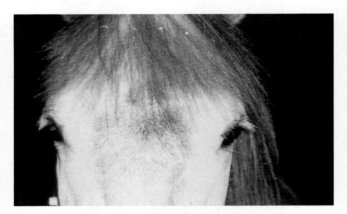

FIGURE 7-18 Adult horse in the United Kingdom with the diagnosis of grass sickness; the horse has received a few drops of 0.5% phenylephrine in its left eye. Note the difference in the angles of the eyelashes, indicating loss of sympathetic innervation in the right eyelids and the recovery in the left eyelids. (We thank Dr. Caroline Hahn for the use of this slide).

The cause of the sweating in the horse has been the subject of considerable debate.[4] Some relate it to denervation hypersensitivity, but it occurs so immediately that this idea seems unlikely. Equine sweat glands have a sympathetic cholinergic form of innervation, but they are also very sensitive to circulating norepinephrine and are responsive to changes in blood flow. It is our opinion that the sudden vasodilation that occurs in the skin of horses that suddenly lose their sympathetic innervation increases the blood flow to the denervated area, and excessive sweating results from the exposure of this area to the circulating norepinephrine or possibly from the increased blood flow itself. This same area of vasodilation is hyperthermic, which may be palpated in the ear and can be determined and localized using thermography.[38] A focal area of sweating may be helpful in localizing spinal cord or peripheral nerve lesions in the horse. If a caudal thoracic fracture causes an extensive transverse lesion in one or two adjacent spinal cord segments, the severe pelvic limb paresis and ataxia may be accompanied by a focal band of sweating coursing transversely on both sides of the trunk. This sweating is due to the focal loss of function of the preganglionic sympathetic neurons in the spinal cord or associated ventral roots and proximal spinal nerves.

Figs. 7-19 through 7-21 show a 16-year-old Quarter horse gelding that had been lame in the left thoracic limb for a few days, reluctant to lower his head to eat, and sweating over the entire left side of his head and neck to a line just cranial to his scapula. This precise pattern of sweating was obvious on examination. He was so reluctant to move that it was difficult to tell whether the left thoracic limb lameness was the result of discomfort, lack of support, or both. In the left eye, there was a smaller palpebral fissure, slight miosis, and equivocal elevation of the third eyelid. Decreased air flow was detected at the left naris on expiration. Based on your knowledge of the anatomy of the sympathetic GVE-LMN, you should be able to determine the location of this lesion. See Fig. 7-1, which shows the schematic representation of the GVE sympathetic neuronal innervation of the eye (head). Our rule is that when we

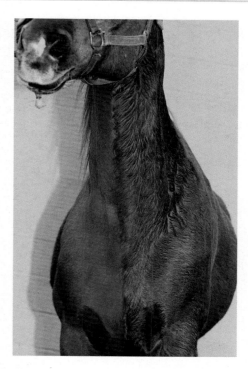

FIGURE 7-20 The same horse as in Fig. 7-19, showing the sharp medial border of the sweating in the neck.

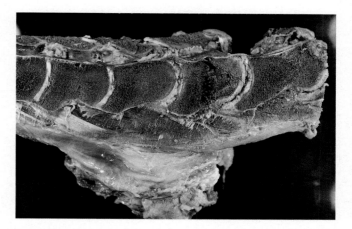

FIGURE 7-21 Same horse as in Figs. 7-19 and 7-20, showing the pathologic fracture of the C6 vertebral body and the ventral projection of the carcinoma that involved the left cervical sympathetic trunk and vertebral nerve.

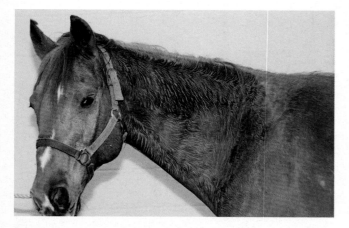

FIGURE 7-19 A 16-year-old Quarter horse with a neoplasm involving its left vertebral nerve and cervical sympathetic trunk in the craniodorsal thorax. The area of sweating due to sympathetic denervation correlates with the distribution of these sympathetic nerves. The sweating was limited to the entire left side of the head and neck. The caudal border of the sweating represents the caudal border of the cutaneous innervation of the C6 cervical spinal nerve.

diagnose Horner syndrome, we always look first for a lesion in some part of this LMN. In some cases there are other clinical signs to help you localize the lesion in this LMN (Table 7-2). For example, an associated facial paralysis or peripheral vestibular signs would suggest otitis media-interna. A sudden onset of a complete GSE-LMN paralysis in one thoracic limb, with extensive analgesia, would suggest brachial plexus root avulsion. A sudden onset of right-side hemiplegia with flaccid paralysis of the thoracic limb and spastic paralysis of the ipsilateral pelvic limb would suggest a spinal cord lesion on the right side of the cervical intumescence that includes the first three thoracic segments. However,

TABLE 7-2 Horner Syndrome: Summary of Lesions

Location	Lesion	Associated Neurologic Deficit
Cervical spinal cord	Focal myelopathy External injury Fibrocartilage emboli Intervertebral disk extrusion	Spastic tetraplegia, dyspnea Spastic hemiplegia: ipsilateral HS
T1-T3 spinal cord	Focal myelopathy External injury Fibrocartilage emboli* Neoplasm Diffuse myelomalacia	Tetraparesis and ataxia or tetraplegia with LMN deficit in thoracic limbs, and UMN and GP deficits in pelvic limbs Diffuse LMN signs and loss of nociception with diffuse myelomalacia
T1-T3 ventral roots, proximal spinal nerves	Avulsion of roots of brachial plexus Lymphoma†	LMN paresis or paralysis of the ipsilateral thoracic limb with variable loss of nociception
Cranial thoracic sympathetic trunk, cervicothoracic ganglion, middle cervical ganglion	Lymphoma Nerve sheath neoplasm Abscess	None, if confined to the trunk or ganglia
Cervical sympathetic trunk	Injury by surgery, jugular venipuncture, dog bites Neoplasm: nerve sheath, lymphoma, thyroid adenocarcinoma	None, if unilateral; bilateral lesions interfere with laryngeal and esophageal functions because of the associated vagal nerve involvement
Tympanic (middle ear) cavity in small animals	Otitis media Neoplasm	Clinical signs of peripheral vestibular system dysfunction: ipsilateral ataxia, head tilt, abnormal nystagmus, facial paresis or paralysis, facial tetanus
Cranial cervical ganglion: internal carotid nerve	Guttural pouch mycosis in horses	Dysphagia, ipsilateral laryngeal hemiparesis: hemiplegia, facial paresis or paralysis
Retrobulbar	Injury, abscess Neoplasm	Varies with degree of involvement of optic and oculomotor nerves, which influence pupillary size and vision (optic)

GP, General proprioception; HS, Horner syndrome; LMN, lower motor neuron; UMN, upper motor neuron

*de Lahunta A, Alexander JW: Ischemic myelopathy secondary to fibrocartilaginous embolism in nine dogs, *J Am Anim Hosp Assoc* 12:37-48, 1976.
†Fox JG, Gutnick MJ: Horner syndrome and brachial paralysis due to lymphosarcoma in a cat, *J Am Vet Med Assoc* 160:977, 1972.

there are also long portions of this GVE-LMN innervation that are not accompanied by any other nerves to help us localize the lesion. Consider the long cervical sympathetic trunk that is at risk for injury by dog bites, aggressive intravenous punctures, and compression by a thyroid neoplasm. I (Eric Glass) have missed the diagnosis of a significantly large thyroid neoplasm that caused Horner syndrome in a very unkempt Old English sheepdog.

Severe spinal cord lesions that interrupt the UMN that controls the GVE sympathetic LMN pathway result in a sympathetic paralysis similar to an LMN paralysis. This will not be seen without obvious signs of cervical spinal cord disease. A horse with a sudden onset of severe right hemiparesis caused by a midcervical lateral funicular lesion will have Horner syndrome and will sweat on the entire right side of its body because of the loss of GVE-LMN activity in *all* the preganglionic sympathetic neurons. Figs. 7-22 through 7-24 and Video 11-10 in Chapter 11, equine spinal cord disease, show examples of this in a horse with a *Sarcocystis neurona* myelitis. A focal infarction of one half of the cervical spinal cord in a dog as the result of fibrocartilaginous emboli causes hemiplegia and sympathetic paralysis of the entire right side of its body, but only the Horner syndrome will be observed. The only way to determine that there is a UMN loss of the sympathetic innervation along the entire right side of this dog's body would be to measure the skin temperature to detect the hyperthermia resulting

from vasodilation. If the spinal cord lesion is bilateral and severe enough to cause miosis, this is a life-threatening lesion because the UMN for respiration will also be compromised. An animal can survive with a focal lesion from the C1 to C5 spinal cord segments that transects one half of the spinal cord, but the same severity of lesion bilaterally

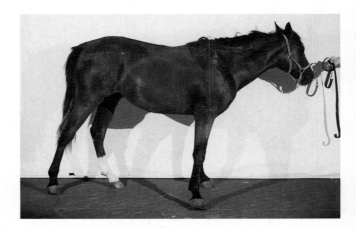

FIGURE 7-22 An 18-month-old standardbred mare with the anatomic diagnosis of right-side C6-T2 spinal cord segments. The mare exhibits sweating on the entire right side of her body. The lesion was focal myelitis caused by the protozoal agent *S. neurona*.

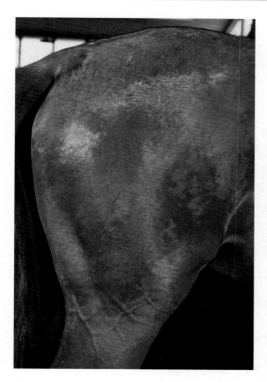

FIGURE 7-23 Right pelvic limb of the horse in Fig. 7-22, showing the sweating in the entire right pelvic region and pelvic limb.

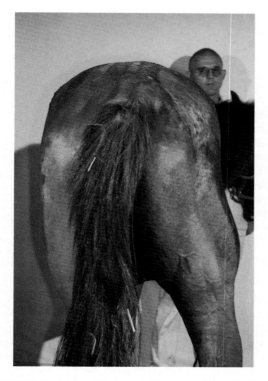

FIGURE 7-24 Caudal view of the horse in Figs. 7-22 and 7-23, showing the sweating limited to the right side.

causes respiratory paralysis and death. If you are presented with a dog that was suddenly found recumbent and unable to move its limbs, and your anatomic diagnosis is C1 to C5 spinal cord segments, be sure to look at the eyes; if the pupils are miotic, the prognosis must be guarded, and emergency treatment is necessary. We have seen unilateral or bilateral Horner syndrome in dogs that have severe acute C1 to C5 spinal cord lesions caused by having been hit by cars or by gunshot wounds.

Return to the anatomic diagnosis of the Quarter horse with the clinical signs just described (see Figs. 7-19 through 7-21). The sweating had a very precise pattern and there were no obvious spinal cord signs to suggest a lesion in preganglionic neurons in the cranial thoracic spinal cord. The sympathetic paralysis of the head can be explained by a lesion lying anywhere from the ventral roots of the first three thoracic spinal nerves, through their rami communicans, through the cranial thoracic sympathetic trunk, through the cervicothoracic and middle cervical ganglia, through the cervical sympathetic trunk, to the cranial cervical ganglion and its branches. The caudal border of the sweating in the neck was the caudal border of the skin innervated by the sixth cervical spinal nerve. The question you must answer is; What supplies the sympathetic postganglionic axons to the cervical spinal nerves from C2 through C6? The answer is that they are supplied by the vertebral nerve, which is a branch of the cervicothoracic ganglion that follows the vertebral artery into the transverse foramen of C6 and continues cranially through these foramina to C1 (Fig. 7-25). These are all postganglionic axons in the vertebral nerve whose cell bodies are in the cervicothoracic ganglion. As this nerve passes between each cervical vertebra it supplies a ramus to the cervical spinal nerve at each of the intervertebral foramina. The anatomic site where these two pathways diverge is in the cranial dorsal thorax at the level of the cervicothoracic ganglion. This horse was euthanized, and a large, poorly differentiated carcinoma was located on the left side of the longus colli muscle in the cranial dorsal thorax, obliterating any evidence of these sympathetic nerves and ganglia. The neoplasm had invaded the T1 vertebral body, which had fractured and was the cause of the extreme discomfort seen in this horse. The primary source of the neoplasm was not found.

A similar case was reported in a 20-year-old gray thoroughbred-Percheron gelding that was examined for sweating on the right side in the same location as the Quarter horse just described, but the caudal border of the sweating was a transverse line from the caudal angle of the scapula to the elbow and included all of the right thoracic limb. The skin in this area felt warm, and thermography was used to confirm the hyperthermia that was present in the same area. The owner had also noted faster hoof growth in the right thoracic limb digit. The hyperthermia and increased hoof growth presumably related to the vasodilation caused by the sympathetic denervation. The anatomic diagnosis was the same as that of the Quarter horse, except that it was on the right side, and the lesion included the branches of the cervicothoracic ganglion that join the ventral branches of spinal nerves C7, C8, T1, and T2 that form the brachial plexus to innervate the thoracic limb. Thoracic radiographs showed increased density in

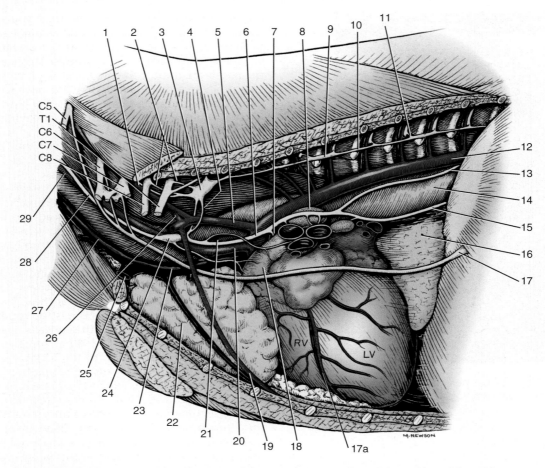

FIGURE 7-25 Thoracic autonomic nerves; left lateral view, lung removed. *RV,* Right ventricle; *LV,* left ventricle.

1. Vertebral artery and nerve
2. Communicating rami from cervicothoracic ganglion to ventral branches of cervical and thoracic spinal nerves
3. Left cervicothoracic ganglion
4. Ansa subclavia
5. Left subclavian artery
6. Left vagus nerve
7. Left recurrent laryngeal nerve
8. Left tracheobronchial lymph node
9. Sympathetic trunk ganglion
10. Sympathetic trunk
11. Ramus communicans
12. Aorta
13. Dorsal branch of vagus nerve
14. Esophagus
15. Ventral trunk of vagus nerve
16. Accessory lobe of right lung (through caudal mediastinum)
17. Phrenic nerve to diaphragm
17a. Paraconal interventricular artery, vein, nerve
18. Pulmonary trunk
19. Internal thoracic artery and vein.
20. Brachiocephalic trunk
21. Cardiac autonomic nerves
22. Thymus
23. Cranial vena cava
24. Middle cervical ganglion
25. Left subclavian vein
26. Costocervical trunk
27. External jugular vein
28. Vagosympathetic trunk
29. Common carotid artery

the craniodorsal thorax, and a cytologic examination of the pleural effusion revealed mesothelial cells containing melanin, so a presumptive melanoma was diagnosed.[27] We have seen lymphosarcoma occur at this site in cats and cause Horner syndrome, but we did not recognize the signs of hyperthermia that may have been present in the neck and possibly in the thoracic limb on the same side as the Horner syndrome.

The concept of pharmacologic testing to determine whether a lesion is in the preganglionic sympathetic neuron or the postganglionic neuron is similar to that described for the parasympathetic system, but it utilizes direct- and indirect-acting sympathomimetic drugs.[5] However, possibly because of our inexperience, we have not found this method to be reliable, so we look to imaging procedures to make this determination.

CASE EXAMPLE 7-1

Signalment: 9-year-old male Irish setter, Leavitt

Chief Complaint: Unable to use the pelvic limbs

History: About 3 weeks prior to this examination, Leavitt was presented to a veterinarian with the complaint of a stiff gait in the pelvic limbs. This veterinarian decided that the gait disorder was due to hip dysplasia and performed a pectineal myotomy. He also noted Horner syndrome in the left eye. Despite the surgery, the gait disorder progressed until the dog could not get up unassisted.

Examination: **Video 7-2** shows that when helped to stand, there was total paralysis of the left pelvic limb and only occasional movement of the right pelvic limb. Note how the trunk swayed to the side when he was assisted only by tail support. There were no postural reactions in the pelvic limbs, but the tone and spinal nerve reflexes as well as nociception were all normal in these limbs. He walked readily with the thoracic limbs, but the strides were short, especially in the left thoracic limb. He had difficulty hopping well with the left thoracic limb, and it was mildly hypotonic. There was slight atrophy in that limb when compared with the normal right thoracic limb. The left cutaneous trunci reflex was consistently absent, regardless of where the thoracolumbar stimulus was made. There was Horner syndrome in the left eye.

Anatomic Diagnosis: Bilateral cranial thoracic spinal cord segments at about the level of the third thoracic segment, with extension on the left side into the first two thoracic and last cervical spinal cord segments

The basis for the pelvic limb signs is described in Chapter 10, concerning small animal spinal cord disease, but a bilateral lesion anywhere between the third thoracic and the third lumbar spinal cord segments could account for the deficit as the result of dysfunction of the UMN and general proprioceptive systems. The presence of Horner syndrome suggests that this same lesion has involved the first three thoracic segments or their spinal nerve roots on the left side. The loss of the motor component of the left cutaneous trunci reflex implicates in the lesion the left-side gray matter or the ventral roots at the C8 and T1 spinal cord segments. These segments are the source of the neurons that comprise the lateral thoracic nerve, which innervates the cutaneous trunci muscle. The mild loss of muscle tone and the atrophy in the left thoracic limb suggest a mild disorder of the GSE-LMN on the left side in the cervical intumescence or its spinal nerve roots. The swaying of the trunk when supported also suggests a more cranial thoracic spinal cord lesion. This is explained in Chapter 10.

Differential Diagnosis: Neoplasm, intervertebral disk protrusion-extrusion, fibrocartilaginous embolic myelopathy (FCEM), myelitis

A neoplasm is the most presumptive diagnosis here, based on the age of the patient, the slowly progressive clinical signs of a focal lesion, and the presence of a large palpable mass on the left side of the cranial thorax. Near the end of the video, it can be seen when the left thoracic limb is protracted and the mass is outlined by my (AD) finger. The Horner syndrome was present when the dog was first examined by the referring veterinarian, and the patient exhibited only pelvic limb stiffness; these facts suggest that the mass developed in the left cranial dorsal mediastinum and grew into the left side of the vertebral canal, compressing the spinal cord just caudal to the cervical intumescence. An intervertebral disk protrusion-extrusion is uncommon at this level and would be unlikely to cause Horner syndrome, especially as the first clinical sign. FCEM is a vascular compromise that is sudden in onset and rarely progresses for more than 24 hours. Viral, fungal, bacterial, and granulomatous myelitis are less common causes of focal

lesions and would not be expected to remain this focal during the 3 weeks of progression of clinical signs.

Based on this assessment and the presence of the palpable thoracic wall mass, thoracic radiographs were obtained. They showed, in addition to the mass in the left thoracic wall, diffuse pulmonary neoplastic metastases (Figs. 7-26 and 7-27). This dog was euthanized, and at necropsy the mass was found to have expanded into the craniodorsal thorax covered by parietal pleura. It obliterated the cranial thoracic sympathetic trunk and cervicothoracic ganglion and extended into the vertebral canal, where it compressed

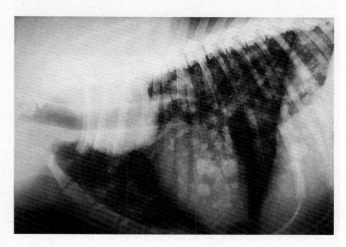

FIGURE 7-26 Lateral radiograph of the dog in this case example. Note the large radiodense mass related to the cranial thorax and the numerous pulmonary metastases.

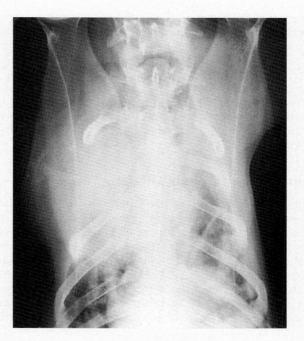

FIGURE 7-27 Dorsoventral radiograph of the dog in this case example. Note the large radiodense mass in the left side of the dog's thorax (right side of figure) and the lysis of the left second and third ribs.

(Continued)

CASE EXAMPLE 7-1—cont'd

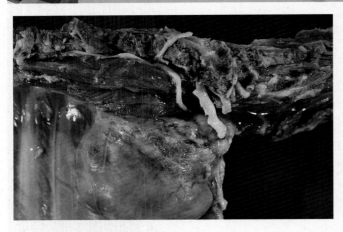

FIGURE 7-28 Gross necropsy specimen of the dog in this case example. It shows the medial surface of the left cranial thoracic wall with ribs 4 and 5 on the left of the photo, just caudal to the large mass that has obscured the cranial thoracic sympathetic trunk and displaced the ventral branches of the T1 and C8 spinal nerves that contribute to the brachial plexus.

the spinal cord (Fig. 7-28). It was diagnosed as a chondrosarcoma. Sometimes, Horner syndrome is an incidental event unrelated to the chief complaint of the patient, but you should make every effort possible to be sure that it is an incidental finding. That mistake in this case cost the dog an unnecessary surgery. I (EG) emphasize, when speaking to our interns and residents, that the Horner syndrome in itself is not a problem, but it is a red flag for a potentially more serious problem.

Idiopathic Horner syndrome is a diagnosis of exclusion when all of your ancillary studies are inconclusive about the cause of Horner syndrome. This is most common in dogs, and there may be an increased risk for it in the golden retriever breed. Many of these cases respond spontaneously if you are patient.

Anisocoria

Anisocoria is the occurrence of unequal or asymmetric pupils. Very slight differences are common and of no significance. It is worth noting that determining which pupil is miotic or mydriatic can sometimes be a challenge, even for the most astute clinician. It may help to compare the pupils in both a lighted and a darkened room. In a lighted room, a dilated pupil resulting from a GVE oculomotor neuron deficit is more obvious because the normal pupil is more constricted in the room light. In a darkened room, a miotic pupil caused by a sympathetic nervous system deficit is more obvious because the normal pupil is more dilated due to the lack of light. There are many causes of anisocoria, and not all are related to disorders of the GVE-LMN innervation of the iris muscles. Box 7-1 contains a list of some of the causes of anisocoria.

Pupils in Acute Brain Disease

Pupillary abnormalities are common following head trauma and severe acute midbrain vasculopathies, and they commonly accompany severe acute prosencephalic disorders, such as thiamin deficiency encephalopathy (polioencephalomalacia) and lead poisoning in ruminants (Fig. 7-29). Severe bilateral miosis is a clinical sign of an acute diffuse brain disorder that in itself may not be of any localizing value. The return of the pupils to normal size and response to light is a favorable prognostic clinical sign and indicates recovery from brain disorders, especially those caused by trauma. In patients with intracranial trauma or vascular compromise, progression from bilaterally miotic to bilaterally mydriatic pupils that are unresponsive to light is a poor prognostic clinical sign because

BOX 7-1 Causes of Anisocoria

MYDRIATIC PUPIL

1. A unilateral GVE oculomotor neuron lesion with ipsilateral mydriasis that is unresponsive to light directed into either eye.
2. Severe unilateral retinal or optic nerve lesions may result in a slight ipsilateral mydriasis that responds only to light directed into the normal eye. If the normal eye is covered, the pupil in the affected eye fully dilates.
3. Age-related iris atrophy is a degenerative disorder, especially in old dogs. Response to light is variable but often the response is poor to absent.
4. A mydriatic drug administered for a fundic examination.
5. Ingestion of a species of belladonna plant that contains atropine.
6. Glaucoma that is an increase in intraocular pressure due to deficient absorption of aqueous with an ipsilateral mydriasis unresponsive to light.
7. Unilateral cerebellar lesions, especially those that affect the cerebellar medullary nuclei, may result in a mydriatic pupil on the same side or the opposite side from the lesion, depending on the nucleus involved.

MIOTIC PUPIL

1. A unilateral GVE sympathetic neuron lesion with ipsilateral miosis. The affected pupil constricts more in bright light and dilates slightly in reduced light. The anisocoria may be more pronounced when examined in the dark.
2. Unilateral iritis with swelling in the iris.
3. Unilateral ocular disorders such as keratitis that cause discomfort may activate ophthalmic nerve sensory neurons, resulting in an oculopupillary reflex (V-III) that causes ipsilateral miosis.

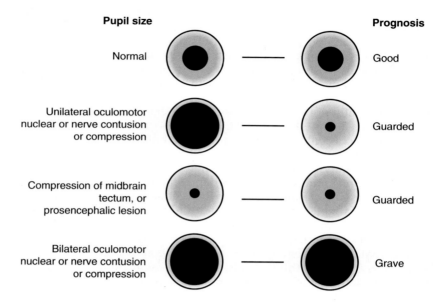

Pupil size			Prognosis
Normal			Good
Unilateral oculomotor nuclear or nerve contusion or compression			Guarded
Compression of midbrain tectum, or prosencephalic lesion			Guarded
Bilateral oculomotor nuclear or nerve contusion or compression			Grave

FIGURE 7-29 A schematic diagram showing the sizes of the pupils in association with head trauma.

it indicates that the secondary hemorrhage and edema are advancing in the brainstem, and the GVE oculomotor neurons associated with the rostral midbrain are unable to function. Intramedullary brainstem hemorrhage is a common lesion in severe head trauma (Figs. 7-30 and 7-31). The same pupillary changes can follow cerebral swelling and herniation of the occipital lobe ventral to the tentorium, causing compression and displacement of the midbrain, oculomotor nerve, or both. Following head trauma, pupillary changes may occur hourly and must be continually evaluated to determine whether the lesion is progressing or whether the treatment is being effective. See the diagram in Fig. 7-29 of pupil sizes and prognosis in intracranial injury.

The cause of unilateral or bilateral miotic pupils in acute prosencephalic disease probably represents the facilitation of these GVE oculomotor neurons as the result of their release from inhibition by prosencephalic UMNs. Whether a loss of the activity of the UMN for the sympathetic system plays a role in producing this miosis is unknown, but there are no other signs of sympathetic paralysis in the head. Experimental studies in dogs have shown that mild compression of the rostral midbrain causes miosis. Continued compression causes mydriasis. This same progression from miosis to mydriasis may occur in the acute brain swelling and herniation of the occipital lobes that causes midbrain compression.

Protrusion of the Third Eyelid

The third eyelid (membrana nictitans) may protrude for a number of reasons. In all animals, this protrusion is a passive event. The third eyelid passively protrudes any time the eyeball is actively retracted by contractions of the retractor bulbi muscle (VI) or the rectus muscles (III, VI). If you press on the eyeball through the upper eyelid, the third eyelid will passively protrude. In the cat, there are also slips of striated muscle from the lateral rectus and levator palpebrae superioris muscles that attach to the two extremities of the third eyelid and can actively contribute

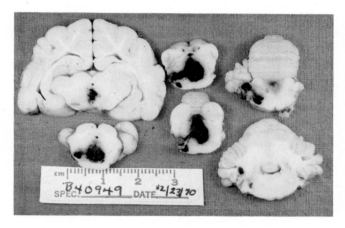

FIGURE 7-30 Transverse sections of the brain of a young adult domestic shorthair that was struck in the head by a vehicle. Note the extensive hemorrhages in the midbrain and pons. This cat was tetraplegic and comatose and had bilateral dilated unresponsive pupils.

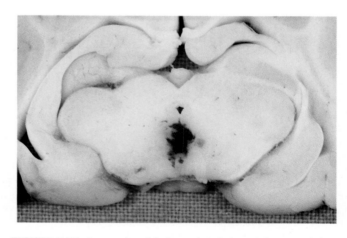

FIGURE 7-31 Close-up view of the hemorrhage in the rostral mesencephalon at the level of the oculomotor nuclei, where the preganglionic parasympathetic neuronal cell bodies are located.

to its protrusion. A constant partial protrusion of the third eyelid occurs in Horner syndrome because of the loss of the GVE sympathetic innervation of the orbitalis smooth muscle that normally keeps it retracted. Brief, rapid, passive protrusions (flashing of the third eyelid) occur in the disease tetanus owing to the effect of the tetanus toxin on the neurons that innervate the extraocular muscles. This is especially noticeable in a horse with this disease. Cerebellar medullary lesions that affect the cerebellar nuclei may occasionally cause a protruded third eyelid, but the clinical signs of cerebellar ataxia predominate. With facial paralysis, the eyelids cannot close to blink when the animal is threatened, as when being tested for its menace response. However, the eyeball retraction that occurs causes a rapid protrusion of the third eyelid. This may be the only indication in your examination that the animal is visual in that eye. Cats with severe systemic disease that are depressed often have bilateral persistent protrusion of the third eyelids. This may result from severe dehydration and depression or from a generalized decrease in sympathetic tone. Sympathomimetic drugs increase the orbitalis muscle tone in the eyelids of these sick cats and cause the third eyelids to retract. The protrusion usually disappears when the cat recovers from its systemic disease. Bilateral protrusion may occur in animals with severe cachexia because of the loss of orbital fat. Bilateral protrusion may also be seen as one of the many clinical signs observed in cats and dogs with dysautonomia, which is a presumptive toxic neuronopathy.[28,29,48] The nature and source of the toxin are unknown. Severe atrophy of the muscles of mastication resulting from trigeminal nerve denervation or chronic myositis indirectly causes passive enophthalmos and therefore passive protrusion of the third eyelid.

■ CONTROL OF MICTURITION

Control of micturition is a complex but essential subject that must be mastered in order to make correct anatomic diagnoses and administer effective treatment. It involves centers in the brainstem, sensory and motor pathways in the spinal cord, sympathetic and parasympathetic GVE-LMNs in the spinal cord, and peripheral nerves as well as GVA neurons in the same peripheral nerves.[17,35] We describe the functional anatomic components of continence and the storage of urine and of the act of evacuation of urine. Fig. 7-32 is a schematic drawing of the neuroanatomy of bladder function.

Sacral Parasympathetic GVE-LMN

The sacral portion of the parasympathetic division of the GVE-LMN has the preganglionic neuronal cell bodies located in the lateral gray column of the sacral spinal cord segments.[26,30,31,37] Their axons course with the ventral roots to the spinal nerves, where they leave the ventral branches of these sacral spinal nerves as separate branches that unite to form the single pelvic nerve on each side of the lateral surface of the rectum. These preganglionic parasympathetic axons in the pelvic nerve are joined by the hypogastric nerve, which carries sympathetic postganglionic axons to form the pelvic plexus. This pelvic plexus is associated with the prostatic or vaginal artery that is located near the entrance to the pelvic cavity and courses beside the rectum toward the neck of the bladder (Fig. 7-33). The parasympathetic preganglionic axons synapse on the neuronal cell bodies of the parasympathetic postganglionic axons that are located in the pelvic plexus (pelvic ganglion) or in the wall of the urogenital organs, rectum, or descending colon. The postganglionic

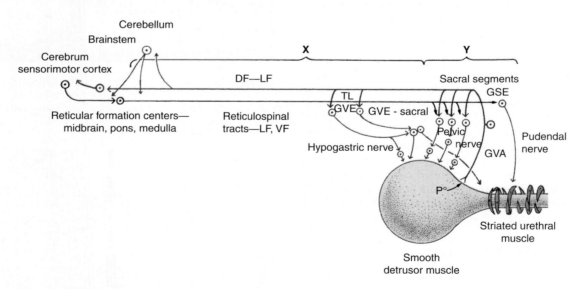

FIGURE 7-32 Neuroanatomy of bladder function. *DF,* Dorsal funiculus; *GSE,* general somatic efferent; *GVA,* general visceral afferent; *GVE;* general visceral efferent; *LF,* lateral funiculus; *TL,* thoracolumbar; *VF,* ventral funiculus.

Lesion at **X**: UMN lesion:
Spinal cord reflex bladder
1. No voluntary control—loss of bladder sensation
2. Retention (brief)—distention—overflow
3. Reflex micturition occurs with frequent voiding anywhere, initiated by abdominal pressure—slight residual remains

Lesion at **Y**: LMN lesion:
Denervated bladder
1. No voluntary control—loss of bladder sensation
2. Retention—distention—overflow—incontinence
3. In time small, brief contractions of bladder muscle occur via an intramural reflex activity—incomplete—large residual remains

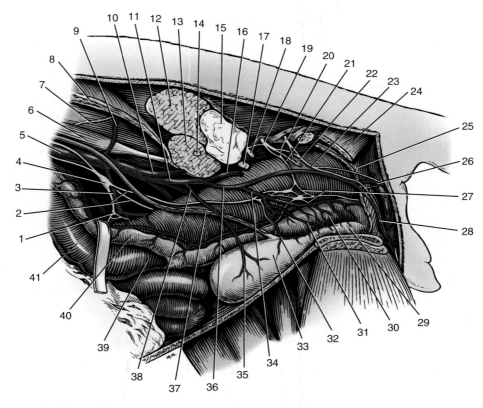

FIGURE 7-33 Autonomic nerves and vessels of pelvic region, left lateral view.

1. Caudal mesenteric plexus
2. Right and left hypogastric nerves
3. Caudal mesenteric artery
4. Caudal mesenteric ganglion
5. Aorta
6. Psoas minor
7. Lateral cutaneous femoral nerve
8. Abdominal oblique muscles
9. Deep circumflex iliac artery
10. External iliac artery
11. Internal iliac artery
12. Quadratus lumborum
13. Iliopsoas
14. Femoral nerve
15. Sacroiliac articulation
16. Caudal gluteal artery
17. Lumbar nerves 6 and 7
18. First sacral nerve
19. Second sacral nerve
20. Third sacral nerve
21. Pelvic nerve

22. Caudal cutaneous femoral nerve
23. Pudendal nerve
24. Coccygeus
25. Levator ani
26. Perineal nerve and artery
27. Pelvic plexus
28. Artery and nerve to clitoris
29. Urethra
30. Vagina
31. Urethral branch of vaginal artery
32. Caudal vesicle artery
33. Bladder
34. Vaginal artery
35. Cranial vesicle artery
36. Internal pudendal artery
37. Ureter and urethral branch of vaginal artery
38. Umbilical artery
39. Uterine artery
40. Uterine horn
41. Descending colon

parasympathetic axons innervate the muscarinic cholinergic receptors on the smooth muscle throughout the wall of the bladder. This smooth muscle is also known as the detrusor muscle; it contracts when stimulated by the parasympathetic neurons. This system is active during urination.

Lumbar Sympathetic GVE-LMN

The cell bodies of the preganglionic sympathetic neurons are located in the lateral gray column in the first four or five lumbar spinal cord segments.[37] Their axons leave these segments through the ventral roots and enter the spinal nerve. As that nerve emerges from the intervertebral foramen, these axons branch off the spinal nerve in a communicating ramus that connects to the lumbar portion of the longitudinal sympathetic trunk. Most of these preganglionic axons destined to innervate the bladder leave the lumbar sympathetic trunk in lumbar splanchnic nerves that course to the caudal mesenteric artery and terminate in the caudal mesenteric ganglion, which is located about halfway along this artery as it courses to the descending colon. In this ganglion, the preganglionic sympathetic axons synapse on the cell bodies of the postganglionic axons. Many of the latter leave the caudal mesenteric ganglion in two hypogastric nerves that pass caudally in the mesocolon to reach the prostatic or vaginal artery on each side. Here the hypogastric nerve intermixes with the pelvic nerve to form the pelvic plexus (see Fig. 7-33). Some of the postganglionic axons terminate in the pelvic ganglion located in the pelvic plexus. These synapses are with the alpha-2 adrenoreceptors on the dendritic zones of the cell bodies of parasympathetic postganglionic axons. When these alpha-2 receptors are stimulated, the parasympathetic postganglionic neuron is inhibited from generating an impulse and thus prevents detrusor muscle contraction. Other sympathetic postganglionic axons follow the branches of the prostatic or vaginal artery to the neck of the bladder, where they have two distributions. One group terminates on the smooth muscle that functions as the internal sphincter located at the neck of the bladder. There are alpha-2 adrenoreceptors on this smooth muscle that initiate contraction when stimulated by the sympathetic nerve's impulse.[39] This action contributes to continence and the storage of urine. The other group of sympathetic postganglionic axons is distributed to the detrusor muscle and terminates on beta receptors in the muscle cell membrane. When these receptors are stimulated, the smooth muscle is inhibited from contracting. This action allows for further expansion of the bladder wall for urine storage. All of this sympathetic innervation is active during the storage of urine.

Sacral GSE-LMN

The sacral segments provide the motor innervation of the urethralis muscle, which is a striated muscle that surrounds the pelvic urethra.[32] This muscle is sometimes referred to as the external sphincter of the bladder. The GSE-LMN cell bodies are located in the ventral gray column of the sacral segments. The axons course through the ventral roots, enter the spinal nerves, continue in their ventral branches, and follow their contribution to the sacral plexus located in the pelvic cavity. These GSE axons leave the sacral plexus in the pudendal nerve and follow its branches to the urethralis muscle, where they innervate the nicotinic cholinergic receptors. Stimulation of these GSE-LMNs provides the voluntary contraction of this muscle that is necessary to maintain continence and storage of urine.

General Visceral Afferent Neurons

The dendritic zones of GVA neurons are located in the wall of the bladder and urethra.[44] They are mechanoreceptors (A-delta) that respond to stretch and distention. Their axons travel through the pelvic nerve and enter the sacral segments of the spinal cord through the segmental dorsal roots. Their cell bodies are located in the sacral spinal ganglia associated with these dorsal roots. These GVA axons terminate on neurons in the dorsal gray column in these sacral segments. Some GVA axons may follow the pathway described for the sympathetic GVE-LMN innervation of the bladder. These axons terminate in the dorsal gray column of the first four or five lumbar spinal cord segments.

Brainstem Centers

Collections of neurons that are primarily in the pontine reticular formation function in the storage and evacuation of urine.[23] They are referred to as centers for micturition. They receive afferent information from spinal cord tracts that originate in the spinal cord segments where the GVAs terminate on neurons in the dorsal gray column. The axons of these dorsal gray column neurons enter the white matter and course cranially in the spinal cord to terminate in the pontine centers. The axons of the neurons in the pontine centers pass caudally in the spinal cord white matter, primarily in reticulospinal tracts, to terminate in the gray matter of the segments where the GVE-LMNs and GSE-LMNs that innervate the bladder and urethra are located. These caudally projecting spinal cord pathways function as the UMN for bladder control by facilitating or inhibiting the appropriate LMNs.

Continence and Storage of Urine

To maintain continence and store urine, it is necessary for the storage center in the pons to send impulses through the reticulospinal tracts to facilitate the activity of the lumbar sympathetic innervation to the bladder and urethra as well as to facilitate the sacral GSE innervation to the urethralis muscle.[15] At the same time, a component of these reticulospinal neurons functions to inhibit the sacral parasympathetic innervation of the detrusor muscle. As urine initially accumulates in the bladder, GVA receptors are activated. They project to the lumbar spinal cord to activate the sympathetic pathway that terminates on the beta adrenoreceptors of the detrusor muscle to inhibit its contraction and allow for bladder expansion and increased storage capacity. As urine leaks out of a distended bladder into the urethra, sensory neuron receptors are stimulated. They project to the sacral spinal cord segments through the pudendal nerve and reflexively increase the stimulus to the GSE neurons that innervate the urethralis muscle. At the same time, the activation of a conscious pathway through the spinal cord and brainstem to the sensory cerebral cortex makes the animal aware of this urethral stimulus. The animal responds by generating a conscious voluntary motor effort to contract this urethralis muscle via reticulospinal pathways to the sacral GSE neurons that innervate it. You now have a description of the neuroanatomy of an experience that we all have on a frequent basis and, thankfully, it functions well under most circumstances.

Micturition, Urination

As bladder volume increases, it exceeds the threshold of GVA mechanoreceptors in the bladder wall that respond to stretch and distention. Impulses travel over these sensory neurons via the pelvic nerves into the sacral spinal cord segment dorsal gray columns to initiate activity in a pathway that projects cranially to the pontine micturition center in the reticular formation as well as to a thalamic nucleus that projects to the sensory area of the cerebral cortex so that the animal is aware of the distended bladder. The micturition center is stimulated directly by this spinal cord pathway or indirectly from the motor cortex in the cerebrum via the internal capsule and crus cerebri. Collaterals of this cranially projecting spinal cord pathway also project to the cerebellum. Activation of the pontine micturition center results in the transmission of impulses in reticulospinal tracts in the spinal cord white matter. Some of these neurons terminate in the lumbar segments, where they are inhibitory to the sympathetic preganglionic neurons. Others enter the sacral segments, where they are facilitory to the parasympathetic preganglionic neurons and inhibitory to the GSE neurons that supply the urethralis muscle. This activity generated by the pontine micturition center reverses the facilitation and inhibition responsible for urinary continence and results in evacuation of the bladder. Some texts refer to this pathway that includes the spinal cord tracts and pontine centers as the detrusor reflex, but we prefer to limit this term to the conventional usage of reflex as an arc between the organ innervated and the spinal cord segments that contain the involved neurons. Including a UMN pathway in a reflex is a confusing concept. It is important to recognize that these pontine centers can function without cerebral input.

Urinary Incontinence

Urinary incontinence is the result of lesions that can occur in any portion of the anatomic pathways concerned with the storage and evacuation of urine.[33,40] The quality of the incontinence depends on the specific anatomic level of the lesion and its severity and duration. It is important to remember that incontinence includes both the leaking of urine and the inability to urinate. Failure to recognize this will lead to inappropriate anatomic diagnosis and treatment.

Lower Motor Neuron Bladder

A LMN bladder results from lesions in the sacral spinal cord segments, sacral spinal nerves, pelvic nerves and sacral plexus, or pudendal nerves. The bladder distends with urine, so if there is no resistance in the atonic urethralis muscle, urine continually overflows and dribbles from the urethral orifice. Usually the bladder is easily evacuated manually. The only resistance to this overflow is the tone in the internal urethral sphincter. Occasionally this may cause some resistance to manual evacuation of the bladder. Associated with the sacral spinal cord segment or sacral spinal nerve lesion, there usually is an atonic anus and lack of a perineal reflex. This is not present if the lesion is limited to the pelvic nerves. Reflex urinary evacuation cannot develop with these lesions. It is possible for a very limited reflex evacuation to occur, with the reflex developing entirely in the wall of the bladder, if that wall is healthy. Only very small amounts of urine are evacuated. It is critical to avoid prolonged, excessive distention of the bladder because it leads to atonia and the bladder's inability to contract.

Treatment includes bethanechol to stimulate the muscarinic receptors in the detrusor muscle and phenoxybenzamine to block the sympathetic alpha receptors in the smooth muscle of the internal sphincter.

Upper Motor Neuron Bladder

An UMN bladder results from lesions cranial to the sacral segments that interrupt the cranially projecting sensory (GVA) and caudally projecting motor (UMN) pathways. This is most common and severe in cases of transverse thoracolumbar spinal cord lesions. These lesions prevent any voluntary micturition, and bladder distention is severe. An inconstant leakage of urine may occur. The bladder wall feels turgid, and there is significant resistance to manual evacuation of the bladder because of the tone in the internal and external (urethralis muscle) sphincters. There may be increased resting tone in the latter due to the loss of inhibitory pathways that help control the activity of the GSE-LMNs in the sacral segments. The direct innervation of the bladder by sensory and motor neurons is still intact. In days to weeks, a variable degree of reflex micturition develops. Bladder distention stimulates GVA neurons that course to the sacral segments via the pelvic plexus and pelvic nerves, where they reflexively activate the parasympathetic preganglionic neurons to the detrusor muscle and inhibit the GSE-LMNs to the urethralis muscle. This permits partial evacuation of the bladder as long as the detrusor muscle is healthy. This reflex is involuntary and can occur spontaneously, without the animal's being aware it is happening, or it may be stimulated by slight abdominal pressure such as that which occurs when you pick up the paralyzed small animal. This is a very common cause of urine soiling of the examiner's clothes!

Treatment includes phenoxybenzamine to block the sympathetic alpha receptors in the smooth muscle of the internal sphincter, bethanechol to stimulate the detrusor muscle, and diazepam or dantrolene to block the striated urethralis muscle. Bethanechol should not be used until the internal sphincter and the striated urethralis muscles are appropriately relaxed. Bethanechol used prematurely may result in urinary bladder rupture.

Cerebral lesions do not directly interfere with the functioning of the micturition centers in the brainstem but may cause a loss of learned habits of micturition. The patient may exhibit normal urination but without regard to where it is performed. Be aware that this incontinence may mimic a urinary bladder and urethra (lower urinary tract) disorder, especially in cats. Normally, the cerebellum has an inhibitory effect on micturition, and cerebellar lesions may cause increased frequency of urination, but this complaint is rarely recognized. The owner is much more concerned about the ataxic gait.

A common cause of incontinence is incompetence of the urethra. The underlying cause is unknown. Micturition is normal, but during urine storage, leakage of urine occurs. This most commonly occurs in older spayed female dogs. Their owners complain that a spot of urine is left when the dog gets up from sleeping. Treatment with estrogen or testosterone may increase the sensitivity of urethral alpha receptors to increase internal sphincter tone, or these receptors can be stimulated directly using an alpha adrenergic agonist such as phenylpropanolamine.

■ CONTROL OF DEFECATION

Defecation is dependent on neuroanatomic structures similar to those utilized for micturition. The sacral spinal cord segment parasympathetic preganglionic neurons provide facilitory LMN innervation to the descending colon and rectum via the pelvic nerve and postganglionic neurons within the wall of these portions of the digestive tract. The L1 to L4 or L5 lumbar spinal cord segment sympathetic preganglionic neurons provide LMN innervation to the descending colon, rectum, and internal anal sphincter via the postganglionic neurons in the caudal mesenteric ganglion, caudal mesenteric plexus, hypogastric nerves, and pelvic plexus (see Fig. 7-33). The sympathetic innervation to the descending colon and rectum is inhibitory, whereas it is facilitory to the internal anal sphincter. The sacral spinal cord segment GSE-LMN innervates the striated external anal sphincter muscle via the sacral plexus and the caudal rectal branch of the pudendal nerve. There are cranially projecting sensory spinal cord tracts to a poorly localized brainstem center for defecation as well as to thalamic nuclei for relay to the sensory cerebral cortex. UMN pathways involve the motor cortex and reticulospinal tracts.

Lesions that cause dysfunction in the sacral components of this innervation cause a neurogenic sphincter incontinence involving continual leakage of feces, without the patient's being aware of the event.[34] This is a common clinical sign seen with the lumbosacral syndrome that was described in Case Example 5-10. Usually there is only a moderate retention of fecal material. Some involuntary fecal evacuation may still occur; it probably represents intrinsic reflex activity within the wall of the bowel. This occurs without the patient's assuming a posture for defecation. If retention is significant and persists without continual manual evacuation, a secondary megacolon may occur. Failure to defecate in cases of LMN disorders is more of a problem in the horse than in small animals.

Spinal cord lesions that are cranial to the sacral spinal cord segments and severe enough to cause paraplegia or severe paraparesis may cause loss of voluntary control over defecation. However, these lesions usually do not result in obstruction of the flow of bowel contents. Although some retention occurs, involuntary reflex fecal evacuation usually follows. Occasionally, with small localized spinal cord lesions cranial to the sacral segments, the chief complaint is fecal incontinence, and pelvic limb gait deficits are mild.[11,12] These dogs act unaware that defecation is occurring and pass feces while they are lying down or walking. These lesions, which are often in the dorsal portion of the involved spinal cord segment, are assumed to interfere primarily with the cranially projecting sensory pathway for defecation. Fecal incontinence has been reported in dogs with syringohydromyelia.

Examples of lesions that involve the LMN for micturition and defecation were described in Chapter 5, and lesions that involve the spinal cord tracts cranial to the LMN are described in Chapters 10 and 11.

PARASYMPATHETIC GVE-LMN OF THE MEDULLA: FACIAL, GLOSSOPHARYNGEAL, VAGUS, AND ACCESSORY NEURONS

The nuclei in the medulla that contain the preganglionic neuronal cell bodies of these GVE-LMNs are located in a column that is dorsal, adjacent to the floor of the fourth ventricle and lateral to the position of the hypoglossal nucleus. This column extends from the level of the facial nucleus to the obex (Fig. 7-34).

The parasympathetic nucleus of the facial nerve is the most rostral in this column. The axons of these preganglionic neuronal cell bodies join the facial GSE motor neurons and enter the internal acoustic meatus. Within the facial canal in the petrous portion of the temporal bone, some of these axons branch off the facial nerve in the major petrosal nerve. This nerve passes through the temporal bone and emerges on the pterygoid muscles, where it synapses on the

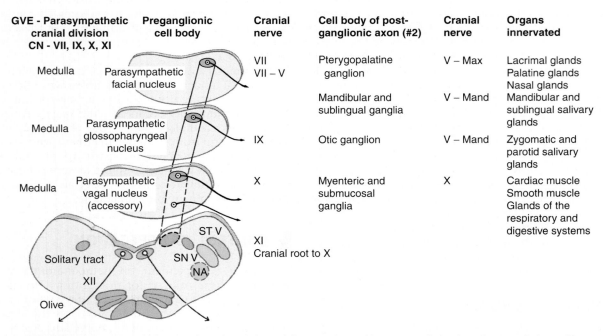

FIGURE 7-34 Parasympathetic GVE nuclear column in the medulla. *NA,* Nucleus ambiguus; *SN V,* spinal nucleus of V; *ST V,* spinal tract of V.

cell bodies of postganglionic neurons in the pterygopalatine ganglion. From this ganglion, postganglionic axons join branches of the trigeminal nerve to innervate the lacrimal gland, and the gland of the third eyelid, palatine, and nasal glands.

Distal to the origin of this branch and still within the facial canal, other preganglionic axons branch off the facial nerve in the chorda tympani. This nerve courses through the tympanic cavity and emerges rostral to the oval foramen to join the lingual nerve, which is a branch of the mandibular nerve from the trigeminal nerve. These preganglionic axons synapse in the sublingual and mandibular ganglia, which are adjacent to the salivary glands; they, in turn, are innervated by the postganglionic axons of the cell bodies in these ganglia. Be aware that occasionally the inflammation associated with otitis media may involve these preganglionic axons in the major petrosal nerve and cause failure of secretion by the glands that produce the aqueous portion of the tear secretion, resulting in keratitis sicca. I (EG) have observed a dog with the classic signs of a severe trigeminal neuritis that also developed a keratitis sicca. It resolved as the dog recovered the use of its jaw. This can be explained by the involvement of the postganglionic axons that join the lacrimal nerve, a branch of the ophthalmic nerve from the trigeminal nerve, or by involvement of the zygomatic branches of the maxillary nerve that reaches these tear-secreting glands. The involvement of this parasympathetic innervation can be determined by the Schirmer tear test. Lesions of the facial nerve that occur after it emerges from the stylomastoid foramen cannot affect this parasympathetic innervation.

The parasympathetic nucleus of the glossopharyngeal nerve is just caudal to the parasympathetic nucleus of the facial nerve. The axons of these preganglionic neuronal cell bodies join the GSE axons from nucleus ambiguus to form the motor component of the glossopharyngeal nerve, which enters the jugular foramen. Within the short space between this foramen and the tympanooccipital fissure, these preganglionic axons leave the glossopharyngeal nerve in the tympanic nerve and course through the tympanic cavity as part of the tympanic plexus. They are continued from the plexus in the minor petrosal nerve that terminates at the otic ganglion just ventral to the oval foramen and the mandibular nerve from the trigeminal nerve that emerges from it. These preganglionic axons synapse in the otic ganglion on the cell bodies of the postganglionic axons. The latter join branches of the mandibular nerve to innervate the parotid and zygomatic salivary glands.

The parasympathetic nucleus of the vagus nerve is a long nucleus that comprises the majority of this nuclear column. Older literature refers to this nucleus as the dorsal motor nucleus of the vagus.[22] It is just dorsolateral to the hypoglossal nucleus and slightly longer. It is medial to the solitary tract and nucleus that is part of the GVA system that makes up a large component of the vagus nerve (see Figs. 2-14 and 2-15).[21] The axons of these parasympathetic preganglionic neuronal cell bodies join the GSE axons from the nucleus ambiguus to form the motor component of the vagus nerve, which enters the jugular foramen and emerges from the tympanooccipital fissure. The GVE parasympathetic preganglionic axons course caudally in this nerve, where it is associated with the cervical sympathetic trunk in the carotid

sheath. They continue through the mediastinum, where they follow branches of the vagus to the heart muscle, lungs, and esophagus.[10] Within these organs, the preganglionic axons synapse with the cell bodies of the postganglionic axons that innervate the cardiac muscle or the smooth muscle and glands in the lungs and esophagus. The remaining preganglionic axons continue into the abdomen in the dorsal and ventral vagal trunks, where they primarily follow the blood vessels to the abdominal organs. They synapse on the cell bodies of the parasympathetic postganglionic axons within the wall of the organ innervated. Within the wall of the digestive tract, this innervation becomes part of the enteric nervous system, which is an extremely complex and autonomous system. The gastrointestinal system can carry out its major functions without this extrinsic innervation. Smooth muscle contractions occur using the intrinsic reflex activity of the enteric neurons. This extrinsic parasympathetic innervation provides what control the CNS has over the enteric nervous system. In a sense, this is a LMN acting as a UMN for regulation of gastrointestinal function.

The cell bodies in the most caudal portion of the parasympathetic nucleus of the vagus nerve have axons that join the GSE axons from the most caudal portion of the nucleus ambiguus. They emerge from the medulla as the cranial roots of the accessory nerve. They join to form the internal branch of the accessory nerve. The latter joins with the external branch to form the accessory nerve that enters the jugular foramen. Within the short space between the jugular foramen and the tympanooccipital fissure, these parasympathetic preganglionic axons join the vagus nerve and are distributed with the preganglionic axons already in the vagus nerve.

The enteric nervous system is a challenge to study but worth the effort.[6-8] Disorders of the enteric nervous system are infrequently studied. As we learn more about its complexities and apply ourselves more vigorously to investigating its abnormalities, we may find more solutions to various gastrointestinal disorders, especially some of the causes of colic in horses.[9]

▮ DYSAUTONOMIA

The one disorder that diffusely affects the GVE-LMN, including the enteric components, is dysautonomia. This disorder has been recognized and studied in horses for many years, especially in the United Kingdom, where it is most common and is known as grass sickness.[36] We are not aware that this disorder has been diagnosed in horses in North America that have never traveled to the United Kingdom. A similar disorder occurs in cats in the United Kingdom, where it is known as the Key-Gaskell syndrome (Fig. 7-35).[45,48] However, more recently a similar dysautonomia has been recognized in young adult dogs that are located mainly in rural areas in Missouri and Kansas.[28,29] Although a neurotoxin is suspected as the causative agent, this has yet to be proven. Degenerative lesions are widely distributed in GVE ganglia, including the enteric components, but they also occur in spinal ganglia and in selected neuronal populations in the CNS.[20] Clinical signs reflect the diffuse involvement of both the parasympathetic and sympathetic components of the GVE system. Dogs and cats exhibit dilated pupils that are

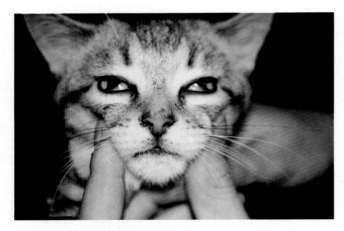

FIGURE 7-35 A 5-month-old domestic shorthair with 4 days of clinical signs suggestive of the diagnosis of dysautonomia. Note the paradoxic ocular signs with dilated, unresponsive pupils (parasympathetic denervation) and bilateral protrusion of the third eyelids and smaller palpebral fissures (sympathetic denervation).

unresponsive to light, protrusion of the third eyelid, dry oral and nasal mucosae, dysphagia, megaesophagus, vomiting, diarrhea or constipation, incontinence of urine and feces, and bradycardia. Horses can die acutely of gastrointestinal stasis and gastric reflux or have a chronic course with intermittent colic. Pharmacologic testing may help to support the diagnosis.[18] There is no specific therapy, and spontaneous recovery is uncommon.

COMPLEX REGIONAL PAIN SYNDROME, REFLEX SYMPATHETIC DYSTROPHY

A clinical syndrome that involves dysfunction of the peripheral cutaneous distribution of sympathetic nerves is currently referred to as complex regional pain syndrome.[43] Previously, it had been called reflex sympathetic dystrophy. The syndrome consists of chronic pain with localized hyperalgesia, which is increased responsiveness to noxious stimuli, and allodynia, which is increased responsiveness to nonnoxious stimuli. Clinical signs of dysregulation of the cutaneous sympathetic innervation include either hyperthermia or hypothermia, hyperhydrosis or hypohydrosis, and edema. Trauma of some sort is usually a precipitating event at some time in the history of the patient. The pathogenesis is poorly understood. This syndrome has been reported in the horse and dog.[14,24]

REFERENCES

1. Acheson GH: The topographical anatomy of the smooth muscle of the cat's nictitating membrane, *Anat Rec* 71: 297-311, 1938.
2. Acland GM, Irby NL, Aquirre GD: Sudden acquired retinal degeneration in the dog: clinical and morphological characterization of the "silent retinal" syndrome, *Trans Am Coll Vet Ophthalmol* 15:86-104, 1984.
3. Barlow CM, Root WS: The ocular sympathetic path between the superior cervical ganglion and the orbit in the cat, *J Comp Neurol* 91:195, 1949.
4. Bell M, Montagna W: Innervation of sweat glands in horses and dogs, *Br J Dermatol* 86:160, 1972.
5. Bistner S, et al: Pharmacologic diagnosis of Horner syndrome in the dog, *J Am Vet Med Assoc* 157:1220, 1970.
6. Burns GA: The taenia of the equine intestinal tract, *Cornell Vet* 82:187-212, 1992.
7. Burns GA, Cummings JF: Equine myenteric plexus with special reference to the pelvic flexure, *Anat Rec* 230:417-424, 1991.
8. Burns GA, Cummings JF: Neuropeptide distribution in the colon, cecum and jejunum of the horse, *Anat Rec* 236: 341-350, 1993.
9. Burns GA, Karcher L, Cummings JF: Equine myenteric ganglionitis: a case of chronic intestinal pseudo-obstruction, *Cornell Vet* 80:53-63, 1990.
10. Carveth SW, et al: Esophageal motility after vagotomy and myomectomy in dogs, *Surg Gynecol Obstet* 114:31, 1962.
11. Cerda-Gonzalez S, Olbe NJ: Fecal incontinence associated with epidural spinal hematoma and intervertebral disk extrusion in a dog, *J Am Vet Med Assoc* 228:230-235, 2006.
12. Chen AV, et al: Fecal incontinence and spinal cord abnormalities in seven dogs, *J Am Vet Med Assoc* 227:1945-1951, 2005.
13. Christensen K: Sympathetic and parasympathetic nerves in the orbit of the cat, *J Anat* 70:225-232, 1936.
14. Collins NM, et al: Suspected complex regional pain syndrome in two horses, *J Vet Intern Med* 20:1014-1017, 2006.
15. Edvardsen P: Nervous control of urinary bladder in cats. I. The collecting phase, *Acta Physiol Scand* 72:157, 1968.
16. Firth EC: Horner syndrome in the horse: experimental induction and case report, *Eq Vet J* 19:9, 1978.
17. Fletcher TF, Bradley WE: Neuroanatomy of bladder-urethra, *J Urol* 119:153, 1978.
18. Fox JG, Gutnick MJ: Horner syndrome and brachial paralysis due to lymphosarcoma in a cat, *J Am Vet Med Assoc* 160:977, 1972.
19. Hahn CN, Mayhew IG: Phenylephrine eyedrops as a diagnostic test in equine grass sickness, *Vet Rec* 147: 603-606, 2000.
20. Hahn CN, Mayhew IG, de Lahunta A: Central neuropathology of equine grass sickness, *Acta Neuropathol* 102:153-159, 2001.
21. Harding R, Leek BF: The locations and activities of medullary neurons associated with ruminant forestomach motility, *J Physiol* 219:587, 1971.
22. Keer FWL: Function of the dorsal motor nucleus of the vagus, *Science* 157:451, 1967.
23. Kuru M, Iwanaga T: Ponto-sacral connections in the medial reticulospinal tract subserving storage of urine, *J Comp Neurol* 127:241, 1966.
24. LaBarre A, Coyne BE: Reflex sympathetic dystrophy in a dog, *J Am Anim Hosp Assoc* 35:229-231, 1999.
25. Mayhew IG: Horner syndrome and lesions involving the sympathetic nervous system, *Eq Pract* 2:44, 1980.
26. Morgan C, Nadelhaft I, de Groat WC: Location of bladder preganglionic neurons within the sacral parasympathetic nucleus of the cat, *Neurosci Lett* 14:189, 1979.
27. Murray MJ, et al: Signs of sympathetic denervation associated with a thoracic melanoma in a horse, *J Vet Intern Med* 11:199-203, 1997.
28. O'Brien DP: *Dysautonomia in dogs* (website): www.cvm. missouri.edu/neurology/. Accessed April 11, 2008.
29. O'Brien DP, Johnson GC: Dysautonomia and autonomic neuropathies, *Vet Clin No Am Sm Anim Pract* 32:251-265, 2002.
30. Oliver JE Jr, Bradley WE, Fletcher TF: Identification of preganglionic parasympathetic neurons in the sacral spinal cord of the cat, *J Comp Neurol* 137:321, 1969.

31. Oliver JE Jr, Bradley WE, Fletcher TF: Spinal cord representation of the micturition reflex, *J Comp Neurol* 137:329, 1969.
32. Oliver JE Jr, Bradley W, Fletcher TF: Spinal cord distribution of the somatic innervation of the external urethral sphincter of the cat, *J Neurol Sci* 10:11, 1970.
33. Oliver JE Jr, Selcer RR: Neurogenic causes of abnormal micturition in the dog and cat, *Vet Clin North Am* 4:517, 1974.
34. Oliver JE Jr, Selcer RR: Neurogenic disorders of the rectum and anal sphincter, *Vet Clin North Am* 4:551, 1974.
35. Petras JM, Cummings JF: Sympathetic and parasympathetic innervation of the urinary bladder and urethra, *Brain Res* 153:363, 1978.
36. Pirie R: Grass sickness, *Clin Tech Eq Pract* 5:30-36, 2006.
37. Purington PT, Oliver JE Jr: Spinal cord origin of innervation to the bladder and urethra of the dog, *Exp Neurol* 65:422, 1979.
38. Purohit RC, McCoy MD, Bergfield WA III: Thermographic diagnosis of Horner syndrome in the horse, *Am J Vet Res* 41:1180-1182, 1980.
39. Rohner TJ, et al: Contractile responses of dog bladder neck muscle to adrenergic drugs, *J Urol* 105:657, 1971.
40. Rosen AH, Ross L: Diagnosis and pharmacologic management of disorders of urinary continence in the dog, *Compend Cont Ed* 3:601, 1981.
41. Rosenblueth A, Bard P: The innervation and function of the nictitating membrane in the cat, *Am J Physiol* 100:537, 1932.
42. Smith JS, Mayhew IG: Horner syndrome in large animals, *Cornell Vet* 67:529, 1977.
43. Stanton-Hicks M, Janig W, Hassenbusch S: Reflex sympathetic dystrophy: changing concepts and taxonomy, *Pain* 63:127-133, 1995.
44. Sundin T, Carlsson C-A: Reconstruction of the severed dorsal roots innervating the urinary bladder: an experimental study in cats. I. Studies on the normal afferent pathways in the pelvic and pudendal nerves, *Scand J Urol Nephrol* 6:176, 1972.
45. Symonds HW, et al: A cluster of cases of feline dysautonomia (Key-Gaskell syndrome) in a closed colony, *Vet Rec* 136:353-355, 1995.
46. Thompson JW: The nerve supply to the nictitating membrane of the cat, *J Anat* 95:371, 1961.
47. Valentine BA, et al: Suprasellar germ cell tumors in the dog: a report of five cases and review of the literature, *Acta Neuropathol* 76:94-100, 1988.
48. Valevets-University of Glasgow, Feline Dysautonomia (Key-Gaskell syndrome) Study Group (website): www.valevets.co.uk/dysautonomia/. Accessed April 11, 2008.

8 UPPER MOTOR NEURON

PYRAMIDAL SYSTEM

HISTOLOGY OF THE CEREBRAL CORTEX

EXTRAPYRAMIDAL SYSTEM

Telencephalon
Cerebral Cortex
Basal Nuclei
Diencephalon
Mesencephalon
Reticular Formation
Rhombencephalon

UPPER MOTOR NEURON FUNCTION

Neuromuscular Spindles
Gait Generation

CLINICAL SIGNS OF UPPER MOTOR NEURON DISEASE

Paresis
Spasticity
Hyperreflexia
Release from Inhibition
Decerebrate and Decerebellate
Rigidity
Extrapyramidal Nuclear Lesions

UNCONTROLLED INVOLUNTARY SKELETAL MUSCLE CONTRACTIONS

Muscle
Inherited Congenital Myotonia
Acquired Myotonia
Nervous System
Tetanus
Tetany
Myoclonus
Movement Disorder

The upper motor neuron (UMN) is the motor system that is confined to the central nervous system (CNS) and is responsible for the initiation of voluntary movement, the maintenance of muscle tone for support of the body against gravity, and the regulation of posture to provide a stable background upon which to initiate voluntary activity. Traditionally, it has been divided into pyramidal and extrapyramidal components. This separation is more significant in primates, in which the pyramidal system is more highly developed and has more important functions than have been observed in domestic animals.

The pyramidal system consists of neurons whose cell bodies are located predominantly in the motor area of the cerebral cortex and whose axons descend through the white matter of the cerebrum and brainstem, including the pyramid on the ventral surface of the medulla. The pyramid is named for its pointed shape in primates. It contains only the projection pathway of the pyramidal system's neurons. Their telodendron is in the gray matter of the caudal brainstem and the spinal cord. The latter is an uninterrupted monosynaptic corticospinal pathway from the cerebrum to the spinal cord by way of the pyramids of the medulla.

In contrast, the extrapyramidal system consists of neurons that originate in the cerebral cortex, including the motor area, and descend into the brainstem directly or by way of basal (subcortical) nuclei. Synapse occurs with additional neurons in the basal nuclei and brainstem nuclei. Axons of these neurons course caudally from specific brainstem nuclei into the spinal cord without traversing the pyramids of the medulla. The telodendron of the brainstem neuron is in the gray matter of the spinal cord. This is a multineuronal, multisynaptic corticospinal pathway. The pyramidal and extrapyramidal systems overlap anatomically and function together. The extrapyramidal system is of much greater importance in the domestic animal. The two systems will be considered together as the UMN in all clinical discussions.

PYRAMIDAL SYSTEM

The development of the pyramidal system is directly related to the capacity of an animal to perform skilled movements. In primates, its termination in the spinal cord is most dense in the areas of the lateral portion of the ventral gray column in which the cell bodies of the general somatic efferent (GSE) lower motor neuron (LMN) to muscles of the digits are located. Here, it may synapse directly on the dendritic zone of the alpha motor neuron (GSE). This anatomic arrangement occurs in primates and in the raccoon, two unrelated species that possess considerable manipulative ability in their thoracic limb digits.[1] The pyramidal system is poorly developed in domestic animals, especially in the horse, ox, and sheep. In the horse, this system makes a sizable contribution to the facial nuclei, the location of the GSE-LMNs that innervate muscles for lip movement, suggesting that these muscles of prehension perform the most highly skilled activity in this species. This system also terminates in the spinal cord dorsal gray column, where it influences the activity of ascending sensory systems.

The cell body of the pyramidal system neuron is located in the cerebral cortex. The majority are located in the motor area in the frontal lobe or the adjacent parietal lobe (Fig. 8-1). In primates, this involves primarily the precruciate gyrus.

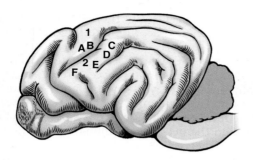

FIGURE 8-1 Topography of the cerebral motor cortex.

1. Postcruciate gyrus
   A. Pelvic limb
   B. Thoracic limb
2. Rostral suprasylvian gyrus
   C. Ear
   D. Eyelid
   E. Masseter, temporal muscles
   F. Lateral cervical muscles

In carnivores, it overlaps on the sensory area, where it is limited to the postcruciate and rostral suprasylvian gyri.[12,19,39] In ungulates, the motor area is located medially along the frontal lobe in the region of the precruciate gyrus. Electrophysiologic stimulation studies have shown that these motor areas can be subdivided into the regions of the body that are innervated by LMNs receiving impulses from the pyramidal system neurons that originate in these specific parts of the motor cortex. This is referred to as a somatotopic organization, in which the various portions of the body are represented topographically on specific regions of the cerebral gyri. The homunculus drawn on the surface of the human cerebrum depicts this phenomenon. Regions involved with more highly skilled functions have a larger representation in this motor area. Muscles with small motor units also have a larger area of representation. The primary motor area of one cerebrum serves the musculature on the contralateral side of the body. In the carnivore, the postcruciate gyrus is related to the innervation of the appendicular musculature.[12,17] The suprasylvian gyrus is related to the motor function of the cervical muscles and the muscles of specific areas of the head. In addition to these motor areas, there are components of the pyramidal system that have cell bodies in the premotor area, the somesthetic area, and related association areas.

Many of these pyramidal system cell bodies are large and are referred to as giant pyramidal cells or Betz cells.[39] They are located in lamina V of the cerebral cortex of the gyri that comprise the motor area of the cerebral cortex. The axons of these cell bodies descend through the white matter of the brain in the following order: the corona radiata of the gyrus in the motor area, the cerebral centrum semiovale, the internal capsule of the telencephalon and diencephalon, the central portion of the crus cerebri of the mesencephalon, the longitudinal fibers of the pons, and the pyramid of the medulla. At the caudal end of the pyramid, 75% or more of these axons cross in the pyramidal decussation and pass through the gray matter to the dorsal portion of the lateral funiculus (see Figs. 2-16 and 2-17). The decussation is not visible on the ventral surface of the medulla because it occurs as the crossing fibers course dorsally into the parenchyma of the junction between the medulla and the first cervical spinal cord segment. These crossed pyramidal system axons form the lateral corticospinal tract medial to the cranial projecting spinocerebellar tracts in the dorsolateral funiculus.[90] In the dog, as the lateral corticospinal tract courses caudally, about 50% of these axons terminate in the cervical spinal cord gray matter, 20% in the thoracic spinal cord gray matter, and 30% in the lumbosacral spinal cord gray matter. Most synapse on interneurons in the ventral gray column that influence the GSE-LMNs located here.[53,63,68] Pyramidal system neurons that have their cell bodies in the somesthetic cerebral cortex synapse on neurons in the dorsal gray column to influence the activity of projection sensory systems. The remaining 25% or less of the pyramidal axons in the medulla continue caudally without crossing and enter the ventral funiculus adjacent to the ventral median fissure where they comprise the ventral corticospinal tract. The axons in this tract course caudally to about the level of the midthoracic spinal cord segments. Prior to terminating in the gray matter along this course, these axons cross to the opposite side. Their synapses are similar to those described for the axons of the lateral corticospinal tract. In cats, this pyramidal system serves the entire spinal cord gray matter. In ungulates, the entire pyramidal system is confined primarily to the cervical spinal cord segments.[10,11]

In addition to the pyramidal system corticospinal axons, other pyramidal system axons terminate in the brainstem to synapse in nuclei of cranial nerves with GSE-LMNs. These are called corticonuclear axons. Corticoreticular neurons synapse in a component of the reticular formation.

The pyramidal system axons are organized regionally in the various portions of the central white matter where they are located. In the crus cerebri, the pyramidal system comprises the projection axons in the center of this crus. The axons to the lumbosacral intumescence (pelvic limb) are lateral. Those projecting to the cervical intumescence (the thoracic limb) are in the middle, and those projecting to the brainstem nuclei (the head muscles) are medial. In the cat, the pyramid in the medulla has been mapped according to the muscle groups affected by its axons.[39,94]

Disturbances in the pyramidal system demonstrate the differences in the roles this system plays in primates compared with its roles in domestic animals. Lesions in the cerebral components of this system in humans cause paralysis of the contralateral voluntary muscle activity that is especially evident in the hands and feet and involves the muscles used in highly skilled functions. In dogs and cats examined a few days after experimental surgical removal of the frontoparietal lobes (motor area), no defect is seen in the gait when the animal walks on a level surface. However, these animals do have a deficiency in their responses to testing of postural reactions in the contralateral limbs. This is most readily appreciated when the hopping responses are tested. Similarly, experimental surgical sectioning of the canine pyramidal system axons in the crus cerebri does not affect the gait.[47] A variety of naturally occurring cerebral lesions in this same area in all species of domestic animals present with a similar clinical syndrome of gait preservation and deficiency of contralateral postural reactions. Because these lesions usually also involve the conscious projections of the general proprioceptive and visual systems, such lesions are discussed in Chapters 9 and 14, with examples in the latter chapter.

HISTOLOGY OF THE CEREBRAL CORTEX

The cerebral cortex is made up of an elaborate organization of neural structures with innumerable connections that form the basis for the numerous functions allotted to it. They include consciousness, intellect, emotion, behavior, perception, and control of somatic and visceral motor functions. They are performed by the reciprocal relationship between the cerebral cortex and the rest of the central and peripheral nervous systems.

The cerebral cortex is the layer of gray matter that covers the white matter of each cerebral gyrus. This cortex varies from 1.5 to 4 mm in thickness and is situated between the pia mater on the surface and the underlying white matter, which it covers. This white matter is the corona radiata of the neocortex. The cortex contains neuronal cell bodies of many different sizes and shapes, axons, telodendria, dendritic zone processes, neuroglial cells, and an abundance of blood vessels, especially capillaries (Fig. 8-2 and 8-3). The neurons in the cortex constitute a system of chains of interrelated neurons. The cortex is a laminated structure based on the organization of the processes (myeloarchitectonics)

or based on the arrangement of the cell bodies (cytoarchitectonics). When viewed according to the organization of the cell bodies, as many as six layers can be recognized (see Fig. 8-2). The extent to which each of these six laminae is developed varies throughout the cerebrum. In general, the neopallium has six layers and the archipallium (hippocampus) and paleopallium (olfactory cortex) have fewer layers. Some functional significance has been attached to the variation in the neocortical laminations in the different regions of the cerebrum. Maps have been prepared that show the laminar variations that occur throughout the cerebrum. Some include more than 100 different areas based on cytoarchitectonic studies. The cortical lamination of the archipallium and the paleopallium is different from the lamination of the neocortex, and it is different in each one. Specific characteristics of each permit their identification.

In general, the neocortical neuronal cell bodies are of two types. The stellate or granule neuron has a round cell body and short processes that are usually confined to the cortex. The pyramidal neuron has a pyramid-shaped cell body that varies in size and has long processes. The axon of the pyramidal neuron projects from the cortex into the underlying

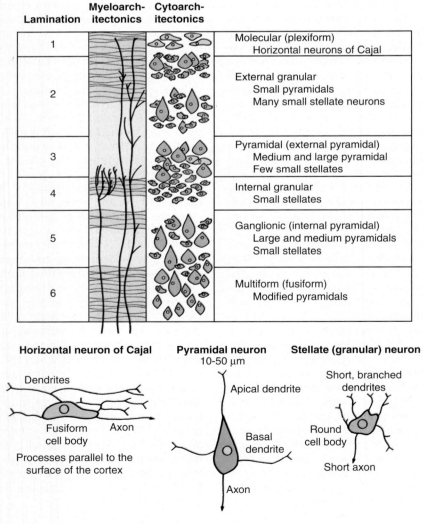

FIGURE 8-2 Histology of the cerebral cortex.

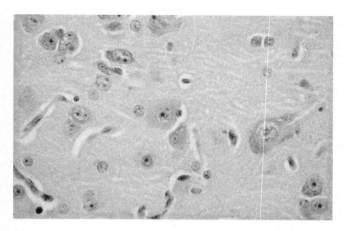

FIGURE 8-3 Microscopic section of dog cerebral cortex. The cells with the recognizable nuclei and cytoplasm are variously sized pyramidal and granular neurons. Most of the small round nuclei without recognizable cytoplasm are astrocytes. There is one small dark oligodendroglial nucleus adjacent to a large pyramidal neuron in the middle. There are a few transverse sections of capillaries in the middle and two longitudinal sections of capillaries in the lower left.

white matter of the corona radiata as an associative axon coursing to another cortical area in the same cerebrum, or as a commissural axon that crosses to a cortical area in the opposite cerebrum, or as a projection axon that projects to nuclear areas in the brainstem or spinal cord. The corticospinal neuron is an example of the last type. Each area of cerebral cortex receives axons from other cortical areas in the same cerebrum (association), from the opposite cerebrum (commissural), and from the brainstem, especially the thalamus (projection). The study of the arrangement of these processes within the cortex, including the processes of the granule neurons, is referred to as myeloarchitectonics.

In the neocortex, the six layers, from superficial to deep, consist of the molecular layer, external granule layer, pyramidal layer, internal granule layer, ganglion layer, and multiformic layer (see Fig. 8-2). The processes of the molecular and external and internal granule layers are confined to the cortex. Axons from the pyramidal, ganglionic, and multiformic layers compose the cortical efferents that form the association, commissural, and projection pathways.

EXTRAPYRAMIDAL SYSTEM

The extrapyramidal system embraces diverse, scattered groups of interconnected and functionally related structures that form a series of neurons in a multisynaptic pathway from the cerebrum to the LMN of the brainstem and spinal cord (Fig. 8-4). These pathways do not traverse the pyramids of the medulla but function with the pyramidal system by providing tonic mechanisms for the support of the body against gravity and by recruiting spinal reflexes for the initiation of voluntary movement. These functions are performed ultimately by the influence of this UMN system on the alpha and gamma motor neurons (LMN) in motor nuclei in the brainstem and in the ventral gray columns of the spinal cord.

The cell bodies of neurons in the extrapyramidal system are located in nuclei in all divisions of the brain. The more important of them are described for each of the brain divisions, along with the courses of their axons. Only the extrapyramidal nuclei in the mesencephalon and rhombencephalon have axons that descend the spinal cord to influence the activity of the lower motor neurons.

Telencephalon

Neuronal cell bodies in the telencephalon (cerebrum) are located either on the surface in laminae of the cerebral cortex or deep to the surface in subcortical nuclei known as basal nuclei. Some authors refer to these as basal ganglia, but this is a misnomer because ganglia, by definition, are collections of neuronal cell bodies in the peripheral nervous system.

Cerebral Cortex

Extrapyramidal neurons are located in the cerebral cortex throughout the cerebrum but most are in the cortex of the motor area and adjacent gyri of the frontal and parietal lobes. Their axons project to basal nuclei and other extrapyramidal nuclei in the brainstem.

Basal Nuclei

The basal nuclei are subcortical collections of neuronal cell bodies in the cerebrum. They include the septal nuclei and amygdala, which function in the limbic system. The caudate nucleus, nucleus accumbens, putamen, pallidum, and claustrum are extrapyramidal basal nuclei (Figs. 8-5 through 8-7; see also Fig. 8-4) that are generally considered to be involved with motor activity. The putamen and pallidum are referred to as the lentiform nucleus because of their collective overall shape on transverse or dorsal plane sections. The term *corpus striatum* includes the caudate nucleus, nucleus accumbens, pallidum, putamen, and claustrum along with the portions of the internal and external capsules of white matter that are related to these basal nuclei.

The caudate nucleus is located primarily in the floor of the rostral part of the lateral ventricle, medial to the internal capsule (see Fig. 2-2). The large head and most of the body are rostral to the diencephalon. The body narrows as it extends caudally, dorsolateral to the diencephalon and medial to the internal capsule (see Fig. 2-3). It is continued by a small tail that curves ventrally into the temporal lobe of the cerebrum. The tail is C-shaped as it curves around the internal capsule. Dorsally, it is medial to the internal capsule, and ventrally, it is lateral to it. The ventral portion ends just caudal to the amygdala. The caudate nucleus receives axons from extrapyramidal neurons in the cerebral cortex, and many of its axons project to the adjacent pallidum.[94] Nigrostriatal projections are axons of cell bodies in the mesencephalic substantia nigra that project primarily to the caudate nucleus.[88]

The nucleus accumbens is a ventral extension of the head of the caudate nucleus. It surrounds the ventral portion of the rostral horn of the internal capsule.

The lentiform nucleus comprises the pallidum (globus pallidus) medially and the putamen laterally. The two nuclei are separated by an irregular layer of white matter. The nucleus is bounded medially by the internal capsule and laterally by the thin external capsule (see Figs. 2-2 and 2-3). The nucleus begins rostrally in the frontal lobe, where it is separated from the head and body of the caudate nucleus by the internal capsule. It extends caudally through the parietal lobe and into the

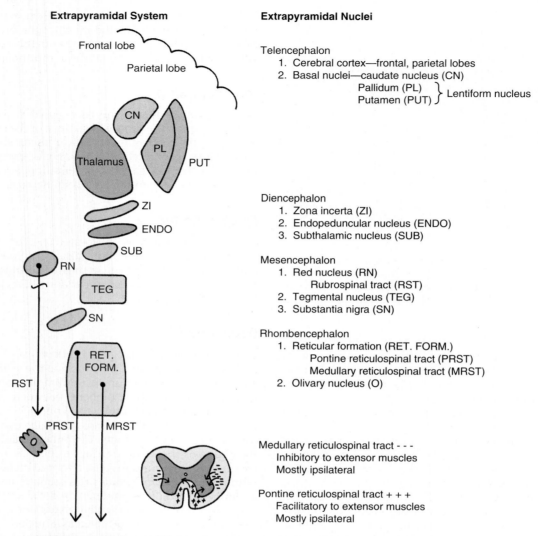

Extrapyramidal System

Frontal lobe

Parietal lobe

CN

PL

Thalamus   PUT

ZI

ENDO

SUB

RN

TEG

SN

RET. FORM.

RST

PRST   MRST

O

Extrapyramidal Nuclei

Telencephalon
1. Cerebral cortex—frontal, parietal lobes
2. Basal nuclei—caudate nucleus (CN)
   Pallidum (PL) }
   Putamen (PUT) } Lentiform nucleus

Diencephalon
1. Zona incerta (ZI)
2. Endopeduncular nucleus (ENDO)
3. Subthalamic nucleus (SUB)

Mesencephalon
1. Red nucleus (RN)
   Rubrospinal tract (RST)
2. Tegmental nucleus (TEG)
3. Substantia nigra (SN)

Rhombencephalon
1. Reticular formation (RET. FORM.)
   Pontine reticulospinal tract (PRST)
   Medullary reticulospinal tract (MRST)
2. Olivary nucleus (O)

Medullary reticulospinal tract - - -
   Inhibitory to extensor muscles
   Mostly ipsilateral

Pontine reticulospinal tract + + +
   Facilitatory to extensor muscles
   Mostly ipsilateral

FIGURE 8-4 The extrapyramidal system. A curved line that crosses a neuronal axon means that it crosses the median plane in the brain.

temporal lobe to a level caudal to the amygdala in the pyriform lobe, where the ventral portions of the lateral ventricle and hippocampus are located. The pallidum is medial to the putamen and is interspersed in the lateroventral portion of the rostral horn of the internal capsule, which gives it a reticulated pattern. The endopeduncular nucleus is a medioventral extension of the pallidum that is most obvious where it is positioned between the internal capsule and the optic tract (see Fig. 2-3). The putamen is the largest portion of the lentiform nucleus and is lateral to the pallidum. It blends with the internal capsule and caudate nucleus rostral to the pallidum and is separated laterally from the claustrum by the external capsule.

The claustrum forms a long thin plate lateral to the external capsule (see Fig. 2-3). It extends from the level of the head of the caudate nucleus rostrally to the level of the ventral extent of the lateral ventricle in the temporal lobe caudally. A very thin layer of white matter, the extreme capsule, separates part of this plate from the neocortex of the lateral aspect of the cerebrum. The ventral portion of the claustrum blends with the adjacent neocortex.

A feedback circuit is provided by a multisynaptic pathway from the neocortical extrapyramidal neurons to the caudate nucleus, to the pallidum, to the ventral rostral nucleus of the thalamus, to the neocortex (Fig. 8-8). At the time of cortical initiation of voluntary movement, such a circuit provides a modifying control mechanism. Certain specific thalamic nuclei serve to project information from the brainstem to the cerebrum. The ventral rostral thalamic nucleus is an example of such a projection nucleus for the extrapyramidal system.

Diencephalon

The extrapyramidal nuclei are located in the ventrolateral section of the thalamus, which is referred to as the subthalamus (Fig. 8-9). The endopeduncular nucleus was described with the pallidum, from which it is a medial extension between the optic tract and the internal capsule. It extends caudally, lateral to the hypothalamus (see Fig. 2-3). The zona incerta is a narrow nucleus located dorsomedial to the ventral thalamic portion of the internal capsule and lateral to the external medullary lamina of the thalamus. It extends through most of the subthalamic section (see Fig. 2-4). The subthalamic nucleus is in the caudal thalamus, caudal to

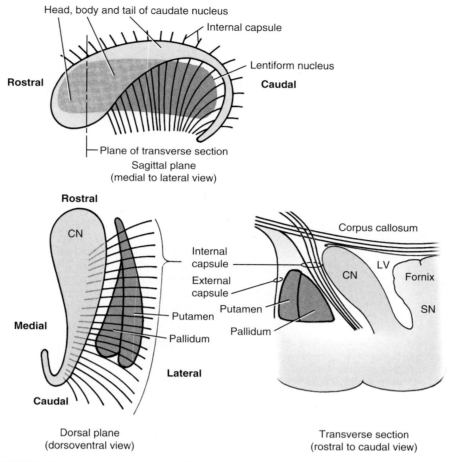

FIGURE 8-5 Extrapyramidal nuclei of the telencephalon. *CN,* Caudate nucleus; *LV,* lateral ventricle; *Pl,* pallidum; *SN,* septal nuclei.

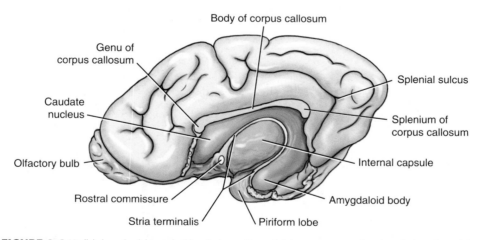

FIGURE 8-6 Medial view of a right cerebral hemisphere with medial structures removed to show the lateral ventricle. The rostral horn of the ventricle is bounded laterally by the *caudate nucleus,* and the distal part of the temporal horn is bounded laterally by the *amygdala;* elsewhere, the ventricle is bounded laterally by white matter.

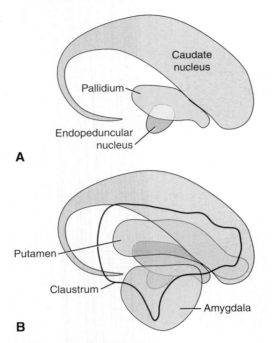

A

B

FIGURE 8-7 Projected profiles of telencephalic basal nuclei as viewed laterally in a right cerebral hemisphere. **A,** Medially positioned nuclei. The pallidum overlaps the dorsal part of the more medially positioned endopeduncular nucleus. **B,** Laterally positioned nuclei are added in darker shading. Only a perimeter is shown for the claustrum, the most lateral basal nucleus. The nucleus accumbens, located ventral to the rostral end of the caudate nucleus, is not shown.

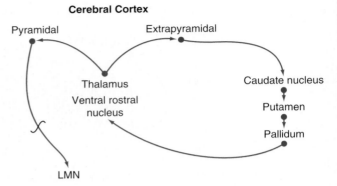

FIGURE 8-8 Schematic diagram of extrapyramidal pathways in the prosencephalon.

the endopeduncular nucleus on the dorsomedial surface of the crus cerebri (see Fig. 2-4). All three of these nuclei are connected to the extrapyramidal nuclei in the telencephalon and caudal brainstem by afferent and efferent axons, but no axons project directly to the spinal cord.

Mesencephalon

There are two well-defined extrapyramidal nuclear areas in the midbrain: the substantia nigra and the red nucleus (Fig. 8-10). The substantia nigra is so named because its cell bodies contain a melanin pigment that increases with age and is macroscopic in some species.[55] This nucleus can be found throughout the length of the mesencephalon dorsal to the crus cerebri and ventral to the tegmentum (see Figs. 2-5 through 2-7). It is bounded rostrally by the subthalamic nucleus. Many of the substantia nigra neurons

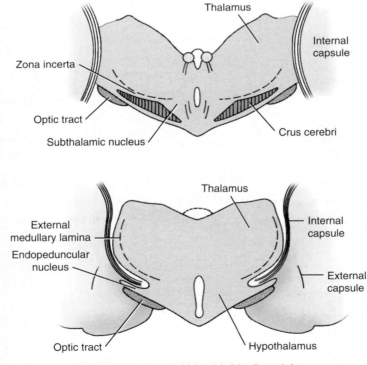

FIGURE 8-9 Extrapyramidal nuclei of the diencephalon.

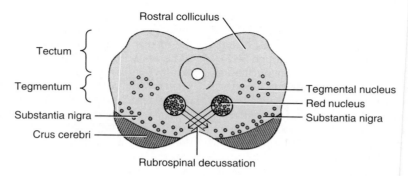

FIGURE 8-10 Extrapyramidal nuclei of the mesencephalon.

project rostrally to the caudate nucleus. Dopamine, which is synthesized by the substantia nigra neurons, is secreted as the neurotransmitter at this level. This is referred to as the nigrostriatal system.[86]

The red nucleus is a well-defined round nucleus in the tegmentum at the level of the rostral colliculi and ventrolateral to the oculomotor nucleus (see Figs. 2-6 and 2-7). It receives a group of afferent axons from the ipsilateral motor area of the neocortex by way of the internal capsule and crus cerebri. Axons of the cell bodies in the red nucleus immediately decussate at the level of this nucleus in the tegmentum and course caudally as the rubrospinal tract. This tract courses from the ventrolateral mesencephalon through the pons and medulla into the lateral funiculus of the spinal cord (see Fig. 2-17). Here the tract is closely associated with the lateral corticospinal tract deep to the superficially positioned cranially projecting spinocerebellar tracts in the dorsal portion of the lateral funiculus. The rubrospinal tract extends through the entire spinal cord. Its axons terminate on interneurons in the ventral gray column of the spinal cord. These interneurons, in turn, influence the activity of the GSE alpha and gamma LMNs. This corticorubrospinal tract is organized somatotopically.[72,74] The neurons in the thoracic limb area of the motor cortex project to the dorsal part of the red nucleus. The neurons in this dorsal part of the red nucleus project to the ventral gray column of the spinal cord segments that innervate the contralateral thoracic limb muscles. Corticorubral neurons from the pelvic limb region of the motor cortex synapse in the ventral part of the red nucleus, whose neurons project to the ventral gray column of the spinal cord segments that innervate the contralateral pelvic limb muscles.[46] The red nucleus neurons are predominantly facilitory to motor neurons of flexor muscles and therefore function in the initiation of protraction of the limbs in gait generation.[48]

Rubronuclear axons course with the rubrospinal axons and at various levels leave the rubrospinal tract as it courses through the caudal brainstem. The rubronuclear axons synapse in the cranial nerve nuclei that contain GSE-LMNs.

The red nucleus also participates in a feedback circuit between the neocortex and the cerebellum (see Fig. 13-20). A significant number of neurons in the neocortex project their axons to the ipsilateral pontine nucleus. The axons of these pontine cell bodies cross in the transverse fibers of the pons to enter the cerebellum via the contralateral middle cerebellar peduncle. Synapses occur in the cerebellar cortex; they are described in Chapter 13, which discusses the

cerebellum. Ultimately, the neural impulses from the cerebellar cortex activate a cerebellar nucleus whose axons emerge from the cerebellum in the rostral cerebellar peduncle. These axons cross in the tegmentum of the midbrain, and some of them terminate on neuronal cell bodies in the contralateral red nucleus. The axons of these neurons course to the thalamus and synapse in the ventral rostral nucleus, whose axons project to the neocortex. This is a cerebropontocerebellar-cerebellorubrothalamocortical circuit that begins and ends in the same area of neocortex. There are also connections from the red nucleus to telencephalic basal nuclei.

Reticular Formation

Before describing the components of the extrapyramidal system in the rhombencephalon, it is necessary to define the reticular formation. The reticular formation is a collection of neuronal cell bodies of various sizes and a plethora of processes that form an ill-defined meshwork in the central core of the brainstem. It extends from the medulla to the caudal diencephalon. Many functions are attributed to the reticular formation. One major function is the role it plays in activating the cerebral cortex to establish the awake state and the level of consciousness. This is referred to as the ascending reticular activating system and is described in Chapter 19, which concerns the diencephalon. The reticular formation is also involved in the various neural connections that induce sleep. Several groups of reticular formation neurons make up the brainstem centers that are involved in the caudally projecting UMN control of respiration, cardiovascular function, voluntary excretions, swallowing, vomiting, and muscle tone and voluntary movement. The extrapyramidal system is involved in this caudally projecting pathway that influences the GSE- and GVE-LMNs involved in voluntary and involuntary motor activity.[62]

Rhombencephalon

A pontine and a medullary nucleus are components of the reticular formation that have a major role in the UMN extrapyramidal control of weight support and the generation of gait. Studies in the cat have defined an area of the reticular formation in the pons that exerts a facilitory influence on spinal cord GSE neurons that innervate extensor muscles by way of a reticulospinal tract (see Figs. 2-9 and 2-10).[68,69] This pontine reticulospinal tract courses mostly in the ipsilateral ventral funiculus. Similarly, an area of the medullary reticular formation has an inhibitory influence on spinal cord GSE neurons that innervate extensor muscles by way of a medullary reticulospinal tract that courses primarily in the central portion of the ipsilateral lateral funiculus (see Figs. 2-11 through 2-15). These pontine and medullary reticular formation nuclei are activated predominantly by corticoreticular pathways from the contralateral cerebral hemisphere. These corticoreticular axons cross the midline of the brainstem at the level of the reticular formation nuclei. Most of the axons of the cell bodies in these pontine and medullary reticular formation nuclei make up the pontine reticulospinal tract and the medullary reticulospinal tract that course caudally in the ipsilateral ventral and lateral funiculi, respectively. Thus, this pathway permits one cerebral hemisphere to control predominantly the motor activity in the opposite side of the body. This contralateral influence is observed in both the motor and the sensory systems.

The olivary nucleus is considered an extrapyramidal nucleus in the medulla. It is located ventrally in the medulla from a level caudal to the facial nucleus to a level caudal to the obex and rostral to the pyramidal decussation. It is dorsolateral to the pyramids and medial lemniscus and medial to the hypoglossal axons that are coursing ventrolaterally (see Figs. 2-14 and 2-15). It is composed of three nuclear groups that at some levels have the appearance of fingers directed ventrolaterally. This extrapyramidal nucleus receives afferent axons from many of the extrapyramidal nuclei in the telencephalon, diencephalon, and mesencephalon. Its efferent axons project primarily to the contralateral portion of the cerebellum. These axons leave the olivary nucleus and immediately cross the midline dorsal to the pyramids, intermingle with the axons in the medial lemniscus, and continue rostrally in a dorsolateral position to enter the caudal cerebellar peduncle, where they are distributed to the cerebellum. This is a major source of extrapyramidal system projection to the cerebellum. An extrapyramidal system feedback circuit also exists between the cerebrum and the cerebellum via this olivary nucleus (Fig. 8-11; see also Fig. 13-20).

In this description of the extrapyramidal portion of the UMN, the final motor pathways by which this system exerts influence over the GSE-LMN are the rubrospinal and the pontine and medullary reticulospinal tracts. Many other brainstem tracts also course to the spinal cord and influence muscle tone and activity by their connections in the spinal cord ventral gray columns. These include the vestibulospinal tracts, the medial longitudinal fasciculus, and the tectospinal tract. Some texts include these tracts with the description of the extrapyramidal system. However, in this text they will be considered with the various systems that have their own anatomic components and functional attributes separate from but interrelated with the extrapyramidal system. Most of these tracts influence the GSE-LMN through interneuronal connections in the spinal cord gray matter where these extrapyramidal system tracts terminate. In addition, there are long spinal interneurons that course in both directions in the spinal cord and participate with the UMN in the control of the LMN.

A comparison of the development of the UMN tracts in the human, cat, and horse craniocervical spinal cords reveals the decrease in importance of the pyramidal system (corticospinal tract) and the increase in the contribution of the extrapyramidal system (rubrospinal tract) in the domestic animal (Fig. 8-12).

UPPER MOTOR NEURON FUNCTION

The functions of the UMN can be summarized as follows: (1) the initiation of voluntary activity of the motor system; (2) the maintenance of muscle tone to support the body against gravity and to establish the posture upon which the voluntary activity can be performed; and (3) the control of the muscular activity associated with the visceral functions—respiratory, cardiovascular, and excretory.

Neuromuscular Spindles

Neuromuscular spindles have a significant role in the function of the UMN. This system carries out its function by influencing the activity of the alpha and gamma motor neurons in the ventral gray columns of the spinal cord. The activity of the neuromuscular spindles in modulating muscle tone involves their control over the stretch reflexes in which the neuromuscular spindles play a major role as a sensory organ. These spindle organs are located in the belly of skeletal muscle (Fig. 8-13). They are spindle-shaped structures composed of intrafusal

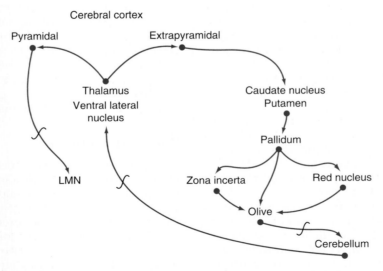

FIGURE 8-11 Schematic diagram of extrapyramidal pathways in the brain.

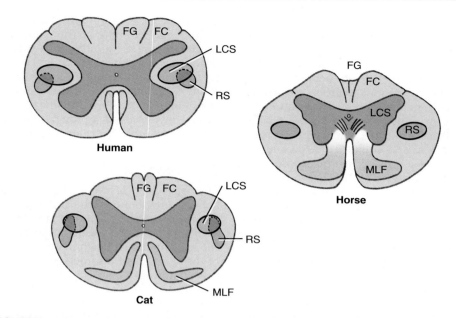

FIGURE 8-12 Comparison of first cervical spinal cord segment in the human, the cat, and the horse. *FC,* Fasciculus cuneatus; *FG,* fasciculus gracilis; *LCS,* lateral corticospinal tract (crossed pyramidal tract); *MLF,* medial longitudinal fasciculus; *RS,* rubrospinal tract.

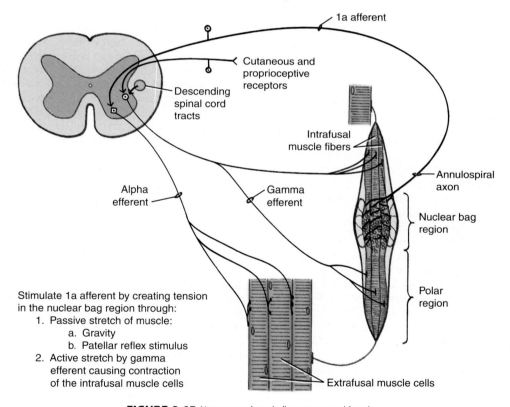

FIGURE 8-13 Neuromuscular spindle anatomy and function.

fibers that are very small, modified striated muscle cells. They are positioned in parallel with the large extrafusal muscle cells in which the spindles are located. A connective tissue capsule encloses the small group of intrafusal fibers and is attached to the endomysium of the adjacent extrafusal fibers. Within the spindle, there are two types of intrafusal fibers. The nuclear bag fiber is interrupted near its middle by a nonstriated dilation containing most of the cell's nuclei. The nuclear chain fiber

has no central dilation, although most of its nuclei are accumulated near the middle of the fiber. These features create for the spindle a central distended nuclear region augmented by a lymph space that envelops the middle portion of the intrafusal fibers. The poles of the spindle are tapered and contain the contractile striated portion of the intrafusal fibers.

The intrafusal fibers are innervated in the polar regions by small myelinated neurons whose cell bodies are in the ventral gray column of the spinal cord intermingled with the larger GSE neurons. These small neurons are called gamma efferent neurons; the larger GSE neurons are referred to as alpha efferent neurons. The gamma efferent neurons are further divided into plate and trail gamma efferent neurons.

The two types of gamma efferent neurons are named according to the forms of their terminations on the intrafusal fiber. The gamma plate neurons terminate on the nuclear bag intrafusal muscle fibers within the neuromuscular spindle. The nuclear bag region is surrounded by the annulospiral dendritic processes of a sensory neuron whose axon is large, and this neuron is classified as 1a. Their cell bodies are in a spinal ganglion, and the axons enter the spinal cord via the dorsal root, where they traverse the dorsal gray column and enter the ventral gray column. There they synapse directly on a GSE alpha motor neuron of an extensor muscle, causing its contraction. This is described as a tonic gamma loop mechanism, and it is responsible for maintaining normal muscle tone. Impulses are stimulated in the annulospiral dendritic zone of the 1a afferent by any action that stretches the nuclear bag region of the spindle. This occurs passively through the stretch of the extensor muscle by gravity or actively through a brief tap on the tendon of the muscle by a blunt instrument, as in the patellar reflex. Active stretching of the nuclear bag results from the contraction of the intrafusal fibers mediated by the gamma efferent neurons.

The gamma trail neurons terminate on the polar areas of the nuclear chain intrafusal fibers in the neuromuscular spindle. Group II sensory neurons innervate the central nuclear region of these fibers, and their dendritic zones respond to the active contraction of the nuclear chain muscle cells. These group II sensory neurons terminate in the spinal cord ventral gray columns on interneurons that are inhibitory to the GSE alpha neurons that innervate flexor muscles. This is referred to as the phasic gamma loop, or flexor reflex gamma loop, and it functions with the UMN to initiate flexor reflexes in the generation of the gait.

Posture is maintained against the steady force of gravity by this neuromuscular spindle activity. The force of gravity stretches extensor muscles and the nuclear bag region of their spindles. The 1a afferent is stimulated; in turn, it stimulates the GSE alpha efferent neuron to cause contraction of the extrafusal fibers of that extensor muscle. Collaterals of the same 1a afferent stimulate interneurons in the ventral gray column that are inhibitory to the GSE neurons that innervate those muscles that are antagonists of the action of the extensor muscle. The activity of this stretch, or myotatic reflex, maintains a constant low-level state of contraction, which provides for muscle tone. Other collaterals of the 1a afferents are involved in cranial projection of general proprioceptive pathways to the cerebellum and somesthetic cortex, which provides these higher centers with information about the state of muscle contraction to be used in the proper coordination of motor activity. The UMN extrapyramidal system influences the activity of these myotatic reflexes by its caudally projecting spinal cord axons that terminate on gamma efferent cell bodies in the ventral gray column.

Golgi tendon organs are the receptors that house the dendritic zones of the 1b sensory neurons that are located in tendons. They have a higher threshold to the stimulus of stretching muscles than the 1a annulospiral afferents. The 1b sensory neurons are stimulated when the tendon is stretched by contraction of the extrafusal fibers in the muscle that are continuous with this tendon. Within the ventral gray column of the spinal cord, the 1b afferent axons synapse on interneurons that are inhibitory to the GSE alpha motor neurons innervating the contracting muscle as well as synapsing on interneurons that are facilitory to the GSE alpha motor neurons innervating the antagonist of this muscle, thus lowering the threshold to stimulus. This inverse myotatic reflex provides for smooth skeletal muscle activity and protects against the overstretching of tendons.

Gait Generation

The interaction of these UMN pathways, the ventral gray column interneurons, the alpha and gamma efferents, and the neuromuscular spindles are all critical factors in postural support and the generation of gait. This is critical for the student and clinician to understand because knowledge of the various gait disorders is the basis for making the correct anatomic diagnosis in the majority of the neurologic disorders in patients.

Locomotion, or gait generation, can be divided into two components: a postural phase and a protraction (swing) phase. The postural phase requires the facilitation of neurons that innervate antigravity extensor muscles. This is the weight-supporting action of muscles. The protraction phase requires the facilitation of neurons that innervate flexor muscles to initiate movement and the facilitation of neurons that innervate extensor muscles to complete the movement. Both of these phases require the UMN recruitment of spinal reflex mechanisms via the activation of what neurophysiologists refer to as the central pattern generators. The central pattern generator is the network of interconnected interneurons in the spinal cord gray matter that modulates motor neuron activity for the generation of gait. These interneurons function between the UMN and the GSE-LMN and between spinal nerve afferents and the GSE-LMN. The role of the UMN in this gait generation is mediated through the central pattern generator. The central pattern generators located in the spinal cord intumescences are the ones most involved with the gait generation.

Although a locomotor pattern can occur as the result of spontaneous activity of the central pattern generator, especially for the pelvic limbs, it is not useful for the patient's locomotion. This is called "spinal walking" and may occur many weeks after a transverse spinal cord lesion that interrupts all of the UMN pathways cranial to that generator. For normal locomotion, the UMN pathways are responsible for stimulating, via the central pattern generators, the appropriate GSE-LMNs that induce the postural and protraction phases of locomotion.

The complexity of this neural arrangement is profound. For learning purposes, it is useful to attempt to translate the arrangements into the functional roles of individual brainstem nuclei and spinal cord tracts, but any such description is obviously an oversimplification of a complex system. In the domestic animal, the roles of the motor cortex of the cerebrum and the corticospinal tracts in locomotion are relatively minimal compared with those roles in primates; this observation is based on the observation that experimental removal of this portion of the cerebrum and natural disorders that interfere with its function do not affect gait generation.

The extrapyramidal system brainstem nuclei caudal to the diencephalon are considered to be the most important

UMN systems necessary for gait generation (Fig. 8-14). The postural phase of the gait is dependent on the activation of antigravity extensor muscles and the inhibition of the flexor muscles. This is the responsibility of the pontine reticular formation nuclei and pontine reticulospinal tracts. The vestibulospinal tract also contributes to this function. The initiation of protraction requires the activation of flexor muscles and the inhibition of extensor muscles to elevate the limb from the ground. This is a function of the medullary reticular formation nuclei and their medullary reticulospinal tracts and of the red nuclei and the rubrospinal tracts. As the protraction phase is completed, the activation of these systems shifts back to the activation of extensors muscles and inhibition of flexor muscles. Further support for the role of the UMN system in locomotion is provided by observation of the results of experimental or natural lesions.

Experimental lesions that selectively destroy the motor cortex, the lentiform nucleus, or the caudate nucleus do not affect gait generation. Experimental or natural lesions that destroy the frontoparietal cortex or the adjacent portion of the internal capsule do not interfere with gait generation, but the postural reactions are deficient in the contralateral (opposite-side) limbs. However, the components of the UMN system affected here are mixed with components of the conscious portion of the general proprioceptive (GP) system, which are also necessary for postural reactions to be normal. We consider that cerebral lesions do not interfere with gait generation but do result in delayed hopping responses in the contralateral limbs as a result of the loss of function of both the UMN and the conscious GP systems located there. This should not be referred to solely as a hemiparesis because the GP system is also involved in the lesion. Case examples are described after the discussion of the GP sensory system in Chapter 9. The only exception to this is that with acute, especially traumatic, cerebral lesions, mild contralateral hemiparesis and loss of general proprioception may be observed in the gait for 2 to 3 days following the onset of the lesion. After that, the gait will be normal, but the contralateral postural reactions will be deficient.

Progressing caudally in the brainstem, experimental surgical ablation of one red nucleus does not induce any gait interference. However, most natural lesions that involve the red nucleus in the midbrain on one side also affect the adjacent pontine reticular formation, which interferes with gait generation and causes hemiparesis. When the lesion affects the pontine and medullary reticular formation UMN nuclei or tracts, the hemiparesis is observed in the ipsilateral (same-side) limbs. Lesions on one side of the medulla or cervical spinal cord cranial to the C5 segment that affect the UMN cause a similar ipsilateral hemiparesis or hemiplegia.

Inquisitive students always ask: Where do unilateral lesions shift from affecting primarily the contralateral limbs to affecting the ipsilateral limbs? We do not know the exact level but believe that it is close to the caudal midbrain. Unilateral prosencephalic UMN lesions cause no loss of gait generation but do cause deficient postural reactions in the contralateral limbs. UMN lesions in the brainstem caudal to the midbrain cause gait deficit, ipsilateral hemiparesis, and postural reaction deficits in those limbs. A severe unilateral caudal medullary UMN lesion may cause ipsilateral hemiplegia. An infarct

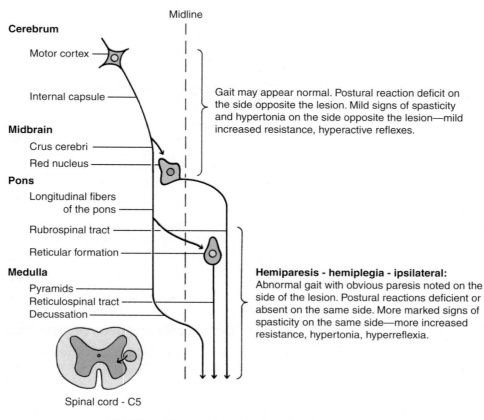

FIGURE 8-14 Diagram of UMN pathways for voluntary movement.

in one side of the cervical spinal cord cranial to the C5 segment caused by fibrocartilaginous emboli will cause complete UMN paralysis—spastic hemiplegia of the ipsilateral limbs. Case examples are presented in Chapter 10, Small Animal Spinal Cord Disease.

CLINICAL SIGNS OF UPPER MOTOR NEURON DISEASE

Paresis

Disorders that interfere with the ability of the UMN to initiate gait generation result in paresis. Paresis by definition is weakness, but the quality of this UMN paresis differs significantly from the quality of LMN paresis. Incomplete LMN disorders interfere with the ability of the patient to support weight but not with initiation of the gait. These patients hop fast if their weight is held up, and they have enough LMN function to try to hop. UMN disorders result in a delay in protraction of the limb when trying to walk or hop or in the complete absence of any protraction.

Subacute or chronic lesions of the prosencephalon do not affect the gait, but postural reactions are delayed in the limbs that are contralateral to a unilateral lesion. This delay in postural reactions is due to the interference with both the prosencephalic UMN pathways and the conscious pathway for GP. It is common to read descriptions that refer to this as a hemiparesis. This is incorrect because the GP system is also involved, and it is misleading because the gait is normal. We believe that the terms *hemiparesis* and *ataxia* should be used only when the gait is abnormal and not when the only abnormality observed is a delay in the postural reactions. In peracute (being hit by a car or receiving a gunshot wound, or following surgery or infarction) unilateral frontoparietal lesions, there is a mild visible contralateral hemiparesis and ataxia for 2 to 3 days following the injury. After that, the gait is normal on a level surface, but the postural reactions are delayed. These latter clinical signs should be described as normal gait with abnormal postural reactions.

Spasticity

The UMN pathways contain axons that are responsible for both activation and inhibition of extensor and flexor muscles via the central pattern generators. However, most lesions that affect the UMN result in the release of antigravity extensor muscles from inhibition, which supports the major role of the UMN in this inhibitory activity. The release of extensor motor neurons from inhibition results in hypertonia, or spasticity, of the extensor muscles. This can be observed in the stiff nature of the impaired gait and the increased resistance to passive manipulation of the limbs. Thus, the quality of UMN paresis is spastic paresis or paralysis. Recall that in LMN disorders, there is a flaccid paresis or paralysis. A classic example of what happens when the LMN never receives any UMN influence is described in Chapter 3 in the section on spinal cord malformations. See Video 3-4, which shows the Simmenthal calf that has no cranial lumbar spinal cord; note the extreme pelvic limb spasticity and the stereotypic spinal reflex walking movements. This certainly emphasizes the role of the UMN in the inhibition of antigravity extensor motor neurons.

Hyperreflexia

The same release from inhibition can be seen in the spinal reflexes, especially the patellar tendon reflex, in which it is more brisk than normal or occasionally is repetitive after a single stimulus, known as clonus. Flexor reflexes may be hyperactive or even be repetitive following a single noxious stimulus. The crossed extensor reflex is another form of release from inhibition due to a UMN disorder. This is normal in a standing animal and is used to support weight when the weight is taken off the opposite limb. It is abnormal when present in a recumbent animal but is easily confused with voluntary movement if the animal is able to struggle to move away from a noxious stimulus. It is best observed in a patient that has a serious enough UMN lesion to result in the absence of any voluntary movement. This abnormal reflex is seen when a mild noxious stimulus causes flexion of the limb stimulated and extension of the opposite limb or crossed extension. In our opinion, the presence of this reflex is just another clinical sign of UMN disinhibition and has no prognostic value. In severely disinhibited lumbosacral LMNs, a single noxious stimulus may induce what is referred to as a mass reflex. Following a single noxious stimulus to a digit, that limb or both pelvic limbs repeatedly flex three or four times, and the tail may flex without further stimuli. A single noxious stimulus to the tail may elicit repeated tail and pelvic limb flexion and even urination.

With UMN lesions, the quality of the paresis varies with the severity of the lesion and the specific tracts involved in the lesion. In most situations, if there is no disturbance to the gray matter of the intumescences, the spinal cord lesion that affects the UMN results in normal to hyperactive spinal reflexes and normal to increased muscle tone in the limbs caudal to the lesion. Any atrophy that occurs in chronic lesions is caused only by disuse. Many case examples of patients with spinal cord disease are presented in Chapters 10 and 11.

Release from Inhibition

A fundamental principle of the development of neurons is their ability to generate and transmit electrochemical impulses to other neurons or to effector organs. This fundamental activity requires significant inhibition to result in smooth, regulated muscle action. A complete loss of this inhibition at the prosencephalic level results in a seizure, which is the ultimate example of uncontrolled-uninhibited release of neuronal activity. Other examples of less fulminating uninhibited spontaneous neural discharge include decerebrate or decerebellate rigidity, tetanus, and tetany that represent uninhibited innervation of antigravity muscles and various forms of myoclonus and movement disorders. The extrapyramidal system plays a major role in most of these examples of spontaneous involuntary muscle contractions.

Decerebrate and Decerebellate Rigidity

The classic example used by neurophysiologists to demonstrate the role of the extrapyramidal system in the control of motor tone is the phenomenon of decerebrate rigidity. When the brainstem is transected between the rostral and caudal colliculi of the midbrain, an uninhibited extensor tonus of the antigravity muscles is produced. The head and neck are markedly extended dorsally, which is known as opisthotonus, and all four limbs in the quadriped are rigidly extended. This is explained as a release mechanism. The myotatic reflexes involving the extensor muscle LMNs have been released from the effects of the descending inhibitory UMN pathways. The facilitory centers in the pontomedullary reticular formation and the vestibular system can function autonomously, whereas the inhibitory centers in the pontomedullary reticular formation require continual input from the cerebral cortex, basal nuclei, and cerebellum in order to function. This experimental midbrain transection removes all of the prosencephalic input, causing the imbalance that is observed as a release phenomenon or decerebrate rigidity. The alpha and gamma LMNs that innervate extensor muscles have been released from the influence of the caudally projecting UMN spinal cord tracts. The vestibulospinal tracts also contribute their facilitory influence to that of the reticulospinal tracts. A similar release phenomenon occurs after surgical ablation of portions of the cerebellum, especially those that include the rostral vermis and adjacent hemisphere. In this decerebellate rigidity, there is opisthotonus and extensor rigidity of the thoracic limbs, but the pelvic limbs are often held in extension though flexed at the hips (Fig. 8-15). Brainstem lesions that cause decerebrate rigidity also usually involve the ascending reticular activating system and cause serious deficits in the patient's sensorium, including coma, whereas a patient with a rostral cerebellar vermal lesion that causes decerebellate rigidity has a normal sensorium. It is our experience that most natural disorders that result in opisthotonus and extensor rigidity involve the cerebellum more than the brainstem but many involve both areas. When presented with a patient that has opisthotonus and some degree of extensor rigidity, you can reliably assume that some portion of the lesion involves structures in the caudal cranial fossa, with the exception of a patient with tetanus, which is described later.

Video 8-1 shows an 8-year-old male working mixed-breed coonhound with a history of 3 to 4 weeks of progressive loss of his normal performance that began with difficulty in using the pelvic limbs and progressed to the thoracic limbs. At the time he was presented for examination, he was unable to get up. Note his severe disorientation and his tendency to assume a posture of opisthotonus associated with extensor rigidity of his limbs. Occasionally the pelvic limbs are held in a flexed hip position. His spastic tetraparesis is worse on the left side. His abnormal nystagmus is caused by the involvement of the vestibular system in the lesion. The anatomic diagnosis was a disorder of the structures located in the caudal cranial fossa: the cerebellum, pons, and medulla. The major disorders to be considered in the differential diagnosis of this progressive syndrome include neoplasia and inflammation (granulomatous meningoencephalitis; viral, protozoal, and fungal infection; abscess). Radiographs showed an extramedullary mass lesion centered in the tentorium cerebelli. At necropsy this was diagnosed as a osteogenic sarcoma that severely compressed the central region of the cerebellum and the underlying pons and medulla. See Case Example 21-3 for a complete description of this case and photos of the radiograph and lesion.

See Figure 8-15, which shows an 8-month-old brown Swiss heifer that, in the course of 24 hours, became blind, paretic, and ataxic, and by 36 hours had become recumbent and obtunded and assumed the posture of decerebellate rigidity seen here. The anatomic diagnosis is a diffuse brain disorder. This heifer has a diffuse metabolic encephalopathy due to a thiamin deficiency; the lesion is referred to as polioencephalomalacia. This posture is caused by the effects of the metabolic disorder on the antigravity inhibitory mechanisms in the cerebellum, pons, and medulla.

Extrapyramidal Nuclear Lesions

There is limited information about specific clinical signs that relate to diseases that cause focal extrapyramidal nuclear lesions. Students often ask, for example, what happens when the caudate nucleus or the substantia nigra is destroyed, and we do not have a reliable answer other than that there may be some disturbance of the motor systems or no clinical signs at all. We offer three motor-type disturbances for consideration.

1. A propulsive activity. A common sign of prosencephalic disorders is the occurrence of propulsive activity, usually continuous pacing in a circle or standing with the head and neck turned to one side, pleurothotonus. Usually these animals turn or circle in the direction of the side of a unilateral prosencephalic lesion but not always. This is sometimes referred to as the adversive syndrome, meaning the tendency to turn toward the lesion. The specific location of the lesion responsible for this propulsive action is unknown. Most are in the frontal or parietal lobe or the rostral thalamic region and are thought to involve a disturbance in the normal circuitry from the cerebral cortex to the basal nuclei to the thalamus and back to the cerebral cortex. Substantia nigra lesions are occasionally reported to produce this kind of propulsive activity.

2. A movement disorder. These disorders are described in the next section in the discussion of uncontrolled involuntary muscle contractions. Their pathogenesis is poorly understood, but a disturbance in the motor circuitry as just described is often implicated in the origin of these movement disorders.

3. Nigropallidal encephalomalacia. This is a disorder observed only in horses when two groups of extrapyramidal nuclei

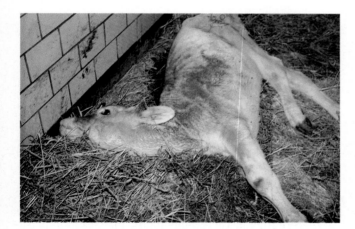

FIGURE 8-15 A brown Swiss heifer exhibiting the clinical signs of decerebellate rigidity with opisthotonus and extensor rigidity of the limbs and with hip flexion due to diffuse metabolic encephalopathy caused by thiamin deficiency. The brain lesion is referred to as polioencephalomalacia.

undergo necrosis.[23] Horses that consume the plant called yellow star thistle *(Centaurea solstitialis)* or Russian knapweed *(Centaurea repens)* for a period of a few weeks suddenly develop acute bilateral necrosis of the substantia nigra and globus pallidus (Figs. 8-16 and 8-17). Most of the clinical signs observed involve dysfunction in prehension and swallowing due to spastic paresis of the jaw, lips, and pharyngeal muscles. These horses become depressed and inactive and die of starvation. Occasionally there may be some mild propulsive activity of the head muscles, but no gait propulsion or movement disorder is observed. A toxic compound has been identified in

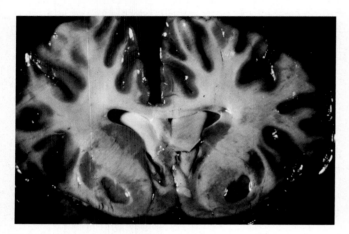

FIGURE 8-16 Transverse section of the cerebrum of an adult horse with nigropallidal encephalomalacia. Note the bilateral cavitation where necrosis occurred in the pallidum.

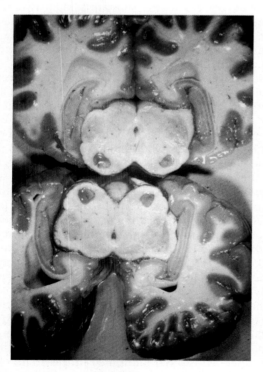

FIGURE 8-17 Transverse section of the brain at the level of the mesencephalon in an adult horse with nigropallidal encephalomalacia. Note the bilateral cavitation where necrosis occurred in the substantia nigra.

C. solstitialis that is similar to dopaminergic neurotoxins that have been studied in humans.[75] This bilateral nuclear necrosis is readily diagnosed by magnetic resonance (MR) imaging.[76]

UNCONTROLLED INVOLUNTARY SKELETAL MUSCLE CONTRACTIONS

In human neurology, any discussion of the extrapyramidal system nuclei includes a consideration of numerous movement disorders. Some of these are well-defined degenerative diseases such as Huntington chorea with caudate nuclei lesions or Parkinson disease with substantia nigra lesions. Many of these uncontrolled spontaneous movements are poorly understood, and there is no adequate classification scheme that can be applied to veterinary medicine. The following is a classification of uncontrolled involuntary muscle contractions that we have developed for veterinary medicine.[26] These are uncontrolled spontaneous contractions of voluntary skeletal muscle that occur involuntarily in the conscious patient. This classification excludes contractions that are part of a seizure disorder. We are well aware that some movement disorders are difficult to differentiate from simple partial seizures in which the patient is still conscious. In addition, although we have included this group of disorders in the UMN chapter, some of these disorders involve primarily other areas of the nervous system and muscle. Box 8-1 shows an outline of this classification.

BOX 8-1 Uncontrolled Involuntary Skeletal Muscle Contractions

I. Muscle
  A. Myotonia
II. Nervous system
  A. Tetanus
  B. Tetany
  C. Myoclonus
    1. Sporadic
    2. Repetitive
      a. Constant
      b. Action-related
        (1) Congenital
        (2) Acquired
      c. Postural
      d. Episodic
      e. Resting
  D. Movement disorder

Muscle

Disorders of the muscle cell membrane may result in persistent repetitive muscle cell contractions without relaxation following a physiologic stimulus. This is the definition of myotonia. It represents a muscle cell membrane disorder. There are inherited and acquired forms of myotonia.

Inherited Congenital Myotonia

The inherited forms of myotonia are often referred to as congenital myotonia, but the myotonic signs are not necessarily present at birth. They usually are first observed at a few weeks of age. From a historical viewpoint, the most well-known myotonia is that which occurs in the goat; it has been recognized since the late 1800s but was not diagnosed as myotonia until the mid-20th century.[14,15] The sudden onset of diffuse extensor muscle rigidity following an abrupt stimulus that often caused collapse of the patient was incorrectly referred to as fainting disease or epilepsy. This disorder is now known to be the result of a sarcolemmal chloride channel defect inherited as an autosomal dominant gene with incomplete penetrance. The clinical signs first occur at a few weeks of age and do not progress significantly. The degree of myotonia is variable; some goats collapse and others remain standing during the brief episode. Unique to this caprine disorder is that following the episode of myotonia, the affected goat completely recovers and remains refractory to another episode for about 30 minutes. Descriptions in the 1800s did not define the breeds involved but mentioned only that they were common in the central eastern states of Tennessee and Kentucky. Today, this disorder is most common in the Pygmy breed. This caprine myotonia is similar to the inherited myotonia of humans known as Thomsen disease. A similar myotonia has been reported in Shropshire lambs, and I (Alexander de Lahunta) have observed it in a Montadale lamb.

Video 8-2 shows a 1-year-old Pygmy goat that exhibited myotonia when startled after a period of rest but was able to remain standing. **Video 8-3** shows a 4-month-old female Montadale lamb with more severe myotonic episodes that caused collapse. Note the rapid recovery. Neurologic examinations were always normal. When this ewe was 1 month old, the owner noted that the lamb would walk with a stiff gait when she first got up. More recently, when she was bumped by an adult, she would fall over, with all four limbs extended, in a way that is similar to what you observe in this video.

In the dog, the two most common breeds in which this inherited form of myotonia occurs are the chow chow and the miniature schnauzer.[31,91,92] Very thorough studies by Dr. Charles Vite at the University of Pennsylvania of the miniature schnauzer disorder determined this to be due to a sarcolemmal chloride channel abnormality that is inherited as an autosomal recessive gene. The offending gene has been identified, and a polymerase chain reaction test is currently in use to determine the carrier dogs. **Video 8-4** shows three 6-month-old miniature schnauzer littermates that exhibit this inherited form of myotonia. Note their hesitancy to come out of the cage, which suggests that they are aware that this will cause a myotonic episode. Also note that the clinical signs nearly resolve briefly while they move around the kennel. (We thank Dr. Charles Vite for this video.)

Affected chow chows were first described in Australia and subsequently have been diagnosed worldwide with this disorder, but the physiologic and genomic basis remains to be determined.[31] In both of these breeds of dogs, like the goat and sheep, the myotonia can be elicited by a sudden movement by the relaxed animal, especially if the resting animal is startled. Unlike the goats and sheep, the dogs do not fully recover between episodes, and a variable degree of stiffness

persists in the gait. This is more obvious in the chow chows than in the miniature schnauzers. **Video 8-5** shows Tonie, a 4-month-old chow chow with this inherited myotonia. Note how severe the myotonia is when he first comes out of the cage on being aroused in the morning after a night's rest. A brief period of apnea may occur at this time. The clinical signs rapidly improve but never disappear as they do in the goats and sheep. His coat was clipped to show off the remarkable muscle hypertrophy that is common in this disorder (Figs. 8-18 through 8-20). In some dogs, treatment with procainamide or mexiletine may provide some relief, but the clinical signs will not resolve. A similar early-onset myotonia that may be inherited has been reported in other breeds of dogs, in the domestic shorthair cat, and in the horse.[60,83,85] Cats are diffusely affected, whereas some forms

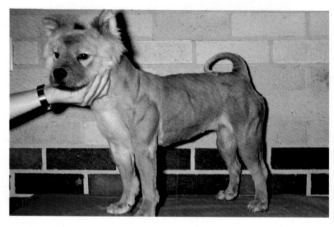

FIGURE 8-18 A 1-year-old chow chow with congenital myotonia. Note the remarkable whole-body muscle hypertrophy.

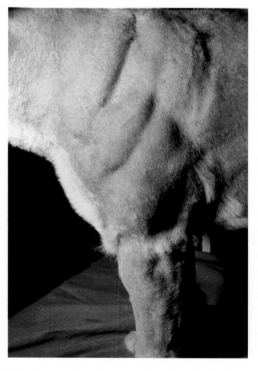

FIGURE 8-19 Close-up view of the muscle hypertrophy in the thoracic limb of the dog in Fig. 8-18.

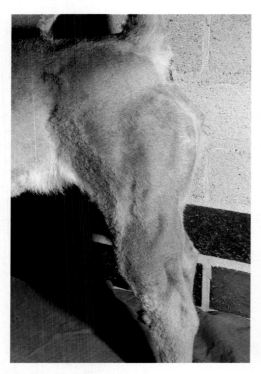

FIGURE 8-20 Close-up view of the muscle hypertrophy in the pelvic limb of the dog in Figs. 8-18 and 8-19.

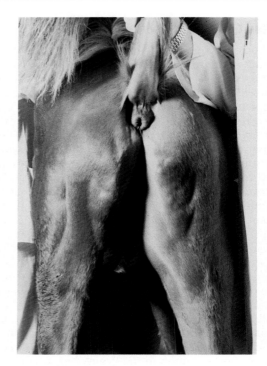

FIGURE 8-22 Another view of the horse in Fig. 8-21.

of myotonia in the horse are very mild and are most obvious in the caudal thigh muscles, where dimpling is readily produced and persists (Figs. 8-21 and 8-22). This focal muscle dimpling produced by tapping the surface of the body is a characteristic feature of myotonia. Myotonia also occurs in horses with inherited hyperkalemic periodic paralysis.[81]

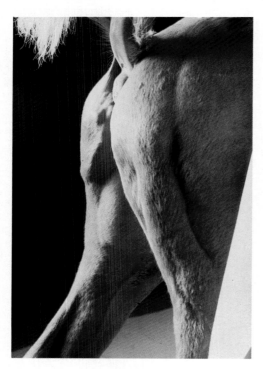

FIGURE 8-21 An 8-month-old standardbred with congenital myotonia that caused myotonic dimples in the caudal thigh muscles.

Video 8-6 shows Rascal, a 4-month-old male domestic shorthair kitten that has always walked with a stiff gait and has very large muscles that can be appreciated only by handling this kitten. The diagnosis of myotonia is supported by electromyography (EMG) studies during which you can see the characteristic myotonic discharges on the oscilloscope and hear their waxing and waning dive-bomber-like sounds. Serum muscle enzymes are normal in these cats. A female half sister of this kitten had the same disorder. An autosomal recessive inheritance is suspected but not proven in the domestic shorthair cat.[85] In male cats that are a few months of age, there is a muscular dystrophy that causes a similar slow, stiff gait and remarkable muscle hypertrophy. However, this is a disease that involves muscle cell necrosis, and the serum muscle enzymes are all significantly elevated. This dystrophinopathy is described in Chapter 5.

A form of congenital myotonia that may be inherited has been observed in Brazilian Murrha buffalo by Dr. Alex Borges at São Paulo State University and Jose Barbosa at Para University, Brazil. These cattle are similar to the goat in that when the myotonic episodes occur, they may fall but the fall is followed by complete recovery for a short period of time before another episode may occur. Muscle hypertrophy is remarkable as these calves grow. The genomic basis for this disorder is currently under study. **Video 8-7A** shows three heifers with this disorder and **Video 8-7B** shows a similarly affected calf.

A form of myotonia may contribute to the gait abnormality observed in a number of myopathic disorders for which paresis is the most significant clinical sign. An example of this is the dystrophinopathy that is inherited in male golden retrievers and has been seen in numerous breeds as an X-linked recessive spontaneous mutation.[51,87] This disorder is described in Chapter 5 and can be seen in Videos 5-16, 5-17, and 5-18, which show affected golden retrievers.

Myotonia may contribute to the stiffness seen in young farm animals that have dietary deficiencies of vitamin E or selenium (see Case Example 5-22).

Acquired Myotonia

Acquired myotonia is most commonly observed in older dogs with hyperadrenocorticoidism that can be caused by a pituitary abnormality, an adrenal cortical neoplasm, or prolonged corticosteroid administration.[36] The myopathic disorder causes a persistent characteristic gait stiffness associated with significant muscle hypertrophy. Complex repetitive discharges, or pseudomyotonia, are observed on EMG evaluation. On EMG, this form of myotonia starts and stops abruptly, without the waxing and waning that is seen in "true" myotonia. The pathophysiology of the muscle disorder responsible for this is not well understood. Considering the large number of dogs that have hyperadrenocorticoidism, this clinical entity is relatively rare. If untreated, the disorder can progress to become severe enough to make the patient be unable to stand and walk. In addition, treatment of hyperadrenocorticoidism does not necessarily result in recovery from this muscle disorder. This is a good example of a gait disorder that fits the saying "seeing is believing." The following videos show dogs with this myopathic disorder. All of these dogs had long histories over many months of slowly progressive gait stiffness that was diagnosed as unexplained lameness and was commonly blamed on chronic arthritis. The dogs were treated with corticosteroids! As a rule, these dogs are referred to a specialty practice without a diagnosis.

Video 8-8: Porky is a 9-year-old castrated male miniature poodle.

Video 8-9: Tangy is an 8.5-year-old dachshund.

Video 8-10: Sarah is a 13-year-old female dachshund.

Video 8-11: Zetti is a 12-year-old miniature poodle.

Video 8-12: Taffy is a 7-year-old miniature poodle. At the end of this video is the EMG study. Listen to the abrupt start and stop of the complex repetitive discharges.

Nervous System

Neuronal causes of involuntary skeletal muscle contractions involve spontaneous uncontrolled discharge of motor neurons. The resulting clinical signs can be grouped into four categories: tetanus, tetany, myoclonus, and movement disorders.

Tetanus

Physiologic tetanus is the clinical sign of sustained contraction of muscles without relaxation that most commonly affects extensor (antigravity) muscles. The degree of persistent extensor muscle contraction is variable among patients and is due to the disinhibition of extensor motor neurons. This clinical sign is most commonly caused by the neurotoxin produced by infection with the bacterium *Clostridium tetani*. This toxin interferes with the interneuronal release of the inhibitory neurotransmitter glycine in the spinal cord ventral gray column and gamma-aminobutyric acid in brainstem motor nuclei. By strict definition tetanus is a clinical sign, although the term is commonly used for the

disease caused by infection by *C. tetani* and its production of tetanospasmin. The clinical sign of tetanus also occurs in the thoracic limbs of Australian cattle dogs that have an inherited polioencephalomyelopathy due to degeneration of interneurons in the cervical intumescence.[13] See Case Example 21-12.

The disease tetanus occurs in all domestic animals and humans. Be sure that your vaccination status is current! *C. tetani* produces spores that are very resistant and can persist for long periods in the environment. When spores gain entrance to an anaerobic environment in an animal's tissues, they convert to the vegetative form and produce a neurotoxin, tetanospasmin, in 4 to 8 hours. An area of tissue damage resulting from trauma or surgery is ideal for this production. The toxin gains access to motor neurons at their telodendrons at the neuromuscular junctions and binds to the axonal gangliosides, where it is transported to the spinal cord within a few hours.[77,82] The toxin passes from the GSE neuronal cell bodies to the adjacent inhibitory neurons at their synaptic sites. There the toxin binds to and enters the interneuron, called a Renshaw cell. This toxin is a zinc endopeptidase that cleaves the cell membrane protein necessary for the release of the inhibitory neurotransmitter and therefore blocks the release of the inhibitory neurotransmitter, glycine or gamma-aminobutyric acid. The toxin usually remains bound to the interneuron for 3 or more weeks. In most cases the toxin spreads rapidly within the CNS, or the toxin may circulate through the vascular system to neuromuscular junctions and thereby gain access to other areas of the CNS. Although this tetanospasmin can bind to other neurons, the major site is on the inhibitory interneurons that synapse on the alpha motor neurons that innervate the antigravity extensor muscles. The site where clinical signs first are seen usually reflects where the toxin first gained entrance to the CNS. If the infection occurred in a wound in the pelvic limb, the clinical signs will first occur in that pelvic limb, followed rapidly by signs in the opposite pelvic limb, then the trunk and thoracic limbs, and finally the neck and head. If a puppy becomes infected in a wound in its mouth, the clinical signs of tetanus will occur in the head and neck first and spread caudally from there. In most cases the clinical signs reflect diffuse and rapid spread of the toxin in the CNS. However, occasionally the clinical signs remain localized to the area where the toxin first entered the CNS. This is called focal tetanus, which you can observe in some of the case examples that follow this brief description of the disease.

Usually clinical signs occur about 5 to 10 days after wound infection.[16] In the most severe form of the disease, the animal is recumbent, with opisthotonus and extensor rigidity in all four limbs (Fig. 8-23), rigid facial and masticatory muscles that prevent prehension, and mouth opening, called lock jaw. In humans, the facial expression created by the tetanic facial muscles is referred to as risus sardonicus, which means "scornful laughter" (Figs. 8-24 through 8-26). Rarely, the CNS neuronal disinhibition causes a seizure. Death occurs as the result of tetanus of the respiratory muscles. In mild diffuse tetanus, the patient remains standing, with its neck and tail extended and its ears and lips drawn back in contraction; it walks slowly, with a very stiff gait (Fig. 8-27). There is no ataxia because the toxin has no effect on sensory systems or the cerebellum. Spasms of the extraocular muscles that cause the eyeball to retract

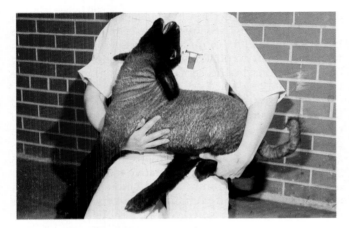

FIGURE 8-23 Tetanus in a young lamb, causing opisthotonus and extensor rigidity of the limbs.

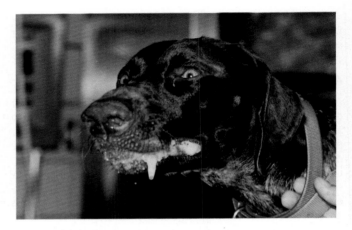

FIGURE 8-26 Risus sardonicus in a coonhound with tetanus.

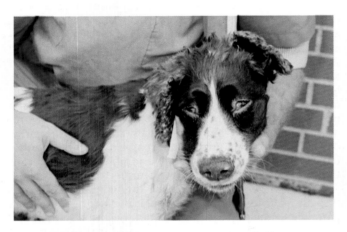

FIGURE 8-24 Risus sardonicus in a Brittany spaniel with tetanus.

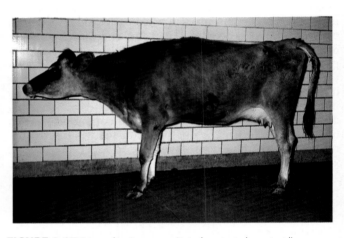

FIGURE 8-27 Tetanus in a Jersey cow. Note the retracted ears, taut lips, extended neck, and elevated tail.

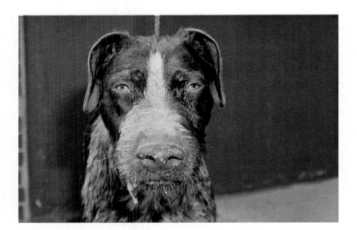

FIGURE 8-25 Risus sardonicus in an Airedale terrier with tetanus.

result in protrusion of the third eyelid. This is often the initial clinical sign observed by owners of dogs with tetanus.[16] This is especially evident in horses, in which it can readily be elicited by a menacing gesture. Bloat may occur in cattle. All of these clinical signs are exacerbated by activity or excitement, and the rate of axonal transport is thought to be increased by neuronal activity.

Although this disease occurs in all domestic animals, the horse appears to be the most susceptible and the dog and cat the least susceptible.[4,50] It is commonly fatal in horses and young farm animals. Treatment should consist of rest in a quiet environment. It may also help to plug the patient's ears with cotton to avoid distractions and excitement. Sedation of the patient may be helpful. Examine the patient carefully for the infected wound, which commonly cannot be found. In cattle, a common site of infection is the uterus, with metritis. Any external wound should be débrided and the patient should receive antibiotics and antitoxin locally and intravenously. The antitoxin has little effect on the toxin that has already bound to the interneurons, but it should prevent further neurotoxin from entering the nervous system. Supportive nursing care is critical to keep the patient adequately nourished and to assist with the excretions. You must be patient, because it may take weeks for recovery to occur. The following videos show examples of tetanus in various species of domestic animals.

Video 8-13 shows Krystal, a 3-month-old female rottweiler, that over 7 days progressed from exhibiting an abnormally stiff facial expression to stiffness in the thoracic limbs to stiffness in the pelvic limbs to recumbency. The video was made on the ninth day of clinical signs. The portion of the video in which you see her brought out of the cage the second time was made 1 week after the first portion. Note the return of function in the pelvic limbs. The last portion of the video, showing Krystal outdoors, was made 6 days later. Note the recovery of function in all limbs but the persistence of the facial muscle signs. The progress of recovery reversed the initial progress of the clinical signs. No wound was found, but the progression of clinical signs suggests that the source of infection may have been infection of an oral cavity lesion possibly related to teething or chewing a sharp object. Younger dogs that develop tetanus are more likely to have more severe clinical signs than older dogs. In a study of 35 dogs with tetanus, the 28-day survival rate was 77%.[15]

Video 8-14 shows Chopper, an adult male mongrel farm dog who, after being missed for a few days, was found in an empty holding tank. In trying to climb out of the steel tank, he had injured all of his paws. They were treated, and about 1 week later he developed a stiff gait, as seen in this video. Note the absence of ataxia! Note the stiffness of the entire body. Note the involvement of the head muscles for facial expression and jaw function. He slowly improved and had recovered in about 3 weeks.

Video 8-15 shows Tags, a 4-month--old spayed female Australian shepherd with 4 days of progressively stiff gait and no evidence of any ataxia. She recovered over the next 3 weeks.

Video 8-16A shows Charlie, a 1-year-old male Shetland sheepdog that over 24 hours became unable to use his left thoracic limb, and 24 hours later he lost the use of his right thoracic limb. See the owner's video and note that both thoracic limbs exhibit tetanus. This video was made 4 weeks after the sudden onset of these clinical signs, and there had been no change. **Video 8-16B** shows Charlie and a control dog playing in the snow. This video was made 6 weeks after Video 8-16A. The last portion of Video 16B, where Charlie is indoors again, was made 6 weeks later, and you can see that he has recovered the use of his right thoracic limb and occasionally uses his left thoracic limb. His recovery from this focal form of tetanus took about 5 months.

Video 8-17 shows Scout, a 6-month-old castrated male domestic shorthair that rapidly developed the signs you see on this video 7 days after surgery for castration. Note the tetanus confined to the pelvic limbs and trunk, which correlates with infection of the surgical wound. His clinical signs did not progress any further, and he recovered over the next 2 to 3 weeks.

Videos 8-18A and 8-18B show Gunner, an adult castrated male domestic shorthair that was attacked by a dog and severely bitten in the left pelvic limb. These wounds were treated surgically and about 2 weeks later the owner observed an abnormal posture of the left pelvic limb. The video was made 1 month after the surgery. This is another example of focal tetanus related to the site of infection. Gunner recovered completely 1 month after this video was made, or 6 weeks after the clinical signs were first observed.

Video 8-19 shows an adult horse exhibiting the clinical signs of tetanus. Note the stiff gait without any ataxia, the stiff neck, elevated tail, abnormal ear posture, and third eyelid elevation, which is seen when the head was elevated. This horse died a few days after this video was made.

Video 8-20 shows a 1-month-old Holstein that developed a stiff gait and became recumbent over a few days. This calf died a few days later of respiratory distress and arrest.

Video 8-21 shows a 1-month-old lamb exhibiting the clinical signs of tetanus. Note the tail-docking surgical wound, which was probably the site of infection and the source of the neurotoxin tetanospasmin. This lamb expired a few days later.

Tetany

Tetany is the clinical sign of sustained contraction of muscles, usually extensors, that is variably intermittent and is related to varying degrees of relaxation of affected muscles. In strychnine intoxication, the toxin interferes with the release of the inhibitory neurotransmitter glycine from spinal cord interneurons, but the degree of extensor muscle contraction varies in the affected patient. This is tetany because the extensor muscle contraction decreases in the relaxed patient but can be exacerbated by any abrupt stimulation that causes the patient to move suddenly.

An inherited congenital tetany occurs in polled Hereford calves.[7,20,43] The tetany is present at birth and causes the calf to be recumbent. These calves always maintain a degree of increased extensor muscle contraction, but any stimulus induces a marked degree of extensor rigidity of the limbs and trunk. Opisthotonus is uncommon. When picked up, these calves have the appearance of and the feel of a wooden sawhorse (Fig. 8-28). This disorder is common in Australia, where Dr. Peter Harper and his colleagues have identified a mutation in the gene responsible for the assembly of the alpha-1 subunit of the glycine receptor on spinal cord extensor motor neuronal cell membranes.[71] This genetic mutation is inherited as an autosomal recessive gene. The abnormal glycine receptors are the basis for the disinhibition seen in these calves. The studies of the pathogenesis of this tetanic disorder are exemplary but unfortunately, the disorder has been labeled as an inherited congenital bovine myoclonus. It is our opinion that this is an inappropriate use of the term *myoclonus*, which we define later. We believe these calves have inherited congenital tetany. **Video 8-22** shows a 6-week-old polled Hereford that has exhibited this inherited tetany since birth.

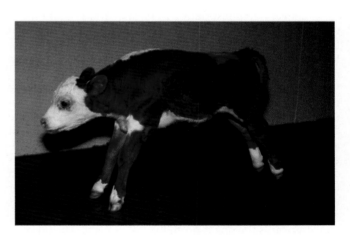

FIGURE 8-28 Newborn Hereford calf with inherited congenital tetany after being placed in a standing position and unable to move.

A neurologic disorder similar to that in these polled Hereford calves occurs in related families of Labrador retrievers and has been described as "familial reflex myoclonus."[33] We believe the clinical sign exhibited by these affected puppies is tetany. **Video 8-23** shows two affected Labrador retriever puppies of a litter of eight produced by the mating of a father and daughter. An autosomal recessive inheritance is suspected but not proven. In addition to litters of this breed, we have observed similar clinical signs of congenital tetany in a litter of cocker spaniels and in lambs. None of these animals have any recognizable structural disorder on microscopic examination of the nervous system. Glycine receptor studies have not been performed on these dogs. A similar inherited glycine receptor abnormality is described in humans as a cause of startle disease, or hyperexplexia.[79] In these patients, an external stimulus usually induces sudden contraction of primarily antigravity muscles.

A presumptive inherited tetany has been published as a myoclonus in Peruvian pasos, in which a deficiency of spinal cord neuronal glycine receptor function was determined.[40] The tetanic episodes and occasionally just myoclonus are stimulus induced. Some of these foals are able to stand and walk. The glycine deficiency has been determined to be worse in the more severely affected recumbent animals.

A form of congenital tetany occurs in newborn Egyptian Arabian foals that have a color-dilution hair coat.[30,65] Breeders have referred to this as the "lavender Arabian foal syndrome," and it is considered lethal. These foals are recumbent at birth and have normal sensorium, but any effort to right themselves elicits severe extensor rigidity of all limbs as well as of the trunk and neck, producing opisthotonus. At times their muscles are remarkably relaxed between episodes, but these foals are never able to stand. They act disoriented and occasionally have abnormal nystagmus. Their occasional thrashing movements mimic seizure activity. We believe that the most prominent clinical sign is episodic tetany and that this is not a seizure disorder. Electroencephalographic studies are needed to better define the clinical signs. This form of tetany is very different from that seen in the Hereford calves in that it is only one of the clinical signs exhibited by these foals. There are no microscopic lesions in the nervous system. Limited study supports the theory of autosomal recessive inheritance of a gene linked to coat color. **Video 8-24** shows a 1-day-old Arabian foal that has been recumbent since delivery. Its sensorium was normal and it could nurse well. **Video 8-25** shows another newborn Arabian foal with the same disorder The veterinarian with this foal is the late Dr. Henry Fanelli, a veterinary practitioner in Montana who recently published his experience with this disorder.[30]

The cavalier King Charles spaniels have an episodic neurologic disorder referred to as episodic falling, hypertonicity, or tetany.[45] We describe this disorder here under the clinical sign but also include it in the category of movement disorders. The terms *tetany* and *dystonia of antigravity extensor muscles* are interchangeable here. This disorder consists of episodes of tetany of the pelvic limbs and trunk or of all four limbs that may cause the patient to fall or to stand with a rigid posture that has been referred to as "deer stalking." It can last from a few seconds to a few minutes, and afterwards the dog is normal in all respects. The onset of this disorder occurs at about 3 to 4 months of age. Episodes may be precipitated by stress or excitement. This disorder

also has some resemblance to hyperexplexia in humans who have a glycine receptor abnormality. There are no histologic lesions in the nervous systems of these dogs. Glycine receptor studies have not been done. No treatment has been entirely satisfactory, but some relief has been observed with the administration of clonazepam or acetazolamide. **Video 8-26** shows a 4-month-old cavalier King Charles spaniel that exhibits this disorder. **Video 8-27** shows a 6-month-old pit bull exhibiting similar clinical signs. These episodes have been present since it was a young puppy. Between the episodes, this dog is entirely normal, but that is not shown on this video.

Focal Tetany: Spastic Paresis and Spastic Syndrome. A form of focal tetany that is presumed to be inherited has been recognized in numerous breeds of cattle. It has been referred to as spastic paresis, or Elso heel.[6] Elso was a Scandinavian bull that was implicated many years ago in disseminating this disorder in Europe, where it is most common. The disease is uncommon in North America, though it occurs occasionally, primarily in the Holstein and Angus breeds. The inheritance is considered to be a polygenic disorder of low heritability. The tetany is limited to the tarsal extensors in the caudal crus that are innervated by the tibial nerve. One or both pelvic limbs are involved, and the onset usually occurs between a few weeks and 6 months of age. The earliest clinical sign is stiffness in the affected pelvic limbs when the calf is walking. The tarsus is more extended than normal, causing the appearance of a "straight hock." As the clinical signs progress, when protraction is first initiated in the affected limb, the tarsus and stifle suddenly overextend and the calf attempts to advance the limb by hip flexion, with the other joints held in extension. The stifle extension is presumed to be secondary to the tarsal extension because of the effect of the reciprocal apparatus and the role of the peroneus tertius. These signs of focal tarsal tetany disappear when the calf lies down and relaxes. They occur only when the limb is moved. As the disorder slowly worsens, the affected limbs may abruptly extend caudally and swing like pendulums during attempts to walk. Each time the hoof touches the ground, the limb briskly extends caudally. The clinical signs may become so severe that the calf cannot stand to walk. The disorder appears to cause the calf considerable discomfort because it becomes inactive and prefers to lie down; subsequently, it loses weight.

No gross or microscopic lesions are recognized in the tibial nerves or in their components in the spinal cord segments. Physiologic studies have implicated hyperactivity of the gamma efferent neurons that innervate the intrafusal muscle fibers in the neuromuscular spindles of the gastrocnemius muscle. Transection of the 1a afferent neuronal axons in the dorsal roots that are associated with the origin of the tibial nerve stop the clinical signs.[25] Selective procaine anesthesia of the gamma efferent neuronal axons in the ventral roots associated with the origin of the tibial nerve also stop the clinical signs.[27,28] The basis for the hyperactivity of these gamma efferent neurons is unknown. Therefore, this disorder is considered to be an idiopathic functional disorder involving the myotatic reflex mechanism for the gastrocnemius muscle.

In Europe, where this disease is common in many breeds, affected calves are treated surgically to allow them to gain market weight in a period of time that is still profitable. Treatment consists of either denervation of the gastrocnemius muscle in the proximal crus or transection of the gastrocnemius tendon at its attachment to the calcaneus.[8] No affected animal or its parents should be used in breeding. **Video 8-28** shows a 5-month-old Holstein with the clinical signs of this focal tetany in the left pelvic limb; the signs have been slowly progressing for 1 month.

Spastic syndrome is a somewhat similar focal tetany that affects adult cattle and that owners refer to as crampiness or stretches. It is most common in the Holstein and Guernsey breeds; the onset occurs between 3 and 7 years of age. The clinical signs are most evident in confined cattle and are associated with attempts to stand up or a sudden movement of the standing animal after a period of relaxation. The disorder is characterized by episodes of marked caudal extension of the pelvic limbs that prevents protraction of the limbs. This tetany may also be evident in the extensor muscles of the lumbar vertebrae. Usually these clinical signs last from a few seconds to several minutes but occasionally they are prolonged. The signs disappear when the animal lies down but can be aggravated by stress or excitement. They persist for the life of the animal and may slowly progress to prevent the animal from being able to stand up. In limited necropsy studies of affected patients, no gross or microscopic lesions have been found in the nervous system. It is presumed to be a functional disorder that may represent a primary disturbance of the myotatic reflex mechanism similar to the focal tetany observed in young cattle (described earlier) and called spastic paresis in the literature. This adult syndrome is thought to be inherited as a single recessive factor with incomplete penetrance. Despite this knowledge, this focal tetany can be found in many older bulls that are regularly used in artificial insemination facilities.

Myoclonus

Myoclonus is the clinical sign of a sudden contraction of a group of muscle cells, followed by immediate relaxation. Sporadic and repetitive forms are observed.

Sporadic Myoclonus. Sporadic myoclonus can be benign or a form of seizure disorder. Benign sporadic myoclonus is a sudden contraction of a group of muscles causing, for example, a limb to move suddenly or the facial muscles to twitch, but it is a single event and is not repeated in the immediate time period. The cause is unknown. Sporadic myoclonus that is repeated over a period of minutes to hours may be a form of a simple partial seizure due to a prosencephalic disorder that is often but not necessarily structural in origin. Idiopathic forms are less common. These patients need to be studied like those with any other seizure disorder and treated with anticonvulsants. See Chapter 18.

Video 8-29 shows Teak, a 15-year-old castrated male dachshund that for 2 weeks exhibited sporadic myoclonus that was increasing in frequency. The owner took Teak to an ophthalmologist because she thought Teak's eyes hurt. It was recommended that Teak be studied for a seizure disorder. The outcome of that case is unknown.

Video 8-30 shows Dakota, a 12-year-old castrated male golden retriever, exhibiting sporadic myoclonus that represents a simple partial seizure disorder.

Video 8-31 shows a stray cat that was rescued from a fire and taken to an emergency hospital for severe dyspnea. The dyspnea had been improving over 2 days, when the neurologic signs observed on this video first occurred. These clinical signs included blindness, with normal bilateral pupil size that responded well to light, and frequent sporadic myoclonus of one thoracic limb or the entire neck and trunk. It was assumed that this sporadic myoclonus was a simple partial seizure due to a prosencephalic disorder resulting from the toxic effects of smoke inhalation but delayed for a few days. This delay is observed in humans following similar exposure to house-fire smoke and varies from a few days to months. This cat spontaneously recovered over the next 7 to 10 days.

Repetitive Myoclonus. Repetitive myoclonus can be constant during both action and rest and even during sleep, or it can be action-related and observed only when the patient is awake and contracting muscles to maintain its posture or to move.

Constant Repetitive Myoclonus. This is a unique syndrome that we have seen only in dogs and most often in dogs that have been infected with the canine distemper virus and have developed some degree of encephalomyelitis.[9] We have also seen this constant repetitive myoclonus in a dog with lead poisoning in which the myoclonus resolved with chelation therapy.

This myoclonic syndrome is usually limited to one or two limbs, occasionally the jaw, and less often the whole body. Whatever group of muscles is involved does not change in the affected dog. The muscle contractions occur rhythmically, one or a few seconds apart and are most obvious in the resting animal. They occur during activity but are usually masked by the action involved. They continue in the recumbent resting state and commonly during sleep. It is hypothesized that this is a functional disorder in the environment of the LMN cell bodies innervating the myoclonic muscles and is caused by some form of pacemaker mechanism that results in the rhythmic stimulation of the participating LMNs. The myoclonus persists despite transection of the spinal cord cranial to the involved intumescence. In many affected dogs, the myoclonus can be stopped by intravenous lidocaine or oral procainamide. When the procainamide is stopped, the myoclonus returns. Microscopic lesions in the environment of these LMNs are very mild or absent.

The role played by the distemper virus in inducing the syndrome is unknown. Usually dogs that have a myoclonic syndrome also have other neurologic deficits due to the destructive effects of the virus. In the older literature, repetitive myoclonus was commonly called canine chorea, which is a misnomer. In chorea, the myoclonic muscle groups continually change in the affected patient. This is described with movement disorders.

Video 8-32 shows Trevor, a 3-month-old male Saint Bernard, that began to exhibit constant repetitive myoclonus in the pelvic limbs the day after his second vaccination for canine distemper. Simultaneously, he developed difficulty walking with the pelvic limbs. In addition to the pelvic limb myoclonus, he exhibits a mild spastic paresis and ataxia in the pelvic limbs, which is characteristic of a mild spinal cord lesion between the T3 and L3 spinal cord segments. Slow hopping in the left thoracic limb implicates a mild lesion in the left side between the C1 and C5 spinal cord segments or in the left side of the caudal brainstem or the right prosencephalon. The myoclonus implicates the L4 to S1 spinal cord segments. Such a multifocal distribution of lesions is typical of an inflammatory lesion in a young dog. Canine distemper is a common cause of such an inflammation in dogs, and the presence of the myoclonus strongly supports this presumptive diagnosis. Trevor was euthanized and this diagnosis was confirmed at necropsy.

Video 8-33 shows a 5-year-old castrated male German shepherd that was adopted at 1 year of age. At that time, he was suffering from a respiratory and gastrointestinal disorder. He recovered from this illness but shortly afterwards developed constant repetitive myoclonus of the masticatory muscles. Although he was examined by a number of veterinarians, no diagnosis was made. At 5 years of age, he was presented to the Dental Service at the University of Pennsylvania because of the deviation of his teeth caused by the chronic myoclonus, which was still present. He exhibited no other neurologic signs. Intravenous lidocaine stopped the myoclonus, and he was placed on an oral dosage of procainamide that maintained elimination of the myoclonus.

Video 8-34 was made of a dog in Mexico that exhibited the same kind of masticatory muscle myoclonus. The tape was made by Cornell students who were in Mexico to assist in a spay-neuter clinic, and this dog was one of their patients. The affected dog is being held by Dr. Katherine Goldberg (Cornell 2004).

Action-Related Repetitive Myoclonus. As a rule, this form of myoclonus diffusely affects skeletal muscle and is rapid, with many contractions and relaxations per second, producing what is commonly described as a tremor. The more active the patient is, therefore recruiting more LMN stimulations, the more rapid is the myoclonus or tremor. It entirely disappears in the totally relaxed or sleeping patient. Action-related myoclonus is sometimes referred to as intention tremors and is related to a cerebellar disorder. However, if the myoclonus is due to a cerebellar disorder, there will be obvious signs of a cerebellar ataxia, and the myoclonus, or tremors, will be limited to the head and neck. A diffuse whole-body, action-related myoclonus or tremor cannot be produced by a lesion that is limited to the cerebellum. In our experience, it requires a diffuse disorder that can be structural, affecting myelin or neurons, or can be functional, caused by toxicity or a neurotransmitter disorder. Congenital and acquired forms of repetitive action-related myoclonus have been observed.

Congenital Action-Related Repetitive Myoclonus (Congenital Tremor). This is most commonly caused by a diffuse abnormality of CNS myelination—a hypomyelination or dysmyelination. The tremors are observed at birth or as soon as the animal can stand and walk. They are related to action and are not present when the patient is resting or sleeping. These congenital myelin disorders have been studied extensively in pigs, in which viral causes (hog cholera, swine fever, circa); inherited causes (Landrace, British Saddle Back); and toxic causes (trichlorfon from 43 to 65 days of gestation) have been identified.[42]

Video 8-35 shows a newborn pig with diffuse congenital action-related repetitive myoclonus (congenital tremors) due to hypomyelination of unknown cause. Note that when the pig is totally relaxed as it tries to sleep, the tremors stop.

In sheep and cattle, the in utero infection by certain strains of the bovine virus diarrhea virus causes hypomyelination. In sheep, the fleece is abnormal and these lambs have been referred to as "hairy shakers" with Border disease.[5,21,54] Occasionally, affected calves and lambs grow out of the problem, presumably by eventually producing sufficient myelin to allow normal neuronal conduction to occur.

Video 8-36 shows a 4-day-old Holstein calf that has been unable to stand since birth and exhibits diffuse tremors whenever it exerts itself. These tremors disappear when the calf is completely relaxed. A diffuse hypomyelination was diagnosed at necropsy, and an in utero infection with a bovine virus diarrhea virus was presumed.

Video 8-37 shows a 3-day-old Hereford calf with a history and clinical signs identical to those of the calf in the previous video. At necropsy, this calf had microscopic evidence of a diffuse edema of the gray and white matter throughout the CNS. These are the lesions published as being congenital cerebral edema by Dr. Robert Jolly and presumed to be caused by an autosomal recessive genetic abnormality.[44,49] This shows the value of a necropsy diagnosis in that the means of preventing more of these cases differs significantly between the two disorders.

Hypomyelination causing congenital tremors in dogs has been reported in many breeds, but no viral cause has yet been identified. In some breeds, an inherited basis has been documented. This includes a sex-linked recessive gene in male springer spaniels and an autosomal recessive gene in Samoyeds, both of which are lethal.[24,29,37,38] However, in most descriptions, the inherited basis is presumed but not confirmed. We have observed a congenital tremor in Dalmatian puppies that is a coarse tremor producing a bouncing movement primarily in the pelvic limbs and trunk, from which recovery occurred in a few weeks. The family incidence suggested an autosomal recessive inheritance. We have recently seen a similar disorder in a litter of golden retrievers. Hypomyelinogenesis causing congenital tremors is reported in rat terrier puppies and is associated with goiter and hypothyroidism secondary to a genetic mutation.[70]

Video 8-38 shows a 6-week-old female Samoyed that has been unable to stand since birth and exhibits a severe whole-body tremor whenever she tries to move. Note that the more excited she gets, the worse the tremor is. A diffuse CNS hypomyelination was diagnosed at necropsy. She was representative of similar puppies born in six related litters over a 3-year period in Peterborough, New Hampshire. An inherited abnormality was strongly suspected as the cause.

Video 8-39 shows a litter of 6-week-old Dalmatian puppies. At 3 weeks of age, five puppies exhibited a coarse tremor of the pelvic limbs and trunk, which was exacerbated by movement. By 6 weeks, two of these puppies had nearly recovered. Note that the clinical signs are still present in three of the puppies at 6 weeks of age. By a few weeks later, these three puppies had also fully recovered.

Video 8-40 shows two kittens of a litter of three with these clinical signs, but no further studies were done to determine the cause of the tremors. Congenital tremors due to hypomyelinogenesis was documented in Siamese kitten littermates.[84]

Action-related repetitive myoclonus (tremors) may accompany disturbances of neuronal function. A congenital diffuse central axonopathy has been described in Quarter horse foals; it caused coarse tremors that were most pronounced in the pelvic limbs and trunk and created a bobbing, bouncing action similar to that of the Dalmatian puppies previously described.[78] We have also observed a similar central axonopathy and coarse action-related tremor most pronounced in the pelvic limbs in newborn Holstein calves. These foals and calves need assistance to stand and walk. The tremors disappear when they are resting or recumbent. Pedigree study of the affected foals and calves suggest that these are inherited disorders.

Video 8-41 shows a Quarter horse foal studied at Purdue University that exhibits the tremors associated with a central axonopathy. **Video 8-42** shows a 2-month-old Holstein calf studied at Cornell University that is representative of 6 of 24 calves born in one season on a farm in Pennsylvania. At necropsy, these calves were seen to have diffuse central axonopathy.

Action-related myoclonus commonly accompanies other neurologic signs in animals with diffuse neuronal storage disorders. These inherited enzyme deficiencies usually do not produce neurologic signs until a few weeks of age or occasionally much later and rarely at birth. Globoid cell leukodystrophy is caused by an inherited enzyme deficiency that results in demyelination.[32] Clinical signs of spinal cord or cerebellar dysfunction occur at a few weeks of age and progress, often including whole-body tremor.

A late-onset oligodendroglial dysplasia occurs in bull mastiffs, producing progressive spinal cord white matter clinical signs at a few months of age that reflect a C1 to C5 anatomic diagnosis.[61] These dogs also develop a mild diffuse whole-body tremor that distinguishes this diffuse myelin disorder from the more common focal compressive cervical spinal cord lesions.

Acquired Action-Related Repetitive Myoclonus. This is observed most commonly in dogs as an acute-onset diffuse whole-body tremor that is nonprogressive and usually responds within a few days to a few weeks to immunosuppressive levels of corticosteroids. Continuous alternate-day therapy may be needed to prevent recurrence. Only occasionally, a mild vestibular or cerebellar ataxia or other neurologic signs accompany the diffuse tremor. This disorder is most common in the small white breeds such as Maltese and West Highland white terriers; it is the basis for the name white shaker syndrome. However, this disorder can occur in any breed and in a dog of any coat color. The larger dog breeds are less commonly affected. Imaging studies are usually normal. Occasionally we have seen evidence of a mild meningoencephalitis on MR imaging. Cerebrospinal fluid (CSF) may be normal or contain a slight elevation of lymphocytes and protein. The few microscopic studies of the CNS show very mild nonsuppurative meningoencephalitis consisting of a few scattered lymphocytic perivascular cuffs in the leptomeninges, parenchyma, or choroid plexus with no associated structural parenchymal lesions. The nature of the lesion and the response to immunosuppressive therapy suggest that this is an autoimmune disorder. Possibly the involved epitope is a neurotransmitter or its cell membrane receptor. There is a precedent for an autoimmune reaction directed against a biochemical compound. The stiff man syndrome in humans is an autoimmune disease directed against glutamic acid decarboxylase, which is an enzyme necessary for the synthesis of gamma-aminobutyric acid, an inhibitory neurotransmitter.[80] In this syndrome there

are progressive persistent muscle spasms in the pelvic limbs due to a central neuronal disinhibition. The following videos show examples of acquired action-related myoclonus. All of these dogs suddenly developed diffuse whole-body tremor that was most prominent when you picked them up and they struggled and tensed their muscles. You could feel their entire bodies vibrate. Occasionally this tremor includes an ocular tremor, known as opsoclonus. This is a form of rapid pendular nystagmus in which the excursions of each eye are of equal speed and distance. Disorders of the vestibular system cause a jerk nystagmus in which each eye has a slow movement in one direction and a fast movement in the opposite direction. All of these dogs had normal neurologic examinations except for the diffuse tremors. All of these dogs responded to corticosteroid therapy over a period of a few days. Cyclosporin has also been used successfully in some of these patients.

Video 8-43 shows Chambers, a 17-month-old female West Highland white terrier that had these tremors for 6 weeks. Note the one episode of disorientation when he struggles to stand.

Video 8-44 shows Misty, a 1-year-old spayed female West Highland white terrier that had diffuse tremors for a few days.

Video 8-45 shows Sasha, a 1.5-year-old spayed female Maltese terrier that had a diffuse tremor for a few days.

Video 8-46 shows Pooh, a 1-year-old spayed female miniature pinscher that had diffuse tremors for 10 days and experienced no change over that period of time.

Video 8-47 shows a 3-year-old spayed female miniature pinscher that had diffuse tremors for a few hours.

The most common disorder that initially resembles this autoimmune inflammation and must be differentiated from it is a toxicity. Many neurotoxins initiate a diffuse whole-body, action-related tremor as the first clinical sign of intoxication. Depending on the nature of the toxin and the amount of exposure, the patient may recover or may progress to other CNS signs, including seizures and coma followed by death. These toxins include metaldehyde (snail bait), pyrethrins, lead, hexachlorophene, chlorinated hydrocarbons, organophosphates, and numerous mycotoxins. A common intoxication that causes an acute onset of severe diffuse tremors is the ingestion of penitrem A, a mycotoxin produced by *Penicillium* species of mold that grow on contaminated bread products and refrigerated products such as cottage cheese.[2,93] In this mycotoxicosis, multiple dogs in a household may develop similar signs after ingesting the same contaminated food product. Macadamia nuts contain a tremorogenic toxin that produces diffuse whole-body tremor in animals that ingest them.[41]

Video 8-48 shows a 6-year-old castrated male golden retriever that had been at a camp beside a pond in the Maine woods with one other dog. Both dogs were found one morning shaking all over, as can be seen in the video. Both were treated with activated charcoal and general anesthesia and recovered. A toxicity was the presumed cause, but the toxin was not identified.

Postural Repetitive Myoclonus. Postural repetitive myoclonus involves muscle activity and therefore could be considered as action-related, but this form appears to be limited to postural muscles involved with weight support and is absent during voluntary movements. It occurs primarily in two forms: one affects the head and neck postural muscles of relatively young dogs; the other occurs in the pelvic limbs of aged dogs. In addition, a unique and severe form of postural myoclonus is pronounced in all the postural muscles of young-adult Great Dane dogs.

An episodic, rapid repetitive myoclonus occurs most commonly in young adult (6 months to a few years) Doberman pinschers and English bulldogs. It is also quite common in boxers and French bulldogs. This myoclonus is a disorder of the relaxed patient and is unassociated with anxiety or stress. It involves primarily the neck muscles and causes a rapid tremor of the head and neck. The movement can be vertical or horizontal and appears to be present only when the head and neck are in a supporting position. It disappears when the dog is distracted by a toy or food, during eating, during any intentional activity, and when the dog lies down so that the head and neck are resting on a supporting surface. The tremor appears to depend on a specific degree of muscle tension in the neck before it occurs, suggesting that it involves some physiologic disturbance of the stretch reflex mechanism. Neuromuscular spindles are abundant in the neck muscles. This disorder is not progressive and is not associated with the development of any other neurologic signs. For unknown reasons, these tremors commonly occur sporadically for 1 to several weeks and then stop for a few weeks or months before recurring again. We have not recognized any pattern in their occurrence. CSF and imaging studies of the head and neck are normal. There are no reports of electrodiagnostic testing, muscle or nerve biopsies, or CNS microscopic study. No studies have been done on the possible inheritance of this disorder. It can occur in any breed and in mixed breeds but certainly predominates in the breeds mentioned earlier, in which the term *head bobbers* is commonly used to describe the condition. This tremor syndrome may have some similarity to benign postural tremors in humans, which are referred to as essential tremors. The cause of this human disorder is poorly understood, but an abnormality of the stretch reflex mechanism has been invoked. No well-designed results of therapeutic drug studies have been published on the canine disorder. However, anticonvulsants, including phenobarbital and potassium bromide, are, not surprisingly, ineffective in treating patients, in our experience. The following videos show examples of this disorder.

Video 8-49 shows Zack, a 3-year-old castrated male Doberman pinscher. Note how the tremors stop when he rests his head and neck on the blanket.

Video 8-50 shows Tiffany, a 2.5-year-old female English bulldog with a history of two periods of head and neck tremors 2 months apart.

Video 8-51 shows Rocky, a 15-month-old male English bulldog. Note that when he picks up the toy, the head and neck tremors stop.

Video 8-52 shows an adult spayed female beagle. This is testimony that myoclonus occurs in the relaxed patient.

In older dogs, a benign, rapid, postural, repetitive myoclonus, tremor, occasionally develops in the pelvic limbs. Rarely are all four limbs affected. This tremor is evident only in the relaxed standing dog and disappears or is completely masked during voluntary movement and disappears in the

recumbent dog that is therefore not supporting weight. This postural myoclonus can be elicited in a dog that is resting in lateral recumbency by applying pressure to the plantar surface of the paw. Like the head bobbers described earlier, this tremor appears to require a certain degree of tension in the limb muscles, suggesting a role of the stretch reflex mechanism in this disorder. No physiologic or pathologic studies have been published on this disorder. Although the intensity of the tremor may progress slightly with age, there is no indication that it causes any discomfort, and it does not interfere with the dog's function and thus does not require any therapy. The following videos show this postural form of myoclonus.

Video 8-53 shows Bumper, a 9.5-year-old Malamute cross-breed.

Video 8-54 shows Candide, a 13-year-old spayed female miniature schnauzer. Note how the slow, steady pressure on the plantar surface of the paw elicits the tremor.

An orthostatic postural repetitive myoclonus, tremor, occurs in young-adult Great Dane dogs.[35] It is observed only when the dog stands at rest or when it is attempting to lie down or posture to drink, eat, or excrete. It becomes severe during efforts to lie down, causing this effort to be prolonged, during which the dog constantly moves and shifts its weight between its limbs. Once the dog is recumbent, it relaxes and the tremor disappears. There is no evidence of any tremor when the dog is walking or running, and the affected dog does not become fatigued. The tremor immediately disappears when the standing dog is picked up and therefore is not supporting any weight. The neurologic examination is normal, as are all the imaging studies, CSF evaluations, and muscle and nerve biopsies. EMG recordings in the awake standing animal show a constant frequency of 13 to 16 Hz that disappears when the dog lies down. This is the basis for the diagnosis of orthostatic postural tremor in humans, which is described as possibly a "functional CNS disorder involving a supraspinal generator." It is possible that a unique disorder of the spinal cord stretch reflex mechanism is as valid a consideration. Maybe this reflects our bias as clinicians and not as neurophysiologists. Based on limited observation of these affected dogs, the tremors slowly increase in intensity with time. An inherited basis is suspected in the Great Dane breed. Drug therapy studies are limited and have been inconclusive to date. Phenobarbital and gabapentin may give some relief.

Video 8-55 shows Dino, a 22-month-old castrated male Great Dane with a history of 6 months of slowly progressive trembling. It was first noticed in the thoracic limbs when he was eating and then spread to involve the pelvic limbs, especially when posturing to urinate. Note that the tremors are present only when he tries to lie down; once he is recumbent, the tremors cease and he is completely relaxed. He can stand up normally and trot off with no clinical signs, and exercise does not fatigue him.

Episodic Repetitive Myoclonus. Episodic nonpostural repetitive myoclonus is a rare observation in dogs that can also be classified as a movement disorder. This is a poorly understood event that has generated numerous terms, the most common of which is myokymia. In human medicine, *continuous muscle fiber activity* is a more recent term that is applied to a group of hereditary and acquired conditions of peripheral nerve origin.[3,89] Myokymia is the most common clinical sign and is defined as undulating vermiform movements of the overlying skin due to contraction of small bands of muscle fibers. With EMG, the individual motor unit potentials fire at a rate of 5 to 150 Hz. In limited observations in dogs, these myokymic events clinically resulted in stiffness of the limbs followed by collapse into lateral recumbency, with rigid limbs and delayed muscle relaxation. In these dogs the events were stimulated by exercise or excitement. Hyperthermia was commonly observed. These episodes can last from a few minutes to a few hours, between which the dog is normal. In humans, continuous muscle fiber activity is considered to represent hyperactivity of peripheral nerve axons and is not usually associated with any recognizable neuropathy. The term *neuromyokymia* has been used by some authors to implicate the role of the neuronal axon in this disorder.[56] An axonal channel defect may be responsible, because many human patients have circulating antibodies to voltage-gated potassium channels in the peripheral nerve axons. As we gain more experience with this seemingly rare canine disorder, we may have to alter its classification. Treatment options are limited; procainamide and mexiletine are reasonable choices.

Shivers is primarily an equine disorder that is most common in the draft horse breeds, especially those that are used regularly for strenuous work.[88] It can occur at any age and affects primarily the muscles of the pelvic region, pelvic limbs, and tail. The clinical signs consist of repetitive myoclonic twitches or quivering of the gluteal and tail muscles, especially when the horse is made to move backwards. The tail may exhibit extensor muscle myoclonic jerks. When the horse stands at rest, the clinical signs usually resolve but recur when backed-up again. Occasionally when backed-up, the affected horse overflexes a pelvic limb and hold it in that position for a few seconds. The clinical signs may remain unchanged for a long period of time or may progress slowly. The cause of this disorder is unknown. The few microscopic studies of the nervous system of affected horses have disclosed no recognizable lesions. Some of these horses have had muscle lesions caused by polysaccharide storage disease, but the role of this muscle disease in causing shivers is unknown and its significance is a subject of considerable debate by those investigating the disorder.[88]

There is no useful ancillary diagnostic procedure. A muscle biopsy should be done to determine whether the horse has polysaccharide storage disease because that may be helped by dietary treatment. There is no specific treatment for shivers. Inheritance is suspected to be involved in the pathogenesis of this disorder, but the genetic pattern is unknown. It is best to avoid breeding affected horses or their parents. With the limited information that we have on this disorder, it is difficult to know where to place it in the classification of uncontrolled voluntary movements. We have decided to consider it a form of episodic repetitive myoclonus until further studies suggest otherwise.

Video 8-56 shows Jerry, a 14-year-old Belgian with this episodic repetitive myoclonus called shivers; it had been present for several months. Note the quivering tail. The gluteal myoclonus is difficult to see in the video. Note the occasional overflexion of the pelvic limbs and less often of the right thoracic limb. It is important to do a complete orthopedic examination to identify any cause of discomfort

in affected horses. Polysaccharide storage disease was diagnosed in Jerry on the basis of a biopsy of the biceps femoris muscle. Necropsy showed no microscopic lesions in any of the peripheral or central components of the nervous system.

Resting Myoclonus. A myoclonus present only during rest, similar to that seen in humans with degeneration of the substantia nigra in Parkinson disease, has not been recognized in domestic animals. Horses that ingest the toxin present in yellow star thistle develop acute degeneration of the substantia nigra and globus pallidus but do not exhibit a resting tremor.[23] No resting tremor occurs as part of the clinical syndrome seen in Kerry blue terriers and Chinese crested dogs, with their cerebellar cortical abiotrophy and degeneration of the substantia nigra and caudate and olivary nuclei.[25,64]

Movement Disorder

A movement disorder is defined as an episodic sudden involuntary contraction of a group of skeletal muscles in a conscious patient with a normal sensorium during rest or activity. Various terms have been used for the varying forms of these paroxysmal movements.

- Chorea is an abrupt, nonsustained contraction of different groups of muscles in the same patient.
- Dystonia is a sustained involuntary contraction of a group of muscles.
- Tetany is a sustained contraction of extensor muscles that is variably intermittent.
- Athetosis is a prolonged contraction of trunk muscles causing a bending or writhing motion.
- Ballism is an abrupt contraction of limb muscles causing a flailing movement of the limb.

In humans, the pathogenesis of many of these movement disorders is unknown. Some well-defined movement disorders are related to disease of specific extrapyramidal nuclei, such as the caudate nuclei in Huntington chorea and the resting myoclonus that occurs with the substantia nigra lesions in Parkinson disease. Others are unassociated with any recognizable CNS lesion but are thought to be related to a dysfunction in the normal circuitry among the motor cortex, the cerebral extrapyramidal nuclei, the thalamus, and the motor cortex. The dysfunction is commonly considered to represent some disorder of neuronal ion channels and is referred to as an ion channelopathy.[52]

In veterinary medicine, movement disorders have been described in a number of dog breeds. For many years an episodic disorder of muscle contraction has been recognized in Scottish terriers and called Scottie cramps.[22,58,59] See **Videos 8-57 and 8-58.** It is our opinion that this is a movement disorder. These involuntary movements usually require a degree of exercise or stress before they occur. They consist of a combination of chorea and dystonia in one or more limbs in the same dog. These muscle contractions can be severe enough to cause the dog to fall. No microscopic lesions have been found in the nervous system of these affected dogs. A deficiency of serotonin activity in the spinal cord gray matter has been implicated in the pathogenesis of this movement disorder.[57,67] The disorder is presumed to be inherited as an autosomal recessive gene.[54] Other movement disorders that may be familial have been recognized in the cavalier King Charles spaniel (tetany, hypertonicity, deer-stalking)[45]; the bichon frise[66]; the soft-coated Wheaton spaniel (personal observation); and the Norwich terrier.[34] A classic severe form of movement disorder was described in two unrelated litters of boxers in which movements were defined as paroxysmal dystonic choreoathetosis (see Video 8-64).[73] MR imaging was normal in these dogs. We have seen what we believe are forms of movement disorders in individual dogs of numerous breeds. In some instances, when the involuntary movement is repeated in the same group of muscles, it may be difficult to differentiate a movement disorder from a simple partial seizure disorder. This is particularly true for the Chinook seizures (personal communication, D. O'Brien, University of Missouri) and the border terrier episodes that are referred to as Spike's disease.[18] If imaging studies and CSF evaluation are normal, an electroencephalographic study (where reliably available) or an anticonvulsant drug trial may be necessary to help differentiate these disorders. It is our opinion that when the diagnosis of movement disorder is suspected, MR imaging is warranted to determine the possible presence of extrapyramidal nuclear lesions. We are not aware that such a relationship has been published to date. A neurotransmitter or ion channel disorder would not be visible on MR images. The movement disorder described in the cavalier King Charles spaniels may be defined as a tetany or a dystonia involving the sudden contraction of the extensor muscles of the pelvic limbs or of all four limbs that is intermittent. There is some resemblance between this disorder and the hyperexplexia in humans caused by a glycine receptor abnormality. This should be investigated in this breed. The following videos show various examples of these movement disorders.

Video 8-57 shows Shamus, a young adult male Scottish terrier that is seen going for a walk after playing in the yard for about 10 minutes. He was normal during that time.

Video 8-58 shows Fergus, a castrated male Scottish terrier. His movement disorder began at 6 months of age, and the video shows him at 3 and 6 years of age with no significant change in the disorder, which is intermittent.

Video 8-59 shows the 4-month-old cavalier King Charles spaniel that was described in the discussion of tetany as a clinical sign. His episodic tetany or extensor muscle dystonia is a form of movement disorder.

Video 8-60 shows TJ, a 6-year-old cavalier King Charles spaniel that had been exhibiting an episodic head tilt with cervical torticollis that occasionally caused him to fall and roll in the direction of the torticollis. Note on the video the sudden change in direction of the head tilt/torticollis. Imaging was recommended for this dog to be sure there was no syringohydromyelia that this breed is at risk for developing secondary to an occipital bone malformation. This study was not performed.

Video 8-61 shows Holly, a 10-year-old spayed female bichon frise that excelled as a pet therapy dog in her neighborhood. Note the dystonic chorea affecting multiple limbs in a varying pattern. These events had been occurring for 2 years with unpredictable frequency.

Video 8-62 shows Shaggy, a 2-year-old castrated male soft-coated Wheaton terrier. The episodic movement disorder seen on the video had been occurring for the past 4 months with increasing frequency.

Video 8-63 shows a 5-month-old castrated male German shepherd with a recent onset of the dystonic choreiform movements seen on the video. Note the haphazard multiple limb involvement. With this disorder, a fall into a pond may be life-threatening!

Video 8-64 shows a group of 5- and 9-month-old boxer dogs from two unrelated litters exhibiting profound examples of severe movement disorder. The onset occurred between 9 and 16 weeks of age, and the frequency varied significantly among individual animals, from 3 to 10 times a day to 1 to 2 times a month. Their movements were described as paroxysmal dystonic choreoathetosis. (We thank Dr. I. K. Ramsey of the University of Cambridge for providing us with this video.)

It is obvious that it is difficult to classify all of these uncontrolled involuntary movements into specific entities. We have tried to provide some order where we believe there is considerable lack of understanding.

REFERENCES

1. Amann J: *The organization of spinal motoneurons and their relationship to corticospinal fibers in the raccoon* (Procyon lotor), PhD dissertation, Ithaca, NY, 1971, Cornell University.
2. Arp LH, Richard JL: Intoxication of dogs with the mycotoxin penitrem A, *J Am Vet Med Assoc* 175:565, 1979.
3. Auger RG: Continuous muscle fiber activity: *Sem Neurol* 11:258-266, 1991.
4. Baker JL, Waters DJ, de Lahunta A: Tetanus in two cats, *J Am Anim Hosp Assoc* 24:159-164, 1988.
5. Barlow RM, Dickinson AG: On the pathology and histochemistry of the central nervous system in Border disease of sheep, *Res Vet Sci* 6:230-237, 1965.
6. Bijlveld K, Hartman W: Electromyographic studies in calves with spastic paresis, *Tijdschr Diergeneesk* 101:805, 1976.
7. Blood DC, Gay CC: Hereditary neuraxial edema of calves, *Aust Vet J* 47:520, 1971.
8. Bouckaert JH, DeMoor A: Treatment of spastic paralysis in cattle: improved denervation technique of gastrocnemius muscle and postoperative course, *Vet Rec* 79:226, 1966.
9. Breazile JE, Blaugh BS, Nail N: Experimental study of canine distemper myoclonus, *Am J Vet Res* 27:1375-1379, 1966.
10. Breazile JE, Swafford BC, Biles AR: Motor cortex of the horse, *Am J Vet Res* 27:1605, 1966.
11. Breazile JE, Swafford BC, Thompson WD: Study of the motor cortex of the pig, *Am J Vet Res* 27:1369, 1966.
12. Breazile JE, Thompson WD: Motor cortex of the dog, *Am J Vet Res* 28:1483, 1967.
13. Brenner O, de Lahunta A, Summers BA: Hereditary polioencephalomyelopathy of the Australian cattle dog, *Acta Neuropathol* 94:64-66, 1997.
14. Brown GL, Harvey AM: Congenital myotonia in the goat, *Brain* 62:24, 1939.
15. Bryant SH: Myotonia in the goat, *Ann N Y Acad Sci* 317:314-325, 1979.
16. Burkitt JM, et al: Risk factors associated with outcome in dogs with tetanus: 38 cases (1987-2005), *J Am Vet Med Assoc* 230:76-83, 2000.
17. Buxton DF, Goodman DC: Motor function and the corticospinal tracts in the dog and raccoon, *J Comp Neurol* 129:341, 1967.
18. Canine epileptiform cramping syndrome: *Spike's disease: border terrier* (website): www.borderterrier-cecs.com/index. htm. Accessed February 8, 2008.
19. Chambers WW, Liu CN: Corticospinal tract in the cat, *J Comp Neurol* 108:23, 1957.
20. Cho DY, Leipold HW: Hereditary neuraxial edema in polled Hereford calves, *Pathol Res Pract* 163:158, 1978.
21. Clarke GL, Osburn BI: Transmissible congenital encephalopathy of lambs, *Vet Pathol* 15:68-82, 1978.

22. Clemmons RM, Peters RI, Meyers KM: Scotty cramp: a review of cause, characteristics, diagnosis and treatment, *Compend Cont Ed* 2:385-388, 1980.

23. Cordy DR: Nigropallidal encephalomalacia in horses associated with ingestion of yellow star thistle, *J Neuropathol Exp Neurol* 13:330, 1954.

24. Cummings JF, Summers BA, de Lahunta A, Lawson C: Tremors in Samoyed pups with oligodendroglial deficiencies and hypomyelination, *Acta Neuropathol* 71:267-277, 1986.

25. de Lahunta A, Averill DR Jr: Hereditary cerebellar cortical and extrapyramidal nuclear abiotrophy in Kerry Blue terriers, *J Am Vet Med Assoc* 168:1119, 1976.

26. de Lahunta A, Glass EN, Kent M: Classifying involuntary muscle contractions, *Compend Cont Ed* 28:516-530, 2006.

27. DeLey G, DeMoor A: Bovine spastic paralysis: results of surgical desafferentation of the gastrocnemius muscle by means of spinal dorsal root resection, *Am J Vet Res* 38:1899, 1977.

28. DeLey G, DeMoor A: Bovine spastic paralysis: results of gamma efferent suppression with dilute procaine, *Vet Sci Comm* 3:289, 1980.

29. Duncan ID: Abnormalities of myelination of the central nervous system associated with congenital tremor, *J Vet Intern Med* 1:10-23, 1987.

30. Fanelli HH: Coat color dilution lethal ("lavender foal syndrome") a tetany syndrome of Arabian foals, *Eq Vet Ed* 17:260-263, 2005.

31. Farrow BRH, Malik R: Hereditary myotonia in the chow chow, *J Sm Anim Pract* 22:451-465, 1981.

32. Fletcher TF, Kurtz HI, Low DG: Globoid cell leukodystrophy (Krabbe type) in the dog, *J Am Vet Med Assoc* 149:165-172, 1966.

33. Fox JG, Averill DA, Hamlett M: Familial reflex myoclonus in Labrador retrievers, *Am J Vet Res* 45:2367-2370, 1984.

34. Furber, R: Norwich terriers, *Vet Rec* 115:46, 1984 (letter).

35. Garosi LS, Rossmeisl JH, de Lahunta A: Primary orthostatic tremor in Great Danes, *J Vet Intern Med* 19:606-609, 2005.

36. Greene CE, Lorenz MD, Munnell JF: Myopathy associated with hyperadrenocorticism in the dog, *J Am Vet Med Assoc* 174:1310-1315, 1979.

37. Griffiths IR, Duncan ID, McCulloch M: Shaking pups: a disorder of central myelination in spaniel dogs. Part II. Ultrastructural observations on the white matter of the cervical spinal cord, *J Neurocytol* 10:847, 1981.

38. Griffiths IR, et al: Shaking pups: a disorder of central myelination in the spaniel dog. Part 1. Clinical, genetic, and light microscopic observations, *J Neurol Sci* 50:423-433, 1981.

39. Groos WP, et al: Organization of corticospinal neurons in the cat, *Brain Res* 143:393, 1978.

40. Gundlach AL, Kortz G, Burazin CD: Deficit of inhibitory glycine receptors in spinal cord from Peruvian pasos: evidence for an equine form of inherited myoclonus, *Brain Res* 628:263-270, 1993.

41. Hansen SR: Weakness, tremors and depression associated with macadamia nuts, *Vet Human Toxicol* 42:18-21, 2000.

42. Harding JD, Done JT, Harbourne JF: Congenital tremor type A111 in pigs and hereditary sex-linked cerebrospinal hypomyelinogenesis, *Vet Rec* 92:527-529, 1973.

43. Harper PAW, Healy PJ, Dennis JA: Inherited myoclonus of polled Hereford calves (so-called neuraxial edema): a clinical, pathological and biochemical study, *Vet Rec* 11:59-62, 1986.

44. Hazlett M, et al: Congenital brain edema in two Hereford calves, *Can Vet J* 41:882, 2000.

45. Herrtage ME, Palmer AC: Episodic falling in the cavalier King Charles spaniel, *Vet Rec* 112:458-459, 1983.

46. Hongo T, Jankowska E, Lundberg A: The rubrospinal tract. 1. Effects on alpha-motor neurons innervating hind limb muscles in cat, *Exp Brain Res* 7:334, 1969.

47. Hukuda S, Jameson SW: Experimental cervical myelopathy. III. The canine corticospinal tract: anatomy and function, *Surg Neurol* 1:107, 1973.

48. Ingram WR, Ranson SW: Effects of lesions in the red nuclei in cats, *Arch Neurol Psychiatr* 28:483, 1932.

49. Jolly RD: Congenital brain edema in Hereford calves, *J Pathol* 114:199, 1974.

50. Killingsworth C, et al: Feline tetanus, *J Am Anim Hosp Assoc* 13:209-215, 1977.

51. Kornegay JE, Tuler SM, Miller DM: Muscular dystrophy in a litter of golden retriever dogs, *Muscle Nerve* 11:1056-1064, 1988.

52. Kulman DM: The neuronal channelopathies, *Brain* 125: 1179-1195, 2002.

53. Lassek AM, Dowd LW, Weil A: The quantitative distribution of the pyramidal tract in the dog, *J Comp Neurol* 51:153, 1930.

54. Markson LM, Terlecki S, Shand A: Hypomyelinogenesis congenita in sheep, *Vet Rec* 71:269, 1959.

55. Marsden CD: The development of pigmentation and enzyme activity in the nucleus substantiae nigrae of the cat, *J Anat* 19:175, 1965.

56. Mertens HG, Zschocke S: Neuromyotomie, *Klinis Wochensch* 43:917-925, 1965.

57. Meyers KM, Dickson WM, Schaub RG: Serotonin involvement in a motor disorder of Scottish terrier dogs, *Life Sci* 13:1261-1274, 1973.

58. Meyers KM, et al: Hyperkinetic episodes in Scottish terrier dogs, *J Am Vet Med Assoc* 155:129, 1969.

59. Meyers KM, Padgett GA, Dickson WM: The genetic basis for a kinetic disorder of Scottish terrier dogs, *J Hered* 61:189, 1970.

60. Montagna P, Liquori R, Monari L: Equine muscular dystrophy with myotonia, *Clin Neurophysiol* 112:294-299, 2001.

61. Morrison JP, Schatzberg S, Summers BA: Leukodystrophy of bull mastiff dogs resembling Charolais ataxia (oligodendroglial dysplasia), *Vet Pathol* 43:29-35, 2006.

62. Nyberg-Hansen R: Sites and mode of termination of reticulospinal fibers in the cat, *J Comp Neurol* 124:71, 1965.

63. Nyberg-Hansen R, Brodal A: Sites of termination of corticospinal fibers in the cat: an experimental study with silver impregnation methods, *J Comp Neurol* 120:369, 1963.

64. O'Brien DP, Johnson GS, Schnabel RD: Genetic mapping of canine multisystem degeneration and ectodermal dysplasia loci, *J Hered* 96:727-734, 2005.

65. Page P, et al: Clinical clinicopathologic, post mortem examination findings and familial history of 3 Arabians with lavendar foal syndrome, *J Vet Intern Med* 20: 1491-1494, 2006.

66. Penderis J, Franklin JM: Dyskinesia in an adult bichon frise, *J Sm Anim Pract* 42:24-25, 2001.

67. Peters RI Jr, Meyers KM: Precursor regulation of serotonergic neuronal function in Scottish terrier dogs, *J Neurochem* 29:753, 1977.

68. Petras JM: Afferent fibers to the spinal cord: the terminal distribution of dorsal root and encephalospinal axons, *Med Serv J Can* 22:668, 1966.

69. Petras JM: Cortical, tectal and tegmental fiber connections in the spinal cord of the cat, *Brain Res* 6:275, 1967.

70. Pettigrew R, et al: CNS hypomyelinatioin in rat terrier dogs with congenital goiter and a mutation in the thyroid peroxidase gene, *Vet Pathol* 43:1023-1029, 2006.

71. Pierce KD, Handford CA, Morris R: A nonsense mutation in the alpha subunit of the inhibitory glycine receptor associated with bovine myoclonus, *Molec Cell Neurosci* 17:354-363, 2001.

72. Pompeiano O, Brodal A: Experimental demonstration of somatotopical origin of rubrospinal fibers in the cat, *J Comp Neurol* 108:225, 1957.

73. Ramsey IK, Chandler KE, Franklin RJ: A movement disorder in boxer dogs, *Vet Rec* 144:179-180, 1999.

74. Rinvik E, Walberg F: Demonstration of a somatotopically arranged corticorubral projection in the cat: an experimental study with silver methods, *J Comp Neurol* 120:393, 1963.

75. Sanders SG: A putative neurotoxin in nigropallidal encephalomalacia and other Parkinson-like disease, *Proc Am Coll Vet Intern Med* 20:386-388, 2002.

76. Sanders SG, Tucker RL, Bagley RS: Magnetic resonance imaging features of equine nigropallidal encephalomalacia, *Vet Radiol Ultrasound* 42:291-296, 2001.

77. Schwab ME, Thoenen H: Electron microscopic evidence of a transsynaptic migration of tetanus toxin in spinal cord motoneurons: an autoradiographic and morphometric study, *Brain Res* 105:213, 1976.

78. Seahorn TL, Fuentealba IC, Illanes OG: Congenital encephalomyelopathy in a quarter horse, *Eq Vet J* 23:394-395, 1991.

79. Shiang R, Ryan SG, Zhu Z: Mutations in the alpha-1 subunit of the inhibitory glycine receptor causes the dominant neurologic disorder, hyperexplexia, *Nature Genet* 5:351-358, 1993.

80. Solimena M, Folli F, Aparisi R: Autoantibodies to GABA-ergic neurons and pancreatic beta cells in stiff man syndrome, *N Eng J Med* 322:1555-1560, 1990.

81. Spier SJ, Carlson GP, Holliday TA: Hyperkalemic periodic paralysis in horses, *J Am Vet Vet Med Assoc* 197:1009-1017, 1990.

82. Spring-Mills E, Elias JJ: Tetanus toxin: direct evidence for retrograde intra-axonal transport, *Science* 188:945, 1975.

83. Steinberg S, Botelho S: Myotonia in a horse, *Science* 137:979-980, 1962.

84. Stoffregen DA, et al: Hypomyelination of the central nervous system of two Siamese kitten littermates, *Vet Pathol* 30:388-390, 1993.

85. Toll J, Cooper BJ, Altschul M: Congenital myotonia in 2 domestic cats, *J Vet Intern Med* 12:116-119, 1998.

86. Usunoff KG, et al: The nigrostriatal projection in the cat. Part I. Silver impregnation study, *J Neurol Sci* 28:265, 1976.

87. Valentine BA, Cooper BJ, de Lahunta A: Canine X-linked muscular dystrophy, *J Neurol Sci* 88:69-91, 1988.

88. Valentine BA, et al: Clinical and pathological findings in two draft horses with progressive muscle atrophy, neuromuscular weakness and abnormal gait characteristic of shivers syndrome, *J Am Vet Med Assoc* 215:1661-1665, 1999.

89. Van Ham L, Bhatti S, Polis R: Continuous muscle fiber activity in six dogs with episodic myokymia, stiffness and collapse, *Vet Rec* 15:769-774, 2004.

90. Verhaart WJC: The pyramidal tract: its structure and function in man and animals, *World Neurol* 3:43, 1962.

91. Vite CH, Cozzi F, Rich M: Myotonic myopathy in a miniature schnauzer: case report and data suggesting abnormal chloride conductance across muscle membrane, *J Vet Intern Med* 12:394-397, 1998.

92. Vite CH: Myotonia and disorders of altered muscle cell membrane excitability, *Vet Clin North Am Sm Anim Pract* 32:169-187, 2002.

93. Walter SL: Acute penitrem A and roquefortine poisoning in a dog, *Can Vet J* 43:372-374, 2002.

94. Webster KE: The cortico-striatal projection in the cat, *J Anat* 99:329, 1965.

9 GENERAL SENSORY SYSTEMS: GENERAL PROPRIOCEPTION AND GENERAL SOMATIC AFFERENT

SENSORY SYSTEMS

GENERAL PROPRIOCEPTION

Spinal Nerve General Proprioception
*General Proprioceptive Pathways
for Reflex Activity and Cerebellar
Transmission*
*General Proprioceptive Pathways to
the Somesthetic Cortex for Conscious
Perception*
Cranial Nerve General Proprioception
Reflex Activity
Conscious Pathway

Clinical Signs
Diseases

GENERAL SOMATIC AFFERENT SYSTEM

Spinal Nerve General Somatic Afferent System
*Reflex General Somatic Afferent
Pathway*
Cutaneous Area, Autonomous Zone
Anatomy of the Flexor Reflex
*General Somatic Afferent Pathway
for Conscious Perception*
Cranial Nerve

*Reflex General Somatic Afferent
Pathway*
*General Somatic Afferent Pathway
for Conscious Perception*
Clinical Signs
Diseases
Canine Sensory Neuropathy
Sensory Ganglioradiculitis
Facial Hypalgesia or Analgesia
Pain Syndromes

SUMMARY OF SPINAL CORD PATHWAYS

SENSORY SYSTEMS

A sensory system is characterized by a peripheral afferent neuron with a dendritic zone that is commonly modified to form a receptor organ; an axon that courses into the gray matter of the central nervous system (CNS); a cell body in a ganglion of the peripheral nervous system; and a centrally located relay nucleus and tract that courses primarily to a specific thalamic nucleus that relays to a specific area of the cerebral cortex. Each type of sensory stimulus, or sensation, is known as a modality, a form of energy that is converted by the receptor organ into a neuronal impulse. These modalities include touch, temperature, movement, chemicals, pressure, light, and sound, which inform the CNS of the features of the external and internal environments of the body. In some instances there is a specific structural neuroanatomic pathway for a modality, such as light and sound. Most receptor organs have a low threshold for a certain modality but still can be stimulated by other modalities. This form of energy to which a receptor organ is most sensitive is referred to as the adequate stimulus. Anatomically there are encapsulated and nonencapsulated receptor organs. The dendritic zone of the encapsulated receptor is associated with a well-developed connective tissue capsule of which there are many varieties. These connective tissue modifications provide the structural features necessary for that receptor to be most sensitive to one specific modality or energy form, although the receptor is not limited to that modality. Several forms of energy may excite that receptor. Even without a connective tissue modification, the nonencapsulated receptors exhibit low thresholds of sensitivity to one specific modality. The histologic features do not necessarily restrict the receptor to sensitivity to one specific modality. Nevertheless, they are classified as thermoreceptors, mechanoreceptors, chemoreceptors, and photoreceptors on the basis of their adequate stimulus.

Receptors have been classified according to their location in the body. Exteroceptors are located on or near the surface of the body and are sensitive to changes in the external environment that affect the body surface. They include the general somatic afferent (GSA) neurons for touch, temperature, pressure, and noxious stimuli; and special somatic afferent (SSA) neurons for light and sound. Proprioceptors are sensitive to movement and include those for general proprioception that are diffusely located in the internal mass of the body in muscles, tendons, and joints and the receptors for special proprioception located in the labyrinth in the inner ear. Interoceptors are located within the viscera of the body and are sensitive to changes in the internal environment. They include the general visceral afferent (GVA) neurons for body temperature, blood pressure, gas concentration, pressure, and movement in body viscera; and the special visceral afferent (SVA) neurons for the chemical energy concerned with taste and smell.

The use of the term *pain* is badly abused. I (Alexander de Lahunta) was guilty of this in the first two editions of this book, before Dr. Ralph Kitchell of the University of California set me straight. Pain is *not* a sensory modality. We do not give a patient a pain stimulus. We do not test for pain. We test for what we interpret as a painful response by stimulating the patient with a noxious stimulus. We test for nociception, which is the patient's perception of this noxious stimulus. Pain is the subjective cerebral response of the patient to the stimulation of a variety of receptors referred to as nociceptors. This group of receptors is nonselective in the form of energy that elicits its maximal response, but the stimulus threshold for these modalities is high. The intensity of the stimulus required to evoke an impulse from these receptors is at a level that is potentially destructive to the tissue. It requires a high-intensity excitation by mechanical (the pressure of tissue forceps), electrical (a cattle prod), or chemical stimuli. These are noxious stimuli, and the behavioral response observed is nociception, or what we interpret to be pain. The latter varies significantly among individual patients in terms of their response to the same noxious stimulus. Consider the different responses you would expect in reaction to moderate compression of the digits by forceps in a high-strung Chihuahua and in a laid-back collie dog.

GENERAL PROPRIOCEPTION

General proprioceptive (GP) neurons constitute a sensory system that detects the state of the position and the movement in muscles and joints.[16] Two basic pathways are described for this system. One is the pathway for segmental reflex activity and for transmitting proprioceptive information to the cerebellum. The other is the conscious proprioceptive pathway that involves the transmission of proprioceptive information to the sensory somesthetic cerebral cortex. These pathways are considered separately for the spinal nerves and cranial nerves.

Spinal Nerve General Proprioception

For all the spinal nerves, the GP afferent neuron has its dendritic zone in a muscle, tendon, or joint. The 1a afferent in neuromuscular spindles and the 1b afferent in Golgi tendon organs are examples of such receptors. The axons course proximally in peripheral nerves to the spinal nerve and through the spinal ganglion associated with the dorsal root of that spinal nerve. The cell body of that GP afferent is in the segmental spinal (dorsal root) ganglion. The axon continues in the dorsal root to enter the spinal cord along the dorsolateral sulcus.

General Proprioceptive Pathways for Reflex Activity and Cerebellar Transmission

Reflex Activity. The GP axons enter the dorsal gray column of the spinal cord segment. Some axons (1a from a neuromuscular spindle) synapse directly on the general somatic efferent (GSE) alpha motor neuron in the ventral gray column to complete a reflex arc. Others (1b from a Golgi tendon organ) indirectly influence an alpha motor neuron and complete the reflex arc by synapsing on an interneuron (Fig. 9-1). The activity of some interneurons influences GSE alpha motor neurons in other spinal cord segments by passing cranially and caudally in the fasciculus proprius of the lateral funiculus. Recall that this pathway comprises the white matter that is immediately adjacent to the gray matter throughout the spinal cord. It is also referred to as the propriospinal fiber system, which connects adjoining and distant spinal cord segments. This provides a means of interrelating neural activity within the spinal cord.

Cerebellar Transmission from Trunk and Pelvic Limbs. These transmissions are shown in Figs. 9-1 through 9-3.[20,30,38]

Dorsal Spinocerebellar Tract. The GP axon enters the dorsal gray column and synapses on a neuronal cell body on the medial aspect of the base of the dorsal gray column. This is in the nucleus thoracicus (nucleus dorsalis, nucleus of the dorsal spinocerebellar tract, Clarke nucleus).[21,44] Most of the axons of these cell bodies enter the lateral funiculus of the same side of the spinal cord (ipsilateral) and pass cranially on the surface of the dorsal portion of the lateral funiculus in the dorsal spinocerebellar tract. Here this tract is lateral to the upper motor neuron (UMN) pathways, which includes the lateral corticospinal, rubrospinal, and medullary reticulospinal tracts. The nucleus thoracicus extends from approximately the eighth cervical to the fourth lumbar spinal cord segments in the cat. The GP afferents from the pelvic limbs must course cranially to the cranial lumbar segments to synapse in this nucleus. The dorsal spinocerebellar tract passes cranially through the entire spinal cord to the medulla, where it joins the caudal cerebellar peduncle by way of the superficial arcuate fibers on the surface of the medulla (Fig. 9-4; see also Figs. 2-13 through 2-15). It is distributed primarily to the cerebellar cortex of the vermal and paravermal lobules.

Ventral Spinocerebellar Tract. The GP axon enters the dorsal gray column and synapses on cell bodies near its base laterally. These cell bodies form a continuous column from the cranial thoracic spinal cord segments through the lumbar and sacral segments. Most axons of these cell bodies cross to the opposite-side lateral funiculus by way of the ventral white commissure. In the contralateral lateral funiculus, they form the ventral spinocerebellar tract[23,32] on the surface of the lateral funiculus ventral to the dorsal spinocerebellar tract. The ventral spinocerebellar tract courses cranially through the entire spinal cord. It continues through the medulla on its lateral side and enters the pons, where it joins the rostral cerebellar peduncle and courses caudally through it into the cerebellum (see Fig. 9-4). Within the cerebellum, most of these axons cross back to the side from which they originated from their cell bodies, and they terminate primarily in the vermal and paravermal lobules.

Cerebellar Transmission from Thoracic Limbs and the Cervical Region

Cuneocerebellar Tract. This cuneocerebellar tract contains GP axons from the dorsal roots of the spinal nerves from C1 to T8. It provides a GP cerebellar pathway from the thoracic limbs[38] similar to the dorsal spinocerebellar tract from the pelvic limbs.[31] The GP axons in the dorsal roots enter the spinal cord along the dorsolateral sulcus and continue dorsal to the dorsal gray column to enter the lateral portion of the dorsal funiculus without synapse. This is the fasciculus cuneatus. The GP axons pass cranially in the fasciculus cuneatus to the caudal medulla, where they terminate by forming synapses with neuronal cell bodies in the lateral cuneate nucleus (see Figs. 9-1 through 9-4; see also Figs. 2-14 and 2-15). This nucleus is located dorsally in the medulla, dorsolateral to the parasympathetic nucleus of the vagus nerve. It is ventromedial to the caudal cerebellar peduncle, rostral to the level of the obex, and caudal to the caudal vestibular nucleus. Axons of the

Cervical region and thoracic limbs

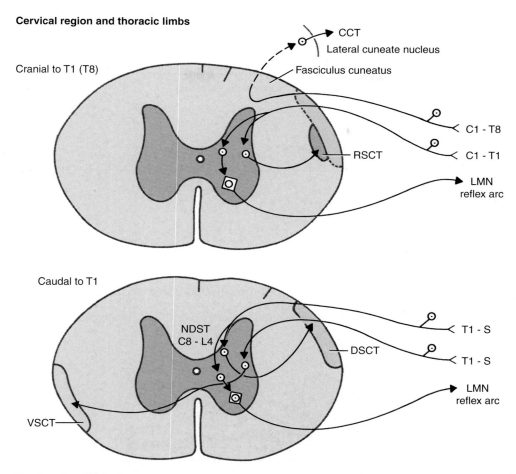

FIGURE 9-1 GP pathways for reflex action and to the cerebellum-spinocerebellar pathways. *CCT,* Cuneocerebellar tract; *DSCT,* dorsal spinocerebellar tract; *LMN,* lower motor neuron; *NDST,* nucleus of dorsal spinocerebellar tract—C8-L4 (cat); *RSCT,* cranial (rostral) spinocerebellar tract; *VSCT,* ventral spinocerebellar tract.

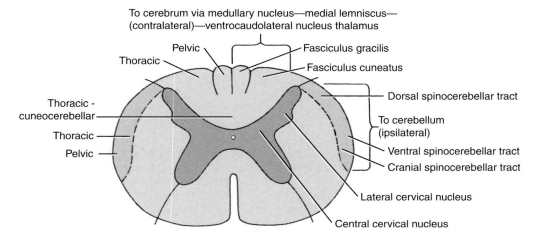

FIGURE 9-2 GP pathways at the second cervical spinal cord segment.

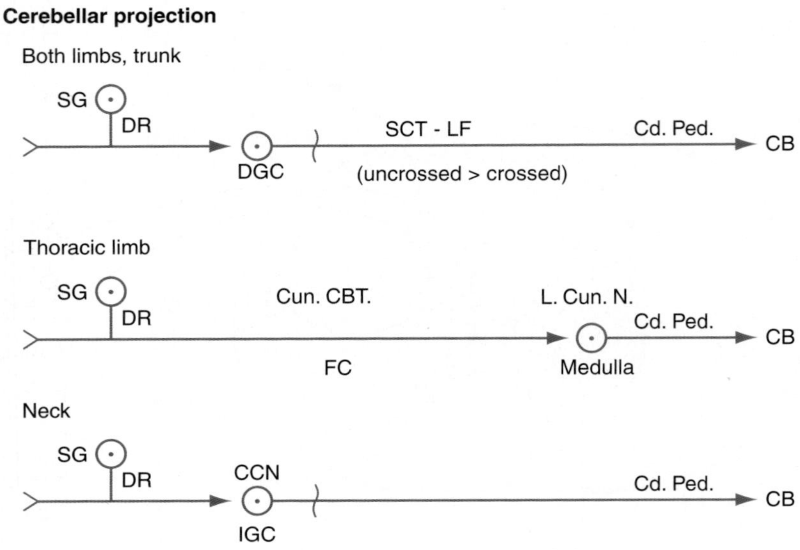

Cerebellar projection

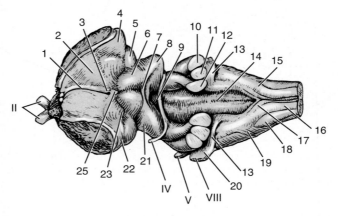

FIGURE 9-3 Cerebellar projection. *CB,* Cerebellum; *CCN,* central cervical nucleus; *Cd. Ped.,* caudal cerebellar peduncle; *Cun. CBT.,* cuneocerebellar tract; *DGC,* dorsal gray column; *DR,* dorsal root; *FC,* fasciculus cuneatus; *IGC,* intermediate gray column; *L. Cun. N.* lateral cuneate nucleus; *LF,* lateral funiculus; *SCT,* spinocerebellar tract; *SG,* spinal ganglion; *l,* crossed pathway.

FIGURE 9-4 Dorsal view of the brainstem. *II,* Optic nerves; *IV,* trochlear nerve; *V,* trigeminal nerve; *VIII,* vestibulocochlear nerve.

1. Stria habenularis thalami	10. Middle cerebellar peduncle	19. Superficial arcuate fibers
2. Dorsal aspect of thalamus	11. Caudal cerebellar peduncle	20. Left ventral cochlear nucleus
3. Habenular commissure	12. Rostral cerebellar peduncle	21. Brachium of caudal colliculus
4. Lateral geniculate nucleus	13. Acoustic stria	22. Optic tract
5. Medial geniculate nucleus	14. Dorsal median sulcus in fourth	23. Brachium of rostral colliculus
6. Rostral colliculus	ventricle	24. Cut surface between cerebral
7. Commissure of caudal colliculi	15. Lateral cuneate nucleus	hemisphere and brainstem
8. Caudal colliculus	16. Fasciculus cuneatus	25. Pineal body-epiphysis
9. Crossing of trochlear nerve fibers	17. Nucleus gracilis	
in rostral medullary velum	18. Spinal tract of trigeminal nerve	

neuronal cell bodies in the lateral cuneate nucleus enter the adjacent caudal cerebellar peduncle and pass into the cerebellum.

Cranial (Rostral) Spinocerebellar Tract. For this thoracic limb GP pathway, the GP axons in the dorsal roots associated with the cervical intumescence enter the dorsal gray column and synapse on neuronal cell bodies near its base in the centrobasilar nucleus.[42] The axons of these cell bodies enter the ipsilateral lateral funiculus and course cranially, medial to the ventral spinocerebellar tract (see Fig. 9-2).

They continue into the medulla and pons, where they enter the cerebellum through both the caudal and the rostral cerebellar peduncles.

Cervicospinocerebellar Pathway. The central cervical nucleus is located in the intermediate gray column of the first four cervical spinal cord segments.[15,28,37] It receives GP axons in dorsal roots from cervical spinal ganglion neuronal cell bodies that are thought to be concerned primarily with general proprioception from the neck (see Fig. 9-3). The axons from the neuronal cell bodies in this nucleus cross to the contralateral lateral funiculus. They continue cranially into the medulla and enter the cerebellum through the caudal cerebellar peduncle.

Cervicospinovestibular Pathway. For the vestibular special proprioceptive system to function, it needs afferents from the GP system in the neck muscles. They are provided by the spinovestibular tract in the ventral funiculus. This tract receives axons from the ipsilateral dorsal gray column, and it terminates in the medullary caudal vestibular nucleus.

This brief description gives some indication of the complexity of this sensory system and should serve to provide some humility when you are attempting to make an accurate anatomic diagnosis. The student and clinician should appreciate that these spinocerebellar pathways provide the cerebellum, predominantly ipsilaterally, with information about where the limbs, trunk, and neck are located in space, both during movement and during a fixed posture. This information is critical for the cerebellum in its role of regulating the posture, tone, locomotion, and equilibrium. A practical lesson that should come out of this is that a unilateral cervical spinal cord lesion causes primarily a GP ataxia on the same side as that lesion.

General Proprioceptive Pathways to the Somesthetic Cortex for Conscious Perception

Fasciculus Gracilis and Fasciculus Cuneatus. These fasciculi located in the dorsal funiculus contain axons that conduct impulses from receptors sensitive to a number of modalities, some of which are concerned with general proprioception. These GP axons are in the dorsal roots of all the spinal nerves. Each dorsal root enters the spinal cord at the dorsolateral sulcus. The GP axons concerned with conscious proprioception pass dorsal to the dorsal gray column and without synapsing enter the dorsal funiculus and course cranially. The GP axons from the pelvic limbs and the trunk caudal to about the level of the sixth thoracic spinal cord segment course cranially in the medial portion of this funiculus in the fasciculus gracilis (see Figs. 9-5 and 9-6; see also Figs. 9-2 and 9-4).[36] Cranial to this level, the GP axons are situated more laterally and comprise the fasciculus cuneatus (see Fig. 2-17). The dorsal funiculus is organized somatotopically so that the GP axons from the more caudal levels are positioned in the dorsal funiculus more medially. At progressively more cranial levels, the GP axons are contributed to a more lateral aspect of this funiculus. Thus the cervical GP axons are the most lateral in the funiculus. As these GP axons course cranially, many leave this pathway to terminate in the adjacent spinal cord gray matter.

Nucleus Gracilis and Medial Cuneate Nucleus. The GP axons that reach the caudal medulla in the fasciculus gracilis terminate by synapsing on neuronal cell bodies in the nucleus gracilis (see Figs. 9-4 through 9-6).[26,39] This nucleus is located in a dorsal position, where it begins in the most cranial portion of the fasciculus gracilis. This occurs just caudal to the level of the obex and at the level of the pyramidal decussation. It is adjacent to the dorsal median sulcus and extends rostrally to the level of the obex, where it is dorsal to the parasympathetic nucleus of the vagus nerve and medial to the medial cuneate nucleus (see Figs. 2-16 and 2-17).

The GP axons concerned with conscious proprioception that reach the caudal medulla in the fasciculus cuneatus terminate by synapsing on neuronal cell bodies in the medial cuneate nucleus (see Fig. 9-5).[27,39] This nucleus is dorsal in the caudal medulla just lateral to nucleus gracilis. It is larger than nucleus gracilis and extends rostrally beyond the level of the obex, where it is medial to the caudal portion of the lateral cuneate nucleus (see Figs. 2-15 and 2-16). Remember that the lateral cuneate nucleus is in the cuneocerebellar pathway.

Medial Lemniscus and Ventral Caudal Lateral Thalamic Nucleus. Axons from the neuronal cell bodies in nucleus gracilis and the medial cuneate nucleus course ventrally and transversely through the medulla as the deep arcuate fibers to the opposite side of the median plane (see Figs. 2-14 and 2-15). There they form the medial lemniscus dorsal to the contralateral pyramid and ventromedial to the olivary nucleus (see Figs. 9-5 and 9-6). The medial lemniscus, oriented in a dorsal plane, courses rostrally through the medulla dorsal to the pyramid (see Figs. 2-13 through 2-15). As it passes through the dorsal part of the trapezoid body, it is medial to the dorsal nucleus of the trapezoid body (see Figs. 2-11 and 2-12). In the pons, it is located dorsal to the longitudinal fibers of the pons (see Figs. 2-9 and 2-10). In the mesencephalon, it is ventral in the caudal tegmentum and dorsal to the substantia nigra, and it shifts laterally as it course through the tegmentum of the rostral mesencephalon and into the caudal diencephalon (see Figs. 2-5 through 2-8). The medial lemniscus terminates by synapsing on neuronal cell bodies in the ventral caudal lateral nucleus of the thalamus. This is a specific projection nucleus of the thalamus for sensory systems that enter the spinal cord over the dorsal roots of spinal nerves. It is a poorly defined nucleus located ventrally in the caudal thalamus dorsal to its external medullary lamina. The axons of the neuronal cell bodies in this nucleus join the thalamocortical fibers and enter the internal capsule and centrum semiovale to be distributed to the somesthetic cortex of the cerebral hemisphere.

The somesthetic cortex is described classically as being located in the parietal lobe of the cerebrum, caudal to the cruciate sulcus.[2,25] In the dog, it overlaps with the motor cortex because it is located in the caudal part of the postcruciate gyrus and the rostral suprasylvian gyrus. There is a somatotopic organization of the medial lemniscus, the ventral caudal lateral nucleus of the thalamus, and the somesthetic cortex (see Figs. 9-5 and 9-6). All sensory systems project to localized regions of the cerebral cortex called primary sensory areas. Five of these are well established: auditory, visual, olfactory, gustatory, and somesthetic. The somatotopic organization of the somesthetic cerebral cortex reflects the density of receptor organs in the various regions of the body. For example, the prehensile organs of the animal (the nose and lips of the pig and horse, the lips and tongue of the dog, the forepaws of the raccoon and cat, the hand of the primate) have an abundance of receptor organs for this function and a correspondingly large area of representation in the somesthetic cortex.[1,2]

Although this dorsal funiculus pathway is emphasized in neurology texts as being concerned primarily with the conscious perception of general proprioception, in reality it is much more complex and functions with other sensory modalities. In addition, there are other pathways for transmitting general proprioception to a level of conscious perception. These include pathways that utilize the lateral cervical nucleus and nucleus Z.

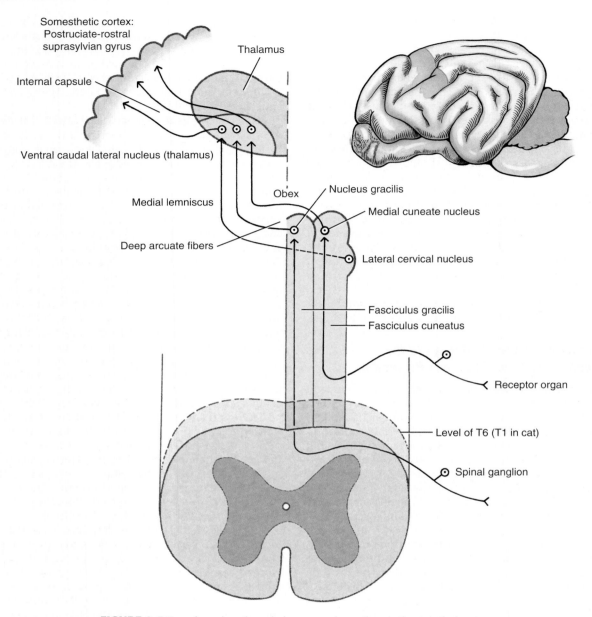

FIGURE 9-5 General proprioception, spinal nerve conscious pathway to the somesthetic cortex.

Lateral Cervical Nucleus. The lateral cervical nucleus projects from the lateral side of the dorsal gray column in the first two cervical spinal cord segments. Primarily, it receives axons from the spinocervical tract that is located in the ipsilateral lateral funiculus.[6,9-11,47,51] The neuronal cell bodies of these spinocervical tract axons are located in nucleus proprius, which is in the middle portion of the ipsilateral dorsal gray column that extends the entire length of the spinal cord. GP axons in all the dorsal roots have access to these neurons in the dorsal gray column.

The neurons in the lateral cervical nucleus serve as the third set of neurons in this spinocervicothalamic pathway.[22] The axons of the neuronal cell bodies in this lateral cervical nucleus course cranially and cross to the opposite side in the caudal medulla, where they join the medial lemniscus. Their course in the medial lemniscus to the ventral caudal lateral thalamic nucleus and from there to the somesthetic

cortex is similar to that of the deep arcuate fibers that enter the medial lemniscus. The lateral cervical nucleus is somatotopically organized, with pelvic limb afferents synapsing in the dorsolateral aspect of the nucleus and thoracic limb afferents synapsing in the ventromedial aspect. In the dog and cat this nucleus has a major role in the conscious projection of tactile sensation.

Nucleus Z. Nucleus Z is a small nucleus located at the rostral aspect of nucleus gracilis in the caudal medulla. It receives axons from the lateral funiculus that originate from ipsilateral dorsal gray column neuronal cell bodies located in spinal cord segments caudal to the cervical intumescence. Nucleus Z also receives collateral branches from axons in the dorsal spinocerebellar tract. The axons of neuronal cell bodies in nucleus Z cross in the caudal medulla to join the contralateral medial lemniscus, where their course to the thalamus and somesthetic cortex is described earlier.

Cerebral projection

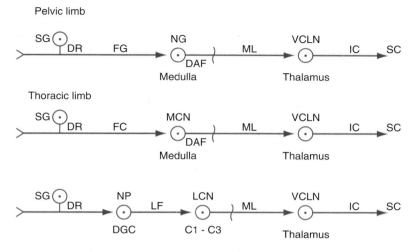

FIGURE 9-6 Cerebral projection. *C1-C3,* Cervical spinal cord segments; *DAF,* deep arcuate fibers; *DGC,* dorsal gray column; *DR,* dorsal root; *FC,* fasciculus cuneatus; *FG,* fasciculus gracilis; *IC,* internal capsule; *LCN,* lateral cervical nucleus; *LF,* lateral funiculus; *MCN,* medial cuneate nucleus; *ML,* medial lemniscus; *NG,* nucleus gracilis; *NP,* nucleus proprius; *SC,* somesthetic cortex; *SG,* spinal ganglion; *VCLN,* ventral caudal lateral nucleus of thalamus; *l,* crossed pathway.

Once again, the student and clinician should appreciate the complexity that has been introduced here but should also understand the following clinical observations:

1. As clinicians, we cannot localize lesions to individual CNS tracts concerned with posture and locomotion, and we cannot reliably distinguish lesions that affect the conscious GP pathway from those that affect the unconscious GP pathways to the cerebellum. Therefore, the clinical term *conscious proprioception* should not be used because it is not accurate.

2. There is no reliable test that clearly distinguishes the loss of general proprioception from the loss of UMN function. The two systems are closely related throughout the CNS, and most lesions affect the two systems simultaneously.

3. Determining the location of lesions in the UMN and GP systems is limited to regional anatomic diagnoses. They include the prosencephalon, the pons and medulla, the cerebellum, and the four divisions of the spinal cord (C1-5, C6-T2, T3-L3, and L4-Cd). The details of making these anatomic diagnoses are found in the subsequent chapters.

Cranial Nerve General Proprioception

Consideration of the GP system located in the cranial nerves is primarily an anatomic exercise because there is not much of clinical importance here that we have recognized. Most of these GP receptor organs are located in the muscles of mastication, in facial and extraocular muscles, and in the temporomandibular joints. The axons from these receptors course to the brainstem primarily in the three branches of the trigeminal nerve. All of these GP axons in the ophthalmic, maxillary, and mandibular nerves course through the trigeminal ganglion, which is located in the petrous portion of the temporal bone and enter the pons with the trigeminal nerve. In the pons, these GP axons form the mesencephalic tract of the trigeminal nerve that courses rostrally along the lateral border of the central gray substance of the fourth ventricle and mesencephalic aqueduct. Although the

rule is that cell bodies of afferent neurons are located in ganglia in the peripheral nervous system, these GP neurons are an exception to this rule and have their cell bodies within the CNS. They are located in the mesencephalic nucleus of the trigeminal nerve in a narrow band on the lateral border of the central gray substance throughout the mesencephalon. These are very large pyramid-shaped cell bodies that are readily recognizable. On microscopic examination of brain sections, recognizing a single row of these large cell bodies informs you that you are looking at the mesencephalon.

Reflex Activity

For reflex function, the axons may pass from the mesencephalic nucleus directly to the adjacent GSE nuclei of cranial nerves to synapse on an alpha motor neuron (Fig. 9-7). Other mesencephalic nucleus axons may synapse in the pontine sensory nucleus of the trigeminal nerve which, in turn, may synapse on a GSE neuron in a cranial nerve nucleus.

Conscious Pathway

GP axons from neuronal cell bodies in the mesencephalic nucleus of the trigeminal nerve enter the adjacent pontine sensory nucleus of the trigeminal nerve where they synapse on neuronal cell bodies in this nucleus. This pontine sensory nucleus is located in the caudal pons and rostral medulla, where it is positioned between the trigeminal nerve and its GSE motor nucleus. It is ventromedial to the middle and rostral cerebellar peduncles. The axons of these cell bodies in the pontine sensory nucleus cross through the ventral portion of the reticular formation to join the contralateral trigeminal lemniscus (quintothalamic tract), which joins the medial lemniscus and courses rostrally to the caudal thalamus. These axons terminate by synapsing on neuronal cell bodies in the ventral caudal medial nucleus of the thalamus. The thalamic nuclear axons join the thalamocortical fibers and course through the internal

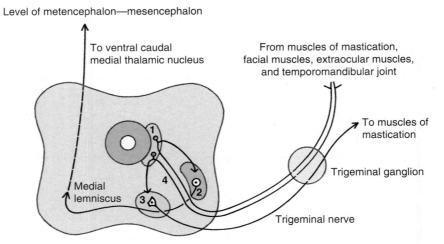

FIGURE 9-7 Trigeminal proprioceptive pathways.
1. Nucleus of the mesencephalic tract of the trigeminal nerve
2. Pontine sensory nucleus of the trigeminal nerve
3. Motor nucleus of the trigeminal nerve
4. Mesencephalic tract of the trigeminal nerve

capsule, centrum semiovale, and corona radiata to reach the somesthetic cortex. The involvement of the mesencephalic nucleus of the trigeminal nerve in the GP innervation of head muscles may be limited to the muscles of mastication. Retrograde studies using horseradish peroxidase have shown that the afferent neurons that supply the dog's tongue have no cell bodies in the mesencephalic nucleus. The cell bodies of the intramuscular neurons of both the intrinsic and extrinsic tongue muscles are located in the first cervical spinal ganglia, the distal ganglia of the vagus, and the trigeminal ganglia. Other studies in the sheep and pig have shown that the neuronal cell bodies of the afferent neurons of their extraocular muscles are all in the trigeminal ganglia.

Clinical Signs

Ataxia and incoordination are synonyms for the principal clinical sign observed with lesions that affect the GP system that enters the CNS from spinal nerves. Many case studies have been published in which the patient is described as being ataxic and incoordinated, as though these were two different deficits—which they are not! There are three qualities of ataxia: general proprioceptive ataxia, vestibular ataxia, and cerebellar ataxia. The use of the terms *sensory ataxia* and *motor ataxia* is inaccurate and confusing and should be avoided. GP ataxia is a result of the lack of kinesthesia, the lack of the sense of motion, or the lack of awareness of the position of the neck, trunk, and limbs in space. When we are evaluating the posture and gait of a patient, we always ask ourselves: Does this animal know where its limbs are, relative to its body? If the answer is no, then there is likely to be a deficit in the animal's GP system. A common mistake is to refer to a patient with only lower motor neuron (LMN) signs as being ataxic.

We have already stressed that focal lesions usually affect the UMN system and the GP system at the same time, and it is often difficult to distinguish the GP ataxia from the UMN paresis; it is not necessary to do this. Remember that we are trying to make an anatomic diagnosis of which level of the CNS is affected by a lesion, not which specific tracts are affected at that level. Nevertheless, the loss of function in the GP system is primarily responsible for the following clinical signs.

The patient may stand with the paws or hoofs placed more lateral than normal or with a base-wide stance or, occasionally, may stand with the dorsal surface of the paw or hoof on the ground surface. On moving, the limb may swing wide to the side and circumduct or abduct more than normal, cross beneath the trunk, or adduct more than normal, sometimes interfering with the opposite limb. There may be a delay in the initiation of protraction of the limb on getting up or while walking. The latter may cause a longer stride than normal. The patient may drag its digits while walking or may walk on the dorsal surface of its paw or hoof, which is often referred to as "knuckling over." Occasionally while walking, a degree of overresponse is seen during flexion of the limb. This causes the limb to be lifted higher than usual, and it may be combined with excessive abduction of the limb. This excessive flexion is often called hypermetria and may be confused with the hypermetria that occurs with cerebellar disorders. This is not surprising, considering that these GP lesions involve the input of the spinocerebellar tracts to the cerebellum. Hypermetria may reflect a loss of the inhibitory influence of the cerebellum on the brainstem UMN nuclei. We address this issue when we describe the clinical signs of cerebellar disease. A common clinical sign of dysfunction of the UMN and GP systems in the cervical spinal cord is a longer thoracic limb stride that hesitates slightly before the paw or hoof lands on the ground surface. Various terms have been used for this sign, including overreaching, floating, and hypermetria. This clinical sign is commonly mistaken for a sign of cerebellar dysfunction. We do not know whether this clinical sign reflects dysfunction of the GP or the UMN system or both, but when present it is very reliable for a cervical spinal cord white matter lesion. See Case Examples 10-4 and 10-5 and Videos 10-27 and 10-32 in Chapter 10, which concerns small animal cervical spinal cord diseases.

As previously indicated, normal postural reactions require that all components of the nervous system be intact. The postural reactions include the hopping or hemiwalking responses, paw or hoof replacement, placing, and the tonic neck test. Any one of these tests will be delayed by lesions in the GP system, but none of them is specific for only that system. In the tonic neck test, with the patient standing in place, the head and neck are fully extended; the normal animal extends its thoracic limbs to maintain its posture. An abnormality is recognized when the paw or hoof is flexed so that the dorsal surface is in a weight-bearing position. Occasionally, it helps to induce this clinical sign if the patient is forced to walk in a head-and-neck-extended position. With prosencephalic lesions, the gait is usually normal and the only abnormality is the delay in postural reactions. The same may be true with very mild caudal brainstem or spinal cord lesions that affect the UMN and GP systems without causing the expected gait deficit that is seen in most cases.

Prosencephalic lesions that involve the frontoparietal cortex and its corona radiata, the associated centrum semiovale, internal capsule, and thalamocortical fibers or thalamic nuclei are readily recognized on the neurologic examination by the presence of a normal gait on a flat surface and a delay in postural reactions, especially the hopping responses, in the limbs on the side opposite from the prosencephalic lesion. With peracute lesions, a mild contralateral hemiparesis and ataxia may be observable in the gait for the first day or two after the peracute traumatic or vascular insult. These lesions affect the prosencephalic components of *both* the UMN and the GP systems.

A unilateral cervical spinal cord lesion between the C1 and C5 spinal cord segments causes an ipsilateral spastic hemiparesis and ataxia with delayed or absent postural reactions in the limbs on the same side as the lesion. A mild delay in postural reactions may be observed in the contralateral limbs because of the small number of GP system neurons from the contralateral side that have axons that cross at their origin to enter a spinocerebellar pathway that courses to the medulla and cerebellum on the same side where the cervical spinal cord lesion is located. Similarly, a few UMN axons cross in the spinal cord segment, where they terminate. They would also be affected by the unilateral cervical spinal cord lesion. However, the predominant gait abnormality and postural reaction deficits will be on the ipsilateral side of the lesion.

Unilateral lesions in the pons and medulla usually produce an ipsilateral spastic hemiparesis and ataxia that can be seen in the gait. Such lesions also produce delayed or absent postural reactions in the same ipsilateral limbs. The ataxia and part of the postural reaction deficit can be explained by the unilateral lesion affecting the spinocerebellar pathways that predominantly are transmitting proprioceptive information from the ipsilateral limbs. However, these lesions also affect the medial lemniscus, which is transmitting conscious GP impulses from the contralateral limbs. We believe that the loss of the spinocerebellar GP pathways causes more deficits in the gait and postural reactions than the loss of the GP conscious pathways. This theory is based on the published results of experimental studies as well as on our study of natural lesions.[48] Experimental sectioning of the dorsal funiculi bilaterally in the dog, cat, and monkey initially resulted in a high stepping gait that was nearly completely compensated for in a 2- to 3-week period.[40] We have observed significant paresis and ataxia in dogs and horses with cervical spinal cord compression associated with cervical vertebral malformation and malarticulation in which there were no microscopic lesions in the dorsal funiculi.

Diseases

Most of the diseases that affect the GP system that originates in spinal nerves also affect other systems and are described with discussion of that system or with discussion of a region of the CNS such as the spinal cord. Spinal cord diseases are addressed in Chapters 10 and 11. Peripheral nerve lesions affect the axons of the first neurons in this system, but the involvement of the GSE-LMN axons predominates the clinical signs. These are discussed in Chapter 5. A unique inflammatory lesion that is limited to the neuronal cell bodies in peripheral ganglia affects only the GP and GSA systems. This ganglionitis is described after the discussion of the GSA system in this chapter.

A rare iatrogenic peripheral neurologic disorder affecting the GP and GSA systems may follow a small animal surgical restraint procedure. If the patient is immobilized on the surgical table by placing ties just proximal to the tarsus, the compression of the sensory branches of the peroneal nerves located there may result in the dog's walking on the dorsal aspects of its digits. At this level, the GSE-LMN axons that innervate the cranial crural muscles have left the peroneal nerves, leaving only GP and GSA axons to be compressed. Hypalgesia or analgesia of the dorsal surface of the paw may accompany this abnormal paw position. The prognosis in these patients depends on the length of time of the compression and on the force applied by the tie.

■ GENERAL SOMATIC AFFERENT SYSTEM

The GSA system is often loosely referred to as the "pain, temperature, touch system." This points out the widespread misuse of pain as a modality, which we address at the beginning of this chapter. The receptor organs, both encapsulated and nonencapsulated, are classified as exteroceptors because they receive their stimuli by physical contact with the external environment. These exteroceptors are further classified as mechanoreceptors, thermoreceptors, and nociceptors on the basis of the form of energy that is their adequate stimulus. Although the neurons in this system are concerned with the perception of changes in temperature, crude and discriminating touch, and various levels of noxious stimuli, it is often difficult to interpret the animal's response to the testing of these modalities. Therefore, the clinical neurologist must be most concerned with the patient's response to noxious stimuli, or nociception.[5]

GSA neurons are found in all the spinal nerves and in many cranial nerves. The role of this system in reflex activity and in the pathways of nociception are described.

Spinal Nerve General Somatic Afferent System

Many of the GSA neurons related to noxious stimuli have dendritic zones that are free endings on the surface of the body. The axons course through the named peripheral nerves, the spinal nerves, and the dorsal roots to enter the spinal cord at the dorsolateral sulcus (Fig. 9-8). Their

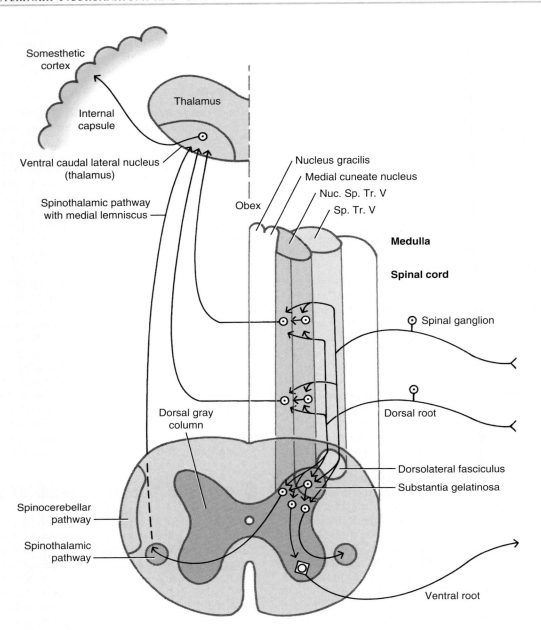

FIGURE 9-8 Spinal cord reflex and conscious perception GSA pathways. *Nuc. Sp. Tr. V.,* Nucleus of spinal tract of trigeminal nerve; *Sp. Tr. V,* spinal tract of trigeminal nerve.

cell bodies are located in the segmental spinal ganglion. Remember that there are no synapses in these sensory ganglia. Within the spinal cord, the GSA axon forms relatively short branches that course cranially and caudally on the surface of the dorsal gray column for a distance of two or three spinal cord segments. The tract that they form there is the dorsolateral fasciculus (Lissauer tract). Collaterals of these axonal branches enter the dorsal gray column all along the segments that are traversed. They provide branches that terminate by synapsing on interneurons located at the apex of the dorsal gray column in an area called the substantia gelatinosa. The axons continue into the middle of this gray column, where they synapse on other interneurons involved with reflex activity or on neurons that project cranially to the brainstem as part of the conscious pathway.

Reflex General Somatic Afferent Pathway

The GSA neuronal axons synapse on interneurons in the spinal cord gray matter, which in turn synapse on GSE alpha motor neurons in the ventral gray column (see Fig. 9-8). Some of these interneuronal axons enter the fasciculus proprius, where they course cranially or caudally to synapse on GSE alpha motor neurons in adjacent segments. The flexor (withdrawal) reflex requires the activation of a large number of GSE motor neurons that are located in a number of adjacent spinal cord segments that comprise the cervical and lumbosacral intumescences. This spread of the initial GSA stimulation is accomplished by the branching of their axons in the dorsolateral fasciculus and via their synapsing on these long interneurons. This reflex requires only the activity of the GSA neurons in the peripheral nerves that are stimulated, the associated spinal cord segments, the GSE axons in the peripheral nerves, and the muscles they innervate. These reflexes are normal or hyperactive in animals in which these spinal cord segments are separated from any communication with the brain by transverse lesions. As an example, review Video 3-4, shown in Chapter 3. It showed the 3-day-old Simmenthal calf in which there was no development of the first three lumbar spinal cord segments. All the movements you see in the pelvic limbs reflect exquisite hyperactivity of the flexor reflexes, for which the isolated lumbosacral intumescence is responsible.

Cutaneous Area, Autonomous Zone

The surface of the body can be mapped according to the distribution of GSA receptor organs that are associated with specific peripheral nerves or with specific dorsal roots. The area for an individual dorsal root is a dermatome. Dermatomal mapping represents the distribution of each dorsal root's GSA neuron's receptor organs on the body surface. This demonstrates the fate of the embryonic dorsal root innervation of the dermatomal portion of the somite. As the somitic dermatome expanded and contributed to the surface of the body, its dorsal root innervation extended with it by way of branches of the spinal nerve and the various named peripheral nerves.

Studies in the dog have shown that each dermatome of the neck and trunk extends from the dorsal to the ventral midline, and there is a craniocaudal overlap of up to three dorsal roots in the lumbosacral region.[19] The cutaneous area is the portion of the surface of the body innervated by GSA neurons in any one specific peripheral nerve. There is considerable overlap of the cutaneous areas of adjacent peripheral nerves. The autonomous zone is the portion of the body surface that is innervated by only one specific peripheral nerve (Figs. 9-9 and 9-10). Not all peripheral nerves have an autonomous zone. An awareness of these autonomous zones is critical for the clinician in determining the severity of a peripheral nerve lesion and thus the prognosis. Knowledge of peripheral nerve cutaneous areas is essential for successful local anesthesia. Because of the contribution of multiple spinal cord segments to the various named peripheral nerves, sensory deficits, like motor deficits, are more obvious with disrupted named peripheral nerves than with a disrupted single spinal nerve or dorsal root.

Anatomy of the Flexor Reflex

The anatomy of the flexor reflex in the thoracic and pelvic limbs is demonstrated in the following examples. Usually the noxious stimulus consists of compression of the base of a digit or a coronary band by forceps. Forceps are usually more reliable than using your fingers because the forceps deliver a constant repeatable pressure. In large animals, a pin, the pointed end of closed forceps, or a ballpoint pen may be a sufficient stimulus in the standing animal. Recumbent large

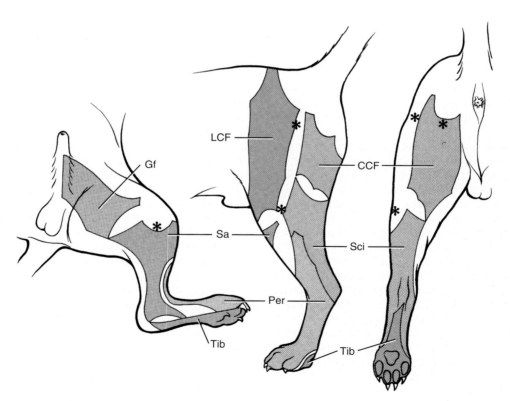

FIGURE 9-9 Autonomous zones of the cutaneous innervation of the pelvic limb. Medial, lateral, and caudal aspects. *CCF,* Caudal cutaneous femoral; *Gf,* genitofemoral; *LCF,* lateral cutaneous femoral; *Per,* peroneal; *Sa,* saphenous; *Sci,* sciatic; *Tib,* tibial. Asterisks indicate palpable bony landmarks: medial and lateral tibial condyles, greater trochanter, and lateral end of tuber ischiadicum. The sciatic nerve autonomous zone is for lesions proximal to the greater trochanter and includes the zones for the peroneal and tibial nerves. For sciatic nerve lesions caudal to the femur, the autonomous zone varies depending on how many of its cutaneous branches are affected.

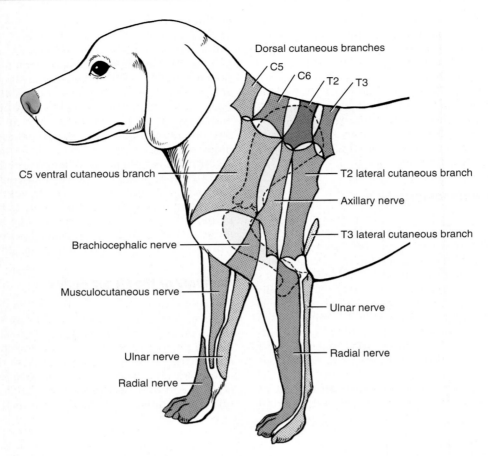

FIGURE 9-10 Autonomous zones of the cutaneous innervation of the thoracic limb.

animals commonly require a more rigorous stimulus, especially in cases of recumbent limbs. Occasionally an electric prod is necessary to assess reflex activity or nociception in recumbent cattle.

Thoracic Limb. A noxious stimulus applied to a digit causes withdrawal of the limb by flexion of the shoulder, elbow, carpus, and digits. Compression of the digits stimulates nociceptors in the radial nerve dorsally (plus the ulnar nerve in digit 5) and in the median or ulnar nerves on the palmar surface. The axons of these nociceptors course proximally in these named peripheral nerves and enter the spinal cord through the dorsal roots of the C7, C8, and T1 spinal cord segments (radial nerve) or through the C8, T1, T2 segments (median and ulnar nerves). Branches of these axons course cranially and caudally over a few segments in the dorsolateral fasciculus. Collaterals synapse on interneurons in the gray matter of the cervical intumescence. These interneurons synapse on GSE-LMNs in the ventral gray column of these segments that have axons that innervate the flexors of the shoulder (ventral roots and spinal nerve ventral branches of C7, C8, T1, and the axillary and radial nerves); flexors of the elbow (ventral roots and spinal nerve ventral branches of C6, C7, C8, and the musculocutaneous nerve); and flexors of the carpus and digits (ventral roots and spinal nerve ventral branches of C8, T1, T2, and the median and ulnar nerves).

The flexor reflex as well as nociception can be used to determine the integrity of the autonomous zone of individual named peripheral nerves. There is no need to

learn the boundaries of any autonomous zone. It is necessary to know only one site that is within the autonomous zone for each peripheral nerve that you want to test. In the thoracic limb, the autonomous zones most commonly tested by us include the skin of the dorsal paw for the radial nerve, the medial surface of the antebrachium for the musculocutaneous nerve, and the caudal surface of the antebrachium for the ulnar nerve (see Fig. 9-10).[35]

Pelvic Limb. A noxious stimulus applied to a digit causes withdrawal of the limb by flexion of the hip, stifle, tarsus, and digits. Compression of digits three to five stimulates nociceptors of the sciatic nerve (the peroneal nerve dorsally and the tibial nerve on the plantar surface). Compression of digits one and two includes the saphenous nerve. From digits three to five, the axons of the nociceptors course proximally in the sciatic nerve and enter the spinal cord through the dorsal roots of the L6, L7, and S1 spinal cord segments. From digits one and two, axons also course proximally in the saphenous nerve, a branch of the femoral nerve, and enter the spinal cord through the dorsal roots of L4, L5, and L6 spinal cord segments. Branches of these axons course cranially and caudally over a few segments in the dorsolateral fasciculus. Collaterals synapse on interneurons in the gray matter of the lumbosacral intumescence. These interneurons synapse on GSE-LMNs in the ventral gray column of most of the lumbar and the first sacral spinal cord segments that have axons that innervate the flexors of the hip (the ventral roots, the spinal nerve ventral branches of L1 to L6, and the femoral nerve); the flexors of the stifle (ventral roots and spinal nerve ventral branches of L6, L7, S1, and the sciatic nerve); the flexors of the tarsus (ventral roots and spinal nerve ventral branches of L6, L7, and the peroneal nerve); and the flexors of the digits (ventral roots and spinal nerve ventral branches of L7, S1, and the tibial nerve).

In the pelvic limb, a site for testing the autonomous zone for the tibial nerve is the skin of the plantar surface of the paw because the peroneal nerve uses the dorsal surface of the paw. To test the saphenous nerve (branch of the femoral nerve L4, L5, L6), use the medial surface of the crus; to test the genito-femoral nerve (L3, L4), use the proximal medial surface of the thigh; to test the caudal cutaneous femoral nerve (S1, S2, S3), use the caudal surface of the thigh; to test the lateral cutaneous femoral nerve (L3, L4, L5), use the craniolateral surface of the thigh. In male dogs, the prepuce can be used to test the genitofemoral nerve (L3, L4), and the skin of the penis to test the pudendal nerve (S1, S2, S3).[24,50] (See Fig. 9-9.)

Testing for the flexor reflex provides you with two responses for the price of one stimulus. The flexor reflex tests both the anatomic components of the reflex arc that were just described as well as the conscious perception pathway, or nociception. It is important for you to appreciate this and to take the time to differentiate between the two responses. When the conscious perception pathway is intact, the normal flexor reflex is more vigorous because of the added voluntary activity of the muscles involved in the reflex arc. Use caution when testing the flexor reflexes in animals in which the nociception pathways are intact so as to avoid being injured and to better assess the integrity of the components of the reflex arc.

General Somatic Afferent Pathway for Conscious Perception

For all the modalities served by the spinal nerve GSA neurons, the GSA axons in the dorsal roots enter the dorsal gray column and synapse on the neuronal dendritic zone or cell body in a specific nucleus or laminar zone (Fig. 9-11; see also Fig. 9-8). The axons of these cell bodies project cranially through a spinal cord funiculus and continue through the brainstem to terminate in the ventral caudal lateral nucleus of the thalamus. These thalamic neuronal cell bodies project axons to the somesthetic cortex for conscious perception of each of the specific modalities.[3-5,25,33,34,41-43]

Nociceptive Pathway. About one half of the afferent axons in cutaneous nerves originate from nociceptors. These receptors are stimulated by strong mechanical, thermal, and occasionally chemical stimuli. Inflammation in the vicinity of the nociceptors releases endogenous substances, such as serotonin, bradykinin, and prostaglandins, that lower the threshold of these nociceptors to noxious stimuli. The axons of these nociceptors are small and unmyelinated or lightly myelinated axons that are classified as A-delta or C-type axons. Their peripheral nerve pathways to the spinal cord segments are similar to those described for the flexor reflexes of the limbs. Collaterals of these axons terminate by synapsing on neuronal dendritic zones or cell bodies located in the various laminae of the dorsal gray column. These laminae are commonly referred to as Rexed laminae after the neuroanatomist responsible for their description. There are 10 laminae. Laminae I through VI are in the dorsal gray column. Neurons that participate in the nociceptive pathway are located in all six of these laminae. These cell bodies provide varying numbers of axons that contribute to spinal cord tracts that are located in all of the funiculi of the spinal cord. Most, but not all, of these axons cross to the opposite side of the spinal cord before coursing cranially in one of the three funiculi to ultimately reach the thalamus. The most significant nociceptive pathway in primates is the lateral spinothalamic tract.[34] It has a similar function in domestic animals, but its significance has been questioned. For this spinothalamic pathway, the neuronal cell body is located in the dorsal gray column. Its axon crosses to the opposite lateral funiculus where it becomes a component of the spinothalamic tract. This spinothalamic tract is in the ventral portion of the lateral funiculus, medial to the ventral spinocerebellar tract in humans and pigs.[5] It is more dorsal in the lateral funiculus of cats. In primates, it is a continuous uninterrupted pathway to the thalamus. In domestic animals, it is a multisynaptic pathway with axons leaving the tract at various levels to enter the spinal cord gray matter and synapse on a neuronal cell body. The axon of this cell body then reenters the spinothalamic tract of the same or the opposite-side lateral funiculus. Ultimately, the axons in this tract continue rostrally through the brainstem to

GSA pathway

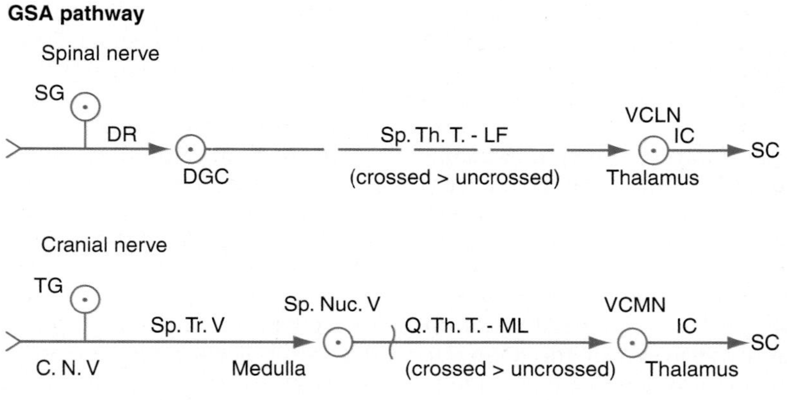

FIGURE 9-11 GSA pathway. *CNV,* Cranial nerve V; *DGC,* dorsal gray column; *DR,* dorsal root; *IC,* internal capsule; *LF,* lateral funiculus; *ML,* medial lemniscus; *Q. Th. T.,* quintothalamic tract; *SC,* somesthetic cortex; *SG,* spinal ganglion; *Sp. Nuc. V,* nucleus of spinal tract of trigeminal nerve; *Sp. Th. T.,* spinothalamic tract; *Sp. Tr. V.,* spinal tract of trigeminal nerve; *TG,* trigeminal ganglion; *VCLN,* ventral caudal lateral nucleus; *VCMN,* ventral caudal medial nucleus; *ʔ,* crossed pathway.

terminate by synapsing on a neuronal cell body in the ventral caudal lateral nucleus of the thalamus. The axons of this thalamic nucleus leave the thalamus via the thalamocortical projection fibers and enter the internal capsule and centrum semiovale, then continuing through a corona radiata to terminate in the somesthetic cerebral cortex of the frontoparietal lobes (see Fig. 9-11). Although nociception is considered to be a function of the somesthetic cerebral cortex, there is evidence that some perception may occur at the level of the thalamus. Video 3-1 in Chapter 3 shows a newborn calf that has no cerebral hemispheres, only a brainstem and cerebellum. This calf showed occasional discomfort when noxious stimuli were applied to its hooves or nasal septum.

As these spinothalamic axons course through the brainstem, collaterals synapse in various nuclei in the reticular formation that function in the ascending reticular activating system. This serves to diffusely activate the cerebral cortex to help maintain the conscious awake state.

Other neuronal cell bodies in the laminae of the dorsal gray column provide axons that use the following pathways to reach the thalamus for relay to the somesthetic cerebral cortex for nociception. The dorsal column postsynaptic pathway consists of dorsal gray column axons that enter the ipsilateral fasciculus gracilis or fasciculus cuneatus, where they course cranially to synapse in nucleus gracilis, the medial cuneate nucleus, or nucleus Z. The axons of these cell bodies cross through the caudal medulla to join the medial lemniscus, which courses rostrally to the thalamus. The spinocervicothalamic pathway consists of dorsal gray column axons that enter the ipsilateral dorsal portion of the lateral funiculus, where they course cranially to terminate in the lateral cervical nucleus in the first two cervical spinal cord segments. Axons from neuronal cell bodies in the lateral cervical nucleus cross to the opposite side to join the medial lemniscus, which courses rostrally to the thalamus. The spinomesencephalic tract is in the ventral funiculus. It receives axons from dorsal gray column neuronal cell bodies that cross at their origin to enter the contralateral spinomesencephalic tract. This tract courses through the caudal brainstem to terminate in various midbrain nuclei and thalamic nuclei.

The GSA conscious perception pathway is obviously extremely complex. We often refer to the entire complex as the spinothalamic system. Important practical points to remember are the following:

1. This system is diffusely distributed in tracts that either anatomically or functionally are in all of the spinal cord funiculi; therefore, it requires a severe transverse lesion that disrupts all of the spinal cord funiculi to cause a complete interruption in nociception and analgesia caudal to the lesion.

2. Because the majority of the axons in this spinothalamic system cross at their origin, a unilateral spinal cord lesion may cause a recognizable decrease in nociception-hypalgesia on the opposite side of the body caudal to the lesion. A lesion that causes a hemisection of the spinal cord, such as a midthoracic infarct resulting from fibrocartilaginous emboli, causes spastic paralysis of the ipsilateral pelvic limb and hypalgesia of the contralateral pelvic limb. In human neurology this is referred to as Brown-Séquard syndrome. Remember that the UMN system crosses predominantly prior to the pons and medulla, and the GSA nociceptor pathway crosses predominantly at its origin in the spinal cord.

3. The predominance of axons that cross at their origin in this nociceptive pathway is supported by lesions that disrupt the prosencephalic components of this pathway on one side. This results in hypalgesia of the contralateral side of the head, neck, trunk, and limbs.

There are numerous neuroanatomic and neurochemical factors that function to modulate the nociceptive system.[5,41-43] Much of the modulation occurs in the dorsal gray column where the primary GSA afferents terminate. Interneurons in the substantia gelatinosa at the apex of the dorsal gray column are inhibitory to the projection pathway neurons in other dorsal gray column laminae. These interneurons are activated by large-diameter myelinated nonnociceptive neurons. This activation modulates the output from the nociceptive projection neurons. Neuronal cell bodies in the periaqueductal gray area of the mesencephalon, the pontine locus ceruleus, and the medullary raphe nuclei all project axons caudally into the spinal cord that terminate in the dorsal gray column to inhibit the nociceptive projection neurons. Some of this inhibition involves the release of serotonin. The nociceptive GSA neuronal cell bodies in the spinal ganglia produce the neurotransmitter substance P, which is released at their telodendria in the dorsal gray column. Substance P is inhibited by the local action of the opiates morphine and enkephalin in the dorsal gray column.

Cranial Nerve

By far, the majority of the GSA system neurons involved with cranial nerves are components of the trigeminal nerve. The GSA axons course from the receptor organs on the surface of the head through the branches of the ophthalmic, maxillary, and mandibular nerves from the trigeminal nerve and through its ganglion, where their cell bodies are located. The trigeminal ganglion is located in the canal for the trigeminal nerve in the rostral part of the petrous portion of the temporal bone. The trigeminal nerve enters the pons through the caudolateral portion of the transverse fibers of the pons as these fibers form the middle cerebellar peduncle. This is just rostral to the origin of the facial and vestibulocochlear nerves (Fig. 9-12; see also Fig. 2-10). Figs. 9-13 and 9-14 show the ventral surface of the brain of an adult sea lion; Fig. 9-15 shows an adult dog for comparison. In the sea lion, note the very large trigeminal nerves that suggest extensive GSA innervation of the head in this species. Also note the large portions of the cerebellar hemispheres that extend laterally over the pons and medulla; they are associated with enlarged transverse fibers of the pons that caudally overlap the trapezoid body. This association is described in Chapter 13, which concerns the cerebellum.

In the brainstem, these GSA axons form the spinal tract of the trigeminal nerve. The tract has a short rostral portion in the pons and a long portion that extends caudally on the lateral side of the medulla (see Fig. 9-4). This tract is shaped like a quarter circle with the concave surface facing medially (see Figs. 2-11 through 2-17). As this tract passes from rostral to caudal, it is medial to the cochlear nuclei in the vestibulocochlear nerve and to the dorsal spinocerebellar tract as the latter enters the caudal cerebellar peduncle through the superficial arcuate fibers. At the obex, this spinal tract of the trigeminal nerve becomes superficial on the lateral side of the medulla between the fasciculus cuneatus dorsally and the dorsal spinocerebellar tract ventrally. The

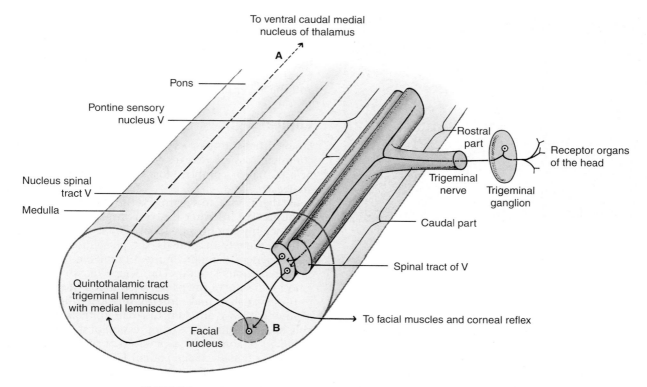

FIGURE 9-12 Trigeminal nerve, GSA pathways. **A,** Conscious pathway; **B,** reflex pathway.

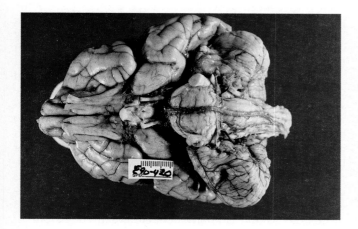

FIGURE 9-13 Ventral surface of the brain of an adult sea lion. Note the large trigeminal nerves, the transverse fibers of pons, and the lateral aspect of the cerebellar hemispheres.

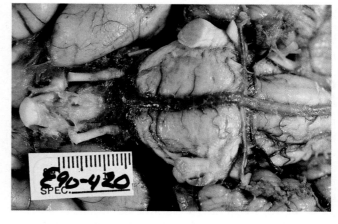

FIGURE 9-14 The same brain as in Fig. 9-13.

spinal tract continues caudally into the first cervical spinal cord segment, where it is continued by the dorsolateral fasciculus (see Figs. 2-15 and 2-16). Throughout this course of the trigeminal spinal tract, a nuclear column is located on its concave medial surface. Rostrally in the pons, this is the pontine sensory nucleus of the trigeminal nerve (see Fig. 2-11). Throughout the medulla and into the first cervical spinal cord segment, it is the nucleus of the spinal tract of the trigeminal nerve (see Figs. 2-12 through 2-17). This nuclear column is similar in shape to the spinal tract of the trigeminal nerve. In the cervical spinal cord, this nucleus is continuous with the substantia gelatinosa of the dorsal gray column. GSA axons in the spinal tract terminate by

synapsing on neurons in the nuclear column medial to this tract. The pontine sensory nucleus is thought to be primarily concerned with mechanoreception. The entire spinal nucleus is concerned with GSA reflex activity and nociception in the head.

Reflex General Somatic Afferent Pathway

Axons of the neuronal cell bodies in this nucleus of the spinal tract of the trigeminal nerve project to GSE-LMN nuclei in the brainstem to complete reflex arcs. A useful example is the palpebral reflex, in which a light touch on the eyelids stimulates GSA receptors whose axons course in branches of

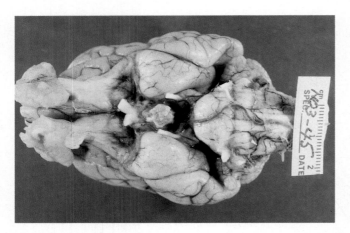

FIGURE 9-15 The ventral surface of a normal dog brain for comparison with Figs. 9-13 and 9-14.

the ophthalmic and maxillary nerves from the trigeminal nerve through the trigeminal ganglion and into the spinal tract of the trigeminal nerve. These terminate by synapsing in the nucleus of this spinal tract. The axons of these neuronal cell bodies course to the adjacent facial nucleus to synapse on GSE-LMNs. The axons of these LMNs course through the facial nerve and its palpebral branches to innervate the orbicularis oculi and cause closure of the eyelids. The corneal reflex has a similar pathway but involves stimulation only of branches of the ophthalmic nerve. If possible, you should avoid evoking this corneal reflex so as not to injure the cornea. If it is absolutely necessary, use a cotton ball or swab to perform the test.

General Somatic Afferent Pathway for Conscious Perception

For nociception, other axons from neuronal cell bodies in the pontine sensory nucleus and the nucleus of the spinal tract of the trigeminal nerve cross predominantly to the opposite side of the brainstem to become associated with the medial lemniscus. These axons are sometimes referred to as the trigeminal lemniscus or the quintothalamic tract. These axons course rostrally to the caudal thalamus to terminate by synapsing on neuronal cell bodies in the specific projection nucleus of the thalamus for the GSA system that is present in cranial nerves. This is the ventral caudal medial nucleus of the thalamus. Axons of the cell bodies in this thalamic nucleus project from the thalamus in the thalamocortical fibers, enter the internal capsule and centrum semiovale, and are distributed through corona radiata to the head region of the somesthetic cerebral cortex (see Figs. 9-11 and 9-12). There is clinical evidence for a predominantly contralateral projection of this trigeminal nerve nociceptive pathway. Unilateral lesions that involve prosencephalic components of this GSA nociceptive pathway cause contralateral hypalgesia. A reliable test for nociception in the head is to lightly touch the mucosa of the nasal septum with the blunt end of closed forceps. This stimulates the ethmoidal nerve, which is a branch of the ophthalmic nerve from the trigeminal nerve. This mucosa is very sensitive;

many animals show no cerebral response to the pinching of various areas of the skin on the head. Sites to test for the autonomous zone for each of the three branches of the trigeminal nerve include the nasal septum mucosa for the ophthalmic nerve, the upper lip for the maxillary nerve, and the lower lip or tongue for the mandibular nerve.

Clinical Signs

Lesions that interfere with GSA function cause a partial or complete loss of reflexes—hyporeflexia or areflexia and/or a partial or complete loss of nociception-hypalgesia or analgesia.

By definition, nociception is the perception of a noxious stimulus. We interpret this response as pain, and it varies considerably among individual animal patients. In humans, and presumably in animals, the perception is modified by past experiences and memories of previous encounters with similar noxious stimuli. The degree of attention and the emotional state of the patient also modify the response. All of these variables make interpreting disruption of the nociceptive pathway difficult. In small animals, the most reliable noxious stimulus is compression of the skin at the base of a digit or compression of a fold of skin on the body surface using forceps. If the patient is cooperative, it is best to lightly grasp a fold of skin before compressing it. Using a sharp pin as a stimulus is often unreliable in small animals but may be effective in horses. In large animals, the blunt end of closed forceps or a ballpoint pen may be sufficient to elicit nociception. In recumbent large animals, an electric prod may be necessary, especially on the recumbent side. In the head, all animals readily respond to lightly touching the nasal mucosa with the blunt end of closed forceps or, in large animals, your finger.

Many publications describe testing for superficial and deep "pain" by varying the degree of compression of the skin, suggesting that there are different nociceptive pathways in animals. We do not feel this is reliable enough to be worth trying to interpret the responses. There is so much difference among individual animal patients that we do not believe we can reliably tell the difference between an animal's response to light compression versus more rigorous compression. In addition, within the spinal cord any difference between the nociceptive pathways of these two degrees of noxious stimuli is poorly defined. We are not aware of any definitive clinical significance in trying to make this nociceptive distinction, so we neither do it ourselves nor advocate doing it.

Nociceptive testing has significant prognostic value in cases of spinal cord or peripheral nerve lesions, especially injuries. A common small animal spinal cord injury occurs when a dog or cat is struck by an automobile, and a thoracic vertebra is fractured. In severe spinal cord injury, there is complete paralysis of motor function, but if nociception is still intact in the pelvic limbs, you know there is a nociceptive pathway through the injury and the spinal cord has not been severed. The prognosis is still guarded but is better than if there was analgesia caudal to the lesion. Remember that your neurologic examination tests only nervous system function, not its structural integrity.

A dog with this traumatic injury that has complete paralysis of motor and sensory function caudal to the lesion may still recover if the dysfunction is due primarily to hemorrhage and edema, which can resolve. Your examination defines only the degree of dysfunction, not the degree of structural damage. The same concept applies to peripheral nerve lesions. If an animal fractures the body of its ilium, which injures the adjacent sciatic nerve, the presence of nociception in the autonomous zone of this nerve indicates that the nerve has not been severed, and the prognosis for recovery is guarded but better than if there was analgesia in this autonomous zone.

Be aware that loss of the GSA innervation of the cornea by the ophthalmic nerve from the trigeminal nerve can result in neurotrophic keratitis.[49] This innervation is necessary for the normal maintenance of the integrity of the cornea. Occasionally, this is the first clinical sign that an owner recognizes in a dog that has a developing malignant nerve sheath neoplasm of the trigeminal nerve.

Diseases

Many of the peripheral nerve disorders that are described in Chapter 5 and involve the GSE-LMN also involve the peripheral nerve components of the GSA system. As a rule, the loss of the GSE-LMN predominates the clinical signs. Chapter 10 includes numerous spinal cord disorders that affect components of the GSA system, especially the conscious perception pathway. Neuropathies that involve predominantly the GP and GSA systems are much less common but have been described. Be aware that animals that exhibit self-mutilation may suffer from a distal sensory neuropathy or a behavioral disorder such as obsessive-compulsive disorder. Two examples of the former are described here.

Canine Sensory Neuropathy

Dr. John Cummings and I (AD) studied a self-mutilation of the digits (acral mutilation) with nociceptive loss in three of a litter of nine English pointers.[12,14] A similar clinical syndrome resulting from autosomal recessive inheritance was described in Czechoslovakian short-haired pointers.[45] At around 3 months of age, these three English pointers began to constantly lick or bite at their paws. This progressed to severe acral mutilation, with necrosis and even loss of digits accompanied by analgesia in some of the digits. Gait, postural reactions, and spinal reflexes were normal. The last were absent when analgesic digits were stimulated. Necropsy of one dog revealed a decrease in size of the spinal ganglia due to a deficiency of neuronal cell bodies that varied from about 20% to 50% of the neuronal cell bodies. There was reduced axonal density in the dorsolateral fasciculus and mild degeneration in dorsal roots, spinal ganglia, and peripheral nerves.

Immunocytochemical stains showed a deficiency of the nociceptive neurotransmitter substance P in the dorsal gray column. We concluded that the acral mutilation was a result of a hypoplasia and slowly progressive postnatal degeneration of GSA neurons.

Two long-haired dachshunds were studied for slowly progressive pelvic limb ataxia, urinary incontinence, episodes of gastrointestinal disturbance, and peripheral nociceptive deficit.[17,18] When the dogs were walking, the pelvic limbs would abduct and overflex on protraction, producing a bouncy type of hypermetric gait. There was a

complete loss of general proprioception. One dog constantly chewed on its penis. All four paws were analgesic in one dog and hypalgesic in the other. There was a generalized hypalgesia over the trunk, neck, and head. Patellar reflexes were normal but flexor reflexes were usually absent due to the loss of GSA function. These signs began shortly after the dogs could first walk and were obvious by 12 weeks of age. After months of slow progression, the clinical signs remained unchanged. Motor nerve conduction was normal but sensory nerve conduction was decreased or absent. Necropsy revealed a distal axonopathy of sensory neurons and loss or degeneration of large myelinated axons and unmyelinated axons. A familial disorder was suspected. Other diseases affecting the GP or GSA systems have been described in the boxer, Pyrenean mountain dog, and Parson (Jack) Russell terrier.

Sensory Ganglioradiculitis

We have studied a number of adult dogs of various breeds that present with a fairly abrupt onset of a gait disorder that is unusual and slowly progresses. The signs are more obvious in the pelvic limbs. There is excessive overflexion of the limbs, along with abduction that creates an abrupt, bouncy type of action. It most resembles a cerebellar gait disorder but the balance is quite well preserved. The ataxia is too extreme for a spinal cord disorder. This gait is very difficult to describe and is best understood by studying the videos. When you examine a dog with this disorder, you usually react by saying, "This gait disorder does not make any sense." Then you hope to find other clinical signs to support the diagnosis of sensory ganglioradiculitis.[8,13,46] These dogs may stand with a base-wide posture. Postural reactions are delayed. Spinal flexor reflexes are normal, but the patellar reflex is commonly depressed or absent. Some asymmetry in these signs may be present. We believe this is a general proprioceptive disorder without any associated motor system involvement.

Other signs that have been observed in some of these dogs involve cranial nerves. They include facial hypalgesia, difficult prehension, gagging due to partial dysphagia, megaesophagus, and masticatory muscle atrophy. At necropsy there is diffuse nonsuppurative lymphoplasmacytic inflammation of multiple spinal and cranial nerve ganglia that extends into the dorsal roots. There is recognizable loss of neuronal cell bodies in these ganglia and wallerian degeneration in the associated dorsal roots and more distal peripheral nerves. The masticatory muscle atrophy is thought to be due to the inflammation in the trigeminal ganglion affecting the GSE-LMN axons that course through this ganglion to enter the mandibular nerve from the trigeminal nerve that innervates these muscles. At present there is no ancillary procedure that is reliable other than a biopsy of a spinal ganglion. Magnetic resonance imaging studies must be more extensively evaluated in this disorder. An autoimmune disorder or possibly a viral infection is considered to be the most likely cause. Too few cases of this disorder are recognized and treated to allow us to recommend any reliable therapy. Pathologists should take note that when they recognize a wallerian-type degeneration that is limited to the dorsal funiculi at *all* levels of the spinal cord, and in the absence of any other spinal cord lesions, the primary lesion is in the spinal ganglia. What you are observing is the wallerian degeneration of the GP conscious pathway axons that directly enter the dorsal funiculi without synapse until they reach the caudal medulla. The following videos show three dogs with this presumptive diagnosis.

Video 9-1 shows Bailey, a 2-year-old castrated male mixed-breed dog with a history of a progressive gait disorder for 6 to 8 weeks. The clinical signs began in the right pelvic limb and spread to the left pelvic limb; more recently, the thoracic limbs had been abnormal. Initially, he was treated for an undiagnosed orthopedic disorder that included chiropractic therapy. He was referred to Eric Glass for study for a spinal cord disorder. Note the pelvic limb asymmetry. Note the loss of patellar reflexes. Whenever you have loss of the patellar reflexes with normal ability to support weight, normal tone, and no atrophy, be aware that the reflex is absent because of loss of the sensory components of the reflex arc. Bailey had no cranial nerve abnormalities. Bailey received corticosteroid therapy for 6 weeks, but no change was seen, and he was followed for 4 years without any remarkable change occurring in his clinical signs.

Video 9-2 shows Max, an 11-year-old male Pomeranian with at least a 1-year history of having difficult walking with the pelvic limbs. Note that the gait is most abnormal in the pelvic limbs, but postural reactions are abnormal in all four limbs. Note the absence of patellar reflexes, with normal tone and no atrophy; the hypalgesic digits, especially in the thoracic limbs; and the analgesia of the nasal septum. The cerebrospinal fluid showed an elevated protein level.

Video 9-3 shows Millie, a 9-year-old spayed female Labrador retriever with several months of a progressive pelvic limb gait disorder that more recently had also affected the thoracic limbs. Note the abrupt hypermetric gait and abnormal postural reactions and the lack of patellar reflexes but normal quadriceps femoris tone and no atrophy. Note the normal flexor reflexes in the pelvic limbs and possible hypalgesia. Not shown is the significant nasal septum hypalgesia that was present.

Facial Hypalgesia or Analgesia

Facial hypalgesia or analgesia is caused by lesions that affect the trigeminal nerve, the trigeminal ganglion, or the trigeminal tract in the pons and medulla. About one third of dogs with idiopathic trigeminal neuritis have unilateral or bilateral facial hypalgesia or analgesia that accompanies the paralyzed dropped jaw. This sensory loss resolves as the jaw function returns. Chapter 6 and Video 6-3 show examples of this disorder. Unilateral partial or complete facial analgesia sometimes accompanies a malignant nerve sheath neoplasm of the trigeminal nerve. Unilateral facial analgesia in an animal following intracranial trauma indicates possible involvement of the spinal tract of the trigeminal nerve in the medulla and, hence, a guarded prognosis. Facial paralysis (cranial nerve VII) and clinical signs of a peripheral vestibular disorder (cranial nerve VIII) are common with otitis media-interna but if there is also facial hypalgesia or analgesia, the anatomic diagnosis is a lesion involving the petrous portion of the temporal bone or an intracranial lesion at that level, not otitis media-interna. A pure sensory neuropathy of the trigeminal nerve is rare but has been reported as a bilateral disorder in a young collie dog.[7] Remember that lesions that affect the ophthalmic nerve from the trigeminal nerve and deafferent the cornea may result in degenerative changes in the cornea. It is referred to as neurotrophic keratitis and consists of edema and erosion of the epithelial cells.[46] This relationship between the cellular metabolism of the cornea and its sensory nerve supply is poorly understood.

Unilateral nasal hypalgesia is a reliable sign of a contralateral prosencephalic disorder. Although the hypalgesia is present over the entire contralateral side of the body, the extreme sensitivity of the nasal septum mucosa makes it a reliable area to test. We review and show examples of the clinical signs that we can test during a neurologic examination that support an anatomic diagnosis of a prosencephalic disorder after we describe the anatomy of the visual system in Chapter 14. Fig. 9-16 combines the pathways seen in Fig. 8-14 (UMN), Fig. 9-5 (GP), Fig. 9-8 (GSA-spinal nerve), and Fig. 9-12 (GSA-cranial nerve). It illustrates the basis for two of the three clinical signs that we recognize in cases of unilateral prosencephalic lesions. A lesion that interrupts the left prosencephalic components of the systems seen here results in a right postural reaction deficit with a normal gait and a right-side hypalgesia. The visual system is added to this in Chapter 14 to illustrate the basis for a contralateral menace deficit.

Pain Syndromes

Neurogenic or neuropathic pain is most commonly related to disturbances of peripheral nerves in which the pain is found in the cutaneous area of the involved peripheral nerve. This is occasionally seen in dogs with unilateral cervical intervertebral disk extrusion-protrusion that compresses a spinal nerve. It is often referred to as a root signature. CNS lesions that cause a patient discomfort or pain include lesions within the dorsal gray column, with loss of inhibition of the neurons involved with nociception; and pontomedullary lesions that interfere with the nuclei of the caudally projecting pathways that are the source of this inhibition. A syndrome referred to as thalamic pain consists of spontaneous discomfort related to a thalamic lesion, often a neoplasm. Loss of the GSA thalamic relay nucleus results in hypalgesia. In this syndrome the clinical sign is hyperalgesia. There is a report of a unilateral thalamic glioma in a dog in which there was spontaneous discomfort on the contralateral side of the body.[29] **Video 9-4,** made by the cat's owner, shows an adult cat that was presented to a referring veterinarian. The cat had a 1-week history of change in behavior that consisted of continual howling and apparent hyperesthesia on normal

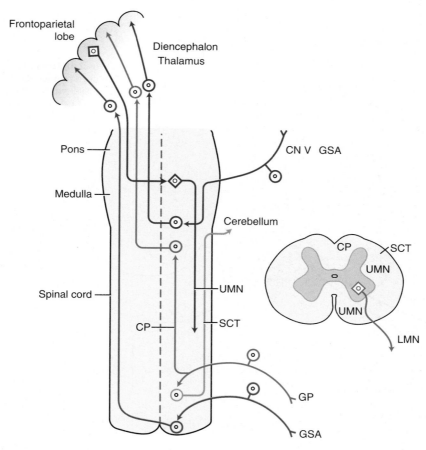

FIGURE 9-16 Diagram of the prosencephalic anatomic pathways for the UMN, GP, and GSA systems. *SCT,* Spinocerebellar tracts.

handling and manipulation. The cat was euthanized and a necropsy diagnosed a diencephalic ependymoma. The mechanism of this "thalamic pain" is poorly understood.

SUMMARY OF SPINAL CORD PATHWAYS

Fig. 9-17 diagrams the spinal cord pathways of the UMN, GP, and GSA systems. If you cover one half of this spinal cord transection and imagine it to be at the level of the C2 segment, you should be able to understand why this patient was exhibiting ipsilateral spastic hemiparesis, GP ataxia, and contralateral hypalgesia of the caudal neck, trunk, and limbs.

Fig. 9-18 shows the pattern of spinal cord degeneration that follows a focal transverse lesion. Understanding this relies on your knowledge of the general position of the cranial and caudal projecting spinal cord pathways and the principle of wallerian degeneration. This principle is especially useful for the pathologist in localizing focal spinal cord lesions by microscopic examination of transverse sections of the spinal cord. Recall that when an axon is transected, the portion of the axon that courses distally to its telodendron degenerates and secondary demyelination follows this axonal degeneration. In Fig. 9-18, the three transverse sections on the right show this pattern of degeneration. The C6 section in the middle is the site of the primary lesion that resulted in diffuse axonal disruption. Disruption of the cranial projecting axons at C6 causes wallerian degeneration in these tracts in all of the transverse sections cranial to C6, to the level where they terminate in a telodendron. This pattern of cranial projecting pathways is seen in the top transverse section of Fig. 9-18. Disruption of the caudally projecting axons at C6 causes wallerian degeneration in these tracts in all of the transverse sections caudal to C6, to the level where these axons terminate in telodendrons in the spinal cord gray matter. This pattern of caudal projecting pathways is seen in the bottom transverse section in Fig. 9-18.

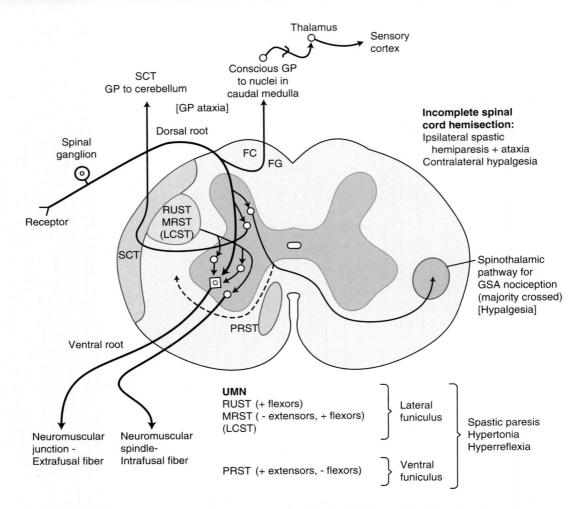

FIGURE 9-17 Diagram of the spinal cord anatomic pathways for the UMN, GP, and GSA systems. The GP includes: *FC,* Fasciculus cuneatus (forelimb); *FG,* fasciculus gracilis (hindlimb); *SCT,* spinocerebellar tracts. *LCST,* Lateral corticospinal tract; *MRST,* medullary reticulospinal tract; *PRST,* pontine reticulospinal tract; *RUST,* rubrospinal tract.

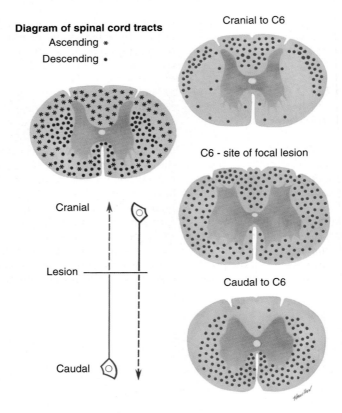

FIGURE 9-18 Pattern of spinal cord degeneration following a focal segmental lesion.

REFERENCES

1. Adrian ED: Afferent areas in brain of ungulates, *Brain* 66:89, 1943.
2. Adrian ED: The somatic receiving area in the brain of the Shetland pony, *Brain* 69:1, 1946.
3. Breazile JE, Kitchell RL: Ventrolateral spinal cord afferents to the brainstem in the domestic pig, *J Comp Neurol* 133:363, 1968.
4. Breazile JE, Kitchell RL: A study of fiber systems within the spinal cord of the domestic pig that subserve pain, *J Comp Neurol* 133:373, 1968.
5. Breazile JE, Kitchell RL: Pain perception in animals, *Fed Proc* 28:1379, 1969.
6. Brodal A, Rexed B: Spinal afferents to the lateral cervical nucleus in the cat: an experimental study, *J Comp Neurol* 98:179, 1953.
7. Carmichael S, Griffiths IR: Case of isolated sensory trigeminal neuropathy in a dog, *Vet Rec* 107:280, 1981.
8. Chrisman CL, et al: Sensory polyganglioradiculoneuritis in a dog, *J Sm Anim Hosp Assoc* 35:232-235, 1999.
9. Craig AD: Spinocervical tract cells in cat and dog, labeled by the retrograde transport of horseradish peroxidase, *Neurosci Lett* 3:173, 1976.
10. Craig AD: Spinal and medullary input to the lateral cervical nucleus, *J Comp Neurol* 181:729, 1978.
11. Craig AD, Burton H: The lateral cervical nucleus in the cat: anatomic organization of the cervicothalamic tract, *J Comp Neurol* 185:329, 1979.
12. Cummings JF, et al: Hereditary sensory neuropathy-nociceptive loss and acral mutilation in pointer dogs, *Am J Pathol* 112:136-138, 1983.
13. Cummings JF, de Lahunta A, Mitchell W J Jr: Ganglioradiculitis in the dog: a clinical, light and electron microscopic study, *Acta Neuropathol* 60:29-39, 1983.
14. Cummings JF, de Lahunta A, Winn SS: Acral mutilation and nociceptive loss in English pointer dogs, *Acta Neuropathol* 53:119, 1981.
15. Cummings JF, Petras JM: The origin of spinocerebellar pathways. 1. The nucleus cervicalis centralis of the cranial cervical spinal cord, *J Comp Neurol* 173:655, 1977.
16. Dietz V: Proprioception and locomotor disorders, *Nature Rev Neurosci* 3:781-790, 2002.
17. Duncan ID, Griffiths IR: A sensory neuropathy affecting long-haired dachshund dogs, *J Sm Anim Pract* 23:381, 1982.
18. Duncan ID, Griffiths IR, Munz M: The pathology of sensory neuropathy affecting long-haired dachshund dogs, *Acta Neuropathol* 58:141, 1982.
19. Fletcher TF, Kitchell RL: The lumbar, sacral and coccygeal tactile dermatomes of the dog, *J Comp Neurol* 128:171, 1966.
20. Grant G: Spinal course and somatotopically localized termination of the spinocerebellar tracts: an experimental study in the cat, *Acta Physiol Scand* 56(suppl):194, 1962.
21. Grant G, Rexed B: Dorsal spinal root afferents to Clarke's column, *Brain* 81:567, 1958.
22. Ha H, Liu CN: Organization of the spinocervicothalamic system, *J Comp Neurol* 127:445, 1966.
23. Ha H, Liu CN: Cell origin of the ventral spinocerebellar tract, *J Comp Neurol* 133:185, 1968.
24. Haghighi SS, et al: Electrophysiologic studies of the cutaneous innervation of the pelvic limb of male dogs, *Am J Vet Res* 52:352-362, 1991.
25. Hamey T, Bromely RB, Woosley CN: Somatic afferent area I and II of dog's cerebral cortex, *J Neurophysiol* 19:485, 1956.
26. Hand PJ: Lumbosacral dorsal root terminations in the nucleus gracilis of the cat: some observations on the terminal degeneration in other medullary sensory nuclei, *J Comp Neurol* 126:137, 1966.
27. Hand PJ, Van Winkle T: The efferent connections of the feline nucleus cuneatus, *J Comp Neurol* 171:83, 1977.
28. Hirai N, Hongo T, Sasaki S: Cerebellar projection and input organizations of the spinocerebellar tract arising from the central cervical nucleus in the cat, *Brain Res* 157:341, 1978.
29. Holland CT, Charles JA, Cortaville PE: Hemihyperesthesia and hyperresponsiveness resembling central pain syndrome in a dog with a forebrain oligodendroglioma, *Aust Vet J* 78:676-680, 2000.
30. Holmquist B, Oscarsson O: Location, course and characteristics of uncrossed and crossed ascending spinal tracts in the cat, *Acta Physiol Scand* 58:57, 1963.
31. Holmquist B, Oscarsson O, Rosen I: Functional organization of the cuneocerebellar tract in the cat, *Acta Physiol Scand* 58:216, 1963.
32. Hubbard JI, Oscarsson O: Localization of the cell bodies of the ventral spinocerebellar tract in lumbar segments of the cat, *J Comp Neurol* 118:199, 1962.
33. Hudson AJ: Pain perception and response: central nervous system mechanisms, *Can J Neurol Sci* 27:2-16, 2000.
34. Kennard MA: The course of ascending fibers in the spinal cord of the cat essential to the recognition of painful stimuli, *J Comp Neurol* 100:511, 1954.
35. Kitchell RL, et al: Electrophysiologic studies of cutaneous nerves of the thoracic limb of the dog, *Am J Vet Res* 41:61-76, 1980.
36. Landgren S, Silfvenius H: Projection to cerebral cortex of group 1 and muscle afferents from the cat's hind limb, *J Physiol* 200:353, 1969.
37. Matsushita M, Hosoya Y, Ikeda M: Anatomical organization of the spinocerebellar system in the cat as studied by retrograde transport of horseradish peroxidase, *J Comp Neurol* 184:81, 1979.
38. Matsushita M, Ikeda M: The central cervical nucleus as cell origin of a spinocerebellar tract arising from the cervical spinal cord: a study in the cat using horseradish peroxidase, *Brain Res* 10:412, 1975.
39. Matzke HA: The course of the fibers arising from the nucleus gracilis and nucleus cuneatus of the cat, *J Comp Neurol* 84:439, 1951.
40. McCormack M, Dubrovsky B: Impairment in limb action after dorsal funiculi section in cats, *Exp Brain Res* 37:31, 1979.
41. Melzack R: The perception of pain, *Sci Am* 204:41, 1961.
42. Melzack R, Wall PD: Pain mechanisms: a new theory, *Science* 150:971, 1965.
43. Muir WW, Woolf CJ: Mechanisms of pain and their therapeutic implications, *J Am Vet Med Med Assoc* 219:1346, 2001.
44. Petras JM, Cummings JF: The origin of spinocerebellar pathways. II. The nucleus centrobasalis of the cervical enlargement and the nucleus dorsalis of the thoracolumbar spinal cord, *J Comp Neurol* 173:693, 1977.
45. Pivnik L: Zur vergleichenden Problematik einiger akrodystrophischer Neuropathien bei Menschen und Hund, *Schweiz Arch Neurol Neurochir Psychiatr* 112:365, 1973.
46. Porter B, et al: Ganglioradiculitis (sensory neuropathy) in a dog: clinical, morphologic and immunohistochemical findings, *Vet Pathol* 39:598-602, 2002.
47. Rexed B, Brodal A: The nucleus cervicalis lateralis, a spinocerebellar relay nucleus, *J Neurophysiol* 14:399, 1951.

48. Reynolds PJ, Talbott RE, Brookhart JM: Control of postural reactions in the dog: the role of the dorsal column feedback pathway, *Brain Res* 40:159, 1972.

49. Scott DW, Bistner SI: Neurotrophic keratitis in a dog, *Vet Med Sm Anim Clin* 68:1120, 1973.

50. Spurgeon TL, Kitchell RL: Electrophysiological studies of the cutaneous innervation of the external male genitalia of the male dog, *Anat Histol Embryol* 11:289-306, 1982.

51. Truex RC, et al: The lateral cervical nucleus of cat, dog and man, *J Comp Neurol* 139:93, 1970.

10 SMALL ANIMAL SPINAL CORD DISEASE

NEUROLOGIC EXAMINATION

Gait
Postural Reactions
Spinal Reflexes
Cranial Nerves

SUMMARY OF POSSIBLE CLINICAL SIGNS RELATED TO SPINAL CORD LESIONS

Lumbosacral: Fourth Lumbar to Fifth Caudal
   Spinal Cord Segments
Thoracolumbar: Third Thoracic to Third
   Lumbar Spinal Cord Segments
Caudocervical: Sixth Cervical to Second
   Thoracic Spinal Cord Segments
Craniocervical: First Cervical to Fifth
   Cervical Spinal Cord Segments
Schiff-Sherrington Syndrome and
   Spinal Shock

SMALL ANIMAL THORACOLUMBAR SPINAL CORD DISEASES

Paraplegia
   CASE EXAMPLE 10-1
      Fibrocartilaginous Embolic Myelopathy
   CASE EXAMPLE 10-2
Monoplegia
   CASE EXAMPLE 10-3

CASE EXAMPLE 10-4
Paraparesis and Ataxia
   CASE EXAMPLE 10-5
      Nephroblastoma
      Vertebral Malformation
      Myelitis
      Discospondylitis
      Multiple Cartilaginous Exostosis
   CASE EXAMPLE 10-6
      Intervertebral Disk Extrusion-Protrusion
   CASE EXAMPLE 10-7
      Lymphoma
   CASE EXAMPLE 10-8
      Degenerative Myelopathy
      Subarachnoid Diverticula
      Degenerative Joint Disease
   CASE EXAMPLE 10-9
      Afghan Hound Myelinolysis
      *Spondylosis Deformans and Dural
         Ossification*

SMALL ANIMAL CERVICAL SPINAL CORD DISEASES

Tetraplegia
   CASE EXAMPLE 10-10
   CASE EXAMPLE 10-11
      Hypervitaminosis A
   CASE EXAMPLE 10-12
      Progressive Compressive Cervical Myelopathy

*Vertebral Malformation and
   Malarticulation*
C2-C3 Meningeal Fibrosis
Tetraparesis, Hemiparesis, Ataxia
   CASE EXAMPLE 10-13
   CASE EXAMPLE 10-14
   CASE EXAMPLE 10-15
   CASE EXAMPLE 10-16
      *Inherited Encephalomyelopathy-
         Polyneuropathy*
      *Other Inherited Disorders in the
         Rottweiler Breed*
   CASE EXAMPLE 10-17
Tetraparesis-Ataxia: LMN Thoracic Limbs, UMN
   Pelvic Limbs—"Two-Engine"
   CASE EXAMPLE 10-18
   CASE EXAMPLE 10-19
Hemiplegia, Hemiparesis, Ataxia
   CASE EXAMPLE 10-20
   CASE EXAMPLE 10-21
Tetraparesis-Ataxia: Thoracic Limbs
   CASE EXAMPLE 10-22
Multifocal-Diffuse Paresis, Ataxia
   CASE EXAMPLE 10-23
Neck Discomfort
   CASE EXAMPLE 10-24
      Canine Meningeal Polyarteritis

The objective of this chapter is first to review the method and interpretation of the neurologic examination as it relates to localizing lesions in the spinal cord in small animals, and second, to present case studies that illustrate examples of these in the four regions of the spinal cord.

NEUROLOGIC EXAMINATION

The complete neurologic examination is described in Chapter 20. The components referable to the spinal cord are reviewed here. There are five parts to the neurologic examination:

1. Examination of gait and posture
2. Postural reactions
3. Muscle tone, size, and spinal reflexes
4. Cranial nerves
5. Sensorium

Careful examination of all of these is necessary to determine whether a lesion is confined to the spinal cord and at what level. Remember that, as described in Chapter 5, spinal reflexes require only the specific peripheral nerves and the spinal cord segments with which they connect, whereas postural reactions depend on the same components as the spinal reflexes plus the cranial projecting general proprioceptive (GP) pathways in the spinal cord white matter to the brainstem, cerebellum, and frontoparietal cerebrum and the caudal projecting upper motor neuron (UMN) pathways that return from the cerebrum and brainstem and comprise tracts in the white matter of the spinal cord that terminate in the cervical and lumbosacral intumescences. These postural reactions test the integrity of nearly the entire peripheral and central nervous systems. By themselves, postural reactions are relatively non-localizing for a lesion.

Gait

The clinical signs of UMN and GP dysfunction are described in Chapters 8 and 9, and it is emphasized that most gait abnormalities involving these systems reflect a combination of UMN (spastic paresis) and GP (ataxia) clinical signs because of their close anatomic relationship. It also is strongly urged that differentiation between the clinical signs caused by disruption of these two systems is of no practical value. With spinal cord lesions that affect the UMN and GP systems between spinal cord segments T3 and L3, there is a tendency to describe the pelvic limb gait as just ataxic or occasionally just paretic. In reality, the gait abnormality usually reflects a dysfunction of both systems and should be referred to as pelvic limb ataxia and paresis or paraparesis and pelvic limb ataxia. The same rule holds for cervical spinal cord lesions that occur between spinal cord segments C1 and C5: tetraparesis (quadriparesis) and ataxia of all four limbs. The terms *paraplegia* and *tetraplegia* should be used only when there is absolutely no voluntary movement in the pelvic limbs or in all four limbs, respectively. To observe ataxia, there has to be voluntary movement. Therefore, the term *ataxia* is inappropriate for a paraplegic or tetraplegic animal. Patients that are recumbent in the pelvic limbs (T3-L3 lesion) or in all four limbs (C1-C5 lesion) and show no voluntary movement when picked up and moved along the ground surface while suspended but exhibit some voluntary limb movement when recumbent should be described as nonambulatory paraparetic or tetraparetic. The same terminology applies to lesions that involve the lumbosacral or cervical intumescence, except that the quality of the paresis reflects a lower motor neuron (LMN) dysfunction.

The gait should be examined in a place where the patient can move freely, leashed or unleashed, and where the ground surface is not slippery. The floor of many examining rooms is too small and too slippery for an adequate evaluation of the gait. In some patients with vertebral column injury and spinal cord contusion that are ataxic and paretic, moving the patient on a slippery surface may cause it to fall, and further injury may result. The availability of a corridor and an indoor-outdoor carpet is very helpful for this examination.

I (Eric Glass) use a covered outdoor area to evaluate neurologic patients. It has a specialized surface that is used in many playgrounds. This surface is soft and provides excellent traction for paretic and ataxic patients. The material, Vitriturf (Hanover Specialties, Hauppauge, NY), is commercially available and easily installed. It is important to evaluate the gait while you lead the patient and while an assistant leads the patient, in a straight line as well as in circles in each direction.

A patient with lesions that affect the pontomedullary or spinal cord UMN and GP systems and is still able to walk unassisted exhibits a delay in the onset of protraction, which is the swing phase of the gait; a stiff quality of movement; and often a longer stride, due to a delay in the termination of protraction. In the thoracic limbs, this causes a floating, overreaching action, with the limb in extension. It is important to recognize the extension of the thoracic limb joints and the prolongation of the protraction, which causes the paw to be placed on the ground farther cranially than normal. This is in contrast to the thoracic limb gait in a cerebellar disorder, where the protraction is abrupt and all the limb joints flex, causing the limb to move more dorsally toward the neck. As protraction is completed, the limb is commonly misdirected. This difference in the thoracic limb gait between a UMN-GP system dysfunction and a cerebellar dysfunction is difficult to describe but should be obvious when you study the videos of these disorders. (See Chapter

13 for a description of the gait of a cerebellar disorder.) In UMN-GP system disorders, on protraction, the affected limb may abduct excessively, especially on turns, when it is often referred to as circumduction. The limb may also adduct excessively before it supports weight. This may appear as a crossing of the limbs as they are advanced. Often, the dorsal surface of the paw will scuff the ground on protraction or the patient will support its weight on the dorsal surface of the paw. Occasionally a pelvic limb is flexed excessively on protraction, creating a hypermetria in the gait. The trunk may also appear to be unstable and to sway as the patient walks, especially on turns. Remember that these clinical signs reflect dysfunction in both the UMN and the GP systems. There is ample opportunity in the disease section of this chapter to visualize on videos what is described here.

Many clinicians use a grading system to assess the degree of pelvic limb function as an aid in determining the prognosis and to evaluate response to therapy. This was originally designed for dogs with thoracolumbar spinal cord injury resulting from intervertebral disk extrusions. This is a common disorder in dogs in which numerous surgical procedures have been performed over many decades. However, it is applicable to any spinal cord lesion at any level. Grade 0 refers to a patient with no voluntary movement in the pelvic limbs and therefore is paraplegic. Grade 5 refers to a patient with normal pelvic limb function. Patients with functional grades 1 and 2 are unable to stand in the pelvic limbs without assistance. When you hold the patient up by grasping the base of the tail, and only very slight movements of the pelvic limbs occur, this patient would receive a grade of 1 for its function. If voluntary movements readily occur but are delayed, awkward, and poorly placed, the degree of function would be grade 2. A patient with grade 3 function is able to stand up in its pelvic limbs without assistance but has great difficulty and is able to walk but with significant paresis and ataxia. A patient with grade 4 function readily stands up unassisted and exhibits only mild paresis and ataxia in its gait. These are grades of function, not grades of paresis and ataxia. When we describe a grading system that is used for horses (see Chapter 11), it refers to grades of dysfunction and is used primarily for horses with cervical spinal cord disease.

Postural Reactions

The degree of functional deficit dictates the need for postural reaction testing. The postural reactions are always absent in all limbs of a tetraplegic patient and in the pelvic limbs of a paraplegic patient. However, in the paraplegic patient it is very important to evaluate carefully the gait and postural reactions in the thoracic limbs so as to avoid missing a multifocal disorder. For example, a young dog may present to you with a progressive pelvic limb dysfunction that has become paraplegic, but you determine it also has hopping deficits in the thoracic limbs. This strongly suggests a multifocal anatomic diagnosis and a presumptive diagnosis of an inflammatory disorder such as canine distemper myelitis.

You were introduced to postural reactions in Chapter 5 as they relate to examining patients with neuromuscular disorders. It is critical to remember that postural reactions essentially require that all components of the peripheral nervous system and the central nervous system (CNS) that affect the limb you are testing be intact.

There is no test for just the UMN or just the GP system. Although a number of these postural reactions are described in the neurologic literature, in our experience the most reliable postural reaction is the patient's ability to hop laterally on one limb. After that would be the paw replacement test. Hemiwalking is most useful when your patient is too large for you to be comfortable evaluating the hopping responses. Placing of the limbs is useful only in the small-sized patients and when the hopping responses are equivocal.

The following is the sequence of my (Alexander de Lahunta) examination of the patient after evaluating its gait. Be sure to know the name of your patient and talk to it continuously to ensure its cooperation. Make its environment as nonthreatening as possible. In the hospital, I always performed my examinations on a rug or a floor with a rubber surface. Straddle the patient, with both you and the patient facing in the same direction, and palpate all of its neck, trunk, and limb muscles from cranial to caudal to determine whether there is any atrophy. After you palpate each limb, flex and extend it to determine both the muscle tone and the range of motion of the joints. If there is significant joint disease that restricts the range of motion, it contributes to the gait disorder. When you place the limb back in its supporting position, place it on the dorsal aspect of the paw and observe how readily the patient returns the paw to its normal position. This is the paw replacement test. Remember, despite what you may hear from your colleagues or read in the literature, that this is *not* a test for conscious proprioception. No such test exists. Be aware that some dogs are normally quite slow to replace the paw.

To test thoracic limb hopping, with your left hand, elevate the abdomen just enough to take the weight off the pelvic limbs. Put your left elbow on your left thigh to take the stress off your back. With your right hand, pick up the right thoracic limb and hop the patient on its left thoracic limb to the left. You should not have to move your pelvic limbs. Stand still. When you have hopped the patient to the left as far as it is comfortable, change hands so that your right hand elevates the patient's abdomen and pelvic limbs and your right elbow is resting on your right thigh. With your left hand, pick up the patient's left thoracic limb and hop the patient to the right on its right thoracic limb. Keep repeating this back and forth until you are comfortable that the responses are normal or abnormal. As you stand over the patient looking down the lateral aspect of the limb that is being hopped, as soon as the shoulder region moves laterally over the paw, the paw should move. Any delay in this is abnormal. The hopping movements should be smooth and not irregular or excessive. The paw should never drag or land on its dorsal surface. Carefully compare one thoracic limb with the other.

For pelvic limb hopping in patients that are not too large, stand beside the patient's left side and place your left forearm and hand between its thoracic limbs so that you can elevate the thorax to take the weight off its thoracic limbs. With your right hand, pick up the patient's left pelvic limb and push the patient to its right side so that it has to hop on the right pelvic limb. Then change sides and repeat this for the left pelvic limb. The responses should be brisk and smooth but will not be quite as fast as in the thoracic limbs. Abnormalities are the same as those described for the thoracic limbs. In large patients, the same observations may be made by just standing beside the patient, picking up the pelvic limb on that side, and pushing the pelvic region away from you so that the patient has to hop on the opposite pelvic limb. This can usually be done with the patient standing still on its thoracic limbs. Repeat this on each side until you are comfortable with the responses observed. As you perform these hopping responses, you will also appreciate the degree of muscle tone that is present in the limbs.

In very large patients, these same hopping responses can be evaluated by hemiwalking the patient. Stand beside the patient and pick up both the thoracic and pelvic limbs on that side. Push the patient away from you and observe the hopping responses in both limbs on the opposite side. Change sides and repeat this on the opposite side, and be sure that you compare the thoracic limbs with each other and the pelvic limbs with each other.

In small patients in which the hopping responses are difficult to interpret, it may be useful to test the placing response. Pick the patient up and bring its thoracic limbs to the edge of a table or chair so that the dorsal surface of the paw contacts the front surface of the object. The normal patient will immediately place its paws on the horizontal surface of the table or chair. Test both limbs at the same time as well as individually. Repeat this for the pelvic limbs. Be sure to test this response while holding the patient from each side. Occasionally, for some unknown reason, a normal patient does not respond with the limbs on the side on which it is being held. It may also be useful to block the patient's vision during this test by extending its neck so that it cannot see the projecting surface of the object you are using for the test.

In cooperative patients, when you are not sure of the thoracic limb function, it may help to wheelbarrow the patient with its neck held in extension. With your right (or left) forearm, elevate the abdomen of your patient so that the pelvic limbs are no longer supporting weight. With your other hand, hold the neck in extension and move the patient forward. In this posture, vision is compromised and there is a greater need for general proprioceptive function. In cases of mild nervous system lesions, this may cause the animal to scuff the dorsal surface of its paws or to overreach on protraction.

Spinal Reflexes

The patient should be placed in lateral recumbency. Usually you will need an assistant to help hold the patient in this position. For cats and toy breeds of dogs, I (AD) find it useful to sit on the floor with my back against the wall and my knees flexed, with the patient placed between my thighs and with its back resting on my thighs. This is useful not only to evaluate muscle tone and spinal reflexes but also to perform the cranial nerve examination. Most patients tolerate this position quite well, and it allows you to control the patient easily.

Flex and extend each limb to further appreciate the degree of muscle tone that you already assessed in the standing position and during the testing of the postural reactions. The only tendon reflex that I (AD) perform is the patellar reflex, which is an assessment of the femoral nerve and spinal cord segments L4, L5, and L6. The detailed anatomy of these tendon reflexes is described in Chapter 5. These tests should be performed before testing the flexor reflexes, in which a noxious stimulus is used. Test the flexor reflexes using a pair of forceps for compressing the skin at the base of the digits. Initially, exert just enough compression to obtain a flexor response or evidence of nociception. These flexor reflexes test various components of the spinal cord segments that comprise the lumbosacral or cervical intumescence and the related peripheral nerves that supply the limb being tested. The detailed anatomy of these reflexes is described in Chapters 5 and 9. Remember that these flexor reflexes test not only the reflex arc but also determine the integrity of the nociceptive pathway to the somesthetic cerebral cortex. The latter is very important in evaluating the level of severe focal spinal cord lesions as well as in making a prognosis for those lesions. Be sure to test all of these reflexes with the patient in both left and right recumbency.

When this testing has been completed and the patient is returned to the standing position, perform the cutaneous trunci reflex. (You may see this reflex referred to as the panniculus reflex, but that is a misnomer because the panniculus adiposus is a layer of fat in the trunk region and is not responsible for this cutaneous reflex; see Fig. 5-9.) Using your forceps, gently probe or squeeze the skin along the dorsal midline, starting at the level of the pelvis, and repeat this stimulus over each vertebra until you observe the cutaneous trunci contracting on both sides. In many normal small animals this may not occur until about the midlumbar region, and in a very few normal animals, it will not occur at all. The forceps pressure stimulates impulses in the dorsal branches of the spinal nerves that supply the area stimulated. Because of the short caudal distribution of these dorsal branches, each spinal nerve supplies the skin for a distance of about two vertebrae caudal to the intervertebral foramen, where the spinal nerve emerges from the vertebral canal. The general somatic afferent (GSA) neurons that are stimulated synapse in the respective dorsal gray column on long interneurons whose axons enter the adjacent fasciculus proprius bilaterally but predominantly on the contralateral side, in our opinion. Here these axons course cranially to the C8 and T1 spinal cord segments to terminate in the ventral gray columns by synapsing on the general somatic efferent (GSE) neurons that innervate the cutaneous trunci

via the brachial plexus and the lateral thoracic nerve. Recall that this reflex is lost in injuries that cause avulsion of the roots of the spinal nerves that supply the brachial plexus. In these patients, compression of the skin at any level along the trunk elicits only a cutaneous trunci reflex on the side that is opposite from the affected thoracic limb. This reflex is also helpful in determining the level and prognosis of a severe transverse spinal cord lesion such as an injury resulting from a vertebral column fracture or an intervertebral disk extrusion. Similar to nociception, it requires a bilateral transverse lesion to interfere with the pathway of these long interneurons. This cutaneous reflex is especially helpful in patients that are very stoic and respond poorly to most any noxious stimulus to any part of their body.

Cranial Nerves

The examination of cranial nerves is described in Chapters 6 and 7. When presented with a patient that exhibits clinical signs of spinal cord disease, the cranial nerve examination is important for determining whether the spinal cord signs are part of a multifocal disease process. It is also important to determine whether the spinal cord lesion is at a level where it can interfere with the sympathetic pathway to the head and cause Horner syndrome. That syndrome is observed when the cranial nerves are examined.

SUMMARY OF POSSIBLE CLINICAL SIGNS RELATED TO SPINAL CORD LESIONS

The spinal cord is divided into four regions on the basis of the clinical signs that are exhibited when any one of these four regions is affected (Fig. 10-1).

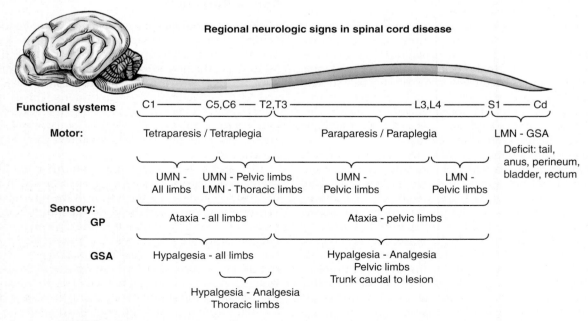

FIGURE 10-1 Regional neurologic signs in spinal cord disease. *GP,* General proprioceptive; *GSA,* general somatic afferent; *LMN,* lower motor neuron; *UMN,* upper motor neuron.

Lumbosacral: Fourth Lumbar to Fifth Caudal Spinal Cord Segments

A. Complete necrosis from the L4 through the five caudal spinal cord segments
  1. Flaccid paraplegia: no weight support and no voluntary movement of the pelvic limbs and tail
  2. Normal thoracic limbs
  3. Neurogenic atrophy in nonacute lesions
  4. Atonia: in pelvic limbs, anus, and tail, dilated anus
  5. No postural reactions in the pelvic limbs
  6. Areflexia: patellar, flexor, and perineal reflexes
  7. Analgesia: pelvic limbs, perineum, tail, and penis
B. Partial necrosis of gray and white matter between the L4 and the five caudal spinal cord segments
  1. Flaccid paraparesis and ataxia of pelvic limbs
  2. Normal thoracic limbs
  3. Mild neurogenic atrophy in nonacute lesions
  4. Hypotonia or normal tone in the pelvic limbs
  5. Postural reactions in the pelvic limbs attempted but abnormal
  6. Hyporeflexia or areflexia: patellar and flexor reflexes
  7. Hypalgesia or normal nociception: pelvic limbs, tail, and perineum

Thoracolumbar: Third Thoracic to Third Lumbar Spinal Cord Segments

A. Complete necrosis at a focal site between the third thoracic and third lumbar spinal cord segments
  1. Spastic paraplegia: normal reflex weight support if held up in a standing posture but no voluntary movement of the pelvic limbs or tail; normal thoracic limbs. With peracute transverse lesions, the thoracic limbs may be hypertonic and held in extension (Schiff-Sherrington syndrome). With cranial thoracic spinal cord lesions, it may be difficult for the patient to stand up on its thoracic limbs from a recumbent position, and there may be loss of trunk support when the patient is suspended by the base of the tail and made to walk on the thoracic limbs. The trunk may abnormally sway to the side.
  2. No neurogenic atrophy
  3. Normal tone or hypertonia (spasticity) in the pelvic limbs
  4. No postural reactions in the pelvic limbs
  5. Reflexes are normal or hyperactive: patellar (+2 or +3) and flexor
  6. Crossed extension may be observed with the flexor reflex
  7. Analgesia caudal to the level of the lesion by about two spinal cord segments
  8. Absent cutaneous trunci reflex caudal to the level of the lesion by about two spinal cord segments
B. Partial necrosis of gray and white matter at a focal site between the third thoracic and third lumbar spinal cord segments
  1. Spastic paraparesis and ataxia of pelvic limbs, with normal thoracic limbs
  2. No neurogenic atrophy
  3. Normal tone or hypertonia (spasticity) in the pelvic limbs
  4. Postural reactions attempted but abnormal in pelvic limbs

  5. Reflexes are normal or hyperactive: patellar (+2 or +3) and flexor
  6. Crossed extension possibly observed with the flexor reflex
  7. Hypalgesia or normal nociception caudal to the level of the lesion

Note: Lesions that affect only the white matter from L4 to L6 or L7 may produce similar clinical signs.

Caudocervical: Sixth Cervical to Second Thoracic Spinal Cord Segments

Complete necrosis of these segments may cause death due to loss of respirations. Partial necrosis of gray and white matter between the sixth cervical and second thoracic spinal cord segments.
  1. Tetraparesis and ataxia of all four limbs or nonambulatory tetraparesis and ataxia or tetraplegia
  2. Thoracic limb deficits that may be worse due to the loss of ability to support weight
  3. Short strides in the thoracic limbs with long paretic and ataxic strides in the pelvic limbs: a "two-engine gait"
  4. Thoracic limb neurogenic atrophy with nonacute lesions
  5. Postural reactions attempted if not tetraplegic and are abnormal in all four limbs; thoracic limb responses may be worse
  6. Reflexes depressed or absent in the thoracic limbs and normal or hyperactive in the pelvic limbs; lesions confined to the white matter at this level have normal to hyperactive thoracic limb reflexes
  7. Crossed extension may occur with the pelvic limb flexor reflexes
  8. Hypalgesia or normal nociception in all four limbs or only hypalgesia in the thoracic limbs
  9. Miosis, ptosis, protruded third eyelid, and enophthalmos with lesions between T1 and T3

Craniocervical: First Cervical to Fifth Cervical Spinal Cord Segments

Complete necrosis of these segments causes death due to loss of respirations. Partial necrosis of gray and white matter at a focal site between the first and fifth cervical spinal cord segments.
  1. Spastic tetraparesis and ataxia of all four limbs or nonambulatory spastic tetraparesis and ataxia or spastic tetraplegia; recumbent patients, when held up, exhibit hypertonia and support their weight by hyperactive extensor tone. This differentiates them from patients that are tetraplegic due to neuromuscular disorders that cause flaccid paralysis and that are atonic in all their muscles.
  2. No neurogenic muscle atrophy in chronic lesions.
  3. Postural reactions abnormal in all four limbs if they can be performed at all.
  4. Reflexes in all four limbs are normal or hyperactive.
  5. Crossed extension may occur with the flexor reflexes.
  6. Hypalgesia is possible caudal to the level of the lesion but is rarely determined; most cranial cervical lesions that are severe enough to cause analgesia caudal to the lesion cause death due to the loss of respirations.

Most compressive lesions that affect the cranial cervical spinal cord segments cause more obvious clinical signs in the pelvic limbs than in the thoracic limbs. Explanations for this include the following: lesions that compress from the periphery of the spinal cord affect primarily the superficial tracts, which contain cranially coursing GP pathways from the pelvic limbs (Fig. 10-2); the pelvic limbs are further removed from the center of gravity, which is just caudal to the thoracic limbs; more UMN pathways terminate in the cervical intumescence than in the lumbosacral intumescence. Occasionally a cervical spinal cord lesion causes more obvious clinical signs in the thoracic limbs. This is seen with caudocervical lesions that affect the gray matter in the intumescence, causing LMN signs in the thoracic limbs. With more craniocervical lesions, this occurs when the spinal cord lesion affects the tracts closer to the gray matter and spares the more superficial tracts. These are predominantly UMN pathways to the cervical intumescence. A glial neoplasm that arises in the gray matter and grows peripherally toward the surface of the spinal cord will do this as will a midline intervertebral disk protrusion that compresses the spinal cord dorsally and laterally, making the spinal cord form a tent shape over the compressing mass. This disparity in clinical signs is also seen in many dogs with an atlantoaxial subluxation.

Be aware that lesions that affect the first two or possibly three cervical spinal cord segments may also cause clinical signs of vestibular system dysfunction. This presumably results from the interruption of the spinovestibular tracts that carry GP impulses from the first three cervical spinal nerves, which are important in the orientation of the head to the neck.

There are two additional important concepts to remember when dealing with spinal cord lesions. First, lesions in the intumescences that affect the gray matter as well as the white matter present with the clinical signs of loss of the gray matter; that is, LMN clinical signs. You cannot observe UMN or GP clinical signs unless the LMN is intact. Second, a focal lesion between the C1 and C5 or T3 and L3 spinal cord segments that affects both the white matter and the gray matter causes clinical signs referable only to the white matter lesion; that is, UMN and GP clinical signs. Loss of the gray matter in a segment that innervates only the axial muscles cannot be determined by a physical neurologic examination. Only a careful electromyographic study may reveal the denervation of a segment of axial muscles.

Bladder and occasionally rectal dysfunction commonly accompanies spinal cord lesions. These lesions were described, along with the anatomy involved, in Chapter 7. Lesions in the sacral segments result in LMN incontinence in urine and feces; UMN incontinence is common with severe lesions of the cervical and thoracolumbar spinal cord segments. This incontinence is a primary concern in your treatment of the patient.

Schiff-Sherrington Syndrome and Spinal Shock

These two separate clinical disorders often present at the same time in a patient and appear to be exceptions to the rules that we have established for UMN and LMN disorders. They occur only with peracute, usually transverse, spinal cord lesions between the T3 and L3 spinal cord segments. Fractures of the vertebral column are the most common cause of such lesions. Others include infarction caused by fibrocartilaginous emboli and the myelopathy associated with peracute intervertebral disk extrusions. These patients exhibit persistent severe extension of the thoracic limbs in most postures because of disinhibition of the extensor motor neurons in the cervical intumescence. However, when these patients are held up, the thoracic limb gait is normal except for a mild stiffness. These clinical signs represent the Schiff-Sherrington syndrome.[79] The disinhibition is not the result of dysfunction in a UMN pathway, which is why these patients can walk so well with the thoracic limbs when the trunk and pelvic limbs are supported. The disinhibition is the result of a sudden loss of the axons in a long interneuronal pathway that originates from neuronal cell

FIGURE 10-2 Transverse section of cervical spinal cord. The more superficial location of pelvic limb spinocerebellar tracts may explain the more profound pelvic limb ataxia that is often observed with compressive lesions. *CCB,* Cuneocerebellar tract; *FC,* fasciculus cuneatus; *FG,* fasciculus gracilis; *SCB,* spinocerebellar tracts; *UMN,* upper motor neuron.

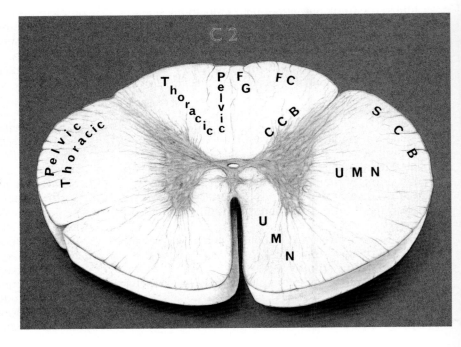

bodies primarily in the gray matter of the L1 to L5 spinal cord segments. These interneurons are referred to as border cells because they are located in the dorsolateral border of the ventral gray column of the lumbar spinal cord segments.[89] Their axons course cranially in the fasciculus proprius and terminate by synapsing on thoracic limb extensor LMNs in the cervical intumescence (Fig. 10-3). Their normal function is to inhibit these extensor motor neurons. This extensor release phenomenon is observed only with peracute severe lesions, and it spontaneously resolves in about 10 to 14 days. The presence of the Schiff-Sherrington syndrome indicates a severe lesion and a guarded prognosis but does not indicate that recovery cannot occur.

The severe peracute thoracolumbar spinal cord lesion that is responsible for the Schiff-Sherrington syndrome usually causes paraplegia because of the complete interruption in function of the UMN pathways, and it usually causes analgesia caudal to the lesion because of interruption of the nociceptive pathways. As a rule, with progressive transverse spinal cord lesions, paraplegia occurs before analgesia, suggesting that the nociceptive pathways are the most resistant to spinal cord compression and ischemia. However, in these severe peracute transverse thoracolumbar spinal cord lesions in which the Schiff-Sherrington syndrome is present, there usually is severe pelvic limb hypotonia. If you examine this patient within a few hours of the onset of the paraplegia, there may be absent or very depressed pelvic limb tone and spinal reflexes. These paradoxical LMN-like pelvic limb signs in a patient with a UMN pathway interruption represent what is called spinal shock.[88] In primates, spinal shock causes areflexia and atonia for 2 to 3 weeks. In domestic animals, the areflexia is observed for only a few hours after the onset of the lesion, but the hypotonia persists for 10 to 14 days, when it is replaced by normal tone

at first and then by hypertonia. The reasons a UMN lesion causes LMN signs are poorly understood. One explanation is that the sudden loss of the UMN synapses, indirectly via interneurons or directly on the dendritic zones or the cell bodies of the alpha motor neurons, causes such a disruption to that LMN cell body that it cannot function for a variable period of time. In primates, more of these UMN pyramidal system synapses are directly on the LMN, which may explain the difference in reaction among species that is observed here. Some studies have found an excessive accumulation of the inhibitory neurotransmitter glycine in the lumbosacral intumescence in these patients.[86] The basis for the release of glycine is unknown. It is important to understand this unique combination of clinical signs that results from a focal lesion in the UMN and GP systems and not make an anatomic diagnosis of a multifocal disorder.

In a recumbent patient that has a fracture and should not be manipulated, the basis for these clinical signs can be determined through minimal handling of the patient. With the patient lying on the floor, a table, or a stretcher, provide a rigorous noxious stimulus to a digit of a pelvic limb; no movement occurs or there is just a mild reflex flexion if it is a few hours after the onset of clinical signs. Note the bilateral pelvic limb hypotonia. Provide very minimal compression of a digit of one of the hyperextended thoracic limbs or just a light squeeze of that forepaw with your hand, and note the immediate vigorous voluntary withdrawal of the limb. This tells you that you have a transverse thoracolumbar spinal cord lesion with Schiff-Sherrington syndrome in the thoracic limbs and spinal shock in the pelvic limbs. By providing forceps compression of the skin on the midline of the back as a noxious stimulus, starting in the caudal lumbar region and progressing cranially, a line of analgesia and/or a cutaneous trunci reflex can be found that locates the focal

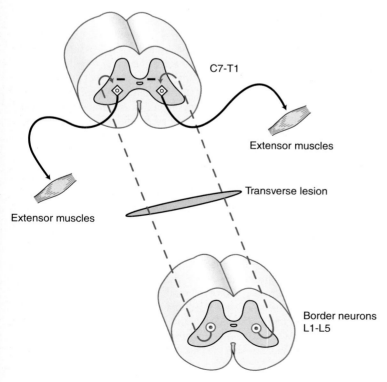

C7-T1

Extensor muscles

Extensor muscles

Transverse lesion

Border neurons
L1-L5

Schiff-Sherrington Syndrome

FIGURE 10-3 Schematic diagram depicting the cranial projecting pathway that, when interrupted, results in the Schiff-Sherrington syndrome.

lesion, and imaging studies can be pursued with no further manipulation of the patient. If the patient does not have a fracture, its ability to walk with the thoracic limbs when supported differentiates the Schiff-Sherrington syndrome from a severe cervical spinal cord lesion.

(For a complete description of disorders that affect the lumbosacral spinal cord segments or the peripheral nerves associated with these segments, see the case examples of neuromuscular disease in Chapter 5.)

SMALL ANIMAL THORACOLUMBAR SPINAL CORD DISEASES

Paraplegia

CASE EXAMPLE 10-1

Signalment: 8-year-old spayed female boxer, Brittney

Chief Complaint: Unable to use the pelvic limbs

History: The day before this dog was videoed, the owner left her home at 11 AM, leaving Brittney in the house. On returning at 3 PM, she found Brittney unable to stand on her pelvic limbs.

Examination: Video 10-1 shows the flaccid paraplegia and the hyperextended thoracic limbs but normal voluntary use of these limbs. Note the atonia and areflexia in the left pelvic limb and the mild hypotonia and hyporeflexia in the right pelvic limb. Note the analgesia of the left pelvic limb except for the proximal medial thigh area. Not shown are the normal tail, anal tone, and perineal reflex.

Anatomic Diagnosis: L4 to S1 spinal cord segments, worse on the left side

The thoracic limbs exhibit the Schiff-Sherrington syndrome resulting from the sudden loss of function of the lumbar spinal cord neuronal cell bodies of the long interneurons that normally inhibit thoracic limb extensor motor neurons. However, the pelvic limbs' clinical signs are not due to spinal shock because they are so asymmetric, and the left pelvic limb areflexia had persisted for 24 hours when this examination was done. The intact nociception from the proximomedial thigh area indicates sparing of the genitofemoral nerve, which arises from the L3 and L4 spinal cord segments. The right pelvic limb paralysis represents a mixture of loss of function of the UMN and GP systems in the white matter and mild loss of GSE LMN function, all of which could occur in these segments.

Differential Diagnosis: Fibrocartilaginous embolic myelopathy (FCEM); intervertebral disk extrusion; neoplasia

External injury was excluded by the history. Based on the acute onset of clinical signs and the signalment, FCEM and intervertebral disk extrusion are the two most presumptive diagnoses. The absence of any discomfort is more likely with FCEM, but exceptions are common. It is important to make this distinction in the clinical diagnosis because an extruded intervertebral disk commonly requires immediate surgery.

Ancillary Procedures: Radiographs of the lumbar and sacral vertebrae were normal. A myelogram and a computed tomography (CT) scan with a myelogram (see Video 10-1) showed a mild intramedullary swelling of the lumbosacral intumescence. The CT images are from the body of the L3 vertebra through the body of the L5 vertebra.

Because of the guarded prognosis, the owner of Brittney requested euthanasia. Necropsy confirmed extensive infarction scattered through the caudal lumbar and cranial sacral spinal cord segments. The gray matter was more extensively affected on the left side. There were numerous fibrocartilaginous emboli in spinal cord blood vessels associated with these lesions.

FIBROCARTILAGINOUS EMBOLIC MYELOPATHY

FCEM is a spinal cord lesion that is common in dogs but is uncommon in other species of domestic animals.* It is most common in young adult dogs of the larger breeds but it can occur as young as 3 months of age and it is common in the miniature schnauzer, Labrador retriever, and boxer breeds, in our experience. The clinical signs are peracute in onset and usually stabilize within 24 hours. Rarely, clinical signs may progress for 48 hours. Following that, there is no further progression or there is improvement, depending on the degree of ischemia or infarction that has occurred. The source of the fibrocartilage is assumed to be the intervertebral disk that is undergoing degeneration. This embolic fibrocartilage has the same collagen type that is found in the nucleus pulposus. How this degenerate fibrocartilage gains access to the spinal cord vasculature remains speculative. These emboli are more common in small arteries but also can be found in veins. Arteriovenous anastomoses do occur in the blood supply of the spinal cord and have been implicated in the distribution of the emboli. Protrusion of degenerate disk material into the adjacent ventral internal vertebral venous plexus has occasionally been observed at necropsy. It has been suggested that the normally avascular intervertebral disk is invaded by new growth of arteries when degeneration occurs in the annulus fibrosis and this is a route for these emboli to enter the arterial vasculature. We find this mechanism difficult to accept. In humans, degenerate intervertebral disk material can protrude into the adjacent vertebral body where there is ready access to the blood vessels in the marrow of the vertebra. One route of venous drainage from this marrow is into the ventral internal vertebral venous plexus within the vertebral canal. These intramedullary protrusions are referred to as Schmorl nodes. They are rare, or at least rarely identified in dogs, which may be because of dogs' quadruped posture and the thick layer of cortical bone that is adjacent to the intervertebral disk. Reverse venous blood flow may be involved in the distribution of these emboli. Whenever an animal strains by contracting its trunk muscles with the glottis closed, the increased pressure in the thorax and abdomen interferes with the venous return to the heart and forces the venous blood into the vertebral venous plexus. This is the Valsalva maneuver, and it may play a role in the ability of these emboli to gain access to the spinal cord vasculature. The involvement of the intervertebral disk as the source of these emboli is also supported by the observation that these lesions occur primarily in the spinal cord. One report of brainstem lesions with fibrocartilaginous emboli indicated a possible source of emboli from cervical intervertebral disks.[5] Magnetic resonance (MR) imaging often shows intervertebral disk degeneration at the level of the FCEM lesion in the spinal cord. These FCEM lesions can be unilateral or bilateral at any level of the spinal cord, and they affect various combinations of the gray and white

---

*References 5, 14, 23, 32, 35, 37, 42, 53, 61, 95, 110, 111.

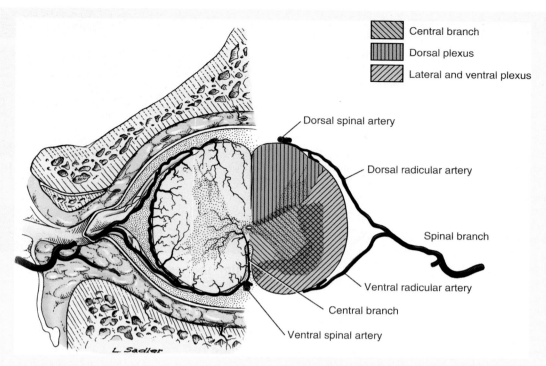

FIGURE 10-4 Arterial vasculature of the canine spinal cord. The lesion distribution following fibrocartilaginous embolism often reflects occlusion of multiple arteries.

matter. The lesions are usually limited to a few adjacent spinal cord segments. There are many examples in the following case examples that involve the various regions of the spinal cord. Caudal brainstem signs are rare and probably are associated with emboli arising from the cervical intervertebral disks.

Because of the extensive collateral circulation to the spinal cord (Fig. 10-4), multiple blood vessels must be compromised to cause the degree of infarction and severe clinical signs seen in dogs similar to Brittney. This suggests that a sudden shower of emboli must occur at one time. At necropsy, these emboli can be found in many blood vessels in or near the lesions. Usually, this shower affects the blood vessels to a few adjacent spinal cord segments and the associated lesions often are scattered and asymmetric within these segments. Thus, the clinical signs are usually focal and often asymmetric, as seen in Brittney. FCEM may be much more common than we realize and not be extensive enough to cause clinical signs or cause only transient clinical signs. Most veterinarians have had the experience of being called by a distraught owner who has just found their pet dog collapsed and unable to stand, but by the time the dog arrives at the hospital for examination, the dog is walking normally. We believe that some of these transient episodes of collapse may be due to transient spinal cord ischemia caused by FCEM.

Many dogs in which you make this clinical diagnosis will recover spontaneously. This is more common in dogs with paresis and ataxia due to interruption of the UMN and GP pathways. The more severe the involvement of the gray matter in the intumescences, the more guarded the prognosis. As a rule of thumb, if there are no signs of improvement in 10 to 14 days after the onset of clinical signs, it is unlikely that any recovery will occur. In a few patients, after an initial mild improvement, there may be a period of weeks before they rapidly regain the ability to walk. We

usually tell owners that it may take up to 10 weeks before final improvement occurs.

An interesting observation is that FCEM is very rare in the chondrodystrophic breeds in which the chondroid metaplastic form of intervertebral disk degeneration is so common. FCEM also is observed in dogs as young as 3 months of age in which you do not expect intervertebral disk degeneration to occur. In these young dogs, the source of cartilage may be the vertebral growth plates. Often, there is an associated history of mild trauma such as a sudden fall or vigorous playing and jumping as with catching a frisbee. This relationship between young age and vigorous handling is associated with FCEM in young feeder pigs; it occurs during their transportation in crowded trucks.

The three primary disorders that can cause an acute onset of relatively nonprogressive spinal cord dysfunction are external injury by objects in the environment, most commonly vehicles; internal injury resulting from intervertebral disk extrusions; and vascular compromise resulting from FCEM. The history usually permits substantiation or exclusion of external injury. Lacking that, vertebral column radiographs should provide that answer. To differentiate between the other two causes of these clinical signs, evidence of discomfort by the patient is more suggestive of an intervertebral disk extrusion than of FCEM, but exceptions are common for both of these disorders. Ultimately, immediate imaging is necessary because a diagnosis of an intervertebral disk extrusion usually requires emergency surgery. Myelograms in dogs with FCEM are helpful only in the small percentage of dogs in which intramedullary swelling is extensive. MR imaging is much more reliable in detecting the spinal cord edema that accompanies the ischemia or infarction caused by the fibrocartilaginous emboli.[25] Be aware that MR imaging that is done in the first 24 to 48 hours after the embolic shower occurs may occasionally be normal.

CASE EXAMPLE 10-2

Signalment: 3-year-old female Labrador retriever, Brandy

Chief Complaint: Unable to stand in the pelvic limbs

History: Brandy was an indoor dog in which the owner observed a sudden loss of the ability to walk with the left pelvic limb, followed in a few hours by collapse of the right pelvic limb.

Examination: Video 10-2 was made 12 hours after the onset of the pelvic limb dysfunction. Note the paraplegia with thoracic limb hyperextension but normal voluntary movements in the thoracic limbs. Note the pronounced pelvic limb hypotonia but intact spinal reflexes. Note the line of analgesia at about the thoracolumbar junction.

Anatomic Diagnosis: Focal caudal thoracic transverse spinal cord lesion with Schiff-Sherrington syndrome in the thoracic limbs and spinal shock in the pelvic limbs

Differential Diagnosis: FCEM, intervertebral disk extrusion, neoplasia

The owner's history of this dog's clinical signs is sufficient to deny any external injury. It was difficult to determine how much of this dog's struggling was due to discomfort, frustration, or dislike of the examiners. An acute intervertebral disk extrusion is less likely than FCEM in a 3-year-old Labrador retriever, due to its young age.

No ancillary studies were performed in Brandy, and with no clinical signs of improvement after a few days, the owners elected euthanasia. Necropsy revealed extensive ischemic and hemorrhagic infarction in the caudal thoracic spinal cord segments, with numerous fibrocartilaginous emboli in both arteries and veins. No intervertebral disk material was found on opening the ventral internal vertebral venous plexus in the area of the involved spinal cord segments, and a median plane section of the vertebral column did not reveal any recognizable intervertebral disk material in the marrow of the vertebral bodies.

The following videos show two more examples of the Schiff-Sherrington syndrome.

Video 10-3 shows Spanky, an 11-year-old male mixed-breed dog that was riding in a car that skidded on ice and struck a guard rail. Radiographs (shown in the video) revealed a fracture in the spinous process of the T6 vertebra and a collapsed intervertebral disk space between the T5 and T6 vertebrae, with no displacement. The video was made 4 days after the injury. Note the pelvic limb hypertonia and hyperreflexia and therefore no evidence of any spinal shock. Note the presence of nociception in the pelvic limbs, indicating that the spinal cord lesion has not caused a complete transverse dysfunction. A body cast was applied and Spanky regained the ability to walk with his pelvic limbs in about 5 weeks.[72]

Video 10-4 shows a 6-year-old Parson (Jack) Russell terrier that was struck by an automobile and suffered a moderately displaced fracture of the L3 vertebra. The video shows the radiographs. Note the clinical signs of Schiff-Sherrington syndrome but the absence of any spinal shock.

In our experience, Schiff-Sherrington syndrome and spinal shock are rare in cats. The following three videos show cats with thoracolumbar vertebral column fractures that caused a transverse spinal cord dysfunction with peracute paraplegia and analgesia caudal to the lesion.

Video 10-5 shows Poison, an 8-year-old castrated male domestic shorthair that was struck by a vehicle 2 days before the video was made. Note the crossed extension in the pelvic limbs and the pelvic limb flexion when the tail was compressed with forceps. The latter is referred to as a mass reflex, which is another manifestation of hyperreflexia. Radiographs (see the video) showed a fracture at the articulation between the L3 and L4 vertebrae, with at least 50% displacement. Poison was euthanized and the necropsy showed that at the site of the fracture and displacement, there was only a sleeve of dura remaining. The parenchyma of the spinal cord at this site had been completely crushed and displaced into the adjacent spinal cord segments (Fig. 10-5).

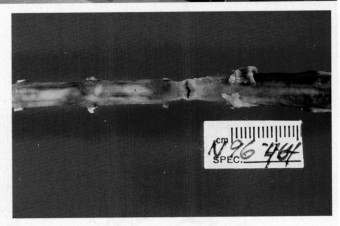

FIGURE 10-5 Lumbar spinal cord of the cat in Video 10-5, showing a crease in the dura at the level of the fracture site. At this site there is only a sleeve of dura, and the parenchyma has been entirely displaced into the adjacent spinal cord segments.

Video 10-6 shows George, an adult Siamese cat that was found beside the road unable to use his pelvic limbs. Radiographs (see the video) showed a fracture at the articulation between the T13 and L1 vertebrae, with slight displacement. Note the pelvic limb flexion when the tail was compressed with forceps. This is an example of a mass reflex. George was euthanized and necropsy revealed hemorrhage and necrosis that involved all of the transverse section of the spinal cord at the level of the fracture (Fig. 10-6).

The spinal cord lesions resulting from injury caused by external trauma include the physical disruption of the high-risk spinal cord parenchyma as compared with the more resistant dural layer of meninges. See Fig. 10-6, which shows this severe spinal cord lesion. A contused spinal cord exhibits hemorrhage, edema, and necrosis due to compromise of the spinal cord's vasculature. Following the traumatic event, there is continued degeneration of the injured spinal cord that progresses for a few hours, usually less than 24 hours. The basis for this is the subject of intense research directed at determining ways to treat these patients to prevent this progressive spinal cord destruction. Areas of interest include the release of neurotransmitters, such as toxic levels of glutamate, excessive accumulation of calcium ions, free

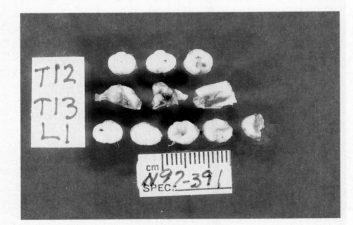

FIGURE 10-6 Transverse sections of the spinal cord of the Siamese cat in Video 10-6, showing the hemorrhage and necrosis at the site of the displaced fracture.

radical species, nitrous oxide, and the release of various amines that cause vasoconstriction and subsequent ischemia and infarction.

Video 10-7 shows an 8-week-old Siamese kitten that was found beside the road by Society for the Prevention of Cruelty to Animals employees. Radiographs (see the video) showed a fracture at the T8-T9 vertebral articulation, with complete displacement through the vertebral canal. No owner was located. Despite the peracute

paraplegia and analgesia caudal to the lesion, there were no signs of the Schiff-Sherrington syndrome or spinal shock. A medicine resident adopted the kitten, knowing that there would be no improvement in the clinical signs. The fracture was reduced and stabilized and a cart was made for the kitten (see the video). When the resident took a permanent position in Alaska, the then young adult cat was doing fine and enjoying life in a larger cart.

Monoplegia

CASE EXAMPLE 10-3

Signalment: 3-year-old castrated male malamute, Drake
Chief Complaint: Unable to use the left pelvic limb
History: After a 5-mile run with his owners, Drake was in their home when he suddenly lost the ability to move his left pelvic limb. He was examined by a local veterinarian and then referred to Cornell University, where his disorder was filmed on the second day of the dysfunction, which had not changed since the onset.
Examination: Video 10-8 shows the spastic monoplegia limited to the left pelvic limb. The right pelvic limb gait was normal, but the limb showed some difficulty with the hopping response.
Anatomic Diagnosis: A focal lesion on the left side, between the T3 and L3 spinal cord segments

Do not confuse this anatomic diagnosis with sciatic nerve paralysis, which looks much different. Review Video 5-44 of the collie dog Keane, described with Case Example 5-15; Keane has a left sciatic nerve injury due to a pelvic fracture. Dogs with sciatic nerve deficits

can always advance the limb by hip flexion, and there is hypotonia of the crural muscles.
Differential Diagnosis: FCEM, intervertebral disk extrusion, neoplasia

External injury was excluded based on the history and on the knowledge that such localized unilateral signs would be very unusual for an external spinal cord injury. The lack of any discomfort at the onset of the paralysis or during the examination is more suggestive of FCEM than of an intervertebral disk extrusion. An intervertebral disk extrusion would be unlikely in a 3-year-old nonchondrodystrophic breed. However, it can best be ruled down by imaging. Radiographs and a myelogram were normal, which supported a presumptive FCEM lesion.

On the video, you can follow the spontaneous recovery. The section of the video where Drake is walking indoors after you see his vigorous response to a noxious stimulus was made 1 week later, and the section outdoors was made 3 weeks after the initial filming.

CASE EXAMPLE 10-4

Signalment: A 6-year-old castrated male Labrador retriever, Penfield
Chief Complaint: Unable to use the right pelvic limb
History: The owners were playing ball with Penfield in a local park when he suddenly yelped and stopped using his right pelvic limb.
Examination: This examination took place the day after the onset of the clinical signs, which had not changed. **Video 10-9** shows that this dog's clinical signs are the mirror image of those observed in Drake in Case Example 10-3. Penfield exhibits a spastic monoplegia of his right pelvic limb.
Anatomic Diagnosis: Focal lesion on the right side of the spinal cord between the T3 and L3 spinal cord segments
Differential Diagnosis: The diagnosis is the same as that described for Drake in Case Example 10-3. The indication of discomfort when the initial clinical signs occurred is suggestive of a possible intervertebral disk extrusion. Radiographs and a myelogram diagnosed a unilateral right-side intervertebral disk extrusion between the L3 and L4 vertebrae. This was removed via a hemilaminectomy, and Penfield was walking with the right pelvic limb after about 3 weeks.

The following two videos show the same two clinical disorders that are described in this case example and Case Example 10-3.

Video 10-10 shows Dude, a 3-year-old male miniature schnauzer that had been outdoors unconfined during the night and was found in the morning unable to use his left pelvic limb. From your study of this video you should make the anatomic diagnosis of a focal spinal cord lesion on the left side between the T3 and L3 spinal cord segments. The differential diagnosis is the same as in this case example and Case Example 10-3 but must include external injury because the history cannot rule it out. The absence of any reluctance to try to walk as well as of any discomfort when palpated and the presence of extensive unilateral signs all suggest that external injury is unlikely. The young age of this dog suggests that a unilateral intervertebral disk extrusion is also less likely. In addition, this breed is at some risk for the development of fibrocartilaginous emboli. Radiographs and a myelogram were normal, which made FCEM the most presumptive diagnosis. Within 2 to 3 weeks, without specific therapy, Dude was walking well in the left pelvic limb. Figure 10-7 shows the kind of FCEM lesion that explains these clinical signs but from which recovery would not occur.

(Continued)

CASE EXAMPLE 10-4—cont'd

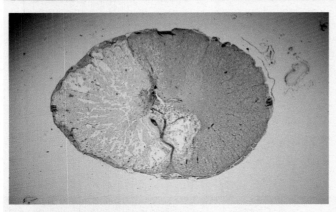

FIGURE 10-7 Transverse section of the T13 spinal cord segment of a 3-year-old Saint Bernard with a left pelvic limb spastic monoplegia due to a fibrocartilaginous embolism that caused ischemic infarction of the left half of the spinal cord. A similar anatomic but less severe lesion was presumed to have occurred in Drake in Video 10-8 and in Dude in Video 10-10.

Video 10-11 shows Beaver Dam, an 8-year-old spayed female mixed-breed dog that was presented because of difficulty using the left pelvic limb. This dysfunction began when the dog fell down a flight of stairs and had not changed significantly since that time. From your study of the video, you should make the same anatomic and differential diagnosis as for Dude in the previous video. The video of Beaver Dam shows the radiographs, myelogram, and CT imaging, which diagnosed intervertebral disk extrusions at the L1-L2, and L3-L4 vertebral articulations. The owner elected to treat the dog medically, and no follow-up on its success is available.

Paraparesis and Ataxia

CASE EXAMPLE 10-5

Signalment: 5-month-old male Labrador retriever, Cassidy

Chief Complaint: Unable to walk normally with the pelvic limbs

History: About 4 weeks before examination at Cornell University, this dog was on a camping trip in the Adirondacks when the owners first noticed that Cassidy occasionally stumbled with his left pelvic limb. Within the next week he was also stumbling with the right pelvic limb. This pelvic limb dysfunction slowly progressed until the time of this examination.

Examination: Video 10-12 shows the monoplegia of the left pelvic limb and grade 2 monoparesis and ataxia of the right pelvic limb, with absent postural reactions. Cranial nerves and thoracic limb function were all normal. Note the mild hypertonia and normal spinal reflexes for the pelvic limbs and the normal nociception.

Anatomic Diagnosis: A focal or diffuse lesion between spinal cord segments T3 and L3, worse on the left side

With normal nociception, there is no reliable way to localize a focal lesion between these segments using the physical neurologic examination. Be aware that there could be multiple or diffuse lesions in this anatomic area that would explain the clinical signs that were observed in this dog.

Differential Diagnosis: The following diagnoses are limited to those spinal cord disorders that could cause a progressive lesion within these thoracolumbar spinal cord segments of a dog: neoplasm, vertebral malformation, myelitis, discospondylitis, multiple cartilaginous exostosis, intervertebral disk extrusion-protrusion, degenerative myelopathy.

NEPHROBLASTOMA

Although we tend to relegate neoplasia to older dogs, there are many exceptions to this, and one of them occurs at this location in dogs. Nephroblastoma is a unique intradural, extramedullary (extraaxial)

neoplasm that occurs in young dogs, usually between spinal cord segments T10 and L2 (Figs. 10-8 through 10-10).[91] Most of our experience and reports in the literature involve dogs younger than 3.5 years of age, many of them only a few months old. There are numerous reports, mostly in the European literature, that describe this neoplasm as an ependymoma.[58,92,109] In the first two editions of this text, I (AD) recognized that this was not intramedullary and therefore was not an ependymoma, and I called it a neuroepithelioma based on the morphology of the cells and the abundance of tubular elements in the neoplasm. Since then, we have recognized tubular structures that resemble renal glomeruli and have diagnosed this neoplasm as a

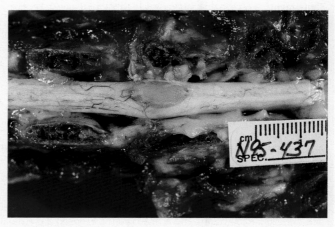

FIGURE 10-8 A nephroblastoma in a 5-month-old Labrador retriever at the level of the T13 spinal cord segment.

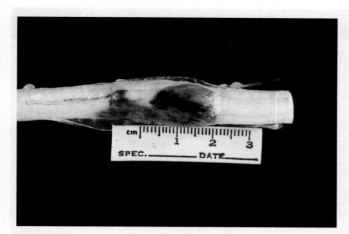

FIGURE 10-9 A nephroblastoma in a 10-month-old German shepherd at the level of the T12 spinal cord segment, with the dura reflected.

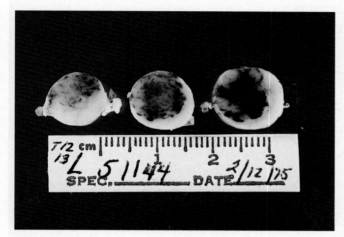

FIGURE 10-10 A transverse section of the nephroblastoma in Fig. 10-9. The nephroblastoma is intradural but extramedullary. Note the marked spinal cord compression.

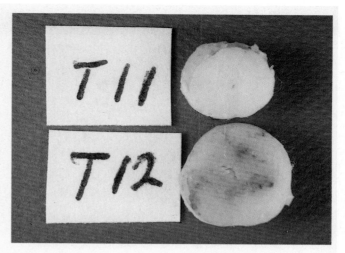

FIGURE 10-11 A nephroblastoma in the T12 spinal cord segment of a 6-month-old German shepherd.

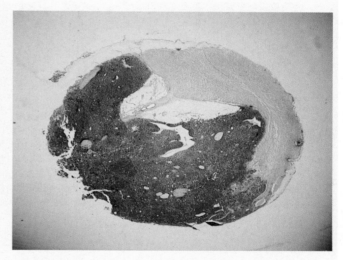

FIGURE 10-12 A microscopic section of the nephroblastoma in the dog in Fig. 10-11. The nephroblastoma is growing in the subarachnoid space, compressing the spinal cord to the right side.

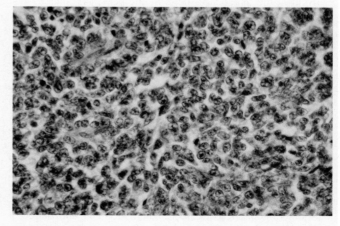

FIGURE 10-13 A microscopic section of the diffuse blastemal epithelial cells of a nephroblastoma.

presumptive nephroblastoma. It is an embryonic neoplasm that may arise from mesonephric tubules. This is supported by the positive immunocytochemical staining of the neoplastic cells for a polysialic acid marker of this tumor; the test was developed in children by Dr. J. Roth in Switzerland.[78]

In children, this nephroblastoma occurs in the kidney and is called a Wilm tumor. A gene located on chromosome 11 has been identified for this tumor in children. Using antibodies developed for the protein product of this tumor gene, immunocytochemical staining has identified this protein product in the canine neoplasm.[76] The unique location of this neoplasm between spinal cord segments T10 and L2 correlates with the site of embryonic renal development from intermediate mesoderm. This is adjacent to the development of the somitic sclerotomes that envelope the neural tube that forms the thoracolumbar spinal cord. A Wilm tumor has three components, sheets of unorganized epithelial cells referred to as blastemal cells; tubular elements lined by epithelial cells that vary from squamous to cuboidal and some of which form glomerular structures; and a fibrous component that consists primarily of bundles of collagen. The canine neoplasm is made up primarily of the first two components (Figs. 10-11 through 10-15). A nephroblastoma

(Continued)

CASE EXAMPLE 10-5—cont'd

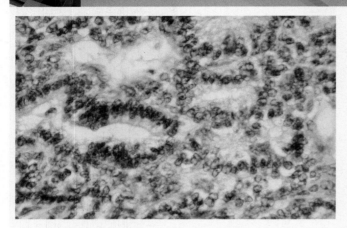

FIGURE 10-14 A microscopic section of the tubular elements of a nephroblastoma.

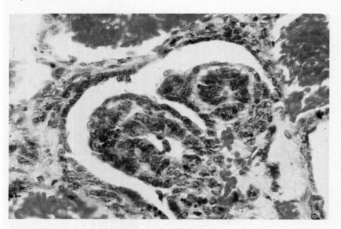

FIGURE 10-15 A microscopic section of a glomeruloid structure in a nephroblastoma.

in this spinal cord location is very rare in children. In dogs, this neoplasm does occur in the kidney but it is much more common adjacent to the spinal cord. There are no reports of this neoplasm being in both locations in the same patient.

Typically, the clinical signs occur in one pelvic limb prior to their occurrence in the other, which reflects the asymmetric location of the neoplasm. We suspect this is a very slowly growing neoplasm and recognize that the spinal cord can be slowly compressed by an extramedullary mass for a long time before the autoregulation of spinal cord vascular perfusion fails and clinical signs occur. Therefore, when these clinical signs occur, be aware that the spinal cord is already very compressed, and if surgery is to be considered it should be done as soon as possible. Often at necropsy, the spinal cord consists only of a thin 1- to 3-mm quarter-moon-shaped shell covering one side of the neoplasm (see Figs. 10-10 through 10-12). When surgeons remove this neoplasm they often see the severely compressed spinal cord slowly start to fill the space where the mass was removed. Postoperative radiation therapy should be done to avoid recurrence of the neoplasm.

Another neoplasm that is more common in cats and can occur at any level of the vertebral canal is lymphoma. In cats it commonly occurs before 1 year of age. Gliomas are less common in the spinal cord of all species and usually occur in older animals.

VERTEBRAL MALFORMATION

Vertebral malformation with kyphosis and secondary spinal cord compression is a realistic consideration in this dog. This vertebral malformation is usually in the midthoracic portion of the vertebral column.[49,67] Although these dogs have the vertebral malformation at birth, the clinical signs of spinal cord compression usually do not occur until a few months of age but prior to 1 year of age. We believe that the kyphosis that causes the spinal cord compression develops at the site of the malformation as the dog grows, and this accounts for the age of onset of the progressive spastic paraparesis and ataxia of the pelvic limbs. Occasionally, on your physical examination of the patient, you can see and palpate the kyphosis. However, it is easy to overlook if you do not take the time to carefully examine the patient for it. This malformation is readily seen on radiographs. It was not visible or palpated in Cassidy. (See Videos 10-15 and 10-16.)

MYELITIS

Myelitis must be a consideration in any patient with progressive spinal cord clinical signs and especially in a young animal. The most common is myelitis caused by the canine distemper virus. Other infectious diseases are caused by the protozoal agents (*Toxoplasma gondii, Neospora caninum*); *Rickettsia* species, and fungal agents.[4] Granulomatous meningoencephalomyelitis is a presumed autoimmune disorder that rarely is limited to a focal lesion in the spinal cord.[28,51] As a rule, these infectious agents cause multifocal lesions, and you should expect that after 4 weeks of progressive thoracolumbar clinical signs, there would be some clinical indication of lesions elsewhere in the CNS. Although these infectious agents can also affect other organs systems, the CNS may be the only system affected. Serology and evaluation of the cerebrospinal fluid (CSF) may be of value in making this diagnosis. Other infectious agents may be more common in different geographic locations.

DISCOSPONDYLITIS

Discospondylitis, also known as intradiscal osteomyelitis, is usually caused by a bacterial or fungal agent.[44,45,52] *Staphylococcus aureus* is the most common isolate. *Streptococcus* species and *Escherichia coli* have also been isolated in this lesion. Be aware that in some southern states, *Brucella canis* has been identified in these infections, and it is contagious to humans. The encroachment of this expanding infection into the vertebral canal can compress the spinal cord, or compression can follow the vertebral instability caused by the infection. Most vertebral column infections are hematogenous, but the source is rarely identified. A migrating plant awn can also be the source of this lesion. The incidence is higher in male dogs, and the incidence in both sexes increases as a dog ages. As a rule, these infected vertebrae cause a great deal of discomfort for the patient, and this is obvious when you palpate the vertebral column. Many of these dogs are depressed, have a fever, and exhibit clinical pathologic changes suggestive of an infection. Cassidy had no systemic signs of an infection and exhibited no discomfort when the vertebral column was vigorously palpated. Any of the imaging procedures (radiography, CT, MR imaging) are useful in making this diagnosis. Be aware that the radiographic changes may lag behind the onset of clinical signs.

MULTIPLE CARTILAGINOUS EXOSTOSIS

Multiple cartilaginous exostosis is an uncommon disorder of young animals that occasionally involves the spinal cord.[30] These exostoses are benign proliferations of cartilage and bone associated with growth plates. They grow by endochondral ossification similar to that of physeal cartilage. These growths are covered by hyaline cartilage and are common in long bones, ribs, and vertebrae. They form large, easily palpable masses at these sites. Those that develop along the vertebral column may invade the vertebral canal and cause an extradural spinal cord compression. These growths are more common in the thoracolumbar vertebral column. As a rule, these exostoses stop growing as the normal growth plates stop their growth. Occasionally, one of them becomes neoplastic and continues to grow. If neurologic signs develop, it occurs prior to 1 year of age. These growths were not palpated in Cassidy.

Intervertebral disk extrusion-protrusion in this breed at this age would be very unlikely. Similarly, although the anatomic diagnosis in Cassidy is compatible with degenerative myelopathy, the age of onset is not. Most of these dogs are at least 5 years old and usually are older than 8 years. The progression of clinical signs is very slow and a monoplegia or paraplegia would be very rare for this disorder. In addition, this degenerative disorder is very rare in this breed. Although the age of onset is appropriate for an inherited degenerative CNS disorder, we are not aware that a disorder that would be compatible with this anatomic diagnosis has been reported in this breed.

Nephroblastoma was the presumptive clinical diagnosis made for Cassidy. Radiographs were normal but a myelogram revealed an intradural extramedullary mass lesion at the level of the vertebral foramen of T13. The myelogram on the video clearly shows the cupping of the contrast as it tries to get by the mass lesion that is in the subarachnoid space. Although this neoplasm is surgically accessible, the duration and severity of the clinical signs indicate that the compression is very severe and the prognosis is guarded. The owner elected to have Cassidy euthanized, and a necropsy confirmed the diagnosis of a nephroblastoma.

Video 10-13 shows another dog with a nephroblastoma. This is Caleb, a 6-month-old castrated male vizsla with a history of 10 days of a rapidly progressive difficulty using his pelvic limbs that started in the right pelvic limb. The video includes the myelogram that shows an intradural extramedullary mass at the level of the thirteenth thoracic vertebral foramen. The mass can be seen on the CT images made from the level of the intervertebral disk between the T12 and T13 vertebrae to the level of the intervertebral disk between the T13 and L1 vertebrae. The neoplasm was removed surgically, and significant improvement in the gait was observed by 1 week postoperatively. It is difficult for the surgeon to remove all of the neoplasm, and we have seen recurrence of the neoplasm occur within a 3-month period. We strongly recommend that this surgical site receive radiation therapy postoperatively.

CASE EXAMPLE 10-6

Signalment: 6-year-old Staffordshire terrier, Sassy
Chief Complaint: Difficulty using the pelvic limbs
History: A week before examination at Cornell University, Sassy was examined by a local veterinarian for a sudden onset of abnormal use of the pelvic limbs, which slowly progressed during this 1-week interval.
Examination: Video 10-14 shows the spastic paraparesis and the pelvic limb ataxia that is fairly symmetric. The pelvic limb hypertonia is severe. Despite being a very stoic dog, Sassy occasionally exhibited discomfort when the lumbar vertebrae were manually compressed.
Anatomic Diagnosis: Focal or diffuse spinal cord lesion between the T3 and L3 segments
Differential Diagnosis: Intervertebral disk extrusion-protrusion, neoplasm, discospondylitis, FCEM, myelitis, degenerative myelopathy, vertebral malformation

Intervertebral disk extrusion-protrusion is the most presumptive diagnosis for Sassy; neoplasm and discospondylitis are the most important to exclude. The sudden onset is less likely with degenerative myelopathy, vertebral malformation, and myelitis. The lack of any other location of clinical signs does not favor myelitis. The sudden onset is compatible with FCEM but not with the history of progression of the clinical signs for 1 week. Degenerative myelopathy is a slowly progressive disorder and is uncommon in this breed. A thoracic vertebral malformation with kyphosis should have shown clinical signs before Sassy was 1 year old. Imaging is necessary to differentiate among the first three differential diagnoses.

INTERVERTEBRAL DISK EXTRUSION-PROTRUSION

Intervertebral disk extrusion or protrusion occurs in all breeds of dogs but is most common in the chondrodystrophic breeds such as the dachshund, Pekingese, French bulldog, basset hound, Welsh corgi, beagle, and American spaniel.[6,12] Endochondral ossification is altered in these dog breeds and is sometimes referred to as a hypochondroplasia.[34] The chemical constituents of

the nucleus pulposus of the intervertebral disk differ between the chondrodystrophic breeds and the nonchondrodystrophic breeds. This is the basis of early onset of a chondroid form of metaplasia that occurs in the chondrodystrophic breeds. Hyalin cartilage replaces the nucleus, and further degeneration leads to calcification of the nucleus.[40,90] These degenerative changes lead to loss of the ability of the intervertebral disk to absorb the normal compressive pressures that occur in the vertebral column. The increased rigidity in the nucleus leads to tears in the annulus and extrusion of the degenerate nuclear material into the vertebral canal. Protrusions consist of proliferated annular fibers secondary to the degeneration of the nucleus and the chronic malarticulation that results between the vertebral bodies. This can be considered a form of degenerative joint disease (DJD) affecting a fibrocartilaginous joint. The metaplasia and degeneration in the chondrodystrophic breeds commences at a few months of age. The shock-absorbing function is compromised enough so that clinical disease related to acute extrusions or more chronic protrusions commonly occur by 2 to 3 years of age. Although not specifically classified as chondrodystrophic breeds, the following breeds are also commonly affected by intervetebral disk extrusion or protrusion at a relatively young age: Lhasa apso, shih tzu, miniature poodle, and cocker spaniel.

In the nonchondrodsytrophic breeds, a fibrous form of metaplasia occurs, resulting in replacement of the nucleus with fibrocartilage. This starts at 4 to 5 years of age and slowly progresses as an aging process. Thus, clinical signs of intervertebral disk extrusion or protrusion in these breeds is usually related to an older age and is rarely seen before 4 to 5 years of age. A similar form of intervertebral disk degeneration occurs in cats as they age. Clinical signs of intervertebral disk extrusion or protrusion are relatively uncommon in cats and most commonly occur in the lumbar region of older cats.[48,50]

In 1952, H. J. Hansen described the pathology of intervertebral disk displacements, and since then many veterinarians have referred to intervertebral disk extrusions as Hansen type I disk and intervertebral

(Continued)

CASE EXAMPLE 10-6—cont'd

disk protrusions as Hansen type 2 disk.[34] Most intervertebral disk extrusions are spontaneous and are not associated with any traumatic event. In dogs, about 80% of thoracolumbar extrusions or protrusions occur between the T10 and L3 vertebrae.[11,29,56] This may relate to the increased motion of the vertebral column at this level compared with the more stable thoracic area. In addition, between the first 10 thoracic vertebrae there is an intercapital ligament that courses across the dorsal surface of the intervertebral disk to connect the heads of the ribs where they articulate with both adjacent vertebrae. This is an added support to the articulation of the vertebral bodies and may help to prevent intervertebral disk extrusion or protrusion between thoracic vertebrae cranial to T10.

These extrusions or protrusions produce varying degrees of compressive myelopathy and ischemia or infarction resulting from interference with the blood supply to the spinal cord. Sudden large extrusions cause acute injuries similar to those of an external traumatic event, with hemorrhage, edema, and necrosis in both the gray and white matter. It is very rare for the extruded material to enter the spinal cord. There is no myelitis in the spinal cord. Inflammation can occur

in the extruded degenerate intervertebral disk material and cause it to enlarge, which accounts for progressive clinical signs in some dogs. At necropsy, small protrusions are commonly found that have not caused neurologic signs, despite some that have caused mild spinal cord compression. Larger protrusions cause focal axonal degeneration and demyelination and progressive clinical signs. At surgery, hemorrhage may sometimes be seen mixed with the extruded intervertebral disk material. Its blue to black color suggests chronicity. Some surgeons refer to this as a "crank-case oil" appearance. This hemorrhage is also readily appreciated on MR imaging.

A third type of presumptive intervertebral disk extrusion is recognized clinically and is best observed in MR imaging. A small percentage of dogs of any breed experience severe external trauma that is commonly associated with motor vehicles. The patient has profound neurologic signs referable to the site of the injury. On MR imaging, there is an obvious collapsed intervertebral disk space and focal changes within the spinal cord parenchyma but without significant compression resulting from the presumptive extruded intervertebral disk (Figs. 10-16 and 10-17).[36] Clinicians refer to these

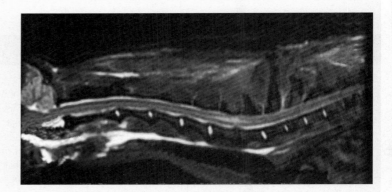

FIGURE 10-16 Sagittal T2-weighted MR image of the neck and cranial thorax of a 7-year-old male Shetland sheepdog that became tetraparetic after being attacked by a larger dog, grasped by the neck, and shaken. Note the loss of hyperintensity of the nucleus pulposus of the intervertebral disk between the C6 and C7 vertebral bodies and the interruption of the adjacent subarachnoid space but without significant evidence of extradural extruded intervertebral disk. Note the hyperintensity of the adjacent spinal cord parenchyma suggesting edema or possible necrosis. Note the enlarged central canal in the spinal cord segments dorsal to the C6 and C7 vertebral bodies. This is an example of a type 3, or "high-velocity," intervertebral disk extrusion.

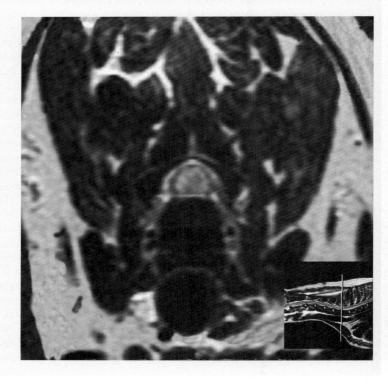

FIGURE 10-17 Axial T2-weighted MR image of the spinal cord at the level of the extruded intervertebral disk between the C6 and C7 vertebrae in the dog in Fig. 10-16. Note the hyperintensity of the central portion of the spinal cord, the thinning of the ventral subarachnoid space, and the lack of significant extradural intervertebral disk material.

as high-velocity disk extrusions, or type 3 disk. Myelography reveals diffuse intramedullary swelling at these sites, which is associated with attenuation of the subarachnoid space. At surgery, the spinal cord appears edematous or slightly bruised. There is minimal evidence of any extruded intervertebral disk material in the extradural space. It is assumed that a small amount of intervertebral disk material has extruded dorsally against the spinal cord at a high velocity, causing severe contusion of the spinal cord without any obvious persistent compression. These observations need to be confirmed and explored further by necropsy study. Video 10-3 may represent a traumatic form of a type 3 intervertebral disk extrusion.

Discomfort is the most common clinical sign observed with intervertebral disk extrusion or protrusion, followed by varying degrees of paraparesis and pelvic limb ataxia. The spinal cord and the intervertebral disk have no GSA innervation. Therefore, the discomfort associated with intervertebral disk extrusion or protrusion is related to the disruption of the highly innervated periosteum or perichondrium associated with the vertebral column and the meninges associated with the spinal cord and the spinal nerves. The latter may be compressed by extrusions or protrusions that occur laterally into the intervertebral foramen. Paraplegia, with or without analgesia caudal to the spinal cord lesion, is the least common clinical presentation, and in a very small percentage of these dogs is associated with a progressive myelomalacia that was described in Case Example 5-14. The grading scheme for the degree of pelvic limb function that was previously described in this chapter was developed to follow the degree of recovery in these dogs using various medical and surgical techniques.

The clinical diagnosis of intervertebral disk extrusion-protrusion is most commonly made by radiographs. For many years, myelography was the gold standard for confirming the diagnosis and for surgical intervention. Now, fortunately, myelography is being rapidly replaced by MR imaging because of its accuracy and the absence of any need to access the subarachnoid space to inject contrast solution.[9,81] MR imaging allows the surgeon to determine accurately the predominant side of the intervertebral disk extrusion and the precise location of the spinal cord edema, unlike myelography. Given our advancements in veterinary medicine, a definitive diagnosis of intervertebral disk extrusion-protrusion should not be made solely on radiographs because many dogs with other diseases have evidence of intervertebral disk degeneration on radiographs. At least a myelogram, and preferably MR imaging, is necessary.

When Sassy, the dog in this case example, was studied, only radiographs were made, and they revealed a significant extrusion of the intervertebral disk between the L3 and L4 vertebrae. The owners elected euthanasia rather than surgery, and this diagnosis was confirmed at necropsy (Figs. 10-18 through 10-20).

Video 10-15 shows Mojo, a 7-month-old castrated male English bulldog that the owners thought had not been walking well in the pelvic limbs for nearly 2 months, and the problem was slowly getting worse. Study the video first. You should have appreciated the mild symmetric (grade 3 to 4) spastic paraparesis and pelvic limb ataxia and have made the anatomic diagnosis of a focal or diffuse lesion between the T3 and L3 spinal cord segments. This alone should generate a differential diagnosis similar to that in Cassidy, the young Labrador retriever in Case Example 10-5. However, you should have observed that in Mojo, there was an abnormal dorsal curvature of the midthoracic vertebral column that was palpated on the video. When you do this palpation, note the abnormal dorsal position of the ribs as they articulate with the vertebrae involved in the kyphosis. This strongly suggests a presumptive diagnosis of a vertebral column malformation

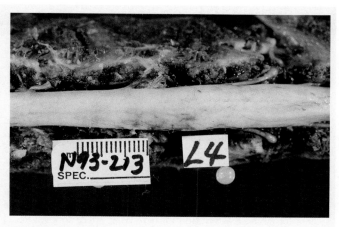

FIGURE 10-18 Gross lesions observed in Sassy, the dog in Video 10-14. The lumbar spinal cord has been exposed by a laminectomy of the lumbar vertebrae. The spinal cord is wider at the L4 level due to an intervertebral disk extrusion between the L3 and L4 vertebrae ventral to the spinal cord.

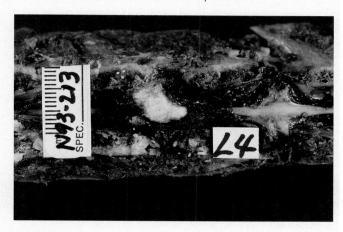

FIGURE 10-19 The same dog as in Fig. 10-18, with the spinal cord removed from the vertebral canal, showing the extruded intervertebral disk between the L3 and L4 vertebrae and hemorrhage resulting from the rupture of the ventral internal vertebral venous plexus.

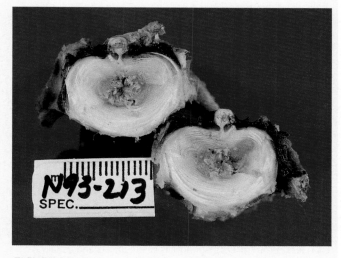

FIGURE 10-20 The same dog as in Figs. 10-18 and 10-19, showing a transverse section of the intervertebral disk between the L3 and L4 vertebrae. Note the degeneration of the nucleus pulposus and its extrusion into the overlying vertebral canal.

(Continued)

with kyphosis and spinal cord compression at that level.[49,67] This was confirmed by radiographs and a myelogram (see Video 10-15) that showed significant spinal cord compression over the elevated ninth thoracic vertebra. At the time of this study there were no reports of successful surgical decompression of a vertebral malformation similar to this. It requires correction of the kyphosis by removal of the elevated vertebral bodies, which is a ventral form of decompression and an onerous task. This was done for Mojo in a procedure that removed the entire ninth thoracic vertebra and took 7 hours. Mojo was worse immediately after surgery as can be seen on the video, but over the following weeks he recovered nearly all of his pelvic limb function and was still doing well 2 years after the surgery. Mojo was a delightful patient for all those who cared for him. What a face to love! Recall that we believe the delay in the onset of clinical signs in dogs with this thoracic vertebral malformation occurs because as the dog grows, kyphosis develops at the site of the malformed vertebral bodies. In time, the kyphosis causes compressive myelopathy in the spinal cord at this site. Remember that spinal cord malformations cause clinical signs to be observed at birth or as soon as the animal is able to walk, and they do not progress. Although the literature suggests that this disorder is more common in the brachycephalic breeds, any breed can be affected. See the description of this disorder following the differential diagnosis for Case Example 10-5. **Video 10-16** shows an 8-month-old beagle from a research laboratory. The dog has progressive spastic

paraparesis and pelvic limb ataxia due to this vertebral malformation. Note the visible elevation of the malformed midthoracic vertebrae. Fig. 10-21 shows the thoracic vertebral radiograph of this dog. The vertebral malformation has often been referred to as a hemivertebra but in reality it is a much more complex vertebral malformation.

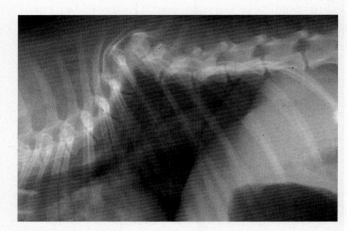

FIGURE 10-21 Lateral thoracic radiograph of the dog in Video 10-16. Note the significant kyphosis at the level of the vertebral malformation.

Signalment: 1-year-old female domestic shorthair
Chief Complaint: Abnormal use of the pelvic limbs
History: Over a 2- to 3-day period this cat rapidly lost the use of its pelvic limbs to the point that it could not stand without help.
Examination: Video 10-17 shows the grade 2 spastic paraparesis and pelvic limb ataxia.
Anatomic Diagnosis: Focal or diffuse lesion between the T3 and L3 spinal cord segments
Differential Diagnosis: Lymphoma, feline infectious peritonitis (FIP) viral myelitis, protozoal myelitis, vertebral malformation, intervertebral disk extrusion-protrusion, discospondylitis, degenerative myelopathy

The most common clinical disorders to cause progressive clinical signs with this anatomic diagnosis at this age are lymphoma and FIP viral myelitis.

Usually a FIP infection causes multifocal signs or primarily caudal brainstem signs. Focal thoracolumbar spinal cord signs are unusual. Similarly, the less common protozoal infection by *T. gondii* usually causes multifocal clinical signs.

Vertebral malformation is uncommon in cats and was not palpated in this cat. Clinical signs of an intervertebral disk extrusion-protrusion are uncommon and are restricted to older cats, especially in the lumbar region. The same applies to degenerative myelopathy, which is even less common. Discospondylitis is rare in cats and usually causes extreme discomfort. Other neoplasms would be uncommon at this age.[71] A myelogram or MR imaging is needed to further support the diagnosis of a lymphoma, and the CSF is usually very altered in cats with FIP and contains high levels of both protein and leucocytes.

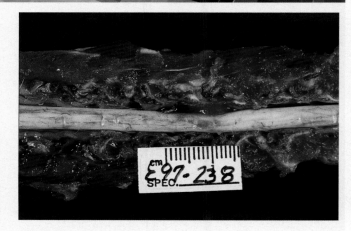

FIGURE 10-22 An extradural lymphoma in a 1-year-old domestic shorthair with clinical signs similar to those in the cat in Video 10-17.

No ancillary studies were done in this cat, and she was euthanized. Necropsy confirmed an extradural lymphoma in the vertebral canal from the T5 to T7 vertebrae, compressing the spinal cord (Fig. 10-22).

LYMPHOMA

Lymphoma is the most common neoplasm to affect the spinal cord in cats and cattle.[70] It is usually located in an extradural position at any level of the vertebral canal but most commonly in the thoracolumbar area. Most lymphomas are restricted to the vertebral foramina of one to three vertebrae. Be aware that the color of the lymphoma can vary from a red to pale yellow appearance. The latter is easily confused with the normal epidural fat that is located in this extradural space. Most of these cats do not have evidence of lymphoma in other body sites except for the bone marrow. In our experience, most, but not all, have serum antibodies for the feline leukemia virus. Because of the possible systemic nature of this neoplasm, it is uncommon for these cats to have the vertebral canal lymphoma removed surgically. Based on my (AD) experience of studying the spinal cords of these cats microscopically, the lesions of compressive myelopathy are often quite mild, and clinical recovery or at least improvement would have been expected with surgical removal of the lymphoma. If surgery is done, it should be followed by a course of radiation therapy as well

as chemotherapy. Remember that occasionally lymphoma infiltrates peripheral nerves and mimics the clinical signs of a nerve sheath neoplasm. (See Case Example 5-6 and Video 6-1 in Chapter 6.) This neoplasm can also develop in the intracranial leptomeninges and infiltrate the adjacent brain parenchyma. This is rare in cats and more common in horses.

Like other slow-growing extradural or intradural extramedullary neoplasms, the spinal cord has usually become significantly compressed before clinical signs occur. We believe that the onset of clinical signs, which can be fairly rapid, is associated with the time when spinal cord autoregulation to maintain normal blood perfusion becomes inadequate. Be aware that occasionally, after ancillary diagnostic procedures that require general anesthesia, the clinical signs may be worse. This may be due to the effect of the anesthesia on the spinal cord blood flow to this already compromised area.

CASE EXAMPLE 10-8

Signalment: An 8-year-old castrated male German shepherd, Sparky
Chief Complaint: Difficulty walking with the pelvic limbs
History: The pelvic limb dysfunction had been slowly progressing for about 5 months; some days were better than others when he walked.
Examination: Video 10-18: Be aware that German shepherd breeders have selected for a sloped back posture that results in increased flexion of the tarsus, which mimics tibial nerve paresis. That posture is normal for this dog.
Anatomic Diagnosis: Focal or diffuse spinal cord lesion between the T3 and L3 segments; we often refer to this gait as a "T3-L3 gait," indicating loss of function of both the UMN and GP systems that control the pelvic limbs.
Differential Diagnosis: The following are all possible causes of a progressive T3-L3 lesion: degenerative myelopathy, intervertebral disk extrusion-protrusion, neoplasm, discospondylitis, myelitis, subarachnoid diverticulum (meningeal fibrosis), DJD of thoracolumbar articular processes.

DEGENERATIVE MYELOPATHY

Degenerative myelopathy is the most presumptive clinical diagnosis based on the information presented here; a chronic intervertebral disk protrusion is the major disorder to be excluded.[2,11,38,39] A prolonged slow progression of a spastic paraparesis and pelvic limb ataxia in a German shepherd over 5 years old is this disorder until proven otherwise. This is a diagnosis of exclusion because, unlike the other disorders in the differential diagnosis, there is no ancillary procedure to confirm degenerative myelopathy. The name *degenerative myelopathy* is redundant because by strict definition a myelopathy is a spinal cord degeneration. It is also very nonspecific because there are many different myelopathies in dogs, and many of them are inherited disorders. Nevertheless, neurologists use the name *degenerative myelopathy* as if it represented a specific clinical disease that is most common in the German shepherd breed but also occurs in other breeds, especially the boxer, kuvasz, and Bernese mountain dog, in our experience. This term refers to a disorder of dogs older than 5 years in which a diffuse axonal necrosis is present primarily in the

lateral and ventral funiculi of the thoracolumbar spinal cord segments. Secondary demyelination and astrogliosis are associated with this axonopathy. There is no pattern to this axonopathy to suggest a dying-back process (Figs. 10-23 through 10-26). Despite the presence of some neuronal cell body degeneration in a few brainstem nuclei, this is insufficient to explain the degree and location of the axonopathy.[46] There may well be a genetic predisposition to the development of this lesion, but the late onset and the lack of confirming pathologic diagnoses has made that difficult to establish.

The initial clinical signs of spinal cord dysfunction are commonly mistaken for the clinical signs of hip dysplasia, which also may be present in a patient with this spinal cord disorder. Occasionally, there is mild asymmetry in the pelvic limb signs. Although the abnormal gait clearly exhibits the clinical signs of loss of function of the UMN and GP systems, in a small percentage (10% to 20%) of these patients, you may find a unilateral or bilateral decrease or loss of the patellar reflex. In the presence of normal or increased pelvic limb tone and no atrophy

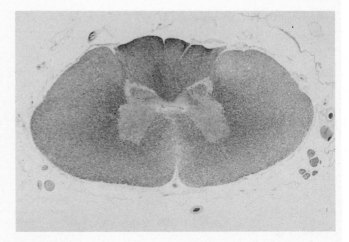

FIGURE 10-23 A microscopic section of the thoracic spinal cord in a dog with degenerative myelopathy stained for myelin. Note the diffuse loss of myelin, which is due to secondary demyelination.

(Continued)

CASE EXAMPLE 10-8—cont'd

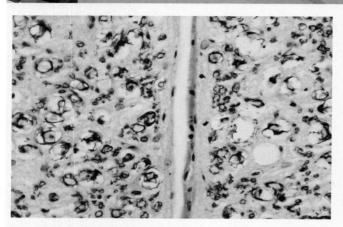

FIGURE 10-24 The same dog shown in Fig. 10-23. This is a microscopic section of the ventral funiculi on either side of the ventral median fissure. Note the marked loss of axons and myelin and their replacement by astrogliosis (the pale areas).

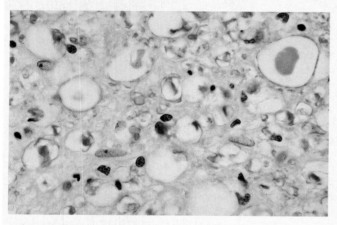

FIGURE 10-25 The same dog as in Figs. 10-23 and 10-24. This is a microscopic section of the ventral funiculus. The vacuoles represent secondary demyelination. There is a lack of axons. A degenerating axon, a spheroid, is at the upper right. The intervening pale area consists of astrocytic processes.

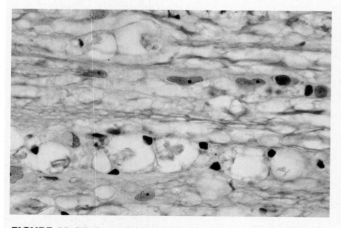

FIGURE 10-26 The same dog as in Figs. 10-23 through 10-25. This is a longitudinal microscopic section showing a chain of ellipsoids reflecting secondary demyelination and containing axonal fragments.

of the quadriceps femoris muscle, this patellar reflex loss is thought to represent dysfunction of the sensory component of the reflex arc. How it relates to the spinal cord axonopathy that is present in this disorder is unknown. It may be part of that process and reflect lesions in the dorsal gray column of the L4 and L5 spinal cord segments that are difficult to recognize. It may relate to the mild neuropathy in the dorsal roots that is commonly observed in necropsies of older dogs that have no neurologic signs or other lesions in the nervous system. This age-related neuropathy is most prominent in the roots of the lumbosacral spinal cord segments.[39] Recall that occasionally the patellar reflex is depressed or absent in older dogs that have no other neurologic signs. Although in this spinal cord disorder, there are commonly lesions of axonopathy in the cervical spinal cord segments, it is very rare to see any neurologic signs in the thoracic limbs. The rate of progression of this axonopathy is variable. It may take 6 to 12 months before the dog is unable to stand without assistance. We have never seen a dog that had this diagnosis confirmed at necropsy progress to paraplegia. Owners are anxious to know when their dogs will be unable to get up, and the question is difficult to answer because of the variation among individual patients.

A number of studies have implicated disorders in the immune system of these dogs, but any relationship to the pathology of this degenerative myelopathy is unproven.[7,103,104] This is not an inflammatory disease of the spinal cord. Attempts to identify evidence of a retrovirus in the lesions have been unsuccessful. There is no treatment for neurons with degeneration of their axons. Because this is a very slow degeneration, the patient may have brief periods of compensation that are thought by owners to represent improvement. Treatment of these patients with the antiinflammatory drug aminocaproic acid has been extensive because of the unfounded publicity it has received, but there is no scientific evidence to support its efficacy as treatment or preventive therapy. With the advent of alternative therapies and the desperation of the owners of these patients, many treatments have been tried, including acupuncture and chiropractic therapy. There is no evidenced-based medicine to support the use of any of these therapies. Fortunately, most of them have not harmed the patients. Vitamins E and B$_{12}$ are frequently used because of their role in other degenerative neurologic disorders in domestic animals and primates, but no studies have established either a deficiency in these vitamins or any response to treatment. Treatment of a group of affected German shepherds for a period of 3 years with the neutroceutical S-adenosylmethionine because of its role as a methyl donor in maintaining CNS myelin and axons was not beneficial. Recent studies support the use of intense physiotherapy in prolonging the length of time the patient remains ambulatory.[47] This involves primarily active exercise, with 5 to 10 minutes of walking at least five times daily, but also includes passive exercise, massage, and hydrotherapy.

Degenerative myelopathy is uncommon in small dog breeds and in cats.[62] When cats have chronic degenerative myelopathy, feline leukemia viral antigen has been found in the spinal cord lesions.[13,65] A similar myelopathy has been reported in two young German shepherd dogs, but its relationship to the older-dog myelopathy is unknown. The Pembroke Welsh corgi is a breed that has been reported to develop a slowly progressive pelvic limb paresis and ataxia without any abnormalities on MR imaging studies. This may be a similar disease to the degenerative myelopathy described above but with more continuous, bilaterally symmetrical and well-defined spinal cord lesions. In a study of 21 affected Pembroke Welsh corgis the median age of onset of paraparesis and pelvic limb ataxia was 11 years. Progression of clinical signs occurred slowly over a median period of 19 months with a median age at euthanasia of 13 years. By the time of euthanasia, many dogs exhibited thoracic limb neurologic abnormalities and were paraplegic. A familial basis was proposed but not proven.[17]

Intervertebral disk extrusion-protrusion certainly is the most significant clinical disorder one must differentiate from degenerative myelopathy, despite the slow and prolonged progression of clinical signs. Slow development of a bulging annulus fibrosis protrusion or the continued proliferation that occurs in extruded degenerate nucleus pulposus could cause this chronic compression. The diagnosis can readily be confirmed by imaging studies. MR imaging is by far the most reliable of these procedures. Be aware that it is common for these older German shepherds that develop degenerative myelopathy also to have one or more mild intervertebral disk protrusions. The experienced clinician recognizes this and avoids unnecessary surgery. In addition, a corticosteroid treatment trial may help to distinguish clinically significant intervertebral disk problems.

Neoplasms typically cause progressive clinical signs, but the duration of the slow progression observed in Sparky is unusual. In fact, neoplasms that affect the spinal cord more often cause rapid onset and progression of clinical signs, as seen in Cassidy in Case Example 10-5. Nevertheless, neoplasia has to be considered a serious possibility. Examples of it include intramedullary glioma, intradural-extramedullary meningioma or nerve sheath neoplasm, and extradural lymphoma or metastatic neoplasm, which may also affect the vertebral body, as in hemangiosarcoma. The diagnosis requires imaging studies.

Discospondylitis would not be expected to cause such a prolonged, progressive course and would be expected to cause significant discomfort in the dog. Myelitis would not be expected to remain so focal for such a length of time.

SUBARACHNOID DIVERTICULA

Subarachnoid diverticula have been reported incorrectly as sub-arachnoid cysts that cause spinal cord compression in dogs. These are not cysts. Although they have the appearance of cysts on myelograms and MR images, the spaces readily fill with contrast during myelography, which supports the idea that they are diverticuli of the subarachnoid space. There is no excuse for continuing to refer to them as cysts when that term is a misnomer. The cause of the diverticulum is unknown. It may be the result of a partial obstruction of the smooth pulsatile flow of CSF. This may be due to fibrosis of the arachnoid trabeculae similar to the lesion that is common at the C2-C3 articulation and is referred to as meningeal fibrosis. The latter is described in Case Example 10-14, cervical spinal cord disorders. It is difficult to prove on microscopic examination of the meninges that are removed surgically to decompress the spinal cord. These biopsies consist of normal connective tissue. Whether the connective tissue is excessive or not is difficult to determine. These diverticula may occur at any level of the spinal cord but commonly are found in the thoracolumbar area. The onset of clinical signs varies from a few months to more than 5 years, and you would not expect the progression to be as slow as it is in this case example. The diagnosis is readily made by myelography or MR imaging.

DEGENERATIVE JOINT DISEASE

DJD in the synovial joints of thoracolumbar vertebrae is commonly observed on radiographs of older dogs but rarely causes spinal cord compression except at the lumbosacral articulation, where it may be a component involved with the compression of the spinal nerve roots at that level. This was described as the lumbosacral syndrome in Chapter 5. However, in young Shiloh shepherds, a DJD in one or more pair of intervertebral synovial joints occurs between the T11 and L2 articulations, which may bilaterally compress the dorsolateral aspect of the spinal cord.[63] Clinical signs of spastic paraparesis and pelvic limb ataxia occur before 1 year of age, usually at a few months of age, and are progressive. The consistent location of this DJD at the thoracolumbar junction of young rapidly growing dogs suggests that at a critical time in their growth, an injury occurs to these joints and results in their malarticulation and subsequent DJD. The proliferation of the articular processes and their joint capsules may encroach far enough into the vertebral canal to compress the spinal cord segments located at these sites. The Shiloh shepherd breed was developed from lines of German shepherds that were selected for their superior size and good disposition. These dogs have exceptionally long trunks. It is our hypothesis that during vigorous exercise and play, the long thoracolumbar vertebral column is at risk for injury at the thoracolumbar junction where there is less support and more mobility. Histologic study of the affected joints shows only the changes expected with DJD. In reviewing radiographs of normal littermates of affected Shiloh shepherds, this lesion was occasionally seen without evidence of any spinal cord compression. The data collected at this time support the theory of an inherited predisposition for the disorder. Sparky was not a Shiloh shepherd, and the onset of his clinical signs occurred much later than would be expected for the Shiloh shepherd disorder.

Radiographs and a myelogram were normal in Sparky, as was the evaluation of his CSF. At the time of that study, MR imaging was not available. In our experience, MR studies in dogs with degenerative myelopathy are normal. Based on these studies, a presumptive diagnosis of degenerative myelopathy was made. No medical therapy was advised. Physical therapy and as much reasonable exercise as possible were recommended.

For other examples of degenerative myelopathy, consider the following videos.

Video 10-19 shows Killian, an 8-year-old castrated male boxer with a history of several months of a slowly progressive difficulty using his pelvic limbs. Note the exacerbation of the gait abnormality when Killian is turning as he walks. Note the bilateral hypertonia but depressed left patellar reflex.

Video 10-20 shows McDuff, an 11-year-old male collie with a history of 6 to 8 months of slowly progressive difficulty using his pelvic limbs. Note the absent left patellar reflex but normal tone and no atrophy in that limb.

Video 10-21 shows Werrig, a 9-year-old spayed female Dalmatian that had exhibited a slowly progressive abnormal pelvic limb gait for 8 months. Werrig exhibits the classic appearance of grade 3 spastic paraparesis and pelvic limb ataxia.

CASE EXAMPLE 10-9

Signalment: An 8-month-old female Afghan hound, Lewis
Chief Complaint: Unable to use the pelvic limbs
History: Lewis was one of three dogs in a litter of six that had developed similar clinical neurologic signs within a period of about 10 days. At 7 months of age, the entire litter was ill with fever, vomiting, and diarrhea over a 2-week period. They recovered from this illness before the neurologic signs began in three of the dogs.
Examination: Video 10-22 shows severe grade 2 spastic paraparesis and pelvic limb ataxia. Note especially the inability to stand up on its thoracic limbs unassisted. Note how the trunk sways to the side as Lewis attempts to stand. When assisted, note the tendency of the trunk to sway to either side yet note the normal thoracic limb gait.
Anatomic Diagnosis: Focal or diffuse lesion between the T3 and L3 spinal cord segments; if this is a focal lesion, then it is likely to be in the more cranial thoracic segments. The difficulty in standing up on the thoracic limbs and the swaying of the trunk are caused by loss of the UMN and GP systems in the cranial thoracic region; these systems normally control the axial trunk muscles. This is not seen when the lesions that involve the UMN and GP systems are located more caudally in the thoracic or in the cranial lumbar spinal cord segments.
Differential Diagnosis: The differential diagnosis is the same as described in the earlier cases of progressive signs of a lesion between the T3 and L3 spinal cord segments. The greatest concern at this age and with the involvement of multiple dogs in the same litter, in which some undefined systemic illness has recently occurred, is the involvement of the CNS with a canine distemper virus infection. The fact that all three dogs had the same spinal cord anatomic diagnosis is unusual; this viral infection usually affects multiple levels of the CNS, especially the brain. Multifocal clinical signs would also be expected of other infectious diseases, such as toxoplasmosis and neosporosis. Remember that before you complete your list of differential diagnoses, you must consider the possibility of inherited degenerative disorders that might explain the anatomic diagnosis in this breed. This is especially indicated when multiple dogs in a litter are affected by the same neurologic signs. A description of just such a disease in the Afghan hound follows.

AFGHAN HOUND MYELINOLYSIS

Afghan hound myelinolytic encephalomyelopathy is inherited as an autosomal recessive gene. It is a unique primary demyelination that causes necrosis of myelin but spares the axons.[3,18,21] It appears to start in the myelin in the midthoracic spinal cord segments and to progress cranially and caudally. The clinical signs begin with mild pelvic limb spastic paresis and ataxia and loss of control of the trunk muscles by 7 to 10 days. They are followed by thoracic limb spastic paresis and ataxia and then recumbency by about 14 to 21 days. The initial onset of clinical signs ranges between 3 and 13 months of age. The myelinolytic lesion is bilaterally symmetric in all of the funiculi but spares the fasciculus proprius. The "naked" demyelinated axons float unsupported in their funiculi among a plethora of lipid-filled macrophages (Figs. 10-27 through 10-30). One of the earliest publications on this disorder erroneously explained this lesion as a

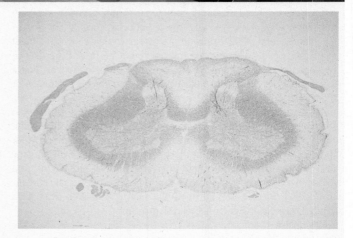

FIGURE 10-27 A microscopic section of the C8 spinal cord segment from a young Afghan hound with myelinolysis. Note the sparing of the fasciculus proprius and the nerve roots.

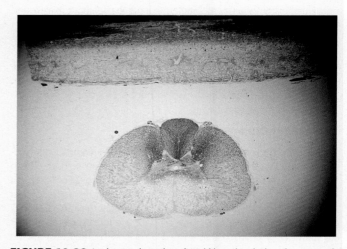

FIGURE 10-28 A microscopic section of a midthoracic spinal cord segment of an Afghan hound with myelinolysis. Note the bilateral symmetry of the lesion.

vascular compromise. You cannot cause a primary demyelination with axonal sparing by means of any known vascular disorder. The unique distribution of this lesion is unexplained. Most of these dogs also have the same primary demyelination of the axons that surround the dorsal nucleus of the trapezoid body. No clinical signs have been associated with the lesion. This inherited myelinolytic disorder was confirmed at necropsy in the dogs in this litter.

SPONDYLOSIS DEFORMANS AND DURAL OSSIFICATION

These are two disorders anatomically associated with the spinal cord that are occasionally considered to be the cause of neurologic signs.

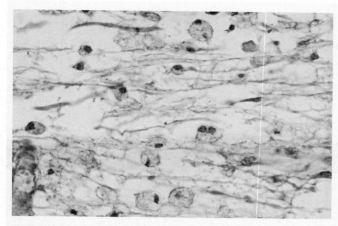

FIGURE 10-29 A microscopic section of a midthoracic spinal cord segment of an Afghan hound with myelinolysis showing "naked" axons coursing through the funiculus and macrophages distributed along the axons, containing the phagocytized myelin.

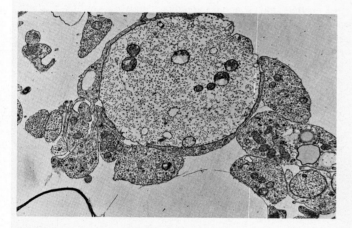

FIGURE 10-30 An electron micrograph (prepared by Dr. John Cummings) of a section of spinal cord similar to that in Fig. 10-29, showing the preserved demyelinated axon. Demyelination is primary in this inherited disorder.

It is our opinion that this is incorrect. Spondylosis deformans is common in the thoracolumbar vertebral column, especially in older large-breed dogs.[55,66] Occasionally, it is seen in young adult dogs. It is most common at the level of the thoracolumbar and lumbosacral articulations. It is a proliferation of bone on the ventral and lateral aspects of the vertebral bodies on each side of the intervertebral disk. There is an increased incidence of intervertebral disk degeneration associated with this spondylosis, but the spondylosis lesion does not extend into the vertebral canal and rarely reaches the level of the intervertebral

foramina. This common disorder may cause some stiffness in the trunk and occasional discomfort but not paresis and ataxia. In well-developed cases, the bony proliferation may fuse ventral to the intervertebral disk, forming a bridge between the two vertebral bodies. An extreme but rare example of this vertebral body bridging is referred to as disseminated idiopathic skeletal hyperostosis (DISH).[69] It is unclear whether spondylosis and DISH are a continuum or two separate diseases. Dogs with DISH have a continuous thick column of bone covering the ventral and lateral sides of the vertebral bodies in the lumbar and a portion of the thoracic vertebral column. I (EG) diagnosed a DISH lesion in a 9-year-old female Babirussa, a wild pig species from Southeast Asia, that had spastic paraparesis and pelvic limb ataxia due to an associated intervertebral disk extrusion. We believe that a fracture in the lumbar portion of the DISH lesion in this Babirussa acted as a fulcrum at an intervertebral disk and resulted in its extrusion.

Dural ossification involves the formation of plaques of bone within the dura that may indent the adjacent spinal cord.[68,105] This dural ossification is a form of metaplasia of the dura. The plaques contain bone marrow. In the older literature the plaques were incorrectly referred to as pachymeningitis. They are most common on the midline of the dura, ventral to the spinal cord in the cranial cervical and lumbar areas of the spinal cord. Fig. 10-31 shows an extreme example of this in a 6-year-old Great Dane in which the dural ossification extended the entire length of the spinal cord. The small indentations of the spinal cord caused by these plaques do not result in any recognizable microscopic lesions, so this dural ossification should not be expected to cause any neurologic signs. Occasionally, these plaques can be recognized on lateral radiographs of the vertebral column as thin, hyperdense lines where they cross an intervertebral foramen.

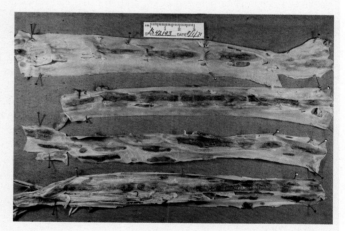

FIGURE 10-31 This is the entire dura from a 6-year-old Great Dane that has been removed from the spinal cord and opened to show the extensive dural metaplasia-ossification located on the inner surface of primarily the ventral aspect of the dura. There were no spinal cord lesions associated with it.

SMALL ANIMAL CERVICAL SPINAL CORD DISEASES

See the description earlier in this chapter and Fig. 10-1 for a summary of the clinical signs that are observed in the two regions of the spinal cord that involve all four limbs. The following case examples demonstrate many of the various disorders that affect the cervical spinal cord.

Tetraplegia

CASE EXAMPLE 10-10

Signalment: 5-year-old castrated male German shepherd, Sam
Chief Complaint: Unable to stand
History: The day before this examination, Sam was found recumbent in his pen. He was alert but unable to stand.

Examination: Video 10-23 shows the tetraplegia, which is defined as no voluntary movement of any limb when supported and when recumbent. Note that the patellar reflexes can be elicited only in the recumbent limb, which is normal in some dogs, and that is why it is necessary to test this reflex in both positions before you consider it to be absent. Crossed extension occurs in the pelvic limbs. Nociception is intact. Remember that analgesia essentially requires a transverse lesion, and in the cervical spinal cord this would cause death due to respiratory paralysis.

Anatomic Diagnosis: Focal or diffuse bilateral lesion of the C1 to C5 spinal cord segments

Differential Diagnosis: External injury, FCEM, intervertebral disk extrusion, neoplasm, myelitis, discospondylitis

Realistically, this acute onset of tetraplegia could be explained by one of the first three differential diagnoses listed; external injury is essentially excluded for Sam by the history. Imaging procedures are needed to differentiate between FCEM and an acute intervertebral disk extrusion and must be done as soon as possible because the latter diagnosis requires immediate surgical treatment. The imaging also diagnoses neoplasm, which would be an unusual cause of such an acute onset of clinical signs. Myelitis and discospondylitis would not be expected to cause such an acute onset of such severe clinical signs.

Radiographs and a myelogram were performed on Sam. The video shows the intramedullary swelling in the spinal cord within the vertebral foramen of C3. The presumptive diagnosis of FCEM was made. MR imaging is the preferred imaging for this diagnosis but was not available when Sam was studied. While hospitalized, Sam remained recumbent and developed the ability to move his limbs in a few days. He was discharged and remained recumbent for 10 days after the onset of clinical signs. The end of the video shows Sam able to stand and walk 3 weeks after the onset of his presumptive vascular disorder.

Video 10-24 shows Molly and Snowball, who are both tetraplegic. This is a unique opportunity to observe two tetraplegic dogs, one caused by a diffuse LMN disorder and the other caused by a focal cervical UMN-GP system lesion. The anatomic diagnosis is based entirely on the evaluation of muscle tone and spinal reflexes. Molly is the gray-colored 11-year-old spayed female miniature schnauzer with a 10-day history of progressive paresis that began with pelvic limb lameness that was initially diagnosed as arthritis. Snowball is the all-white 8-year-old mixed-breed who was presented unable to stand after being struck by a car. She was tetraplegic when presented, but by the time the video was made 7 days later, she had regained some voluntary movement in the left limbs. The anatomic diagnosis in Molly is diffuse neuromuscular disease. See Case Example 5-1 for a discussion of the differential diagnosis. A presumptive diagnosis of polyradiculoneuritis was made for Molly, and her therapy consisted of nursing care. Molly first began to move her limbs 6 weeks after this examination, and it was 3 months before she could stand and walk. Radiographs of Snowball taken before she was videoed showed no fracture but a possible narrowing of the intervertebral disk between the C2 and C3 vertebrae. Snowball was able to stand and walk 3 weeks after the injury. Be aware that the most common cervical vertebra to fracture is the cranial aspect of the body of C2 (Fig. 10-32). This may be the result of the physical stress that is placed there, where the dens articulates with the atlas. The latter acts as a fulcrum when there is forced flexion of the head and neck. In addition, the presence of two growth plates in the cranial portion of the body of the axis may be a risk factor for a fracture there (see Fig. 10-34). These dogs usually exhibit extreme discomfort. It is less common for trauma at this site to tear the transverse ligament of the atlas and the dorsal atlantoaxial ligament, resulting in a subluxation.

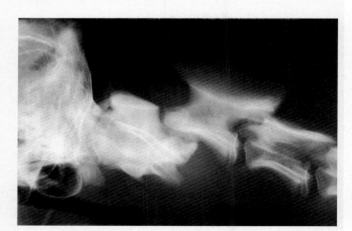

FIGURE 10-32 A cervical radiograph of a 5-month-old dog that was struck by a car and suffered a fracture of the cranial aspect of the axis at the level of the growth plates on either side of the intercentrum 2 ossification center. Note the large space between the dorsal arch of the atlas and the spine of the axis due to the dorsal displacement of the portion of the axis caudal to the fracture.

CASE EXAMPLE 10-11

Signalment: 13-year-old castrated male domestic shorthair, Curtis
Chief Complaint: Unable to stand
History: A week before examination, Curtis suddenly developed difficulty walking, which rapidly progressed to recumbency. He had been blind for a number of months due to retinopathy.
Examination: Video 10-25 shows the tetraplegia with extensive hypertonia in all four limbs and the pelvic limb crossed extension.
Anatomic Diagnosis: Focal or diffuse lesion between the C1 and C5 spinal cord segments
Differential Diagnosis: Ischemic myelopathy, FCEM, neoplasm, intervertebral disk extrusion, myelitis, discospondylitis, vertebral malformation

A neoplasm and a compromise of the spinal cord blood supply are the two most presumptive diagnoses. The latter rarely progresses as did the clinical signs in this cat unless there were repeated episodes of vascular compromise. FCEM does occur in cats, but the more common cause of CNS vascular compromise in cats is hypertensive vasculopathy. The retina and the CNS are the most common organs to be affected by hypertension. Blood pressure should be assessed routinely in your examination of cats with any acute CNS disorder. An acute intervertebral disk extrusion is certainly compatible with this history and anatomic diagnosis but is a less common disorder in the cat. The acute onset and focal clinical signs make myelitis caused

by the FIP virus or *T. gondii* unlikely. Discospondylitis is uncommon in cats and is less likely to cause an acute onset of clinical signs. Vertebral malformations are rare in cats and would not be expected to cause clinical signs at that age.

Curtis was determined to have chronic renal disease and markedly elevated blood pressure. No further studies were performed. Curtis was euthanized, and necropsy showed numerous areas in the cervical spinal cord with ischemic lesions. In the absence of any fibrocartilaginous emboli, they were assumed to be related to the hypertension. The chronic retinopathy was also thought to result from the same hypertension.

HYPERVITAMINOSIS A

Be aware that cats that are continually fed a diet that contains high levels of vitamin A, such as raw liver, may develop extensive bone proliferation related to synovial joints.[27,80] These exostoses may become extensive enough to fuse the entire cervical vertebral column, limb joints and, ultimately, the entire vertebral column. Clinical signs of cervical discomfort and rigidity are common. Neurologic deficits relate to spinal nerve entrapment at intervertebral foramina and compression of the cervical spinal cord. The lesion is obvious on radiographs.

CASE EXAMPLE 10-12

Signalment: 10-year-old female Doberman pinscher, Mary
Chief Complaint: Unable to stand
History: Mary had a progressive gait abnormality in all four limbs for a few weeks; in the last week it rapidly progressed to recumbency.
Examination: Video 10-26 shows the tetraplegia with severe hypertonia. You can feel this hypertonia just by lifting the dog up and placing her limbs on the floor. Why is the thoracic limb extensor hypertonia not the Schiff-Sherrington syndrome?
Anatomic Diagnosis: Focal or diffuse lesion between the C1 and C5 spinal cord segments

This is not the Schiff-Sherrington syndrome because the dog has no voluntary movement in its thoracic limbs. The hypertonia and tetraplegia exist because of the loss of the UMN tracks that are cranial to the cervical intumescence and control thoracic limb tone and function.
Differential Diagnosis: The following diagnoses are causes of progressive lesions at this anatomic site: neoplasm, intervertebral disk extrusion or protrusion, vertebral malformation-malarticulation, C2-C3 meningeal fibrosis, myelitis, discospondylitis, syringohydromyelia.

PROGRESSIVE COMPRESSIVE CERVICAL MYELOPATHY

Progressive compressive myelopathy is a common cervical spinal cord lesion that is secondary to a primary disorder that compromises the space available in the vertebral canal. These disorders more commonly cause progressive tetraparesis or hemiparesis and ataxia. The following is a brief review of the causes, and examples will follow.
1. Intervertebral disk extrusion or protrusion. This vertebral column disorder is described earlier in this chapter in Case Example 10-6, the section on thoracolumbar spinal cord disease. In the cervical region, the intervertebral disk between the C2 and C3 vertebral bodies is

the most common site where this occurs (Fig. 10-33). A chronic protrusion is common in the caudal cervical intervertebral disks, where it results from chronic malarticulation (see the later discussion).
2. Neoplasm. This category includes extradural neoplasms, such as lymphoma or metastatic neoplasms, including hemangiosarcoma

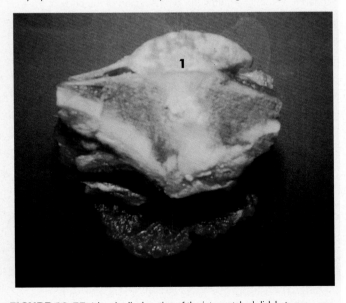

FIGURE 10-33 A longitudinal section of the intervertebral disk between portions of the C2 and C3 vertebral bodies of a 10-year-old boxer with clinical signs similar to those of Mary in Video 10-26. Note the large proliferated, extruded intervertebral disk, dorsally (1).

(Continued)

CASE EXAMPLE 10-12—cont'd

and intradural-extramedullary neoplasms, such as meningiomas and nerve sheath neoplasms. Spinal cord meningiomas are most common at the C1 and C2 level, in our experience. An intramedullary glioma is the least common neoplasm at this site.
3. Vertebral malformation-malarticulation. There are congenital and acquired forms of this disorder.

VERTEBRAL MALFORMATION AND MALARTICULATION

Congenital vertebral malformation is uncommon in the cervical vertebrae except possibly for the atlantoaxial subluxation seen in the toy breeds, where the dens is absent. However, this may not be a malformation. An occiptoatlantoaxial malformation has been reported in a dog and a cat.[99,102]

Atlantoaxial Subluxation

Atlantoaxial subluxation is a dorsal displacement of the cranial aspect of the body of the axis into the vertebral canal because of the lack of the dens.[19,33,75] It is most common in the toy and miniature breeds of dogs, or "purse dogs." The absence of the dens is caused either by the degeneration of the dens that was present at birth or by malformation, an aplasia in which the dens fails to develop. Most authors refer to this as an aplasia or a hypoplasia without any scientific proof. The dens is derived from the ossification center of the axis referred to as centrum 1 (Fig. 10-34).[100,101] Intercentrum 1 is the ossification center for the ventral arch (body) of the atlas. Ossification of centrum 1 forms the cranial articular surface of the axis body and the dens. Most dogs also have a very small ossification center called the centrum of the proatlas that forms the small apex of the dens. This fuses with the ossification center of centrum 1 at 3 to 4 months. Ossification is first seen in centrum 1 at 3 weeks of age and fuses caudally with the ossification of intercentrum 2 of the body of the axis at 7 to 9 months. Intercentrum 2 is a narrow ossification center between the ossification centers of centrum 1 and centrum 2. The latter forms the central region of the body of the axis. A narrow caudal epiphyseal ossification center completes the body of the axis. If centrum 1 fails to develop, the entire cranial portion of the body of the axis that articulates with the atlas would be absent, not just the dens. We believe it is more likely that the dens, which is present at birth, undergoes a progressive degeneration at a few months of age so that only the cranial articular surface of the axis is left to form the atlantoaxial joint. This process may be similar to that of necrosis of the femoral head, which occurs in these same small breeds and is called Legg-Perthe disease.[57] The pathogenesis of this disease is thought to be related to the early development of the sex hormones in these breeds.

The normal alignment of the atlas and axis is dependent on the dens and cranial articular surface of the axis being held in contact with the caudal articular foveae of the atlas by the transverse ligament of the atlas, which is attached on both sides of the ventral arch of the atlas and passes dorsal to the dens. In addition, the thick dorsal atlantoaxial ligament between the dorsal arch of the atlas and the spine of the axis contributes to this joint stability. The clinical signs of a subluxation usually occur between 6 and 18 months of age but occasionally later. The loss of the dens may precede the subluxation by a considerable period of time if the dense connective tissue of the dorsal atlantoaxial ligament resists the instability between the atlas and axis. This delay would be much less likely if the cartilaginous centrum 1 failed to develop a dens at birth. The degree of activity of the patient may influence how long the dorsal atlantoaxial ligament is able to resist stretching excessively to cause the subluxation. When subluxation occurs, the cranial surface of the body of the axis rotates dorsally into the vertebral canal. A dog in this situation has an intact transverse ligament that is forced from its normal dorsal plane into a transverse plane as the subluxation occurs (Fig. 10-35). A rare congenital absence of the transverse ligament of the atlas has been reported.[98]

The atlantoaxial subluxation is usually first recognized on lateral cervical radiographs by the increased space between the dorsal arch of the atlas and the spinous process of the axis, which appears to project dorsally (Fig. 10-36). This increased space is where the dorsal atlantoaxial ligament has been stretched. It may be difficult to observe the lack of the dens on a lateral radiograph because of the superimposition of the wings of the atlas. If the head is carefully rotated a few degrees it will expose the cranial articular surface of the axis without its dens. Ventrodorsal or open-mouth craniocaudal views may also show the lack of a dens, but care must be taken to avoid excessive manipulation of such a patient in which the cervical spinal cord is already compromised. MR imaging is especially useful in these dogs because it may determine the degree of gliosis and atrophy of the spinal cord in chronic cases, which is useful prognostic information.

The clinical signs vary from reluctance to have the head touched through severe neck discomfort, and mild tetraparesis and ataxia to tetraplegia. These patients should be handled with extreme care, and all manipulation of the atlantoaxial joint should be avoided. The clinical signs may worsen after exercise, especially if the paresis and ataxia cause the dog to fall and flex its neck excessively. Be aware that if you anesthetize such a dog for imaging or subsequent surgery, there will be no muscle tone to help prevent further subluxation. Remember that no animal can survive a severe cervical spinal cord compression at this level because of the interference with the reticulospinal pathways necessary for respiration. The use of a thick cotton neck wrap for a

FIGURE 10-34 Diagram of canine atlas and axis showing ossification centers and approximate times, in months, of closure of the growth plates observed radiographically, ventrodorsal view. *C1,* Centrum 1; *C2,* centrum 2; *CP,* centrum of proatlas; *CdE,* caudal epiphysis; *IC1,* intercentrum 1; *IC2,* intercentum 2.

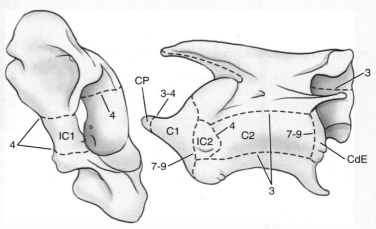

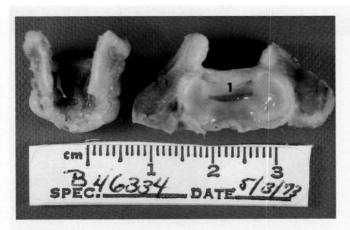

FIGURE 10-35 Necropsy specimen of a 3-month-old toy poodle that was tetraplegic due to atlantoaxial subluxation. The axis is on the left, with no visible dens. The atlas is on the right, showing its caudal surface and the abnormal transverse plane of the ligament of the dens (1) that was forced into this position by the displaced cranial articular surface of the axis.

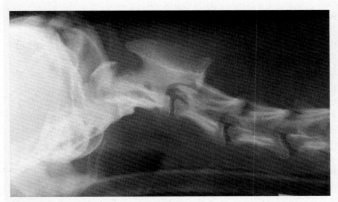

FIGURE 10-36 Cervical radiograph of a 6-month-old miniature poodle, showing the dorsal subluxation of the axis due to the absence of the dens.

cast may help to avoid increased trauma to the compressed spinal cord during your diagnostic manipulations.

Realistic treatment requires surgery. Many procedures have been described, and the choice is somewhat dependent on the age of the patient and the degree of ossification of the atlas and axis. It must be remembered that the surgeon is often faced with a severely compromised cervical spinal cord, and it is difficult to perform the surgical manipulations that are necessary for repair without causing further spinal cord compression, which may be lethal for the patient.

Acquired Vertebral Malformation-Malarticulation

Acquired vertebral malformation-malarticulation has a plethora of names in the literature that refer to the cervical vertebral disorders that are thought to cause the gait disorder seen in large-breed dogs that many refer as the "wobbler syndrome." You should avoid this terminology because any partial cervical spinal cord lesion can cause a wobbly gait. It is our belief that these acquired vertebral malformations and malarticulations are secondary to osteochondrosis that is a common developmental bone disorder in rapidly growing large-breed dogs and horses. In dogs, it appears to be responsible for

two age-related forms of this vertebral disorder: a vertebral foramen stenosis in young dogs and a degenerative disorder in older dogs.*

Stenosis

Stenosis of one or more cervical vertebral foramina occurs most commonly in young large-breed dogs, especially Doberman pinschers, Great Danes, and basset hounds.[74,108] Clinical signs occur at a few months of age, usually before 1 year. The bone surrounding the vertebral foramen fails to resorb sufficiently to enlarge the foramen to accommodate the growing spinal cord. Stenosis occurs at either end of the foramen or on both sides of the vertebral articulation (Figs. 10-37 through 10-41). It usually affects multiple cervical vertebrae caudal to C2. The cervical vertebral lesion as well as the

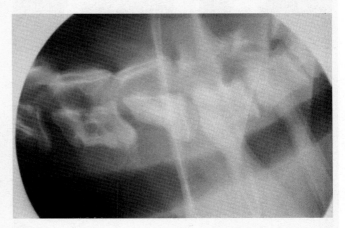

FIGURE 10-37 Cervical radiograph of a malformed C7 vertebra with a narrow cranial orifice to the vertebral foramen in a 6-month-old Great Dane.

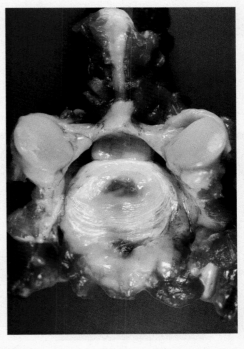

FIGURE 10-38 Cranial surface of the C7 vertebra seen in Fig. 10-37 after disarticulation to show the compressed spinal cord in the narrow cranial orifice to the vertebral foramen.

*References 15, 22, 24, 60, 73, 74, 77, 96, 107, 108.

(Continued)

CASE EXAMPLE 10-12—cont'd

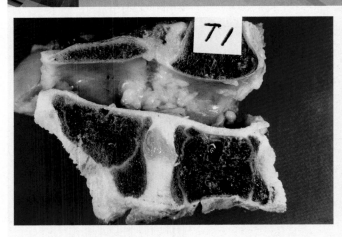

FIGURE 10-39 Longitudinal section of the C7 vertebra seen in Figs. 10-37 and 10-38.

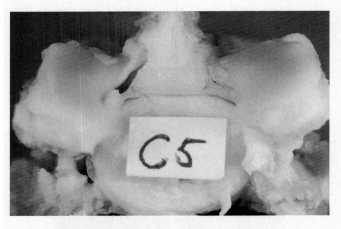

FIGURE 10-40 Cranial surface of the disarticulated C5 vertebra in a 5-month-old Doberman pinscher. Note the narrow cranial orifice to the vertebral foramen, the compressed spinal cord, and the thickened yellow ligament resting on the dorsal surface of the spinal cord.

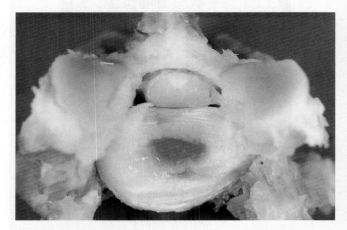

FIGURE 10-41 Cranial surface of the C4 vertebra from the same dog as in Fig. 10-40. Note the normal space around the spinal cord as compared with that in Fig. 10-40. The discoloration of the dorsal funiculi represents the wallerian degeneration of these cranial projecting pathways, which were disrupted by the compression at the level of the C5 spinal cord segment.

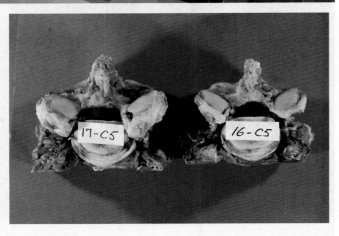

FIGURE 10-42 Cranial surface of the disarticulated fifth cervical vertebrae from two littermate Great Dane puppies. Number 17, on the left, came from a puppy that was allowed to eat ad lib, whereas Number 16, on the right, came from a puppy that was fed 25% less than Number 17. Note the failure of bone resorption around the cranial orifice of the vertebra in the puppy fed ad lib.

typical synovial joint lesions of osteochondrosis have been produced experimentally in Great Dane puppies by allowing unrestricted feeding on a diet that gives them a high energy level and a high level of calcium (Fig. 10-42).[43] If the clinical signs are recognized early, some improvement may occur if the patient's diet is restricted in its energy-giving and calcium levels and the activity of the patient is restricted too. Surgery is not as good an option when there are multiple sites of compression.

Degenerative Joint Disease

DJD occurs in the caudal cervical vertebrae (C5-C6, C6-C7) of middle-aged to older large-breed dogs, especially Doberman pinschers.[22,60,82,83,96] We believe this is the result of chronic malarticulation at these joints that represents the effects of osteochondrosis when these patients were young dogs. The major source of compression in most dogs is the proliferation and protrusion of the annulus fibrosis (Figs. 10-43 through 10-45). Other sources

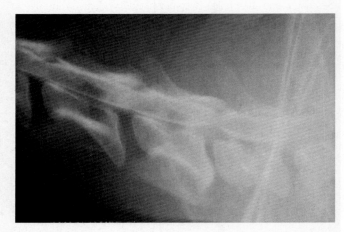

FIGURE 10-43 Cervical myelogram of an 8-year-old Doberman pinscher with clinical signs similar to those of Hilde in Case Example 10-18, Video 10-39. Note the narrow intervertebral disk space between the C6 and C7 vertebrae and the elevation of the ventral contrast line due to the protrusion of the intervertebral disk.

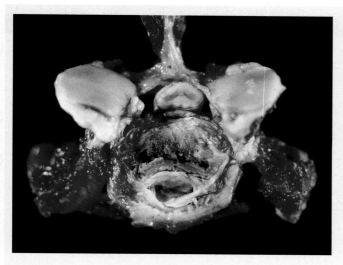

FIGURE 10-44 Cranial surface of the disarticulated C7 vertebra. Note the severe degeneration of the intervertebral disk and the dorsal proliferation of the annulus fibrosis, compressing the spinal cord. The discoloration of the gray matter represents the chronic compression that has caused the loss of the neuronal cell bodies and their replacement by astrocytes. This gray matter lesion is responsible for the atrophy of the lateral scapular muscles that is common in these dogs.

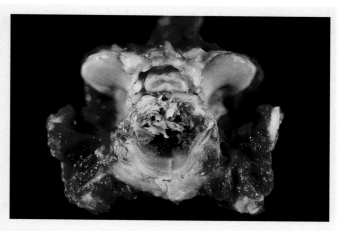

FIGURE 10-45 Caudal surface of the C6 vertebra in the dog in Figs. 10-43 and 10-44, showing the same changes as described in Fig. 10-44.

include proliferation of the articular processes and their joint capsules, the yellow ligament, and the dorsal longitudinal ligament. Rarely, a synovial cyst may be associated with the joint capsule proliferation. (See Case Examples 10-13 and 10-18, cervical spinal cord disease for examples of this disorder.) Many names have been given for this lesion but the most common is caudal cervical spondylomyelopathy. In horses this DJD primarily affects the articular processes. Occasionally, DJD primarily affects the articular processes of the caudocervical vertebrae of young adult large, breed dogs causing a dorsolateral compression of the spinal cord.

C2-C3 MENINGEAL FIBROSIS

Meningeal fibrosis is a lesion that is seen in young large-breed dogs, especially the rottweiler, Bernese mountain dog, and Labrador retriever, and is poorly understood.[8] This fibrosis causes thickening of the dura

and presumably of the arachnoid and its trabeculations because there is commonly an associated subarachnoid space diverticulum on the dorsal aspect of the spinal cord at this level. The spinal cord lesion is a compressive myelopathy that is thought to be secondary to the meningeal fibrosis. Surgery is a challenge because of the thickness of the articular processes at this level, and the chronicity of the spinal cord lesion commonly interferes with recovery. Respiratory distress and failure are possible after decompression and should be discussed with the owner prior to surgery.

The clinical signs exhibited by Mary, the Doberman pinscher in Case Example 10-3, are too severe to be caused by syringohydromyelia or discospondylitis and too focal to be infectious myelitis. Focal granulomatous meningomyelitis is unlikely. This presumably autoimmune disorder is described in a later chapter. Mary's age of 10 years would make a C2-C3 meningeal fibrosis unlikely. Imaging studies are needed to differentiate among neoplasm, intervertebral disk extrusion-protrusion, and vertebral malformation-malarticulation. Myelography revealed an extensive intramedullary mass lesion in the C2 and C3 spinal cord segments. Mary was euthanized, and at necropsy this mass was diagnosed as a malignant glioma.

Tetraparesis, Hemiparesis, Ataxia

CASE EXAMPLE 10-13

Signalment: 15-month-old male Bernese mountain dog, Gus
Chief Complaint: Abnormal stumbling gait
History: For almost 1 year his gait has seemed progressively more abnormal. A veterinarian had diagnosed a cerebellar disorder and thought it might be due to a cerebellar cortical abiotrophy.
Examination: Video 10-27 shows the slight delay in protraction and the longer strides in all four limbs, but they are easier to see in the thoracic limbs. The thoracic limbs, appear to overreach or float at the end of protraction before they are placed on the ground. Note the extension in these limbs when they overreach. Tone was increased in all four limbs

and the spinal reflexes were normal to increased. Note, at the end of the video, that the significant postural reaction deficits can be determined by hemiwalking the dog, which is easier to do in such a large dog.
Anatomic Diagnosis: A focal or diffuse lesion between the C1 and C5 spinal cord segments

This gait is characteristic of a dysfunction of the UMN and GP systems in the cervical spinal cord and is often mistaken for a cerebellar hypermetria. In the latter the protraction is more sudden, causing an abrupt movement and the limb exhibits a more flexed posture. **Video 10-28** shows a comparison with a 3-month-old Labrador retriever

(Continued)

CASE EXAMPLE 10-13—cont'd

that has a cerebellar cortical abiotrophy. Note the abrupt, excessive "bursty" limb movements in this puppy.

Differential Diagnosis: For a focal progressive disorder: malformation-malarticulation, C2-C3 meningeal fibrosis, discospondylitis, intervertebral disk extrusion-protrusion, neoplasm, syringohydromyelia, myelitis

The age and progressive history are most compatible with a malformation-malarticulation or a C2-C3 meningeal fibrosis. These two disorders are described in Case Example 10-12. It would be unlikely for a discospondylitis to be so slowly progressive and to not cause some obvious discomfort. A primary degeneration of the nucleus pulposus with extrusion or protrusion would be very unusual at this age in this breed. Unlike the possible findings in the thoracolumbar spinal cord, we are not aware of any neoplasm that is common at this age at this site. Be aware that both intramedullary and extramedullary neoplasms do occur in young animals but they are not common. We have not observed this degree of cervical spinal cord dysfunction with a cervical syringohydromyelia. The long course with focal clinical signs would be unusual for an inflammatory disease. There is no inherited myelopathy reported for this breed.

Radiographs and a myelogram diagnosed stenosis of the vertebral foramina at the C5-C6 articulation. The owners elected euthanasia and a compressive myelopathy was diagnosed at this level.

The following videos show examples of young dogs with cervical vertebral foraminal stenosis.

Video 10-29 shows a 6-month-old spayed female Doberman pinscher that exhibits the overreaching action of the thoracic limbs, especially as she slowly turns. Radiographs showed a mild foraminal stenosis of the C3 to C6 vertebrae. She improved with restriction of her diet and her activity.

Video 10-30 shows a 7-month-old Great Dane with nonambulatory spastic tetraparesis and ataxia caused by foraminal stenosis at the C5-C6 articulation.

Video 10-31 shows Kodiak, a 2-year-old castrated male German shepherd with a history of 5 months of a slowly progressive gait disorder. You should make the anatomic diagnosis of a focal or diffuse lesion between the C1 and C5 spinal cord segments. Kodiak also shows decreased range of motion when either thoracic limb is flexed, and both elbows are enlarged due to chronic degenerative joint disease. He has mild atrophy of the lateral scapular muscles, which could result from disuse associated with his elbow disease or from denervation if his cervical spinal cord disease is more caudal in the white matter and includes the ventral gray columns or the spinal nerves of either the C6 or C7 spinal cord segments. The differential diagnosis for this anatomic diagnosis in Kodiak is the same as is described for Gus in this case example. Radiographs (see the video) show DJD of the synovial joints at the C5-C6 and C6-C7 articulations. The dorsoventral view shows the proliferation of the articular processes medially into the vertebral canal, and the myelogram confirms the spinal cord compression at both of these articulations.

CASE EXAMPLE 10-14

Signalment: A 5-month-old male Bernese mountain dog, Max

Chief Complaint: Abnormal stumbling gait

History: For the past month Max had exhibited a progressive gait abnormality in all four limbs.

Examination: Video 10-32 shows the similarity in clinical signs between Gus in Case Example 10-13 and Max in this case example.

Anatomic Diagnosis: Focal or diffuse lesion between the C1 and C5 spinal cord segments

Differential Diagnosis: See the list of disorders for Gus in Case Example 10-13 and the discussion presented there.

A myelogram diagnosed a C2-C3 meningeal fibrosis with a subarachnoid diverticulum. This study is shown on the video. The first myelogram was made after contrast was introduced into the subarachnoid space between the L5 and L6 vertebrae, and the second myelogram was made after an injection of contrast at the cerebellomedullary cistern. MR imaging is especially useful in making this diagnosis. Max was euthanized, and this diagnosis was confirmed at necropsy.

The following videos show three additional dogs with this C2-C3 meningeal fibrosis causing compressive cervical myelopathy.

Video 10-33 shows Reba, a 2-year-old female rottweiler with a 10-month history of a slowly progressive gait disorder. This dog exhibits the most remarkable thoracic limb overreaching that we have observed with a cervical spinal cord lesion. In contrast to the gait exhibited by dogs with diffuse cerebellar disease, note the marked extension of these limbs as they are protracted. A laminectomy

was performed to remove the area of meningeal fibrosis, and Reba improved over the following weeks.

Video 10-34 shows Yagar, a 10-month-old castrated male rottweiler with a 2-month history of a progressive gait disorder that was diagnosed as a cerebellar disorder, and a cerebellar cortical abiotrophy was suspected. The owner requested a second opinion because no evidence of cerebellar abiotrophy had been published about this breed. Based on your study of this video you should make the anatomic diagnosis of a C1 to C5 focal or diffuse lesion. Subsequent radiographs with a myelogram diagnosed a C2-C3 meningeal fibrosis.

Video 10-35 shows Clementine, a 14-month-old spayed female Labrador retriever with a slowly progressive gait abnormality for 5 to 6 months, with no evidence of any discomfort and no response to corticosteroid therapy. Note that the deficit in the thoracic limbs is worse than that in the pelvic limbs. Two examinations are shown in this video, as well as MR images of the lesion taken between the two examinations. Surgical decompression was performed by removing the caudal aspect of the spinous process of C2 and the laminae of the caudal aspect of C2 and the cranial aspect of C3. The meninges and associated diverticulum were removed from the spinal cord at this surgical site. After several weeks, Clementine recovered from the surgery and improved. Clementine has been followed clinically for a number of years and has shown no adverse effects resulting from the laminectomy and removal of the dura-arachnoid.

CASE EXAMPLE 10-15

Signalment: 13-month-old castrated male mixed-breed dog, Sammy
Chief Complaint: Abnormal stumbling gait
History: The owner thought that Sammy's gait abnormality had started about 6 months before this examination and had definitely become worse during that period.
Examination: Video 10-36: Study this video and make your anatomic diagnosis.
Anatomic Diagnosis: A focal or diffuse lesion between the C1 and C5 spinal cord segments
Differential Diagnosis: See the list of disorders for Gus in Case Example 10-13 and the discussion that followed.

The video shows the radiographs that revealed a mineralized mass between the dorsal aspect of C2 and C3. The myelogram shows the severity of the spinal cord compression at that site. The mass was removed surgically and diagnosed as osteochondralcalcinosis (calcinosis circumscripta, tumoral calcinosis).[1] The dorsal aspect of the atlantooccipital and atlantoaxial sites are the most common sites of this lesion, but it has been reported at other levels of the vertebral column. After the surgery, Sammy was tetraplegic for several days but made nearly full recovery over the ensuing weeks.

CASE EXAMPLE 10-16

Signalment: 5-month-old castrated male rottweiler, Hans
Chief Complaint: Abnormal gait and difficult breathing
History: When Hans was about 8 weeks old, the owner recognized that his pelvic limb gait seemed abnormal. When he was 12 weeks old, he began to exhibit some difficulty breathing, especially when exercised or excited. By then, his pelvic limb gait was worse, and at 4 months of age, he occasionally stumbled with his thoracic limbs. The owner also stated that Hans occasionally "lost his meal," and the description seemed to fit regurgitation, not vomiting.
Examination: Video 10-37 shows the mild clinical signs in the thoracic limbs—the prolonged stride and mild overreaching when the limb is advanced. The thoracic limb hopping responses are also slower than normal. Note the inspiratory dyspnea that Hans shows during this examination with his gasping for air and the marked abdominal movement associated with contraction of the diaphragm. Also note the sunken appearance of the eyes and the protruded third eyelids bilaterally.
Anatomic Diagnosis: A focal or diffuse lesion between the C1 and C5 spinal cord segments and the recurrent laryngeal and vagal nerves
Differential Diagnosis: For the spinal cord lesion, the differential diagnosis is the same as the three case examples that were listed and briefly discussed for Gus in Case Example 10-13. In addition to those, an inherited myelopathy has been reported in the rottweiler breed; it is associated with a neuropathy that is most pronounced in the recurrent laryngeal nerves and some of these dogs have a megaesophagus or microphthalmia bilaterally. Hans exhibits all of these features.

INHERITED ENCEPHALOMYELOPATHY-POLYNEUROPATHY

Inherited encephalomyelopathy-polyneuropathy is a preferred term for a disorder first published in 1997 to describe neuronal vacuolation and spinocerebellar degeneration in young rottweiler dogs and defined as an autosomal recessive genetic disorder.[26,54,97] The name these authors gave to this degenerative disorder is incomplete and refers only to the most pronounced lesions in the spinal cord. The spinal cord lesion consists of a bilateral symmetric axonopathy with secondary demyelination and astrogliosis, which is most pronounced in the lateral and ventral funiculi. This lesion is not limited to the spinocerebellar tracts. Many tracts are affected, including the UMN tracts, which is why the gait disorder is typical for a dysfunction of the GP and UMN systems. The thoracolumbar segments are most affected, which possibly suggests where the degenerative lesion first

develops and explains why the clinical signs are first observed in the pelvic limbs. Vacuolation of neuronal cell bodies is scattered through the spinal cord and brain with no other evidence of any microscopic abnormality of these neurons. The brains of these dogs test negative for prion protein. A neuropathy is prominent in the recurrent laryngeal nerves and scattered in other long nerves. There is significant denervation atrophy of all the intrinsic laryngeal muscles except for the cricothyroideus (Figs. 10-46 and 10-47). The clinical signs begin at about 6 to 8 weeks of age and can start either with inspiratory dyspnea or paraparesis and pelvic limb ataxia. Some of the dogs that first exhibited the signs of laryngeal paralysis had had laryngeal tie-back surgery to improve their breathing before the clinical signs were first observed in the pelvic limbs. It is paramount that the veterinary surgeon be aware of this disorder and counsel the owner appropriately before surgery. All dogs progress in a few weeks to tetraparesis and ataxia in all four limbs. Some dogs develop megaesophagus and regurgitate, and some dogs have bilateral microphthalmia. These small eyes appear to be sunken into the orbits, and therefore the third eyelids become prominent. There is no Horner syndrome in these dogs. A few dogs have been reported to exhibit clinical signs of dysfunction of the cerebellum or the vestibular system, but this has not been our experience.

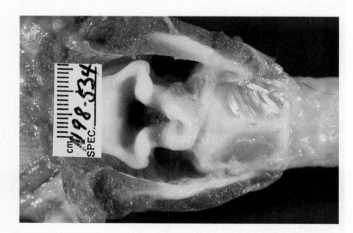

FIGURE 10-46 Dorsal surface of the larynx from a 5-month-old rottweiler with inspiratory dyspnea due to inherited encephalomyelopathy-polyneuropathy. Note the severe denervation atrophy of both dorsal cricoarytenoideus dorsalis muscles.

(Continued)

CASE EXAMPLE 10-16—cont'd

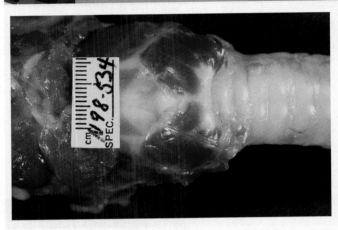

FIGURE 10-47 Ventral surface of the larynx of the same dog as in Fig. 10-46, showing the normal cricothyroideus muscles.

OTHER INHERITED DISORDERS IN THE ROTTWEILER BREED

In addition to this inherited disorder, there are at least six other presumably inherited degenerative disorders of the nervous system that have been reported in the rottweiler breed. In our experience, the disorder that we have described in Hans, inherited encephalomyelopathy-

polyneuropathy, is by far the most common one that we currently see in this breed. The following is a brief description of the others.

1. Neuroaxonal dystrophy is an axonopathy that causes the clinical signs of progressive cerebellar disorder and has an onset between 1 and 2 years of age.[16,20]
2. Leukoencephalomyelopathy is a primary demyelination that causes progressive cervical spinal cord signs that start between 1.5 and 3.5 years of age.[31,87,106]
3. Motor neuron disease causes progressive diffuse LMN signs starting at about 4 weeks of age but does not cause any dyspnea.[84,85]
4. Polyneuropathy (axonopathy) causes progressive diffuse LMN signs, including inspiratory dyspnea starting at about 2 months of age. Cataracts may also be observed. All the lesions are limited to the peripheral nerves in these dogs.[59]
5. A distal neuropathy has been reported in mature rottweilers, with clinical signs of diffuse LMN disease starting between 1 and 4 years of age. Dyspnea has not been reported in these dogs.[10]
6. A Duchenne type of muscular dystrophy, a dystrophinopathy, has been reported in male rottweilers. This is a progressive, diffuse myopathy that starts at about 8 weeks of age but does not cause any dyspnea.

We have recently studied two littermate boxers from western Canada that had the same clinical and pathologic disorder as the rottweiler in Case Example 10-16.

CASE EXAMPLE 10-17

Signalment: A 3.5-year-old spayed female miniature schnauzer, Tasha
Chief Complaint: Abnormal use of the right pelvic limb
History: The owner noticed that over a few hours, Tasha became lame in the right pelvic limb. The video was made 4 days later, and the owner thought that Tasha had already exhibited some improvement.
 Examination: Video 10-38 shows the examination.
Anatomic Diagnosis: A focal or diffuse lesion on the right side between the C1 and C5 spinal cord segments.

You should have recognized a spastic hemiparesis and ataxia of the right limbs and noticed the mild overreaching of the right thoracic limb and the slow hopping responses in that limb. The veterinarian who

saw Tasha on the day when her clinical signs first began recognized that both right limbs were abnormal.
Differential Diagnosis: FCEM, intervertebral disk extrusion-protrusion

External injury was excluded because of the history. An intervertebral disk extrusion-protrusion would be unusual in this breed at this age, and the lack of any discomfort was more suggestive of FCEM. This is a breed that is at risk for FCEM. The asymmetric clinical signs as well as the spontaneous improvement are most compatible with FCEM. Based on this evaluation, no ancillary procedures were performed, and Tasha completely recovered over the following two weeks.

Tetraparesis-Ataxia: LMN Thoracic Limbs, UMN Pelvic Limbs—"Two-Engine"

CASE EXAMPLE 10-18

Signalment: A 9-year-old spayed female Doberman pinscher, Hilde
Chief Complaint: Abnormal stumbling gait
History: The gait abnormality had been progressing for about 6 weeks.
 Examination: Video 10-39 shows the difference in length of stride between the pelvic and the thoracic limbs. This is often referred to as

a "two-engine" gait. In the hopping responses, I (EG) am supporting most of the dog's weight in the initial thoracic limb hopping, which shows a better response than when I (EG) have Hilde support all of her weight. Note the atrophy of the lateral scapular muscles. Note the tendency of Hilde to hold her neck slightly flexed and her reluctance to move it freely.

Anatomic Diagnosis: The C6 or C7 spinal cord segments

The pelvic limb clinical signs are clearly due to a dysfunction of the UMN and GP systems. The thoracic limb clinical signs are a paradox because the short-strided gait and the lateral scapular atrophy are LMN signs, and the marked hypertonia is a UMN clinical sign. The poor hopping responses when Hilde had to support all of her weight suggest a LMN component of the deficit. This mixture of clinical signs indicates a caudocervical spinal cord lesion with involvement of both the gray and the white matter. It is typical for a focal lesion at either the C5-C6 or C6-C7 articulation. Remember that the lateral scapular muscles are innervated by the suprascapular nerve that is formed by the ventral branches of the C6 and C7 spinal nerves. The denervation atrophy relates to the loss of GSE LMNs in either the C6 or C7 spinal cord segments (see Fig. 10-44).

Differential Diagnosis: The most common cause of this anatomic diagnosis, with its unique combination of UMN-GP and LMN clinical signs, is the DJD form of cervical vertebral malformation-malarticulation. A proliferation and protrusion of the annulus fibrosis is usually the major structure involved in the spinal cord compression (see Figs. 10-43 through 10-45). This is often associated with collapse of the intervertebral disk space and the development of enthesophytes in the adjacent vertebral bodies. A Doberman pinscher that is more than 5 years of age is at risk for this disorder. Be aware that a lesion in the cranial thoracic vertebrae that causes discomfort, such as a neoplasm, may also cause a short-strided thoracic limb gait, but the hopping responses will be normal.[64] Discospondylitis or a neoplasm of the vertebrae are such considerations. The flexed neck posture and limited movement are commonly seen in this DJD disorder. Significant resistance is commonly shown by the patient to attempts to manipulate the neck, but these dogs rarely exhibit the extreme discomfort often seen in dogs with acute intervertebral disk extrusion. Imaging studies are necessary to further define the clinical diagnosis. See the video for the radiographs and myelogram that were performed on Hilde, the dog in this case example; they show the changes described earlier at the C6-C7 articulation and the associated extradural compression of the spinal cord.

Videos 10-40A and B shows Tigger, a 12-year-old male Ibizan hound at its kennel in Texas. Tigger had a lesion similar to that of Hilde, and it caused a slowly progressive gait disorder. Video 10A was made a few weeks after the onset of clinical signs, and Video 10B was made about 3 months later, just prior to euthanasia. Tigger's tissues were sent to us for study because the owner was a breeder of Ibizan hounds and wanted to make sure that his dog did not have the presumably inherited axonopathy that we have recognized in this breed. This axonopathy is described in Chapter 13; it causes clinical signs within the first few weeks of life. These clinical signs have a cerebellar quality. See Video 13-37 to appreciate the difference from Tigger.

Video 10-41 shows Hoosier, an 8-year-old castrated male Dalmatian with a history of 2 months of a progressive gait abnormality along with some discomfort when he gets up and down. Note that Hoosier exhibits a two-engine type of gait similar to that seen in Hilde. However, his hopping responses in the thoracic limbs are normal. The anatomic diagnosis was cranial thoracic spinal cord segments. The radiographs and myelogram (see video) show a neoplasm within the body of the second thoracic vertebra that is compressing the spinal cord. We attributed the short-strided thoracic limb gait to the discomfort caused by this bone neoplasm. At necropsy, it was diagnosed as a chondrosarcoma.

CASE EXAMPLE 10-19

Signalment: A 16-year-old spayed female domestic shorthair, Izzy
Chief Complaint: Abnormal gait
History: Izzy had exhibited a progressive gait abnormality for 6 to 8 weeks.
Examination: Video 10-42 shows the two-engine type of gait. Hopping responses were slow in all four limbs, and muscle tone and spinal nerve reflexes were normal. There was moderate atrophy of the muscles in both thoracic limbs.
Anatomic Diagnosis: C6 to T2 spinal cord segments

The short strides in the thoracic limbs are a clinical sign of dysfunction of their LMN innervation.
Differential Diagnosis: Neoplasia, intervertebral disk extrusion-protrusion, discospondylitis, myelitis

Neoplasia is the most presumptive clinical diagnosis for this anatomic site at this age and with such a slow progression.[69] Lymphoma is the most common feline neoplasm that affects the spinal cord and it usually is an extradural mass lesion.[70] As a rule, it occurs in younger cats. At this age, a glioma is a strong consideration. An intervertebral disk extrusion-protrusion is uncommon but is a consideration at this age. Vertebral discospondylitis is rare in cats. Myelitis caused by the FIP virus or *T. gondii* is not likely to remain so focal for this period of time and is less common at this age.

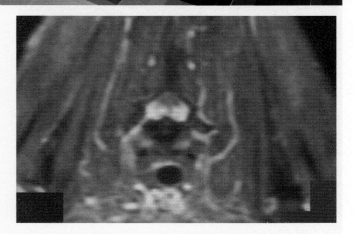

FIGURE 10-48 T1-weighted MR image with contrast at the level of the T1 spinal cord segment of the cat in this case example. Note the bilateral enhancement and enlargement of the ventral roots.

MR imaging showed a contrast-enhanced mass lesion bilaterally associated with the first thoracic spinal nerve roots, with compression of the spinal cord at that level (Fig. 10-48). An infiltrating form of

(Continued)

CASE EXAMPLE 10-19—cont'd

lymphoma was suspected. Izzy was euthanized, and at necropsy the bilateral mass lesions were malignant nerve sheath neoplasms of the first thoracic spinal nerve roots (Figs. 10-49 through 10-51). This is a rare neoplasm in cats to affect the peripheral nerves at the level of the spinal cord. Note the close correlation between the gross lesion and the MR images. Compare this with the neoplasms in Figures 10-52 and 10-53, which show a lymphoma infiltrating cranial thoracic spinal nerve roots and nerves bilaterally.

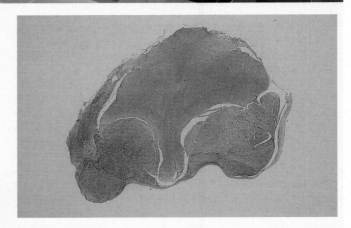

FIGURE 10-51 Microscopic section of the T1 spinal cord segment seen in Fig. 10-50, showing bilateral neoplasms primarily in the ventral roots. Note how well this correlates with the MR image in Fig. 10-48. This neoplasm was a nerve sheath neoplasm, which is rare in cats, especially in spinal nerve roots.

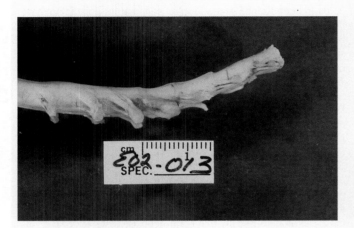

FIGURE 10-49 The spinal cord of the cat in this case example, from the sixth cervical to the fifth thoracic segments. Note the enlargement of the T1 spinal nerve roots.

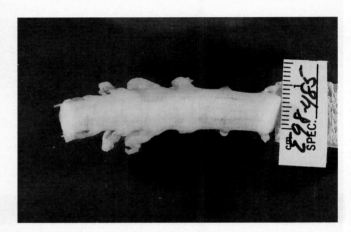

FIGURE 10-52 Dorsal surface of the spinal cord, from the C5 to the T2 spinal cord segments. This is from a 1-year-old domestic shorthair with progressive clinical signs similar to those of Izzy, the cat in Video 10-42. Note the enlargement of the C8 spinal nerve roots.

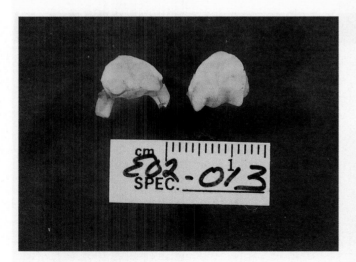

FIGURE 10-50 Transverse section of the C8 and T1 spinal cord segments of the cat in Fig. 10-49. The round bulges of the nerve roots at C8 are the normal spinal ganglia. A mass lesion obliterates the ventral roots on both sides of the T1 spinal cord segment, and these enlargements compress the spinal cord.

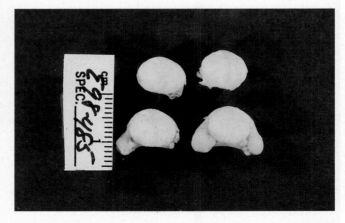

FIGURE 10-53 Transverse section of the C8 spinal cord segment in Fig. 10-52. The enlargement of the nerve roots is due to an infiltrating lymphoma. This is a more common lesion in the cat than the nerve sheath neoplasm.

Hemiplegia, Hemiparesis, Ataxia

CASE EXAMPLE 10-20

Signalment: A 3-year-old spayed female border collie, Welch

Chief Complaint: Unable to stand and walk

History: Welch was confined to her home and was normal when the owners left for work but was found unable to stand when they returned 8 hours later.

Examination: **Video 10-43** shows the right-side hemiplegia and the difference in the quality of the paralysis between the spastic right pelvic limb and the flaccid right thoracic limb. Nociception was normal in the right pelvic limb and mildly hypalgesic in the right thoracic limb. She had a sympathetic paresis (Horner syndrome) that was visible in the right orbital structures.

Anatomic Diagnosis: The right side of the cervical intumescence (C6 to T2 spinal cord segments)

The gray matter lesion accounts for the marked LMN clinical signs and the mild clinical signs of GSA dysfunction in the right thoracic limb. The white matter lesion accounts for the severe UMN clinical signs in the right pelvic limb. When the patient cannot protract the limb, you cannot evaluate the GP spinal cord pathways. The Horner syndrome could be due to the gray matter lesion extending into the first three thoracic spinal cord segments and interfering with the right preganglionic GVE sympathetic neurons, or it may be the result of the right-side lateral funicular lesion in the caudal cervical spinal cord segments interfering with the UMN pathway for the sympathetic system.

Differential Diagnosis: FCEM, intervertebral disk extrusion-protrusion, neoplasm

External injury was excluded because these signs developed while Welch was confined to her home. FCEM is the most presumptive clinical diagnosis, based on the sudden onset of the paralysis and no indication of any progression of clinical signs in the limbs on the left side over the 2 days before this examination. A unilateral intervertebral disk extrusion would be less likely at this age in this breed, and the sudden onset of such severe focal clinical signs would be unusual for a neoplasm.

Cervical vertebral radiographs were normal but a myelogram showed a mild intramedullary swelling of the caudocervical spinal cord segments that was thought to represent edema or hemorrhage associated with the ischemic myelopathy. No change was observed over the next 10 days, and Welch was euthanized. At necropsy, the right side of the cervical intumescence felt soft and had a slight discoloration. Transverse sections of the preserved spinal cord showed hemorrhages and softening of the gray and white matter on the right side of the C6, C7, and C8 spinal cord segments (Fig. 10-54). On microscopic examination this gross lesion represented a severe hemorrhagic and ischemic necrosis of most all of the gray matter and adjacent white matter of the lateral funiculus, with some involvement of the dorsal and ventral funiculi, all on the right side of these spinal cord segments (Figs. 10-55 through 10-58). Numerous arteries and veins contained fibrocartilaginous emboli. There were no recognizable lesions in the first three thoracic spinal cord segments, suggesting that the Horner syndrome was caused by the lateral funicular lesion disrupting the UMN pathway of the sympathetic system.

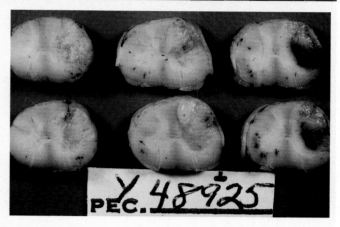

FIGURE 10-54 Transverse sections of the C6 to C8 spinal cord segments of the dog in this case example, showing the hemorrhage and softening due to necrosis on the right side.

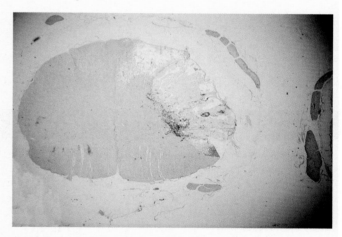

FIGURE 10-55 Microscopic section of the C8 spinal cord segment of the dog in Fig. 10-54. Note the sharp borders of the ischemic infarct. Compare this with Fig. 10-54.

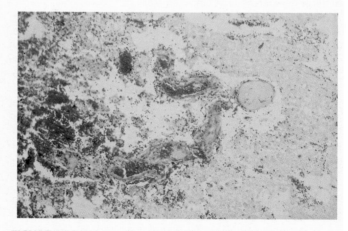

FIGURE 10-56 Microscopic section of the deep portion of the right lateral funiculus of the C8 spinal cord segment seen in Fig. 10-55, showing both hemorrhagic and ischemic necrosis. Note the round structure on the right of center, and see Fig. 10-57.

(Continued)

CASE EXAMPLE 10-20—cont'd

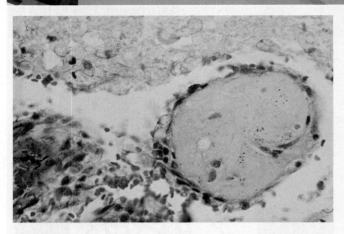

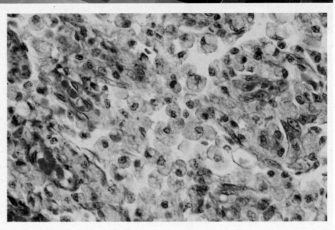

FIGURE 10-57 Microscopic section of the round structure seen in Fig. 10-56. This is a fibrocartilage embolus in an enlarged blood vessel.

FIGURE 10-58 Another area of the same lesion shown in Fig. 10-56, showing a plethora of macrophages phagocytizing the necrotic parenchyma. There is no recognizable parenchyma here.

CASE EXAMPLE 10-21

Signalment: A 5-year-old female Labrador retriever, Kassie

Chief Complaint: Difficulty walking

History: Five days before this examination, Kassie suddenly lost the ability to walk normally with the left pelvic limb. That was followed 2 hours later by left thoracic limb dysfunction, and she was recumbent when examined a few hours later by a local veterinarian. This veterinarian also recognized that the left pupil was smaller than the right pupil. Kassie had regained the ability to stand and walk by the time she was referred to Cornell University.

Examination: Video 10-44 shows the two-engine type of gait but only in the left limbs. The left thoracic limb LMN clinical signs are more pronounced than they were in Hilde in Case Example 10-18. Note the hypertonia in the left pelvic limb and the hypotonia in the left thoracic limb. The pupils were symmetric and normal in size and response to light. No discomfort was elicited on manipulation of the neck.

Anatomic Diagnosis: C6 to T2 spinal cord segments on the left side

The left pupillary miosis observed by the local veterinarian was either a UMN partial sympathetic paresis or involvement of the GVE LMN in the first thoracic spinal cord segment. The hemiparesis here has a LMN quality in the thoracic limb and a UMN quality in the pelvic limb.

Differential Diagnosis: FCEM, intervertebral disk extrusion, neoplasm

External injury was excluded because these clinical signs were all observed by the owner of Kassie in an enclosed environment.

FCEM is the most presumptive clinical diagnosis in Kassie, based on the sudden onset, the progression over only a few hours, and the spontaneous improvement over the 5 days before this examination.

Kassie's age warrants consideration of a unilateral intervertebral disk extrusion. No imaging was done on Kassie, and she continued to improve without therapy.

Video 10-45 shows Pepper, a 3-year-old castrated male miniature poodle who exhibited a sudden onset of difficulty using the left pelvic limb. That was followed in a few hours by difficulty in the left thoracic limb. On the initial examination there was no voluntary movement in the left pelvic limb. The video was made 3 days after the onset of the abnormality. Note the short strides in the left thoracic limb and the fair hopping when her weight was supported. Pepper is a smaller version of Kassie and has the same anatomic and differential diagnoses, but the lesion involves less of the gray matter than in Kassie because there is no loss of muscle tone. I (EG) made another interesting observation in Pepper when I carefully evaluated nociception in the limbs and trunk on both sides and found it to be slightly but consistently decreased on the right side. This right-side hypalgesia can be explained by the crossing of the nociceptive pathway at its origin in the spinal cord. The interruption of this pathway at the level of C6 on the left caused the right-side hypalgesia caudal to this level. MR imaging showed an intramedullary hyperintensity on the T2-weighted images that was limited to the left side of the C6 and C7 spinal cord segments, suggesting edema associated with FCEM (Figs. 10-59 and 10-60). MR imaging is especially useful in diagnosing FCEM because it is noninvasive compared to myelography. Pepper continued to improve spontaneously and made a full recovery.

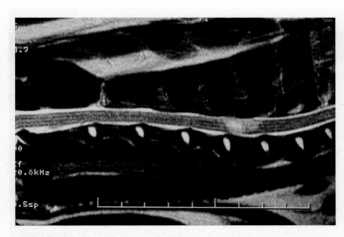

FIGURE 10-59 Sagittal T2-weighted MR image of the neck of the dog in Video 10-45. The intramedullary hyperintensity over the body of the C6 vertebra is assumed to be edema associated with ischemic myelopathy due to fibrocartilaginous emboli.

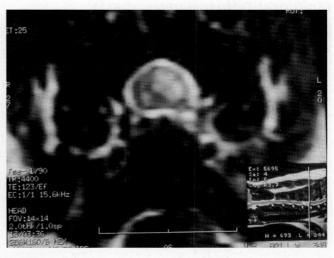

FIGURE 10-60 Axial T2-weighted MR image of the neck of the dog in Video 10-45, showing the presumptive edema predominantly on the left side of the C7 spinal cord segment (right side of image) primarily in the region supplied by the dorsolateral superficial plexus.

Tetraparesis-Ataxia: Thoracic Limbs

CASE EXAMPLE 10-22

Signalment: A 6.5-year-old spayed female mixed-breed, Olive
Chief Complaint: Unable to walk
History: About 2 weeks before this examination Olive began to stumble on her right thoracic limb. Over the next week it became worse, and the left thoracic limb also became affected. At presentation she could not use either thoracic limb.
Examination: Video 10-46 shows the disparity in her ability to use the thoracic versus the pelvic limbs. Note the thoracic limb hypertonia and intact spinal reflexes. Nociception was considered to be normal, as was the cutaneous trunci reflex.
Anatomic Diagnosis: A focal or diffuse lesion between the C1 and C5 spinal cord segments that affects primarily the central region of the spinal cord at this level.

This specific location explains the profound disparity between the more severely affected thoracic limbs and the mildly affected pelvic limbs.
Differential Diagnosis: Intervertebral disk extrusion-protrusion, neoplasm, myelitis

An intervertebral disk extrusion-protrusion that occurs on the midline through the dorsal longitudinal ligament and compresses the spinal cord on its ventral midline causes the spinal cord to "tent" over the compressing mass, and the central portions of the spinal cord will be more seriously affected than the peripheral components that are more commonly compressed. Central lesions of the cervical spinal cord cranial to the C6 segment appear to affect predominantly the UMN tracts that are projecting to the ventral gray columns of the cervical intumescence. An extramedullary neoplasm at the same ventral midline site could cause the same compression. An intramedullary neoplasm that developed in the center of the spinal cord and expanded peripherally is another consideration. A myelitis that is localized to the central portion of the spinal cord white

matter could also cause this anatomic diagnosis (canine distemper viral myelitis, protozoal myelitis, granulomatous meningomyelitis). FCEM was excluded from consideration because of the 2 weeks of progressive clinical signs. Imaging studies and CSF evaluation are needed to differentiate between these disorders.

A myelogram and a CT with contrast in the CSF showed a diffuse intramedullary swelling of the spinal cord segments from C3 to C6. Olive was euthanized and a necropsy revealed this diffuse swelling to be a form of glioma called gliomatosis cerebri, which is a rare neoplasm to find in the spinal cord. It infiltrated the gray matter and adjacent white matter, sparing the peripheral portion of the white matter in all the funiculi (Fig. 10-61).

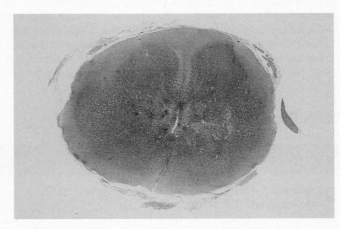

FIGURE 10-61 Microscopic section of the C3 spinal cord segment of Olive, the dog in Video 10-46, showing the diffuse glial neoplasm centrally located, with sparing of the peripheral tracts.

Multifocal-Diffuse Paresis, Ataxia

CASE EXAMPLE 10-23

Signalment: A 9.5-week-old female cairn terrier, Puppy
Chief Complaint: Stumbling in the pelvic limbs
History: Puppy was from a litter of three in which the other two dogs were males and were normal. When Puppy was 7 weeks old, she appeared to be stiff in the pelvic limbs when she walked. She often stood base-wide and occasionally stumbled with the pelvic limbs. Since then, the pelvic limb gait abnormality had slowly worsened.

 Examination: Video 10-47 shows Puppy's gait abnormality.

Anatomic Diagnosis: A focal or diffuse lesion between the C1 and C5 spinal cord segments or multifocal lesions that include one or more lesions between the T3 and L3 spinal cord segments as well as the C1 to C5 segments; plus there may be some involvement of the cerebellum.

The gait is compatible with a cervical spinal cord white matter lesion; this assessment is based on the overreaching of the thoracic limbs on protraction, with extended thoracic limbs, and on the clinical signs of spastic paraparesis and ataxia in the pelvic limbs. The thoracic limb hopping responses are slightly delayed for a dog of this size and appear too hypertonic, and too stiff. Watch the thoracic limbs carefully during the hemiwalking and note the delayed protraction and hypermetric response, with excessive elbow flexion that suggests a cerebellar disorder. Not shown on the video is an occasional brief head tremor and a slight balance loss. These cerebellar signs are very subtle and easily overlooked or considered insignificant. If the initial clinical signs affected only the pelvic limbs, as described by the owner, they may be explained by a diffuse white matter lesion that began in the T3 to L3 spinal cord segments, by the development of the first lesion of a multifocal disorder, or by the initial clinical signs of a focal cervical spinal cord disorder before they appear in the thoracic limbs.

Differential Diagnosis: The following disorders are considerations for a progressive multifocal or diffuse CNS disorder: infectious encephalomyelitis (canine distemper virus); protozoal agents (*T. gondii, N. caninum*); fungal agents (*Cryptococcus neoformans*); rickettsial agents; autoimmune granulomatous meningoencephalomyelitis; and inherited enzyme disorder causing a storage disease (globoid cell leukodystrophy).

Remember to consider in your differential diagnosis any disorder that may be inherited in the breed of your patient. Globoid cell leukodystrophy (Krabbe disease in children) is a disorder that is most common in the West Highland white terrier and the cairn terrier. It is inherited as an autosomal recessive gene and results in a deficiency of the lysosomal enzyme galactosylceramidase 1 (beta galactocerebrosidase). Most inherited enzyme disorders that affect lysosomal degradative enzymes within neurons result in the accumulation of substrate of the deficient enzyme in the neurons. The subsequent enlargement of these neuronal cell bodies is the basis for the term *storage disease*. In this leukodystrophy, the lack of galactosylceramidase results in the accumulation of psychosine (galactosylsphingosine), which is toxic to oligodendrocytes and Schwann cells and causes a primary demyelination. Neurons appear normal. The globoid cells are the macrophages that are filled with phagocytized myelin remnants (Fig. 10-62). Clinical signs first occur between 3 and 7 months of age and can begin as a T3 to L3 spinal cord disorder, as in Puppy, and progress to cervical spinal cord and cerebellar clinical signs; or the first clinical signs may reflect cerebellar dysfunction that then progresses to clinical signs of spinal cord involvement. Following the discovery of the gene mutation in children with Krabbe disease, the same gene mutation was found in these two breeds of dogs that have a similar disorder. A polymerase chain reaction test is now available for testing blood leucocytes for this gene mutation. It not only confirms the diagnosis in an affected patient but also determines carrier animals, which will help to prevent further propagation of the disease. This test was performed on Puppy's blood and it confirmed the diagnosis of globoid cell leukodystrophy. This disease will slowly progress over many months and ultimately result in recumbency, dementia, blindness, and death by 1 to 2 years of age. Puppy was euthanized, and a necropsy revealed the characteristic lesions of this inherited disorder.

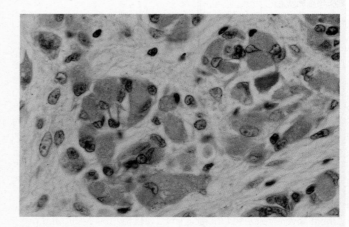

FIGURE 10-62 Microscopic section of the white matter lesion in a cairn terrier with globoid cell leukodystrophy. The dark cells clustered around blood vessels are the globoid cells. These are macrophages that contain phagocytized myelin debris.

Neck Discomfort

CASE EXAMPLE 10-24

Signalment: A 7.5-year-old spayed female Dalmatian, Squirt
Chief Complaint: Discomfort
History: Many weeks of episodes of discomfort, especially with any movement of her neck

 Examination: Video 10-48 shows the partially flexed posture of the neck, the neck rigidity, and the occasional flexion of the right thoracic limb while standing. The last aspect is referred to as a root signature. The gait is normal, as are the postural reactions and spinal reflexes.

Anatomic Diagnosis: Cervical spinal cord meninges and/or spinal nerve roots, spinal nerves

Differential Diagnosis: Cervical intervertebral disk extrusion-protrusion, cervical vertebral discospondylitis, cervical vertebral neoplasia, meningitis, intracranial neoplasia

Squirt's history and clinical signs are most typical of an intervertebral disk extrusion-protrusion. The components of the intervertebral disk are not innervated, but the perichondrium that covers the annulus fibrosis and the adjacent periosteum and meninges are innervated and are the source of discomfort when they are disrupted or inflamed. Discospondylitis can be the cause of extreme discomfort, as can neoplasms of the vertebrae. Meningitis is often overlooked because it is a less common cause of cervical discomfort in small animals. In small ruminants, pigs, and foals, meningitis is most commonly caused by a hematogenous bacterial infection. This is much less common in small animals. The most common cause of meningitis in young dogs is an autoimmune disorder. Occasionally, neck discomfort is related to an intracranial neoplasm that involves the meninges directly or by displacing the brain secondary to brain swelling with or without the development of a cervical spinal cord syrinx.

Cervical radiographs of Squirt showed a narrowed space for the intervertebral disk between the C5 and C6 vertebral bodies; refer to the video. A myelogram showed an interruption in the ventral contrast line at this articulation, supporting the diagnosis of an intervertebral disk extrusion.

CANINE MENINGEAL POLYARTERITIS

Canine meningeal polyarteritis, autoimmune meningitis, immune-mediated meningitis, steroid-responsive meningitis-arteritis, beagle pain syndrome, sterile meningitis of boxers, necrotizing meningeal arteritis, and canine juvenile polyarteritis syndrome are all names for the same noninfectious disorder, which is the most common cause of meningitis in young dogs (usually younger than 2 years).[41,64,93,94] It is more common in the larger breeds; boxers and Bernese mountain dogs are especially at risk. It is also a problem in large colonies of beagles used in research laboratories. A sudden onset of extreme discomfort is the most common clinical sign. As a rule there are no neurologic deficits, but these patients are commonly depressed and usually have a fever. They have an appearance similar to that seen in Video 10-48 of Squirt. The discomfort is manifested by extreme reluctance to move, neck rigidity, a short-strided and stiff gait when the patient moves, and uncontrollable screaming when the patient is handled. As the CNS parenchyma becomes involved, the clinical signs reflect the segmental area affected by the lesion. This is more common in dogs that have a protracted course, with repeated episodes of the disorder. The meningeal lesion is an extensive suppurative leptomeningitis associated with severe arteritis and fibrinoid necrosis of the arterial wall. Subarachnoid hemorrhage is common in this lesion. Spinal cord meninges are more severely affected than the brain meninges. Similar arterial lesions are occasionally seen in the thyroid, heart, and mediastinum. We have seen one 2-year-old Labrador retriever with an acute onset of paraplegia and analgesia caudal to the midthoracic level that had this meningeal polyarteritis and a focal subarachnoid hemorrhage that severely compressed the cranial thoracic spinal cord (Figs. 10-63 through 10-67). A blood count usually shows leucocytosis with neutrophilia. The CSF clearly reflects this lesion in marked elevation of protein and leucocytes, mostly neutrophils (hundreds to thousands of neutrophils/cmm). These neutrophils are nondegenerate. Xanthochromia is common in the CSF. No infectious agents have been isolated from the CSF. IgA is elevated in both the serum and the CSF, which supports a primary immune-mediated meningeal disorder. The cause of the immune system dysregulation is unknown. In some dogs, these clinical signs may resolve spontaneously after 2 to 11 days of discomfort and fever. However, these clinical signs commonly recur after a variable period of

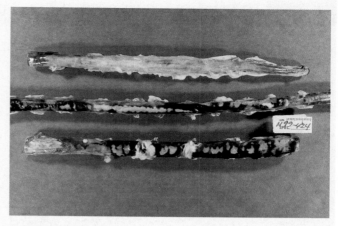

FIGURE 10-63 Dorsal surface of the spinal cord of a 2-year-old Labrador retriever with severe meningeal polyarteritis and diffuse subarachnoid hemorrhage.

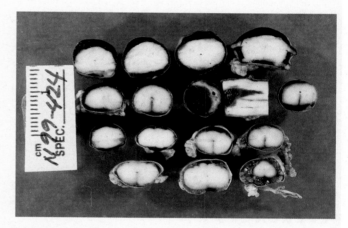

FIGURE 10-64 Transverse sections of the spinal cord seen in Fig. 10-63. Note the diffuse subarachnoid hemorrhage. In the third section from the left, in the middle row, note the massive hemorrhage causing severe compression of the spinal cord. It is at the level of the T4 spinal cord segment. This is an unusual lesion in this meningeal disorder, and it caused paraplegia.

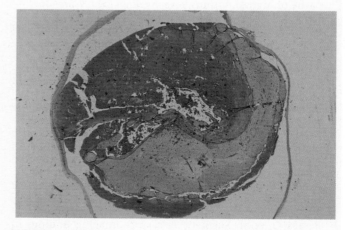

FIGURE 10-65 Microscopic section of the T4 spinal cord segment seen in Fig. 10-64. Note the extensive compression of the spinal cord to the right side.

(Continued)

CASE EXAMPLE 10-24—cont'd

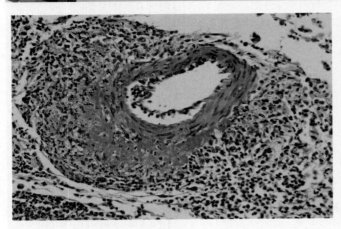

FIGURE 10-66 Microscopic section of the T4 spinal cord segment showing subarachnoid hemorrhage and meninges filled with inflammatory cells, most of which were neutrophils. Note the blood vessel exhibiting fibrinoid necrosis related to vasculitis.

a few days to months. Most dogs respond well to immunosuppressive levels of corticosteroid therapy, which often has to be continued by alternate-day therapy to avoid recurrence of the clinical signs. A less severe, protracted form occurs in dogs with repeated episodes of this disorder. Occasionally, juvenile dogs with immune-mediated polyarthritis also have meningeal polyarteritis.

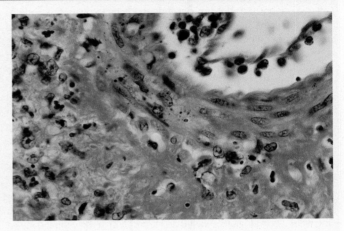

FIGURE 10-67 Microscopic section of the blood vessel wall in Fig. 10-66 exhibiting fibrinoid necrosis.

Bacterial meningitis is uncommon in small animals. As a rule, infection with rickettsial, bacterial, and fungal agents is bloodborne and involves the meninges prior to invading the parenchyma. None of these microorganisms have a specific predilection for the nervous system. Lethargy, discomfort, and fever are the most common clinical signs prior to involvement of the parenchyma. CSF pleocytosis is usually neutrophilic, but it is often difficult to culture the infections agent from the CSF. MR images may reveal meningeal enhancement.

REFERENCES

1. Alden C, Dickerson TV: Osteochondromatosis of the cervical vertebrae in a dog, *J Am Vet Med Assoc* 168:142, 1976.
2. Averill DR Jr: Degenerative myelopathy in the aging German shepherd dog: clinical and pathologic findings, *J Am Vet Med Assoc* 162:1045, 1973.
3. Averill DR Jr, Bronson RT: Inherited necrotizing myelopathy of Afghan hounds, *J Neuropathol Expt Neurol* 36:734, 1977.
4. Averill DR, Jr, de Lahunta A: Toxoplasmosis of the canine nervous system: clinicopathologic findings in four cases, *J Am Vet Med Assoc* 159:1134, 1971.
5. Axlund TW, et al: Fibrocartilaginous embolic encephalomyelopathy of the brainstem and midcervical spinal cord in a dog, *J Vet Intern Med* 18:765-767, 2004.
6. Ball MU, et al: Patterns of occurrence of disk disease among registered dachshunds, *J Am Vet Med Assoc* 180:519, 1982.
7. Barclay KB, Haines DM: Immunohistochemical evidence for immunoglobulin and complement deposition in spinal cord lesions in degenerative myelopathy in German shepherd dogs, *Can J Vet Res* 58:20-24, 1994.
8. Baum F, de Lahunta A, Trotter EJ: Cervical fibrotic stenosis in a young rottweiler, *J Am Vet Med Assoc* 201:1222-1224, 1992.
9. Besalti O, et al: Magnetic resonance imaging findings in dogs with thoracolumbar intervertebral disk disease: 69 cases (1997-2005), *J Am Vet Med Assoc* 228:902-908, 2006.

10. Braund KG, et al: Distal sensorimotor polyneuropathy in mature rottweiler dogs, *Vet Pathol* 31:316-326, 1984.
11. Braund KG, Vandevelde M: German shepherd dog myelopathy: a morphologic and morphometric study, *Am J Vet Res* 39:1309, 1978.
12. Brown NO, Helphrey ML, Prata RG: Thoracolumbar disk disease in the dog: a retrospective analysis of 187 cases, *J Am Anim Hosp Assoc* 13:665, 1977.
13. Carmichael KP, Bienzle D, McDonnell JJ: Feline leukemia virus-associated myelopathy in cats, *Vet Pathol* 39:536-545, 2002.
14. Cauznille L, Kornegay JN: Fibrocartilaginous embolism of the spinal cord in dogs: review of 36 histologically confirmed cases and retrospective study of 26 suspected cases, *J Vet Intern Med* 10:241-245, 1996.
15. Chambers JN, Betts CW: Caudal cervical spondylomyelopathy in the dog: a review of 20 clinical cases and the literature, *J Am Anim Hosp Assoc* 13:571, 1977.
16. Chrisman CL, Cork LC, Gamble DA: Neuroaxonal dystrophy in rottweiler dogs, *J Am Vet Med Assoc* 184:464-467, 1984.
17. Coates JR, et al: Clinical characterization of a familial degenerative myelopathy in Pembroke Welsh Corgi dogs, *J Vet Intern Med* 21:1323-1331, 2007.
18. Cockrell BY, et al: Myelomalacia in Afghan hounds, *J Am Vet Med Assoc* 162:362, 1973.
19. Cook JR, Oliver JE Jr: Atlanto-axial luxation in the dog, *Compend Cont Ed* 3:242, 1981.
20. Cork LC, et al: Canine neuroaxonal dystrophy, *J Neuropathol Expt Neurol* 42:286-296, 1983.

21. Cummings JF, de Lahunta A: Hereditary myelopathy of Afghan hounds: a myelinolytic disease, *Acta Neuropathol* 42:173, 1978.
22. de Lahunta A: Progressive cervical spinal cord compression in Great Dane and Doberman pinscher dogs (a wobbler syndrome). In Kirk RW, editor: *Current veterinary therapy V: small animal practice*, Philadelphia, 1974, Saunders.
23. de Lahunta A, Alexander JW: Ischemic myelopathy secondary to presumed fibrocartilaginous embolism in nine dogs, *J Am Anim Hosp Assoc* 12:37, 1976.
24. Denny HR, Gibbs C, Gaskell CJ: Cervical spondylopathy in the dog: a review of thirty-five cases, *J Sm Anim Pract* 18:117, 1977.
25. De Risio L, et al: Magnetic resonance imaging findings and clinical associations in 52 dogs with suspected ischemic myelopathy, *J Vet Intern Med* 21:1290-1298, 2007.
26. Eger CE, et al: Progressive tetraparesis and laryngeal paralysis in a young rottweiler with neuronal vacuolation and axonal degeneration: an Australian case, *Aust Vet J* 76:733-737, 1998.
27. English PB: A case of hyperostosis due to hypervitaminosis A in a cat, *J Sm Anim Pract* 10:207, 1969.
28. Fankhauser R, et al: Reticulosis of the central nervous system in dogs, *Adv Vet Sci Comp Med* 16:35, 1972.
29. Fundquist B: Thoraco-lumbar disk protrusion with severe spinal cord compression in the dog. I. Clinical and pathoanatomic observations, with special reference to the rate of development of symptoms of motor loss, *Acta Vet Scand* 3:256, 1961.
30. Gambardella PC, Osborne CA, Stevens JB: Multiple cartilaginous exostoses in the dog, *J Am Vet Med Assoc* 166:761, 1975.
31. Gamble DA, Chrisman CL: A leukoencephalomyelopathy of rottweiler dogs, *Vet Pathol* 21:274-280, 1984.
32. Gandini G, et al: Fibrocartilaginous embolism in 75 dogs: clinical findings and factors influencing the recovery rate, *J Sm Anim Pract* 44:76-80, 2003.
33. Geary JC, Oliver JE Jr, Hoerlein BF: Atlanto-axial subluxation in the canine, *J Sm Anim Pract* 8:577, 1967.
34. Ghosh P, et al: A comparative clinical and histochemical study of the chondrodystrophoid and onchondrodystrophoid canine intervertebral disk, *Vet Pathol* 13:414, 1976.
35. Gilmore DR, de Lahunta A: Necrotizing myelopathy secondary to presumed or confirmed fibrocartilaginous embolism, *J Am Anim Hosp Assoc* 23:373-376, 1987.
36. Griffiths IR: A syndrome produced by "explosions" of the cervical intervertebral disks, *Vet Rec* 87:737, 1970.
37. Griffiths IR: Spinal cord infarction due to emboli arising from the intervertebral disks in the dog, *J Comp Pathol* 83:225, 1973.
38. Griffiths IR, Duncan ID: Chronic degenerative radiculomyelopathy in the dog, *J Sm Anim Pract* 16:461, 1975.
39. Griffiths IR, Duncan ID: Age changes in the dorsal and ventral lumbar nerve roots of dogs, *Acta Neuropathol* 32:75, 1975.
40. Hansen HJ: A pathologic-anatomical study on disk degeneration in the dog, *Acta Orthoped Scand Suppl* 11:202, 279-291, 1952.
41. Harcourt RA: Polyarteritis in a colony of beagles, *Vet Rec* 102:519, 1978.
42. Hayes MA, et al: Acute necrotizing myelopathy from nucleus pulposus embolism in dogs with intervertebral disk degeneration, *J Am Vet Med Assoc* 173:289, 1978.
43. Hedhammer A, et al: Overnutrition and skeletal disease: an experimental study in growing Great Dane dogs, *Cor Vet Suppl* 5:64, 1, 1974.
44. Henderson RA, et al: Discospondylitis in three dogs infected with Brucella canis, *J Am Vet Med Assoc* 165:451, 1974.
45. Hurov L, Troy G, Turnwald G: Discospondylitis in the dog: 27 cases, *J Am Vet Med Assoc* 173:275, 1978.
46. Johnston PE, et al: CNS pathology in 25 dogs with chronic degenerative radiculomyelopathy, *Vet Rec* 146:623-633, 2000.
47. Kathmann S, et al: Daily controlled physiotherapy increases survival time in dogs with suspected degenerative myelopathy, *J Vet Intern Med* 20:927-932, 2006.
48. King AS, Smith RN: Disk protrusions in the cat: distribution of dorsal protrusions along the vertebral column, *Vet Rec* 72:335, 1960.
49. Kneckt CD, Blevins WE, Raffe MR: Stenosis of the thoracic spinal canal in English bulldogs, *J Am Anim Hosp Assoc* 15:181, 1979.
50. Knipe MF, et al: Intervertebral disk extrusion in six cats, *J Fel Med Surg* 3:161-168, 2001.
51. Koestner A, Zeman W: Primary reticulosis of the central nervous system, *Am J Vet Res* 23:381, 1962.
52. Kornegay JN: Canine discospondylitis, *Compend Cont Ed* 1:930, 1979.
53. Kornegay JN: Ischemic myelopathy due to fibrocartilaginous embolism, *Compend Cont Ed* 2:402, 1980.
54. Kortz GD, et al: Neuronal vacuolation and spinocerebellar degeneration in young rottweiler dogs, *Vet Pathol* 34:296-302, 1997.
55. Levine GJ, et al: Evaluation of the association between spondylosis deformans and clinical signs of intervertebral disk disease in dogs: 172 cases (1999-2000), *J Am Vet Med Assoc* 228:96-100, 2006.
56. Levine JM, et al: Association between various physical factors and acute thoracolumbar intervertebral disk extrusion or protrusion in dachshunds, *J Am Vet Med Assoc* 229:370-375, 2006.
57. Ljunggren G: Legg-Perthes disease in the dog, *Acta Orthoped Scand Suppl* 95:1, 1967.
58. Luttgen PJ, Bratton GR: Spinal cord ependymoma: a case report, *J Am Anim Hosp Assoc* 12:788, 1976.
59. Mahony OM, et al: Laryngeal paralysis-polyneuropathy complex in young rottweilers *J Vet Intern Med* 12:330-337, 1998.
60. Mason TA: Cervical vertebral instability (wobbler syndrome) in the Doberman, *Aust Vet J* 53:440, 1977.
61. Massalgi HJJ, Jaffe KM: Fibrocartilaginous embolism: an uncommon cause of spinal cord infarction: a case report and review of literature, *Arch Phys Med Rehabil* 85:153-157, 2004.
62. Mathews NS, de Lahunta A: Degenerative myelopathy in an adult miniature poodle, *J Am Vet Med Assoc* 11:1213-1214, 1985.
63. McDonnell JJ, et al: Thoracolumbar spinal cord compression due to vertebral process degenerative joint disease in a family of Shiloh shepherd dogs, *J Vet Intern Med* 17:530-537, 2003.
64. Meric SM, Perman V, Hardy RM: Corticosteroid-responsive meningitis in ten dogs, *J Am Anim Hosp Assoc* 21:677, 1985.
65. Mesfin GM, Kusem HD, Parker A: Degenerative myelopathy in a cat, *J Am Vet Med Assoc* 176:62, 1980.
66. Morgan JP: Spondylosis deformans in the dog, *Acta Orthoped Scand Suppl* 96:1, 1967.
67. Morgan JP: Congenital anomalies of the vertebral column of the dog: a study of the incidence and significance based on radiographic and morphologic study, *J Am Vet Radiol Soc* 9:21, 1968.
68. Morgan JP: Spinal dural ossification in the dog: incidence and distribution based on radiographic study, *J Am Vet Radiol Soc* 10:43, 1969.
69. Morgan JP, Stavenborn M: Disseminated idiopathic skeletal hyperostosis (DISH) in a dog, *Vet Radiol Ultrasound* 32:65, 1991.

70. Northington JW, Juliana MM: Extradural lymphosarcoma in six cats, *J Sm Anim Pract* 19:409, 1978.

71. O'Brien D, Parker AJ, Tarvin G: Osteosarcoma of the vertebra causing compression of the thoracic spinal cord in a cat, *J Am Anim Hosp Assoc* 16:497, 1980.

72. Olby N, et al: Long-term functional outcome of dogs with severe injuries of the thoracolumbar spinal cord: 87 cases (1996-2001), *J Am Vet Med Assoc* 222:762-769, 2003.

73. Olsson S-E, Stavenborn M, Hoppe F: Dynamic compression of the cervical spinal cord: a myelographic and pathologic investigation in Great Dane dogs, *Acta Vet Scand* 23:65, 1982.

74. Palmer AC, Wallace ME: Deformation of the cervical vertebrae in basset hounds, *Vet Rec* 80:430, 1967.

75. Parker AJ, Park AD: Atlanto-axial subluxation in small breeds of dogs: diagnosis and pathogenesis, *Vet Med* 68:1133, 1973.

76. Pearson GR, Gregory SP, Charles AK: Immunohistochemical demonstration of Wilm's tumor gene product WT 1 in a canine "neuroepithelioma" providing evidence for its classification as an extrarenal nephroblastoma, *J Comp Pathol* 116:321-327, 1997.

77. Raffe MR, Knecht CD: Cervical vertebral malformation: a review of 36 cases, *J Am Anim Hosp Assoc* 16:881, 1980.

78. Roth J, Blaha I, Bitter-Suermann D: Blastemal cells of nephroblastomatosis complex share an onco-developmental antigen with embryonic kidney and Wilms' tumor: an immunocytochemical study on polysialic acid distribution, *Am J Pathol* 133:596-608, 1988.

79. Ruch TC: Evidence of the nonsegmental character of spinal reflexes from an analysis of the cephalad effects of spinal transection (Schiff-Sherrington phenomenon), *Am J Physiol* 114:457, 1936.

80. Seawright AA, English PB, Gartner RJW: Hypervitaminosis A and deforming cervical spondylosis of the cat, *J Comp Pathol* 77:29, 1967.

81. Seiler G, et al: Staging of lumbar intervertebral disk degeneration in nonchondrodystrophic dogs using low-field magnetic resonance imaging, *Vet Radiol Ultrasound* 44:179-184, 2003.

82. Seim HB, Withrow SJ: Pathophysiology and diagnosis of caudal cervical spondylo-myelopathy with emphasis on the Doberman pinscher, *J Am Anim Hosp Assoc* 18:241, 1982.

83. Sharp N, et al: Computed tomography in the evaluation of caudal cervical spondylomyelopathy of the Doberman pinscher, *Vet Radiol Ultrasound* 36:100-108, 1995.

84. Shell LG, Jortner BS, Leid MS: Spinal muscular atrophy in two rottweiler littermates, *J Am Vet Med Assoc* 190:878-880, 1987.

85. Shell LG, Jortner BS, Leid MS: Familial motor neuron disease in rottweiler dogs: neuropathologic studies, *Vet Pathol* 24:135-139, 1987.

86. Simpson RK, Robertson CS, Goodman JC: Glycine: an important potential component of spinal shock, *Neurochem Res* 18:887-892, 1993.

87. Slocombe RF, Mitten R, Mason TA: Leukoencephalomyelopathy in Australian rottweiler dogs, *Aust Vet J* 66:147-150, 1989.

88. Smith PM, Jeffrey ND: Spinal shock-comparative aspects and clinical relevance, *J Vet Intern Med* 19:788-793, 2005.

89. Sprague JM: Spinal "border cells" and their role in postural mechanisms (Schiff-Sherrington phenomenon), *J Neurophysiol* 16:464, 1953.

90. Stigen O: Calcification of intervertebral disks in the dachshund: radiographic study of 115 dogs at 1 and 5 years of age, *Acta Vet Scand* 37:229-237, 1996.

91. Summers BA, de Lahunta A, McKentee M: A novel intradural-extramedullary spinal cord tumor in young dogs, *Acta Neuropathol* 75:402-410, 1988.

92. Teuscher E, Cherrstrom EC: Ependymoma of the spinal cord in a young dog, *Schweiz Tierheilk* 116:461, 1974.

93. Tipold A, Jaggy A: Steroid responsive meningitis-arteritis in dogs: long-term study of 32 cases, *J Sm Anim Pract* 35:311, 1994.

94. Tipold A, Vandevelde M, Zurbriggen A: Neuroimmunological studies in steroid-responsive meningitis-arteritis in dogs, *Res Vet Sci* 58:103, 1995.

95. Toro-Gonzalez G, et al: Acute ischemic stroke from fibrocartilaginous embolism of the middle cerebral artery, *Stroke* 24:738-740, 1993.

96. Trotter EJ, et al: Caudal cervical vertebral malformation-malarticulation in Great Danes and Doberman pinschers, *J Am Vet Med Assoc* 168:917, 1976.

97. Van den Ingh TSGAM, Mandigers PJJ, Van Nes JJ: A neuronal vacuolar disorder in young rottweiler dogs, *Vet Rec* 142:245-247, 1998.

98. Watson AG, de Lahunta A: Atlanto-axial subluxation and absence of the transverse ligament of the atlas in a dog, *J Am Vet Med Assoc* 195:235-237, 1989.

99. Watson AG, de Lahunta A, Evans, HE: Morphology and embryological interpretation of a congenital occipto-atlanto-axial malformation in a dog, *Teratology* 38:451-460, 1988.

100. Watson AG, Evans HE: The development of the atlas-axis complex in the dog, *Anat Rec* 184:558, 1976.

101. Watson AG, Evans HE, de Lahunta A: Ossification of the atlas-axis complex in the dog, *Anat Histol Embryol* 15:122-138, 1986.

102. Watson AG, Hall MA, de Lahunta A: Congenital occipto-atlanto-axial malformation in a cat, *Compend Cont Ed* 7:245-252, 1985.

103. Waxman FJ, Clemmons RM, Henrichs DJ: Progressive myelopathy in older German shepherd dogs. II. Presence of circulating suppressor cells, *J Immunol* 124:1216, 1980.

104. Waxman FJ, et al: Progressive myelopathy in older German shepherd dogs. I. Depressed response to thymus-dependent mitogens, *J Immunol* 124:1209, 1980.

105. Wilson JW, Greene HJ, Leipold HW: Osseous metaplasia of the spinal dura mater in a Great Dane, *J Am Vet Med Assoc* 167:75, 1975.

106. Wouda W, Van Nes JJ: Progressive ataxia due to central demyelination in rottweiler dogs, *Vet Quart* 8:89-97, 1986.

107. Wright F, Palmer AC: Morpholgical changes caused by pressure on the spinal cord, *Pathol Vet* 6:355, 1969.

108. Wright F, Rest R Jr, Palmer AC: Ataxia of the Great Dane caused by stenosis of the cervical vertebral canal: comparison with similar condition in the basset hound, Doberman pinscher, ridgeback and thoroughbred horse, *Vet Rec* 18:697, 1973.

109. Zachary JF, O'Brien DP, Ely RW: Intramedullary spinal ependymoma in a dog, *Vet Pathol* 18:697, 1981.

110. Zaki F, Prata RG: Necrotizing myelopathy secondary to embolism of herniated intervertebral disk material in the dog, *J Am Vet Med Assoc* 165:1080, 1976.

111. Zaki F, Prata RG, Werner LL: Necrotizing myelopathy in a cat, *J Am Vet Med Assoc* 169:228, 1976.

NEUROLOGIC EXAMINATION

Gait and Posture
Postural Reactions
    Head Elevation
    Circling
    Swaying
    Backing
Spinal Nerves
    Muscle Atrophy
    Cutaneous Reflexes
    Tail, Anus, and Perineum
    Patellar Reflex
    Flexor (Withdrawal) Reflexes
Cranial Nerves
    Laryngeal Adduction
    Neck Discomfort

SUMMARY OF CLINICAL SIGNS AT SPECIFIC AREAS OF THE SPINAL CORD

Lumbosacral: Fourth Lumbar through the Caudal Spinal Cord Segments
Thoracolumbar: Third Thoracic to the Third Lumbar Spinal Cord Segments

Caudocervical: Sixth Cervical to the Second Thoracic Spinal Cord Segments
Craniocervical: First Cervical to the Fifth Cervical Spinal Cord Segments
Grading System for Horses

EQUINE SPINAL CORD DISEASE

CASE EXAMPLE 11-1
    Cervical Vertebral Malformation-Malarticulation
    Equine Degenerative Myeloencephalopathy
    Diskospondylitis
CASE EXAMPLE 11-2
    Equine Protozoal Myelitis
CASE EXAMPLE 11-3
    Equine Herpesvirus-1 Myelopathy
CASE EXAMPLE 11-4
    Neoplasm-Melanoma at T17
    T17 Fracture in a Foal
    Cervical Scoliosis–Parelaphostrongylus Tenuis

FARM ANIMAL SPINAL CORD DISEASE

CASE EXAMPLE 11-5
    P. Tenuis Myiasis
    Vertebral Malformation

CASE EXAMPLE 11-6
    Caprine Arthritis Encephalitis Virus
    Copper Deficiency-Enzootic Ataxia
    Organophosphate Toxicity
CASE EXAMPLE 11-7
    Hepatic Encephalomyelopathy in a Calf
    Brown Swiss Myelopathy
    Charolais Leukodystrophy
CASE EXAMPLE 11-8
    T4 Fracture in a Cow
CASE EXAMPLE 11-9
    Rabies Myelitis
    Lumbosacral Discospondylitis in a Cow
CASE EXAMPLE 11-10
CASE EXAMPLE 11-11

NEUROLOGIC EXAMINATION

In this chapter, the term *large animal* refers to the horse, ox, sheep, goat, pig, and the Camelidae. The neurologic examination of large animals is similar to that of small animals, with adjustments that are necessary to accommodate the size of the patient. Five components of the examination include (1) gait and posture, (2) postural reactions, (3) spinal nerves, (4) cranial nerves, and (5) sensorium. See Chapter 20 for a description of the complete examination. Only specific components that relate to spinal cord disease are reviewed here.

Gait and Posture

Observe the standing animal for the position of its head, neck, trunk, and limbs, being especially observant for a head tilt, lowered position of the neck, trembling, and tail position. Evaluate the gait on a surface that is not slippery. Walking the patient on macadam or concrete not only makes the evaluation difficult, but it is also dangerous for a paretic and ataxic patient. Most deficits can be observed at a slow straight walk and on turns as you observe the patient from one side. Subtle deficits may require walking the patient over a low obstacle such as a curb or walking on a slope, if available. Occasionally, trotting the patient is helpful. Turning the patient loose in a paddock may also be useful to observe the patient when it changes the speed of its gait and adjusts to making sudden turns. We rely almost entirely on observing the walking gait from one side as the patient is being led by an assistant, and then we repeat this part of the examination while leading the patient ourselves. Note any delay in the onset of protraction (the swing phase), the ability to support weight, length of the strides, the tendency to overreach with the limb extended, scuffing of the digit or digits, swinging the limb outwards (abduction) or inwards (adduction), swaying of the trunk and pelvis, and the range of neck movements. Spasticity may make the limbs appear stiff and cause the hoof to strike the ground surface abruptly, causing an audible slapping noise on a hard surface. Be aware of breed differences in their normal gait. For example, do not confuse the neurologic sign of overreaching in the thoracic limbs with the normal high action of the Paso Fino and Tennessee Walking Horse breeds.

Postural Reactions

The postural reactions as described for small animals can be performed on small pigs, calves, foals, most goats and sheep, crias, and some adult Camelidae. The hopping, hemiwalking, and hoof replacement tests are the most reliable. If your patient is cooperative, it is possible to pick up one limb and lean into the patient to force it to hop on the opposite limb. In most adult horses and cattle, this task is difficult to do and to evaluate and is obviously stressful for you to perform. It also can be dangerous in a patient that has neurologic dysfunction. We do not routinely use this test in large patients.

For larger patients that are cooperative, the following maneuvers require more neurologic function of the upper motor neuron (UMN) and general proprioceptive (GP) systems to be normal and may elicit or exacerbate clinical signs that may not be appreciated while just observing the patient walk in a straight line. These maneuvers include head elevation and circling and swaying of the patient.

Head Elevation

After walking your patient with its head in its normal posture, lift the patient's head with the shank or just by the halter until you have the head elevated as far as possible and your patient is still willing to walk. As you continue walking your patient, this exercise may elicit or exacerbate the tendency of the patient to overreach or float with the thoracic limbs at the end of the protraction phase of the gait. Sometimes the affected patient will scuff its hoof at the onset of protraction or even buckle onto the dorsal surface of the digit or digits and stumble.

Circling

In our opinion, circling your patient 8 to 10 times in each direction is by far the most useful manipulation to detect subtle neurologic abnormalities, especially those that affect the UMN and GP systems. This part of the examination should be performed by an attendant, as well as yourself. These circles should be fairly small tight circles, with the person holding the lead located in the center of the circle. Remember that anytime you pull the lead toward you, the pelvic limbs will move away from you. Besides making the patient start to circle, this method is a good way to prevent someone getting kicked! The normal animal will step around briskly with relatively short strides and will not pivot on a limb or step on itself. All movements will be smooth and regular. A normal patient will act as if it knows exactly where its digits are located. The patient with spinal cord disease that involves the UMN and GP systems will pivot on the inside limb, which is held in place and not protracted. If the lesion is severe, the patient may collapse or nearly collapse with this maneuver. With mild lesions, an obvious delay will occur in the onset of protraction in the limb or limbs on the inside (concave side) of the circle, creating a pivoting motion on the digits. At the same time the opposite or outside pelvic limb may flex and abduct excessively as it is protracted, which creates a wide swinging motion termed *circumduction*. The outside thoracic limb may appear stiff and swing across cranial to the supporting inside limb as the patient attempts to circle. The outside thoracic limb may step on the supporting limb.

Recall from the previous chapters on the UMN and GP systems that we cannot distinguish between the clinical signs caused by dysfunction of these two systems (see Fig. 10-2). Because of their close anatomic relationship, these two systems are usually affected together with spinal cord lesions, and differentiating between them is unnecessary. Our objective is to recognize a deficit of the UMN and GP systems together and determine the level of the spinal cord where these systems are affected.

Swaying

The standing or walking patient that can be easily pulled by the tail to either side or is easily pushed to either side is suggestive of paresis. This test is best performed with the patient walking while you pull the tail toward you. This test may also accentuate an ataxia that accompanies the paresis because the patient may stumble as it adjusts to the change in posture on being pulled to one side. Some variation exists in how much a horse will resist this effort, which makes your interpretation quite subjective. This effort to determine paresis can be accomplished more forcefully by vigorously pulling both the tail and the head lead toward you simultaneously. Paresis may also be detected by firmly squeezing the patient along the trunk, causing it to extend its vertebral column. The paretic animal may sink excessively, buckle its digits, or even collapse on the ground.

Backing

Cooperative patients that have spinal cord disease may have difficulty backing up and will appear awkward or very slow to protract a limb. If the deficit is severe, animals will not protract either pelvic limb and may collapse on them.

Spinal Nerves

Spinal nerves are evaluated by assessing the patient's muscle tone and size and spinal nerve reflexes. This examination is performed in small pigs, calves, foals, crias, and most goats and sheep in a similar manner to small animals where you can straddle them and manipulate and palpate their entire limbs and then place them in lateral recumbency to test the patellar and withdrawal reflexes. In the standing large animal, you are limited to examination of muscle size by vision and palpation, evaluating tail and anal tone and the perineal reflex, performing the cutaneous reflexes, and determining nociception from the skin throughout the neck, trunk, limbs, tail and perineum. Realistically, if the patient can stand and walk, you can assume that its spinal reflex function in the limbs is intact. In the recumbent large animal, you can manipulate the limbs to determine muscle tone, and you can test the patellar and withdrawal reflexes in the nonrecumbent limbs. Evaluating these factors in the recumbent limbs is very difficult because of all the weight that is on them and especially if the patient has been recumbent for any length of time.

Muscle Atrophy

Muscle atrophy is a clinical sign of lack of nourishment, disuse, or denervation. Denervated muscles atrophy rapidly. Neurogenic atrophy is faster and more complete than disuse atrophy, although these types may be difficult to differentiate in some patients. A good example of neurogenic atrophy is the diffuse atrophy that accompanies equine motor neuron disease (EMND). Horse owners will complain of a rapid loss of weight despite an excellent appetite in their animal. Remember that a loss of any component of the lower motor neuron (LMN) will result in denervation atrophy. These components include the neuronal cell body in the ventral gray column as in motor neuron disease, the ventral roots, and spinal nerves as in chronic polyneuritis or any part of the peripheral nerve in its course to the muscle as in radial nerve injury.

Cutaneous Reflexes

Cutaneous reflexes are especially responsive in the horse, in which tapping the skin with the blunt end of closed forceps or the end of a ballpoint pen or other hard object will elicit contractions of the skin all along the side of the animal. In the neck, this event is caused by the contraction of the cutaneous colli muscle innervated by the facial nerve. In the trunk, the cutaneous trunci muscle is innervated by the lateral thoracic nerve from the brachial plexus and the C8 and T1 spinal cord segments. The sensory component of these skin reflexes involves the general somatic afferent (GSA) neurons in the peripheral nerves that innervate the area of skin that you stimulate and long interneurons within the spinal cord that course to the C8 and T1 spinal cord ventral gray column for the cutaneous trunci and to the facial nucleus in the medulla for the cutaneous colli. These cutaneous reflexes are readily elicited in most normal horses. Some farm animals may require vigorous stimulation to obtain the reflex, and occasionally it cannot be elicited in some normal animals. Remember that this same skin stimulation will also elicit activity in the nociceptive pathway to the prosencephalon, and you should limit the degree of stimulus to prevent injury. Focal loss of cutaneous sensitivity is unusual because of the large overlap of cutaneous areas. Focal loss of cutaneous nociception is observed in the region of the tail, anus, and perineum in polyneuritis equi or sacrocaudal fractures in cattle from being ridden by other cattle. It is easy to be misled by what you first believe is an area of hypalgesia or even analgesia. Be sure to repeat the stimulation numerous times before considering it a reliable observation. Nociception is very difficult to evaluate in the recumbent large animal. The patient will often fail to respond to the same stimulus to which it would respond if standing. Sometimes, if this factor is especially important in your interpretation of the anatomic diagnosis or establishing a prognosis, careful use of a cattle prod as a stimulus is helpful.

Tail, Anus, and Perineum

Tail, anus, and perineum are readily evaluated by manipulation of the tail, palpation of the anus, and stimulation of the skin of the perineum. Loss of tone in the tail implicates the caudal nerves and caudal spinal cord segments. A loss of tone in the anus implicates the sacral plexus, sacral nerves, and sacral spinal cord segments. The perineal reflex consists of closure of the anus and flexion of the tail after stimulating the skin of the perineum and therefore tests both the caudal and sacral nerves and their spinal cord segments. In the standing horse, evaluate these areas with caution. You can stand beside the pelvic limb and slip your hand under the tail, which you can elevate to check for tone and palpate the anus, which is very tight in the normal horse and tightens further when palpated.

Patellar Reflex

The patellar reflex is the only tendon reflex that is reliable in large animals, and it can be elicited only in the recumbent, relaxed patient. The pleximeter can be used in the smaller animals. In the horse and ox, the lateral side of your hand with your digits extended can be used to strike the intermediate patellar ligament. Hold the pelvic limb as relaxed as possible and in partial flexion. This test evaluates the L4 and L5 spinal cord segments, spinal nerve roots, and ventral branches and the femoral nerves. With LMN lesions, this reflex will be decreased or absent. With UMN lesions, it will be normal or exaggerated.

Flexor (Withdrawal) Reflexes

The flexor withdrawal reflexes are usually elicited by compressing the skin of the coronary band region or the bulb of the hoof with forceps. Occasionally, in recumbent large animals, this test may require the use of an electric prod. In the pelvic limb the flexion that is elicited is a function of the sensory and motor components of the sciatic nerve and the L6, S1, and S2 spinal cord segments, spinal nerve roots, and ventral branches. Flexion of the hip, however, is a function of the femoral nerve and most of the lumbar spinal cord segments, spinal nerve roots, and ventral branches. In the thoracic limb, the flexor reflex involves several specific peripheral nerves and the C6 to T2 spinal cord segments, spinal nerve roots, and ventral branches. The afferent neurons that are stimulated will depend on the site of the stimulus. The coronary band or bulb regions are innervated by the median and ulnar nerves in the horse plus the radial nerve in the other large animals. The flexion of the joints is mediated through the LMNs that are located in all of the nerves derived from the brachial plexus, which includes the radial, axillary, musculocutaneous, median, and ulnar nerves. These reflexes will all be preserved with transverse spinal cord lesions that are cranial to the spinal cord segments involved in the reflex.

Remember that the noxious stimulus that is used to elicit these flexor reflexes also tests the nociceptive pathway through the spinal cord and brainstem to the cerebrum. A transverse lesion between the T3 and L3 spinal cord segments will interrupt these nociceptive pathways, resulting in analgesia caudal to a line that is approximately two vertebrae caudal to the level of the spinal cord lesion. This same lesion will interrupt the long interneurons involved in the cutaneous trunci reflex that course cranially in the fasciculus proprius. The level where you can first elicit this cutaneous trunci reflex will be the same as the line of analgesia.

Cranial Nerves

The cranial nerve examination is important for detecting multifocal lesions and for evaluating spinal cord lesions that affect the first three thoracic spinal cord segments and cause a sympathetic paralysis, called *Horner syndrome*, which was described in Chapter 7. With severe lateral funicular lesions in the cervical spinal cord segments, a UMN paralysis of the entire sympathetic innervation will occur on the ipsilateral side of the body including the head. In horses, this paralysis will be apparent by the ipsilateral whole-body sweating that will occur. A focal lesion between the T1 and L4 spinal cord segments that destroys the intermediate gray column will cause a focal area of sweating where the skin is deprived of its sympathetic innervation.

Laryngeal Adduction

Some equine clinicians test one additional reflex—the laryngeal adduction reflex—using the slap test.[40] This test requires the integrity of all of the cervical and the cranial thoracic spinal cord segments, the nucleus ambiguus in the medulla, and the vagal and recurrent laryngeal nerves. The test is performed by standing beside the neck of the horse with one hand grasping the larynx. With the other hand, a brisk slap is delivered to the saddle area of the thorax. In the normal animal, this action will elicit a brief closure of the glottis by adduction of the vocal folds, which you will feel with the hand that is grasping the larynx or you can observe with an endoscope. You will feel the larynx move when this adduction occurs. The anatomic pathway involved with this response starts with the stimulation of cutaneous branches of cranial thoracic spinal nerves that synapse on long interneurons in the ipsilateral dorsal gray column. Most of the axons of these long interneurons cross to the opposite-side fasciculus proprius and course cranially to the medulla, where they synapse on GSE LMN cell bodies in the nucleus ambiguus that is contralateral to the side that is slapped. The axons of these neuronal cell bodies enter the vagus nerve and course caudally to the thorax, where they leave the vagus nerve in the recurrent laryngeal nerve to course cranially to the larynx, where they innervate the intrinsic muscles that function to close the glottis. Based on this pathway, unilateral cervical spinal cord lesions that involve the lateral funiculus may cause this slap reflex to be absent when tested on the side opposite from the lesion. Bilateral cervical spinal cord lesions may cause a bilateral loss of this reflex. Be aware that many long-necked horses have a left-side laryngeal paresis from a neuropathy in the left recurrent laryngeal nerve, which can cause this slap reflex to be absent when performed on the horse's right side. This reflex test requires considerable practice and experience to perform well, which is something that we have not done and therefore do not believe that we can rely on this reflex to help identify cervical spinal cord lesions.

Neck Discomfort

Neck discomfort should be assessed in any patient in which you suspect a cervical spinal cord lesion. As a rule, it is not present in horses with static or dynamic cervical spinal cord compression from stenosis of the vertebral foramina. It is most common in horses that have degenerative joint disease (DJD) of the articular processes at the synovial joints. If the discomfort is severe, you will see a lack of neck motion as the horse turns at the end of a walk or when being circled. The horse that keeps the neck rigid during a turn is often called "weathervaning" the neck. If you do not observe this result, stand in front of the horse and slowly move its head and neck to each side to determine the range of motion and whether any resistance exists on one or both sides. You may be able to attract the horse to make this movement using a carrot as a stimulus. For more vigorous assessment, stand beside the horse and, using the halter, pull the head towards you while you press with the fist of your other hand on

the vertebral bodies to apply pressure to the neck as it is flexed. Perform this exercise on both sides. With unilateral degenerative synovial joint lesions, the horse usually exhibits more discomfort when the neck is flexed laterally away from the side where the lesion is located.

SUMMARY OF CLINICAL SIGNS AT SPECIFIC AREAS OF THE SPINAL CORD

The spinal cord is divided into four regions based on the clinical signs that are exhibited when any one of these four regions are affected. See Fig. 10-1, which also applies to these large animals.

Lumbosacral: Fourth Lumbar through the Caudal Spinal Cord Segments

Normal thoracic limbs
Paretic and ataxic pelvic limbs with short strides from decreased ability to support weight to paraplegia
Decreased or absent tail, anal, and pelvic limb tone and spinal reflexes; atrophy of pelvic limb muscles
Hypalgesia or analgesia of the tail, anus, and pelvic limbs caudal to the cranial border of the lesion
Urinary incontinence and obstipation

Thoracolumbar: Third Thoracic to the Third Lumbar Spinal Cord Segments

Normal thoracic limbs
Pelvic limb spastic paresis (paraparesis) and ataxia to spastic paraplegia
Normal tail and anal tone and reflexes and normal to increased pelvic limb tone and reflexes; no neurogenic atrophy
Hypalgesia or analgesia caudal to the cranial border of the lesion
Focal sweating in horses
Urinary incontinence

Caudocervical: Sixth Cervical to the Second Thoracic Spinal Cord Segments

Ataxia and paresis of all four limbs (ataxia and tetraparesis) to tetraplegia
Pelvic limb spasticity and thoracic limb flaccidity
Normal or increased pelvic limb tone and reflexes
Decreased to absent thoracic limb tone and reflexes; thoracic limb atrophy
Hypalgesia to analgesia caudal to the cranial border of the lesion
Hypalgesia may be more pronounced in the thoracic limbs
Horner syndrome plus sweating of the entire side of the body in horses

Craniocervical: First Cervical to the Fifth Cervical Spinal Cord Segments

Ataxia and spastic paresis of all four limbs (ataxia and tetraparesis) to tetraplegia; ataxia and spastic paresis may be more obvious in the pelvic limbs

Normal or increased tone and reflexes in all four limbs

Hypalgesia caudal to the cranial border of the lesion

Horner syndrome and sweating of the entire side of the body in horses

Grading System for Horses

In an attempt to quantify the neurologic signs for comparative diagnostic purposes, for prognosis, and to follow the course of the disease with or without treatment, Dr. Ian Mayhew developed a grading system for cervical spinal cord disorders in horses based on the degree of neurologic deficit present in the patient.[50] This system differs from the grading system used in small animals with thoracolumbar lesions, which grades the degree of function present in the patient. In small animals, the degree of spinal cord damage and resultant clinical signs are used for surgical selection, as well as for prognosis and to follow the course of the disorder.

Grade 0: Normal strength and coordination

Grade 1: Normal gait when walking straight; slight deficit on walking in tight circles or walking with the neck and head extended or when pulled by the tail (sway)

Grade 2: Mild spastic tetraparesis and ataxia at all times and especially during the manipulations described for grade 1

Grade 3: Marked spastic tetraparesis and ataxia with a tendency to buckle and fall on vigorous circling, backing, or swaying

Grade 4: Spontaneous stumbling, tripping, and falling

Grade 5: Recumbent, unable to stand

EQUINE SPINAL CORD DISEASE

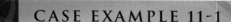

CASE EXAMPLE 11-1

Signalment: 2-year-old male Thoroughbred

Chief Complaint: Abnormal pelvic limb gait

History: Ten days before this examination, the horse suddenly began to sway and stumble in the pelvic limbs, and this dysfunction has progressed slightly since the onset. During these 10 days, the horse received treatment for a presumptive protozoal infection with no effect.

Examination: See **Video 11-1**. The horse exhibits most of the clinical signs that were described for a disorder affecting the UMN and GP systems in the cervical spinal cord. Note the tendency to delay and occasionally buckle at the onset of protraction with the thoracic limbs, as well as overreaching (floating) before the end of protraction. Most owners do not recognize this thoracic limb overreaching and complain only about the pelvic limb gait abnormality.

Anatomic Diagnosis: Focal or diffuse spinal cord lesion between the C1 and C5 segments

Differential Diagnosis: Malformation-malarticulation, equine degenerative myeloencephalopathy, equine protozoal myelitis, diskospondylitis

External injury and vascular compromise were excluded because of the history of progression of clinical signs and the lack of any circumstance in the environment of this patient that would account for any external injury. Neoplasia is rare in the vertebral canal or spinal cord of horses and especially at this age. We have never seen an extruded or protruded intervertebral disk in a horse of any age, and reports are rare. Be aware that infections with the rabies and West Nile viruses can first produce clinical signs of spinal cord disease. Rabies always progresses very fast, and most horses will develop intracranial signs and be recumbent in approximately 4 days and dead by 10 days. West Nile encephalomyelitis progresses at a variable rate from acute, similar to rabies, to a very chronic progression or even recovery from mild clinical signs.

CERVICAL VERTEBRAL MALFORMATION-MALARTICULATION

Cervical vertebral malformation-malarticulation is a very common disorder in horses that causes a compressive myelopathy. This condition was described for dogs in Chapter 10 and will be repeated here for the horse. Remember that the primary disease is the cervical vertebral column malformation and malarticulation. The compressive myelopathy is secondary because the spinal cord is in the way of and compromised by the stenosis (Fig. 11-1). Congenital and acquired forms of this disorder have been found.

Congenital Occiptoatlantoaxial Malformation

Congenital vertebral malformation is uncommon. An inherited malformation that involves the occipital and cranial cervical somites occurs in the Arabian breed and is termed *occiptoatlantoaxial malformation* (OAAM).[57,87] This condition is presumed to be inherited as an autosomal-recessive genetic disorder. In this malformation the factors that determine the formation of the occipital bone, the atlas, and the axis have been affected such that the atlas is occipitalized and fused by fibrocartilage to the occipital bone. The caudal portion of the atlas, which should consist of articular fovea, has a more rounded appearance similar to occipital condyles. The axis has a more atlas-like appearance and has transverse processes that tend to resemble the wings of the atlas. The malformed axis usually forms a false joint in thickened connective tissue ventral to the fused atlas. This defect involves the development of the sclerotomal portions of the occipital and cranial cervical somites. Clinical signs reflect the compression that occurs to the cervical spinal cord within a reduced foramen in the atlas or occasionally, the malformation has occurred without spinal cord compression. Foals may be born recumbent and unable to stand if the spinal cord compression is severe at birth. If assisted to stand, they exhibit a severe spastic tetraparesis and ataxia and readily fall, especially if they extend their neck to nurse. Occasionally, an audible click will be heard at the site of the malformation when the head is moved. This sound most likely represents movement at the luxated atlantoaxial joint. Other foals with this malformation may not show clinical signs until a few weeks or months of age. Progression of these signs usually follows. This delay in clinical signs probably reflects the failure of the vertebral foramina of the malformed atlas or axis to remodel to accommodate the enlarging spinal cord. As a rule, the clinical signs of spastic paresis and ataxia are quite profound in all four limbs. An important diagnostic feature is the abnormal neck posture. The head and neck are more extended than normal and have a stiff appearance. Careful palpation will diagnose this abnormality, given that no movement will be noted at the normal position of the atlantooccipital joint, and the normally palpable broad transverse processes (wings) of the atlas are reduced to small stubs of bone (Fig. 11-2). Radiographs will reveal the extent of the

(Continued)

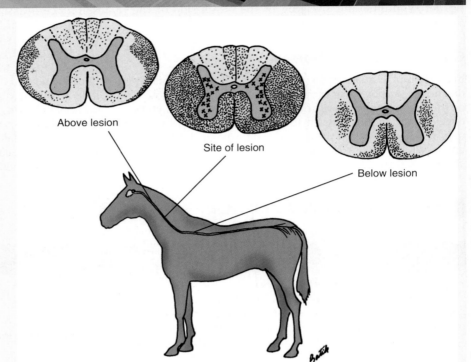

Above lesion

Site of lesion

Below lesion

FIGURE 11-1 The pattern of neuropathologic lesions that occur with compressive myelopathy associated with cervical vertebral malformation-malarticulation. The portions of the lesions in the transverse sections cranial and caudal to the focal compression reflect the Wallerian degeneration of the cranial and caudal projecting pathways, respectively.

malformation and a myelogram is necessary to diagnose the specific location and degree of spinal cord compression (Figs. 11-3, 11-4).

See **Video 11-2** that shows a 6-month-old Arabian with this malformation. Note the severe gait disorder, the extended neck posture, and the inability to flex the atlantooccipital joint

We have seen a variation of this malformation in one half-Arabian foal that remained recumbent after birth in which an attempt was made to develop two atlantes and two axes.[23] One atlas was reduced in size and fused to the occipital bone. The other atlas was approximately normal size and shape and articulated cranially with the occipitalized

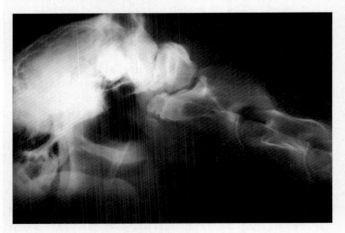

FIGURE 11-2 Lateral cervical radiograph of the 6-month-old Arabian seen in Video 11-2. Note the small atlas fused by fibrocartilage to the occipital bone. Note the elongated dens and cranial articular surface of the axis displaced ventral to the ventral arch (body) of the atlas. The radiodensity ventral to the displaced dens is ossification in the adjacent connective tissue.

atlas. It articulated caudally with an enlarged axis that had a very long narrow cranial portion in the position of the dens and cranial part of the body. Study of the numerous growth plates indicated the formation of two fused axial bodies. The elongated cranial portion projected into the vertebral canal and compressed the spinal cord.

Acquired Vertebral Malformation-Malarticulation

Acquired vertebral malformation-malarticulation is most commonly termed the *wobbler syndrome*.* Realistically, this term is nonspecific and should be avoided because any cervical spinal cord lesion will make a horse wobble! So many abbreviations have been used to indicate this disorder that they just cause confusion. Therefore we will avoid using any of these abbreviations in the following discussion. In our opinion, these acquired cervical vertebral malformations and malarticulations are primarily secondary to osteochondrosis, a common developmental bone disorder in rapidly growing animals such as the horse. This disorder is multifactorial, which has all the features that are so prominent in the race horse industry: (1) selecting for the genes, which will foster rapid growth, (2) providing feed that is high in calcium and energy to encourage this rapid growth, and (3) placing these animals as soon as possible into a vigorous training program to make them winners as 2-year-old horses. Nothing could be worse for these young athletes! Two forms of this vertebral disorder are observed: (1) a vertebral foramen stenosis in the younger horse and (2) a degenerative disorder of the synovial joints that is usually in older horses, but the age is quite variable here.

Stenosis

Stenosis of one or more vertebral foramina occurs in young horses from approximately 4 to 24 months of age. This abnormality is most

*References 26, 28, 34, 37, 55, 56, 61, 69, 71, 82-85.

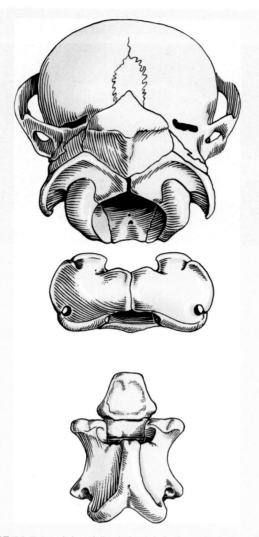

FIGURE 11-3 Dorsal view of disarticulated skull, atlas, and axis of a normal foal.

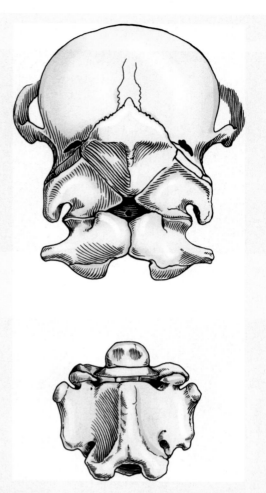

FIGURE 11-4 Dorsal view of the skull of an Arabian foal with OAAM with the small atlas fused to the occipital bone and the disarticulated axis with broad transverse processes. Note the small pointed transverse processes of the atlas. Palpation of these and the lack of atlantooccipital motion is supportive of this diagnosis.

common in male Thoroughbreds, but any breed and sex can be affected. As a rule, stenosis affects the middle cervical vertebra from C3 to C6 and is caused by failure of the bone that surrounds the vertebral foramen to resorb sufficiently to enlarge the foramen enough to accommodate the growing spinal cord (Figs. 11-5 through 11-8). Stenosis occurs at either end of the vertebral foramen or on both sides of the articulation. A prominent feature is the dorsal projection of the caudal epiphysis, which narrows the caudal opening of the vertebral foramen (Fig. 11-9). One or more vertebrae may be affected in a single horse. This lesion has been produced experimentally in Great Dane puppies fed an unrestricted diet, and it has been prevented in Thoroughbred foals by restricting their diet in its calcium and energy content, as well as volume, and restricting the foal's exercise.[28,56]

Two categories of this stenotic lesion have been described—a static form and a dynamic form. Normal functional anatomy and disease often defy strict classification, thus overlap is common here, but consideration of these two categories may help in determining what therapy to consider.

Static and Dynamic Stenosis

Static stenosis is indicated when myelographic evidence is found of significant spinal cord compression on both the normally extended

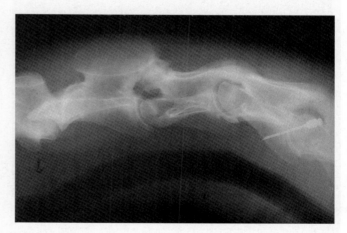

FIGURE 11-5 Lateral cervical radiograph of a 6-month-old Thoroughbred with a static stenosis at the C3-C4 articulation.

(Continued)

CASE EXAMPLE 11-1—cont'd

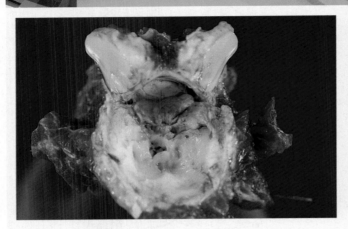

FIGURE 11-6 Caudal aspect of the C3 vertebra seen in the radiograph in Fig. 11-5 after disarticulation at necropsy. Note the compression of the spinal cord in the caudal orifice of the vertebral foramen.

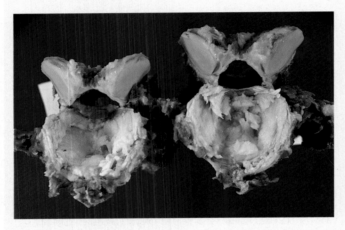

FIGURE 11-7 Caudal aspect of the C3 and C4 vertebrae from the horse in Fig. 11-5 after disarticulation and preservation. Note the narrow caudal orifice of the vertebral foramen of the C3 vertebra on the left compared with the normal caudal orifice of the C4 vertebral foramen on the right.

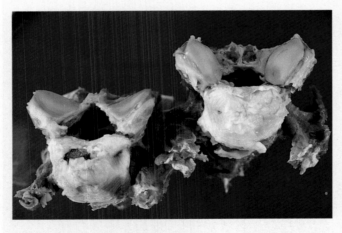

FIGURE 11-8 Cranial aspect of the C3 and C4 vertebrae from the horse in Fig. 11-5 after disarticulation and preservation. Note the narrow cranial orifice of the vertebral foramen of C4 on the right compared with the normal cranial orifice of the vertebral foramen of C3 on the left.

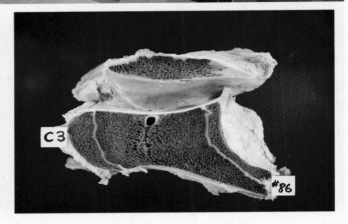

FIGURE 11-9 Section of the C3 vertebra on the median plane. Note the narrow caudal orifice of the vertebral foramen and the elevation of the vertebral body at the level of the caudal epiphysis.

(neutral) and the flexed radiographic views of the cervical vertebrae. Dynamic stenosis implies an instability at one or more articulations and is diagnosed when significant spinal cord compression is visible only on the radiographic view of the myelogram made when the neck is flexed. Several measurements have been described for determining whether a clinically significant stenosis is present in the cervical vertebrae. In many horses, this diagnosis can be made with lateral cervical vertebral radiographs of the standing horse that is lightly sedated with its neck in its normal resting position. Occasionally, the malarticulation is very severe and obvious without any measurements. More common are characteristics observed that suggest a stenosis, and these characteristics gain more significance in the presences of measurements that indicate a narrow vertebral canal at some point. The radiographic features that suggest a stenosis include:

1. A slight subluxation between vertebrae with increased flexion or dorsal angulation between adjacent vertebrae that is best seen between the bodies on either side of the intervertebral disk
2. A prominent caudal epiphysis that projects dorsally into the vertebral foramen
3. A caudal extension of the vertebral arch over the articulation (see Figs. 11-5 through 11-9)

The measurements of the size of the vertebral foramina are expressed as a ratio to prevent errors associated with the size of the patient and the distance between the origin of the x-rays and the patient. The minimal sagittal diameter for the vertebral foramen of a vertebra is made by measuring the height of the vertebral foramen at its most narrow point. The minimal sagittal diameter ratio is determined by dividing this measurement of the minimal sagittal diameter of the foramen by the maximal sagittal diameter of the vertebral body, which is at the cranial aspect of the vertebral body. These measurements must be made perpendicular to the ventral surface of the vertebral foramen. A study in 1994 considered a ratio below 0.52 for C4 and C5 and below 0.56 for C6 and C7 to be abnormal.[61] Greater ratio values are considered normal.

This radiographic study may be sufficient to make the presumptive diagnosis of cervical vertebral compressive myelopathy (see Fig. 11-5). If this diagnosis is less certain, or if surgical therapy is a consideration, cisternal myelography is required, and the patient must be placed under general anesthesia. Myelography is necessary to distinguish between a static and a dynamic stenosis. When viewing the myelogram, be aware that, in a lateral cervical vertebral radiograph with the neck flexed, the ventral contrast column will always be thinned over the articulations. This view clearly shows the large normal range of motion that occurs between adjacent cervical vertebrae. A rule of thumb that is often used as a guide is that most horses with a significant stenosis will exhibit a 50% decrease in the height of the dorsal contrast column at the articulation when compared with the height in the middle of the vertebral foramen. A recent study, which was correlated with a necropsy diagnosis of the lesion and its location, indicated that a 70% decrease was more reliable when the neck was flexed.[82] A more accurate measurement is to compare the total height of the dural tube (from the ventral surface of the ventral contrast column to the dorsal surface of the dorsal contrast column) where it is the smallest at the articulation with the same measurement of the maximal diameter of this tube in the middle of the vertebral foramen. A decrease of 20% or more at the articulation suggests a significant stenosis. In a static stenosis, evidence on a myelogram will show significant stenosis with the neck in its neutral extended position, as well as the flexed position. In a dynamic stenosis, significant stenosis is evident only on the flexed neck view. A dynamic stenosis may be prevented by surgical arthrodesis of the affected cervical vertebrae. Unfortunately at this time, magnetic resonance (MR) imaging is not routinely performed in horses because of their size.

Degenerative Joint Disease

DJD of the synovial joints at the articular processes is the other form of vertebral malformation-malarticulation that can result in spinal cord compression. This osteoarthropathy is more common in older horses but has been seen in yearlings. This lesion usually occurs in the more caudocervical vertebral articulations. We believe that this degeneration is the result of chronic malarticulation at these joints that represents the effects of osteochondrosis when these patients were young or an injury followed by malarticulation. This degeneration was observed in the study of the Great Dane puppies fed an unrestricted diet. Horses that have the stenotic or degenerative lesions have an increased incidence of osteochondrosis of synovial joints in their limbs. Spinal cord compression occurs when the proliferation of the articular processes and joint capsules extends into the vertebral foramen. Occasionally, a synovial cyst develops associated with the degenerate joint capsule and contributes to the compression. Because of their dorsolateral location, these osteoarthropic lesions may show evidence of spinal cord compression on myelograms with the neck extended. If this DJD only occurs on one side, the compression and the clinical signs may be mildly asymmetric. As a rule, when a horse exhibits discomfort on neck movements, this degenerative joint lesion is usually present (Figs. 11-10 through 11-16).

With either form of this malformation-malarticulation, the clinical signs may be sudden in onset and exhibit a variable progression, or the clinical signs may develop and progress slowly over a period of weeks to months. When they develop slowly, owners often believe their horse is lame from an orthopedic disorder. No medical therapy exists for these patients. For many years, surgical arthrodesis of the vertebral bodies has been used especially for the patients with a dynamic stenosis.[83-85] Arthrodesis has also been performed on horses with DJD to stop the movement at the joints that malarticulate, which provides opportunity for resolution of some of the soft- and hard-tissue proliferation. Surgery has been most effective for horses with the stenotic form of this disorder. Most surgeons believe they can improve the clinical signs by at least one grade, and numerous mildly affected racehorses have gone back to racing. Obviously, the owner needs to

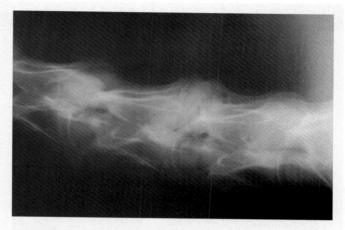

FIGURE 11-10 Lateral cervical radiograph of a 5-year-old Thoroughbred, showing DJD of the synovial joints at the C5-C6 articulation.

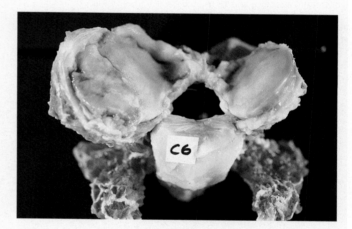

FIGURE 11-11 Cranial aspect of the disarticulated C6 vertebra of the horse in Fig. 11-10. Note the asymmetry of the articular processes, the disruption of the articular cartilage of the right cranial articular process and its thick joint capsule.

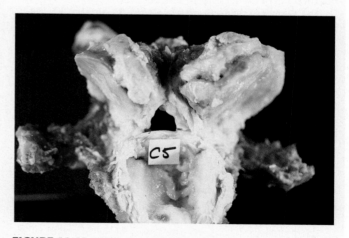

FIGURE 11-12 Caudal aspect of the disarticulated C5 vertebra of the horse in Fig. 11-10. This bone articulated with the bone in Fig. 11-11. Note the narrow caudal orifice of the vertebral foramen and the soft-tissue structure in this foramen on the right side, which is a synovial cyst.

(Continued)

CASE EXAMPLE 11-1—cont'd

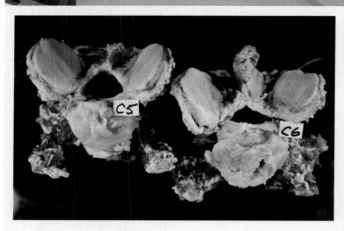

FIGURE 11-13 Disarticulated C5 and C6 vertebrae from a 2-year-old Thoroughbred with DJD of the synovial joints that caused a compressive myelopathy associated with the reduced size of the cranial orifice of the C6 vertebral foramen.

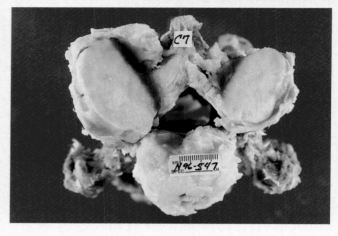

FIGURE 11-15 Cranial aspect of the C7 vertebra of the horse in Fig. 11-14. Note the narrowing of the right side of the cranial orifice of the vertebral foramen.

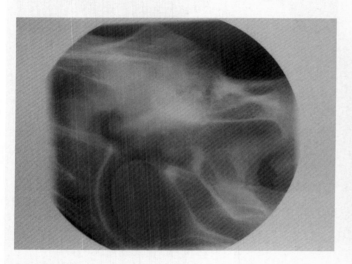

FIGURE 11-14 Lateral radiograph of the C6-C7 articulation in the 6-year-old Dutch Warmblood horse seen in Video 11-7. Note the extensive DJD of the synovial joints at the articular processes.

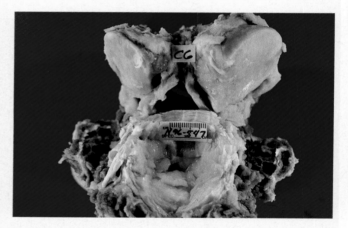

FIGURE 11-16 Caudal aspect of the disarticulated C6 vertebra of the horse in Fig. 11-14. Note the similar narrowing of the right side of the caudal orifice of the vertebral foramen related to the remarkably thickened right caudal articular process.

be informed of the potential danger associated with riding a patient who may appear to be recovered but may well have permanently lost enough axons at the site of the compression to cause the animal to stumble when in a stressful situation. A normal neurologic examination in no way guarantees a normal spinal cord! It is one thing to repair a large-breed dog surgically with this disorder so that it can walk up and down stairs without assistance, but a human life is put in danger when a surgically repaired horse is put back into service. On the racetrack, many human lives are put at risk when one of these operated horses is loaded into the starting gait. The veterinary surgeon, as well as the owner of the patient, must accept the responsibility for the consequences of this risk.

This disorder can be prevented by slowing the rate of growth of foals by altering their diet and structuring a less-vigorous training program while these horses are young. Can you imagine a racehorse trainer

recommending a restricted diet and less vigorous training program? Nonetheless, rest assured, it will work to reduce the occurrence of this disorder. A study was done on large breeding farms in Kentucky in which the foals were radiographed starting at 3 months of age.[28,56] Radiographic changes were graded, and horses that were considered to be at risk for developing this cervical vertebral disorder were placed on both a restricted diet and a restricted exercise program. These management changes resulted in a significant decrease in the incidence of this bone disorder on these farms.

EQUINE DEGENERATIVE MYELOENCEPHALOPATHY

Equine degenerative myeloencephalopathy is a diagnosis that is much less common than it was 10 to 15 years ago.* The two terms used to name this disease are redundant, given that a myeloencephalopathy

*References 22, 24, 25, 52, 54, 55, 60.

is a degeneration by strict definition. Nevertheless, we will keep this name to be consistent with the literature. The primary lesion is a diffuse axonopathy throughout the white matter of the spinal cord that predominates in the superficial tracts of the dorsolateral and the ventral funiculi, but all portions are affected with the least lesions in the dorsal funiculi (Fig. 11-17). This axonopathy is accompanied by a secondary demyelination and astrogliosis (Figs. 11-18 through 11-21). In addition, loss of neuronal cell bodies and spheroid development is extensive in the lateral cuneate nuclei, with variable spheroid development in the nucleus of the dorsal spinocerebellar tract (nucleus thoracicus) in the spinal cord dorsal gray column, nucleus gracilis, the medial cuneate nucleus, the olivary nuclei, reticular formation, and the vestibular nuclei in the brainstem. This brainstem nuclear lesion is the reason for including encephalopathy in the name of this disorder. In addition, an accumulation of lipopigment occurs in the endothelial cells of capillaries in the spinal cord and the pigment epithelium and outer layers of the retina, similar to older horses with motor neuron disease.[22] These lesions are now thought to be the result of a deficiency in the availability of vitamin E in the diet or a disorder in its metabolism. In addition, some evidence has been found to support a possible familial basis for this disorder.[48] On two large horse farms, the incidence of this disorder was significantly reduced when the pregnant mares and their foals were supplemented with vitamin E. Where serum vitamin E levels have been studied, these have only been reduced in clinically affected horses less than 1 year of age.[25] Foals raised in stables and on dirt paddocks with no access to green feed are at risk for developing this disorder. Young zebras raised in captivity in a similar environment have been diagnosed with this disorder.[60] As a rule, this lesion develops only in young horses. Older horses with vitamin E deficiency develop the GSE LMN degeneration of EMND. We believe that the remarkable decrease in this diagnosis parallels the decrease in the diagnosis of EMND because horse owners are more aware of the need for vitamin E supplementation, especially when a source of green feed is limited. Similar myelopathic lesions occur in nutritional deficiencies in other

species of domestic animal. A good example is copper deficiency in small ruminants. Copper levels are normal in the tissues of these affected horses. The onset of clinical signs in affected horses is reported to vary from birth to 2 years. However, most affected foals are only a few months of age when these clinical signs first occur in the pelvic limbs. Those horses considered to be first affected after 1 year of age may well have had prior clinical signs that were not recognized. The clinical signs of spastic paraparesis and pelvic limb ataxia slowly progress to the thoracic limbs. If an affected horse is monitored for many months, the progression seems to cease before the affected horse becomes unable to stand. These clinical signs are identical to those caused by the malformation-malarticulation disorder. Radiographs are required to diagnose the latter. No radiographic abnormalities are noted in the cervical vertebrae of horses with degenerative myeloencephalopathy. In a prolonged case of this disorder, a fundic examination may possibly show a yellow discoloration if the lipopigment accumulation in the retina has been extensive. Vitamin E supplementation of affected horses will stop the progression of the clinical signs but will not improve them because this condition is an axonopathy, which cannot resolve, nor can these axons be effectively replaced. The disorder can be prevented by supplementation of the pregnant mare and her foal at birth.

This diagnosis is very unlikely for the Thoroughbred in this case example because of the sudden onset of clinical signs in a 2-year-old horse. Only the anatomic diagnosis is compatible.

See **Video 11-3**. This video shows is a 1-year-old female Arabian horse that has had a recognizable gait abnormality that has been slowly progressing for 6 months. Radiographic study of the cervical vertebrae was normal. She was euthanized, and degenerative myeloencephalopathy was confirmed at necropsy.

Equine protozoal myelitis is the most common inflammatory disease of the central nervous system (CNS) of horses, especially the spinal cord. It can occur anywhere in the spinal cord with lesions in white and gray matter. It often has a multifocal distribution.

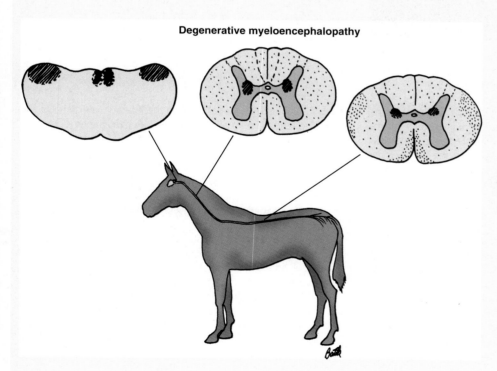

Degenerative myeloencephalopathy

FIGURE 11-17 The pattern of the neuropathologic lesions of equine degenerative myeloencephalopathy.

(Continued)

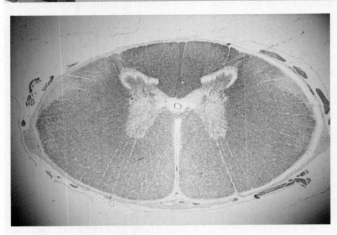

FIGURE 11-18 Microscopic transverse section of a midthoracic spinal cord segment of a horse with degenerative myeloencephalopathy stained with Luxol fast blue for myelin. Note the bilateral symmetry of the secondary demyelination of the superficial tracts in the lateral and ventral funiculi. The myelin has been replaced by astrogliosis.

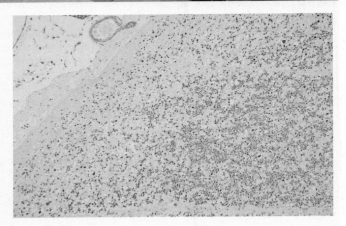

FIGURE 11-20 Microscopic section of the same site as Fig. 11-19 with an immunocytochemical stain for neurofilaments. Note the reduction of axons where the myelin was depleted in Fig. 11-19.

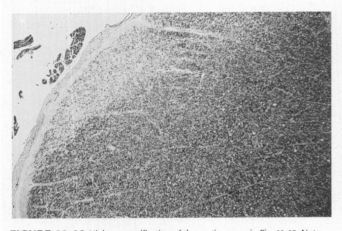

FIGURE 11-19 Higher magnification of the section seen in Fig. 11-18. Note the secondary demyelination and astrogliosis in the area of the superficial tracts in one dorsolateral funiculus. These would predominantly be spinocerebellar tracts.

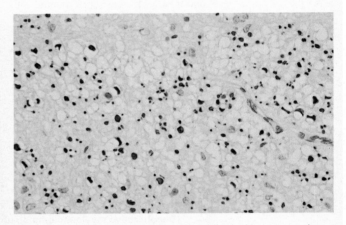

FIGURE 11-21 Higher magnification of the section in Fig. 11-20. Note the reduction of axons. The intervening nonstained tissue consists of astrocytic processes.

If these inflammatory lesions occurred bilaterally in one cervical spinal cord segment or were randomly scattered through several cervical spinal cord segments so that both sides were affected at some point between the C1 and C5 spinal cord segments, the clinical signs would be compatible with those observed in this case example. This protozoal disease is described in Case Example 11-2.

DISKOSPONDYLITIS

Diskospondylitis is a disease most commonly observed in foals that have experienced a bacterial infection and have been septic. Although this disease can occur at any level in the vertebral column, the caudal cervical vertebrae appear to be at some risk for this infection.

The mass effect of the abscess associated with this infection or the subluxation of the unstable fibrocartilaginous joint causes spinal cord compression. These foals usually hold their neck stiff and exhibit discomfort when the neck is handled. They often have a fever and may have neutrophilia in their complete blood count (CBC). Cerebrospinal

fluid (CSF) is usually normal because the infection is external to the dura. The lesion can usually be observed on radiographs. Computed tomographic (CT) and MR imaging can also be used to make the diagnosis if the foal is small enough. If you use general anesthesia for restraint, be extremely cautious of manipulating the neck of these patients because the involved articulation will be very unstable when muscle tone is absent. This diagnosis would be unlikely in the horse in this case example because of its age and lack of any systemic clinical signs of an infection.

See **Video 11-4** of Gabriel. This video shows a 1-month-old Percheron colt that became lame at 3 days of age with a swollen tarsus and he had a fever. Suppurative tarsitis was diagnosed, and he improved on antibiotic therapy. Ten days later the fever returned. He had difficulty standing, and his gait became stiff. Study the video, and make your anatomic diagnosis. The anatomic diagnosis was a focal or diffuse spinal cord lesion between the C1 and C5 segments. The radiographs and CT scans (see video) show a diskospondylitis at the C6-C7 articulation. The CT images are from the middle of C5 to the middle of C7. Note the subluxation on the CT reconstruction. The foal was unable to stand after this procedure, and the subluxation likely occurred during the CT procedure when the foal was anesthetized. The lateral radiographic view of this standing foal was sufficient to make this clinical diagnosis. The clinical signs showed the compressive effect of the infection on the white matter at this site and not the gray matter.

Radiographs of the horse in this case example revealed a stenosis between the C3 and C4 cervical vertebrae and DJD of the synovial joints at the C5-C6 articulation. A myelogram showed spinal cord compression related to the DJD at the C5-C6 articulation. Surgical arthrodesis of the vertebral bodies was performed at this articulation. No follow-up results are available.

See the following videos to appreciate the clinical signs of equine cervical vertebral malformation-malarticulation in several horses. After studying these videos, you should feel comfortable in recognizing the anatomic diagnosis of a C1-C5 spinal cord lesion.

 Video 11-5 shows a 4.5-month-old Quarter horse colt that was found down suddenly in the paddock 3 weeks before this examination. A gait abnormality was recognized when he was assisted to stand, and this abnormality had progressed slightly since then. The radiographs with a myelogram (see video) show a dynamic stenosis at the C3-C4 and C4-C5 articulations, but especially the latter, where the total dural tube diameter is reduced in size greater than 20% when the neck is flexed.

Video 11-6 shows a 1-year-old Standardbred colt with an abnormal gait that was found when he was on pasture. These clinical signs may have been present and not recognized for a few days. He was placed in a stall, and the clinical signs became worse over the week before he was presented for this examination. Radiographs showed abnormal vertebral foramina measurements, indicating stenosis at the C3-C4 and C4-C5 articulations and DJD at the C6-C7 articulation. No myelogram was performed because the owner did not consider surgery as an option. The horse was euthanized, and at necropsy, a compressive myelopathy was found in the spinal cord at the site of the C4-C5 articulation.

 Video 11-7 shows a 6-year-old Dutch Warmblood mare with a very slowly progressive gait disorder for 6 months. For the first few months, only an orthopedic disorder in the pelvic limbs was considered but could not be diagnosed. Acupuncture, chiropractic adjustments, and corticosteroid injections into the epaxial muscles were all ineffective. On the video, the gait disorder obviously represents a dysfunction of the UMN and GP systems in the cervical spinal cord. Radiographs (see video) show DJD at the C5-C6 and C6-C7 articulations. This horse was euthanized, and a necropsy diagnosis was made of a compressive myelopathy at the level of the C6-C7 articulation (see Figs. 11-14 through 11-16).

 Video 11-8 shows a 6-year-old Thoroughbred gelding that fell on an icy road 10 months before this examination. A gait abnormality was observed approximately 5 months later and had been slowly progressing since that time. Radiographs (see video) showed mild DJD at the C4-C5 articulation and severe degenerative synovial joint lesions at the C5-C6 articulation. He was euthanized, and a necropsy showed a compressive myelopathy at the level of the C5-C6 articulation. In this horse, the initial fall may have injured these articular processes, which caused malarticulation and the subsequent development of these degenerative lesions.

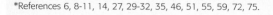

CASE EXAMPLE 11-2

Signalment: 14-month-old Thoroughbred colt, Twain

History: Eleven days before this examination, this colt suddenly became lame in the right thoracic limb, and a shoulder or radial nerve injury was suspected. However, the clinical signs worsened and included abnormal use of the right pelvic limb.

Examination: See **Video 11-9**. When this horse was circled to its right, you sensed that he might fall on you because of lack of normal support in the right thoracic limb. Note the occasional tendency to buckle in the right thoracic limb and the way he flips the digit forward to land on the sole of the hoof. This is different from overreaching with the limb in extension.

Anatomic Diagnosis: Focal lesion in the right C6 to T2 spinal cord segments

The right thoracic limb clinical signs were predominantly that of a LMN paresis and ataxia. The actions described previously reflected a partial deficiency of radial nerve function. The right pelvic limb clinical signs were all caused by UMN paresis and GP ataxia.

Differential Diagnosis: Equine protozoal myelitis (EPM), cervical vertebral malformation-malarticulation, equine degenerative myelo-encephalopathy, diskospondylitis

External injury, fibrocartilaginous embolic myelopathy, and equine herpesvirus-1 myelopathy were not considered because of the history of progressive clinical signs. Neoplasia was not considered because of the age of this horse and the rarity of this particular diagnosis in the equine CNS. Equine viral myelitis was considered unlikely because of the focal nature of the clinical signs limited to the spinal cord and the duration of clinical signs for rabies and Eastern equine viral encephalitis.

EPM is the most presumptive clinical diagnosis for this Thoroughbred, primarily because of the asymmetry of the clinical signs that included involvement of the gray matter (LMN). This degree of asymmetry would be very unusual for a malformation-malarticulation disorder. Unilateral DJD of a synovial joint may cause a mild asymmetry but not to this degree and not with the LMN clinical signs because of gray matter involvement. Sudden onset, asymmetric signs, and clinical signs of gray matter disease do not occur in degenerative myeloencephalopathy. The asymmetry, age, lack of discomfort, and lack of fever would make a diskospondylitis unlikely.

EQUINE PROTOZOAL MYELITIS

EPM and encephalitis is the most common CNS inflammatory disease in the horse (Fig. 11-22).* Estimates suggest that approximately 50% of all horses in the United Sates are infected based on serum antibody assays for what presumably is the most common protozoal agent involved, *Sarcocystis neurona*. The incidence varies among states,

---

*References 6, 8-11, 14, 27, 29-32, 35, 46, 51, 55, 59, 72, 75.

(Continued)

CASE EXAMPLE 11-2—cont'd

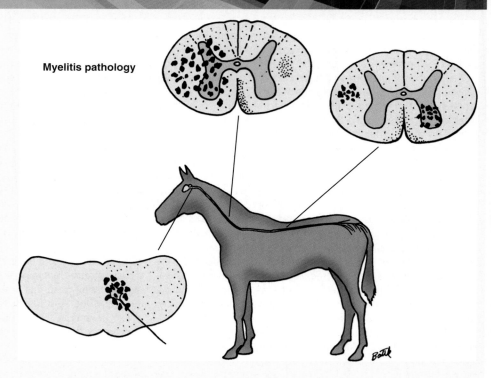

Myelitis pathology

FIGURE 11-22 The pattern of the neuropathologic lesions of EPM and encephalitis.

and, in some areas, the incidence increases to 80% in older horses. Antibody levels increase with the age of the horse, suggesting reexposure to the protozoa or the horse has a chronic persistent infection that continually stimulates the immune system and places this horse at risk for clinical illness.[10] *Neospora hughesi* has also been implicated in a few horses, primarily in the West Coast states.[51] This disease is not contagious as it cannot be passed directly between horses.

The normal life cycle of *S. neurona* requires a primary and intermediate host. The most recent field and laboratory studies implicate the opossum as the most likely primary host. This assumption correlates well with the disease being limited to the Americas, where the opossum is also located. This disease is not seen in European horses that have not traveled to the Americas. Several species of North and South American opossums have been identified as its definitive host. The natural intermediate hosts that have been identified include the raccoon, striped skunk, and nine-banded armadillo. The horse is an aberrant intermediate host in which the life cycle cannot be completed. In the normal life cycle, the *S. neurona* merozoite that is encysted in the muscle of the intermediate host is ingested by the opossum, where it invades the intestinal epithelium. Sexual reproduction takes place in this epithelium, resulting in the production of oocysts, which enter the intestinal lumen and sporulate to form sporocysts. Each sporocyst forms four sporozoites and passes in the feces into the external environment, where they are ingested by the intermediate host. The sporozoite invades the intestinal epithelium and associated arterial endothelial cells of the intermediate host. Asexual reproduction by schizogony takes place in these endothelial cells, resulting in the production of merozoites that are released into the bloodstream and migrate to the muscles where they encyst. When the intermediate host dies and the muscles are eaten by the opossum, the cycle is completed. The horse becomes infected when

it eats feed that has been contaminated by the feces of the opossum that contain infective sporozoites. These sporozoites are presumed to invade the intestinal epithelium. Where asexual reproduction occurs and how the organism reaches the CNS is unknown. Schizogony is seen in the CNS, but whether it also occurs in intestinal or other extraneural vascular endothelium is unknown. Merozoites have occasionally been found in CNS endothelial cells. Cysts have not been reported in the muscles of the horse, but these have not been adequately studied for this possibility. The assumption is that the CNS infection is usually hematogenous, with merozoites circulating free in the bloodstream or in infected lymphocytes. However, some unique cases have been found in which focal motor nuclear lesions in the CNS make a route over peripheral nerves that innervate infected muscle a strong possibility. See Case Example 6-2. *N. hughesi* presumably has a similar life cycle involving primary and intermediate hosts that have yet to be identified.

All breeds of horses are susceptible to this infection. The few horses that develop lesions are thought to have been subject to some form of stress such as transportation, training, showing, pregnancy, or some other change in their environment that might lead to stress-related immunosuppression. The last of these circumstances is a common factor in protozoan infections. Both humoral and cellular immunity are thought to be involved in the resistance of the horse to the development of lesions. The disease occurs at any age, but it is most common in the young adult between 1 and 5 years of age. The onset of clinical signs is variable from acute with a rapidly progressive course to slow, followed by a chronically progressive, course. The former is more common. The clinical signs are extremely variable because they depend on the anatomic location of the lesions in the CNS. The acute lesion consists of a nonsuppurative inflammation with parenchymal necrosis associated with extensive edema and occasionally hemorrhage. This may be extensive enough to be observed on transverse sections of the preserved brain and spinal cord as a gross enlargement and discoloration of the affected site in the CNS. The inflammation is mostly lymphoplasmacytic with numerous macrophages and scattered eosinophils, neutrophils, and multinucleated giant cells. Astrocytic scarring is common in chronic lesions. In untreated horses, the merozoites and schizonts may be found in macrophages and neurons or occasionally free in the parenchyma (Figs. 11-23 through 11-32). Immunocytochemistry is now available to confirm this diagnosis and differentiate *S. neurona* from the much less common *N. hughesi*. The lesion is often well developed in one area of the CNS, where parenchymal necrosis is extensive, but the inflammation may also be quite widespread in the meninges and parenchyma without necrosis. Lesions occur in both the gray matter, as well as the white matter, and are often asymmetric in distribution. Occasionally, the lesion is almost limited to the gray matter, which may result in an observable area of focal muscle atrophy. Asymmetry of clinical signs and focal muscle atrophy are clinical signs that are highly suggestive of this diagnosis. The most common location of the lesion is in the spinal cord followed by the

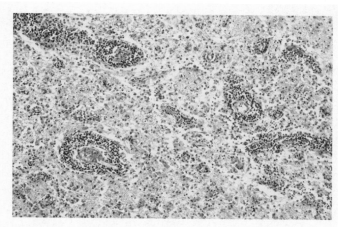

FIGURE 11-25 Higher magnification of the area seen in Fig. 11-24. Note the thick perivascular cuffs and the extensive inflammation throughout the white matter parenchyma.

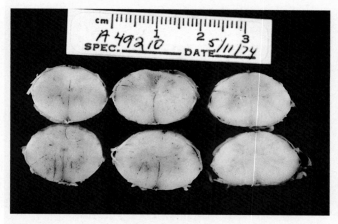

FIGURE 11-23 Transverse sections of preserved thoracolumbar spinal cord segments from a 2-year-old Standardbred with progressive spastic paraparesis and pelvic limb ataxia. The two transverse sections on the right are grossly normal. Note the discoloration of the other transverse sections due to extensive inflammation seen in the next five figures.

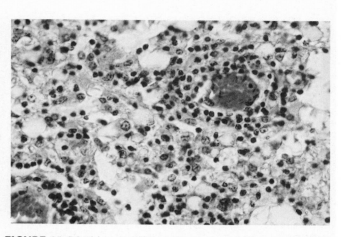

FIGURE 11-26 Higher magnification of the area seen in Fig. 11-25. Note the nonsuppurative quality of the inflammation.

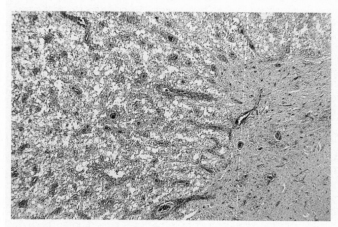

FIGURE 11-24 Microscopic section of the L3 spinal cord transverse section present in Fig. 11-23. Note the extensive inflammation in the deep portion of one lateral funiculus and the adjacent gray matter.

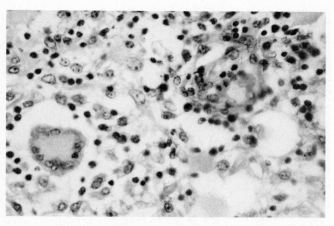

FIGURE 11-27 Higher magnification of the area seen in Fig. 11-25. Note the multinucleated giant cell in the nonsuppurative inflammation.

(Continued)

CASE EXAMPLE 11-2—cont'd

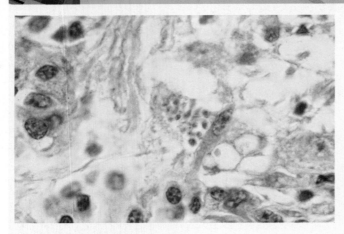

FIGURE 11-28 Higher magnification of the area seen in Fig. 11-25. Note the collection of protozoal agents.

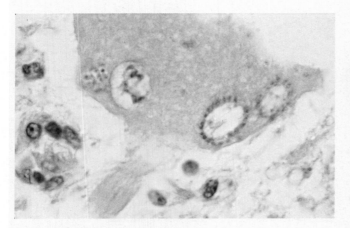

FIGURE 11-29 A neuronal cell body in the spinal cord gray matter of a horse with protozoal myelitis. Note the axon hillock and the four intracytoplasmic structures. The two on the right are protozoal schizonts (asexual division). On the left of the hillock is the nucleus, and next to that is a collection of protozoal organisms that probably consists of merozoites on the margin of a schizont.

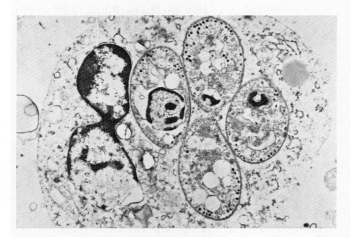

FIGURE 11-30 Electron photomicrograph of a macrophage in the spinal cord of a horse with protozoal myelitis containing four merozoites.

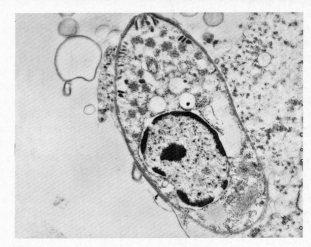

FIGURE 11-31 Electron photomicrograph of a single merozoite in the spinal cord lesion of a horse with protozoal myelitis.

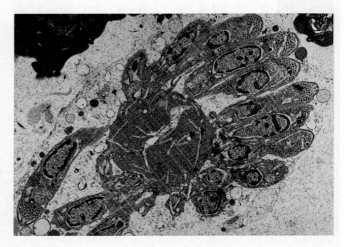

FIGURE 11-32 Electron photomicrograph of a protozoal schizont in the process of endopolygeny to produce merozoites by asexual reproduction. These three electron photomicrographs were made in 1975 before this protozoal agent was identified as *S. neurona*.

caudal brainstem; it is least common in the prosencephalon. As with most inflammatory diseases, the anatomic diagnosis is completely dependent on the location of the lesion in the CNS, and the differential diagnosis depends entirely on the anatomic diagnosis.

CSF is often normal despite the presence of inflammation in the leptomeninges. Occasionally, mild elevations are noted in protein and lymphocytes and macrophages. A polymerase chain reaction (PCR) test on the CSF for this organism's DNA will be positive only in the small percentage of horses in which the organism is present in the subarachnoid space. Therefore the PCR test is impractical. Western blot immunoassay for antibodies in the CSF is usually positive for horses with this disease, but false positives are common because obtaining a CSF sample from the lumbosacral subarachnoid space without some blood contamination is difficult. This test will be positive for the serum antibodies in the CSF if the blood contamination is so small that the CSF only contains eight red blood cells (RBCs)/mm[3].[59] This factor makes the interpretation of any antibodies in the CSF unreliable. Cisternal CSF is less likely to have blood contamination but requires general anesthesia to obtain. Remember that many horses are infected and have serum antibodies but only a very few have the disease and produce intrathecal antibodies. The absence of any serum antibodies makes the presence of this disease highly unlikely. Be aware that these antibodies are passively transferred from the mare to her foal in the colostrum, and up to 9 months may be required for these serum antibodies to disappear from the foal's serum, although the mean time is 4.5 months.[13] After infection, these antibodies can be detected for many years, even after removal from an endemic area. No definitive antemortem test exists for the diagnosis of this inflammatory disease. The antemortem diagnosis is most dependent on the presence of serum antibodies for *S. neurona*, the anatomic diagnosis, and the best judgment of the experienced clinician. Difficulty occurs when horses are presented for subtle gait abnormalities in which the orthopedic examination is unrewarding. Many of these horses have been treated for protozoal myelitis with or without finding antibodies for *S. neurona* in CSF from a lumbosacral sample that is frequently blood contaminated. We firmly believe that this diagnosis has often been made without justification because treatment is available. However, we also recognize that obtaining this justification is sometimes very difficult. Treatment consists of the oral administration of folate inhibitor drugs. The most common of these has been a combination of sulfadiazine and pyrimethamine. More recently, this combination has been replaced by one of the following antiprotozoal drugs: pontazuril, diclazuril, toltrazuril, or nitazoxanide. Intravenous dimethyl sulfoxide is often used to reduce the vasogenic edema in acutely affected horses. Success of treatment depends on the severity and location of the lesions. Published results suggest that approximately 60% of horses with moderate to severe clinical signs will improve after treatment with any of the approved medications, and 10% to 20% will make a complete recovery. Long-term therapy for 3 to 6 months may be necessary to prevent relapses. Some investigators have recommended following the recovery with repeated analysis of the CSF for antibodies and terminating the treatment when these disappear from the CSF. However, the common contamination of the CSF with serum antibodies makes this recommendation difficult to support. Owners must be advised of the risk of using any presumably recovered patient for riding activity! Prevention of this disease depends on avoiding exposure to opossums and their fecal contamination of the feed. Although this goal is difficult to achieve on pastures, at least the stored hay and grain can usually be protected from this source of contamination. A vaccine is available.

For other examples of horses with clinical signs of myelitis caused by *S. neurona*, see Video 5-52 in Chapter 5 and Video 6-11 in Chapter 6.

Video 11-10 shows an 18-month-old Standardbred mare that suddenly became lame in the right thoracic limb 10 days before this examination. Within a few days the gait was abnormal in the right pelvic limb. She occasionally fell when she moved suddenly to her right side, and she needed assistance to stand. The day before this examination, it was noted that she would sweat on the entire right side of her body, including the head. (See Figs. 7-22 through 7-24 in Chapter 7.) Note that the gait abnormality in this horse in Video 11-10 is similar to that of this case example (Video 11-9). In addition, whole-body sweating was noted on the right side and a mild atrophy of the right lateral scapular muscles. The anatomic diagnosis is the same as this case example (focal C6-T2). The whole-body, right-side sweating is the result of a loss of the sympathetic system UMN pathways in the right lateral funiculus. The age of the horse and the sudden onset of asymmetric clinical signs, including muscle atrophy, all make protozoal myelitis the most presumptive diagnosis and justifies therapy. With no response to treatment after 7 days, this mare was euthanized, and a necropsy confirmed the diagnosis of protozoal myelitis lesions primarily on the right side of the C6-C8 spinal cord segments.

Video 11-11 shows Duke, a 4-year-old castrated male Belgian, that suddenly had difficulty walking. Duke was kept out on pasture during the day with three other Belgians and was brought into the barn in the evenings. One evening, he did not show up at the pasture gate with the others and was found reluctant to move, and when urged, his gait was abnormal. The video was made the next day. Note the right hemiparesis and ataxia, similar to this case example (Video 11-9) and the horse in Video 11-10. The anatomic diagnosis was a focal or diffuse lesion on the right side of the cervical spinal cord, but we debated whether the cervical intumescence was involved. The right thoracic limb clinical signs probably represent a combination of LMN and UMN and GP system dysfunction. Less tendency to overreach with that limb than to have difficulty supporting weight was noted.

With no more than 1 day of clinical signs, considering progression of signs in the differential diagnosis was impossible. Therefore the differential diagnosis would include those described for this case example, as well as the acute, nonprogressive disorders related to infection with the equine herpesvirus-1 or ischemic myelopathy caused by fibrocartilaginous emboli. Neck injury in a horse of this size was considered highly unlikely. Duke's function was to pull wagons and sleighs filled with adults and children for various celebrations. The owner believed that the liability was too great to continue to use Duke regardless of the outcome of his clinical signs, and he was euthanized. At necropsy, numerous foci of ischemic myelopathy were present in the right side of the C6-C8 spinal cord segments associated with fibrocartilaginous emboli in small arteries. Not enough is known about this syndrome in the horse to predict the outcome.[78] However, in dogs, many of these patients will spontaneously make a full recovery.

CASE EXAMPLE 11-3

Signalment: 15-year-old female Quarter horse, Furlong
Chief Complaint: Difficulty walking with the pelvic limbs
History: Furlong was used as a school horse in the morning. Late that afternoon, she suddenly began to sway and stumble in the pelvic limbs. She was hospitalized late that evening.

Examination: See **Video 11-12** made 8 hours after the sudden onset without any significant change in the clinical signs. The examination was limited by the severity of her pelvic limb paresis and ataxia. Note the hypotonic tail and anus. During the examination, urine was excreted in brief bursts. On rectal examination a distended bladder was palpated.

(Continued)

CASE EXAMPLE 11-3—cont'd

Anatomic Diagnosis: Focal or diffuse lesion between the T3 and L3 spinal cord segments and the sacrocaudal segments

The thoracic limbs appeared to be normal. The sacrocaudal clinical signs were mild.

Differential Diagnosis: Equine herpesvirus-1 myelopathy, EPM, fibrocartilaginous embolic myelopathy, viral myelitis (rabies, West Nile)

The environment of this horse excluded consideration of an external injury. Neoplasia affecting the spinal cord of horses is rare and less likely to cause such an acute onset of clinical signs. A sudden intervertebral disk extrusion is also very rare in adult horses. Diskospondylitis is more common in foals and less likely to cause a sudden onset of clinical signs.

EQUINE HERPESVIRUS-1 MYELOPATHY

Equine herpesvirus-1 myelopathy is the most presumptive clinical diagnosis. This viral strain is the most common cause of a vasculitis that affects the blood vessels of the CNS and reproductive tract of adult horses.* The latter results in abortion. Clinical signs of involvement of the respiratory system with rhinopneumonitis are occasionally found. Equine herpesvirus-4 is the common cause of rhinopneumonitis in young horses. Spinal cord lesions and clinical signs are the most common when the nervous system is affected by equine herpesvirus-1. Brainstem and prosencephalic lesions and clinical signs do occur but are rare. Clinical signs are always acute in onset and rarely progress for more than 2 to 3 days, which is typical for a vascular compromise. The clinical signs are usually symmetric, but asymmetric signs can occur as well. Viremia follows infection via the respiratory system, and infected leucocytes circulate to the vasculature of the nervous system. The primary viral-induced lesion is the result of this virus infecting the endothelial cells of the blood vessels in the nervous system, resulting in vasculitis and thrombosis. This vascular compromise causes ischemic or hemorrhagic degeneration (myelopathy) of the nervous system parenchyma. Inflammation is confined to the blood vessels, primarily in the leptomeninges. The clinical signs usually reflect the white matter lesions, which, in Furlong, the mare in this case example, were most severe in the thoracolumbar spinal cord segments. The severity of the clinical signs is determined by the summation of the ischemic lesions that are scattered through the white matter of the spinal cord. Individual ischemic lesions often have a linear appearance in the white matter that corresponds to the area supplied by a compromised penetrating artery from the vascular plexus on the surface of the spinal cord. See Fig. 10-4 for the anatomy of the spinal cord blood supply and Figs. 11-33 through 11-41 for the lesions. Mild sacrocaudal signs are common with this disorder but are difficult to correlate with lesions in these segments. The incontinence more likely reflects the involvement of the spinal cord tracts necessary for micturition, but the hypotonia and possibly hypalgesia of the tail, anus, and perineum remain poorly explained. Cervical spinal cord lesions cause spastic tetraparesis and ataxia similar to horses with the malformation-malarticulation disorder. When cervical spinal cord lesions are extensive, the patient will go down and be unable to stand (see Fig. 11-38). Once this recumbency occurs, the horse is rarely able to stand again. Horses that remain standing after 3 days have a fair to good prognosis for spontaneous recovery. This status probably reflects the absence of ischemic necrosis (infarction) and the resolution of edema that may have developed at the sites of the ischemia. The severity of the clinical signs and the prognosis reflect

*References 7, 13, 38, 39, 41-43, 49, 68, 74.

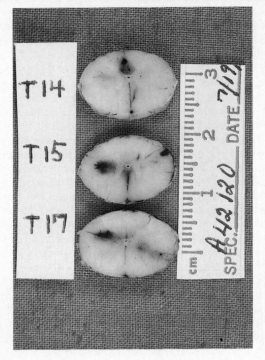

FIGURE 11-33 Transverse sections of the preserved spinal cord from a 4-year-old horse with the clinical diagnosis of equine herpesvirus-1 myelopathy. Note the linear nature of the discolorations that represent ischemic and hemorrhagic infarction in the territory supplied by the penetrating arteries in which vasculitis and thrombosis has occurred primarily in the meningeal vascular plexus. Note this normal vascular pattern in Fig. 10-4.

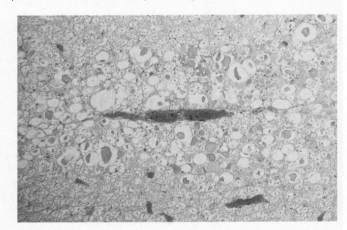

FIGURE 11-34 Microscopic section of one of these ischemic infarcts. Note the orientation of the lesion along the blood vessel, the numerous spheroids (axonal swellings), and the swelling of the myelin sheaths. Note the lack of inflammation, which is usually limited to the wall of the blood vessels in the meninges.

the degree of vascular compromise to the CNS parenchyma. In mild cases that improve rapidly in approximately 7 days, the clinical signs may reflect only dysfunction in axonal depolarization caused by the energy loss as a result of the ischemia. With more severe ischemia, edema and axonal spheroids develop in the parenchyma, which

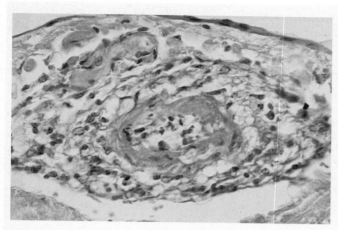

FIGURE 11-35 Microscopic section of a meningeal artery exhibiting vasculitis and vessel wall degeneration.

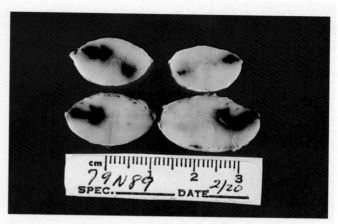

FIGURE 11-38 Transverse sections of preserved cervical, thoracic, and lumbar spinal cord segments from an adult horse with the clinical diagnosis of equine herpesvirus-1 myelopathy. This horse became recumbent over a 12-hour period.

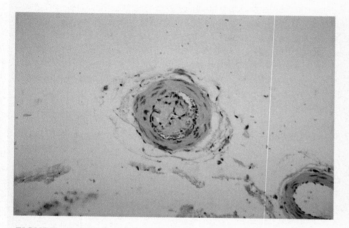

FIGURE 11-36 Microscopic section of a meningeal artery containing a thrombus.

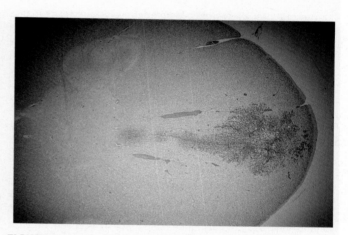

FIGURE 11-39 Microscopic section of a hemorrhagic infarct in the spinal cord of the horse in Fig. 11-38.

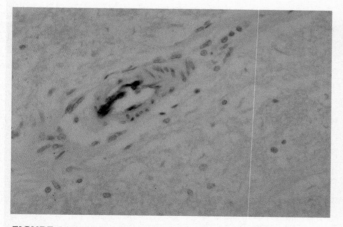

FIGURE 11-37 Microscopic section of a meningeal artery stained immunocytochemically for equine herpesvirus-1, which is visible in the endothelium of the vessel wall.

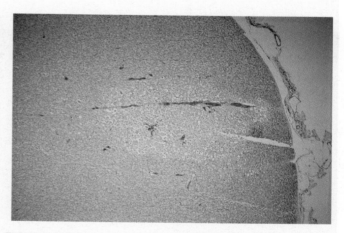

FIGURE 11-40 Microscopic section of an ischemic infarct in the spinal cord of the horse in Fig. 11-38.

(Continued)

CASE EXAMPLE 11-3—cont'd

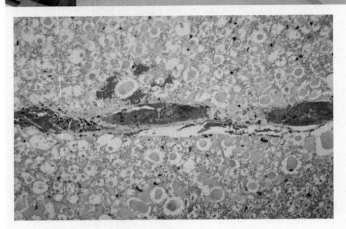

FIGURE 11-41 Higher magnification of the ischemic infarct in Fig. 11-40. Note the numerous spheroids.

may resolve over a few weeks. More extensive vascular compromise results in infarction, which is permanent. Most infected horses are mildly depressed. This disease often affects multiple horses on the same premises, and be aware that if you hospitalize such a horse, you place your other hospitalized patients at risk for this infection. Isolating infected patients is extremely important because they can readily pass the virus to other horses in aerosols of nasopharyngeal secretions or on feed, equipment, or the hands and clothes of individuals contaminated by these secretions that are in their environment. Fever commonly precedes and may accompany the clinical signs of CNS infection and may be useful in determining early infection of a horse before the onset of clinical signs.

Diagnosis can be supported by demonstrating the presence of viral DNA or antigen in the buffy coat of serum or nasal secretions by PCR evaluation. Virus may be isolated from nasopharyngeal secretions. CSF often is xanthochromic, with an elevated protein level and a normal to slight elevation of the leucocyte count. No evidence-based data have been found to support specific antiviral therapy. Nursing care with special attention to the evacuation of urine is the most effective treatment. The results of vaccination to prevent the neurologic form of this disease have not been satisfactory.

When an outbreak occurs on a farm, 1 to 6 weeks may pass before the clinical signs are seen in the last horse to be infected. Be aware that this virus often causes a persistent infection that may reactivate when the infected horse is stressed by such activities as excessive athletic exercise, transportation, or changes in farm management. Recrudescence may occur in a horse that has recovered from the clinical signs of this infection in its nervous system.

EPM is a strong candidate for the anatomic diagnosis in Furlong. It can be ruled down by isolation of equine herpesvirus-1 or identifying its DNA in nasal secretions or the absence of antibodies in the serum for *S. neurona*. The combination of a gait disorder typical of a lesion in the T3 to L3 spinal cord segments plus urinary incontinence and mild tail and anal hypotonia is very characteristic of a mild to moderate infection with the equine herpesvirus-1 virus. As a rule, you would expect the clinical signs of a protozoal infection to continue to progress after the onset.

Fibrocartilaginous embolic myelopathy (FCEM) causes a similar ischemic or hemorrhagic myelopathy of a few adjacent spinal cord segments with a sudden onset of clinical signs that rarely progress after 24 hours. It occurs in adult horses but is rare and would unlikely cause the unique anatomic diagnosis, as observed in Furlong. In addition, no fever is noted in animals that have FCEM, and multiple animals are not affected on the same farm, as often happens with equine herpesvirus-1 myelopathy. No ancillary procedure has been developed to support the diagnosis of FCEM in this horse because this region cannot be reliably imaged.

Viral myelitis must be an initial consideration before you have time to observe whether the clinical signs will be progressive. Rapid progression to recumbency in 4 to 5 days would be expected with rabies myelitis. West Nile viral myelitis usually causes progressive clinical signs, but this circumstance can vary considerably between infected horses. The most reliable way to rule down these causes of viral myelitis is to determine the presence of the equine herpesvirus-1 virus in the patient.

The horse in this case example did not improve over the next few days and was euthanized. A necropsy confirmed the diagnosis of ischemic myelopathy associated with vasculitis with herpesvirus-1 identified in the endothelial cells by immunocytochemistry.

CASE EXAMPLE 11-4

Signalment: 14-year-old female Oldenburgh Warmblood, Charisma
Chief Complaint: Abnormal pelvic limb gait
History: Charisma was a grand prix jumper whose performance began to decrease 3 months before this examination, and her pelvic limb function began to deteriorate at that time. All orthopedic examinations were normal.
 Examination: See **Video 11-13**. Note that the thoracic limbs are normal, and if you were leading this horse, you would better appreciate the severity of the pelvic limb paresis and ataxia. If this horse were turned vigorously, she would go down and need help to stand.
Anatomic Diagnosis: Focal or diffuse spinal cord lesion between the T3 and L3 spinal cord segments
Differential Diagnosis: Neoplasm-melanoma, EPM, intervertebral disk extrusion-protrusion, diskospondylitis

Equine herpesvirus-1 myelopathy and FCEM were excluded only because they cause an acute onset of nonprogressive neurologic

signs. The prolonged course of this anatomic diagnosis made a viral myelitis most unlikely.

NEOPLASM-MELANOMA AT T17

Metastatic melanoma is the most presumptive clinical diagnosis for Charisma based on her age, color, and primarily the presence of melanomas in her perineal area.[79] Other extramedullary neoplasms compressing the spinal cord are uncommon.[80] In the absence of these recognizable melanomas, a slowly progressing protozoal myelitis would be a strong consideration, providing that she had serum antibodies for *S. neurona*. Intervertebral disk extrusion-protrusion is rare in horses, even at this age. Diskospondylitis is uncommon at this age, would unlikely be this chronic, and should cause considerable discomfort.

Charisma was too large for imaging studies. A vaccine was made for her melanoma with which she was treated unsuccessfully. When

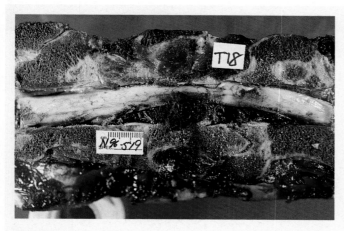

FIGURE 11-42 Dorsal view of the extradural melanoma compressing the spinal cord in the vertebral foramen of T17 in the 14-year-old Oldenburgh Warmblood in this case example.

she became unable to stand on the pelvic limbs even when assisted, she was euthanized. At necropsy, melanomas were found diffusely distributed through the thoracolumbar axial muscles, and an extradural melanoma was present in the vertebral foramen of T17, which displaced and compressed the adjacent spinal cord (Fig. 11-42).

T17 FRACTURE IN A FOAL

See **Video 11-14** of a 1-month-old Thoroughbred colt that was found down at pasture after a severe thunderstorm. The video was made approximately 24 hours later. Manipulation of the colt was restricted because a fracture was suspected. Note the extension of the thoracic limbs but also their vigorous voluntary movement along with neck flexion while the colt remained recumbent. Note also the absence of any voluntary movements with the pelvic limbs. This thoracic limb extension is caused by Schiff-Sherrington syndrome. This syndrome is described in Chapter 10. No evidence was found of any spinal shock in this colt. Note the preserved muscle tone and spinal reflexes in the pelvic limbs, tail, and anus and the analgesia caudal to a line at the level of the caudal thoracic vertebrae. A caudal thoracic spinal cord transverse lesion was diagnosed, and radiographs revealed a compression fracture of T17 with displacement into the vertebral canal. Decompressive surgery revealed a severe hemorrhage and softening of the spinal cord at the fracture site, and the colt was euthanized. A lack of bone density in foals and young farm animals places them at risk for fractures when they fall. Presumably, this foal's injury was related to a fall associated with the excitement caused by the thunderstorm.

CERVICAL SCOLIOSIS—PARELAPHOSTRONGYLUS TENUIS

See **Video 11-15** of Thor, a 2-year-old castrated mixed-breed horse with the chief complaint of a "bent neck." The abnormal curvature of the neck was first observed 5 days before this examination, and a mild gait abnormality was suspected for approximately 2 days. In the video, note the scoliosis of the cervical vertebrae with the concavity on the left side. Also note the mild clinical signs of UMN and GP dysfunction in the right limbs and the analgesia of the right side of his neck. By the time this video was made, Thor had developed a strong objection to our testing of his analgesia, which extended from approximately the level of his atlas to the midthoracic trunk on the right side only.

Scoliosis is an uncommon clinical sign in the adult horse.[81] Most publications that describe the basis for scoliosis in animals indicate that

it is the result of denervation of the muscles on one side of the neck, and the scoliosis is the result of the unopposed muscle contractions on the opposite side, the side toward which the scoliosis is directed. This assumption is reasonable, and to explain the scoliosis in Thor, a necropsy should reveal a lesion in the right ventral gray column or the intramedullary axons of the right ventral roots. The right side area of analgesia would require a right-side dorsal gray column lesion from approximately C2 to approximately T10, and the right-side UMN and GP system dysfunction requires at least a mild right-side white matter lesion at some level in the cervical spinal cord segments. We have observed scoliosis in four other horses that had cervical spinal cord lesions confined to the area of the dorsal gray column of multiple segments on one side. No ventral gray column lesions were noted. The concavity of the scoliosis was always opposite to the side of the lesion, which meant that their necks flexed laterally away from the side of the lesion. A similar clinicoanatomic relationship has been observed in humans and experimental animals. The assumption is that this lesion interferes with the afferents from neuromuscular spindles that are involved with the stretch reflexes necessary to maintain muscle tone. The disparity in muscle tone would account for the deviation of the cervical vertebrae to the side opposite to the lesion. A dorsal gray column lesion over multiple segments would cause an ipsilateral hypalgesia or analgesia. The extension of this lesion into the adjacent lateral funiculus would explain the mild right-side spastic hemiparesis and ataxia observed in Thor. The lesion that we have observed in all of these horses consisted of a continuous nonsuppurative inflammation associated with scattered areas of necrosis centered in the dorsal gray column with variable extension into the adjacent white matter. A few eosinophils were present in the inflammation, which has the appearance of a parasitic tract lesion similar to what we commonly see in small ruminants and Camelidae caused by the migrating larvae of *Parelaphostrongylus tenuis*. In these species the lesions are not confined to the dorsal gray column. The life cycle of this parasite is described with the spinal cord diseases of ruminants in this chapter.

Thor was euthanized, and this inflammatory destructive lesion was found in the dorsal gray column and adjacent white matter on the right side of the spinal cord from C2 to the caudal thoracic spinal cord segments. In the C5 spinal cord segment, transverse sections of a parasite were found and identified as a protostrongylid nematode, presumably a larva of *P. tenuis* (Figs. 11-43 through 11-47).[81]

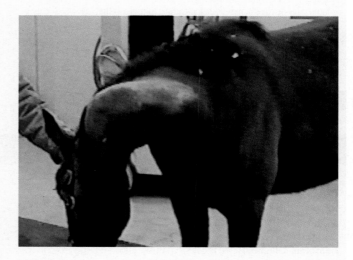

FIGURE 11-43 A yearling Dutch Warmblood with severe right cervical scoliosis for 2 weeks.

(Continued)

CASE EXAMPLE 11-4—cont'd

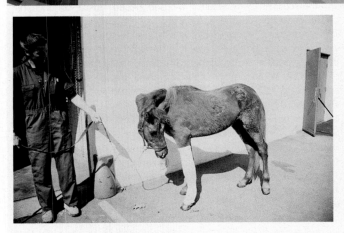

FIGURE 11-44 A 19-month-old Arabian with severe left cervical scoliosis for 8 months.

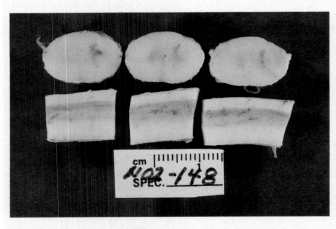

FIGURE 11-45 Transverse sections of the C3, C4, and C5 spinal cord segments from the horse in Fig. 11-44 with the left cervical scoliosis. Note the discoloration of the right dorsal gray column in the transverse sections. The three longitudinal sections were made in the sagittal plane of the right dorsal gray column. This discoloration reflects the chronic astrogliosis that followed the tissue necrosis and inflammation associated with a presumptive migrating larva.

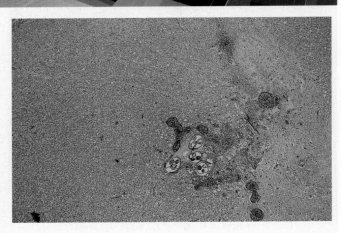

FIGURE 11-46 Microscopic section of the right dorsal gray column in the C5 spinal cord segment from Thor, the 2-year-old mixed breed seen in Video 11-15 with the severe left cervical scoliosis. Note the inflammation and the transverse sections of a nematode larva.

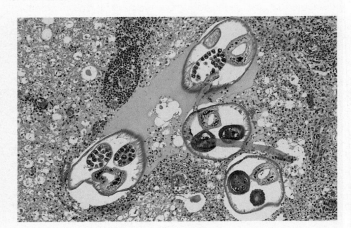

FIGURE 11-47 Higher magnification of the lesion seen in Fig. 11-46. This parasite was identified as a protostrongylid nematode that is most likely *P. tenuis*.

FARM ANIMAL SPINAL CORD DISEASE

CASE EXAMPLE 11-5

Signalment: 3-year-old castrated male llama, Rocky
Chief Complaint: Abnormal use of the pelvic limbs
History: The difficulty using the pelvic limbs developed rapidly over 3 days, and he now needs assistance to stand in the pelvic limbs.
 Examination: See **Video 11-16**.
Anatomic Diagnosis: A focal or diffuse lesion in the spinal cord between the T3 and L3 segments

Differential Diagnosis: *P. tenuis* myiasis, diskospondylitis, vertebral malformation, intervertebral disk extrusion-protrusion, neoplasm

Because of the 3 days of progressive clinical signs, external injury was excluded. We have not diagnosed FCEM in any ruminant or Camelidae. In this species, myiasis with the larvae of *P. tenuis* is by far the most presumptive clinical diagnosis for this alpaca, given that it is a very common disease in the northeastern states where the white tail deer are so common. Diskospondylitis is a worthy consideration and would require radiography for confirmation. Clinical signs of spinal cord compression by a vertebral malformation usually occur before 1 year of age. Both intervertebral disk extrusion-protrusion and neoplasia are rare in this species and would not be expected at this age. We have not made these diagnoses in any species of Camelidae.

P. TENUIS MYIASIS

P. tenuis infection is a common disorder of sheep, goats, and Camelidae.* Although *P. tenuis* infection is rare in cattle, it has been reported.[33] It has recently been described in the horse.[81] (See Video 11-15 in the section on equine spinal cord diseases in this chapter.) Clinical signs can reflect parasite migration in any part of the CNS, but spinal cord signs are most commonly observed. *P. tenuis* is a protostrongylid nematode, the primary host of which is the white tail deer, where the parasite is called the *meningeal worm*. The intermediate host is a slug or snail. *P. tenuis* is present in North America wherever the white tail deer are located. The small ruminant or Camelidae is an aberrant primary host in which the life cycle is not completed.

In the normal life cycle, the first-stage larva is passed in the feces of the primary host, the white tail deer. This first-stage larva enters the footpad of the intermediate host, the slug, or snail. Over the next 2 to 3 weeks, two molts occur, resulting in the formation of the infective third-stage larva. The white tail deer eats the infected slug or snail or ingests their slime secretions that contain the third-stage larva, which contaminates the grass eaten by the primary host. The third-stage larva enters the intestinal epithelium and migrates through the intestinal wall into the mesentery or into the peritoneal cavity. The migratory route from there to the vertebral canal is unknown. The third-stage larva enters the spinal cord and is thought to develop in the dorsal gray column to a fourth-stage larva. It then migrates into the subarachnoid space and enters the cranial cavity, where it molts into a fifth-stage larva, which is the adult form of the parasite. The adult is a long, very thin, threadlike structure located in the intracranial subarachnoid space or a venous sinus. Copulation occurs, and the eggs are deposited into a venous sinus, where they circulate as emboli to the lungs, where they lodge in capillaries and become incorporated into granulomas. The eggs hatch and release first-stage larvae that escape from the granuloma and penetrate the alveoli. They enter the airway and migrate by mucociliary action to the pharynx, where they are swallowed and ultimately excreted by the white tail deer. When the third-stage larva is ingested by the aberrant primary host (the sheep, goat, alpaca, llama, rain deer, caribou, moose, fallow, or mule deer), the larva penetrates the intestinal wall and migrates via an unknown route to the spinal cord. The larva enters the spinal cord, where it migrates, causing necrosis and nonsuppurative inflammation with eosinophils. Migration and lesions may occur in the brainstem. The life cycle is interrupted at this stage. When large quantities of third-stage larvae were fed to sheep and goats, the shortest time between the feeding and the observation of clinical neurologic signs was 11 days (Figs. 11-48 through 11-51).

Clinical signs most commonly reflect the development of spinal cord lesions at any level. Brainstem signs occasionally occur, but cerebral signs are rarely observed. Despite what we have observed in horses that have this parasite, scoliosis is uncommon in these ruminant and Camelidae species.[44] The presence of a pleocytosis in the CSF that contains eosinophils is strongly supportive of this diagnosis. However, the absence of eosinophils in the CSF does not deny the diagnosis. Despite available treatment with various anthelmintics such as fenbendazole or ivermectin, the prognosis is

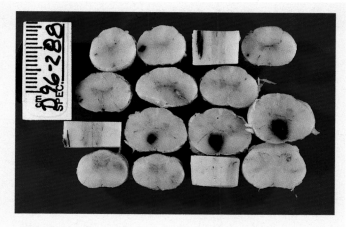

FIGURE 11-48 Transverse sections of the preserved spinal cord of a 5-year-old llama with progressive tetraparesis and ataxia of all four limbs. The discolorations are the result of the hemorrhage and inflammation associated with necrosis caused by a migrating *P. tenuis* larva.

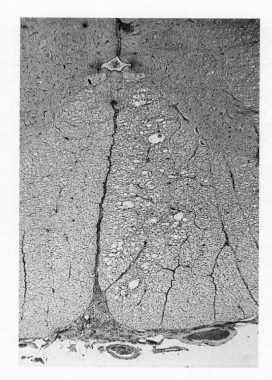

FIGURE 11-49 Transverse microscopic section of the ventral funiculi of a thoracic spinal cord segment from an adult sheep with *P. tenuis* larval myiasis. Note the inflammation in the ventral meninges and the destruction in one ventral funiculus where the larva migrated.

guarded. The best prevention is to avoid exposure of the aberrant primary host to the feces of the white tail deer. When this is not practical, rigorous preventative therapy with anthelmintics such as ivermectin every 30 to 45 days from spring to fall may prevent the development of CNS lesions.

For other examples of this parasitic infection, see the following videos.

*References 1-4, 30, 44, 45, 53, 86.

(Continued)

CASE EXAMPLE 11-5—cont'd

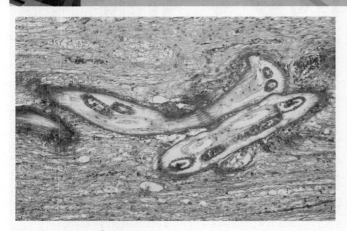

FIGURE 11-50 Longitudinal microscopic section of a *P. tenuis* larva in the thoracic spinal cord of an adult sheep.

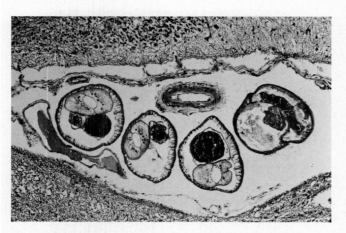

FIGURE 11-51 Transverse sections of one or more *P. tenuis* larvae adjacent to the cerebellum in an adult sheep.

 Video 11-17. This video shows an adult female Toggenburg with 2 weeks of a progressive gait abnormality in all four limbs resulting in recumbency. She was the tenth goat on the farm to be affected with primarily spinal cord signs over the last few weeks in the late summer and early fall. Note the nonambulatory tetraparesis and the presence of enough spasticity for this doe to support herself unassisted. Your anatomic diagnosis should be a focal or diffuse lesion in the spinal cord between the C1 and C5 segments. Her lumbosacral CSF sample contained numerous eosinophils.

Video 11-18. This video shows a group of adult llamas that were fed third-stage larvae as part of an experiment on the pathogenesis and diagnosis of *P. tenuis* myiasis. Note the one adult llama with the mild neurologic signs. Also note her tendency to overreach with the thoracic limbs, indicating that at least one lesion is located in the cervical spinal cord between the C1 and C5 segments. The more severe pelvic limbs signs may still be caused by the cervical spinal cord lesion or may reflect another lesion between the T3 and L3 spinal cord segments.

Video 11-19. This video shows Marie, an adult female llama, with a 1-week history of progressive difficulty using her pelvic limbs. Compare her thoracic limb gait with the previous llama in Video 11-18. Marie's thoracic limb function is normal. Her anatomic diagnosis should be a focal or diffuse spinal cord lesion between the T3 and L3 segments. Eosinophils were present in her lumbosacral CSF sample.

Video 11-20. This video shows Dolly, a 2-year-old female alpaca with a rapid onset of a "bump on the left side of her neck" approximately 10 days before this examination during which little change in the neck posture was noted. The "bump" on her neck is a cervical scoliosis that is similar to the horses we have studied with scoliosis that have a parasitic tract lesion in their dorsal gray column on one side that we believe is caused by the migration of *P. tenuis* in this species. Dolly did not exhibit any other neurologic signs. We did not detect any hypalgesia or analgesia in her neck. The scoliosis with the convexity on the right suggest a left-side gray matter lesion in the C1-C5 spinal cord segments. Her CSF had a pleocytosis with numerous eosinophils. Despite how common this parasitic myiasis is in the CNS of Camelidae, sheep, and goats, scoliosis is an uncommon sign in these species.

VERTEBRAL MALFORMATION

Video 11-21. This video shows Buddy, a 4-month-old male Alpaca cria, with a 3-week history of progressive pelvic limb dysfunction resulting in paraplegia. Note the mass reflexes that a noxious stimulus elicited. Nociception was severely compromised, but we were not sure if analgesia was present in the pelvic limbs. The anatomic diagnosis was a focal or diffuse spinal cord lesion between the T3 and L3 segments. Radiographs showed a vertebral malformation with kyphosis that was responsible for severe spinal cord compression.

CASE EXAMPLE 11-6

Signalment: 3-month-old female Toggenburg goat
Chief Complaint: Unable to stand
History: She suddenly was observed to drag her right pelvic limb, which rapidly progressed within 1 day to difficulty using both pelvic limbs, and the following day, she was unable to stand. She was presented on the third day recumbent and unable to stand.
Examination: See **Video 11-22**. This kid is alert and responsive and has normal cranial nerves. Note the nonambulatory tetraparesis with no voluntary limb movement when held up but vigorous pelvic limb movement in response to a noxious stimulus when recumbent. Also note that the patellar reflexes were present and normal only in one recumbency. The explanation for this circumstance is unknown, but it emphasizes the importance to always test them in both recumbencies before considering them to be absent. Note the discomfort that occurred on flexing the neck when pressure was applied to the caudal cervical vertebrae. Also note the thoracic limb hypotonia, the abnormal withdrawal reflexes, and the mild bilateral atrophy of the lateral scapular and triceps muscles.

Anatomic Diagnosis: A focal spinal cord lesion between the C6 and T2 segments or multifocal spinal cord lesions that include these segments

The mild thoracic limb hypotonia, the lack of their withdrawal from a noxious stimulus, and, instead, an extension of the limbs and a mild bilateral atrophy of the lateral scapular and triceps muscles all suggest a LMN component to their paresis. This mild evidence and the lack of any voluntary effort to move the limbs when held up also implicates the UMN system in the severe paresis.

Differential Diagnosis: Myelitis caused by the caprine arthritis encephalitis virus, *P. tenuis* myiasis, diskospondylitis, vertebral malformation, copper deficiency (enzootic ataxia), organophosphate toxicity

CAPRINE ARTHRITIS ENCEPHALITIS VIRUS

Caprine arthritis encephalitis (CAE) is a multisystem viral disease of goats caused by a lentivirus, a type-C retrovirus that is related to the visna virus of sheep.[17-21,77] In addition to causing a demyelinating leukoencephalitis of young goats, this virus causes pneumonitis, arthritis, and mastitis of older adult goats. The virus is transmitted not only from an infected doe to her kid in the colostrum and milk, but also by direct contact transmission. The neurologic disease usually occurs between 1 and 6 months of age, is acute in onset, and is rapidly progressive. Lesions can be focal, multifocal, or diffuse in the CNS, with the spinal cord most commonly affected. The caudal brainstem is occasionally affected but rarely the prosencephalon. Although the initial action of the virus is to cause a primary demyelination, this phase is rapidly followed by an extensive inflammatory response that is considered to be a cell-mediated immunopathologic response. This inflammation is nonsuppurative, with massive accumulations of mononuclear cells in a perivascular location, as well as throughout the involved parenchyma, where necrosis is extensive. Lesions predominate in the white matter, but extensions into the adjacent gray matter also occur. Focal lesions are often recognized on gross examination of the preserved spinal cord or brain. Slight enlargement of the affected area will be noted, and on transverse section, this area will be firm with a yellow to tan discoloration (Figs. 11-52 through 11-57). Usually, the extent of the neurologic dysfunction results in euthanasia. If the patient is allowed to survive, the progress of the disease may cease, but any significant recovery rarely occurs. The anatomic diagnosis is determined by the location of the lesions.

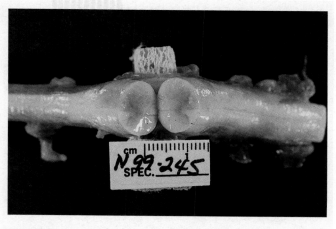

FIGURE 11-53 Same specimen as in Fig. 11-52 after making a transverse section through the lesion.

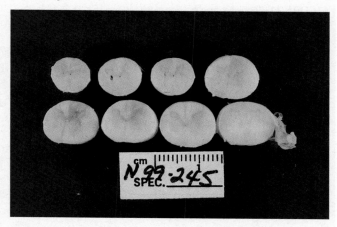

FIGURE 11-54 Transverse sections of the preserved spinal cord seen in Figs. 11-52 and 11-53. Note the diffuse discoloration, primarily of the white matter.

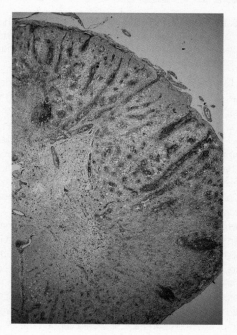

FIGURE 11-55 Microscopic section of half of a cervical spinal cord segment in a kid with CAE. Note the extensive inflammation and necrosis.

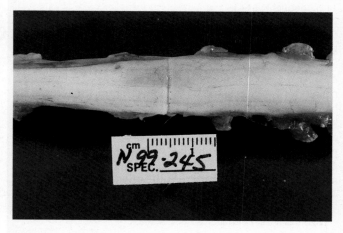

FIGURE 11-52 Dorsal view of the cervical intumescence of the goat in Video 11-22. Note the swelling and discoloration of the intumesence.

(Continued)

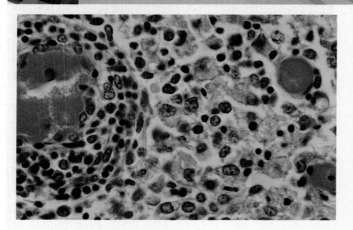

FIGURE 11-56 Higher magnification of the section in Fig. 11-55. Note the extensive nonsuppurative inflammation and the abundance of macrophages.

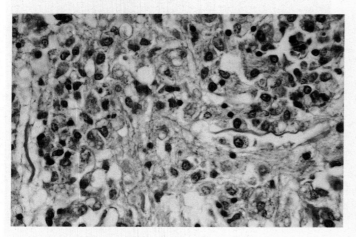

FIGURE 11-57 Higher magnification of the lesion seen in Fig. 11-55. Note the macrophages adjacent to a demyelinated axon. The CAE retrovirus causes a primary demyelination. However, the immune response results in the inflammation that causes the necrosis.

The diagnosis is dependent on determining the presence of serum antibodies to this virus. Herd infection is common because this virus can persist without causing disease. Therefore the presence of the serum antibodies indicates only infection and not necessarily the disease as well. The factors that are responsible for the onset of disease in an individual animal are unknown. The CSF reflects the massive inflammation that is present in the CNS lesions that includes the meninges with markedly elevated protein and mononuclear cells. Eosinophils are not part of this inflammation. Thus this diagnosis is supported by the CSF abnormalities and the presence of serum antibodies.

Prevention of this disease is dependent on the elimination of any goat from the herd that contains antibodies for the CAE virus. Before accomplishing this task, any kid born from a doe with these serum antibodies should be immediately removed from this doe at birth and be fed milk from an uninfected doe.

P. tenuis myiasis is a strong candidate for the clinical diagnosis in this kid. Only the age makes a CAE viral myelitis more likely. The presence of eosinophils in the CSF would support the myiasis.

Diskospondylitis is also a strong candidate at this site at this age and with the observation of neck discomfort. CSF should be normal or only slightly altered. Radiographs are usually diagnostic.

Vertebral malformation with secondary compressive myelopathy is uncommon at this site. We have seen a malformation with subluxation at the C2-C3 articulation in a few goats.

COPPER DEFICIENCY-ENZOOTIC ATAXIA

Copper deficiency-enzootic ataxia is seen as an acquired disease in young sheep and goats and occasionally pigs, with an onset of a slowly progressive paraparesis and pelvic limb ataxia at 2 to 4 months of age.* Clinical signs are symmetrical and usually reflect a UMN-quality paresis and a GP system ataxia. Occasionally, LMN signs are observed. As the disease progresses, the thoracic limbs will become involved. The lesion is a dying-back axonopathy of CNS neurons and a secondary demyelination and astrogliosis in the spinal cord. In the kid in this case example, the rapid progression of the clinical signs and the focal nature of the anatomic diagnosis make copper deficiency an unlikely diagnosis.

ORGANOPHOSPHATE TOXICITY

Organophosphates may cause a delayed form of toxicity that results in a symmetric spastic paraparesis and pelvic limb ataxia.† These clinical signs may not occur until 3 to 5 weeks after using an organophosphate anthelmintic. Haloxon has been most frequently implicated, but other triorthocresyl phosphate forms may also exhibit this delayed form of toxicity. As a rule, the clinical signs occur rapidly and then remain static and limited to the pelvic limbs. Some sheep may be resistant to this toxicity based on the level of their plasma esterase. A similar organophosphate-induced spinal cord disorder occurs in cattle. By the time that the clinical signs are recognized, significant reduction of the serum cholinesterase levels does not usually occur.

In the kid in this case example, CAE viral antibodies were in the serum, and the CSF contained 246 mg/dl of protein (normal <40), 76 RBCs/mm³, and 315 white bloods cells (WBCs)/mm³ (normal <5), with 72% macrophages and 28% lymphocytes. CAE myelitis was considered to be the presumptive clinical diagnosis. This kid was euthanized, and this diagnosis was confirmed at necropsy (see Figs. 11-52 through 11-54).

See the following videos of other goats with CAE viral myelitis.

Video 11-23. This video show a 3-month-old female Toggenburg kid with 3 days of a progressive gait disorder. From your study of this video, you should have recognized a right-side spastic hemiparesis and ataxia. Patellar reflexes were brisk, and flexor reflexes were normal, as was nociception. Based on this information, you should have made the anatomic diagnosis of a right-side focal spinal cord lesion between the C1 and C5 segments. The rapid course of a focal, asymmetric lesion at this age strongly implicates a diagnosis of CAE myelitis. Serum antibodies for the CAE virus were found, and the CSF contained 40 mg/dl of protein, 7 RBCs/mm³, and 23 WBCs/mm³, with 100% mononuclear cells. This kid was euthanized, and the diagnosis of CAE myelitis was confirmed at necropsy. Figs. 11-58 and 11-59 show the unilateral midcervical spinal cord CAE myelitis that caused this spastic hemiparesis and ataxia.

*References 12, 15, 16, 58, 67, 77.
†References 5, 50, 62, 66, 73, 88.

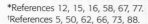

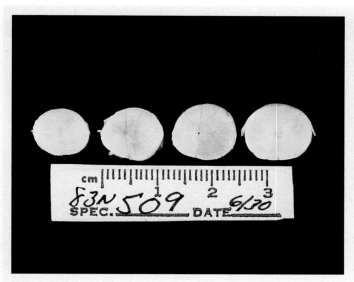

FIGURE 11-58 Transverse sections of the preserved spinal cord from a young goat with a right spastic hemiparesis and ataxia of its right limbs.

Video 11-24. This video shows a 2-month-old female Toggenburg with 10 days of a progressive gait disorder resulting in recumbency 4 days before this examination. Note the spastic tetraplegia. Your anatomic diagnosis should be a focal or diffuse spinal cord lesion between the C1 and C5 segments. The rapid clinical course and age of this patient make CAE myelitis a strong consideration for the clinical diagnosis. Serum antibodies for this virus were found, and the CSF contained 655 mg/dl of protein, 54 RBCs/mm³, and 73 WBCs/mm³, with 75% monocytes and 25% lymphocytes. She was euthanized, and a diffuse nonsuppurative myelitis was diagnosed in numerous spinal cord segments that was compatible with a diagnosis of CAE myelitis.

Video 11-25. This video show Maggie, a 9-year-old female mixed-breed goat with a 2-month history of an initial acute onset and rapid

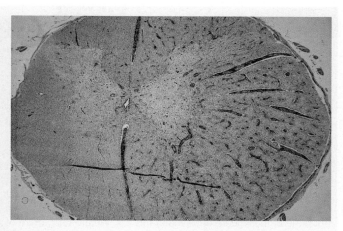

FIGURE 11-59 Microscopic section of the third transection from the left in Fig. 11-58. Note the swelling and inflammation of the right side and the correlation with the clinical signs. This is a CAE viral-induced lesion.

progression of loss of pelvic limb function. This phase was followed by some improvement and then regression of clinical signs. Note the severe spastic paraparesis (grade 1 using the small animal scale) and pelvic limb ataxia and the normal function of the thoracic limbs. Your anatomic diagnosis should be a focal or diffuse spinal cord lesion between the T3 and L3 segments. Differential diagnosis includes *P. tenuis* myiasis, myelitis caused by the CAE virus, diskospondylitis, and neoplasm. The serum contained antibodies for the CAE virus. The CSF contained 155 mg of protein/dl, 2 RBCs/mm³, and 22 WBCs/mm³, with 90% lymphocytes and 10% monocytes. This inflammatory response in the CSF and the absence of eosinophils make a CAE viral myelitis the most presumptive clinical diagnosis in this goat. However, this goat was older than most goats that we see with this disease, and the absence of eosinophiles in the CSF does not rule out *P. tenuis* myiasis. No further studies were conducted to confirm the diagnosis.

CASE EXAMPLE 11-7

Signalment: 2-month-old female Holstein
Chief Complaint: Abnormal gait
History: The gait abnormality had been slowly progressing for at least 2 weeks.
Examination: See **Video 11-26**. Note the delay in the onset of protraction and the long strides in all four limbs with the overreaching action in the thoracic limbs, especially on turning.
Anatomic Diagnosis: Focal or diffuse spinal cord lesion between the C1 and C5 segments
Differential Diagnosis: Diskospondylitis or vertebral canal abscess, lymphosarcoma, hepatic encephalomyelopathy

These progressive clinical signs at this age are most commonly caused by a hematogenous bacterial infection causing a diskospondylitis or an abscess that has developed within the vertebral canal or adjacent to the vertebral column with extension into the vertebral canal. Lymphosarcoma most commonly occurs in the extradural space of adult cattle at any level of the vertebral canal and causes a

compresssive myelopathy.[36,70] This type is termed the *enzootic form of lymphosarcoma,* which is caused by the bovine leukemia virus in cattle that are usually older than 4 years. A sporadic form occurs in cattle younger than 3 years but is much less common. In this 2-month-old calf, no fever was noted, nor were any systemic signs of an infection in the CBC. CSF was normal. Radiographs were normal as was the CSF evaluation.

HEPATIC ENCEPHALOMYELOPATHY IN A CALF

The owner of this heifer calf elected euthanasia. Necropsy showed no gross lesions of any component of the CNS, but the liver was small. On microscopic examination the changes in the liver supported a portosystemic shunt, which had been overlooked at the necropsy. The entire CNS had an extensive dilation of the myelin sheaths, which was especially profound in the spinal cord. With diffuse liver dysfunction that causes neurologic signs from hepatic

(Continued)

CASE EXAMPLE 11-7—cont'd

encephalopathy, two microscopic changes can be seen in the CNS. All species show a change in the nuclei of the astrocytes that reflects their reaction to the increased levels of circulating ammonia and other metabolites not cleared by the liver. In human neuropathology, these abnormal astrocytes are termed *Alzheimer astrocytes*. The other CNS lesion of hepatic encephalopathy that is observed in all species except the horse is a fluid accumulation within the myelin lamellae, causing a dilation of the myelin sheaths that is sometimes called *polymicrocavitation*. This myelin lesion is most extensive in cattle and was severe enough in the spinal cord of this calf to explain the clinical signs that were observed. As a rule, you would expect to observe episodic prosencephalic signs in this metabolic disorder, but none of these were observed in this calf. We are now aware of calves studied at other hospitals that exhibited cervical spinal cord signs with a portosystemic shunt and similar CNS lesions. These shunts are most common in dogs that exhibit episodic clinical signs of prosencephalic dysfunction with no indication of any spinal cord dysfunction. The extent of the myelin sheath dilation in the CNS in dogs with hepatic encephalopathy is much less than in cattle. This bovine case was an eye opener for us, a live-and-learn case that keeps one humble.

 See **Video 11-27** of a 1-month-old female Holstein that became unable to stand in the pelvic limbs over a 1-week period. The severe spastic paraparesis and pelvic limb ataxia justify the anatomic diagnosis of a focal or diffuse spinal cord lesion between the T3 and L3 segments. Radiographs (see video) show a diskospondylitis at the T13-L1 articulation with a compression fracture of T13.

 See **Video 11-28**. This video shows a 6-year-old Holstein cow with 5 days of a progressive gait abnormality. Study the video. The cranial nerve examination was normal. Your anatomic diagnosis should be a focal or diffuse spinal cord lesion between the C1 and C5 segments. The two most common causes of progressive focal spinal cord disease in Holstein cattle are diskospondylitis in young animals and lymphosarcoma in older cattle. This cow was euthanized, and a necropsy showed an extradural lymphosarcoma compressing the spinal cord in the foramen of C4.

BROWN SWISS MYELOPATHY

Be aware that many inherited neurologic disorders of the CNS of Brown Swiss cattle have been discovered. An autosomal-recessive inherited motor neuron disease, often called *spinal muscular atrophy*, was described in Chapter 5. The term *weaver* has been used for a slowly progressive degenerative myeloencephalopathy that is inherited as an autosomal-recessive genetic disorder.[63,76] This neurologic disorder is an axonopathy with secondary demyelination and astrogliosis and with onset of UMN and GP system dysfunction in the pelvic limbs at 5 to 8 months of age. After weeks of progression, clinical signs of mild thoracic limb dysfunction may be noted. These cattle become unable to stand on the pelvic limbs by 18 to 36 months of progression. A congenital axonopathy has also been described in Brown Swiss calves that are born down unable to stand with clinical signs of diffuse UMN and GP system dysfunction and lesion distribution similar to the late-onset axonopathy just described.[47] Some of these calves exhibit opisthotonus and extensor rigidity. Whether the late-onset axonopathy and the congenital axonopathy are the same disease process remains to be determined.

CHAROLAIS LEUKODYSTROPHY

In Charolais cattle, a diffuse CNS white matter oligodendroglial dysplasia occurs that causes a slowly progressive spastic paraparesis and pelvic limb ataxia with an onset between 1 and 2 years of age.[64] These clinical signs of spinal cord disease slowly progress from the pelvic limbs to the thoracic limbs, and recumbency can follow. Female cattle exhibit an unusual rhythmic pulsatile form of urination. Charolais leukodystrophy appears to be a disorder of paranodal myelin, with whorls of hypertrophic oligodendroglial cell membrane and cytoplasm developing at the nodes of Ranvier. These plaques of myelin dysplasia are most common in the spinal cord funiculi, cerebellar medulla, optic tracts, internal capsule, and corpus callosum. The prevalence is presumed to be the result of an inherited disorder in the Charolais breed. However, we have seen the same lesion in an 18-month-old Hereford that was culled in the surveillance for bovine spongiform encephalopathy at a western New York packing plant because of a gait abnormality.

CASE EXAMPLE 11-8

Signalment: 1-year-old female Holstein
Chief Complaint: Abnormal gait
History: This heifer was one of a small group of heifers on a partially wooded rented pasture where they were observed only sporadically. At one of these observations, it was noticed that this heifer had an abnormal gait.
 Examination: See **Video 11-29**. Note the difference in the protraction phase of the gait between the pelvic and thoracic limbs.
Anatomic Diagnosis: Focal cranial thoracic spinal cord segments. This gait fits the pattern of what is termed a *two-engine gait*, which was described in Chapter 10. The pelvic limb dysfunction clearly indicates an interruption in the UMN and GP systems that normally control their voluntary movements. As a rule, the short strides in the thoracic limbs

reflect loss of a portion of their LMN innervation of extensor muscles necessary for weight support. This loss would be explained by a mild lesion in the C6 to T2 spinal cord segments involving both the gray and white matter. However, the short-strided thoracic limbs may also reflect a cranial thoracic lesion that causes discomfort or causes a loss of the UMN system that controls axial muscles at a cranial thoracic level. In this video, you should have recognized that when this heifer stood up after being down or when she tried to prevent herself from falling after stumbling, the thoracic limb strength that she exhibited was remarkable and did not exhibit any indication of a LMN paresis.
Differential Diagnosis: Because of the limited observation of this heifer, the nature of the onset and course of these clinical signs was unknown.

Fracture, diskospondylitis or abscess in the vertebral canal, lymphosarcoma

T4 FRACTURE IN A COW

The last two diagnoses were briefly described in Case Example 11-7. No ancillary procedures were available for further study of this heifer. She was euthanized, and a necropsy diagnosed a fracture of the T4 vertebra, with partial displacement into the vertebral canal. Microscopic examination of the vertebral body showed no evidence of osteomyelitis. The authors thank Dr. Brian Farrow of Sydney, Australia, for this video.

See **Video 11-30**. This 3-year-old female Angus was found down at pasture. If you just observe this cow *over the fence,* you will have no indication of the anatomic location of the neurologic disorder. In the initial portion of the video, her recumbent posture might suggest opisthotonus and extensor rigidity, or the thoracic limb extension might suggest the Schiff-Sherrington syndrome. With the help of the hip lifter, her paraplegia is obvious, and she has normal use of her thoracic limbs, head, and neck, which still supports the possibility of the Schiff-Sherrington syndrome. Spinal nerve reflexes were difficult to evaluate in the pelvic limbs because of the hypertonia; they were intact in the tail and anus. Hypalgesia was severe caudal to the cranial lumbar area. Radiographs revealed a fracture of the L3 vertebra with displacement into the vertebral canal.

CASE EXAMPLE 11-9

Signalment: 5-year-old female Holstein
Chief Complaint: Abnormal use of the pelvic limbs
History: This cow's ability to use her pelvic limbs deteriorated over 5 days, resulting in her inability to stand on the fourth day.
Examination: See **Video 11-31**. Before this video was made, when the pelvic limbs were assisted with the hip lifter, she was able to stand with her thoracic limbs. Note the repetitive flexion exhibited in both pelvic limbs that alternates between the two limbs. This flexion resembles an equine *stringhalt* action, as well as the continuous action seen with the myoclonic syndrome in dogs. Remember that in horses and, to a lesser degree, in cattle the anatomic reciprocal apparatus functions in the pelvic limbs. Therefore any stifle flexion will result in simultaneous flexion of the tarsus and fetlocks. Tail tone was mildly depressed, but the perineal reflex was intact. Nociception seemed depressed in the sacrocaudal nerve distribution. The bladder was enlarged on rectal examination.
Anatomic Diagnosis: Lumbosacrocaudal spinal cord segments

The repetitive stringhalt-type myoclonic action suggests a disturbance of inhibition in the ventral gray columns in the caudal lumbar and sacral segments. Assessing the cranial extent of the spinal cord lesion was not possible.
Differential Diagnosis: Lymphosarcoma, diskospondylitis, rabies myelitis

Extradural lymphosarcoma is the most common cause of clinical signs of spinal cord dysfunction at any level in the adult cow.[36,70] The viral-associated enzootic form would be expected at her age of 5 years. Diskospondylitis commonly occurs at the lumbosacral articulation but can occur at any level of the vertebral column. It is more common in calves and, at the lumbosacral articulation, will only affect the sciatic nerve contribution to the gait unless the infection spreads cranially within the vertebral canal. With a lesion confined to the lumbosacral articulation, this cow should be able to stand and walk. See **Video 11-32** for this comparison.

RABIES MYELITIS

The most common cause of myelitis in cattle is infection with the rabies virus. This neurotropic virus affects neuronal cell bodies

in the gray matter at all levels of the CNS. Clinical signs may initially reflect spinal cord dysfunction, but the disease usually progresses rapidly to cause clinical signs of brainstem and cerebral dysfunction. Clinical signs limited to spinal cord dysfunction are unusual. However, a loss of tail tone is often observed in cattle with intracranial signs of rabies encephalitis. By the time the rapidly progressive disease affects the brainstem, many of the spinal cord signs may be masked.

The CSF contained a normal protein level, with 26 WBCs/mm^3 that consisted of 26% macrophages and 74% lymphocytes. This cow was euthanized, and a necropsy diagnosis was made of a nonsuppurative myelitis scattered through most of the lumbosacrocaudal segments accompanied by viral inclusions in neuronal cell bodies (Negri bodies), which immunocytochemisty confirmed to be rabies virus. *Always* remember rabies when you consider your differential diagnosis in any species!

LUMBOSACRAL DISCOSPONDYLITIS IN A COW

See Video 11-32. This video shows a 2-year-old female Holstein with a rapidly progressive abnormal gait in both pelvic limbs for the previous 4 days. Note the ability to protract the limbs by hip flexion (intact lumbar nerves and segments) and support weight (intact femoral nerves, L4, L5 spinal cord segments) but overflexed tarsi and a tendency to buckle dorsally at the fetlocks (tibial nerve dysfunction, S1, S2 spinal cord segments), loss of tail tone (deficiency of caudal nerves or segments), and possible hypalgesia of anus, perineum, and caudal thighs (deficiency of sacral nerves or segments). The degree of hypalgesia was difficult to assess because of the stoic behavior of this cow. On attempting to obtain CSF at the lumbosacral site, a suppurative exudate was aspirated. Radiographs showed a diskospondylitis of the lumbosacral articulation. This cow was euthanized, and necropsy confirmed the diskospondylitis, as well as extension of the suppurative inflammation into the vertebral canal where it surrounded the sacrocaudal segments and spinal nerves. Two months before this disorder was diagnosed, the tail was removed by elastic band occlusion of its blood supply.

CASE EXAMPLE 11-10

Signalment: 4-month-old female Montadale lamb

Chief Complaint: Inability to stand unassisted

History: This lamb developed difficulty walking with all four limbs 1 week before this examination. Her abnormal gait progressed rapidly and she had been unable to stand unassisted for 2 days. The owner also commented that the right ear had been drooped for approximately 1 month.

Examination: See **Video 11-33**. Note the disparity in the function of the thoracic limbs compared with the pelvic limbs and the loss of muscle tone and withdrawal reflexes only in the thoracic limbs. In the cranial nerve examination, note the absent right eyelid closure when the lids are touched but the eyeball still retracts (sensory nerve V is intact) or when the ewe is menaced (vision is intact). On neck extension in ruminants, the eyeballs do not normally elevate, and sclera is visible in the palpebral fissure, which is the opposite response seen in small animals. In this ewe, the right eyeball elevates on neck extension, which suggests some disturbance in the peripheral or central components of the vestibular system on the right side.

Anatomic Diagnosis: Focal lesion in spinal cord segments C6-T2 plus the right facial nucleus or nerve and possible vestibular system components

The severity of the clinical signs caused by the spinal cord lesion prevents the recognition of any clinical signs that may be in the medulla affecting the UMN and GP systems where the facial nucleus is located. The separation in time between the observation of the facial paresis and the onset of clinical signs of spinal cord dysfunction suggests that these clinical signs may be unrelated.

Differential Diagnosis: Diskospondylitis and otitis media-interna, *P. tenuis* myiasis, listeriosis, copper deficiency and otitis media-interna, selenium toxicity and otitis media-interna

If we consider that the facial paralysis and the suggestion of a vestibular nerve dysfunction are secondary to an otitis media-interna, then a diskospondylitis of the caudal cervical vertebrae is the most presumptive clinical diagnosis that needs to be pursued. *P. tenuis* myiasis is still a strong consideration, but the severity of the LMN clinical signs in the thoracic limbs would be unusual. The rapid clinical course of the spinal cord lesion and the disparity in the dysfunction between the thoracic and pelvic limbs would not be expected with copper deficiency. A sudden onset of LMN dysfunction in all four limbs has been reported in sheep with lesions of poliomyelomalacia similar to those that occur in pigs with selenium toxicity. The lack of LMN dysfunction in the pelvic limbs make this diagnosis very unlikely in this ewe. Listeriosis is very common in ruminants but is a disease that regularly affects the caudal brainstem, and clinical signs of spinal cord dysfunction are rare or unrecognized because of the severity of the pontomedullary lesions. We have never recognized clinical signs of focal spinal cord dysfunction in a ruminant with a necropsy diagnosis of listeriosis, but there are reports from Australia of myelitis caused by this bacterium. Unilateral facial paralysis and vestibular system dysfunction are common clinical signs seen with pontomedullary listeriosis.

Lumbosacral CSF contained 560 mg/dl of protein (normal <40), 893 RBCs/mm^3, and 569 WBCs/mm^3 (normal <5), with

87% macrophages, 13% lymphocytes, and 5% neutrophils. These findings are most compatible with a severe case of listeriosis with extensive meningeal inflammation. Although mild cases of listeriosis may respond to antibiotic therapy, the owner elected to have this ewe euthanized. The diagnosis of listeriosis was confirmed with moderate lesions in the pons and medulla and remarkably extensive necrotizing lesions in the cervical intumescence centered in the gray matter but the inflammation also extended into the nerve roots, which is very unusual for listeriosis. The bacterium, *Listeria monocytogenes,* was immunocytochemically identified in macrophages in the lesion.

See **Video 11-34** of a 4-month-old castrated male mixed-breed lamb that became unable to stand after 3 days of progressive difficulty with walking. Note the severe nonambulatory tetraparesis with increased muscle tone in the pelvic limbs and decreased muscle tone in the thoracic limbs. The withdrawal reflexes and nociception were both reduced in the thoracic limbs. The anatomic diagnosis was a focal lesion between spinal cord segments C6 and T2. The most common presumptive clinical diagnosis is a diskospondylitis or vertebral canal abscess. Although experimental studies support the possibility of *P. tenuis* myiasis at this age, the young age for a natural infection make this diagnosis less likely. Clinical neurologic signs of copper deficiency are observed at this age, but such a rapid onset of tetraparesis and the disparity in the quality of the paresis between the pelvic and thoracic limbs would not be expected. Radiographs (see video) revealed a diskospondylitis at the C5-C6 articulation. The lamb was euthanized, and this diagnosis was confirmed at necropsy.

See **Video 11-35**. This video shows a 2-month-old female mixed-breed lamb that was vaccinated and had her tail docked when she was 2 weeks of age along with a large group of other similar-aged lambs. The following day, it was noticed that this lamb was unable to stand with her pelvic limbs. Two other lambs had difficulty using their pelvic limbs but recovered in a few days. This lamb remained unchanged over the next 6 weeks before this examination. Note the severe spastic paraparesis and the difficulty that this lamb has supporting her trunk when held by the stump of her tail, but note also her normal thoracic limb function. Also note the suggestion of a mild elevation of her cranial thoracic vertebral spinous processes. Your anatomic diagnosis should be a focal cranial thoracic or diffuse lesion in the spinal cord between the T3 and L3 segments that probably involves the more cranial components of this anatomic diagnosis. The sudden onset without progression of clinical signs for 6 weeks suggests a spinal cord injury or vascular compromise. We have not observed FCEM in ruminants, and with the proximity in time of vigorous handling of these lambs just before the observation of their clinical signs makes an injury the most presumptive clinical diagnosis. Radiographs (see video) showed a healed compression fracture of the third thoracic vertebra with a mild degree of kyphosis at the fracture site. The lamb was euthanized, and this diagnosis was confirmed at necropsy.

The bones of foals and young farm animals may be at risk for fracture because of deficient ossification.

CASE EXAMPLE 11-11

Signalment: 2-week-old female mixed-breed pig

Chief Complaint: Abnormal use of the pelvic limbs

History: This pig was found in her pen unable to stand on her pelvic limbs. She was not observed well enough to know whether the onset was sudden with no progression of the clinical signs or if this disorder was progressive. She was normal at birth.

Examination: See **Video 11-36**. Note the elevation of the vertebral column at the thoracolumbar junction.

Anatomic Diagnosis: Focal or diffuse spinal cord lesion between the T3 and L3 segments

Using the small animal grading system, this condition is a severe grade 3 spastic paraparesis and ataxia.

Differential Diagnosis: Vertebral malformation with kyphosis, vertebral fracture with displacement, vertebral abscess with pathologic fracture and displacement, FCEM

All four of these clinical diagnoses occur in pigs and could cause these clinical signs of spinal cord disease. Imaging is necessary to differentiate them. Radiographs showed a vertebral malformation with kyphosis at the T13-L1 articulation and associated narrowing of the vertebral canal.

FCEM occurs in young growing pigs and is often associated with experiences that make trauma a risk, such as during the transportation of large numbers of pigs.[65] The age of these pigs makes the vertebral growth plates a consideration for the source of these emboli (Figs. 11-60 through 11-64). This disorder was described in detail in Case Example 10-1.

Nutritional and toxic forms of myelopathy occur in pigs. These forms cause progressive clinical signs and would be a consideration in this pig in this case example in which the history is unclear. However, these circumstances would not cause the vertebral deformity that was observed in this pig. Copper deficiency causes a rapidly progressive paraparesis and pelvic limb ataxia in 3.5- to 6-month-old pigs that can progress to paraplegia.[57,67] This condition is similar to the disorder that occurs in lambs and kids at that age that is related to copper deficiency. In all of these species, this disorder causes a degeneration of axons and secondary demyelination. Neuronal cell-body degeneration also occurs in widely dispersed areas of the nervous system. Organic arsenicals are

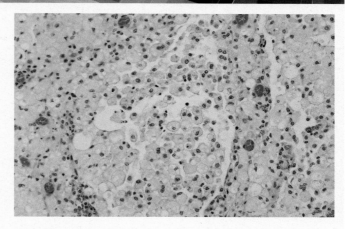

FIGURE 11-61 Higher magnification of an ischemic area in the section in Fig. 11-60. Note the lack of any recognizable parenchyma, which has been replaced by macrophages.

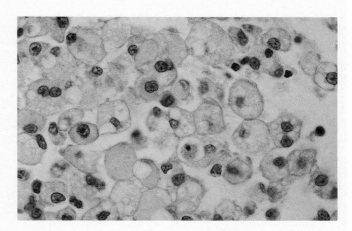

FIGURE 11-62 Higher magnification of the area in Fig. 11-61. Note the lipid-filled macrophages (gitter cells).

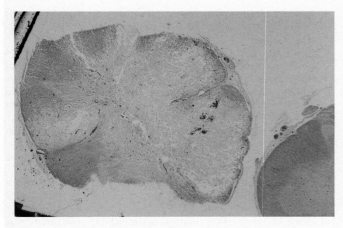

FIGURE 11-60 Microscopic transverse section of a lumbar spinal cord segment from a 5-month-old pig that was found paraplegic following truck transportation. Note the extensive ischemic infarction of gray and white matter.

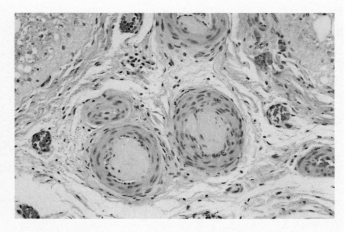

FIGURE 11-63 Higher magnification of the ventral meninges in Fig. 11-60. Note the multiple arteries obstructed with fibrocartilaginous emboli.

(Continued)

CASE EXAMPLE 11-11—cont'd

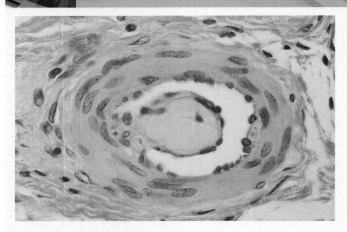

FIGURE 11-64 Higher magnification of the ventral meninges in Fig. 11-60. Note the obstructed artery exhibiting recanalization by the endothelial cells.

sometimes added to the ration of pigs as growth stimulants and to prevent dysentery. Overdose of arsanilic acid initially causes a progressive spastic paraparesis and pelvic limb ataxia,[48] which progresses to involve the thoracic limbs and is followed by recumbency. At necropsy, diffuse degeneration of axons and myelin is noted.

 See **Video 11-37**. This video shows a 10-day-old female mixed-breed pig found in its pen with dysfunction of her pelvic limbs. The nature of the onset and the course of the clinical signs is unknown. Study the video. Your anatomic diagnosis should be a focal or diffuse spinal cord lesion between the T3 and L3 segments. The differential diagnosis includes vertebral malformation, vertebral column and spinal cord injury, vertebral column diskospondylitis or vertebral canal abscess, or a nutritional myelopathy.

Nutritional myelopathy is unlikely at this age with such severe clinical signs in the pelvic limbs. The onset of this disorder is usually between 3 and 6 months. Most vertebral malformations that cause enough kyphosis to compress the spinal cord are usually visible or palpable, as in this case example. Imaging is necessary to differentiate the other diseases. Radiographs showed a compression fracture of the L1 vertebra.

See **Video 11-38**. This video shows a 1-month-old female mixed-breed pig with a history of not using the pelvic limbs for 10 days. Study the video, and note the reluctance to use the pelvic limbs. Therefore you cannot determine if she is unable to use them as a result of a neurologic disorder or is just unwilling to use them because of an orthopedic disorder that causes discomfort. Note that she walks almost entirely on her thoracic limbs by contracting her thoracolumbar epaxial muscles to extend her vertebral column so that the pelvic limbs do not bear any weight. When she is held up, you can see the marked enlargement of both stifles, and the radiographs show the extensive lysis associated with a bilateral stifle infection.

See **Video 11-39**. This video shows a 10-week-old female mixed-breed pig that was noted as having difficulty using her pelvic limbs and exhibiting an unusual action with the right pelvic limb. This problem was initially thought to be a form of myoclonus caused by a spinal cord lesion before we received the pig for examination. Study the video. In our opinion, her neurologic examination was normal, the clinical signs were caused by a lesion affecting the right stifle, and the pig was reluctant to bear weight on that limb. When she leaned to the left to avoid bearing weight on the right pelvic limb, the digits came off the floor, and all the repetitive movements were her attempts to reach the floor with the right pelvic limb digits. If I placed my hand against the plantar surface of the digits, the action stopped. The radiographs show the severe infection involving the right stifle and adjacent tissues. This pig was euthanized, and a necropsy showed a suppurative lesion involving the right stifle. No microscopic lesions were found in the CNS or peripheral nerves in the right pelvic limb.

REFERENCES

1. Alden C, et al: Cerebrospinal nematodiasis in sheep, *Am J Pathol* 99:257, 1975.
2. Anderson RC: The development of Pneumostrongylus tenuis in the central nervous system of white-tail deer, *Pathol Vet* 2:360, 1965.
3. Anderson RC, Lankester MW, Strelive UR: Further experimental studies of Pneumostrongylus tenuis in cervids, *Can J Zool* 44:851, 1966.
4. Anderson RC, Strelive UR: The effect of Pneumostrongylus tenuis (Nematoda: Metastrongyloidea) in kids, *Can J Comp Med* 33:280, 1969.
5. Baker NF, et al: Neurotoxicity of haloxon and its relationship to blood esterases of sheep, *Am J Vet Res* 31:865, 1970.
6. Beech J, Dodd DC: Toxoplasma-like encephalomyelitis in the horse, *Vet Pathol* 11:87, 1974.
7. Bitsch V, Dam A: Nervous disturbances in the horse in relation to infection with equine rhinopnemonitis virus, *Acta Vet Scand* 12:134, 1974.
8. Boy MG, Galligan DT, Divers TJ: Protozoal encephalomyelitis in horses: 82 cases (1972-1986), *J Am Vet Med Assoc* 196:632-634, 1990.
9. Bowman DD, et al: Characterization of Sarcocystis neurona from a thoroughbred with equine protozoal myeloencephalitis, *Cornell Vet* 82:51-52, 1992.
10. Brown CM, et al: Persistence of serum antibodies to Sarcocystis neurona in horses moved from North America to India, *J Vet Intern Med* 20:994-997, 2006.
11. Brown TT Jr, Patton CS: Protozoal encephalomyelitis in horses, *J Am Vet Med Assoc* 171:492, 1977.
12. Chalmers GA: Swayback (Enzootic ataxia) in Alberta lambs, *Can J Comp Med* 38:111, 1974.
13. Charlton KM, et al: Meningoencephalomyelitis in horses associated with equine herpesvirus infection, *Vet Pathol* 13:59, 1976.
14. Cook AG, et al: Interpretation of the detection of Sarcocystis neurona antibodies in the serum of young horses, *Vet Parasitol* 95:187-195, 2001.
15. Cordy DR: Enzootic ataxia in California lambs, *J Am Vet Med Assoc* 158:1940, 1971.

16. Cordy DR, Knight HD: California goats with a disease resembling enzootic ataxia or swayback, *Vet Pathol* 15:179, 1978.

17. Cork LC: Differential diagnosis of viral leukoencephalomyelitis of goats, *J Am Vet Med Assoc* 169:1303, 1976.

18. Cork LC, Davis WC: Ultrastructural features of viral leukoencephalomyelitis of goats, *Lab Invest* 32:359, 1975.

19. Cork LC, et al: Infectious leukoencephalomyelitis of young goats. *J Infect Dis* 129:134, 1974.

20. Cork LC, et al: Pathology of viral leukoencephalomyelitis of goats, *Acta Neuropathol* 29:281, 1974.

21. Cork LC, Narayan O: The pathogenesis of viral leukoencephalomyelitis-arthritis of goats. I. Persistent viral infection with progressive pathologic changes, *Lab Invest* 42:596, 1980.

22. Cummings JF, et al: Endothelial lipopigment as an indicator of alpha tocopherol deficiency in two equine neurodegenerative diseases, *Acta Neuropathol* 56:1433-1439, 1995.

23. de Lahunta A, Hatfield C, Dietz A: Occipitoatlantoaxial malformation with duplication of the atlas and axis in a half Arabian foal, *Cor Vet* 79:185-193, 1989.

24. Dill SG, et al: Factors associated with the development of equine degenerative myeloencephalopathy, *Am J Vet Res* 51:1300-1305, 1990.

25. Dill SG, et al: Serum vitamin E and blood glutathione peroxidase values of horses with degenerative myeloencephalopathy, *Am J Vet Res* 50:166-168, 1989.

26. Dimock WW, Errington BJ: Incoordination of Equidae: wobblers, *J Am Vet Med Assoc* 95:261, 1939.

27. Divers TJ, Bowman DD, de Lahunta A: Equine protozoal myeloencephalitis—recent advances in diagnosis and treatment, *Vet CE Advisor-Vet Med*, Feb(suppl 1):3, 2000.

28. Donawick WJ, et al: Results of low protein, low energy diet and confinement on young horses with wobbles, *Proc Am Assoc Eq Pract* 39:125-127, 1993.

29. Duarte PC, et al: Risk of postnatal exposure to Sarcocystis neurona and Neospora hughesi in horses, *Am J Vet Res* 65:1047-1052, 2004.

30. Dubey JP, et al: Sarcocystis neurona n. sp. (Protozoa: Apicomplexa), the etiologic agent of equine protozoal myeloencephalitis, *J Parasitol* 77:212, 1991.

31. Dubey JP, et al: A review of Sarcocystis neurona and equine protozoal myeloencephalitis (EPM), *Vet Parasitol* 95:89-131, 2001.

32. Dubey JP, et al: Completion of the life cycle of Sarcocystis neurona, *J Parasitol* 86:1276-1280, 2000.

33. Duncan RB, Patton S: Naturally occurring cerebrospinal Parelaphostrongylus in a heifer, *J Vet Diagn Invest* 10: 287-291, 1998.

34. Falco MJ, Whitwell K, Palmer AC: An investigation into the genetics of "wobbler disease" in Thoroughbred horses in Britain, *Eq Vet J* 8:165, 1976.

35. Fayer R, Mayhew IG, Baird JD: Epidemiology of equine protozoal myeloencephalitis in North America based on histologically confirmed cases. A report, *J Vet Intern Med* 4:54-57, 1990.

36. Ferrer J: Bovine lymphosarcoma, *Compend Cont Ed* 2:S235, 1980.

37. Freaser H, Palmer AC: Equine incoordination and wobbler disease of young horses, *Vet Rec* 80:338, 1967.

38. Friday PA, et al: Ataxia and paresis with equine herpesvirus 1 infection in a herd of riding school horses, *J Vet Intern Med* 14:197-201, 2000.

39. Goehring LS, et al: Equine herpesvirus 1-associated myeloencephalopathy in the Netherlands: a four year retrospective study (1999-2003), *J Vet Intern Med* 20:601-607, 2006.

40. Greet TRC, et al: The slap test for laryngeal adductory function in horses with suspected cervical spinal cord disease, *Eq Vet J* 12:127, 1980.

41. Henninger RW, et al: Outbreak of neurologic disease caused by equine herpesvirus-1 at a university equestrian center, *J Vet Intern Med* 21:157-165, 2007.

42. Jackson T, Kendrick JW: Paralysis of horses associated with equine herpesvirus 1 infection, *J Am Vet Med Assoc* 158:1351-1357, 1971.

43. Jackson TA, et al: Equine herpesvirus 1 infection of horses: studies on the experimentally induced neurologic disease, *Am J Vet Res* 38:709, 1977.

44. Johnson AL, Lamm CG, Divers TJ: Acquired cervical scoliosis attributed to Parelaphostrongylus tenuis infection in an alpaca, *J Am Vet Med Assoc* 229:562-565, 2006.

45. Kennedy PC, Whitlock JH, Roberts SJ: Neurofilariosis: a paralytic disease of sheep. I. Introduction, symptomatology and pathology, *Cornell Vet* 42:118, 1952.

46. Kisthardt K, Lindsay DS: Update and review: equine protozoal myeloencephalitis, *Eq Pract* 19:8-13, 1997.

47. Kwiecien JM, et al: Congenital axonopathy in a Brown Swiss calf, *Vet Pathol* 32:72-75, 1995.

48. Leder AE, et al: Clinical, toxicological and pathological aspects of arsanilic acid poisoning in swine, *Clin Toxicol* 6:439, 1973.

49. Little PB, Thorsen J: Disseminated necrotizing myeloencephalitis: a herpes associated neurological disease of horses, *Vet Pathol* 13:161, 1976.

50. Malone JD: Toxicity of haloxon, *Res Vet Sci* 5:17, 1964.

51. Marsh AE, Barr BC, Madigan J: Neosporosis as a cause of equine protozoal myeloencephalitis, *J Am Vet Med Assoc* 209:1907-1913, 1996.

52. Mayhew IG, et al: Equine degenerative myeloencephalopathy: a vitamin E deficiency that may be familial, *J Vet Int Med* 1:45-50, 1987.

53. Mayhew IG, et al: Naturally occurring cerebrospinal parelaphostrongylosis, *Cornell Vet* 65:56, 1976.

54. Mayhew IG, et al: Equine degenerative myeloencephalopathy, *J Am Vet Med Assoc* 170:195, 1977.

55. Mayhew IG, et al: Spinal cord disease in the horse, *Cornell Vet* 68(suppl 6):1, 1978.

56. Mayhew IG, Donawick WJ, Green SL: Diagnosis and prediction of cervical vertebral malformation in Thoroughbred foals based on semiquantitative radiographic indicators, *Eq Vet J* 25:435-440, 1993.

57. Mayhew IG, Watson AG, Heissan JA: Congenital occipitoatlantoaxial malformations in the horse, *Eq Vet J* 10:103, 1978.

58. McGavin MD, Ranby PD, Tammemagi L: Demyelination associated with low liver copper levels in pigs, *Aust Vet J* 38:8, 1962.

59. Miller MM, et al: Effect of iatrogenic blood-contaminated equine CSF on Sarcocystis neurona western blot reactivity and CSF indices, *Proc Am Assoc Eq Pract* 44:138-139, 1998.

60. Montali RJ, et al: Spinal ataxia in zebras, *Vet Pathol* 11:68, 1974.

61. Moore BR, et al: Assessment of vertebral canal diameter and bony malformations of the cervical part of the spine in horses with cervical stenotic myelopathy, *Am J Vet Res* 55: 5-13, 1994.

62. Nicholson SS: Bovine posterior paresis due to organophosphate poisoning, *J Am Vet Med Assoc* 165:280, 1974.

63. Oyster R, Leipold HW, Troyer D: Clinical studies of bovine progressive myeloencephalopathy of Brown Swiss cattle, *Prog Vet Neurol* 2:159-164, 1991.

64. Palmer AC, et al: Progressive ataxia of Charolais cattle associated with a myelin disorder, *Vet Rec* 91:592, 1972.

65. Pass DA: Posterior paralysis in a sow due to cartilaginous emboli in the spinal cord, *Aust Vet J* 54:100, 1978.

66. Perdrizet JA, Cummings JF, de Lahunta A: Presumptive organophosphate–induced delayed neurotoxicity in a paralyzed bull, *Cornell Vet* 75:401-410, 1985.

67. Pletcher JM, Banting LF: Copper deficiency in piglets characterized by spongy myelopathy and degenerative lesions in the great blood vessels, *J S Afr Vet Assoc* 54:43-46, 1983.

68. Purcell AR, et al: Neurologic disease induced by equine herpesvirus 1, *J Am Vet Med Assoc* 175:473, 1979.

69. Rantanen NW, et al: Ataxia and paresis in horses. Part II. Radiographic and myelographic examination of the cervical vertebral column, *Compend Cont Ed* 3:S161, 1981.

70. Rebhun WC, et al: Compressive neoplasms affecting the bovine spinal cord, *Compend Cont Ed* 6:S396-S400, 1984.

71. Reed SM, et al: Ataxia and paresis in horses. Part I. Differential diagnosis, *Compend Cont Ed* 3:S88, 1981.

72. Rooney JR, et al: Focal myelitis and encephalitis in horses, *Cornell Vet* 60:494, 1970.

73. Sanders DE, et al: Progressive paresis in sheep due to delayed neurotoxicity of triaryl phosphates, *Cornell Vet* 75:493-504, 1985.

74. Saxegaard F: Isolation and identification of equine rhinopnemonitis virus (equine abortion virus) from cases of abortion and paralysis, *Nord Vet Med* 18:504, 1966.

75. Simpson CF, Mayhew IG: Evidence for sarcocystis as the etiologic agent of equine protozoal myeloencephalitis, *J Protozool* 27:288, 1980.

76. Stuart LD, Leipold HW: Lesions in bovine progressive degenerative myeloencephalopathy ("Weaver") of Brown Swiss cattle, *Vet Pathol* 22:13-23, 1985.

77. Summers BA, et al: Studies on viral leukoencephalomyelitis and swayback in goats, *Cornell Vet* 70:372, 1980.

78. Taylor HW, Vandevelde M, Firth EC: Ischemic myelopathy caused by fibrocartilaginous emboli in a horse, *Vet Pathol* 14:479, 1977.

79. Traver DS, et al: Epidural melanoma causing posterior paralysis in a horse, *J Am Vet Med Assoc* 170:1400, 1977.

80. Van Biervliet JA, et al: Extradural undifferentiated sarcoma causing spinal cord compression in 2 horses, *J Vet Intern Med* 18:248-251, 2004.

81. Van Biervliet JA, et al: Acquired cervical scoliosis in six horses associated with dorsal grey column chronic myelitis, *Eq Vet J* 36:86-92, 2004.

82. Van Biervliet JA, et al: Evaluation of decision criteria for detection of spinal cord compression based on cervical myelograms in horses: 38 cases (1901-2001), *Eq Vet J* 36: 14-20, 2004.

83. Wagner PC, et al: Surgical stabilization of the equine cervical spine, *Vet Surg* 8:7, 1979.

84. Wagner PC, et al: Evaluation of cervical spinal fusion as a treatment in the equine wobbler syndrome, *Vet Surg* 8:84, 1979.

85. Wagner PC, et al: Ataxia and paresis in horses. Part III. Surgical treatment of spinal cord compression, *Compend Cont Ed* 3:S192, 1981.

86. Whitlock JH: Neurofilariosis, a paralytic disease of sheep. II. Neurophilaria cornellensis n.g.n. sp. (Nematoda filaroidia) a new nematode parasite from the spinal cord of sheep, *Cornell Vet* 42:125, 1952.

87. Whitwell KE: Craniovertebral malformations in an Arab foal, *Eq Vet J* 10:125, 1978.

88. Williams JF, Dade AW, Benne R: Posterior paralysis associated with anthelmintic treatment of sheep, *J Am Vet Med Assoc* 169:1307, 1976.

12 VESTIBULAR SYSTEM: SPECIAL PROPRIOCEPTION

ANATOMY AND PHYSIOLOGY

Receptor
  Crista Ampullaris
  Macula
Vestibulocochlear Nerve: Cranial Nerve
  VIII–Vestibular Division
Vestibular Nuclei
  Spinal Cord
  Brainstem
  Cerebellum

CLINICAL SIGNS OF VESTIBULAR SYSTEM DISEASE

Unilateral Peripheral Vestibular Disease
  Abnormal Posture and Vestibular
    Ataxia
  Normal Nystagmus
  Abnormal Nystagmus
  Postrotatory Nystagmus
  Caloric Nystagmus
  Strabismus
  Postural Reactions
Bilateral Peripheral Vestibular System Disease
Central Vestibular System Disease
  Paradoxical Vestibular System
    Disease

VESTIBULAR SYSTEM DISEASES

Dogs
  CASE EXAMPLE 12-1
    Benign Idiopathic Canine Peripheral Vestibular
    Disease
  CASE EXAMPLE 12-2
    Otitis Media-Interna
  CASE EXAMPLE 12-3
    Neoplasm
  CASE EXAMPLE 12-4
    Neoplasm
    Granulomatous Meningoencephalitis
  CASE EXAMPLE 12-5
    Ischemic Encephalopathy
  CASE EXAMPLE 12-6
    Metronidazole Toxicity
  CASE EXAMPLE 12-7
    Leukodystrophy
Cats
  CASE EXAMPLE 12-8
    Benign Idiopathic Feline Peripheral Vestibular
    Disease
    Otitis Media-Interna
  CASE EXAMPLE 12-9
    Bilateral Otitis Media-Interna
    Congenital Peripheral Vestibular System Disease

  CASE EXAMPLE 12-10
    Neoplasm
    Cuterebra *Larval Myiasis*
  CASE EXAMPLE 12-11
    Feline Infectious Peritonitis Viral
      Meningoencephalitis
    Thiamin Deficiency Encephalopathy
Horses
  CASE EXAMPLE 12-12
    Otitis Media-Interna
    Temporohyoid Osteopathy
    Benign Idiopathic Peripheral Vestibular
      Disease
  CASE EXAMPLE 12-13
    Equine Protozoal Encephalitis
Ruminants
  CASE EXAMPLE 12-14
    Otitis Media-Interna in a Calf
    Otitis with Intracranial Abscess in a Calf
  CASE EXAMPLE 12-15
    Listeriosis in a Cow
  CASE EXAMPLE 12-16
Congenital Nystagmus

The vestibular system is the primary sensory system that maintains the animal's balance, its normal orientation relative to the gravitational field of the earth. This orientation is maintained in the setting of linear or rotatory acceleration or deceleration or tilting of the animal. The vestibular system is responsible for maintaining the position of the eyes, neck, trunk, and limbs relative to the position or movement of the head at any time.

ANATOMY AND PHYSIOLOGY

Receptor

The receptor for special proprioception (SP)—the vestibular system—develops in conjunction with the receptor for the auditory system (special somatic afferent system). They are derived from ectoderm but are contained in a mesodermally derived structure. Together these receptors are the components of the inner ear. The ectodermal component arises as a proliferation of ectodermal epithelial cells on the surface of the embryo adjacent to the developing rhombencephalon. This structure is the otic placode, which subsequently invaginates to form an otic pit and otic vesicle (otocyst) that breaks away from its attachment to the surface ectoderm. This saccular structure undergoes extensive modification of its shape but always retains its fluid-filled lumen and surrounding thin epithelial wall as it becomes the membranous labyrinth of the inner ear. Special modifications of its epithelial surface at predetermined sites form the receptor organs for the vestibular and auditory systems.

Corresponding developmental modifications occur in the surrounding paraxial mesoderm to provide a supporting capsule for the membranous labyrinth. This fluid-filled ossified structure is the bony labyrinth contained within the developing petrous portion of the temporal bone.

These membranous and bony labyrinths are formed adjacent to the first and second branchial arches and their corresponding first pharyngeal pouch and first branchial groove. The first branchial groove gives rise to the external ear canal. The first pharyngeal pouch forms the auditory tube and the mucosa of the middle-ear cavity. The intervening tissue forms the tympanum. The ear ossicles are derived from the neural crest of branchial arches 1 (malleus and incus) and 2 (stapes). These ossicles become components of the middle ear associated laterally with the tympanum (malleus) and medially with the vestibular window of the bony labyrinth of the inner ear (stapes).

Anatomically, the bony labyrinth in the petrous part of the temporal bone consists of three continuous fluid-filled portions (Figs. 12-1 and 12-2). These areas are the large vestibule and the three semicircular canals and the cochlea, which arise from the vestibule. Dilation in one end of each of the bony semicircular canals is the ampulla. All three continuous bony components contain perilymph, a fluid similar to cerebrospinal fluid (CSF), from which it may be derived. In the bony labyrinth are two openings: the vestibular and cochlear windows, which are named according to the components of the bony labyrinth in which they are located. Each opening is covered by a membrane, and the stapes is inserted in the membrane that covers the vestibular window.

The ectodermally derived membranous labyrinth consists of four fluid-filled compartments, all of which communicate (Fig. 12-3; see also Figs. 12-1 and 12-2). These compartments are contained within the components of the bony labyrinth and include the saccule and utriculus within the bony vestibule, the three semicircular ducts within the bony semicircular canals, and a cochlear duct within the bony cochlea. The endolymph contained within the membranous labyrinth is thought to be derived from the blood vessels along one wall of the cochlear duct and is absorbed back into the blood through the blood vessels surrounding the endolymphatic sac. The three semicircular ducts are the anterior (vertical), posterior (vertical), and lateral (horizontal). Each semicircular duct is oriented at right angles to the others. Thus rotation of the head around any plane causes endolymph to flow within one or more of the ducts. Each semicircular duct connects at both ends with the utriculus, which, in turn, connects with the saccule by way of the intervening endolymphatic duct and sac. The saccule connects with the cochlea duct by the small ductus reuniens.

Crista Ampullaris

At one end of each membranous semicircular duct is a dilation called the *ampulla*. On one side of the membranous ampulla, a proliferation of connective tissue forms a transverse ridge called the *crista* (see Figs. 12-1 through 12-3). It is lined on its internal surface by columnar neuroepithelial cells. On the surface of the crista is a gelatinous structure that is composed of a protein-polysaccharide material called the *cupula,* which extends across the lumen of the ampulla. This neuroepithelium is composed of two basic cell types: hair cells and supporting cells. The neurons of the vestibulocochlear nerve are derived from otic placode ectoderm. The dendritic zones of the neurons of the vestibular portion of the vestibulocochlear nerve are in synaptic contact with the base of the hair cells. These hair cells have on their luminal surface 40 to 80 hairs, or modified microvilli (stereocilia), and a single modified cilium (kinocilium). These structures project into the overlying cupula. Movement of fluid in the semicircular ducts causes deflection of the cupula, which is oriented transversely to the direction of flow of the endolymph. This deflection bends the stereocilia, which is the source of the stimulus by way of the hair cells to the dendritic zone of the vestibular neuron that is in synaptic relationship with the plasmalemma of the hair cell.

In one end of each semicircular duct is one membranous ampulla with its crista ampullaris. Because the three semicircular ducts are all at right angles to each other, movement of the head in any plane or angular rotation affects a crista ampullaris and stimulates vestibular neurons. These cristae function in dynamic equilibrium.

The vestibular neurons are tonically active, and their activity is excited or inhibited by deflection of the cupula in different directions. Each semicircular duct on one side is paired with a semicircular duct on the opposite side by their common position in a parallel plane. These synergistic pairs are the left and right lateral ducts, the left anterior and right posterior ducts, and the left posterior and right anterior ducts. When movement in the direction of one of these three planes stimulates the vestibular neurons of the crista of one duct, they are inhibited in the opposite duct of the synergistic pair. For example, rotation of the head to the right causes the endolymph to flow in the right lateral duct such that the cupula is deflected toward the utriculus and the cupula of the left lateral duct is deflected away from the utriculus. This action causes increased activity of vestibular neurons on the right side and decreased activity on the left side, resulting in a jerk nystagmus to the right side, which

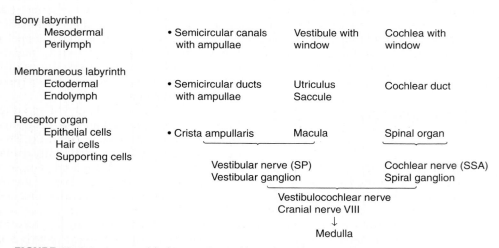

Bony labyrinth			
Mesodermal	• Semicircular canals	Vestibule with	Cochlea with
Perilymph	with ampullae	window	window
Membraneous labyrinth			
Ectodermal	• Semicircular ducts	Utriculus	Cochlear duct
Endolymph	with ampullae	Saccule	
Receptor organ			
Epithelial cells	• Crista ampullaris	Macula	Spinal organ
Hair cells			
Supporting cells			

Vestibular nerve (SP) Cochlear nerve (SSA)
Vestibular ganglion Spiral ganglion

Vestibulocochlear nerve
Cranial nerve VIII
↓
Medulla

FIGURE 12-1 Components of the inner ear. *SP,* Special proprioception; *SSA,* special somatic afferent.

Schematic anatomy of the vestibular system

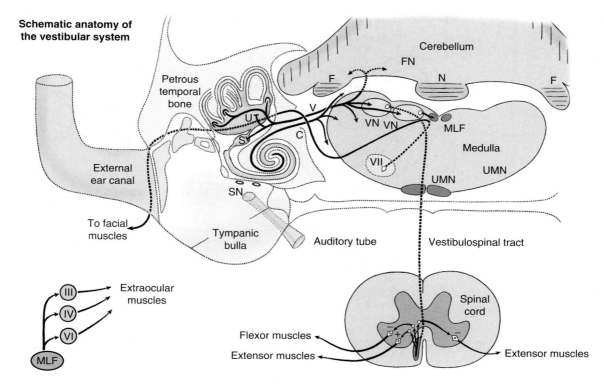

FIGURE 12-2 Schematic anatomy of the vestibular system. *III,* Oculomotor nucleus; *IV,* trochlear nucleus; *VI,* abducent nucleus; *VII,* facial nucleus; *C,* cranial nerve VIII–cochlear portion; *V,* cranial nerve VIII–vestibular portion; *F,* flocculus; *FN,* fastigial nucleus; *MLF,* medial longitudinal fasciculus; *N,* nodulus; *S,* saccule; *SN,* sympathetic neurons; *U,* utricle; *UMN,* upper motor neuron; *VN,* vestibular nucleus.

is an involuntary rhythmic oscillation of the eyes. The anatomic orientation of the stereocilia relative to the kinocilium on the surface of the crista is responsible for the difference in activity relative to the direction of the cupula deflection. Deviation of the stereocilia toward the kinocilium increases vestibular neuron activity. These receptors are not affected by a constant velocity of movement but respond to acceleration or deceleration, especially when the head is rotated.

Macula

The macula is the receptor found in the utriculus and saccule, which are located in the bony vestibule. These maculae are on one surface of each of these saclike structures (see Figs. 12-1 through 12-3). Each macula is an oval-shaped plaque in which the membranous labyrinth has proliferated. The surface of the macula consists of columnar epithelial cells. This neuroepithelium is composed of hair cells and supporting cells. Covering the neuroepithelium is a gelatinous material, the statoconiorum (otolithic) membrane. On the surface of this membrane are calcareous crystalline bodies known as *statoconia (otoliths)*. Similar to the hair cells of the cristae, the macular hair cells have projections of their luminal cell membranes—stereocilia and kinocilia—into the overlying statoconiorum membrane. Movement of the statoconia away from these cells is the initiating factor in bending the stereocilia to stimulate an impulse in the dendritic zones of the vestibular neurons that are in synaptic relationship with the base of the hair cells. The macula in the saccule is oriented in a vertical direction (sagittal plane), whereas the macula of the utriculus is in a horizontal direction

(dorsal plane). Thus gravitational forces continually affect the position of the statoconia relative to the hair cells. These structures are responsible for the sensation of the static position of the head and linear acceleration or deceleration. They function in static equilibrium. The macula of the utriculus may be more important as a receptor for sensing changes in head posture, whereas the macula of the saccule may be more sensitive to vibrational stimuli and loud sounds.

Vestibulocochlear Nerve: Cranial Nerve VIII—Vestibular Division

The dendritic zone of the vestibular portion of cranial nerve VIII is in a synaptic relationship with the hair cells of each crista ampullaris and the macula utriculi and macula sacculi. The axons course through the internal acoustic meatus with those of the cochlear division of this nerve. The cell bodies of these bipolar-type sensory neurons are inserted along the course of the axons within the petrous portion of the temporal bone, where they form the vestibular ganglion (see Fig. 12-3). After leaving the internal acoustic meatus with the cochlear division of the vestibulocochlear nerve, the vestibular nerve axons pass to the lateral surface of the rostral medulla at the cerebellomedullary angle, which occurs at the level of the trapezoid body and the attachment of the caudal cerebellar peduncle to the cerebellum. The vestibular nerve axons enter the medulla between the caudal cerebellar peduncle and the spinal tract of the trigeminal nerve and terminate in telodendria at one of two sites. The majority of them terminate in the vestibular nuclei in the medulla and pons. A few course directly into the cerebellum by way of the

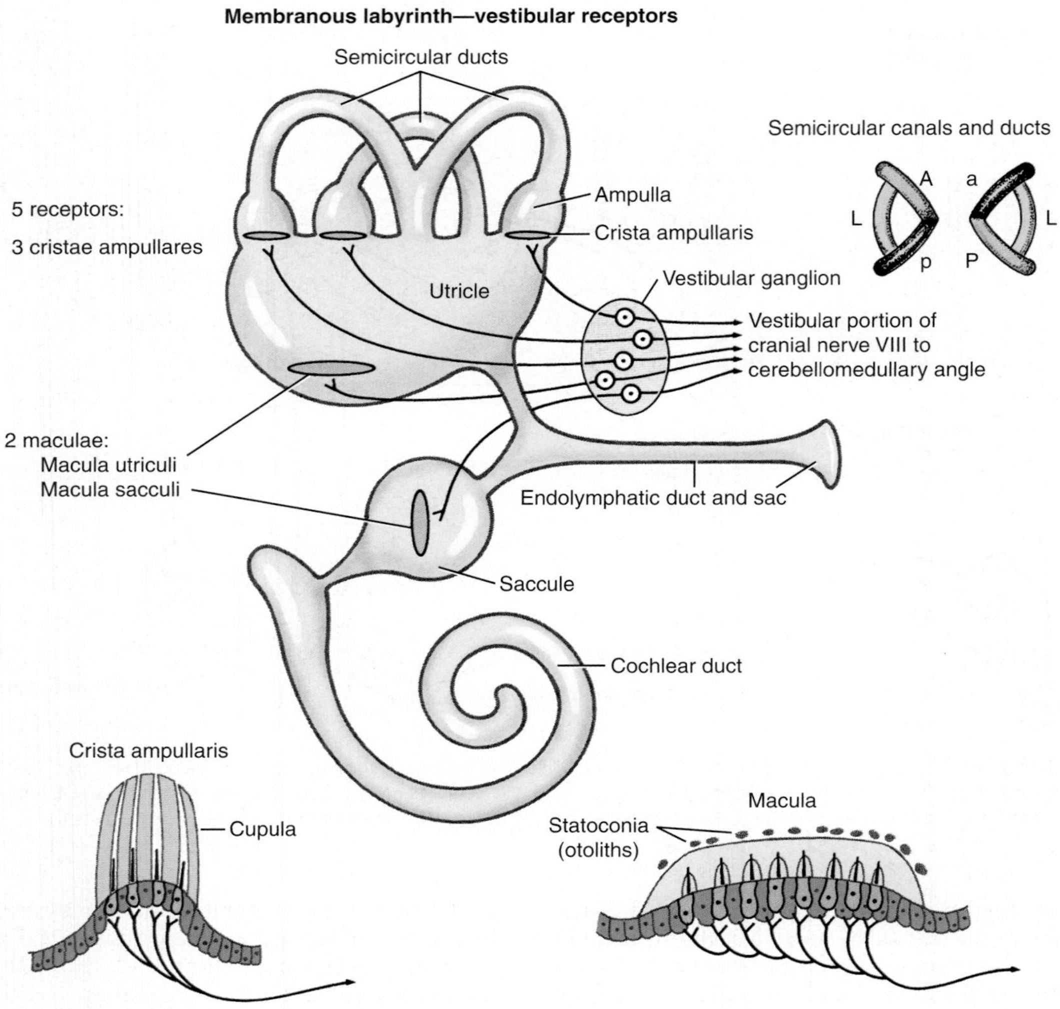

Membranous labyrinth—vestibular receptors

FIGURE 12-3 Special proprioception–vestibular system. Membranous labyrinth–vestibular receptors. *A,* Anterior–vertical plane; *L,* lateral–horizontal plane; *P,* posterior–vertical plane.

caudal peduncle and terminate in the fastigial nucleus in the cerebellar medulla and the cortex of the flocculonodular lobe. These latter axons form the direct vestibulocerebellar tract.

Vestibular Nuclei

On either side of the dorsal part of the pons and medulla adjacent to the lateral wall of the fourth ventricle are four vestibular nuclei (Fig. 12-4; see also Fig. 12-2). From the level of the rostral and middle cerebellar peduncles, they extend caudally to the level of the lateral cuneate nucleus in the lateral wall of the caudal portion of the fourth ventricle. The four nuclei are the rostral, medial, lateral, and caudal vestibular nuclei. They form a continuous column on each side of the pons and medulla. The rostral vestibular nucleus is located medial to the rostral and middle cerebellar peduncles, dorsal to the motor nucleus of the trigeminal nerve in the pons (see Fig. 2-11). The medial and lateral vestibular nuclei are located ventromedial to the confluence of the three cerebellar peduncles with the cerebellum (see Fig. 2-12). They are dorsal to the ventrolateral projection of the facial neurons. The medial nucleus continues caudally adjacent to the caudal vestibular

nucleus in the dorsal medulla to the level of the lateral cuneate nucleus (see Fig. 2-13). The lateral vestibular nucleus is only located at the level of the confluent cerebellar peduncles (see Fig. 2-12). The caudal vestibular nucleus is caudal to the lateral vestibular nucleus and continues caudally to the level of the lateral cuneate nucleus. The caudal cerebellar peduncle is dorsolateral to the caudal vestibular nucleus. The spinal tract of the trigeminal nerve and its nucleus are ventrolateral to the caudal vestibular nucleus in the medulla. These vestibular nuclei receive afferents from the vestibular division of the vestibulocochlear nerve. From the vestibular nuclei are numerous projections, which can be grouped into spinal cord, brainstem, and cerebellar pathways (see Fig. 12-4).

Spinal Cord

The lateral vestibulospinal tract courses caudally in the ipsilateral ventral funiculus through the entire spinal cord. Its axons terminate in all of the spinal cord segments on interneurons in the ventral gray columns (see Fig. 2-17). These interneurons are facilitory to ipsilateral alpha and gamma motor neurons to extensor muscles, inhibitory to the ipsilateral

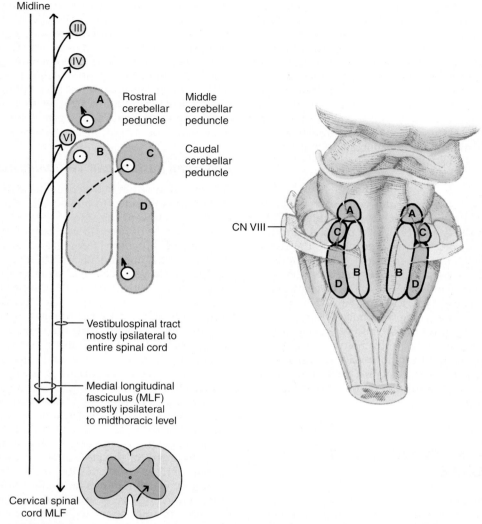

Midline

III

IV

A

Rostral
cerebellar
peduncle

Middle
cerebellar
peduncle

VI

B

C

Caudal
cerebellar
peduncle

D

CN VIII

A

A

C

C

B

B

D

D

Vestibulospinal tract
mostly ipsilateral to
entire spinal cord

Medial longitudinal
fasciculus (MLF)
mostly ipsilateral
to midthoracic level

Cervical spinal
cord MLF

FIGURE 12-4 Vestibular nuclei and tracts. **A,** Rostral vestibular nucleus; **B,** medial vestibular nucleus; **C,** lateral vestibular nucleus; **D,** caudal vestibular nucleus.

alpha motor neurons to flexor muscles, and some interneurons cross to the opposite ventral gray column where they are inhibitory to the contralateral alpha and gamma motor neurons to extensor muscles (see Fig. 12-2). Thus the effect of stimulation of the neuronal cell bodies, the axons of which are in the vestibulospinal tract, is an ipsilateral extensor tonus and contralateral inhibition of this mechanism. The cell bodies of most of the axons in the lateral vestibulospinal tract are located in the lateral vestibular nucleus.

The medial vestibulospinal tract arises from cell bodies in the rostral, medial, and caudal vestibular nuclei and passes caudally in the ipsilateral ventral funiculus of the cervical and cranial thoracic spinal cord segments.[49] These axons terminate on interneurons in the ventral gray columns, which influence the activation of the alpha and gamma motor neurons that innervate primarily neck muscles. In addition, the medial vestibular nucleus projects axons into the medial longitudinal fasciculus, which courses caudally in the dorsal portion of the ventral funiculus through the cervical and cranial thoracic spinal cord segments.[35,36]

Through these spinal cord pathways, the position and activity of the limbs, neck, and trunk can be coordinated with movements of the head.

Brainstem

Neuronal cell bodies in the vestibular nuclei have three general terminations in the brainstem.

1. Axons course rostrally in the medial longitudinal fasciculus (MLF) to terminate in the motor nuclei of cranial nerves VI, IV, and III. Their purpose is to provide coordinated conjugate eye movements associated with changes in the position of the head. In most normal animals, this eye movement can be readily elicited by repeatedly moving the head from one side to the other and observing the jerk nystagmus that is produced. When the brainstem is severely contused by a head injury, these pathways may be disrupted, and eyeball movements cannot be elicited by changing the position of the head. This clinical sign usually indicates a poor prognosis because of the severity of the associated lesion.

2. Axons project into the reticular formation. Some of these axons provide afferents to the vomiting center located there. This pathway is involved with motion sickness.

3. We are all readily aware of any loss of our balance. Balance requires a pathway for conscious perception that involves a relay through a thalamic nucleus. This pathway is not well defined for the vestibular system. It may be closely

associated with the conscious pathway for the auditory system. Axons of neuronal cell bodies in vestibular nuclei course rostrally through the midbrain to terminate in the contralateral medial geniculate nucleus of the thalamus or some other thalamic nucleus. Synapse occurs here, and the axons of the cell bodies in that thalamic nucleus project by way of the internal capsule to the cerebral cortex, probably the cortex in the temporal lobe. Interference with this conscious pathway would explain the occasional observation of clinical signs of a vestibular system dysfunction after an acute prosencephalic lesion.

Cerebellum

Axons of neuronal cell bodies in the vestibular nuclei, in addition to some in the vestibular ganglia, project to the cerebellum through the caudal cerebellar peduncle and terminate mostly in the cortex of the flocculus of the hemisphere and the nodulus of the vermis (the flocculonodular lobe). These axons have collaterals that synapse in the fastigial nucleus, which is the most medial of the three nuclei in the cerebellar medulla (see Figs. 12-2 and Fig. 2-13).

Through these pathways the vestibular system functions to coordinate the position of the eyes, neck, trunk, and limbs with the position and movements of the head. The system maintains equilibrium during active and passive movement and when the head is at rest. Interference with the system results in varying degrees of loss of balance and abnormal head position.

CLINICAL SIGNS OF VESTIBULAR SYSTEM DISEASE

Vestibular system disease produces varying degrees of loss of equilibrium, causing imbalance and a unique quality of ataxia that is designated vestibular ataxia as opposed to general proprioceptive ataxia and cerebellar ataxia. Clinical neurologists think about and describe disorders of the vestibular system as peripheral or central. Only minor differences exist in the clinical signs of vestibular system dysfunction between lesions of this system in the petrous portion of the temporal bone (peripheral) or the vestibular nuclei on one side of the medulla or the vestibular components of the cerebellum (central). The determination of whether the vestibular system signs reflect a dysfunction of the peripheral or central components of the vestibular system is more dependent on recognition of clinical signs caused by the dysfunction of other systems located in the brainstem or cerebellum. As a rule, the most common diseases that affect the peripheral components of the vestibular system are less serious than those that affect the central components. We will first describe the clinical signs of vestibular system dysfunction as they would occur with a complete disruption of the vestibular receptors or vestibular nerve in the petrous portion of the temporal bone. These signs are the clinical signs of peripheral vestibular disease.

Unilateral Peripheral Vestibular Disease

Unilateral disease of the peripheral components of the vestibular system[9] is characterized by an asymmetric ataxia with loss of balance but with preservation of strength. No loss of general proprioception occurs in peripheral vestibular system disease. Therefore these patients know exactly where their limbs are in space, and no paresis is present, thus they can support weight well (normal lower motor neuron [LMN] activity) and move their limbs rapidly (normal upper motor neuron [UMN] activity) to prevent themselves from falling as a result of their balance loss. The clinical signs will be recognized on your observation of the posture and gait of the patient and on your examination of the posture and movement of the eyes.

Abnormal Posture and Vestibular Ataxia

Loss of coordination between the head and the neck, trunk, and limbs is reflected in a head tilt, with the more ventral ear directed toward the side of the vestibular system disorder. The degree of head tilt can vary from just a few degrees that may be difficult to recognize to nearly 45 degrees with the patient having difficulty standing up. To recognize the mild head tilt, you need to observe the patient's head from in front of the patient and with your head at the level of the head of the patient. The neck and trunk will lean, fall, or even roll toward the side of the lesion. The neck and trunk may be flexed laterally with the concavity directed toward the side of the lesion. The patient may tend to circle toward the affected side. These circles are usually small, which will appear as though the patient is falling in that direction. Animals that propulsively circle from prosencephalic lesions have no ataxia or other signs of vestibular system dysfunction and usually walk in wider circles. Occasionally, it may be possible to elicit mild hypertonia in the limbs on the side of the body opposite to the side of the vestibular system lesion. The asymmetry of the ataxia may be explained by the loss of tonic activity in the vestibulospinal tract on the side of the lesion, which removes facilitation of ipsilateral extensor muscles and a source of inhibition of contralateral extensor muscles. The unopposed activity of the contralateral vestibulospinal tract causes the neck and trunk to be forced toward the side of the lesion by excessive unopposed extensor muscle tonus. The entire body will lean, fall, or roll toward the side of the lesion. With peripheral vestibular system disorders, rolling is usually limited to the first 24 to 48 hours after a peracute onset of clinical signs. If the rolling persists longer than that, the lesion more likely involves the central components of the vestibular system. Frequently, the patient falls when it shakes its head. With only the vestibular system affected, these patients will make very rapid and short limb movements in their attempt to maintain their balance. As you evaluate a patient such as this one, you should ask yourself if this patient knows where its limbs are in space. The answer will be definitely *yes* if only the peripheral vestibular system is affected. Patients with vestibular ataxia use their eyes to help maintain their balance. Therefore blindfolding these patients usually makes their vestibular ataxia worse. This tactic is most helpful when you are not sure if the vestibular system is involved in the patient's clinical signs. Be cautious when you perform this test with large animals so that they do not fall and injure themselves or the observers. For horses and cattle, use a folded towel that is slipped under the halter so that it can be readily removed by pulling on one edge of the towel. *Never* tie the blindfold onto the halter. Cats often carry their tails elevated straight dorsally when they have a significant balance loss.

Normal Nystagmus

Nystagmus is an involuntary rhythmic oscillation of the eyes. Eye movements that are equal in each direction indicate a pendular nystagmus, which is uncommon, usually benign, and is associated with congenital visual system pathway abnormalities. Eye movements that are unequal, with a slow movement (slow phase) in one direction and a fast return (quick phase) of the eye to its starting position, indicate a jerk nystagmus, which can be normal or abnormal and reflect a dysfunction in the vestibular system. The direction of the nystagmus, by convention, is ascribed to the direction of the quick or fast phase of the jerk nystagmus. Both eyes are usually affected and usually in the same direction. This jerk nystagmus is a normal response to any rapid movement of the head. Stand over any normal dog and watch its eyes as you move the head in a horizontal-dorsal plane form side to side. You will observe a horizontal jerk nystagmus. As you move the head to the right, both eyes will repeatedly jerk quickly to the right with a slow return to the left. As you move the head to the left, the opposite will happen; both eyes will repeatedly jerk quickly to the left and slowly return to the right. This procedure is termed *normal vestibular* or *physiologic* nystagmus. Some textbooks refer to this response as vestibular-ocular nystagmus, or a doll's eye response. It evaluates not only the vestibular system, which is the sensory arm of this response, but also the medial longitudinal fasciculus in the brainstem and the abducent nerve innervation of the lateral rectus muscle that abducts the eye and the oculomotor nerve innervation of the medial rectus muscle that adducts the eye. If you flex and extend the neck so that the head moves up and down, the same eye movements will occur in a vertical direction. This event is a vertical jerk nystagmus. The quick phase of the nystagmus is always in the direction of the head movement. This response is a normal reflex in which the slow component is initiated by way of the vestibular receptors in the membranous labyrinth and the quick component involves a brainstem center related to the vestibular system. This reflex is important in maintaining visual fixation on stationary points as the body rotates.

Abnormal Nystagmus

When the head is held in its normal extended (neutral) position, or if held flexed laterally to either side or held fully extended at rest, no nystagmus will occur in the normal animal. It normally occurs only when you move the head. With dysfunction of the vestibular system, a jerk nystagmus may be observed. If it is observed when the head is held in its normal extended (neutral) position, it is called a resting or spontaneous nystagmus. If it is induced only by holding the head fixed in lateral flexion or full extension, it is called a positional nystagmus. These events are both forms of abnormal nystagmus. If you are suspicious of the possibility of a vestibular system disorder, looking for positional nystagmus when you place the patient on its back with its neck extended may be useful. Remember that it is normal for nystagmus to occur when you move the head! How do you explain this abnormal nystagmus? If you consider the existence of a continual bilateral stimulation of vestibular neurons that constantly reflects the position or movement of the head and that this provides a balanced tonic stimulation of the vestibular nuclei on each side and from there to the nuclei that innervate the extraocular muscles, then any interruption of this balanced tonic stimulation might result in an alteration at the nuclei of the neurons that innervate extraocular muscles that results in nystagmus. With peripheral vestibular diseases, the imbalance represents a loss of tonic stimulation of the vestibular nuclei from the affected side.

In disorders of the peripheral vestibular system, the abnormal resting or positional nystagmus is directed in a horizontal-dorsal plane or is rotatory but is always directed (quick phase) away from the side of the lesion or head tilt. To determine the direction of a rotatory nystagmus, observe the direction that the 12-o'clock position of the pupil moves during the quick phase. This direction does not change when the position of the head is changed. Occasionally, an abnormal positional nystagmus may appear vertical, especially when the patient is in dorsal recumbency. Previous theories suggested that vertical nystagmus only occurred with disorders of the central vestibular system, but we now believe this idea may be incorrect and oversimplified. Some patients with disorders of the peripheral vestibular system have almost a vertical nystagmus, but careful examination will usually reveal a slight rotatory component. We no longer use vertical nystagmus alone to distinguish peripheral from central vestibular system disease. With disorders of the central components of the vestibular system, the nystagmus may be horizontal, rotatory, or vertical. It may be directed toward or away from the side of the lesion, and it may change in direction with the head held in different positions. Thus the presence of a nystagmus that is directed toward the side of the lesion or head tilt or changes direction with changes in the position of the head are the only reliable features of the abnormal nystagmus that indicate a central involvement of the vestibular system. Many patients with central vestibular system disease will have abnormal nystagmus that is horizontal or rotatory and is directed to the side opposite to the side of the lesion and does not change its direction with changes in head position. Therefore, to determine a disorder of the central vestibular system, you must identify clinical signs of the central lesion that involve other neurologic systems, especially the UMN and general proprioception (GP) systems. Resting nystagmus is more common in acute disorders of the peripheral components of the vestibular system, and the rate of either resting or positional nystagmus tends to be more rapid than when the disorder is in the central components of the vestibular system. Some patients with severe resting nystagmus exhibit a slight head rotation that occurs simultaneously with the nystagmus corresponding to its rate and direction. In addition, a simultaneous eyelid blink may be seen concomitant with the nystagmus, which presumably is a reflex action. These latter two findings are very common in rabbits.

Normal nystagmus requires normal function of the vestibular system components, normal medial longitudinal fasciculus bilaterally, and normal general somatic efferent (GSE) neurons in the abducent, trochlear, and oculomotor nuclei. Abnormal nystagmus indicates a disruption in the normal bilateral balance of sensory information from the peripheral vestibular receptor and the activity of the central components of the vestibular system. No normal or abnormal nystagmus can occur with bilateral loss of function in the peripheral vestibular system, its central components, the medial longitudinal fasciculus, or the GSE motor neurons of the abducent, trochlear, and oculomotor nuclei. Bilateral otitis interna is the most common cause of the complete absence of any normal or abnormal nystagmus.

Postrotatory Nystagmus

If an animal is rotated rapidly, as it accelerates, the labyrinth moves around the endolymph, which deflects the cupula of the crista ampullaris, stimulating the vestibular nerve and thus eliciting eye movements. The quick phase is in the direction of the rotation, but this aspect cannot be seen as the animal is moving. In time, the rotation of the endolymph reaches the same speed of rotation of the labyrinth. At this constant velocity, the cupulae are not deflected. Thus no rotatory stimulus reaches the vestibular nerve, and nystagmus does not occur. When the rotation is suddenly stopped, once again, a disparity occurs in the rotation of the labyrinth and the endolymph. The labyrinth is stationary, and the endolymph continues to flow for a short interval during which it deflects the cupulae. Vestibular neurons are stimulated, and nystagmus occurs. However, the direction of flow is opposite to that which occurred during acceleration, and the quick phase of the nystagmus is directed opposite to the direction of the rotation. The speed and duration of this postrotatory nystagmus are variable but should be approximately equal when the response to rotation is compared for both directions.

Vestibular system disease is suspected when a different response is elicited to spinning in one direction compared with the other. As a rule, when the patient is rotated in a direction opposite to the side of a peripheral receptor lesion, postrotatory nystagmus is depressed. This postrotatory test stimulates both labyrinths. However, the labyrinth on the outside of the rotation, on the side of the head opposite to the direction of rotation, is stimulated more because it is farther away from the axis of rotation, which may explain the abnormal postrotatory nystagmus that is observed with unilateral peripheral vestibular disease. On rotating the patient away from the side of the lesion, the diseased labyrinth is farthest from the axis of rotation. It cannot be stimulated properly because of the lesion, and a depressed postrotatory response may be observed.

This test can be performed only on patients that are small enough to be picked up and held with your elbows extended. It requires two people, the holder and the examiner. The holder directs the head of the patient away from his or her body and spins in a circle as rapidly as possible for 6 to 7 rotations and stops suddenly. The examiner immediately grasps the head of the patient and observes the eyes for nystagmus. The eyes of the holder will show the same postrotatory response. For some large dogs, you can secure them in a rotating desk chair and spin them with the chair. In most small animals, this postrotatory response can be readily elicited. We perform this test only when the clinical signs of a peripheral vestibular disorder are subtle and a need exists for more supportive information or in a patient that is suspected of having a bilateral peripheral vestibular system disorder in which no normal nystagmus will occur; it is not reliable for determining the side of the lesion.

Caloric Nystagmus

The vestibular receptors of each inner ear can be tested separately by using the caloric test. Irrigation of the external ear canal with ice-cold water or warm water for 3 to 5 minutes causes the endolymph to flow in the semicircular ducts. Using cold water, this test normally induces a jerk nystagmus to the side opposite to the ear being stimulated. If the peripheral receptor on the side being stimulated is nonfunctional because of a disease process, no nystagmus will be observed with this caloric test. Covering the patient's eyes may prevent voluntary repression of the response by fixation on an object in the environment of the visual field. This test is useful in humans who can be restrained in an adjustable chair that will permit not only the testing of an individual ear, but also individual semicircular ducts. Most animals need considerable physical restraint to perform this test, and, from personal experience, some normal dogs will not exhibit any nystagmus with prolonged irrigation of the ear canal with cold water. Thus this caloric testing is both unreliable and not practical in our animal patients. We avoid its use.

Strabismus

Strabismus is an abnormal position of the eye relative to the orbit or palpebral fissure that is a clinical sign of loss of innervation to the extraocular muscles and was described with the cranial nerves in Chapter 6. This strabismus is visible in all positions of the head. In the normal small animal, when the head and neck are extended in the tonic neck reaction, the eyes should elevate and remain in the center of the palpebral fissures. With disorders of any component of the vestibular system, this effect may not occur on the side of the lesion, resulting in a *dropped* or ventrally deviated eye that exposes the sclera dorsally. Occasionally, a slight ventral or ventrolateral strabismus is observed without head and neck extension but disappears when the head position is changed. This action will mimic an oculomotor nerve strabismus. However, when you move the head side to side to test for normal physiologic nystagmus, the affected eye will adduct and abduct well, indicating that cranial nerves III and VI are not impaired. This inconstant abnormal eye position is known as *vestibular* strabismus. You should look for this impairment when you hold the head and neck in extension because it may be the only clinical sign observed in mild disorders of the vestibular system. This vestibular strabismus will be on the same side as the lesion in the vestibular system.

In ruminants, it is normal for their eyes to not elevate completely when the head and neck are extended; therefore you expect to see some sclera dorsal to the cornea in these species, but it should be equal on both sides. Horses may exhibit a slight ventral deviation of the eyes when you try to extend their head and neck, but their size makes this observation difficult.

Postural Reactions

The vestibular system is the *only* system involved with movement of the animal that, when deficient, does not interfere with the performance of the postural reactions. Hopping, hemiwalking, placing, and paw or hoof replacement will all be normal. Only the animal's ability to right itself from a recumbent position may be altered, and this action toward the side of the lesion may be exaggerated. In the worst situation, the patient may continually roll in that direction.

The ability to perform these postural reactions (except for righting) is critical to determining whether the vestibular system disorder involves the peripheral or central components of the vestibular system. You need to repeat the hopping responses many times to be comfortable that they are normal in your patient with peripheral vestibular disease. In patients with severe loss of their ability to balance, holding them securely to perform these postural reactions may be difficult. With an acute onset of severe loss of balance, delaying or repeating this part of the neurologic examination after 24 hours may be necessary to allow time for the most severe clinical signs to abate enough so that you can handle the patient for this examination. The ground surface must not be slippery and should provide good traction for the patient. Be careful if you pick up one of these patients because severe disorientation will be initiated, and they will thrash their limbs to seek a supporting surface. If you suddenly pick up a cat with this disorder, you are in danger of being grasped by the struggling patient.

Vomiting as a continuous event is an uncommon clinical sign of vestibular system dysfunction in domestic animals. However, in approximately 25% of animals presented with an acute onset of vestibular system dysfunction, the owners will report observing an episode of vomiting at the onset of clinical signs.

Bilateral Peripheral Vestibular System Disease

When the peripheral components of the vestibular system are dysfunctional bilaterally, such as in a patient with bilateral otitis media-interna, no postural asymmetry is noted. Balance is lost to either side, resulting in the patient assuming a crouched posture closer to the ground surface. They can walk well but are often slow and cautious to prevent falling, especially when they move their heads suddenly. The most characteristic clinical sign is the presence of wide head excursions. When the patient moves its head to either side to look at objects in its environment, the movement is greater than normal, which gives the appearance that it cannot be stopped and the movement is prolonged. These wide head excursions occur to either side and to the same degree and may occasionally be accompanied by a brief staggering movement. Because no functional vestibular receptors or vestibular nerves exist, no stimulus exists to be projected into the brainstem and to the cranial nerves that move the eyes. Therefore no normal or abnormal nystagmus can be observed.

Central Vestibular System Disease

We have already indicated that the only clinical signs of dysfunction of the vestibular system that occur with disorders of the central components of the vestibular system and not with peripheral vestibular system disorders are the presence of an abnormal nystagmus that changes directions when the position of the head is changed and a horizontal or rotatory nystagmus directed toward the side of the head tilt and body deviation.[46] If the nystagmus is absolutely vertical, the disorder is most likely in the central components of the vestibular system. Be aware that what appears to be vertical may have a slight rotary component, which can occur with peripheral vestibular system disorders. The most reliable clinical sign that determines that a lesion exists in

the pons or medulla affecting the vestibular nuclei is an ipsilateral postural reaction deficit or a recognizable spastic hemiparesis and ataxia from involvement of the UMN and GP systems adjacent to these nuclei here in the caudal brainstem. Clinical signs of cerebellar and cranial nerve dysfunction (except for the facial nerve) also implicate a cerebellar or pontomedullary location for the clinical signs of vestibular system dysfunction. Remember that facial paralysis and Horner syndrome can occur along with clinical signs of vestibular nerve dysfunction with diseases of the middle and inner ear in small animals and just facial paralysis in the horse and farm animals. Lesions that involve solely the vestibular nuclei on one side cause ipsilateral clinical signs similar to all the lesions that affect the peripheral components of the vestibular system with the patient's head tilt and loss of balance directed toward the side of the lesion.

Paradoxical Vestibular System Disease

Paradoxical vestibular system disease is a unique syndrome in which the head tilt and loss of balance are directed toward the side *opposite* to the central lesion, which usually involves the caudal cerebellar peduncle. An explanation for this paradox in the direction of the clinical signs of vestibular system dysfunction is based on the rule that the direction of the head tilt and balance loss will be toward the side of the *least* vestibular system activity. When we describe the physiologic anatomy of the cerebellum in Chapter 13, you will learn that the Purkinje neurons that form a single layer of cells in the cerebellar cortex are the only neurons that project their axons from the cerebellar cortex. These neurons are all inhibitory neurons that release gamma-amino butyric acid at their telodendria. Most of these neurons terminate via their telodendria on neuronal cell bodies in the cerebellar nuclei, which are located in the central portion of the cerebellum known as the cerebellar medulla. The neurons in these cerebellar nuclei comprise the majority of the efferent axons that leave the cerebellum to terminate in various brainstem nuclei. An exception to this rule is a small population of Purkinje neurons, most of which are located in the cortex of the folia of the flocculus in the hemisphere and the nodulus in the vermis. The Purkinje neurons of these cortical areas have axons that leave the cerebellum directly as a component of the caudal cerebellar peduncle. They terminate in the vestibular nuclei, where they are inhibitory to the activation of these neuronal cell bodies. A lesion in the caudal cerebellar peduncle interferes with this inhibition, resulting in excessive discharge of vestibular system neurons on that side. The imbalance in vestibular system activation between the two sides is recognized as a head tilt and loss of balance to the side opposite to this lesion because, as a rule, the direction of the head tilt and balance loss will be towards the side with the least activity of the vestibular system. This paradoxical syndrome is in contrast to lesions that cause a loss of activation of the neuronal cell bodies in the vestibular nuclei as seen in disorders of the peripheral components of the vestibular system or within the vestibular nuclei themselves.

Experimental studies support our clinical observations and proposed explanation.[25] Ablation of the caudal cerebellar peduncle dorsal to the medulla on one side will produce a head tilt and balance loss directed toward the side opposite to the lesion with the nystagmus directed toward the side of the lesion. If the vestibular nuclei are included in this lesion, the head tilt and balance loss will be directed toward the side of the lesion, and the nystagmus will be toward the side opposite to the lesion, similar to disorders of the vestibular nerve or its receptors. Similarly, ablation of the flocculus and nodulus within the cerebellum will produce this paradoxical vestibular system syndrome, with the clinical signs directed toward the side opposite to this cerebellar lesion. However, experimental ablation of the fastigial nucleus, a source of activation of the vestibular nuclei, causes ipsilateral vestibular system signs.

In clinical practice, the side of this unilateral lesion will be determined on your neurologic examination by the side of the postural reaction deficit or the side of the hemiparesis and ataxia, which will be ipsilateral to the lesion. The caudal cerebellar peduncle lesion will be contralateral to the direction of the head tilt in paradoxical vestibular system disease. The caudal cerebellar peduncle lesion that causes the paradoxical vestibular system clinical signs also interferes with GP afferents that are entering the cerebellum. Their interruption will cause ipsilateral ataxia and a deficit

in postural reactions. The lesions that affect the caudal cerebellar peduncle and cause the paradoxical vestibular system signs are variable and most commonly include infarcts, neoplasms, and inflammations, in our experience. Most of these lesions, when unilateral, also affect the UMN system to the ipsilateral neck, trunk, and limbs and ipsilateral GSE LMNs in cranial nerves.

Be aware that clinical signs of vestibular system dysfunction will occur if the dorsal roots of the first three cervical spinal cord segments are interrupted. This dysfunction has been observed in experimental animals in which these roots have been transected, presumably caused by the loss of GP afferents from neuromuscular spindles, which are critical for maintaining normal orientation of the head with the neck. Spinal cord lesions at this level that interrupt the spinovestibular tracts may have the same effect. We have observed temporary clinical signs of vestibular system dysfunction in three dogs after resection of extramedullary spinal cord tumors at the level of the C1 and C2 vertebrae, presumably from surgical trauma to these spinal cord segments. These clinical signs resolved in all three dogs within a 3- to 5-day period.

VESTIBULAR SYSTEM DISEASES

Dogs

CASE EXAMPLE 12-1

Signalment: 14-year-old male golden retriever, Sonny
Chief Complaint: Unable to stand up
History: The owners were reading at 7 PM when they heard a thrashing in their bedroom and found Sonny throwing himself around as he tried unsuccessfully to stand. They wrapped him in a blanket and brought him to the hospital, where he was examined and found unable to stand at that time. The video was made 6 hours after the sudden onset of these clinical signs, 5 hours after his hospitalization.
 Examination: See **Video 12-1**. Note how rapidly this dog moves his limbs to maintain his balance and his normal rapid hopping responses. Also note the abnormal spontaneous right nystagmus.
Anatomic Diagnosis: Left peripheral vestibular system (membranous labyrinth, vestibular receptors, vestibular nerve portion of cranial nerve VIII, vestibular ganglion)
Differential Diagnosis: Benign idiopathic canine peripheral vestibular disease, otitis media-interna, ototoxicity

BENIGN IDIOPATHIC CANINE PERIPHERAL VESTIBULAR DISEASE

Benign idiopathic canine peripheral vestibular disease is the most presumptive clinical diagnosis in this patient based on the peracute onset, the age of the dog, and clinical signs limited to the peripheral components of the vestibular system predominantly on one side.[4,42] Whether the cochlear nerve or its receptors are also involved is unknown, given that you cannot reliably diagnose unilateral deafness without the use of electrodiagnostic equipment. Because this disorder is most prevalent in aged dogs, it is often termed *geriatric canine peripheral vestibular disease*. The cause of the disorder is unknown. Microscopic study of euthanized patients are uncommon because most dogs will spontaneously recover, the procedure is not routine in most necropsy laboratories, and the process of decalcification

that is required makes recognition of subtle abnormalities difficult. The rapid recovery suggests that this disease may be a functional disorder, possibly an alteration in the production and absorption of endolymph that causes increased pressure within the membranous labyrinth. This theory has been proposed for the pathogenesis of Meniere disease in humans, which is an episodic disorder of the inner-ear components. Vestibular neuronitis is described in humans with an acute onset of clinical signs of a peripheral vestibular system dysfunction. Spontaneous recovery occurs. A herpesvirus-induced vestibular ganglionitis and an autoimmune inner-ear inflammation have also been proposed in humans. Paroxysmal positional vertigo (dizziness) in humans has been related to one or more statoconia that detach from the statoconiorum membrane and lodge in one of the semicircular ducts. Recovery is associated with specific head position adjustments to dislodge the statoconia. Many of the acute peripheral vestibular diseases of humans are not well understood.[11,17]

The idiopathic canine disorder is rarely observed before 5 years of age. The clinical signs are usually peracute in onset and rapidly improve to near complete resolution by 1 to 3 weeks from the onset. Residual clinical signs are uncommon. A few dogs may have a persistent head tilt. However, recurrences occasionally occur after a variable period of weeks to months. The onset of clinical signs can occur at any time of the year, which differs from a similar clinical syndrome that is seen in cats.

With this rapid spontaneous recovery and without knowing the cause of this disorder, no basis exists for specific treatment. In the first 24 to 48 hours when the clinical signs are severe and incapacitating, treatment with diazepam (Valium) or, to a lesser extent, meclizine (Antivert) may decrease the intensity of the clinical signs. Diazepam or similar drugs are used in a variety of vestibular system disorders in humans. In the past, this disorder was incorrectly diagnosed as a stroke, a brain infarction, which often resulted in the unnecessary euthanasia of the patient. This practice is inexcusable with the present level of veterinary education. Severe clinical signs of vestibular system dysfunction often accompany the development of cerebellar ischemic lesions or infarcts (stroke), but the neurologic examination should support the anatomic diagnosis of a cerebellar disorder.[18,20] In addition, the clinical signs of this predominantly cerebellar disorder may resolve spontaneously or at least improve remarkably. If you are presented with a dog within a few hours of the peracute onset of the clinical signs of a peripheral vestibular disorder, the patient's severe disorientation may make performing a complete neurologic examination impossible. Evaluation of the postural reactions are critical to making the correct anatomic diagnosis. If your anatomic diagnosis of the location of the vestibular system disorder is dependent on the results of your postural reaction testing, we recommend confining the patient to a cage and reevaluating the patient over the next 12 to 24 hours before proceeding with ancillary procedures. Magnetic resonance (MR) imaging to date has been normal in the few patients with this peripheral vestbular system disorder that have been imaged. As MR imaging technology improves and we gain more experience, abnormalities may possibly be found, especially if an inflammatory disorder is present.

Otitis media-interna is your greatest concern in the differential diagnosis when the clinical signs are limited to the peripheral components of the vestibular system.[44] Facial paralysis and Horner syndrome often occur with otitis media-interna in small animals but *never* occur with the benign idiopathic disorder.[3] The peracute onset of severe clinical signs of peripheral vestibular system dysfunction is less common in otitis media-interna. Imaging procedures are the most reliable in supporting the diagnosis of otitis media-interna.

Ototoxicity should be supported by a history of exposure to drugs that affect inner-ear function.[27,32,50,51] Degeneration of the vestibular or cochlear labyrinthine receptors or both may occur with high levels of aminoglycoside antibiotics. These drugs include streptomycin, amikacin, kanamycin, neomycin, gentamycin, and vancomycin. Streptomycin most often affects the vestibular system receptors in cats. The other antibiotics more often affect the cochlear receptors, but both types of receptor are susceptible to degeneration from any of these antibiotics. Clinical signs are usually unilateral but occasionally bilateral clinical signs occur. Spontaneous recovery will

occur only if the diagnosis is made promptly and the exposure period is short before drug removal.

Hypothyroid-induced ischemic neuropathy of the vestibulocochlear nerve is a rare cause of acute clinical signs of a peripheral vestibular system disorder. This diagnosis is supported by clinical laboratory findings of a primary hypothyroidism and severe hyperlipidemia. The ischemic neuropathy may be a result of hypothyroid-induced atherosclerosis or increased blood viscosity involving the labyrinthine artery. This pathogenesis has yet to be confirmed. It is not known if the rapid recovery that follows thyroid supplementation is due to the treatment or spontaneous recovery.

In the southeastern part of the United States where the blue tail lizard is common, many veterinarians believe that acute peripheral vestibular system dysfunction occurs in cats shortly after they eat the tail of this lizard.[1] Additional clinical signs include vomiting, trembling, salivation, and hyperirritability from more diffuse involvement of the nervous system. A few deaths have occurred. Further careful studies of this presumed toxicity are necessary. We have no experience with this unique disorder.

See the following videos for other examples of benign idiopathic canine peripheral vestibular disease.

Video 12-2 shows Iris, a 13-year-old spayed female Norwich terrier who was videoed 24 hours after her sudden onset of severe disorientation, inability to stand, and frequent rolling to the right side. During the videotaping, I (Alexander de Lahunta) could not get the left pelvic limb to hop, but this feature was normal a few hours later. The last portion of the video was made 2 months after the first and shows Iris completely recovered without any treatment.

Video 12-3 shows Sonny, a 12-year-old spayed female mixed breed with a sudden onset of what the owner described as seizure-like activity based on eye shaking and eyelid twitching. However, Sonny was still well aware of her environment, including recognition of the owner. The video was made 18 hours after the onset of clinical signs. Repeating the hopping responses many times was necessary on Sonny before I (AD) was comfortable the responses were normal in this dog with the severe disorientation.

Video 12-4 shows Jute, a 13-year-old female border collie 4 days after a sudden onset of a left head tilt and loss of balance. Initially she could not stand without assistance.

CASE EXAMPLE 12-2

Signalment: 4-year-old castrated male golden retriever, Bozo
Chief Complaint: Head tilt and tearing
History: Eight days before the examination, the owner noticed excessive tearing on the right side of Bozo's face. Four days later, the dog had developed a right head tilt.
Examination: See **Video 12-5**. Note the lack of a right palpebral reflex but the retraction of the eye with the elevation of the third eyelid, the lack of lip and ear tone on the right but the straight philtrum, and note that the clinical signs of peripheral vestibular system dysfunction are limited to the head tilt and abnormal nystagmus. This dog's balance is normal.
Anatomic Diagnosis: Right cranial nerves VII and VIII—vestibular nerve or its labyrinthine receptors
Differential Diagnosis: Right otitis media-interna, neoplasm involving the right temporal bone

OTITIS MEDIA-INTERNA

Otitis media-interna is the most common cause of this combination of cranial nerve dysfunctions.[3,44] However, your neurologic examination must show no postural reaction deficits, which, if present, would indicate a medullary lesion, possibly affecting these two cranial nerves as well. In small animals, the postganglionic sympathetic axons that innervate smooth muscle in the orbit course through or adjacent to the tympanic cavity, where they can be affected by the inflammation in middle-ear infections. Unknown is whether the dysfunction of the peripheral vestibular system requires inflammation within the inner ear or whether the alteration in pressure and temperature caused by the inflammation within the tympanic cavity is sufficient to cause these clinical signs. Otitis media is very common in small animals especially cats and young farm animals, which includes calves,

(Continued)

CASE EXAMPLE 12-2—cont'd

lambs, kids, crias, and pigs (Figs. 12-5 through 12-9). Extension of this infection into the cranial cavity is common when this ear infection is not treated vigorously, and the results of the extension can be lethal. Three anatomic routes for infection can be used to obtain access to the tympanic cavity: (1) from otitis externa, (2) from nasopharyngeal infections extending through the auditory tube, and (3) hematogenous from a bacteremia. Clinical signs can be acute or chronic in onset and progressive. The clinical signs of peripheral vestibular dysfunction are usually less severe than in dogs with the benign idiopathic disorder. The otitis can be bilateral but the neurologic signs unilateral. Otoscopic examination may show changes in the middle-ear cavity with the tympanic membrane ruptured or still intact. However, the otitis media is often undetected with this procedure, and imaging is required for the diagnosis. For years, we have relied on radiographs, but both computed tomographic (CT) and MR imaging are more reliable. CT images are better than MR images to show the degree of bone involvement (see Fig. 12-6). Ideally, treatment should be based on

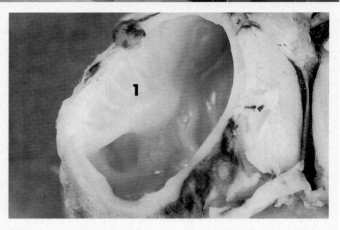

FIGURE 12-7 Normal tympanic bulla in a cat with the ventromedial portion of the tympanic cavity opened to expose the septum bullae (1).

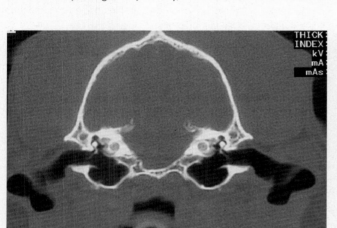

FIGURE 12-5 CT image of a normal dog's head at the level of the tympanic bullae.

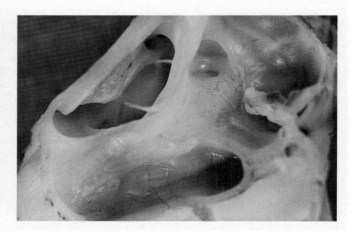

FIGURE 12-8 Same cat as in Fig. 12-7 with the septum bullae partially removed to open the dorsolateral portion of the tympanic cavity and expose the tympanum with the malleus embedded in it.

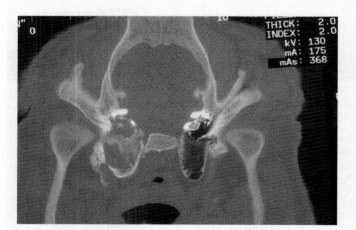

FIGURE 12-6 CT image of a young pig with left otitis media-interna. Note the distortion and destruction of the left tympanic and petrous portions of the temporal bone. This infection was associated with a brainstem abscess. Note the normal right pendular portion of the tympanic bulla, which contains many thin bony laminae. The tympanic cavity is free of these laminae just ventral to the petrous portion of the temporal bone.

isolation of the infectious agent and the use of specific antibacterial or antifungal drugs to which the agent is most susceptible. Remember to avoid the aminoglycoside antibiotics that are ototoxic. Surgery may be required for chronic cases.

Neoplasms occasionally involve the tympanic and petrous portions of the temporal bone. They often arise from the tissues of the external ear canal and invade the temporal bone but primary bone neoplasms occur as well (Fig. 12-10). The anatomic diagnosis might well be identical to that in this dog. As the neoplasm expands medially, brainstem or cerebellar compression (or both) will result with corresponding clinical signs. Diagnosis is dependent on adequate imaging procedures. Squamous cell carcinoma is a common neoplasm that involves the ear of cats.

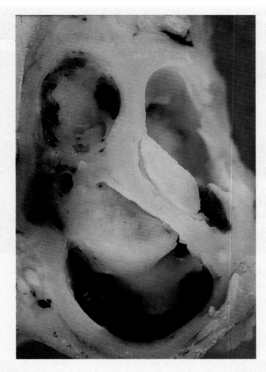

FIGURE 12-9 Same cat as in Figs. 12-7 and 12-8 with the opposite tympanic bulla and septum bullae opened to show suppurative exudate in both portions of the tympanic cavity (otitis media).

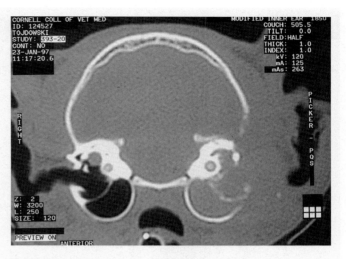

FIGURE 12-10 CT image of the head of an 8-year-old domestic shorthair at the level of the ears. Note the normal right tympanic bulla (left side of image). Also note the thin plate of bone—septum bullae—that partially divides the tympanic cavity into a small dorsolateral and larger ventromedial portion. The two portions communicate near the tympanum. This septum only forms a small ridge in dogs. Note the soft tissue density in the left tympanic bulla and its partial destruction along with destruction of portions of the rest of the temporal bone by a sarcoma.

CASE EXAMPLE 12-3

Signalment: 5.5-year-old female Chesapeake Bay retriever, Splash
Chief Complaint: Head tilt, facial deformity and depression
History: One year before this examination, the owner noticed that Splash had a slight right head tilt; the dog also tended to drool excessively from the right side of her mouth. One month before this examination, the owner noted that the right eye was sunken, and the head appeared to be deformed. For the 2 to 3 weeks before the examination, Splash was depressed and would occasionally stagger and fall.

Examination: See **Video 12-6**. Note the normal gait, and you should have appreciated that the hopping responses on the right side were consistently delayed and lacked the smooth quality seen with the left limbs. Paw replacement was normal. Note the absent right palpebral reflex but intact facial sensation, the elevated right ear with what we thought was increased tone in the right lips, and a very slight deviation of the philtrum to the right. Note the lack of temporal and masseter muscle mass on the right side. Splash resented having her mouth opened, and a mass lesion was palpated on the right side between the transverse process of the atlas and the caudal portion of the mandible. Not seen in the video was a persistent anisocoria with the right pupil always smaller than the left and an abnormal positional nystagmus when she was placed on her back. This nystagmus was vertical or directed to the right side.
Anatomic Diagnosis: Right pons or medulla (or both): right facial neurons, right vestibular system, right motor neurons of the trigeminal nerve, right UMN-GP systems in the pons or medulla (or both)

At the time of this examination, the right facial paralysis observed in this dog is associated with facial tetanus. Presumably the initial clinical signs of vestibular system dysfunction involved the peripheral components, but there is no way to prove this presumption. At the time of this examination, clinical signs of involvement of the UMN and GP systems were noted, most likely in the pons or medulla (or both), which might also affect the vestibular nuclei. The masticatory muscle atrophy implicates the mandibular nerve from the trigeminal nerve or motor nucleus of V in the pons. Otitis media-interna will not affect the trigeminal nerve or its ganglion where it passes through the canal for the trigeminal nerve in the rostral portion of the petrous part of the temporal bone. The thick portion of this bone that separates the tympanic cavity and this nerve prevents this occurrence. However, an erosive neoplasm in the temporal bone knows no boundaries. Presumably, this dog is deaf on her right side, but we cannot determine this loss of function in our physical neurologic examination.
Differential Diagnosis: Neoplasm—intramedullary or extramedullary, abscess—granuloma secondary to otitis media-interna, focal encephalitis—granulomatous meningoencephalitis

NEOPLASM

Based on the 1-year history of very slow progression of clinical signs and the palpation of a mass lesion in the area of the anatomic diagnosis, a neoplasm is the most likely clinical diagnosis. Radiographs determined that a large mass had obliterated most components

(Continued)

CASE EXAMPLE 12-3—cont'd

of the right temporal bone. Splash was euthanized, and necropsy diagnosed this extramedullary temporal bone neoplasm as a basal cell carcinoma (Figs. 12-11 through 12-14).

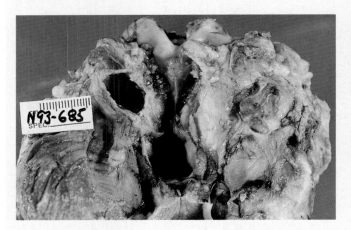

FIGURE 12-11 Ventral view of the head of the dog in Video 12-6 at necropsy with the lower jaw removed. The normal left tympanic bulla has been opened. The comparable right side of the specimen has been obscured and obliterated by the neoplasm.

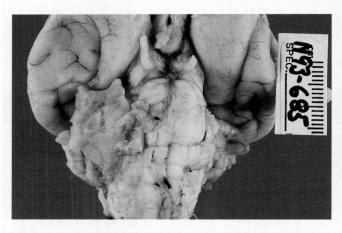

FIGURE 12-12 Ventral view of the preserved brain of the dog in this case example. Note the neoplasm compressing the right side of the caudal brainstem.

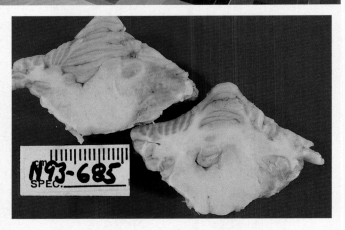

FIGURE 12-13 Transverse section of the brain in Fig. 12-12 at the level of the cerebellum and medulla, showing the extraparenchymal neoplasm at the right cerebellomedullary angle.

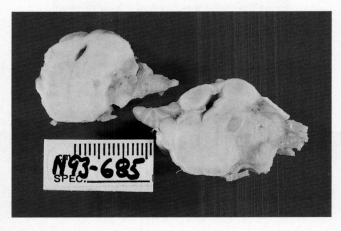

FIGURE 12-14 Transverse section of the brain in Fig. 12-12 at the level of the mesencephalon, showing the neoplasm in the meninges compressing the mesencephalon. This neoplasm is a basal cell carcinoma.

CASE EXAMPLE 12-4

Signalment: 6-year-old spayed female golden retriever, Courtney
Chief Complaint: Difficulty walking and frequent falling
History: Three days before examination, the owner first recognized clinical signs when Courtney fell down the stairs and had difficulty with her balance. The owner blamed the fall as the cause of an injury. However, Courtney developed a left head tilt, and her difficulty with walking progressively worsened. Be aware that neurologic signs associated with a fall are usually the cause of the fall and not the result of it.

Examination: See **Video 12-7**. Note the strong tendency to lean and circle to her left side and the right-side hypermetria with excessive limb flexion most evident in the thoracic limb. The abnormal positional nystagmus was mostly vertical but occasionally rotatory left or right.
Anatomic Diagnosis: Right cerebellum, pons, and medulla

The quality of the hypermetria represents a cerebellar dysfunction based on the excessive flexion of the limb on protraction. In the overreaching form of hypermetria that was described with cervical spinal cord disorders, the thoracic limb is in extension when protracted. See **Video 12-8** described at the end of this case example. The slow hopping and hemiwalking with the right limbs supports a central nervous system (CNS) lesion involving the right UMN or GP systems (or both) in the caudal brainstem or the right side of the cerebellum. The head tilt and loss of balance are directed to the left, which suggests clinical signs of a paradoxical vestibular system disorder, unless multifocal lesions are present, such as right cerebellum and left vestibular nuclei. The clinical signs of a vestibular system disorder are profound. The quality of the gait abnormality, the deficit in postural reactions, and the abnormal nystagmus that changed direction with different head positions all support that the vestibular system involvement is in its central components. This finding indicates unequivocal central vestibular disease![46]

Differential Diagnosis: Neoplasm, inflammation, vascular compromise, malformation, toxicity, hypothyroidism

NEOPLASM

Based on the progressive nature of the clinical signs, neoplasia and focal inflammation are the two most common clinical disorders for consideration in this patient. Neoplasms in the caudal cranial fossa include intramedullary glioma, medulloblastoma (primitive neuroectodermal tumor), choroid plexus papilloma or carcinoma, ependymoma, and extraparenchymal meningioma.

GRANULOMATOUS MENINGOENCEPHALITIS

The most common focal encephalitis to occur in this area of the brain is granulomatous meningoencephalitis (GME).[6,21] The pathogenesis of this disorder is not well understood but is presently considered to be a form of lymphoproliferative disorder that may evolve into a lymphoma. An autoimmune disease has also been proposed. GME tends to be more common in young adult small- to medium-sized breeds, but any breed at any age can be affected. The angiocentric lesions predominate in the white matter and can be diffusely distributed through the brain and spinal cord, occur in multifocal sites, or be primarily located at one site where the perivascular and parenchymal proliferation of lymphoplasmacytic cells and macrophages (histiocytes) can be so extensive as to cause a mass lesion. Lesions in the cerebellum, pons, and medulla are common. A localized form is thought to occur in the optic nerves causing an optic neuritis. Optic neuritis is described in Chapter 14 on the visual system. CSF usually reflects the lesion with marked elevation of protein and nonsuppurative inflammatory cells. MR imaging is the preferred procedure to show these lesions, especially when they are focal. These lesions are hyperintense on T2-weighted and fluid-attenuated inversion-recovery (FLAIR) images. Contrast enhancement is variable. Immunosuppressive drugs such as prednisone or oral cyclosporine and lomustine may be effective at slowing or stopping the progression of the disease and alleviating some of the clinical signs. Focal lesions can be irradiated. Responses to these treatments vary.

Remember that this anatomic site is at risk for developing an abscess or more diffuse suppurative meningoencephalitis associated with extension of an infection from the middle and inner ear.

Vascular compromise causing ischemia or infarction are common in the cerebellum and are usually asymmetric, affecting part or all of one hemisphere and the vermis.[18,20,30] The clinical signs may be very similar to those seen in Courtney. See examples in Chapter 13 on the cerebellum. However, the clinical signs should be acute in onset and not progress over more than 24 hours as a rule. Malformation was included in the differential diagnosis because the caudal cranial fossa is a common site for epidermoid or dermoid cysts to occur.[28] These cysts are thought to be developmental in origin and result from an abnormality when the neural tube folds and closes in this area and separates from the overlying ectoderm. The epithelial lining of these cysts proliferates and secretes, causing the cyst to enlarge and, in time, produce clinical signs from its mass effect. Severe clinical signs of dysfunction in the components of the caudal cranial fossa occur with metronidazole toxicity, but these are usually symmetric and require a history of exposure to this drug.[14] Hypothyroidism has been associated in adult dogs with an acute onset of persistent or progressive clinical signs of a caudal cranial fossa lesion that included involvement of the central components of the vestibular system.[23] In this study, thyroid function evaluations were abnormal and all responded to treatment with levothyroxine. The pathogenesis of the disorder is unknown, although atherosclerosis was suggested in earlier studies.

MR imaging was performed on Courtney and revealed a mass lesion on the right side of the caudal cranial fossa primarily in the right cerebellar hemisphere and the vermis (see video). This finding was interpreted to be an intraparenchymal neoplasm, most likely a glioma. She was euthanized, and no necropsy was performed.

See **Video 12-8**. This video shows Arnie, a 4-year-old bull mastiff with a history of four to five generalized seizures over the previous 3 weeks and 3 days of a head tilt and abnormal gait. Note the right head tilt and drifting to his right side and the overreaching of the left thoracic limb with the limb in extension. This form of hypermetria contrasts with that observed in Courtney, Video 12-7. The prolonged protraction with the limb in extension is a clinical sign of a UMN or GP system disorder, or both. Not seen on the video were the slow hopping responses in the left limbs of Arnie and the abnormal positional nystagmus that changed directions in different positions of the head.

The anatomic diagnosis includes prosencephalon, left cerebellum, pons, and medulla. Seizures are caused by disorders that involve some portion of the prosencephalon. The left UMN-GP systems disorder can be anywhere from the pons through the first to fifth cervical spinal cord segments on the left side. The vestibular system signs are from a CNS lesion that is most likely in the left cerebellum, and these signs are paradoxical vestibular signs. Multifocal lesions are usually either inflammatory or neoplastic. The CSF was normal. MR imaging revealed a small hyperintense lesion in the left diencephalon and a large hyperintense lesion in the left cerebellar hemisphere and the vermis and the left dorsolateral medulla. See the video for the MR images of the cerebellar lesion. In these images, the axial sections alternate between the T2-weighted and proton-density images. The spinal cord was not imaged. Arnie's clinical signs progressed over the next 2 weeks, and he was euthanized. Necropsy diagnosed these areas of MR image hyperintensity as astrocytomas.

CASE EXAMPLE 12-5

Signalment: 9-year-old spayed female border collie, Mercy
Chief Complaint: Head tilt
History: Mercy was presented to Cornell 10 days after an acute onset of inability to stand, thrashing attempts to try to stand, and episodes of neck and thoracic limb extension. Over these 10 days, she improved remarkably but still had a mild head tilt.

Examination: See **Video 12-9**. Note the mild left head tilt, her tendency to drift to the right side, and the slow hopping responses in the right limbs when tested repeatedly. No abnormal nystagmus was noted.
Anatomic Diagnosis: The right side of the cerebellum, pons, and medulla. The head tilt was assumed to be a paradoxical vestibular sign.
Differential Diagnosis: Neoplasm, inflammation, vascular compromise, malformation, toxicity

ISCHEMIC ENCEPHALOPATHY

These diagnoses are the same as those listed for Courtney in Case Example 12-4. However, the acute nontraumatic onset and the steady improvement up to the time of this examination strongly indicated a vascular compromise with ischemic lesions, which were resolving. One week later, Mercy was examined by Eric Glass, who found no neurologic signs, and an MR imaging was normal at that time. These findings indicate a presumptive unilateral cerebellar vascular compromise with ischemia, which completely resolved.[18,20,30] The cause of the vascular compromise is unknown.

CASE EXAMPLE 12-6

Signalment: 6-year-old spayed female Papillon, Dolly
Chief Complaint: Unable to stand
History: Over a few days, Dolly had progressed from difficulty in walking, to difficulty in trying to stand, to tremors of her head.

Examination: See **Video 12-10**. Note the loss of balance with swaying of the body to either side, the difficulty in initiating limb movements, the tendency to assume an opisthotonic posture of the head and neck, the limb hypertonia, the resting vertical nystagmus, and her appearance of disorientation.
Anatomic Diagnosis: Cerebellum, pons, and medulla

These clinical signs are often loosely termed cerebellar-vestibular signs, with the latter a product of involvement of the central components of the vestibular system. They are usually accompanied by some degree of UMN and GP system dysfunction. Head and neck tremors occur with cerebellar disorders. The absolutely vertical nystagmus in combination with the other neurologic signs support a disorder of the central vestibular system components.

Differential Diagnosis: Neoplasm, inflammation, vascular compromise, malformation, toxicity

METRONIDAZOLE TOXICITY

These diagnoses are the same as those listed for Case Examples 12-4 and 12-5. The severity of these clinical signs, their symmetric nature, and the persistent resting abnormal nystagmus are strongly suggestive of metronidazole toxicity.[10,14,38] On questioning Dolly's owner about possible exposure to this drug, we were informed that Dolly had been receiving this drug for 1 month as a treatment for pancreatitis. Further inquiry determined that Dolly was receiving approximately twice the recommended dose of metronidazole. Be aware that dogs that receive recommended doses of this drug are also at risk for this toxicity. As a rule, however, the greatest risk for dogs to develop clinical signs of toxicity occurs when the drug is administered for long periods and especially at excessive doses.

CASE EXAMPLE 12-7

Signalment: 9-month-old female Labrador retriever, Roxy
Chief Complaint: Difficulty with standing and often falls
History: An abnormal gait was first observed at approximately 7 months of age. This phase slowly progressed to difficulty standing and falling to either side, which the owner described as a "drunken gait." Roxy also developed fine tremors of her entire body. The owner described that these clinical signs tended to wax and wane in severity during the day.

Examination: See **Video 12-11**. Note the similarity of these clinical signs to those in Case Example 12-6, Video 12-10, with the poor initiation of limb movements associated with sudden bursts of activity, the inability to coordinate to stand, the episodes of opisthotonus with thoracic limb rigidity, and the fine tremor of the entire body including the limbs. No abnormal nystagmus was noted, and the dog acted alert

and responsive. Note the last portion of the video when the dog is urged to come out of her cage, which occurred approximately 1 hour after the first portion of the video during which the dog was resting in this cage. Note her ability to stand and walk here but with marked difficulty. Roxy was hospitalized the day before this examination, and she was observed to have a generalized seizure in her cage that lasted approximately 1 minute.
Anatomic Diagnosis: Diffuse CNS with a major component involving the cerebellum, pons, and medulla

The clinical signs observed on the video relate to dysfunction in the cerebellum, pons, and medulla similar to Dolly in Case Example 12-6. However, seizures are related to a disorder of some component of the prosencephalon, and the fine whole-body tremors require a diffuse disorder of myelin or axons in the entire CNS.

Differential Diagnosis: Degeneration, toxicity, inflammation

LEUKODYSTROPHY

The slow progression of symmetric clinical signs and the lack of any exposure to a known toxin make toxicity and inflammation less likely. Remember in cases such as this one to look at the breed and ask yourself if any recognized inherited degenerative disorder is described for this breed that causes similar clinical signs. When you search for this data in your textbooks or on the Internet, your answer will be *yes*. In 1975, Dr. Jack McGrath at the University of Pennsylvania described a fibrinoid encephalomyelopathy (Alexander disease) in two 8-month-old littermate Labrador retrievers with clinical signs of a diffuse CNS disorder.[33] This degeneration is a disorder of astrocytes. It is associated with a loss of myelin, especially in the cerebral white matter. Thus this disease is also known as *leukodystrophy*. The abnormal astrocytes are widely distributed in the CNS, but their perivascular density and the myelin loss in the cerebral white matter will appear as a diffuse bilaterally symmetric hyperintensity in T2-weighted and proton-density MR images. In 1985, Dr. Dennis O'Brien described a spongy degeneration of CNS white matter, a leukodystrophy, in Labrador retrievers.[37,52] The onset of clinical signs for the dogs in this report was 4 to 6 months of age. The lesion consists of a separation of the myelin lamellae, causing a dilation of the myelin sheath caused by the accumulation of fluid between lamellae, known as *myelin edema*. It is found throughout the CNS and is especially prominent where large bundles of white matter are found, such as the spinal cord, cerebellar medullary and folial white matter, internal capsule, centrum semiovale, and corona radiata. These lesions are hypointense on T1-weighted MR images and hyperintense on the T2-weighted images. An autosomal-recessive gene inheritance is presumed but is not yet proven. Roxy had a littermate that was euthanized at 4 months of age for generalized seizures, but no necropsy was performed. Roxy was euthanized, and a necropsy confirmed the diagnosis of a leukodystrophy similar to that described by O'Brien.

Cats

CASE EXAMPLE 12-8

Signalment: 3-year-old castrated male domestic shorthair, Reuben
Chief Complaint: Head tilt and loss of balance
History: One late July evening, Reuben's owner let him outdoors for the evening and found him in the morning on the back steps with a head tilt and difficulty walking. Reuben was brought to the hospital that day and videoed the next morning.
Examination: See **Video 12-12**. Note how alert this cat is. Note also his normal quick limb movements as he attempts to maintain his balance. He staggers to either side but more often to the left, which is the side of his head tilt and head turn. In the first portion of the video, when he looks left, note the brief head rotations. These movements correspond to the resting right nystagmus that is present. When you perform the hopping responses in cats, many of them will simply roll over and not respond at all. To prevent this result, hold the cat up and grasp the three limbs that you are not testing, and suddenly lower the cat to the ground with the limb to be hopped extended. As soon as the limb strikes the ground, move the cat laterally on it, and the normal cat will at least give you a few hops before rolling over. Note the elevation of the tail, which is typical of cats with severe balance loss.
Anatomic Diagnosis: Left peripheral vestibular system components
Differential Diagnosis: Benign idiopathic feline peripheral vestibular disease, otitis media-interna, ototoxicity

BENIGN IDIOPATHIC FELINE PERIPHERAL VESTIBULAR DISEASE

Benign idiopathic feline peripheral vestibular disease is the most presumptive clinical diagnosis based on the sudden onset of severe clinical signs of peripheral vestibular system dysfunction with no involvement of the facial nerve or postganglionic sympathetic nerves in the late summer in a young adult cat with access to the outdoors.[7,13] The cause of this disease is unknown. (See the discussion of the similar benign idiopathic canine disorder.) Because this disease in cats occurs at the same time of year as the acute-onset brain disease caused by the myiasis of the larva of a *Cuterebra* sp., some neurologists have hypothesized that this peripheral vestibular syndrome is caused by the migration of this larva in the middle and inner ear. No definitive proof has been found of this occurrence whatsoever. No *Cuterebra* sp. larva have been found in any part of the ear of a cat with or without these clinical signs, and the few necropsies that included study of the inner-ear structures have not found a recognizable lesion. Investigators have reported that this disease can occur in cats that have no access to the outdoors, but these reports are rare. The high incidence of this disorder from late July through September in outdoor cats implies some environmental factor (e.g., insect toxin, toxic spray, plant pollen) that may cause ototoxicity. This factor is unknown. The clinical signs are peracute in onset and typical for a severe dysfunction of the peripheral vestibular system. Although the clinical signs predominate to one side, a bilateral disturbance is suggested by the occasional wide head excursions to either side and the tendency of the cat to stagger in both directions. Fortunately, most of these cats will recover spontaneously. Their vestibular ataxia will be greatly improved by 7 to 10 days, and the head tilt usually resolves by 2 to 4 weeks. Occasionally, a residual head tilt persists. Even recovered cats may exhibit a slight head tilt and balance loss if they are significantly stressed. Without more knowledge of the cause of the pathogenesis of this disorder and the spontaneous recovery, treatment of these cats is unnecessary. However, the use of antibiotics is rational as a treatment for a possible otitis, which is the other most common cause of these clinical signs. Keep these cats in a protected environment while they recover. Rarely does this disorder recur in cats, which is unlike the canine disorder. Experimental surgical ablation of the inner ear of a cat will cause similar clinical signs, including recovery by cerebellomedullary compensation.[9] This disease represents just another of many reasons to keep cats indoors.

OTITIS MEDIA-INTERNA

Otitis media-interna is your other most significant concern for a disorder that would cause this anatomic diagnosis. The presence

(Continued)

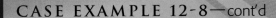

CASE EXAMPLE 12-8—cont'd

of a facial paresis or Horner syndrome would be supportive of this diagnosis because these conditions never occur with the benign disorder just described. Usually the initial clinical signs of peripheral vestibular system dysfunction are not so severe with otitis, but an otoscopic examination should be performed on all of these cats. The most reliable way to diagnose otitis is with imaging, but when presented with a cat such as Reuben in this case example, we would delay imaging unless the patient's recovery was not satisfactory. Ototoxicity obviously requires a history of drug exposure.

 See **Video 12-13**. This video shows a 4-year-old spayed female domestic shorthair with a sudden onset of the clinical signs observed on this video. You should appreciate that all of these clinical signs represent dysfunction in the peripheral components

of the vestibular system. Not shown was the resting right rotatory nystagmus. Note that although the clinical signs are asymmetric with the left head tilt and leaning to the left, this cat has some indication of bilateral dysfunction with the tendency to stagger to either side and the uncontrolled head and neck movements in both directions. This presumptive diagnosis is benign idiopathic feline peripheral vestibular disease.

See **Video 12-14**. This video shows Socks, a 6-month-old castrated male domestic shorthair with a sudden onset of the abnormal gait and posture seen on this video. Your anatomic diagnosis should be right peripheral vestibular system components and left sympathetic innervation to the eye. This finding suggests a bilateral otitis media with the inner ear involved on the right side.

CASE EXAMPLE 12-9

Signalment: 2-year-old female domestic shorthair, Zaro
Chief Complaint: Abnormal head movements
History: Two months before this examination, Zaro was presented to a veterinarian for a sudden onset of a right head tilt and balance loss. These signs were diagnosed as a right peripheral vestibular system disorder. Evidence of right otitis externa was also found. During the next week, the clinical signs progressed to a bilateral loss of balance and what the referring veterinarian described as a "head bob." The head bob and a mild ataxia had persisted unchanged up to the time of this examination.
Examination: See **Video 12-15**. Note the wide head excursions with the inability to stop the head movements to either side. No abnormal nystagmus, no normal physiologic nystagmus, and no postrotatory nystagmus could be generated. This cat was also deaf.
Anatomic Diagnosis: Bilateral peripheral vestibular and cochlear components—cranial nerve VIII

The bilateral, wide, and uncontrolled head excursions are typical of bilateral peripheral vestibular disease. When the inner ear is affected by a disease process bilaterally, deafness can be recognized on your physical neurologic examination.
Differential Diagnosis: Otitis media-interna, ototoxicity

BILATERAL OTITIS MEDIA-INTERNA

Realistically, bilateral otitis involving the inner ear is the only clinical diagnosis we have ever seen as the cause of these clinical signs of acquired bilateral peripheral vestibular system dysfunction. The benign idiopathic disorder can cause bilateral clinical signs, but some asymmetry is most often seen. Radiographs of Zaro showed extensive bilateral changes diagnostic of otitis media. Despite antibiotic therapy and bilateral bulla osteotomy, Zaro's clinical signs remained unchanged.

See the following videos of other cats with bilateral otitis media-interna and clinical signs of bilateral peripheral vestibular nerve and cochlear nerve dysfunction.

Video 12-16. This video shows Fractal, a 12-year-old castrated male domestic shorthair that was anesthetized for surgical treatment of an aural hematoma. While still under anesthesia, both ears were flushed despite no indication of any otitis externa. Be aware that ear flushing procedures can cause complications and should be avoided unless absolutely necessary! On recovery from anesthesia, Fractal exhibited the clinical signs that you see on this video. Fractal did not

startle even with rigorous banging of pans together behind his head as a source of a loud noise, and electrophysiologic testing (brainstem auditory evoked response [BAER]) showed no ability to stimulate a response in the cochlear nerves bilaterally. Ear flushing of any kind can result in what you have seen here, despite any indication of preexisting otitis externa. You cannot assess the tympanum for its barrier function, and small perforations may not be recognized.

Video 12-17. This video shows Magnum, an 8-year-old domestic shorthair with bilateral otitis media-interna.

Video 12-18. This video shows a 10-week-old female domestic shorthair with a 1-week history of losing her balance and what the owner described as "rolling eyes." Two days before this video was made, this kitten began to exhibit wide head excursions. Otitis media-interna was diagnosed in each ear. Treatment for otitis requires long-term oral antibiotics. Surgery is sometimes necessary, especially when the otitis is associated with polyp formation. Corticosteroids should definitely be avoided. We have seen numerous cases of otitis that have been treated with long-term corticosteroids that, secondary to immunosuppression, resulted in an abscess of the petrous portion of the temporal bone and eventual compression of the medulla and pons.

CONGENITAL PERIPHERAL VESTIBULAR SYSTEM DISEASE

Be aware that clinical signs of a peripheral vestibular system disorder are occasionally present at birth or are at least apparent as soon as the affected animal begins to move around and tries to stand and walk. These clinical signs are unilateral or bilateral and often affect both the vestibular nerve and the cochlear nerve or their labyrinthine receptors in the membranous labyrinth. Whether the vestibular system lesions are malformative or an early-onset abiotrophy is unknown. This lesion has been observed in many breeds of small animals with no proof of the presumed inheritance of the disorder. These breeds include the German shepherd,[45] Doberman pinscher, Akita, beagle, English cocker spaniel,[2] and Burmese and Siamese cats. Some of these affected animals improve or even recover in time, presumably from compensation by vestibular system components in the CNS. No microscopic lesions have been recognized in the inner ears of patients that have been studied, but mild lesions of degeneration such as an abiotrophy are difficult to recognize after the process of decalcification of the inner ear that is required to prepare tissue sections for study.

CASE EXAMPLE 12-10

Signalment: 12-year-old spayed female domestic shorthair, Pepi
Chief Complaint: Head tilt and severe balance loss
History: Six weeks before this examination, Pepi was examined for a head tilt and mild loss of balance. Otitis media-interna was diagnosed and treated with antibiotics. Despite 1 month of this therapy, her clinical signs worsened.
Examination: See **Video 12-19**. Study the severe clinical signs of vestibular system dysfunction and determine whether the involvement of this system is central or peripheral or both.
Anatomic Diagnosis: Cerebellum, pons, and medulla, sympathetic innervation to the head

You should have recognized the episodes of opisthotonus and extensor muscle rigidity in the limbs and trunk, the UMN paresis and GP ataxia in the limbs that was worse on the left side, the left facial paralysis, left facial hypalgesia, and the left sympathetic paresis. The last of these signs suggests that, in addition to the caudal cranial fossa brain lesion, a left middle-ear lesion is present or that there is one disorder affecting all of these structures. The latter diagnosis is suspected based on the palpable mass shown at the end of the video on the left side in the angle between the mandible and the transverse process of the atlas. Normally, you should be able to place your finger in a groove between these two structures as on the right side in this cat.
Differential Diagnosis: Neoplasm, inflammation-abscess

NEOPLASM

Based on the assumption that the palpable mass near the area of the anatomic diagnosis is responsible for the clinical signs, a neoplasm or unusually large abscess or granuloma is the most likely clinical diagnosis. Radiographs suggested an aggressive neoplasm, with involvement of all portions of the left temporal bone that compressed the CNS components in the caudal cranial fossa on the left side (Figs. 12-15, 12-16). Pepi was euthanized, and necropsy confirmed this clinical diagnosis. The neoplasm was identified as a squamous cell carcinoma (Figs. 12-17, 12-18).

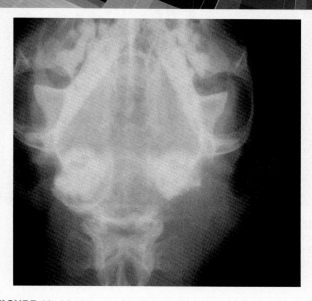

FIGURE 12-16 Dorsoventral radiograph of the head of the cat in Case Example 12-10, Video 12-19, showing the loss of a major portion of the left temporal bone (right side of image) and a soft tissue density in the right tympanic bulla.

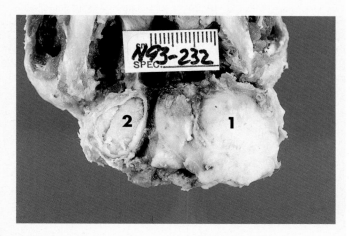

FIGURE 12-17 Ventral surface of the head of the cat in Video 12-19 at necropsy after removal of the lower jaw. Note the massive neoplasm obliterating the left temporal bone (1). Also note the exudate filling the right tympanic bulla (otitis media) (2).

CUTEREBRA LARVAL MYIASIS

See **Video 12-20**. This video shows a 1-year old female domestic shorthair living on a farm in western New York State. Three days before this video was made, she rapidly lost the ability to stand and began to roll to the right side. These signs, as well as the right hemiplegia, can be seen on the video. She had a resting right or vertical nystagmus. Remember that persistent rolling is a clinical sign usually related to dysfunction of the central vestibular system components. The anatomic diagnosis is cerebellum, pons, and medulla. The most likely differential diagnosis for this 1-year-old cat would include three

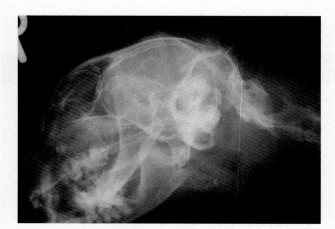

FIGURE 12-15 Lateral oblique radiograph of the head of the cat in Video 12-19. Note the loss of a major portion of the left temporal bone.

(Continued)

CASE EXAMPLE 12-10—cont'd

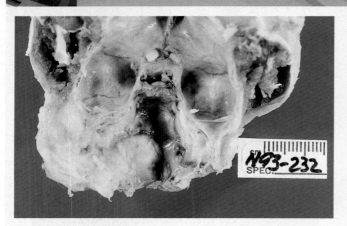

FIGURE 12-18 Same specimen as in Fig. 12-17 to show the floor of the cranial cavity after removal of the brain. Note the neoplasm obliterating the left temporal bone and invading the caudal cranial fossa. The neoplasm was a squamous cell carcinoma.

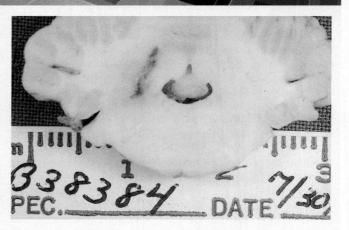

FIGURE 12-19 Rostral surface of a transverse section of the preserved brain of the cat in Video 12-20 at the level of the cerebellum and medulla. Note the area of discoloration in the confluence of the cerebellar peduncles and right cerebellar medulla. This discoloration represents hemorrhage and necrosis caused by the migration of a *Cuterebra sp.* larva.

disorders: (1) Inflammation caused by the feline infectious peritonitis (FIP) virus or the protozoal agent *Toxoplasma gondii*. FIP encephalitis is the most common infection at this site. (2) Myiasis of a larva of the *Cuterebra* sp. of fly. (3) Abscess or suppurative meningoencephalitis secondary to otitis media-interna. CSF contained 89 mg/dl of protein (normal <20) and 289 white blood cells (WBCs)/mm³ that were predominantly neutrophils. This finding supports an inflammation that might relate to any one of these three disorders. This cat was euthanized, and a necropsy diagnosed an extensive larval migration with the dead larva found in the vermis of the cerebellum. The larva was presumed to belong to a species of *Cuterebra* (Figs. 12-19, 12-20). *Cuterebra sp.* myiasis is described in Chapter 14.

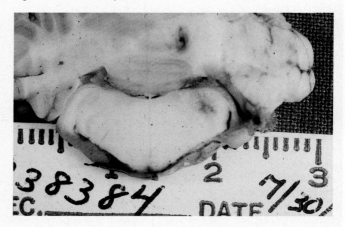

FIGURE 12-20 Caudal surface of a transverse section of the preserved brain of the cat in Video 12-20 just caudal to the transverse section in Fig. 12-19. Note the discoloration of the right dorsolateral medulla and the cerebellar medulla caused by the migration of a *Cuterebra sp.* larva.

CASE EXAMPLE 12-11

Signalment: 8-month-old male Siamese
Chief Complaint: Unable to get up
History: Three months before this examination, this cat developed a gait abnormality in his pelvic limbs that slowly progressed to the thoracic limbs and involved some apparent loss of balance. For the previous few days, he has been unable to stand. During these 3 months, he was examined by the local veterinarian for numerous episodes of depression associated with a chronic fever.

Examination: See **Video 12-21**. Note the disparity in voluntary movements between the thoracic and pelvic limbs. Not shown was an abnormal vertical to horizontal left positional nystagmus.

Anatomic Diagnosis: Diffuse or multifocal including the cerebellum, pons, and medulla and the central portion of spinal cord segments C1 to C5

The history of balance loss and the persistent abnormal positional nystagmus indicates involvement of the vestibular system. The decerebellate posture (Fig. 12-21) indicates a caudal cranial fossa lesion. The tetraparesis and ataxia of all four limbs implicates dysfunction of the UMN and GP systems anywhere from the pons to the C5 spinal cord segment, with possible lesions caudal to this area as well. The more severe UMN paresis in the thoracic limbs indicates that if the lesion involves the C1-C5 spinal cord segments, the lesions are more centrally located in these segments.

Differential Diagnosis: Encephalomyelitis—feline infectious peritonitis (FIP) virus, *T. gondii, Cryptococcus neoformans;* abscess or bacterial or fungal suppurative meningoencephalitis; *Cuterebra* larval myiasis; lymphosarcoma; neuronal storage disease

FELINE INFECTIOUS PERITONITIS VIRAL MENINGOENCEPHALITIS

An inflammatory disease is the most presumptive clinical diagnosis based on the episodes of fever. Infection with the corona virus that causes an exudative peritonitis in cats is termed *feline infectious peritonitis*. Many of these cats that have an exudative peritonitis also have a mild subclinical meningitis. A few cats develop an extensive chronic FIP viral meningoencephalomyelitis with profound neurologic signs and minimal peritonitis.[26,34,43] FIP viral meningoencephalomyelitis is by far the most common infectious disease of the CNS in cats, especially young cats. This abnormality is primarily a surface-oriented disease, which means that the leptomeninges on the external surface of the brain and spinal cord are affected, and the internal ependymal-lined ventricular system is also affected. The latter area includes the choroid plexuses and the central canal of the spinal cord. This disease is an immunopathologic disorder that involves an immune complex–induced vasculitis. The virus can be found in macrophages in the lesion. The degree of accumulation of inflammatory cells can be extensive enough to be seen on gross examination of the CNS, as well as on MR images. Although clinical signs can reflect involvement by this lesion at any level of the CNS, they often relate to the lesions in the area of the cerebellum, pons, and medulla, known as the *caudal cranial fossa*. One study reported pelvic limb paresis, abnormal nystagmus, and seizures as the most common clinical signs observed with this disease. Uveitis may also accompany the neurologic disorder. Clinical signs are slowly progressive and often include partial anorexia and a fever that are unresponsive to antibiotic therapy. The globulin fraction of serum protein is often elevated, and the CSF often is very abnormal, with protein levels even as high as 0.5 to 1.0 g/dl (normal <20 mg/dl) and hundreds of WBCs/mm³ that vary from all mononuclear cells to a high percentage of neutrophils. Serum antibodies against this virus are usually, but not always, present in these cats. However, the antibodies are not specific for this virus but rather for the group of corona viruses.

This disease cannot be differentiated from toxoplasmosis or cryptococcosis based on the neurologic signs. The persistent fever is more typical of an FIP viral infection. As a rule, serum antibodies will be present in cats with toxoplasmosis, and an antigen test will detect cryptococcal organisms in the serum or CSF. These fungal organisms are usually evident in the cytologic examination of the CSF. Cats with an extension of infection from the middle and inner ear may produce evidence of this ear infection on your physical examination and should have recognizable temporal bone lesions on imaging studies. *Cuterebra* myiasis is less likely to cause such a slow progression of neurologic signs or the persistent fever. In addition, *Cuterebra* myiasis is seasonal. Lymphosarcoma most commonly causes an extradural focal compression of the spinal cord but is occasionally within the parenchyma and diffusely distributed through the CNS, primarily in the meninges and the perivascular spaces within the CNS. CSF changes would be expected to be mild and may include lymphocytes, lymphoblasts, or both. Many forms of neuronal storage diseases have been recognized in cats that cause slowly progressive diffuse

neurologic signs of CNS dysfunction. Diffuse whole-body action–related repetitive myoclonus (tremor) is often present with storage diseases along with primarily prosencephalic signs of loss of vision, change in behavior, and seizures. Fevers do not typically occur in storage disorders.

In the cat in this case example, the CSF contained 498 mg/dl of protein and 1144 WBCs/mm³ that were all lymphocytes or monocytes. These findings supported an FIP viral–induced inflammation. The cat was euthanized, and, at necropsy, a very extensive leptomeningitis, choroid plexitis, ependymitis, and associated encephalitis were observed that were characteristic for an infection with the FIP virus (Figs. 12-22 through 12-23).

THIAMIN DEFICIENCY ENCEPHALOPATHY

Be aware that an initial clinical sign of thiamin deficiency in small animals is usually vestibular ataxia.[15,40] However, this phase is usually

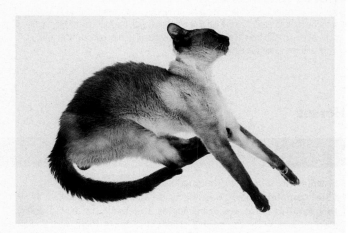

FIGURE 12-21 Cat in Video 12-21, exhibiting a decerebellate posture.

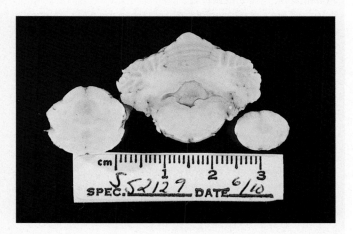

FIGURE 12-22 Transverse sections of the preserved brain of the cat in Fig. 12-21. Note the obliteration of the mesencephalic aqueduct on the left and the central canal of the C1 spinal cord segment on the right. In the center transverse section, note the thickening of the fourth ventricle caudal medullary velum, choroid plexus, and leptomeninges associated with the medulla just caudal to the confluence of the cerebellar peduncles. These areas show inflammatory lesions caused by the FIP virus.

(Continued)

CASE EXAMPLE 12-11—cont'd

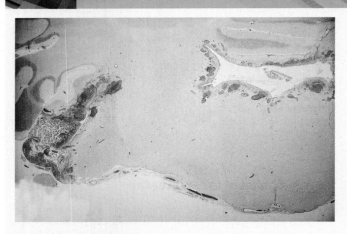

rapidly followed by pupillary dilation and generalized seizures. This condition was more common when cats were fed a fish diet that contained thiaminase. Cooking the animal's food will destroy the thiamin. Also suspected is that prolonged anorexia may lead to a thiamin deficiency sufficient to cause clinical signs. The bilateral symmetric degenerative lesions in the vestibular nuclei, caudal colliculi, oculomotor nuclei, and the lateral geniculate nuclei may be recognized on MR images. The unique anatomy of these lesions was observed on MR images of a dog that led to the diagnosis of a thiamin deficiency of unknown cause.[19] Prompt treatment with thiamin intramuscularly in the early stages of this clinical disorder may lead to complete recovery from this metabolic encephalopathy rather quickly.

FIGURE 12-23 Microscopic section of the brain of the cat in Fig. 12-22 at the level of the confluence of the cerebellar peduncles. Note the discoloration associated with the choroid plexus on the left and associated with the fourth ventricle on the right. Infection with the FIP virus caused this choroid plexitis, ependymitis, and associated periventricular encephalitis.

Horses

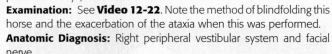

CASE EXAMPLE 12-12

Signalment: 4-year-old Thoroughbred-Trakener gelding
Chief Complaint: Right head deviation and "crooked" face
History: This horse was in training as a dressage horse for the U.S. Olympic team. For the past 3 weeks, the horse displayed a slight head deviation to the right and a tendency to drift to the right. For the previous 4 days, a deviation of the nose to the left was noted.
 Examination: See **Video 12-22.** Note the method of blindfolding this horse and the exacerbation of the ataxia when this was performed.
Anatomic Diagnosis: Right peripheral vestibular system and facial nerve

You should have noted the normal strength and limb placement that this horse exhibits. This horse clearly knows where his limbs are located and has no postural reaction deficits.
Differential Diagnosis: Otitis media-interna, temporohyoid osteopathy, and temporal bone fracture

OTITIS MEDIA-INTERNA

These findings are the classical clinical signs of dysfunction of the vestibular portion of cranial nerve VIII and cranial nerve VII, which, in all species, most commonly relate to a middle- and inner-ear infection. We have not seen a neoplasm of the temporal bone in the horse or a neoplasm of these cranial nerves.

TEMPOROHYOID OSTEOPATHY

A unique bone disorder often accompanies this otitis in horses. This abnormality is a temporohyoid osteopathy, which involves an ankylosis of this joint associated with a proliferation of the long stylohyoid bone and probably the very small tympanohyoid by which

it articulates with the petrous portion of the temporal bone. This circumstance results in a fusion of these bones at the level of the tympanic portion of the temporal bone.[5,16,47] This bony proliferation envelops the tympanic portion of the temporal bone but does not invade the tympanic cavity (see Fig. 6-41.) With this loss of mobility of the hyoid apparatus, a risk of fracture of the petrous portion of the temporal bone exists. The assumption is that the otitis precedes and induces the osteopathy, but no proof has been found. The few microscopic studies on the osteopathy have never shown any indication of an osteomyelitis. The cause of this bone lesion remains unknown and has not been observed in other species. The lesion is unrelated to any disease within the guttural pouch. The assumption is that the ankylosis is secondary to the infection, and the extensive enlargement of the stylohyoid bone is secondary to the immobility of this joint, which prevents normal remodeling of the bone. In some horses, the onset of clinical signs of vestibular nerve dysfunction and the facial paralysis are sudden and thought to be caused by the temporal bone fracture, especially in the few horses that exhibit a brief period of partial dysphagia from presumed involvement of cranial nerves IX and X at the jugular foramen. The latter development cannot be caused by the otitis. Whether otitis was present in these horses before the fracture is unknown. Occasionally, the bone lesion is bilateral, but the neurologic signs have always been unilateral. Radiographs will reveal the enlarged stylohyoid bone with fusion to the temporal bone, but this circumstance prevents evaluation of the middle-ear cavity. The ventrodorsal view is the most reliable view to observe this bone lesion but requires general anesthesia. Although CT imaging is the preferred way to diagnose this disorder and may reveal the fracture when it is present, general anesthesia is required. The enlargement of the stylohyoid bone, as well as the lack of movement at the temporohyoid articulation, can be seen through the wall of the guttural pouch on endoscopic examination. See **Video 12-23** of an endoscopic examination of the guttural pouch of another adult horse that has a left-side stylohyoidosteopathy. The first portion of the video shows the left guttural pouch with the enlarged caudal portion of the stylohyoid bone and the lack of any movement at its articulation with the temporal bone. The last portion of the video shows the right guttural pouch with a normal stylohyoid bone. Note the movement of this bone at its articulation. You may suspect this abnormality during your physical examination by pressing dorsally on the basihyoid bone and assessing the range of motion of the hyoid apparatus, which depends on a mobile tympanohyoid articulation. You will feel resistance in horses with this bone lesion and fusion at this articulation. To prevent fracture related to this bone fusion, a portion of the affected stylohyoid bone is removed, or, more recently, the entire ceratohyoid bone has been removed. The latter surgery is easier to perform and has fewer complications.

The horse in this case example had endoscopic and radiographic evidence of the temporohyoid osteopathy. He was treated for many weeks with antibiotics, made a complete recovery, and was returned to training. Remember that this facial nerve lesion may interfere with tear production, as well as prevent eyelid closure, which places the patient at considerable risk for corneal ulceration, keratitis, or both. You must provide artificial tears for this patient. A temporary tarsorrhaphy may also be employed.

See **Video 12-24**. This video shows an 11-year-old Saddlebred gelding that, 3 days before hospitalization, suddenly experienced a severe loss of balance, with a left head tilt and a left ear droop, and with his nose deviated to the right side. He fell down and fought efforts to get him to stand for 3 days. The video was made on the third day shortly after he was helped to stand. He shows considerable limb trembling in the video, which we believe is related to his prolonged recumbency and muscle compression. Note how rapidly he moves his limbs to compensate for his balance loss. Your anatomic diagnosis should be left cranial nerve VII and the left vestibular portion of cranial nerve VIII. An enlarged stylohyoid bone was observed on endoscopic examination of the left guttural pouch. The assumption was that the sudden onset of these clinical signs was associated with a fracture of the petrous portion of the temporal bone. No CT scanning was available to confirm this diagnosis at the time this horse was studied. Although this horse improved on antibiotic therapy, 2 weeks later, he suddenly had a recurrence of the clinical signs and went down again. The assumption was that, without surgical interruption of the hyoid apparatus, another fracture had occurred. This horse was euthanized, and no necropsy was performed.

BENIGN IDIOPATHIC PERIPHERAL VESTIBULAR DISEASE

See **Video 12-25**. This video shows a 15-year-old Thoroughbred gelding with a peracute onset of balance loss with a right head tilt and a resting rotatory left abnormal nystagmus. The video was made approximately 24 hours after the onset of these clinical signs. Your anatomic diagnosis should be right vestibular portion of cranial nerve VIII. Your differential diagnosis should include otitis media-interna, temporohyoid osteopathy and temporal bone fracture, and benign idiopathic peripheral vestibular disorder. The last of these diagnoses is considered to be the most presumptive because of the acute onset of clinical signs and the absence of any facial nerve deficits. We are not aware of any published report of this benign disorder in the horse. Radiographs of the temporal and stylohyoid bones and guttural pouch endoscopy were all normal. This horse spontaneously completely recovered in approximately a 3-day period. Based on this examination and the rapid resolution of the clinical signs, we presumed that this episode was a possible example of benign idiopathic equine peripheral vestibular disease.

CASE EXAMPLE 12-13

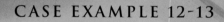

Signalment: 15-year-old Standardbred mare
Chief Complaint: Abnormal gait
History: Three days before this examination, this mare suddenly acted unstable and exhibited a left head tilt. Her unsteady gait worsened over the 3 days.
Examination: See **Video 12-26**.
Anatomic Diagnosis: Cerebellum, pons, and medulla

If you compare the gait of this horse with that of the previously described three horses, you should recognize the significant loss of UMN and GP function in this horse that is not present in the others. This circumstance places the clinical signs of vestibular system dysfunction in this horse within the central components of the vestibular system. The right nasal hypalgesia is best explained by the lesion interrupting the spinal tract of the trigeminal nerve within the pons or rostral medulla.
Differential Diagnosis: Equine protozoal encephalitis; viral encephalomyelitis—rabies, West Nile, eastern equine; equine herpesvirus-1 vasculitis and encephalopathy; abscess; neoplasm

EQUINE PROTOZOAL ENCEPHALITIS

The most presumptive clinical diagnosis of a sudden onset and progression of clinical signs in this area of the brain is an infection with *Sarcocystis neurona*. This disorder is described in Chapter 11. The short period of observation makes rabies and eastern equine encephalomyelitis still strong contenders for this diagnosis, but the lack of any prosencephalic signs makes them less likely. The focal nature and the level of the anatomic diagnosis and the continual progression of the clinical signs make equine herpesvirus-1 infection less likely. The focal sign of facial hypalgesia in the absence of any contralateral prosencephalic signs makes any of these viral diseases unlikely. An abscess from extension of an otitis is unlikely with no initial clinical signs of otitis before the clinical signs of CNS involvement. *Streptococcus equi* abscesses are more common in foals and rare at this age. Focal neoplasms are uncommon in the CNS of horses.

The horse in this case example had serum antibodies for *S. neurona,* which supports exposure to this infectious agent. The CSF contained 51 mg/dl protein (normal <80) but 28 WBCs/mm^3 with 92% lymphocytes and 8% monocytes, which supports a nonsuppurative meningoencephalitis. Although caudal brainstem lesions caused by *S. neurona* have a fair prognosis when treated with antiprotozoal drugs, the owner of this horse elected for euthanasia. At necropsy, extensive necrosis and nonsuppurative inflammation were found in the pons and medulla associated with *S. neurona* organisms.

(Continued)

CASE EXAMPLE 12-13—cont'd

See Videos 12-27 through 12-30 for other examples of varying degree of dysfunction of the central components of the vestibular system with involvement of other systems in the medulla, pons, and cerebellum caused by a nonsuppurative encephalitis as a result of infection with *S. neurona*.

Video 12-27. This video shows a 5-year-old Standardbred gelding that, 10 days before this examination, was in training and unable to maintain his stride in the sulky and drifted to his right side. The gait disorder progressed, and 3 days before this examination the trainer noted a facial asymmetry and a tendency for the horse to circle to his right. Study this video. Note how much effort is needed make him circle to his left, and as soon as I (AD) let up on the lead shank, he veers off to his right side. Note the mild thoracic limb hypermetria with flexion of the joints, which suggests involvement of the cerebellum. Also note the left facial paralysis and atrophy of the left muscles of mastication. Your anatomic diagnosis should be cerebellum, pons, and medulla. The differential diagnosis is the same as that described for the horse in this case example. The lack of any prosencephalic signs after 10 days makes eastern equine encephalomyelitis unlikely. As a rule, rabies encephalomyelitis will cause recumbency in approximately 4 days and death by 7 to 10 days. Equine herpesvirus-1 infection causes an acute onset of clinical signs without progression after approximately 2 days. West Nile viral encephalomyelitis is still a candidate during the summer months when exposure to the carrier mosquitoes exists. However, protozoal encephalitis is still the most presumptive clinical diagnosis for this horse.

This horse was euthanized, and necropsy confirmed the diagnosis of protozoal encephalitis in the cerebellum and caudal brainstem (Figs. 12-24, 12-25).

Video 12-28. This video shows a 9-year-old Standardbred gelding that, for 4 weeks, exhibited slight ataxia when he came out of his stall. He continued racing until 10 days before this examination when he was removed from racing competition because of his progressive gait disorder. Study the video. Note the left head tilt, which indicates a dysfunction in some portion of the vestibular system. Also note that

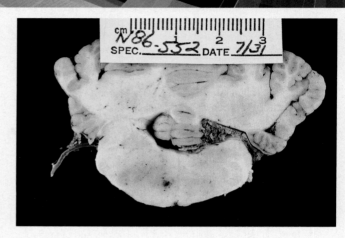

FIGURE 12-25 Caudal surface of a transverse section of the preserved brain of the horse in Video 12-27 just caudal to the transverse section in Fig. 12-24 showing the same lesion.

his gait clearly indicates dysfunction of the UMN and GP systems. The left facial paralysis can be caused by a lesion anywhere from the facial nucleus in the medulla to the stylomastoid foramen, where the facial nerve emerges from the facial canal and forms branches. Only a lesion in the pons and medulla can explain all of these clinical signs. This horse was treated for a presumptive *S. neurona* encephalitis and 1 month later was much improved but not sufficient to allow him to return to racing.

Video 12-29. This video shows a 7-year-old Thoroughbred stallion that, 10 days before this examination, stumbled on coming out of the starting gate. His gait abnormality worsened over the subsequent 10 days. Study the video. Note that the gait disorder represents a dysfunction of the UMN and GP systems that might be at any level between the pons and the C5 spinal cord segment. The severe atrophy of the right muscles of mastication (note the prominence of the right ramus of the mandible and facial crest) indicates that at least part of this lesion is in the pons where the motor nucleus of V is located. The only recognized cause of unilateral atrophy of the muscles of mastication in the horse at this time is an infection with *S. neurona* with loss of these GSE neuronal cell bodies and replacement by astrocytes. No obvious clinical signs of vestibular system dysfunction are noted in this horse. This horse was treated for several weeks with antiprotozoal drugs and recovered his normal gait. This recovery is on the video when snow is seen in the background. Note the absence of recovery of the muscles of mastication because that lesion is permanent.

Video 12-30. This video shows a 10-year-old Appaloosa mare that developed a right head tilt and leaned to the right one day after foaling. Her gait disorder progressed over the next 3 days before this examination. Study the video, and note her mild head tilt and tendency to lean and drift to her right side. However, note the marked clinical signs of dysfunction in the UMN and GP systems that cause her to scuff her hooves and stumble in either direction. She was euthanized, and necropsy confirmed the diagnosis of protozoal encephalitis in the caudal brainstem.

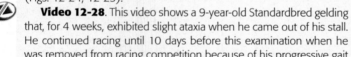

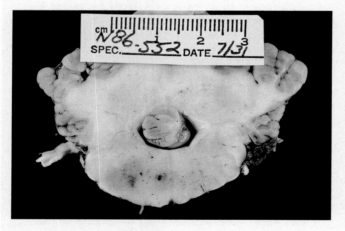

FIGURE 12-24 Caudal surface of a transverse section of the preserved brain of the horse in Video 12-27 at the level of the confluence of the cerebellar peduncles. Note the discoloration on the left side, which was caused by the inflammation and necrosis associated with infection by *S. neurona*.

Ruminants

CASE EXAMPLE 12-14

Signalment: 1-month-old female Holstein

Chief Complaint: Head tilt

History: For the previous few days, this calf has exhibited a mild head tilt and occasionally stumbled.

Examination: See **Video 12-31**. The examiner is indicating loss of tone in the left ear, eyelids, and lips. The left palpebral reflex was decreased, but nociception from the nasal septum was normal.

Anatomic Diagnosis: Left cranial nerve VII and the vestibular portion of cranial nerve VIII

Differential Diagnosis: Otitis median-interna is the only realistic disease to consider in a calf with these clinical signs,[29] which is common in all young farm animals.[39] Similar to dogs and cats, imaging studies will help confirm this diagnosis, with CT being the most reliable. See Video 6-5 for an example of this disorder in another calf and a CT scan of the lesion. These patients should be treated rigorously with antibiotics to prevent extension of the suppurative inflammation into the cranial cavity. These patients with otitis media-interna may exhibit only clinical signs of facial nerve paralysis or only clinical signs of peripheral vestibular system dysfunction.

OTITIS MEDIA-INTERNA IN A CALF

See **Video 12-32**. This video shows two calves from the same farm. The smaller one is 2 months of age, and the larger one is 4 months of age. Both calves have shown clinical signs for approximately 10 days. The smaller calf is alert, responsive, and walks well, but you should recognize a head tilt and ear droop and make the anatomic diagnosis of a right facial (VII) and vestibular nerve (VIII) dysfunction. You should make a presumptive clinical diagnosis of a right otitis media-interna for this calf. This presumption was supported by radiographs that revealed this otitis.

OTITIS WITH INTRACRANIAL ABSCESS IN A CALF

The older calf is depressed and needs assistance to stand and holds its neck in an abnormal extended position. She has a right head tilt, drifts right, and has a left ear droop and no palpebral reflex on the left side but normal eye retraction when the eyelids are stimulated. Your anatomic diagnosis for this larger calf should be pons and medulla because of the depression, difficulty standing, and the neck extension. The left facial paralysis may be caused by the medullary lesion or an otitis media on this side. You should make a presumptive clinical diagnosis of an abscess or suppurative meningoencephalitis at this level that is an extension of an otitis media-interna that may be bilateral. CSF should reflect this suppurative inflammation. This calf was euthanized, and necropsy showed bilateral suppurative otitis media-interna and an abscess and meningitis on the left side of the pons and medulla.

CASE EXAMPLE 12-15

Signalment: 2-year-old female Hereford-Holstein cross

Chief Complaint: Depression and head tilt

History: This cow became depressed and developed a right head tilt approximately 10 days before this examination. She became more depressed and, on occasion, continually walked in circles.

Examination: See **Video 12-33**. Note that this cow's sensorium borders on obtundation. Note also the right head tilt, the paresis of the right facial muscles, muscles of mastication, and tongue muscles.

Anatomic Diagnosis: Pons and medulla—possibly diencephalon. The obtundation suggests the possibility of more than just a caudal brainstem disorder, and the dysfunction of the ascending reticular activating system may be at the level of the diencephalon.

Differential Diagnosis: Listeriosis, rabies, abscess, suppurative meningitis, thrombotic meningoencephalitis

The most common caudal brainstem disorder of adult cattle in the northeast is listeriosis.

LISTERIOSIS IN A COW

Listeriosis is caused by the bacterium, *Listeria monocytogenes*.[8,41] Most affected cattle are over 1 year of age and exhibit various combinations of clinical signs of cranial nerve dysfunction. These signs include facial paralysis, tongue paresis, dysphagia, jaw paresis, and dysfunction of the central components of the vestibular system, along with clinical signs of UMN and GP system dysfunction and loss of their normal sensorium. Some patients continually circle. This circling appears more as a propulsive circling than circling caused by a loss of balance with a vestibular system dysfunction. However, this circumstance is poorly correlated with specific lesion location. Prosencephalic lesions are uncommon with listeriosis yet are the most common cause of propulsive movements. The propulsive circling may possibly occur in these ruminants with listeriosis from involvement of the substantia nigra in the mesencephalon. The prominent caudal brainstem location of this disease reflects the likely route of entrance to the brain for this bacterium. The bacterium enters the body through abrasions and lacerations of the oral mucosa and gains access to the dendritic zones of general somatic afferent (GSA) neurons in the branches of the trigeminal nerve. The bacterium travels retrograde over these axons through the trigeminal ganglion and into the pons, where the fifth cranial nerve attaches to the brainstem. Inflammation occurs in these nerve branches and in the caudal brainstem. Small foci of necrosis filled with neutrophils are scattered primarily through the pons and medulla. Adjacent to these necrotic foci is a nonsuppurative inflammation that includes the meninges. The CSF usually reflects the nonsuppurative component of the inflammation. Rigorous treatment with penicillin will usually improve or resolve the clinical signs in cattle that are still standing. The prognosis is less favorable in small ruminants. Recumbent animals have a poor prognosis regardless of the species. Be aware that this bacterium can affect humans; thus you should, at least, wear protective gloves for this examination and administration of therapy. This organism thrives in poorly prepared silage (pH greater than 5.5), and removal of this as a feed source may prevent further affected animals on the same farm. We have never seen blindness in cattle with listeriosis or cattle with the anatomic diagnosis of a spinal

(Continued)

CASE EXAMPLE 12-15—cont'd

cord location of listeriosis. The latter circumstance may be the result of the lack of lesions in the spinal cord or the masking of these UMN and GP system lesions by the pontomedullary lesions that affect the same systems. See Video 11-33 in Case Example 11-10. This is a lamb with profound spinal cord lesions caused by listeriosis.

Rabies is an unlikely clinical diagnosis because it generally causes recumbency in a few days and death by 7 to 10 days. An abscess or suppurative meningitis (or both) secondary to otitis media-interna is more common in calves and is usually preceded by clinical signs of facial paralysis or peripheral vestibular system dysfunction. Thrombotic meningoencephalitis is caused by the bacterium *Histophilus somni* (*Hemophilus somnus*). This

abnormality is a severe suppurative vasculitis and associated parenchymal necrosis that usually causes a sudden onset of profound brainstem signs or just acute death. Thrombotic meningoencephalitis is an unlikely cause of the more mild brainstem signs with cranial nerve deficits, as seen in the cow in this case example. Lesions may also occur in the prosencephalon and spinal cord. This disease is more common in feedlot cattle in the Midwest than dairy cattle in the northeast.

The CSF in the cow in this case example had 79 mg/dl protein (normal <40) and 31 WBCs/cmm³, all of which were mononuclear cells. Listeriosis was the presumptive clinical diagnosis. This cow was euthanized, and listeriosis was confirmed at necropsy.

CASE EXAMPLE 12-16

Signalment: 9-month-old male Saanen goat

Chief Complaint: Head tilt and abnormal gait

History: Five weeks before this examination, this buck was purchased from a goat herd in Washington State and shipped by air to upstate New York. For the past 3 to 4 weeks, this buck has progressively had more difficulty walking. Recently, he has fallen, with his head extended over his neck and his eyes twitching.

Examination: See **Video 12-34**. Note the right head tilt and abnormal vertical positional nystagmus, the left spastic hemiparesis and ataxia, and the episode of rolling induced by head and neck extension.

Anatomic Diagnosis: Cerebellum, pons, and medulla

The left spastic hemiparesis and ataxia result from UMN and GP system dysfunction on the left side of the pons and medulla. The history suggesting opisthotonus may be an indication of a rostral cerebellar, pons, or midbrain lesion. The right head tilt, abnormal nystagmus, and the rolling episode to the right indicate a paradoxical involvement of the central components of the vestibular system from a lesion in the left cerebellar peduncles or a lesion in the right vestibular nuclei.

Differential Diagnosis: Listeriosis, caprine arthritis encephalitis (CAE) viral encephalitis, *Parelaphostrongylus tenuis* myiasis, abscess, neoplasm

Listeriosis, CAE, and *P. tenuis* myiasis are all common diseases of goats in the Northeast, which can occur at this anatomic site. This goat came from a CAE-free herd in the state of Washington and had no serum antibodies for this viral agent. White tail deer are not indigenous to the state of Washington, and this goat had been in New York State for only 1 week before clinical signs were observed. This time period is too short for this goat to ingest an infected mollusk or the stage-3 larva of *P. tenuis* and develop neurologic signs. Experimentally, the earliest that clinical signs were observed after feeding large quantities of stage-3 larvae to sheep and goats was 11 days. The history reveals no sign of otitis media-interna with neurologic signs to suspect an intracranial extension of that suppurative lesion. In addition, no history of any illness was found to cause a bacteremia that might result in a brain abscess. Neoplasia is rare in goats, especially at this age. Medulloblastoma (primitive neuroectodermal tumor) occurs in the cerebellum of young calves. Listeriosis was considered to be the presumptive clinical diagnosis. The CSF contained 35 mg/dl of protein (normal <40) and 15 WBCs/mm³, with 67% monocytes and 33% lymphocytes. This buck was treated with antibiotics for 10 days but showed no improvement. He was euthanized, and necropsy showed a large well-encapsulated abscess centered in the left cerebellar peduncles and left cerebellar medulla (Fig. 12-26).[22] No source of this focal infection was found. This lesion would have been evident on CT scan or MR imaging.

See **Video 12-35**. This video shows a 4-year-old castrated male Pygmy goat that was found one afternoon with a right head tilt and circling to his left. He was worse the next day when the examination seen in the video was made. Note his severe disorientation, his right head tilt, and a tendency to drift right. Also note that his gait shows only a vestibular ataxia, and note the difficulty with holding this goat stable while trying to evaluate the hopping responses. We concluded that the hopping responses in his right limbs were mildly slow. Note his abnormal resting nystagmus. Not shown was the shift in the direction of the nystagmus with changes in the position of his head. The anatomic diagnosis is right cerebellum, pons, and medulla. The differential diagnosis is the same as that in this case example. This animal is a New York State goat, where the white tail deer are plentiful. CAE is unlikely at this age. Listeriosis and myiasis with the larva of *P. tenuis* are the most presumptive clinical diagnoses for this goat. Listeriosis is the more common cause of these brainstem signs. The CSF contained 170 mg/dl protein (normal <40) and 312 WBCs/mm³, with 52% neutrophils, 17% lymphocytes, 31% macrophages, and no eosinophils. This goat was euthanized and a necropsy diagnosed a necrotizing meningoencephalitis associated with *L. monocytogenes* organisms.

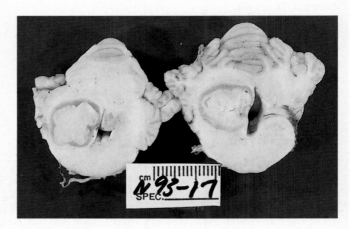

FIGURE 12-26 Caudal surface of a transverse section of the preserved brain of the goat in Video 12-34 at the level of the confluence of the cerebellar peduncles, showing an abscess centered in the left cerebellar peduncles.

Congenital Nystagmus

Congenital pendular resting nystagmus occurs in humans as an inherited abnormality or secondary to congenital lesions in the visual system of the infant, especially the retina, including ocular albinism. The nystagmus is usually pendular, meaning that the eye movements are equal in velocity in both directions and it is very rapid. This nystagmus is benign and does not interfere with vision, given that the brain usually compensates for this presumably at the level of the cerebral cortex.

A congenital rapid pendular nystagmus, which usually resolves spontaneously in a few weeks, occasionally occurs in one or more of a litter of puppies. The cause is unknown.

In the 1970s I (AD) studied a severe congenital nystagmus in an adult female Belgian shepherd (Groenendael) and in three of her six offspring from one litter. In the United States, these dogs are called Belgian sheepdogs. This extreme nystagmus was pendular, which varied in rate but was usually quite rapid. No obvious visual deficiency was noted, and ocular examination was normal. Occasionally, a dog briefly held its head to one side as it was about to jump down from a table level. No ataxia was evident. The head would occasionally oscillate with the nystagmus. Necropsy of the three littermates revealed a complete lack of any optic chiasm (Figs. 12-27 through 12-29). The optic nerve fibers continued into the ipsilateral optic tract uninterrupted and without any indication of decussation. Two of these dogs were 4 years of age at the time of necropsy, and their nystagmus had not changed. On the presumption that this malformation was an inherited disorder, and at the request of a neuroscientist interested in what determines the crossing of axons at the optic chiasm, the owner repeated the mating that produced these three affected dogs, resulting in more achiasmatic puppies with a pendular nystagmus and numerous publications.[24,48] These studies established that the retina is relatively normal in these dogs, and the effect of the autosomal-recessive inherited mutation is most likely exerted outside the retina.

In cattle, a congenital rapid fine pendular nystagmus is observed in many breeds and usually persists for the life of these animals. It does not appear to interfere with vision. As a rule, the farmer is unaware of the nystagmus until a veterinarian observes it on an examination of the animal or when restraining an animal for routine blood testing. These cattle have normal extraocular muscle function and no indication of any vestibular system dysfunction. We are not aware of any structural abnormality in the visual system of these cattle, and they have no indication of any albinism. It is sporadic in occurrence, but a high incidence was seen in one Guernsey herd. The inheritance of this nystagmus is unknown. An

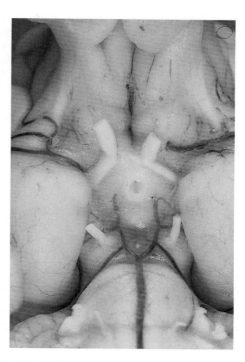

FIGURE 12-28 Ventral surface of the brain of the Belgian shepherd in Fig. 12-27 with congenital nystagmus and a failure of the optic chiasm to develop.

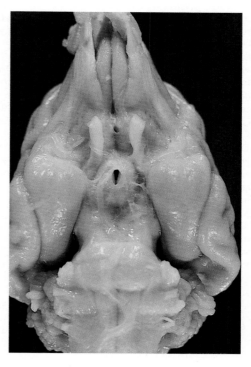

FIGURE 12-29 Ventral surface of the brain of an achiasmatic littermate of the Belgian shepherd in Fig. 12-28.

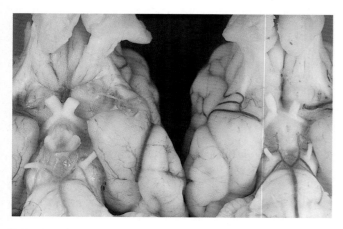

FIGURE 12-27 Ventral surface of the preserved brain of a normal dog on the left and a young adult achiasmatic Belgian shepherd on the right. Note the complete absence of the optic chiasm. This dog exhibited a constant congenital pendular nystagmus.

examination of 2932 cattle seen in 1 month by the ambulatory clinic at Cornell University revealed 15 animals with this pendular nystagmus.[31] See **Video 12-36**. This adult cow has congenital pendular nystagmus, also termed *ocular tremors*.

Congenital rapid fine pendular nystagmus is most often observed in cats with a varying degree of ocular albinism. An abnormality in the retinogeniculate projections and the neuronal organization of the lateral geniculate nucleus have been observed in the Siamese cat and the white Persian tiger. More retinal ganglion neurons project their axons contralaterally in Siamese cats than the normally pigmented feline breeds. No obvious impairment of vision is noted. Many of these cats also have a mild strabismus. This congenital pendular nystagmus also occurs in some cats and cattle with the Chédiak-Higashi syndrome in which pigmentation and melanin granules are abnormal.[12]

Congenital pendular nystagmus may be a result of abnormal sensory input to the system that controls the eye movements related to vision. Some aberration of the architecture of the visual pathway may be the common factor in these patients. The albino cat exhibits excessive contralateral projection of optic nerve axons, and the Belgian shepherds shows complete lack of any contralateral projection.

REFERENCES

1. Adair HS Jr: Blue-tail lizard, *Auburn Vet* 9:117, 1953.
2. Bedford PGC: Congenital vestibular disease in the English Cocker Spaniel, *Vet Rec* 105:530, 1970.
3. Blauch B, Strafuss AC: Histologic relationships of the facial (7th) and vestibulocochlear (8th) cranial nerves within the petrous temporal bone in the dog, *Am J Vet Res* 35:481, 1970.
4. Blauch B, Martin CL: A vestibular syndrome in aged dogs, *J Am Anim Hosp Assoc* 10:37, 1974.
5. Blythe LL, Watrous BJ, Schmitz JA: Vestibular syndrome associated with temporohyoid joint fusion and temporal bone fracture in three horses, *J Am Vet Med Assoc* 185:775-782, 1984.
6. Braund KG, et al: Granulomatous meningoencephalitis in six dogs, *J Am Vet Med Assoc* 172:1195, 1978.
7. Burke EE, et al: Review of idiopathic vestibular syndrome in 75 cats, *J Am Vet Med Assoc* 187:941-943, 1985.
8. Butt MT, et al: Encephalitic listeriosis in two adult llamas (lama glama): clinical presentations, lesions and immunofluorescence of Listeria monocytogenes in brain stem lesions, *Cornell Vet* 81:251-258, 1991.
9. Carpenter MB, Fabrega H, Glinsmann W: Physiological deficits occurring with lesions of the labyrinth and fastigial nucleus, *J Neurophysiol* 22:222, 1959.
10. Caylor KB, Cassimatis MK: Metronidazole neurotoxicosis in two cats, *J Am Anim Hosp Assoc* 37:258-262, 2001.
11. Coats AC: Vestibular neuronitis, *Trans Am Acad Ophthalmol Otolaryngol* 73:395, 1969.
12. Collier L, Bryan GM, Preiur DJ: Ocular manifestations of the Chédiak-Higashi syndrome in four species of animals, *J Am Vet Med Assoc* 175:587, 1979.
13. de Lahunta A: Feline vestibular disease. In Kirk RW, editor: *Current veterinary therapy III*, Philadelphia, 1968, Saunders.
14. Dow SW, LeCouteur RA, Poss ML: Central nervous system toxicosis associated with metronidazole treatment of dogs: five cases (1984-1987), *J Am Vet Med Assoc* 195:365-368, 1989.
15. Everett GM: Observations on the behavior and neurophysiology of acute thiamin deficiency in cats, *Am J Physiol* 141:439, 1944.
16. Firth EC: Vestibular disease and its relationship to facial paralysis in the horse: a clinical study of 7 cases, *Aust Vet J* 53:560, 1977.
17. Gacek RR, Gacek MR: The three faces of vestibular ganglionitis, *Ann Otol Rhinol Laryngol* 111:103-113, 2002.
18. Garosi LS, et al: Results of magnetic resonance imaging in dogs with vestibular disorders: 85 cases (1996-1999), *J Am Vet Med Assoc* 218:385-391, 2001.
19. Garosi LS, et al: Thiamin deficiency in a dog: clinical clinicopathologic and magnetic resonance imaging findings, *J Vet Intern Med* 17:719-723, 2003.
20. Garosi LS, et al: Clinical and topographic magnetic resonance characteristics of suspected brain infarction in 40 dogs, *J Vet Intern Med* 20:311-321, 2006.
21. Gearhart MA, de Lahunta A, Summers BA: Cerebellar mass in a dog due to granulomatous meningoencephalitis, *J Am Anim Hosp Assoc* 22:683-686, 1986.
22. Glass EN, de Lahunta A, Jackson C: Brain abscess in a goat, *Cornell Vet* 83:275-282, 1993.
23. Higgins MA, Rossmeisl JH Jr, Panciera DL: Hypothyroid-associated central vestibular disease in 10 dogs (1999-2005), *J Vet Intern Med* 20:1363-1369, 2006.
24. Hogan D, Williams RW: Analysis of the retinas and optic nerves of achiasmatic Belgian Sheepdogs, *J Comp Neurol* 352:367-380, 1995.
25. Holliday TA: Clinical signs of acute and chronic experimental lesions of the cerebellum, *Vet Sci Commun* 3:259, 1979-1980.
26. Kornegay JN: Feline infectious peritonitis: the central nervous system form, *J Am Anim Hosp Assoc* 16:263, 1978.
27. Lundquist Per-G, Wersall J: Sites of action of ototoxic antibiotics after local and general administration. In Stahle J, editor: *Vestibular function on earth and in space*, New York, 1970, Pergamon.
28. MacKillop E, Schatzberg S, de Lahunta A: Intracranial epidermoid cyst and syringohydromyelia in a dog, *Vet Radiol Ultrasound* 47:339-344, 2006.
29. Maeda T, et al: Mycoplasma bovis-associated suppurative otitis media and pneumonia in bull calves, *J Comp Pathol* 129:100-110, 2003.
30. McConnell JF, Garosi LS, Platt SR: Magnetic resonance imaging findings of presumed cerebellar cerebrovascular accident in twelve dogs, *Vet Radiol Ultrasound* 46:1-10, 2005.
31. McConnon JN, et al: Congenital pendular nystagmus in dairy cattle, *J Am Vet Med Assoc* 182:812-813, 1983.
32. McGee TM, Olszewski J: Streptomycin sulfate and dihydrostreptomycin toxicity, behavioral and histopathological studies, *Arch Otolaryngol* 75:295, 1962.
33. McGrath JT: Fibrinoid leukodystrophy (Alexander's disease). In Andrews EJ, Ward BC, Altman NH, editors: *Spontaneous animal models of human disease*, vol 2, New York, 1979, Academic Press.
34. Montali RJ, Strandberg JD: Extraperitoneal lesions in feline infectious peritonitis, *Vet Pathol* 9:109, 1972.
35. Nyberg-Hansen R: Origin and termination of fibers from the vestibular nuclei descending in the medial longitudinal fasciculus. An experimental study with silver impregnation methods in the cat, *J Comp Neurol* 122:355, 1964.
36. Nyberg-Hansen R, Mascitti TA: Sites and mode of termination of fibers of the vestibulospinal tract in the cat, *J Comp Neurol* 122:369, 1964.

37. O'Brien DP, Zachary JF: Clinical features of spongy degeneration of the central nervous system in two Labrador Retriever littermates, *J Am Vet Med Assoc* 186:1207, 1985.

38. Olson EJ, et al: Putative metronidazole neurotoxicosis in a cat, *Vet Pathol* 42:665-669, 2005.

39. Olson LD: Gross and microscopic lesions of middle and inner ear infections in swine, *Am J Vet Res* 42:1433, 1981.

40. Read DH, Harrington DD: Experimentally induced thiamin deficiency in beagle dogs: clinical observations, *Am J Vet Res* 342:984, 1981.

41. Rebhun WC, de Lahunta A: Diagnosis and treatment of bovine listeriosis, *J Am Vet Med Assoc* 180:395-398, 1982.

42. Schunk KL, Averill DR Jr: Peripheral vestibular syndrome in the dog: review of 83 cases, *J Am Vet Med Assoc* 182:1354-1357, 1983.

43. Slausson DO, Finn JP: Meningoencephalitis and panophthalmitis in feline infectious peritonitis, *J Am Vet Med Assoc* 160:729, 1972.

44. Spreull JSA: Treatment of otitis media in the dog, *J Sm Anim Pract* 5:107-152, 1964.

45. Stirling J, Clarke M: Congenital peripheral vestibular disorder in two German shepherd dogs, *Aust Vet J* 57:200, 1981.

46. Troxel MT, Drobatz KJ, Vite CH: Signs of neurologic dysfunction in dogs with central versus peripheral vestibular disease, *J Am Vet Med Assoc* 227:570-574, 2005.

47. Walker AM: Temporohyoid osteoarthropathy in 33 horses (1993-2000), *J Vet Intern Med* 16:697-703, 2002.

48. Williams RW, Hogan D, Garraghty PE: Target recognition and visual maps in the thalamus of achiasmatic dogs, *Nature* 367:637-639, 1994.

49. Wilson VJ, Wylis RM, Marco LA: Projection to the spinal cord from the medial and descending vestibular nuclei of the cat, *Nature* 215:429, 1967.

50. Winston J: Clinical problems pertaining to neurotoxicity of streptomycin group of drugs, *Arch Otolaryngol* 58:255, 1953.

51. Winston J, et al: An experimental study of the toxic effects of streptomycin on the vestibular apparatus of the cat. I. Central nervous system, *Ann Otol Rhinol Laryngol* 57:738, 1948.

52. Zachary JF, O'Brien DP: Spongy degeneration of the central nervous system in two canine littermates, *Vet Pathol* 22:561-571, 1985.

13 CEREBELLUM

DEVELOPMENT

ANATOMY

    Cerebellar Afferents
        General Proprioception
        Special Proprioception
        Special Somatic Afferent—Visual
          and Auditory
        Upper Motor Neuron
    Cerebellar Efferents
        Cerebellar Cortex
        Cerebellar Nuclei

FUNCTION

CLINICAL SIGNS OF CEREBELLAR DISEASE

CEREBELLAR DISEASES

    Malformation—Abiotrophy
        Dogs
        Cats
        Horses
        Cattle
        Sheep
        Pigs
    Other Cerebellar Diseases
        Inflammation

Neoplasia
Degeneration
Injury
CASE EXAMPLE 13-1
    Neosporosis
CASE EXAMPLE 13-2
    Vascular Compromise
CASE EXAMPLE 13-3
    Neoplasm
CASE EXAMPLE 13-4
    Axonopathy (Hereditary Ataxia)
CASE EXAMPLE 13-5
    Neuronal Storage Disease

DEVELOPMENT

An understanding of the development of the cerebellum is pertinent to the determination of its normal microscopic characteristics and the pathogenesis of the diseases that affect this structure. The cerebellum is the dorsal portion of the metencephalon. The ventral portion is the pons.* The cerebellum develops primarily from the alar plate region of the metencephalon (Fig. 13-1). Its first appearance is a dorsal bulge of the alar plate, which extends the alar plate tissue dorsally and medially in the roof plate, where the growths from each side eventually join each other. The first growth of each alar plate is called the *rhombic lip,* which arises from the side of the rhomboid fossa of the fourth ventricle. This rhombic lip consists of proliferating cells from the germinal layer adjacent to the fourth ventricle.

The undifferentiated cells in this population of germinal layer cells follow one of two pathways. One group differentiates into primitive neurons or glioblasts that migrate into the substance of the rhombic lip. These immature neurons no longer divide but continue to grow and mature. These neurons give rise to the Purkinje neurons that form a layer throughout the cerebellar cortex and the neuronal cell bodies of the cerebellar nuclei found in the medulla of the cerebellum. The second pathway involves actively dividing germinal layer cells that continue to divide as they migrate to the surface of the rhombic lip, where they form a superficial layer termed the *external germinal layer.* As the cerebellar folia develop, these germinal cells will remain on the external surface of these folia. They continue to divide, forming an external germinal layer that is 10 to 12 cells in thickness.[3] Differentiation occurs along the inner aspect of this thick layer of dividing cells, where these cells stop dividing and become primitive neurons or glioblasts that then migrate internally into the substance of the folium. Most of these cells continue past the Purkinje neurons and form the small granule neurons of the granular layer of the cerebellar cortex. This external germinal layer also contributes the few interneurons (stellate neurons) found in the most superficial layers of the cerebellar cortex, the molecular layer, which primarily consists of granule neuronal axons and dendritic zones of Purkinje neurons. Thus the three layers of the definitive cerebellar cortex are from external to internal, the molecular layer, the Purkinje neuron layer, and the granular (granule neuron) layer. The folding of the developing cerebellar cortex produces the cerebellar folia with the folial white matter lamina in the center of each folium. This folial white matter lamina contains the projecting axons of the Purkinje neurons and a plethora of axons of afferent neurons to the cerebellar cortex from the spinal cord and brainstem. After this neuronal development to populate the cerebellum, the remaining germinal layer cells at this level of the neural tube differentiate into a single layer of ependymal cells that form the lining of the fourth ventricle.

Purkinje neurons are formed by differentiation of rhombic lip germinal cells early in embryonic development. The entire population of Purkinje neurons are differentiated over just a few days.[2] They grow and mature as they migrate into the developing cerebellar parenchyma. The total population of Purkinje neurons is well established before the fetus is born. In contrast, the external germinal layer on

---

*References 1-5, 48, 111, 113, 123, 124.

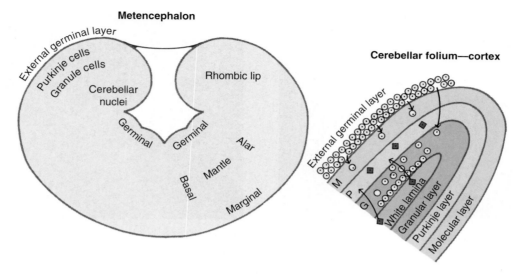

FIGURE 13-1 Development of the cerebellum.

the surface of the folia continues to divide until late in gestation or after birth in some species that includes dogs and cats. The granule cell neurons complete the population of the granular layer after the formation of the Purkinje neurons and before birth in the horse and farm animal species. The process of neuronal migration and organization in these three layers has been studied extensively and involves the cellular action of radially organized astrocytes and the chemical action of growth factor proteins, one of which is known as *brain-derived neurotrophic factor*.[19] This protein has mitogenic influence over the embryonic germinal layer cells and chemotactic effect on their migration. In addition, the leptomeninges adjacent to the developing folia play a role in the organization of the cerebellar cortex.[123] If this layer is disrupted during development, the cortical layers will develop abnormally. In dogs and cats, external germinal layer cell division continues for the first few weeks after birth, and a few granule neurons continue to be formed as late as 10 weeks after birth. The degree of cerebellar development correlates well with the amount of motor function and its degree of coordination that you see in the newborn animal.[55] The newborn animals, such as the foal and the species of farm animals that are able to walk with coordination at birth, have a more completely developed cerebellum than the kitten and puppy or the human baby who are essentially helpless at birth. In humans, as the cerebellum develops after birth, their motor function and coordination for ambulation improve. A direct correlation has been shown between the development of the cerebellar cortex and coordinated mobility in the kitten. The term *altricial* is used for species such as the cat, dog, and human that require a long period of nursing care after birth.

In the calf, the formation of Purkinje neurons is completed by approximately 100 days of gestation. After this differentiation is complete, these Purkinje neurons will grow and mature in conjunction with the continuing development of the cerebellum. In the horse, ox, sheep, goat, llama, and alpaca, the external germinal layer is more active late in gestation and has mostly exhausted its germinal role before birth with the formation of the granule neuronal layer. In the calf, the cerebellar primordium appears at approximately 37 days of gestation. The external germinal layer appears at 57 days of gestation and is maximal in thickness by 183 days, when it is composed of six cell layers. After this phase, it slowly decreases in thickness, reaching a layer that is two cells in thickness by 2 months postnatally and completely disappears by approximately 6 months postnatally. Pathologists should be aware of the presence of this external germinal layer in these young animals and avoid confusing it with meningitis. In the kitten and puppy, the external germinal layer does not reach maximal thickness until the end of the first postnatal week and starts to decrease in size after the second postnatal week. A poorly populated granule neuron layer is present at birth (Fig. 13-4). It grows rapidly in the first few weeks and continues to grow for up to 10 weeks postnatally. External germinal layer cells will persist for as long as 60 to 84 days in the kitten and 75 days in the puppy. When all of the cells have migrated into the molecular and granular layers, only the leptomeninges remain on the surface of the folia adjacent to the molecular layer. Figs. 13-2 through 13-7 illustrate features of this development of the cerebellum.

ANATOMY

The cerebellum consists of a central median region, the vermis, named for the wormlike contortions it presents caudally and a hemisphere laterally on each side of the vermis (Figs. 13-8, 13-9). The cerebellum is divided into two disproportionate regions: (1) the large body of the cerebellum and (2) the small flocculonodular lobe. These two regions are separated by the uvulonodular fissure (see Fig. 13-9). The flocculonodular lobe, also known as the *archicerebellum* or *vestibular cerebellum,* is confined to the ventral aspect of the cerebellum near its center. The nodulus is the most rostral part of the caudal vermis that is adjacent to the fourth ventricle. It connects laterally by a peduncle on each side to

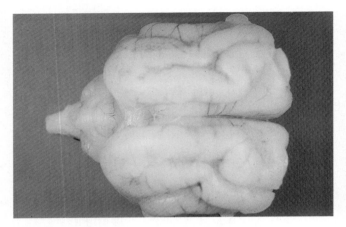

FIGURE 13-2 Dorsal view of a normal 2-day-old puppy brain. Note the degree of development of the cerebral gyri and the relatively small size of the cerebellum.

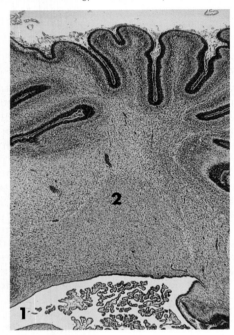

FIGURE 13-3 Transverse microscopic section of a portion of the cerebellum seen in Fig. 13-2. Note the fourth ventricle and a portion of the choroid plexus (1) at the bottom. Note the large cerebellar nucleus in the cerebellar medulla (2) and the thick external germinal layer covering the developing folia.

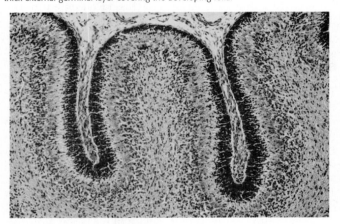

FIGURE 13-4 Higher magnification of the microscopic section seen in Fig. 13-3, showing the developing cerebellar cortex with the prominent densely populated external germinal layer.

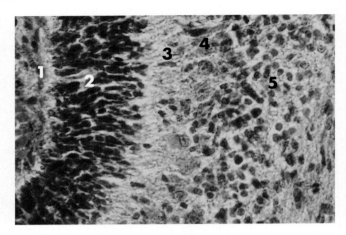

FIGURE 13-5 Higher magnification of the microscopic section seen in Fig. 13-4. The folial sulcus with meninges and capillaries (1) is at the left adjacent to the thick external germinal layer (2). Note the relatively thin molecular layer (3), the row of small Purkinje neurons (4), and the sparsely populated granular layer (5).

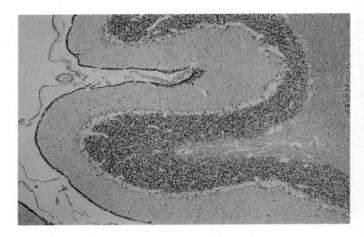

FIGURE 13-6 Microscopic section of a cerebellar folium of a 1-day-old foal. Note the thin external germinal layer and the densely populated granular layer. Compare this figure with those of the 2-day-old dog cerebellum.

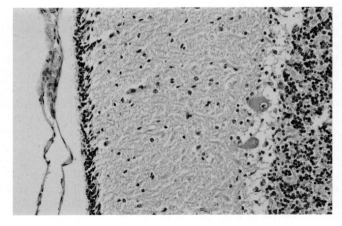

FIGURE 13-7 Higher magnification of the section seen in Fig. 13-6, showing the remnant of the external germinal layer at this age.

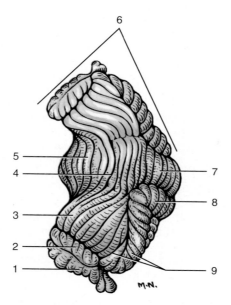

FIGURE 13-8 Dorsolateral view of the cerebellum. The primary fissure (4) divides the cerebellum into rostral and caudal lobes.

1. Ventral paraflocculus
2. Dorsal paraflocculus
3. Dorsal surface of cerebellum
4. Primary fissure
5. Vermis portion of rostral lobe
6. Right cerebellar hemisphere
7. Vermis portion of caudal lobe
8. Paramedian lobule
9. Ansiform lobule

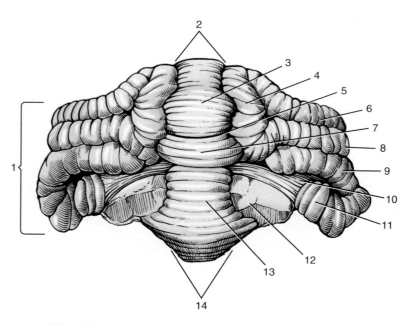

FIGURE 13-9 Cerebellum, ventral surface.

1. Right cerebellar hemisphere
2. Caudal vermis
3. Uvula
4. Paramedian lobule
5. Uvulonodular fissure
6. Ansiform lobule
7. Nodulus
8. Dorsal paraflocculus
9. Ventral paraflocculus
10. Flocculonodular peduncle
11. Flocculus
12. Cerebellar peduncles, cut surface
13. Lingula
14. Rostral vermis

the flocculus, which is a small lobule on the ventral aspect of the cerebellar hemisphere. The much larger body of the cerebellum, consisting of the vermis and two hemispheres, is divided into rostral and caudal lobes by the primary fissure. Within each lobe, the folia are grouped into named lobules that reside in different portions of the vermis and hemispheres.

The cerebellum is attached to the brainstem by three groups of neuronal processes on each side of the fourth ventricle (Fig. 13-10). These processes are the cerebellar peduncles (see Figs. 2-9 through 2-14). Although arranged in a medial to lateral plane, they are named from rostral to caudal based on their connections with the brainstem. The caudal cerebellar peduncle connects the spinal cord and medulla with the cerebellum. It contains primarily afferent processes projecting to the cerebellum. The middle cerebellar peduncle connects the transverse fibers of the pons with the cerebellum, which is entirely afferent to the cerebellum. The rostral cerebellar peduncle connects the cerebellum with the mesencephalon and contains mainly efferent processes passing out of the cerebellum.

When the cerebellum is sectioned transversely or longitudinally, an extensive area of white matter is visible in the center. This area is the cerebellar medulla, which should not be confused with the medulla (oblongata) of the brainstem. The cerebellar medulla has extensions of white matter into the overlying folia. As a group, these extensions appear similar to tree branches and are called the *arbor vitae*. Individually, each is the white lamina of a folium. The arbor vitae are covered by the three layers of the cerebellar cortex. In the cerebellar medulla are situated collections of neuronal cell bodies that comprise the

cerebellar nuclei (see Fig. 2-13). These cell bodies are organized into three nuclei on each side of the median plane. From medial to lateral, these nuclei are the fastigial, interposital, and lateral cerebellar nuclei. For some reason, students have difficulty with this concept of cerebellar nuclei embedded in the white matter of the cerebellar medulla. This arrangement of cerebellar nuclei is directly comparable to the cerebrum, where the neuronal cell bodies are located either on the surface in the cerebral cortex or deep to the surface in basal nuclei. Their arrangement in both the cerebellum and cerebrum is determined by the degree and pattern of migration of the cells from the germinal layer.

The cerebellar cortex, which is composed of three layers, forms the outer portion of each folium and is similar throughout the cerebellum (Fig. 13-11). The folial and sulcal surfaces in the adult are covered by the leptomeninges. Adjacent to these leptomeninges is the most external of the three cortical layers, the relatively cell-free molecular layer. It is composed mostly of the axons and telodendria of granule neurons and the dendritic zones of the Purkinje neurons and a small population of interneurons and astrocytes. The molecular layer covers the middle layer that is a narrow single layer of large flask-shaped neurons, which comprise the Purkinje neuron layer. The deepest of the three layers is the granule neuron (granular) layer. This layer is thick and is composed of a remarkably large number of small neuronal cell bodies and their dendritic zones. This cell layer varies from 5 to 6 neurons thick where the cortex is continuous from one folium to another at the depth of a sulcus to 15 to 20 neurons thick at the top of a folium. Figs. 13-12 through 13-19 illustrate gross and microscopic features of the cerebellum.

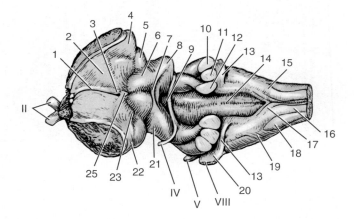

FIGURE 13-10 The brainstem from a dorsolateral perspective. *II,* Optic nerve; *IV,* trochlear nerve; *V,* trigeminal nerve; *VIII,* vestibulocochlear nerve.

1. Stria habenularis thalami
2. Dorsal aspect of thalamus
3. Habenular commissure
4. Lateral geniculate body
5. Medial geniculate body
6. Rostral colliculus
7. Commissure of caudal colliculi
8. Caudal colliculus
9. Decussation of trochlear nerves in rostral medullary velum
10. Middle cerebellar peduncle
11. Caudal cerebellar peduncle
12. Rostral cerebellar peduncle
13. Dorsal cochlear nucleus
14. Median sulcus in fourth ventricle
15. Nucleus cuneatus lateralis
16. Fasciculus cuneatus
17. Fasciculus gracilis
18. Spinal tract of trigeminal nerve
19. Superficial arcuate fibers
20. Ventral cochlear nucleus
21. Brachium of caudal colliculus
22. Optic tract
23. Brachium of rostral colliculus
24. Cut surface of internal capsule
25. Pineal body

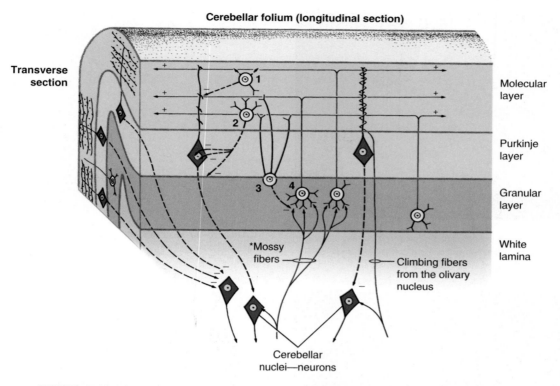

FIGURE 13-11 Microscopic anatomy of the cerebellum. **1,** Stellate cell (outer). **2,** Basket cell. **3,** Golgi cell. **4,** Granule cell. Inhibitory neurons are shown by a broken line; facilitatory neurons are shown by a solid line. *From: Spinocerebellar tracts, cuneocerebellar tracts, pontocerebellar tracts, vestibulocerebellar tracts, reticulocerebellar tracts.

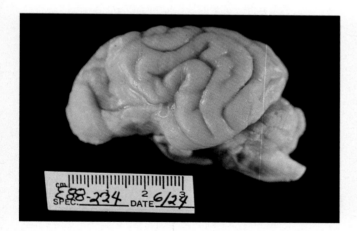

FIGURE 13-12 Lateral view of normal dog brain. Note the relative size of the cerebellum compared with the cerebral hemisphere and caudal brainstem.

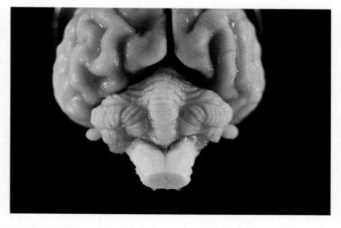

FIGURE 13-13 Dorsocaudal view of normal dog cerebellum. Note the prominent vermis and relatively small hemispheres when compared with some other animals like the bird, bear, sea lion, and primates in Figs. 13-21 through 13-31.

The cerebellar cortex is uniquely organized for the distribution of afferent information (see Fig. 13-11). Two major types of afferents to the cerebellum exist based on the morphology of their telodendrons: mossy fibers and climbing fibers. The more abundant mossy fibers have a widespread origin in the brainstem and spinal cord. As they pass into the cerebellum, collaterals of these axonal processes synapse on the cell bodies and dendritic zones of neurons in the cerebellar nuclei. The main axon continues through the cerebellar medulla into the white lamina of a folium and enters the granular layer, where it terminates on the dendritic zones of the granule neurons. These synapses are sometimes called *glomeruli*. They are adjacent to the small neuronal cell body of the granule neuron. The axon of this granule neuron projects externally through the Purkinje neuronal layer into the molecular layer, where this axon forms two branches that course in opposite directions parallel to the longitudinal axis of the folium. The dendritic zone of the Purkinje neuron is arranged in the molecular layer as a maze of branched axons that are oriented in a flat plane transverse to the axis of the folium. By this arrangement in the molecular layer, the axon of the granule

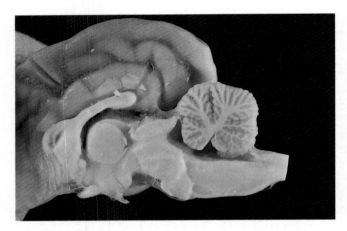

FIGURE 13-14 Median plane longitudinal section of a normal dog brain. Note the cerebellar medulla and the arrangement of the folial white laminae similar to tree branches, the arbor vitae.

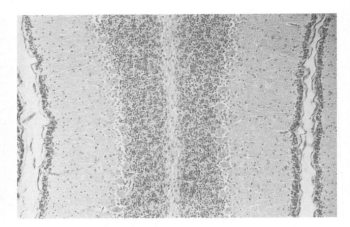

FIGURE 13-17 Microscopic section of a normal single cerebellar folium of a 10-week-old domestic shorthair. Note the remaining external germinal layer on the surface.

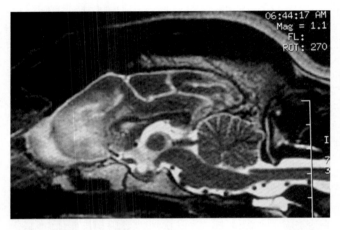

FIGURE 13-15 T2-weighted magnetic resonance image of the median plane of a normal dog brain. Compare this image with Fig. 13-14.

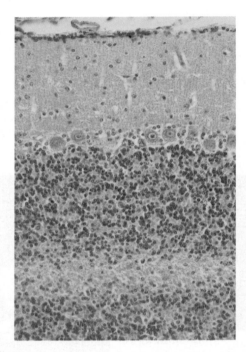

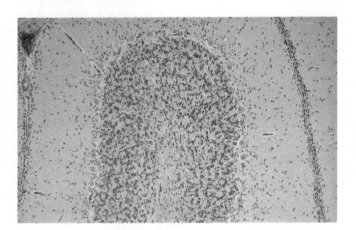

FIGURE 13-16 Microscopic section of a portion of a normal single cerebellar folium of a 1-day-old calf. Note the thin remnant of the external germinal layer.

FIGURE 13-18 Higher magnification of a microscopic section of a portion of a cerebellar folium of a 10-week-old domestic shorthair. Note the thin external germinal layer at the top covering the relatively cell-free molecular layer, the single layer of the large neurons of the Purkinje neuronal layer, and a portion of the cell-dense granular layer at the bottom.

neuron traverses the dendritic zone of numerous Purkinje neurons. Synapse occurs between these processes. This network can be likened to telephone wires (granule neuronal axons) coursing from one telephone pole (dendritic zone of Purkinje neurons) to another. Climbing fibers are the axons of olivary neurons that enter the cerebellum through the

caudal cerebellar peduncle.[34] Collaterals of these axons synapse on neurons in the cerebellar nuclei. The main axon continues through the cerebellar medulla into a white lamina of a folium and passes through the granule neuronal layer and the Purkinje neuronal layer into the molecular layer, where it entwines around the dendritic zone of the Purkinje neuron and terminates there in synapses.

The mossy and climbing fibers are facilitory at their synapse with neurons of the cerebellar nuclei and the granule and Purkinje neurons, respectively.[58] Acetylcholine is the neurotransmitter released at the synapses of the mossy fibers and aspartate at the synapses of the climbing fibers.

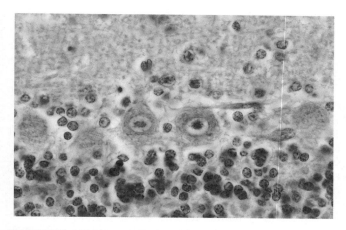

FIGURE 13-19 Higher magnification of the microscopic section seen in Fig. 13-18, showing the single layer of robust Purkinje neurons below the molecular layer and above the granular layer.

The granule neurons are facilitory to the Purkinje neurons with glutamate released at the synapses. Within the molecular layer are stellate neurons (outer and basket) that are inhibitory to the Purkinje neurons. Large stellate neurons (Golgi) are scattered through the granular layer. These neurons are inhibitory to granule neurons.[56] The only axon that projects from the cerebellar cortex (an efferent axon) is that of the Purkinje neuron. These axons pass through the granular layer into the folial white matter lamina and continue into the cerebellar medulla. The majority of these terminate on the dendritic zones of the neurons in the cerebellar nuclei. A small population of Purkinje neuronal axons, the cell bodies of which are primarily located in the flocculonodular lobe, leave the cerebellum through the caudal cerebellar peduncle and terminate on the dendritic zones of neurons in the vestibular nuclei. At all of the telodendria of these Purkinje neurons, the inhibitory neurotransmitter gamma-aminobutyric acid is released.[29] With the exception of these direct cerebellovestibular Purkinje neuronal projections, the efferent axons that project from the cerebellum to the brainstem are all from the cerebellar nuclei.[54] This anatomy supports a major role of the cerebellar cortex in modulating the continual facilitation of the neurons in the cerebellar nuclei via Purkinje neuronal inhibition.

The cerebellum plays a major role in the control of motor activity. Therefore, logically, it must receive afferent information to provide it with knowledge of where the head, neck, trunk, and limbs are in space via connections with the general and special proprioceptive systems. It also needs information on what voluntary motor activity is to occur, and therefore it must receive afferents from the upper motor neuron (UMN) systems. The cerebellum is often called *the great regulator of movement.*

Cerebellar Afferents

General Proprioception

An abundance of spinocerebellar tracts enter the cerebellum primarily through the caudal cerebellar peduncle; a small group enters via the rostral cerebellar peduncle.

Cuneocerebellar tracts from the neck and thoracic limbs enter through the caudal cerebellar peduncle.

Special Proprioception

Vestibulocerebellar axons enter directly from the vestibular portion of cranial nerve VIII or indirectly from the vestibular nuclei via the caudal cerebellar peduncles. Most of the proprioceptive neurons project to the folia of the cerebellar vermis or the adjacent paravermal folia.

Special Somatic Afferent—Visual and Auditory

Tectocerebellar axons enter the cerebellum directly by way of the rostral cerebellar peduncle and project to the head region of the vermis. In addition, axons from the visual and auditory areas of the cerebral cortex project to the pons and synapse on pontine neurons. The axons of these pontine neurons cross in the transverse fibers of the pons and enter the cerebellum through the contralateral middle cerebellar peduncle.

Upper Motor Neuron

The projection of UMN information to the cerebellum is diffuse and complex. Brainstem nuclei involved in this cerebellar projection include the red, pontine, and olivary nuclei and the reticular formation. Many of these nuclei receive projections from the telencephalic basal nuclei and the areas of the cerebral cortex involved with motor function. The red nucleus is the source of rubrocerebellar axons that enter the cerebellum through the rostral cerebellar peduncle. Reticulocerebellar axons enter through the caudal cerebellar peduncle. Many of the extrapyramidal system nuclei of the telencephalon and brainstem project to the cerebellum via the olivary nuclei. The olivary nuclei are located in the ventrolateral portion of the caudal medulla (see Figs. 2-14 and 2-15). They extend rostrally to just caudal to the facial nucleus and caudally to a level just caudal to the obex. The olivary nuclei consist of three components on each side, all of which vary in size throughout the length of the nuclei. Where they are most developed, they have the appearance of three fingers oriented obliquely from dorsomedial to ventrolateral just dorsal to the pyramid and medial lemniscus. The hypoglossal axons course along their lateral border. The axons of the neurons in the olivary nuclei cross the midline and join the contralateral caudal cerebellar peduncle. These axons are the major source of the climbing fibers that enter the cerebellum. The olivary neurons are activated by both the neurons of the UMN system and the spinal cord afferents. The pontine nucleus serves as a major relay nucleus for projection axons from all areas of the cerebral cortex to the cerebellum. This cerebropontocerebellar pathway serves for many functions in addition to the UMN system. The axons of the projection neurons in the cerebral cortex enter the corona radiata of the gyrus where the cortical neurons are located. They continue through the centrum semiovale into the internal capsule, crus cerebri, and longitudinal fibers of the pons. The axons in the cerebropontocerebellar pathway leave the longitudinal fibers of the pons to synapse on ipsilateral pontine neuronal cell bodies. The neuronal cell bodies of the pontine nucleus surround the longitudinal fibers of the pons as the latter courses caudally dorsal to the transverse fibers of the pons (see Figs. 2-9 and 2-10). The axons of the neuronal cell bodies of the pontine nucleus cross the midline where they form the transverse fibers of the pons. They continue into the cerebellum via the contralateral middle cerebellar peduncle. This peduncle projects axons primarily to the folia in the cerebellar hemisphere. A direct relationship exists between the evolution of skilled motor function and the degree of development of the cerebral motor cortex, the pons, and the cerebellar hemisphere. In animals such as the human, who have highly skilled motor activity of the digits, the transverse fibers of the pons are so numerous that they extend caudally and cover the trapezoid body, and the vermis of the cerebellum is partly buried beneath the expanded cerebellar hemispheres (see Figs. 13-23, 13-27, 13-31).

Cerebellar Efferents

Cerebellar Cortex

Purkinje neuronal axons derived mostly from the flocculonodular lobe project directly to the vestibular nuclei via the caudal cerebellar peduncle.

Cerebellar Nuclei

The neurons in the fastigial nucleus project to the vestibular nuclei and reticular formation by way of the rostral cerebellar peduncle. The neurons in the interposital nucleus project

to the red nucleus and the reticular formation by way of the rostral cerebellar peduncle. The neurons in the lateral cerebellar nucleus project to the red nucleus, the reticular formation, the pallidum, and the ventral lateral nucleus of the thalamus, all by way of the rostral cerebellar peduncle.

When the axons in the rostral cerebellar peduncle enter the caudal mesencephalon, most of these cerebellar efferents cross in the ventral tegmental decussation (see Fig. 2-8), occurring at the level of the caudal colliculi caudal to the rubrospinal decussation. These axons cross to terminate in the contralateral red nucleus, ventral lateral thalamic nucleus, or the pallidum. These collections of nuclei participate in a feedback circuit to the cerebral cortex. The most direct pathway is from the neurons in the ventral lateral thalamic nucleus, the axons of which enter the internal capsule via the thalamocortical fibers. They continue through the centrum semiovale into a corona radiata to terminate in an area of the cerebral cortex. A circuitry occurs between the cerebral cortex and the cerebellar cortex that provides immediate feedback from the cerebellum to the cerebrum at the moment when activity is generated in the cerebral cortex. The following example illustrates the structures that participate in this circuitry (Fig. 13-20): Motor cortex of the frontoparietal lobe, corona radiata, centrum semiovale, internal capsule, crus cerebri, longitudinal fibers of the pons, pontine nucleus, CROSS in the transverse fibers of the pons, middle cerebellar

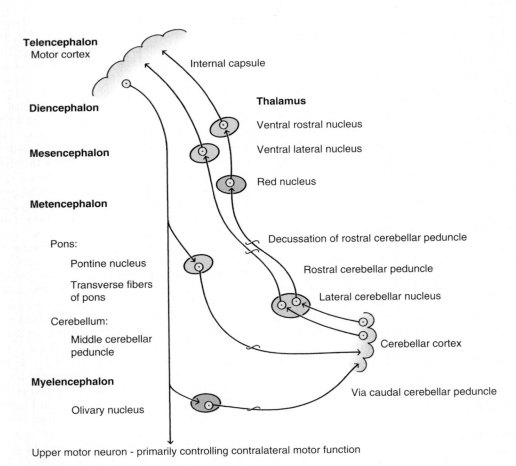

FIGURE 13-20 Role of the cerebellum in control of motor function: feedback circuit to cerebral cortex from the cerebellum.

peduncle, cerebellar medulla, folial white lamina, granular layer neurons, Purkinje neurons, folial white lamina, cerebellar medulla, lateral cerebellar nucleus, rostral cerebellar peduncle, CROSS in ventral tegmental decussation, ventral lateral nucleus of thalamus, thalamocortical fibers, internal capsule, centrum semiovale, corona radiata, and motor cortex of frontoparietal lobe. This model reflects the intimate relationship between the cerebellum and cerebrum and the important role the cerebellum plays in many functions of the cerebrum.

Very few efferent cerebellar axons project to the spinal cord to influence the lower motor neuron (LMN) activity. The cerebellum controls motor activity by its influence on the UMN neuronal cell bodies in the brainstem, the axons of which descend into the spinal cord to regulate LMN activity.

■ FUNCTION

More neurons are found in the cerebellum than in all the remaining areas of the brain combined, and the arrangement of these cells allows for circuitry that makes the action of the cerebellum extremely rapid. Thus the cerebellum has been likened to a computer, with this anatomy being the hardware used for information processing. We tend to limit our understanding of the function of the cerebellum to its role in motor activity because aberrations of this structure are what we see with cerebellar disorders. However, the cerebellum has connections to many regions of the brain, including those involved in sensory systems, cognition, language, and emotions.[95] Consider the immense circuitry between the cerebellum and the cerebrum. The information processing that occurs in the cerebellum allows the cerebellum to be involved in both motor dexterity and mental dexterity. We are just beginning to appreciate the diffuse role the cerebellum plays in various brain functions.

From the perspective of a veterinary clinician, the role of the cerebellum in the control of motor activity is the most significant function to be considered. The cerebellum functions as a regulator, not as the primary initiator, of motor activity. It functions to coordinate and smooth out movements induced by the UMN system, which includes the maintenance of equilibrium and the regulation of muscle tone to preserve the normal position of the body while at rest or during motion. The cerebellum plays a role in all phases of the gait from the initiation through protraction to the termination. In summary, the cerebellar nuclei continually facilitate brainstem neurons, but their activity is regulated by the inhibitory function of the Purkinje neurons in the cerebellar cortex. The degree of activity of these Purkinje neurons is dependent on the afferent information reaching them directly by way of climbing fiber afferents and indirectly via the mossy fiber afferents. A plethora of neurotransmitters is involved in the synapses between these neuronal populations.

In an attempt to correlate structure and function, the cerebellum has been divided topographically in different ways.[27,28] On a phylogenetic basis, the cerebellum can be divided into three regions. The archicerebellum includes primarily the flocculonodular lobe, which is concerned with vestibular system activity. The paleocerebellum includes primarily the vermis of the rostral lobe and adjacent hemisphere and is mostly concerned with spinal cord function

and postural tonus. The neocerebellum includes the vermis of the caudal lobe and most of the cerebellar hemispheres and is more concerned with regulation of skilled movements.

The cerebellum can also be divided into three longitudinal zones of cortex and related nuclei. The medial zone includes the vermis and fastigial nuclei and is concerned with regulating tone for posture and locomotion and equilibrium of the entire body. The intermediate zone includes the paravermal cortex and interposital nuclei and is more concerned with adjusting motor tone and posture to regulate skilled movements. The lateral zone includes the lateral portion of each hemisphere and the lateral nuclei. This zone primarily functions in regulating skilled movements of the limbs. This portion is more highly developed in primates in which skilled limb and hand movements are more common. A similar remarkable development of the cerebellar hemispheres is seen in a few species of exotic animals. Figs. 13-21 through 13-31 show some of the variations in gross morphology of the cerebellum that we have observed in animals.

The rostral portion of the cerebellum is also concerned with the inhibition of LMNs to the antigravity extensor

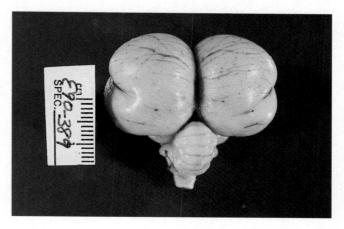

FIGURE 13-21 Figs. 13-21 through 13-31 show some of the variations in the gross morphology of the cerebellum in a few species of animals. Fig. 13-21 is the brain of a great horned owl, which is representative of most avian species where the cerebellum consists only of a vermis. Note the normal absence of any cerebral gyri.

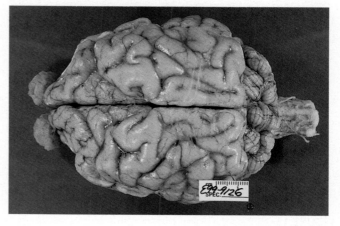

FIGURE 13-22 This is a dorsal view of the brain of an American brown bear. Note the marked width of the cerebellar hemispheres.

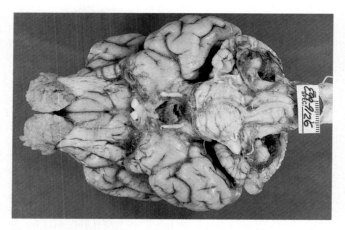

FIGURE 13-23 Ventral view of the brain of the American brown bear. Note the lateral extent of the cerebellar hemispheres and the associated large area composed of the transverse fibers of the pons that cover the trapezoid body.

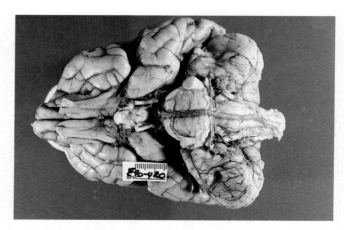

FIGURE 13-26 Ventral view of the brain of a sea lion. Note the large cerebellar hemispheres overlapping the sides of the caudal brainstem.

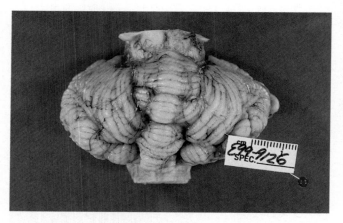

FIGURE 13-24 Dorsal view of the entire cerebellum dissected from the brainstem of the American brown bear.

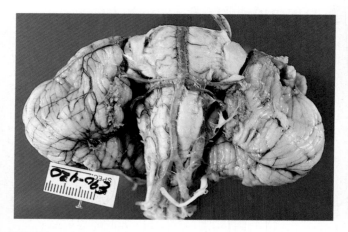

FIGURE 13-27 Ventral view of the caudal brainstem of the sea lion brain. Note the large area occupied by the transverse fibers of the pons and their overlap of the trapezoid body.

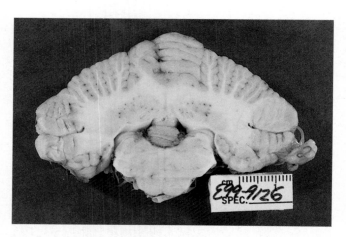

FIGURE 13-25 Transverse section of the American brown bear cerebellum to show the extent of the hemispheres. Note the prominent cerebellar nuclei in the cerebellar medulla.

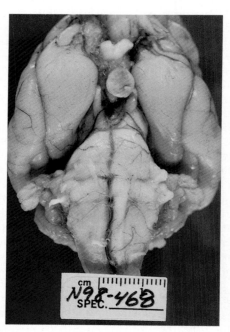

FIGURE 13-28 Ventral view of a normal dog brain for comparison. Compare the lateral extent of the cerebellar hemispheres, the size of the area occupied by the transverse fibers of the pons, and the prominent trapezoid body with the similar anatomy seen in the brains of the American brown bear and the sea lion.

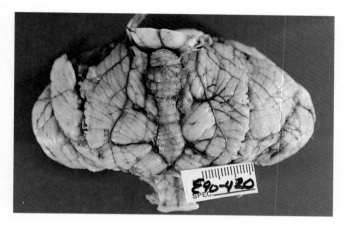

FIGURE 13-29 Dorsal view of the cerebellum of the sea lion brain dissected from the brainstem. Note the large cerebellar hemispheres overlapping on the borders of the vermis.

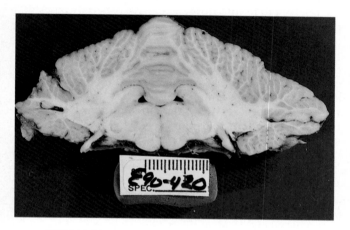

FIGURE 13-30 Transverse section of the sea lion cerebellum.

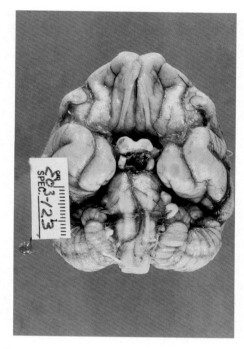

FIGURE 13-31 Ventral view of the brain of a gibbon as representative of a primate species. Note the large cerebellar hemispheres and the associated large area occupied by the transverse fibers of the pons overlapping the trapezoid body.

muscles of the neck and thoracic limbs. It thus participates with the UMN in the support of the body against gravity.

CLINICAL SIGNS OF CEREBELLAR DISEASE

Cerebellar disease does not cause the loss of any single function but rather a general inadequacy of motor response. Cerebellar disorders are often diffuse in the cerebellum and the patient typically exhibits a symmetric cerebellar ataxia. Remember that *ataxia* means "incoordination," and we see three qualities of ataxia: (1) general proprioceptive ataxia (sometimes termed sensory ataxia), (2) vestibular ataxia, and (3) cerebellar ataxia (sometimes called motor ataxia).

Cerebellar disease does not cause paresis. No loss of strength occurs, but in severe disease, the patient may be incapacitated enough by its cerebellar ataxia that it is unable to coordinate its movements to stand. However, strong voluntary movements can be elicited in the recumbent patient. Spasticity and ataxia are most commonly observed in the gait. With severe dysfunction, the patient may be disoriented and fall to either side, forward, or backward. The ataxic gait is characterized by an inability to regulate the rate, range, or force of a movement, which is called *dysmetria*. The manifestation of dysmetria is usually

hypermetria, an overmeasurement in the gait response observed as greater movements of the limbs in all ranges of motion. Flexor actions appear to be especially uninhibited during the gait, which is responsible for the hypermetria. In observing the gait or postural reactions, the threshold for the response appears to be raised. In other words, the onset of the voluntary movement—protraction—is delayed, and the response, once initiated, is exaggerated, creating a "bursty" effect to the movement. After the delay, the limb is raised too high in protraction by excessive joint flexion and is then forcefully returned to the ground surface with excessive joint extension. Inadequate Purkinje neuronal inhibition of the cerebellar nuclei results in this delay in the onset of protraction and the hypermetria that is observed. Be aware of the difference between this cerebellar hypermetria and the form of hypermetria that is seen with C1-C5 lesions that cause dysfunction of the UMN and GP systems that we call *overreaching* or *floating*. The limb has its joints extended during the overreaching protraction with C1-C5 lesions. When the cerebellar ataxia is mild or difficult to recognize in a short-limbed breed such as the Scottish terrier, examining the gait as the patient ascends or descends stairs is helpful. This action will markedly exacerbate the clinical signs of cerebellar dysfunction and frequently cause patients to fall, which often makes them reluctant to go up or down stairs. We refer to this test as the stair test.

The resting posture of the patient may show a broad-based stance with the thoracic limbs and a truncal ataxia, which is a swaying of the body from side to side, forward and backward, or occasionally dorsoventrally. These truncal swaying motions are sometimes called a *titubation*. These motions may appear as gross jerky movements of the entire body. A fine head and neck tremor is characteristic of a cerebellar disorder and is usually augmented by the initiation of voluntary movements, such as when the head is reaching for food or a toy. This tremor is described as an intention tremor, or a form of dysmetria involving the head and neck. Lesions limited to the cerebellum will not cause a diffuse, whole-body tremor, as described in Chapter 8. In severe cerebellar disorders, the patient may lie in lateral recumbency, unable to right itself to stand and with its head and neck extended in a position of opisthotonus.

Muscle tone is usually increased in domestic animals with cerebellar disease. Spinal reflexes are normal or hyperactive. Postural reactions, especially the hopping responses, are delayed and are followed by an exaggerated response. Spasticity may be evident during these responses. Paw or hoof replacement may be normal. With diffuse cerebellar cortical disorders, abnormal positional nystagmus is only occasionally observed. No consistency exists to the direction of the nystagmus, which may also change with different head positions. If the head and neck are extended and then the support is suddenly withdrawn, the head may rapidly descend ventrally beyond the normal neutral position. This action is termed a *head rebound phenomenon* and is a clinical sign of cerebellar dysfunction.

Involvement of the flocculonodular lobe or fastigial nucleus of the cerebellum causes clinical signs of a vestibular system disorder with loss of equilibrium, abnormal nystagmus, bizarre postures, and a broad-based staggering gait with jerky movements and a tendency to fall to either side or backwards. The last of these signs is especially evident if the head and neck are briefly extended and released.

The rostral lobe of the cerebellum is especially inhibitory to the stretch reflex mechanism of antigravity muscles (extensor muscle tone).[116] Lesions in this area may result in opisthotonus with rigidly extended thoracic limbs. In some instances, the pelvic limbs may be flexed forward, ventral to the trunk, by hypertonia of the hypaxial muscles that flex the hips. The combination of extended neck and thoracic limbs with flexed hips is called a *decerebellate posture*. If the rostral lobe lesion involves the ventral lobules, the pelvic limbs may be extended away from the trunk, similar to the thoracic limbs as in a decerebrate posture.

With unilateral lesions, the clinical signs of cerebellar ataxia are ipsilateral with spasticity, hypermetria, and abnormal postural reactions. The disturbance to the vestibular system components of the cerebellum may cause a balance loss and head tilt toward or away from the side of the lesion. Remember what we described in Chapter 12 as the paradoxical central vestibular syndrome that occurs with unilateral cerebellar medullary lesions involving the caudal cerebellar peduncle or flocculonodular lobe of the cerebellum. With these lesions, the clinical signs of vestibular system dysfunction, such as the head tilt, will be contralateral to the lesion. The abnormal nystagmus is usually positional and has no consistency to its direction, which can change with different positions of the head.

Occasionally with unilateral lesions of the fastigial or interposital nuclei, an anisocoria with a dilated pupil may be observed that is slowly responsive to light. The third eyelid may protrude, and the palpebral fissure may be enlarged. The pupillary changes usually occur in the eye that is ipsilateral to an interposital nuclear lesion and contralateral to a fastigial nuclear lesion.[71]

Animals with significant cerebellar disease often fail to respond to the menace test used to evaluate the visual system. In the presence of normal vision and facial muscle function, these animals with cerebellar disease fail to close their eyelids when threatened by a menacing gesture. Varying degrees of this deficit have been observed in all species of domestic animals with diffuse cerebellar lesions, especially deficits that involve the interposital and lateral cerebellar nuclei. The fact that the entire central visual pathway from the retina to the visual cortex, as well as the facial neurons, must be intact for the normal menace response to take place is known. However, the unknown factor is whether the pathway between the visual cortex and the facial nucleus is direct via projection axons from the visual cortex through the internal capsule, crus cerebri, longitudinal fibers of the pons, and corticonuclear fibers to the facial nucleus. Alternatively, the visual cortex may project rostrally to the motor cortex, and the latter projects to the facial nucleus, as just described. Also unknown is whether the rostral colliculus plays any role in this pathway. Where does the cerebellum fit into this scheme? We believe two possibilities exist. Either (1) the pathway responsible for the menace response goes through the cerebellum, or (2) input occurs from the cerebellum to the pathway. In the former instance, the cerebrocortical projection pathway must pass through the cerebellum via the cerebropontocerebellar route, with the cerebellum projecting to the facial nuclei. In the latter instance, the loss of cerebellar activity that normally projects to the cerebral cortex interferes with this menace response at the level of the cerebral cortex, and therefore a pathway through the cerebellum is unnecessary. We have seen unilateral cerebellar lesions in the dog and horse that resulted in a lack of this menace response on the same side as the lesion. If you study Fig. 14-14, you can see why this ipsilateral relationship would be expected. Note that crossing of axons occurs at both the optic chiasm and again at the pons.

CEREBELLAR DISEASES

Malformation—Abiotrophy

The majority of the primary cerebellar diseases that we diagnose in domestic animals are either (1) congenital as a result of an in utero viral infection or, less commonly, a developmental disorder, or (2) they are slowly progressive in young animals, resulting from an inherited cerebellar cortical abiotrophy. Once the anatomic diagnosis is made in these patients, the differential diagnosis is determined by the species and breed of the patient. Rather than present these cerebellar diseases as case examples similar to other chapters, we will describe and illustrate these malformations and abiotrophies primarily by species.

Dogs

Clinical signs of a diffuse cerebellar disorder that is first observed when the puppy tries to stand and walk and is not progressive is most likely the result of a developmental abnormality. These abnormalities are uncommon and have no proven cause in the dog.* No recognized common

---

*References 52, 86, 94, 104, 109, 119.

in utero viral infection in dogs exists that affects primarily the developing cerebellum. If a puppy survives the systemic effects of an infection with the canine herpesvirus in the first week of life, it may be left with a cerebellar ataxia from the effect of the virus on the developing cerebellum.[110] This event is rare. One report has been published of a possible exposure to the canine parvovirus associated with a cerebellar malformation.[118] Cerebellar cortical abiotrophy is common in dogs and affects many breeds, which causes a progressive clinical disorder that usually starts at a few weeks of age. In a few breeds, the onset is at approximately 1 year of age or later. These disorders are inherited disorders that usually involve an autosomal recessive gene.

Malformation. See **Video 13-1**. This video shows Hope, a 3.5-month-old male Labrador retriever. He was presumed to be normal until 2 weeks old when, unlike his littermates, he was unable to stand and would flop from one side to the other. When examined at 1 month of age, he was alert and responsive and would struggle to stand to walk but would constantly lose his balance and fall in all directions. By 3 months of age, he was able to stand and walk a short way but with great difficulty before he fell. The owner made an interesting observation that Hope could swim in the nearby lake much better than he could walk. The referring veterinarian noticed an occasional head and neck tremor. Study the video. These clinical signs are typical of a severe cerebellar disorder with significant involvement of the vestibular components of the cerebellum. The age of onset and the mild improvement over the first few weeks correlate well with an in utero developmental defect in the cerebellum. Little improvement occurred by 4 months of age, and Hope was euthanized. At necropsy the only gross and microscopic lesions involved the cerebellum, most of which was absent (Figs. 13-32 through 13-34). No vermis was noted, and only small asymmetric remnants of the most lateral portions of the hemispheres was observed. Only a thin membrane connected the two hemispheric remnants, and this had small clusters of cerebellar parenchyma in it. Although no perinatal viral disease has been proven in dogs to cause an inflammation of the developing cerebellum resulting in cerebellar hypoplasia and atrophy, this lesion in Hope has

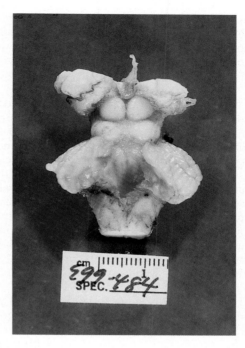

FIGURE 13-33 Dorsal view of the cerebellum and brainstem of the brain seen in Fig. 13-32 with the cerebral hemispheres removed.

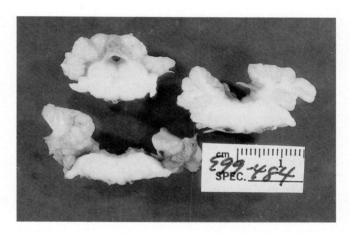

FIGURE 13-34 Transverse sections of the cerebellum, pons, and medulla of the brain seen in Figs. 13-32 and 13-33. Note the severity and asymmetry of the lesion.

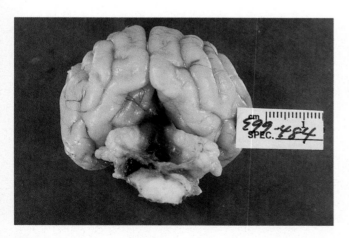

FIGURE 13-32 Dorsal view of the brain of the 3.5-month-old Labrador retriever seen in Video 13-1. Note the absence of primarily the vermal and paravermal portions of the cerebellum.

features similar to that which we see in calves infected in utero with the bovine virus diarrhea virus. Typically in these calves, no evidence was noted after birth of the inflammation that occurred between 100 and 200 days of gestation. A severe in utero compromise of the blood supply from the cerebellar arteries might cause this lesion, but this possibility has not been reported in any domestic animal and would be difficult to prove.

See **Video 13-2**. This video shows a 4-month-old female miniature schnauzer that was unable to stand when her littermates began to walk. By 2 months of age, she could stand and walk a few feet but then would fall to either side. This sign is evident on the video. Not shown are occasional episodes of opisthotonus and extensor rigidity of the limbs. She also occasionally exhibited a mild neck and head tremor. The presence of these clinical signs of cerebellar dysfunction at the time this puppy should be able to stand and walk and the lack of progression of the clinical signs strongly suggests an in utero developmental abnormality. A computed tomographic (CT) scan showed an area of hypodensity on the midline ventral to the tentorium cerebelli centered where the vermis should be located. This dog was euthanized, and necropsy revealed the absence of the entire cerebellar vermis caudal to the primary fissure. This area included the medullary portion with the fastigial nucleus. Microscopic study showed no inflammation. The symmetry of this malformation suggests a primary genetic developmental abnormality rather than a destructive process that a viral agent would produce. In children, partial or complete absence of the cerebellar vermis is called Dandy-Walker syndrome. This syndrome is sometimes accompanied by agenesis of the corpus callosum and other cerebral malformations. No cause has been determined. Dandy-Walker syndrome has been reported in dogs.[94,119]

See **Video 13-3**. This video shows Buddy, a 4-year-old male Samoyed that has exhibited the gait abnormality that you see on this video since he first tried to walk as a puppy. The owners had difficulty training him, but they were devoted to providing him with the best quality of life possible. At 4 years of age, he began to have generalized seizures. Magnetic resonance (MR) imaging was performed as part of his diagnostic study for the seizure disorder. This effort revealed bilateral symmetric lissencephaly and a very small cerebellum. We have observed this same combination of brain malformations in a litter of wire fox terriers and a litter of Irish setters. A similar syndrome occurs in children, which is inherited as an autosomal recessive gene defect. The abnormal gene thought to be involved in neuronal migration is called the *RELN gene*.[50,72,85] This gene codes for the protein reelin, which is involved with neuronal migration during development. Dogs with lissencephaly are typically difficult to train and often develop generalized seizures after one year of age. Buddy's seizures were partially controlled with anticonvulsants.

See **Video 13-4**. The two wire fox terriers in this video were from a litter of three puppies. In the first portion of the video, they are approximately 4 to 5 weeks of age and had never been able to stand to walk. One puppy was euthanized, and necropsy showed a severe cerebellar malformation and bilateral lissencephaly (Fig. 13-35). The cerebellar malformation is responsible for their inability to right themselves to stand and walk. The second portion of the video shows the remaining puppy at approximately 7 weeks of age, and the same dog appears in the last portion of the video at approximately 1 year of age. Three years later the clinical signs of cerebellar dysfunction still had not changed. However, this dog developed generalized seizures at 4 years of age, which presumably reflects the dysplasia associated with the lissencephalic malformation. The cerebellar malformation consisted of a symmetric reduction in its overall size to approximately one third of normal with small blunt folia. These rudimentary folia had no normal cortical organization. Purkinje neurons were haphazardly scattered through clusters of granule neurons. We have observed a similar combination of lissencephaly and cerebellar hypoplasia and dysplasia in a litter of Irish setters (Figs. 13-36 through 13-39).

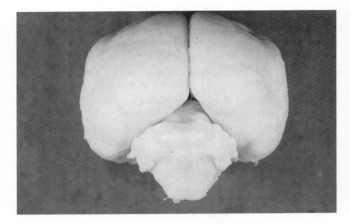

FIGURE 13-35 Dorsal view of the brain of one of the 5-week-old wire fox terrier puppies seen in Video 13-4. The brain was preserved by perfusion. Note the bilateral lissencephaly. Based on the microscopic examination, this cerebellum is hypoplastic and dysplastic. No normal arrangement of the layers of the cerebellar cortex was observed.

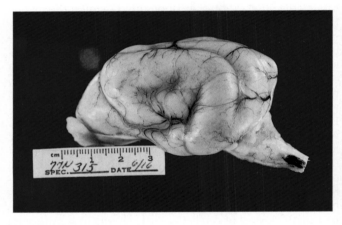

FIGURE 13-36 Lateral view of the brain of a 4-month-old Irish setter that exhibited a nonprogressive cerebellar ataxia since it was able to walk. Note the partial lissencephaly and the small cerebellum that, based on the microscopic examination, is caused by hypoplasia and dysplasia.

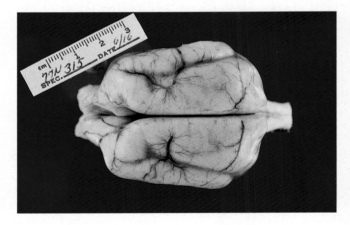

FIGURE 13-37 Dorsal view of the brain of the dog in Fig. 13-36. Note the extent of the lissencephaly and the lack of any visible cerebellum.

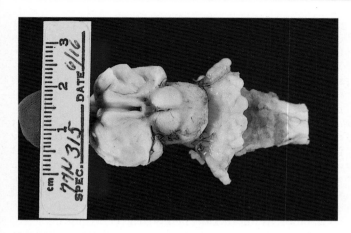

FIGURE 13-38 Brainstem and hypoplastic cerebellum from the dog in Figs. 13-36 and 13-37 after removal of the cerebral hemispheres. Note the symmetry of the cerebellar malformation, which would not be expected if an in utero viral infection was the cause.

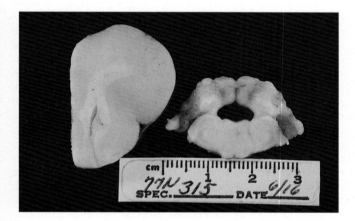

FIGURE 13-39 Transverse sections of one cerebral hemisphere and the medulla from the dog in the previous three figures. Note the thick cerebral cortex, which is called pachygyria, and the severe cerebellar hypoplasia.

Abiotrophy. Cerebellar cortical abiotrophy is usually a postnatal syndrome that occurs in many breeds of dogs.* The affected animal is normal at birth and develops a slowly progressive cerebellar ataxia at a variable time after birth. Most often, this development starts at a few weeks of age after a brief period of normal activity. In a few breeds, the onset of recognizable clinical signs may not occur for a year or more. The rate of progression varies between the breeds that are affected with this disorder. In some breeds, progression is fairly rapid and results in the inability to coordinate to stand. In others, the gait disorder is very mild and does not incapacitate the animal. As a rule, the primary lesion is an intrinsic degeneration of the Purkinje neurons. The term *abiotrophy* describes this form of degeneration. It refers to a cell that dies prematurely as a result of some intrinsic genetically determined abnormality within the cell's metabolic

*References 14, 31-33, 42-47, 67, 69, 70, 87, 92, 102, 103, 125, 129, 130, 132, 134.

system. By definition, abiotrophy (a-bio-trophy) means a lack of (a-) a vital biological substance (bio) necessary for maintenance of that cell (-trophy).[65] Neurons should last for the normal life span of the animal. Any degeneration before this is premature, and if it is caused by some intrinsic defect in that neuron, the degeneration is abiotrophic. The degree of degeneration seen at necropsy depends on how long the degeneration has been progressing. In acute cases, you may see an ischemic type of degeneration in the Purkinje neurons. In chronic cases, no Purkinje neurons may be present, and in their place may be an accumulation of astrocytes that are sometimes called *Bergman astrocytes*. In most animals, the granular layer neurons will also be depleted. This status is thought to be a retrograde form of degeneration because these neurons no longer have any dendritic zones for their synapses once the Purkinje neurons have degenerated. In these chronic cases, astrogliosis will also be present in the cerebellar nuclei that is secondary to the loss of the telodendria of the Purkinje neurons that terminate here. Most breeds have no lesions elsewhere in the brain. The Kerry blue terrier and Chinese crested breeds are exceptions to this rule because they also have degenerative lesions in extrapyramidal nuclei.[42,46,102,103] A cerebellar cortical abiotrophy was first described in Kerry blue terriers in 1976. Since then, a plethora of descriptions have been published of cerebellar cortical abiotrophy in a large number of canine breeds. Where enough data are available, an autosomal recessive form of inheritance has usually been established as the most common cause. Once the anatomic diagnosis of a cerebellar disorder is made, the differential diagnosis for a progressive disorder is abiotrophy, inflammation, cystic malformation, and neoplasia. These patients usually have an onset of clinical signs at an age that is uncommon for neoplasia. Cerebellar medulloblastoma (primitive neurectodermal tumor) is a rare neoplasm seen in young dogs and cattle.[125] Epidermoid or dermoid cysts are uncommon, but the most common site for these cysts to occur is in the caudal cranial fossa, where the cerebellum can be affected by their progressive enlargement as a result of their secretory activity.[96] Inflammation is common at this young age when many of the abiotrophies occur, but its limitation to the cerebellum is unexpected. However, an exception to this rule exists. Neosporosis in young adult dogs has a predilection for the cerebellum.[77] The reason for this predilection is not known, but the slowly progressive clinical signs of a cerebellar disorder that occurs is very similar to those caused by abiotrophy. See Case Example 13-1 that follows in the section on other cerebellar diseases. MR imaging is necessary to help rule out these other diagnoses. The MR images will be normal in the early stages of abiotrophy. In the late stages of chronic abiotrophy, atrophy of the folia is present. The T2-weighted median plane sagittal image is the best image to show an increase in the size of the sulcal spaces between the atrophied folia (Fig. 13-40). Molecular studies are in progress to identify the genomic basis for these inherited abiotrophies, which is necessary for identifying the carrier animals and eliminating them from the breeding programs.

Kerry Blue Terrier. The following discussion is a description of the study to identify a progressive neurologic disorder in the Kerry blue terrier breed that proved to be the result of an inherited cerebellar cortical and extrapyramidal nuclear abiotrophy.[46] It is a dedication to the late Mrs. Zipporah Fleisher of New City, New York, where the

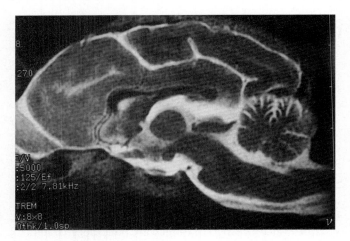

FIGURE 13-40 Median plane T2-weighted MR image of a 15-month-old Kerry blue terrier with cerebellar cortical abiotrophy. Note the atrophy of the folia in the dorsal lobules of the cerebellar vermis.

disease appeared in her kennel in 1967. This study would not have been accomplished without her persistence and dedication to doing what was best for the breed.

The appearance of the first two Kerry blue terriers in Mrs. Fleisher's kennel to exhibit neurologic signs of a cerebellar disorder was in 1967. Gross and microscopic examination of the frozen and thawed brain of one of these dogs showed no inflammation. Because of the suspicion that the neurologic disorder might be inherited, Mrs. Fleisher repeated the mating that produced the first two affected dogs and made three more selective matings of related dogs. By 1970, she had produced 10 affected puppies out of a total of 23 puppies from five litters. Both sexes were affected. All affected dogs had identical neurologic signs and neuronal abiotrophy in selected populations of neurons in the brain. The abiotrophy always affected the Purkinje neurons, and the degeneration in the other populations of neurons varied by the length of time the disorder had progressed before euthanasia. This data strongly supported that this disorder was inherited via an autosomal recessive gene. In 1973, Dr. Terry Holliday diagnosed this clinical disorder in Kerry blue terriers at the University of California-Davis. Pedigree studies of three affected California litters showed common ancestry with the dogs affected in New City, New York. After discovery of these findings in New York and California, affected Kerry blue terriers were diagnosed with this disorder in Texas, Illinois, Canada, and England. In reviewing the canine neurological literature, a 1946 issue of the *Journal of the American Veterinary Medical Association* described a Kerry blue terrier in 1941 with identical clinical signs and pathologic lesions.[101] Identifying a connection between the pedigree of this dog and those studied after 1967 was not possible.

By 1976, all of the affected dogs that were studied had been normal at birth and developed a normal gait at a few weeks of age. They were usually 9 to 10 weeks old when the clinical abnormality began, but a few did not show clinical signs until 16 weeks of age. The earliest clinical signs were a mild intentional head tremor and a slight stiffness in the thoracic limb gait. The gait disorder progressed to an obvious cerebellar ataxia that was initially more obvious in the thoracic limbs. After 3 or 4 months of progression, the ataxia was usually severe, with remarkable bursts of voluntary movement that correlated well with the description of a

sudden onset and overresponse. These dogs never lost their enthusiasm to run and play. This feature will be obvious from the videos that are cited at the end of this description. Most of these affected dogs, after a few months of progressive clinical signs, became unable to stand and would throw themselves around their area of confinement, which justified euthanasia because of their poor quality of life.

Gross loss of cerebellar size was evident only in dogs that had been affected for many weeks. In these chronic cases, the folia appeared narrowed and angular, and the total weight of the cerebellum varied from 6% to 9% of the total brain weight, with 10% to 12% being normal. The earliest microscopic change was the appearance of an ischemic form of degeneration in the Purkinje neurons followed by their disappearance. As the Purkinje neuronal layer became depleted, some loss of the granular layer neurons was observed. Gliosis occurred where the Purkinje neurons were absent, as well as in the cerebellar nuclei. As the disorder progressed, degeneration became evident in the olivary nuclei. This phase was followed by an acute degeneration of the caudate nuclei, and, subsequent to this event, a degeneration of the neurons in substantia nigra occurred bilaterally. No direct anatomic connection exists between all of these populations of degenerating neurons. The granule neuron loss and the degeneration of the olivary nuclei can be explained as a retrograde degeneration, given that the neurons in both of these locations synapse on the Purkinje neurons. The degeneration of neurons in substantia nigra may also be retrograde because many of these neurons synapse on neurons in the caudate nuclei.[13] No direct connections exist between the Purkinje neurons and the neurons in the caudate nuclei. What do the Purkinje neurons and neurons in the caudate nuclei have in common that might explain this unique distribution of lesions? The answer is that they both have receptors for glutamic acid, which is the neurotransmitter released by the granule neurons at Purkinje neurons and by the substantia nigra neurons at the caudate nuclear neurons. Excessive accumulation of glutamate in the vicinity of neuronal cell bodies is toxic and causes an ischemic form of degeneration. The primary abnormality here might be an excessive release or depleted uptake of glutamate. This condition may be a receptor abnormality or may even involve the local astrocytes that participate in the uptake of glutamate. The present assumption is that this condition is an inherited genetic abnormality that involves the molecular nature of the glutamate receptor on these neurons or the mechanism of release or uptake of this neurotransmitter. The same clinical and pathologic disorder occurs in Chinese crested dogs.[103] Molecular studies are now (2007) in progress to identify the responsible gene in these two breeds. The results of this effort will provide a convenient rapid method of identifying carrier dogs that will greatly enhance the ability to make the breed free of this clinical disorder. Figs. 13-41 through 13-52 illustrate these lesions in Kerry blue terriers.

In 1975 the United States Kerry Blue Terrier Club officially recognized this disease as an inherited defect and published a monograph entitled, *Progressive Neuronal Abiotrophy (PNA): A Genetically Inherited Disease in Kerry Blue Terriers*. This resource included the pedigrees of all the affected dogs that had been recognized at that time. Without complete cooperation of the breeders, it is easy for this disease to seem to disappear. Misdiagnosis, cover-up, and lack of a reliable central information gathering can all contribute to an

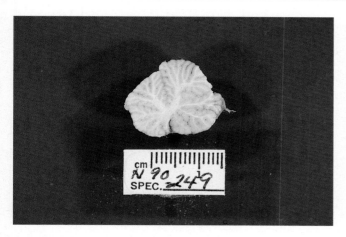

FIGURE 13-41 Median plane longitudinal section of the cerebellar vermis from a Kerry blue terrier with cerebellar cortical abiotrophy affecting primarily the dorsal lobules of the cerebellar vermis. Note the close correlation with the MR image in Fig. 13-40.

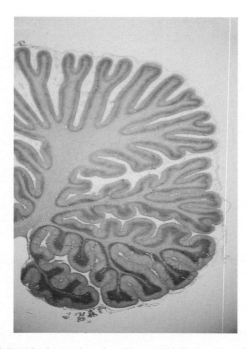

FIGURE 13-42 Microscopic section of the caudal half of a section of cerebellum similar to that seen in Fig. 13-41. Note the sparing of the more ventral lobules. The reason for this consistent lesion topography is unknown.

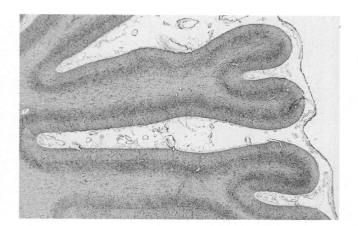

FIGURE 13-43 Higher magnification of the atrophied dorsal lobules seen in Fig. 13-42.

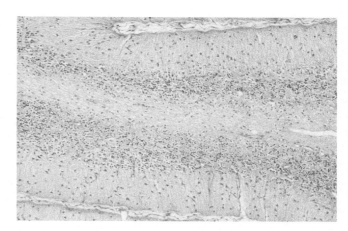

FIGURE 13-44 Higher magnification of the atrophied dorsal lobules seen in Figs. 13-42 and 13-43.

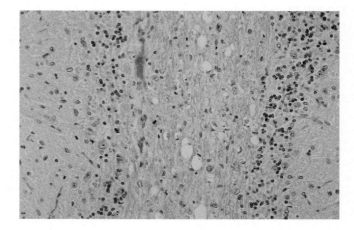

FIGURE 13-45 Higher magnification of a section of a folium similar to that seen in Fig. 13-44. Note the marked absence of both the Purkinje neurons and the granule neurons in the cortex on both sides of the folial white lamina in the center.

apparent decrease in disease incidence. Undoubtedly, this disease occurred between 1941 and 1967 but was simply not properly recognized. Since 1976, scattered diagnoses of this disorder have been made in Kerry blue terriers with a wider range of ages of onset, as well as the degree of progression of the clinical signs. A litter was studied at Iowa State University, where the affected puppies showed their clinical signs at 4 to 5 weeks of age. Dogs studied at Texas A&M University had their onset at 4.5 to 5.5 months of age, and two dogs in Iowa were 8 to 9 months old before any clinical abnormality was recognized. This variation may reflect differences in the mutation of the involved gene. Breeders must not become complacent and believe that this disorder has disappeared. Until molecular studies provide us with the gene that can be used for an accurate antemortem diagnosis, any dog suspected of this disorder must have a necropsy study performed when it is euthanized to confirm the diagnosis. No pedigree should be incriminated for this disorder without a confirmed diagnosis at necropsy.[42,46]

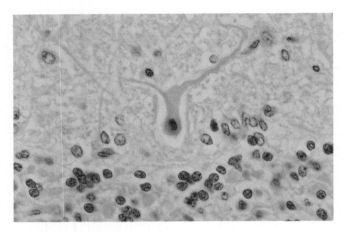

FIGURE 13-46 Higher magnification of the Purkinje neuronal layer of a young affected Kerry blue terrier, showing an ischemic-type degeneration of a Purkinje neuron.

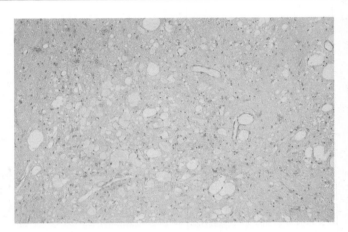

FIGURE 13-49 Microscopic section of the substantia nigra in the mesencephalon from a Kerry blue terrier with cerebellar cortical abiotrophy, showing vacuolar degeneration.

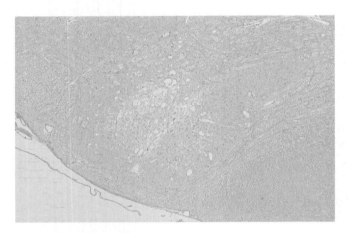

FIGURE 13-47 Microscopic section of the ventrolateral aspect of the caudal medulla of a Kerry blue terrier with cerebellar cortical abiotrophy. Note the vacuolar degeneration of the olivary nucleus.

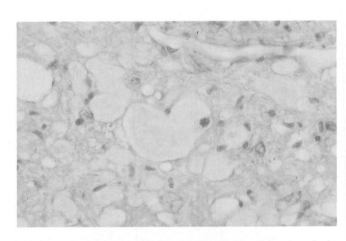

FIGURE 13-50 Higher magnification of the degeneration of the substantia nigra neurons seen in Fig. 13-49.

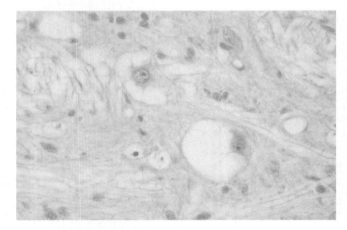

FIGURE 13-48 Higher magnification of the degenerating olivary nucleus seen in Fig. 13-47.

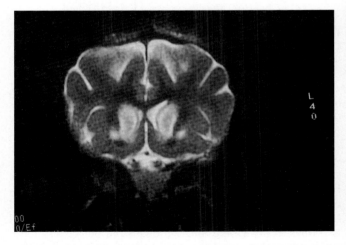

FIGURE 13-51 Axial T2-weighted MR image of a 15-month-old Kerry blue terrier with cerebellar cortical abiotrophy at the level of the cerebral hemispheres just rostral to the diencephalon (see Fig. 2-2). Note the bilateral hyperintensity of the caudate nuclei caused by their necrosis and edema.

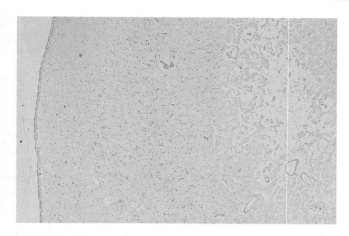

FIGURE 13-52 Microscopic section of a degenerating caudate nucleus in a Kerry blue terrier with cerebellar cortical abiotrophy. The lateral ventricle is on the left.

Currently this Kerry blue terrier and Chinese crested dog inherited disorder is called *canine multiple system degeneration* and has been compared with the human disorder, autosomal recessive juvenile Parkinsonism, which has similar clinical and pathological features. Genetic mapping of the gene locus has been described for these two canine breeds.[103]

See the following videos that show examples of this neuronal abiotrophy in Kerry blue terriers.

Video 13-5. These Kerry blue terriers are from Mrs. Fleisher's kennel in New City, New York. They are the product of the breeding that she carried out to determine the genetic basis for this disorder. The initial portion with my (Alexander de Lahunta) daughter shows three dogs that are approximately 4 months old. The middle portion with the veterinary student shows one of these dogs at approximately 5 months old. The last portion features two dogs (with the group of children) at approximately 6 months old and shows how extensive the progression has been. Note the obvious enthusiasm of the dogs. Certainly, no disruption of their sensorium is seen.

Video 13-6 shows Hobbs, a 6.5-month-old male Kerry blue terrier with progressive clinical signs of a cerebellar disorder for approximately 1 month.

Video 13-7 shows affected Kerry blue terriers that are all from a litter studied at Iowa State University by Dr. Danny Brass. Clinical signs were first observed at 4 to 5 weeks of age and were rapidly progressive. The first portion of the video shows the four affected puppies at 6 week of age. In the middle portion, the three dogs are now 11 weeks of age, and the last portion shows two dogs at 8 months of age. The progression of clinical signs is obvious. The severity of the clinical signs seen here at 8 months of age may reflect the additional loss of function of the extrapyramidal nuclei, which would be degenerate by this age.

Video 13-8 shows Major, a 15-month-old male Kerry blue terrier that was normal until 8 months old when a slight stiffness and ataxia were first observed. MR images of this dog were made at the University of Pennsylvania. These images showed bilateral symmetric degenerative lesions in the caudate nuclei. It is not known when changes can be detected on MR images relative to the onset of clinical signs. The dogs in Videos 13-7 and 13-8 show the extremes in the clinical presentation of this inherited disorder.

Cerebellar cortical Purkinje neuronal abiotrophy has been observed in many breeds of dogs in which the cerebellar lesions are the only brain lesions present. In most of these breeds, an autosomal recessive gene has been proven or presumed to be the form of inheritance. In many of these breeds, molecular studies are in progress to identify the specific genomic basis for the disorder. The following few examples highlight this abiotrophy that we have studied.

Labrador Retriever. **Video 13-9** shows Nutmeg, a 3-month-old female Labrador retriever that was normal when she first began to walk. Her ataxia was first observed at 2 months of age and has progressed to what you see on this video.

In contrast to an onset of clinical signs at a few weeks of age with rapid progression of the clinical signs, a few breeds can be identified in which the onset is delayed to 1 year or more and is very slowly progressive. In the early stages, making the anatomic diagnosis is difficult. The mild cerebellar ataxia can be confused with a spinal cord lesion between the C1 and C5 segments. The breeds in which a late-onset cerebellar cortical abiotrophy has been recognized include the Gordon setter,[33,47,129] Old English sheepdog,[130] Scottish terrier,[134] American Staffordshire terrier (18 months to 9 years),[125] and Brittany spaniel.[69]

Gordon Setter. **Video 13-10**. This video shows a 4.5-year-old male Gordon setter that was referred to Cornell University in 1977 for decompressive surgery for a suspected cervical vertebral malformation-malarticulation disorder. This dog had a history of a slowly progressive gait disorder since he was approximately 2 years old. The young man in the green outfit leading this dog is Dr. John May (Cornell University, 1980) when he was a student. Note the thoracic limb hypermetria with the excessive flexion of the joints, which is a clinical sign of a cerebellar disorder in contrast to the overextension of the joints with cervical spinal cord disease that affects the UMN and general proprioception (GP) systems. Also note the balance loss when the head and neck are extended and released. Balance loss was also observed during the testing of the hopping responses. Not shown was an abnormal positional nystagmus. Our anatomic diagnosis was cerebellum, pons, and medulla. Cerebellar cortical abiotrophy was suspected. The dog was discharged and a few months later was euthanized. Necropsy showed diffuse Purkinje neuronal abiotrophy.

Video 13-11 shows Ruby, a 7-year-old female Gordon setter that developed a slight ataxic gait when she was approximately 9 months old. This gait disorder slowly progressed to the remarkable dysfunction that you see in this video. At the end of the video, note her marked intentional head tremor when she is fed. Not shown was the abnormal positional rotatory to vertical nystagmus.

Dr. Jerrold Bell studied the possible inheritance of this disorder while he was a veterinary student at Cornell University. He was able to trace affected dogs across the United States to the West Coast. When Dr. Bell graduated in 1982, he had identified 52 affected dogs based on necropsies and study of videos. Analysis of the pedigrees established that this cerebellar cortical abiotrophy was caused by an inherited autosomal recessive gene.[47] The late onset of clinical signs, as well as the lack of recognition of mild clinical signs, resulted in many breedings of affected dogs, which helped foster the spread of this disorder. Figs. 13-53 through 13-55 illustrate these lesions in the Gordon setter.

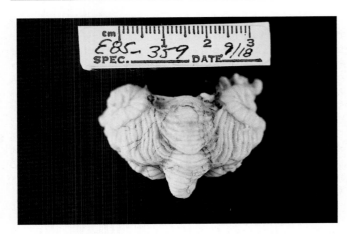

FIGURE 13-53 Dorsal view of the cerebellum of a 6-year-old Gordon setter with cerebellar cortical abiotrophy. Note the atrophied cerebellar folia.

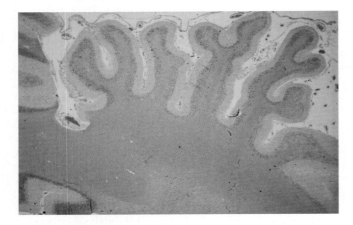

FIGURE 13-54 Microscopic section of the atrophied cerebellar folia seen in the cerebellum in Fig. 13-53.

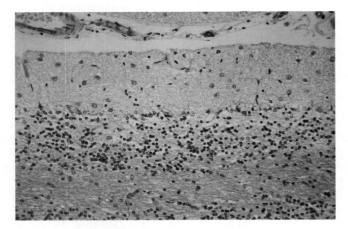

FIGURE 13-55 Higher magnification of the cerebellar cortex of a folium seen in Figs. 13-53 and 13-54. Note the marked loss of Purkinje neurons and granule neurons and the narrowing of the molecular layer.

Old English Sheepdog. **Video 13-12** shows Andy, a 9.5-year-old male Old English sheepdog that was first noticed to have an abnormal gait at 1 year of age, especially when he went up or down stairs. Despite his prancing type of gait, he competed in dog shows until he was 4 years old. The progression of clinical signs was very slow. Cerebellar cortical abiotrophy was not recognized in this breed until the early 1990s. The onset is typically late, varying from 1 to 4 years of age, and the subtle nature of the clinical signs makes them easily confused with a cervical spinal cord lesion. Using the stair test is helpful when evaluating these dogs because this test will markedly exacerbate the cerebellar signs when compared with other anatomic diagnoses. This feature is obvious in this video of Andy. Through the cooperation of dedicated owners and breeders, study of the brains of affected dogs when they died confirmed that the mode of inheritance is an autosomal recessive gene.[130]

Video 13-13 shows Geoffrey, an 8.5-year-old Old English sheepdog that was not noticed to have an abnormal gait until he was 18 months old. As was the case with Andy, the progression of clinical signs was very slow. Note the severe exacerbation of the clinical signs when he attempts to go over the stairs. Because of this difficulty, the owners elected to have him euthanized.

Video 13-14 shows Derrick, a 3-year-old male Old English sheepdog with a slowly progressive gait disorder since he was approximately 1 year old.

Scottish Terrier. **Video 13-15** shows Murphy, a male Scottish terrier that was recognized to have an abnormal gait at approximately 7 months of age that slowly progressed. At the start of this video, Murphy is 2 years old. In the portion of the video that was recorded indoors, he is 6 years old; in the last portion that was recorded outdoors, Murphy is 9 years old. This cerebellar cortical abiotrophy in Scottish terriers is extremely widespread, with affected dogs recognized throughout the United States, in the United Kingdom, and in Africa. In 1995 the Scottish Terrier Club of America reported a 0.5% frequency of this abiotrophy in the breed. Dr. Jerrold Bell determined from pedigree studies that the closest common ancestor was traced back to England in the 1960s. The onset of clinical signs is at a few months of age, and the progression is quite slow. The short limbs of these dogs often makes the recognition of clinical signs of cerebellar dysfunction difficult. In addition, the ataxic gait can be confused with the dystonic movement disorder that is inherited in this breed and is called *Scotty cramps*. This movement disorder is described and illustrated in Chapter 8. A significant difference is that the movement disorder is episodic; thus the dog has many periods with a normal gait. The cerebellar ataxia is always present in the gait of dogs with the abiotrophy. MR imaging has been used to support the diagnosis of this cerebellar cortical abiotrophy in chronically affected dogs.[134] The determination of the genomic basis for this disorder is essential to identify affected and carrier dogs and prevent the perpetuation of this disorder.

Video 13-16 shows Abby, a 4-year-old female Scottish terrier with a progressive gait disorder since approximately 10 months of age. Note the reluctance and the difficulty traversing stairs.

Video 13-17 shows Scott, a 3-year-old male Scottish terrier with a progressive gait disorder since he was 1 year old.

Beagles and Samoyed. In contrast to these postnatal forms of abiotrophy, we have observed beagle and Samoyed puppies with clinical signs of cerebellar dysfunction at the time they could stand to walk. Progression of the clinical signs was not obvious or was minimal. The beagles were affected in all four limbs, but the Samoyeds were most affected in the pelvic limbs. Necropsy revealed diffuse cerebellar cortical abiotrophy in the beagles, with absence of the Purkinje neurons or spheroid development of their axons within the granular layer, which was also reduced in neuronal population. In the Samoyeds spheroid development of Purkinje neuronal axons within the granular layer was the most profound lesion. See **Video 13-18** of these beagle puppies followed by the Samoyed puppies. Both breeds are shown at a few weeks of age and approximately 6 weeks later.

Cats

Malformation

Feline Panleucopenia Virus. In cats, the most common diffuse cerebellar disorder is a congenital malformation. Postnatal cerebellar cortical abiotrophy has been observed but is uncommon in cats.[12] Primary developmental cerebellar malformations are uncommon.[26,114] The congenital malformation that is most common consists of a varying degree of hypoplasia and atrophy caused by a perinatal infection with the feline panleukopenia virus.* This parvovirus has a predilection for rapidly dividing cells, and therefore exposure to this virus at the time of birth puts the cerebellar external germinal layer at risk. Destruction of this layer prevents the formation of the granular layer; thus the name granuloprival hypoplasia. In some kittens, extensive destruction to the parenchyma occurs, with loss of all layers of the cerebellar cortex and much of the cerebellar medulla and nuclei. These severe lesions may be the result of an earlier in utero infection with this virus. The lesions can be experimentally induced by in utero inoculation of virus during gestation.[38] Figs. 13-56 through 13-60 illustrate the lesions seen in this feline disorder. Clinical signs are observed when the kitten first attempts to stand and try to walk. By that time, the development of the cerebellar lesion is completed. Although the disease process does not progress, as the kitten grows and is capable of making more vigorous voluntary movements, the clinical signs may be more obvious. Little compensation occurs, and these clinical signs will be present for the life of the cat. These cats make great pets. They have an excellent quality of life but just need an environment in which they will not get injured when they fall. This disease has an interesting history. It was first recognized as early as the 1880s and until the 1960s was thought to be an inherited disorder, one that was very common in families of unvaccinated farm cats. In 1965, Drs. Kilham and Margolis at Dartmouth Medical College were studying a viral-induced cerebellar disorder in the rat and hamster that caused a cerebellar ataxia in the newborn animals. When the veterinarian in charge of the laboratory animals informed them of this congenital cerebellar ataxia in kittens that he often saw on local farms, they proved that the cat disorder was also viral induced.[88-90] With the help of Dr. Johnson in the United Kingdom,

*References 26, 35-40, 79, 88-91, 97-99, 118, 120.

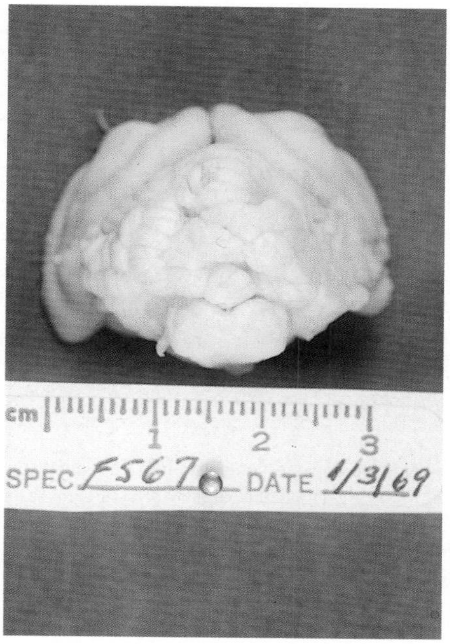

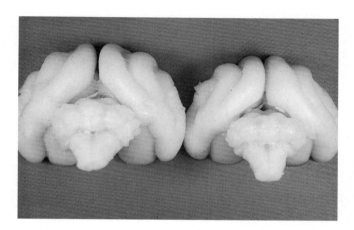

FIGURE 13-56 Caudal view of the normal cerebellum in a cat brain preserved by perfusion. Note its large size relative to the cerebrum.

FIGURE 13-57 Caudal view of the cerebellum in two 6-week-old littermate kittens with cerebellar hypoplasia and atrophy caused by a perinatal infection with the feline panleukopenia virus.

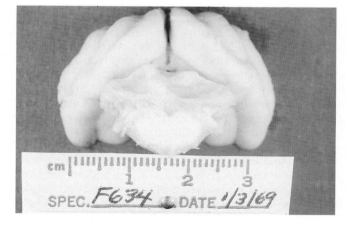

FIGURE 13-58 Caudal view of a 4-month-old kitten with severe cerebellar hypoplasia and atrophy caused by a perinatal infection with the feline panleukopenia virus.

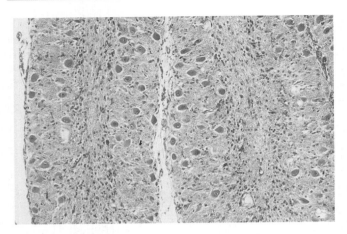

FIGURE 13-59 Microscopic section of two folia from the cerebellum of a kitten in Fig. 13-57. Note the lack of any granular layer and the lack of organization of the Purkinje neurons. This abnormality is granuloprival hypoplasia. Note the loss of the external germinal layer. Compare this figure with the normal kitten folium in Fig. 13-17.

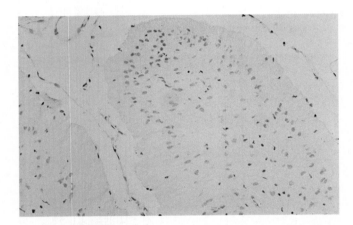

FIGURE 13-60 Microscopic section of a folium from a 3-month-old kitten with cerebellar hypoplasia and atrophy caused by a perinatal infection with the feline panleukopenia virus. Note the absence of any development of a cerebellar cortex. Most of the folium consists of glial cells and afferent processes. Only the absence of the granule neurons is hypoplasia. The loss of Purkinje neurons is caused by degeneration associated with the infection and inflammation.

they showed that the virus was the feline panleukopenia parvovirus.[79] Subsequent studies at Cornell University by Dr. Charles Csiza further confirmed this viral agent as the cause of this congenital cerebellar lesion.[35-40] Whether the natural infection occurs in utero before birth or at or shortly after birth is not known. Using molecular biologic techniques, Dr. Scott Schatzberg reported in 2002 on polymerase chain reaction amplification of parvoviral DNA from archived brain tissues of cats with this cerebellar lesion.[118] This perinatal infection is limited to the developing brain, with most of the lesions being in the cerebellum. No multisystem infection is observed with this virus, as occurs after a few weeks of age. No direct correlation exists between the severity of the clinical signs and the extent of the cerebellar lesions. This viral-induced feline disorder can be prevented by vaccination of queens before pregnancy.

See the following videos for examples of this cerebellar disorder.

Video 13-19 shows three groups of cats, all of which exhibit severe diffuse clinical signs of the cerebellar disorder caused by the perinatal infection with the feline panleukopenia virus. All of these cats have been this way since they were able to try to stand and walk. The first black and white cat is 6 months old. The two orange kittens are 1 month old, and the group of three cats in the grass includes one that is 10 weeks old and two that are 6 months old.

On rare occasion, we have observed nonprogressive cerebellar ataxia that was present since the kittens could try to stand to walk that was clinically identical to those infected perinatally with this virus but in which no gross or microscopic lesions were observed in any part of the central nervous system (CNS). We presumed this condition was a functional disorder or a structural lesion not recognizable with the light microscope. Not enough cases have been observed to define a mode of inheritance. A similar syndrome will be described in calves.

Abiotrophy. Cerebellar cortical abiotrophy is rare in cats compared with dogs and compared with the feline viral-induced cerebellar hypoplasia and atrophy described previously.[12,25,73,121] **Video 13-20** shows a 4-year-old castrated male domestic shorthair that was normal until approximately 18 months old when his gait became hesitant and he began to sway. These clinical signs slowly progressed to what you see on this video. He was euthanized, and necropsy showed nearly complete loss of the Purkinje neurons, with their replacement by astrocytes, a moderate depletion of the granular layer neurons, and an astrogliosis of the cerebellar nuclei but no lesions elsewhere in the brain. This cat also showed some loss of vision starting at approximately 2.5 year of age. By 4 years of age, his vision was very poor, and the pupils were slightly dilated but still responsive to light directed into either eye. Fundic examination showed pronounced tapetal hyperreflexia and attenuated or absent retinal blood vessels. Retinal degeneration was diagnosed and at necropsy was confirmed with a marked loss of photoreceptors. The relationship between the cerebellar cortical abiotrophy and the retinopathy is unknown.

Cerebellar cortical abiotrophy primarily affecting the Purkinje neurons has been described in two Havana brown kittens.[25] These kittens also had a hepatic microcellular dysplasia. The clinical signs of the cerebellar lesion were first observed at 4 and 5 weeks of age and slowly progressed. An inherited disorder is suspected for this syndrome.

Horses

Abiotrophy in Arabians. Cerebellar malformation is rare in foals, and we have not seen a case. Cerebellar cortical abiotrophy occurs most commonly in the Arabian breed or part-Arabian foals.[8,53,108,126,127] Affected horses have been reported in the United States, Australia, and the United Kingdom. Despite the strong presumption since the early 1960s that this malformation is a form of an autosomal recessive inherited disorder, such has not been proven. In affected Arabian foals, the onset of clinical signs is usually from birth to a few months of age. In a very few Arabians, the onset has been delayed until 9 to 24 months. Clinical signs may progress rapidly at first and then after a few months stabilize or slowly progress. We have never seen a patient that became unable to stand. The horse with this diffuse cerebellar cortical lesion has a very unique clinical appearance. The affected horse does not usually have the bursty flexor hypermetria seen in the dog and cat. Spasticity predominates in the gait. When these foals run, a marked swaying of the head and neck from side to side occurs. A head and neck tremor may be the earliest clinical sign observed. Owners will often report that, when they are halter training the foal, its head bobs, and with little stimulation, the foal will rear up, lose its balance, and fall over backwards. Although the gait can somewhat mimic a UMN and GP system dysfunction in the cervical spinal cord, the intentional head tremor and the tendency to rear up with the thoracic limbs in full extension when stimulated excludes this consideration. In addition, horses with this cerebellar cortical abiotrophy lose their menace response. When menaced, the patient will move its head away from the menacing hand without eyelid closure. The eyelids close when they are touched. See the following videos for examples of this cerebellar cortical abiotrophy in Arabian horses.

Video 13-21 shows a 14-week-old Arabian colt that the owner thought was head shy at 1 week of age when she started trying to put a halter on him and he bobbed his head. The head tremor was worse when he was excited, which progressed over the first few weeks. The horse's gait appeared to be too stiff at approximately 10 weeks of age, which also progressed. When the video is first recorded outdoors, the foal first seen on the video is a normal Thoroughbred colt for you to compare with the affected Arabian. Note all the clinical signs that were described for this Arabian cerebellar disorder.

Videos 13-22A and B show an Arabian colt that was videoed in a paddock on its farm at 4 months of age **(A)** and then in the teaching hospital at Cornell University at 8.5 months of age **(B)**. The owner first suspected something was wrong when the colt was approximately 3 months old.

Video 13-23 shows a 6-month-old Arabian filly with progressive clinical signs since approximately 2 months of age.

Video 13-24 shows a young adult Arabian mare, with no history, that was purchased at a horse sale. Her clinical signs speak for themselves. This 16-mm film was made in 1969, converted to video, and then digitized. You can see that the person doing the filming was at some risk of injury! The horse was euthanized, and cerebellar cortical abiotrophy was confirmed at necropsy.

A similar clinical and pathologic syndrome has been reported in Gotland ponies, with the onset of clinical signs from birth to 6 months of age.[17] Clinical signs are slowly progressive, and an autosomal recessive inheritance has been documented for this disease.

Cattle

Malformation

Bovine Virus Diarrhea Virus. In cattle, the most common cause of congenital clinical signs of a cerebellar disorder is the cerebellar malformation caused by the in utero infection of the bovine fetus with the bovine virus diarrhea (BVD)

virus.* The malformation represents the result of both hypoplasia and atrophy. The discovery of this clinical disorder was based on the astute observations of Dr. Robert Kahrs at Cornell University in the 1960s. He studied the medical histories of the herds from which calves had come that were diagnosed at necropsy with this cerebellar malformation.[81] The following discussion is one example of what he found for most of these calves.

On a farm with a herd of 77 cows, an outbreak of diarrhea caused by the BVD virus occurred in 35 cows. Three cows died. Most of the cows were partially anorectic and had decreased milk production. At the time of this illness, 29 cows were pregnant. Nineteen of these cows produced normal calves. Eight cows aborted, and two cows gave birth to calves that, at birth, exhibited the clinical signs of a cerebellar disorder and, at necropsy, showed a cerebellar hypoplasia and atrophy. These cows were pregnant at 46 and 65 days of pregnancy when the illness occurred. Based on these observations, Dr. Kahrs had the large-animal practitioners in New York State collect serum from any calf born with clinical signs of a cerebellar disorder before their consumption of colostrum. All of these serum samples contained antibodies for the BVD virus, indicating infection of the calf when it was a fetus. The next study was to obtain nonimmune cows, breed them, and inoculate them with the BVD virus at 150 days of pregnancy. This experiment resulted in a few calves born with the clinical signs of a cerebellar disorder and the lesions of cerebellar hypoplasia and atrophy similar to what was observed in the natural disease. Another group of nonimmune cows were inoculated with the BVD virus at 150 days of pregnancy, and the fetuses were surgically removed at varying intervals starting at 7 days postinoculation. An acute inflammation was observed in the cerebellum at 17 to 21 days postinoculation with necrosis of the external germinal layer, as well as necrosis of the differentiated cerebellar cortex and folial white matter laminae. By 42 days postinoculation, the cerebellar lesion was complete, and the inflammation was subsiding. Most natural calves born with these lesions were between 100 and 200 days of gestation at the time of the herd illness.

This malformation should not be summarily diagnosed as cerebellar hypoplasia. Only the absence of granular layer neurons represents hypoplasia because the BVD infection destroyed the external germinal layer, which is the origin of this neuronal layer. The massive destruction of the already differentiated Purkinje neurons, the folial white matter laminae, and, in some calves, the cerebellar medulla and nuclei is a degeneration of parenchyma caused by the necrotizing action of the virus and the resulting inflammation. This degeneration results in atrophy. Thus the malformation observed at birth is a combination of hypoplasia and atrophy. The degree of cerebellar lesion in newborn calves varies from a slight gross deformity to almost complete absence of any cerebellar tissue. In the latter case, only a small band of smooth parenchyma may remain over the fourth ventricle where the cerebellum should normally be located. Where folia are present, the cortex is often depleted of varying amounts of its neuronal layers, and the area of the folial white matter lamina is replaced by a cavity. Mild astrogliosis may be the only indication of where a previous cortex existed. Figs. 13-61 through 13-68 illustrate the lesions seen in these calves. Clinical signs of cerebellar

---

*References 15, 20-24, 49, 81-84, 140.

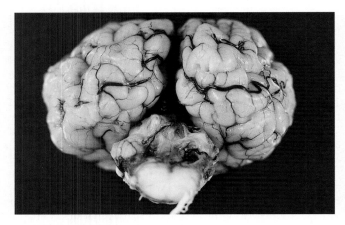

FIGURE 13-61 Dorsal view of a preserved brain of a 2-week-old calf with cerebellar hypoplasia and atrophy caused by the in utero infection with the BVD viral agent. Note the severe lack of cerebellar tissue and its asymmetry.

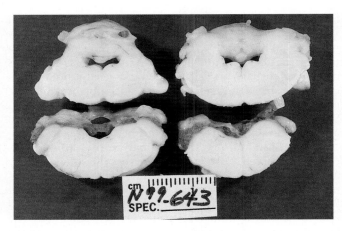

FIGURE 13-64 Transverse sections of the cerebellum, pons, and medulla of the brain seen in Fig. 13-63.

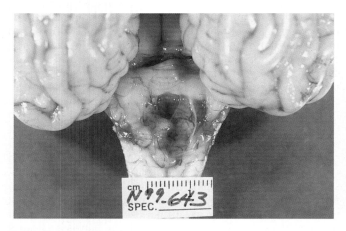

FIGURE 13-62 Dorsal view of the brain of the 3-week-old Holstein calf seen in Video 13-25 directly after its removal at necropsy. Note the similarity to the severe cerebellar lesions seen in Fig. 13-61, a result of the necrosis associated with the inflammation caused by an in utero infection with the BVD viral agent.

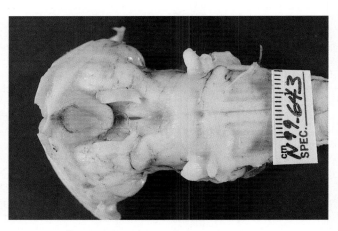

FIGURE 13-65 Ventral surface of the brainstem of the brain seen in Fig. 13-63. Note the very reduced size of the transverse fibers of the pons, which is secondary to the absence of the cerebellar cortex where the axons in the transverse fibers of the pons normally terminate.

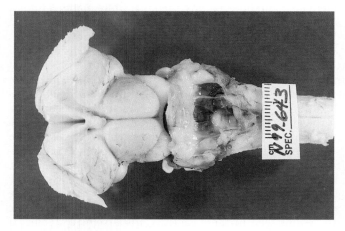

FIGURE 13-63 Dorsal view of the preserved brain seen in Fig. 13-62 after removal of the cerebral hemispheres. Note the narrow band of cerebellar tissue spanning the roof of the fourth ventricle just caudal to the caudal colliculi.

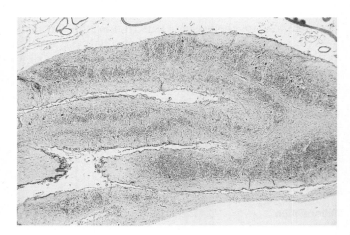

FIGURE 13-66 Microscopic section of a few severely hypoplastic and atrophied folia from a calf with cerebellar lesions similar to those seen in Figs. 13-61 through 13-64. Note the lack of any normal organization of cerebellar cortex.

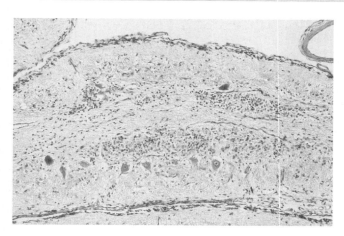

FIGURE 13-67 Higher magnification of a section of one folium seen in Fig. 13-66, showing the marked loss of cortical neurons and the lack of any cortical organization.

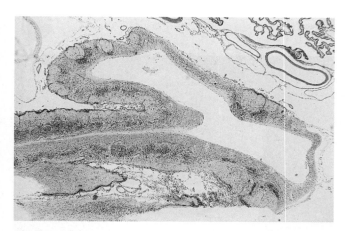

FIGURE 13-68 Microscopic section of another cerebellar folium exhibiting a large cavity in the center where edema and necrosis destroyed the folial white lamina adjacent to the cortex.

dysfunction vary from recumbency with opisthotonus and extensor rigidity of the limbs to a mildly spastic hypermetric unsteady gait and slight head tremor. Abnormal nystagmus occasionally occurs. These calves are alert and responsive and have remarkably strong voluntary movements. The degree of cerebellar lesion does not necessarily correlate with the severity of the cerebellar dysfunction. The clinical signs do not progress after birth. Occasionally, an initially recumbent calf is able to stand after a few days, but its gait remains severely ataxic.

In a few calves with severe cerebellar lesions, cavitated areas can be found scattered through the cerebrum, especially in the occipital lobes. These porencephalic lesions are the result of the inflammation that occurred in that part of the brain. No clinical signs are observed related to these lesions. Ocular lesions have also been observed in spontaneous and experimental examples of this disease. These examples consist of retinal atrophy, cataracts, microphthalmia, retinal dysplasia, and optic neuritis. Some calves are blind at birth, with dilated pupils that are unresponsive to light. At necropsy, these calves have very small optic nerves, optic chiasm, and optic tracts.

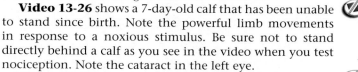

See the following videos for examples of this bovine cerebellar disorder.

Video 13-25 shows a 3-week-old Holstein calf that has been affected with this gait disorder since birth.

Video 13-26 shows a 7-day-old calf that has been unable to stand since birth. Note the powerful limb movements in response to a noxious stimulus. Be sure not to stand directly behind a calf as you see in the video when you test nociception. Note the cataract in the left eye.

Video 13-27 shows three Holstein calves, all from one farm and all born within a 10-day period.

Functional Disorder. Video 13-28 shows two Holstein calves that were unable to stand since birth with very similar clinical signs. The first calf is 1 week old, and necropsy revealed no gross or microscopic lesions. This abnormality is presumed to be a functional cerebellar disorder in which no recognizable structural abnormalities are observed at the level of the light microscope. Functional cerebellar disorder is unrelated to any infection with the BVD virus and may be an inherited disorder. We have seen only a very few of these calves and are unable to define a mode of inheritance. The pathogenesis may be similar to what we described in newborn Arabian foals in Chapter 8. In Chapter 8, we described a congenital tetany with episodes of opisthotonus in recumbent Arabian foals that had a hair coat with a lavender color. Necropsy revealed no recognizable microscopic lesions, and an inherited functional disorder was presumed. The second calf (mostly white) on Video 13-28 is 2 weeks old, and necropsy revealed the gross and microscopic lesions expected with an in utero infection with the BVD virus. Obviously, necropsy is necessary to differentiate these two disorders. Recommendations for preventing further cases are dependent on this information. MR imaging would provide an antemortem differentiation of these two disorders.

The following description is another example of the importance to confirm the basis for the clinical signs of a congenital cerebellar disorder. We studied a Scottish Highland calf that was unable to get up at birth but was alert and, in its attempts to right itself, would exhibit opisthotonus with extensor rigidity of the limbs. It also had an abnormal nystagmus. Clinical signs were similar to those in the calf in Video 13-26. Based on this information, we expected to observe a gross lesion typical of an in utero infection with the BVD virus. Necropsy revealed a symmetric, marked reduction in the overall size of the cerebellum, However, in addition, no trapezoid body was seen on the ventral aspect of the rostral medulla, and the cochlear nuclei were continuous, with a band of parenchyma that extended across the dorsal aspect of the medulla obliterating most of the fourth ventricle. This band was just caudal to the small cerebellar peduncles and was thought to be an abnormal trapezoid body. The corpus callosum was shorter and thinner than normal. This calf also had a tetralogy of Fallot in its heart and aplasia of one kidney and the adrenal on the same side. The brain lesions were considered to be a developmental disorder that could not be caused by an in utero viral infection of the fetus. In this newly established small herd, the three previous calves that were born were down at birth and unable to stand. They were euthanized, and no necropsy was performed. We have observed a similar cerebellar and medullary malformation in an Angus calf and a lamb. Figs. 13-69 through 13-76 illustrate the malformation in these two bovine breeds.

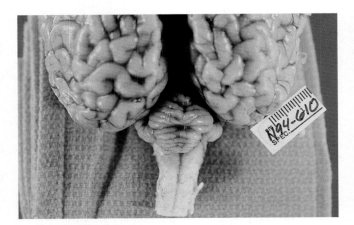

FIGURE 13-69 Dorsal view of the brain of a 1-week-old Scottish Highland calf recumbent from birth with severe clinical signs of a cerebellar disorder. Note the very small symmetric hypoplastic cerebellum.

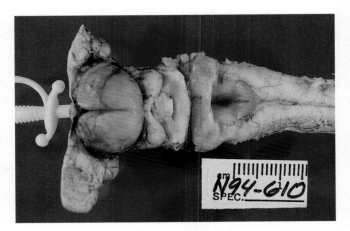

FIGURE 13-72 Dorsal view of the brainstem from the calf in Figs. 13-69 through 13-71. Most of the cerebellum has been removed. A small portion of cerebellum remains just caudal to the caudal colliculi. Caudal to this cerebellar tissue is a band of parenchyma crossing the fourth ventricle. This structure is the trapezoid body, and the small mounds at each end are the cochlear nuclei. At the level of this band of parenchyma, the fourth ventricle consisted of an ependymal-lined space similar to a central canal.

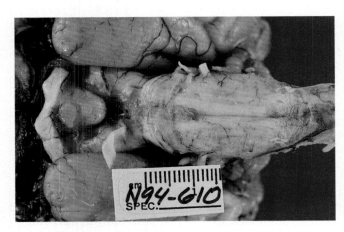

FIGURE 13-70 Ventral view of the brain of the calf in Fig. 13-69. Note the small transverse fibers of the pons and the absence of any trapezoid body.

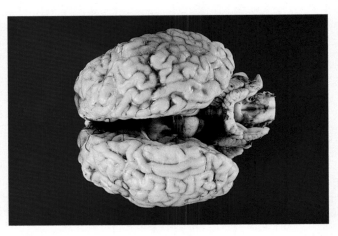

FIGURE 13-73 Dorsal view of the brain of a 1-week-old Angus calf with clinical signs of a severe cerebellar disorder since birth. Note the symmetric cerebellar malformation.

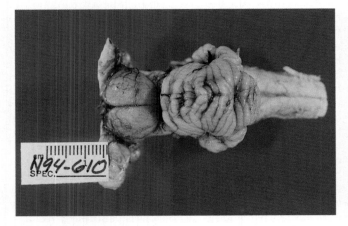

FIGURE 13-71 Dorsal view of the brainstem and hypoplastic cerebellum with the cerebral hemispheres removed from the calf brain in Figs. 13-69 and 13-70. Note the symmetric folial development in the small cerebellum.

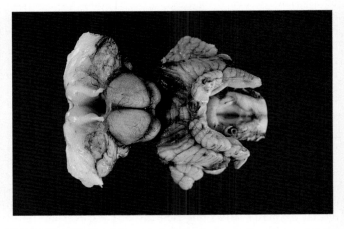

FIGURE 13-74 Dorsal view of the brainstem and cerebellum after removal of the cerebral hemispheres from the brain of the calf in Fig. 13-73. Note the unusual shape of the cerebellum but the symmetry of the malformation.

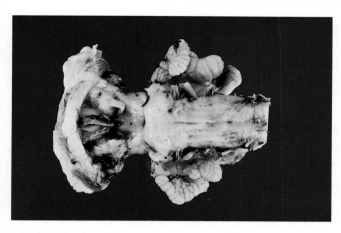

FIGURE 13-75 Ventral surface of the brainstem of the brain in Figs. 13-73 and 13-74. Note the small transverse fibers of the pons and the absence of any trapezoid body.

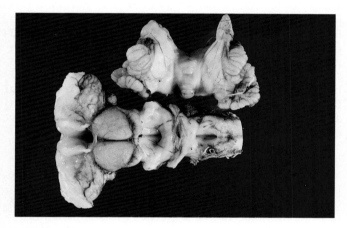

FIGURE 13-76 Dorsal view of the brainstem seen in Fig. 13-74 with the cerebellum detached at its cerebellar peduncles and laid on its dorsal surface beside the brainstem. Note the band of parenchyma crossing the fourth ventricle caudal to where the cerebellum was removed. This band was assumed to be the trapezoid body and the small mounds at either end, and the attached nerve fibers are the cochlear nuclei and vestibulocochlear nerves, respectively. The brains of these two calves in Figs. 13-69 through 13-76 represent a malformation caused by a developmental disorder unrelated to any in utero viral infection and presumably are the result of a genetic disorder.

The in utero infections that were described in Chapter 3 as causes of hydranencephaly also occasionally cause some inflammation and necrosis in the cerebellum resulting in varying degrees of hypoplasia and atrophy. When present, these infections were usually too mild to result in clinical signs of a cerebellar disorder.[66]

Abiotrophy. Cerebellar cortical abiotrophy occasionally occurs in cattle.[30,75,78,138] In the 1970s, we studied a large number of calves from different farms but from the same sire that had a rapid onset of clinical signs of a cerebellar disorder at 3 to 9 months of age.[137] The clinical signs progressed rapidly for a few days and then became static or slowly progressed. Most calves ultimately became unable to stand, but a few remained ambulatory with a severe cerebellar ataxia. Opisthotonus was commonly observed. Their alert sensorium and intact vision, despite a lack

of a menace response, helped differentiate this disorder from a thiamin deficiency–induced polioencephalomalacia, which is a common cause of recumbency and an opisthotonic posture at this age. This diffuse brain disorder caused by thiamin deficiency is described in Chapter 14. Necropsy of the calves with cerebellar cortical abiotrophy showed no gross lesions. Microscopic examination reveals patches of cerebellar cortex with Purkinje neuron abiotrophy. A form of autosomal recessive inheritance was suspected for this disorder. No cases were diagnosed after approximately 1980.

Video 13-29. This video shows a 6-month-old Holstein heifer 3 weeks after the onset of clinical signs of cerebellar cortical abiotrophy. Another form of hereditary cerebellar cortical abiotrophy is reported in Holstein calves but with more extensive neuronal degeneration throughout the brain. The onset of cerebellar ataxia is from 6 weeks to 5 months, and the neurologic signs progress until the calf is unable to stand unassisted.[77]

A suspected, inherited cerebellar hypoplasia and abiotrophy have been reported in Hereford cattle with nonprogressive clinical signs of cerebellar ataxia present at birth.[74] The paucity of Purkinje and granule neurons suggested a developmental arrest resulting in hypoplasia. The cortical gliosis and evidence of degeneration in surviving Purkinje neurons suggested an abiotrophy. However, the entire lesion is just as likely the result of abiotrophy.

A cerebellar cortical abiotrophy is described in Angus calves in Scotland accompanied by a spastic hypermetric ataxic gait.[9-11] The ataxia is preceded by generalized seizures that begin at birth or up to 3 months of age. These seizures are single or multiple and may last for several hours. After numerous episodes of seizures, spasticity and ataxia are evident in the gait. In time, both the seizures and spastic ataxia resolve. By 2 years of age, some of these calves are normal. An inherited basis is proposed for this syndrome. The pathogenesis of this syndrome is unclear, given that no microscopic lesions are described in the prosencephalon to explain the seizures, and the mild cerebellar cortical lesions were presumably self-limiting to allow for the presumed compensation and resultant recovery.

The absence of any further reports suggests that the disorder may have been reduced by a corrective breeding program. A similar cerebellar cortical abiotrophy was described in a 9-month-old Charolais calf that developed seizures and a spastic ataxia at 6 months of age.[30]

See Chapter 3 for a description of an inherited multifocal malformation that was observed in Hereford calves born recumbent and unable to stand.[105] Malformative lesions involved most of the brain segments, including the cerebellum. An autosomal recessive inherited trait was implicated. Cerebellar hypoplasia and multisystem malformations that include the cerebellum have been reported in cattle.[57,61,106]

Sheep

In newborn lambs, severe cerebellar ataxia is described in several breeds in Great Britain that included Welsh and Welsh mountain sheep and in Canada that involved the Corriedale breed.[74,76,130,139] These animals are called daft lambs in England. The ataxia present at birth does not progress despite the evidence that sequential necropsies indicate a progressive degeneration of the cerebellar cortex that is most likely abiotrophy. An autosomal recessive inheritance is proposed for this disorder.

Pigs

Abiotrophy. Our experience with cerebellar disorders in pigs is limited because of the relative paucity of porcine patients in the northeast United States. We are not aware of an in utero viral disease that results in a cerebellar hypoplasia and atrophy similar to the BVD virus in calves. The in utero infection of the fetal pig with the hog cholera, circa, or swine fever viruses causes a diffuse hypomyelinogenesis and a clinical syndrome of congenital tremors as described in Chapter 8. A cerebellar hypoplasia may be included with the lesions that follow in utero infection with the hog cholera virus.[59]

In the early 1970s, a postnatal cerebellar cortical abiotrophy was studied in Yorkshire pigs at Cornell University.[63] Two syndromes were observed that were clinically similar but varied in the nature of the abiotrophy. In one syndrome, 16 pigs were studied from seven litters with related parents on four different farms. These pigs were normal until 3 to 5 weeks of age when a sudden onset of pelvic limb stiffness occurred, followed rapidly by ataxia. The ataxia progressed to the thoracic limbs, and recumbency occurred in a few days. Despite being recumbent, these pigs were extremely alert and struggled vigorously with all limbs to right themselves. Postural reactions were difficult to assess owing to the lack of cooperation of the patient. An abnormal positional nystagmus was present. See **Video 13-30**. The initial portion of the video shows three pigs approximately 2 months old. The two pigs in the middle portion of the video are approximately 3 months old, and the single pig in the last portion is approximately 4 months old. As you can see, once the pigs are recumbent, no obvious change in the clinical signs is observed. Note how alert and responsive these pigs are. Also note their vigorous voluntary limb movements when the pigs are stimulated. This feature is a clue that the major dysfunction in these pigs is their inability to right themselves to stand. They have the desire and the strength but lack the necessary coordination. The abnormal nystagmus emphasizes the vestibular system dysfunction. The most significant brain lesion in these pigs was in the cerebellum and consisted of multiple enlargements of Purkinje neuronal axons, called *spheroids*. These were most pronounced where axons coursed through the granular layer. Loss of Purkinje neuronal cell bodies was minimal. A mild increase appeared to exist in the abundance of these spheroids between pigs necropsied at 2 and 4 months of age.

In the second syndrome, 14 pigs were affected from five litters with related parents. The sudden onset of stiffness and ataxia was between 1 and 4 weeks of age. This phase rapidly progressed to recumbency similar to what was seen in the video of the first syndrome. The cerebellar lesion in these pigs predominated in the vermal and paravermal folia and consisted of complete absence of the external germinal layer and marked loss of Purkinje neurons and granule neurons in the adjacent cerebellar cortex. Viral isolation studies of pigs from both syndromes were unrewarding. The presumption was that the abiotrophy in these two syndromes was most likely an inherited disorder. Since this study, we have not observed any more pigs with either of these two disorders.

Other Cerebellar Diseases

The cerebellum is subject to involvement by the same kind of lesions that affect the adjacent brainstem and other portions of the CNS. These possible diagnoses include inflammations, neoplasms, degenerative disorders, and injury.[107]

Inflammation

The cerebellar white matter and cortex are commonly affected in dogs by the canine distemper virus, which causes demyelination followed by inflammation and necrosis. *Toxoplasma gondii* and *Cryptococcus neoformans* and fungal agents can also involve the cerebellum in dogs and cats. *Neospora caninum* has a predilection for the cerebellum in young adult dogs.[24,77] *Sarcocystis neurona* is an uncommon cause of clinical signs of cerebellar disease in adult horses. In dogs, the white matter of the cerebellar medulla and peduncles is a common site for the autoimmune disorder granulomatous meningoencephalitis.[64] This disorder may be part of a diffuse distribution of this lesion or a focal space-occupying granulomatous lesion limited to this site. The severe meningitis and choroid plexitis in the caudal cranial fossa of cats infected with the feline infectious peritonitis virus may cause clinical signs that include those from a cerebellar origin. The same may occur in any animal but more commonly in young farm animals with bacterial suppurative meningitis or an abscess in the caudal cranial fossa. Parasitic migration may occur through the cerebellum and produce clinical signs of a cerebellar-vestibular disorder. These organisms include *Cuterebra* spp. larvae in cats and *Parelaphostrongylus tenuis* larvae in sheep, goats, and Camelidae. Examples of these infections were described with the vestibular system in Chapter 12. A rare *Hypoderma bovis* larva in the cerebellum of a young horse caused a cerebellar-vestibular disorder (Figs. 13-77, 13-78). In all of these examples, the clinical signs of cerebellar involvement are usually accompanied by other clinical signs suggestive of a multifocal or diffuse disease process.

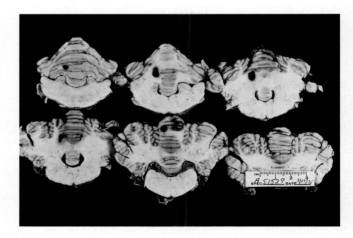

FIGURE 13-77 Transverse section of the cerebellum, pons, and medulla of the brain from a 10-month-old Appaloosa with an acute onset of clinical signs primarily of a vestibular system disorder. Note the hemorrhagic cavity most obvious in the top row of sections.

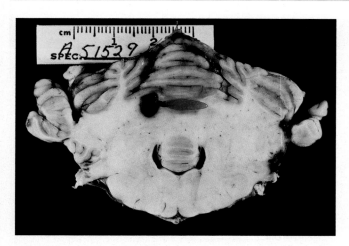

FIGURE 13-78 Higher magnification of the third transverse section in the top row of Fig. 13-77. A *H. bovis* larva was extracted from the lumen of the hemorrhagic cavity.

Neoplasia

Primary and metastatic neoplasms may involve the cerebellum. These neoplasms are often unilateral at the cerebellomedullary or cerebellopontine angle and usually produce clinical signs of cerebellar-vestibular dysfunction, as well as clinical signs of interference with the UMN and GP systems at this level and the various cranial nerves located in the pons and medulla. Medulloblastoma (primitive neurectodermal tumor) occurs in the cerebellum of young dogs and calves and gliomas occur in older dogs.[128] Ependymomas and choroid plexus tumors, as well as meningiomas, may occur at this level.[7,62,141]

Degeneration

Inherited diffuse degenerations such as the various neuronal storage diseases, axonopathies, or leukodystrophies usually include cerebellar lesions, and sometimes the clinical signs of cerebellar dysfunction predominate.[80] Similarly, some species of plants can induce the storage of substrate in neuronal cell bodies by inhibiting a degradative lysosomal enzyme. Lesions are diffuse and include the cerebellum. This circumstance is most common in livestock that graze on these plants. In Australia, ingestion of a species of *Swainsona* can produce an alpha mannosidosis.[51] In Brazil, ingestion of a *Solanum fastigiatum* by cattle produces a neuronal storage disease that profoundly affects the Purkinje neurons in the cerebellum and causes severe cerebellar dysfunction.[115] We have seen a similar disorder in goats in Florida that grazed on *Solanum viarum* (tropical soda apple).[112]

Several plants and fungi have been identified as sources of toxins that produce a diffuse CNS disorder with tremors, hyperexcitability, and ataxia, some of which are cerebellar in origin. These abnormalities are usually functional disorders and are not associated with recognizable lesions.

Vascular compromise of the blood supplied by one rostral cerebellar artery is a common lesion in dogs, resulting in varying degrees of ischemia or infarction.[6,100] The cause of these vascular compromises is unknown, but some may be associated with hypertension, heart disease, hyperadrenocorticoidism, or hypothyroidism. In cats, this abnormality occurs in the distribution of the middle cerebral artery associated with the migration of the larva of a species of *Cuterebra*.

Injury

If the caudal cranial fossa is the main site that receives the major impact of an injury, clinical signs of cerebellar dysfunction may predominate. The domestic animal is capable of remarkable compensation after extensive traumatic lesions of the cerebellar cortex. Lesions that involve the cerebellar nuclei produce more severe deficits and the degree of compensation is less.

CASE EXAMPLE 13-1

Signalment: 3.5-year-old male golden retriever, Kodi
Chief Complaint: Gait abnormality
History: The onset of a slowly progressive gait abnormality is unclear. Between 1 and 2 years of age, Kodi was diagnosed with a cervical spinal cord disorder. Clinical signs were apparently subtle and not clearly defined. At 2.5 years the gait disorder was more obvious and slowly progressed to the time that Kodi was donated to us for study.
Examination: See **Video 13-31**.
Anatomic Diagnosis: Diffuse cerebellum
Differential Diagnosis: Cerebellar cortical abiotrophy, inflammation, neuronal storage disease, neoplasm, malformation—cyst

The slowly progressive symmetric clinical signs of cerebellar dysfunction correlate well with a late-onset cerebellar cortical abiotrophy. We had not observed cerebellar abiotrophy before in golden retrievers and were unaware of any publications of this diagnosis. Encephalitis confined to the cerebellum over this prolonged period seemed unlikely. As a rule, when the cerebellum is involved with an inflammation caused by viral, protozoal, *Rickettsia,* or fungal infections, other areas of the brain or spinal cord will also be involved

and contribute to the clinical signs. The presumably autoimmune disorder granulomatous meningoencephalitis is a reasonable consideration but has the same objections as the infectious diseases. The prolonged clinical course would also make these inflammations less likely. The slowly progressive course and symmetric clinical signs are compatible with a neuronal storage disease, but you would expect some clinical indication of involvement of the prosencephalon over this period. The early age of onset is less likely for a neoplasm except for a medulloblastoma of the cerebellum but the prolonged course of the disorder is even more than you would expect for most neoplasms. A caudal cranial fossa dermoid or epidermoid cyst, as well as a subarachnoid cyst, should be considered.[96] The subarachnoid cyst may be related to the quadrigeminal cistern or the cerebellomedullary angle. A diverticulum of the fourth ventricle may also appear in the area of the quadrigeminal cistern. This cistern is the normal slightly widened subarachnoid space dorsal to the mesencephalic colliculi ventromedial to the occipital lobes. MR imaging is the most reliable ancillary procedure to help with this differentiation but was not available when Kodi was studied. Our presumptive clinical diagnosis

(Continued)

CASE EXAMPLE 13-1—cont'd

before any ancillary procedures were performed was late-onset cerebellar cortical abiotrophy. Cerebrospinal fluid (CSF) evaluation eliminated this consideration because it contained 43 mg/dl of protein (normal <25) and 26 white blood cells/mm³ (normal <5), with 41% lymphocytes, 35% monocytes, 22% neutrophils, and 2% eosinophils. This data supported an inflammatory disease.

NEOSPOROSIS

Kodi was euthanized, and necropsy revealed that the cerebellum was symmetrically reduced in size by approximately two thirds, and its surface was covered by a thick gray membrane obscuring the atrophied folia (Figs. 13-79 through 13-81). Microscopic examination showed severe atrophy of most of the vermal and hemispheric folia. These atrophied folia had no recognizable neurons and consisted entirely of fibrous astrocytes. A nonsuppurative inflammation was prominent in the leptomeninges and scattered through the remaining parenchyma. Associated with this lesion were a few small cysts of protozoal organisms that, with the use of immunocytochemistry, were identified as *N. caninum* (Figs. 13-82 through 13-85).[77] Since

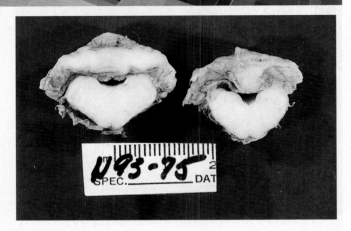

FIGURE 13-81 Transverse sections of the cerebellum, pons, and medulla of the brain seen in Fig. 13-80.

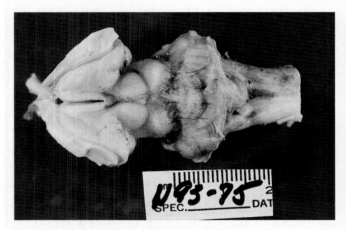

FIGURE 13-79 Caudodorsal view of the brain of the 3.5-year-old golden retriever in Video 13-31. Note the marked atrophy of the cerebellum covered by a thick layer of leptomeninges.

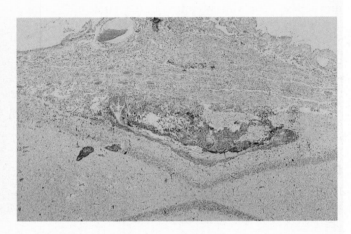

FIGURE 13-82 Microscopic section of the cerebellum from the transverse section seen on the left in Fig. 13-81. Note the severe atrophy of the folia dorsal to the cerebellar medulla.

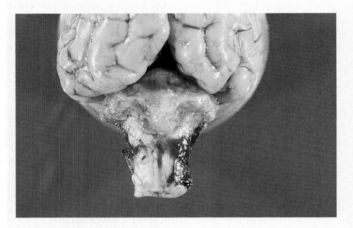

FIGURE 13-80 Dorsal view of the brainstem and cerebellum of the preserved brain seen in Fig. 13-79.

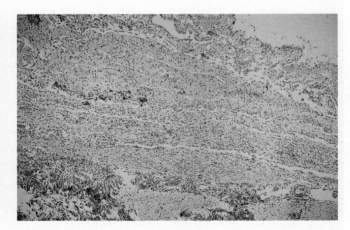

FIGURE 13-83 Higher magnification of the folia seen in Fig. 13-82. Note the inflammation that is still present ventrally and the marked folial atrophy.

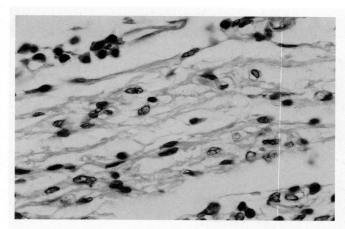

FIGURE 13-84 Higher magnification of one entire atrophic folium seen in Fig. 13-83 that consists solely of fibrous astrocytes.

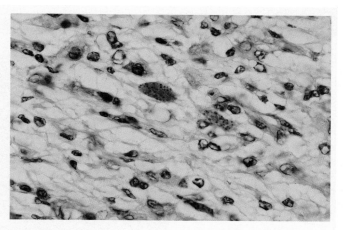

FIGURE 13-85 Higher magnification of a portion of the cerebellar medulla seen in Fig. 13-82. Note the cluster of protozoal organisms in a field of primarily reactive astrocytes. These protozoa were identified as *N. caninum* using immunocytochemistry.

our observation of this case, several publications have been issued of young adult dogs with neosporosis predominantly affecting the cerebellum.[24] Recall that, in Case Example 5-11, we described that in young puppies this organism has a predilection for the long lumbosacral spinal nerve roots, causing a radiculitis.

Recently, we had the opportunity to study MR images sent to us by Dr. Laurent Garosi, a veterinary neurologist in England, of a 9-year-old spayed female West Highland white terrier with a history of 12 months of slowly progressive clinical signs of a cerebellar disorder. These images showed a marked symmetric reduction in the size of the cerebellum

with thickened overlying meninges. No contrast enhancement was used. These images closely resembled the cerebellar lesion seen in Kodi, the dog in this case example (see Figs. 13-79 through 13-81). The presence of serum antibodies for *N. caninum* in this West Highland white terrier supported infection with this protozoal agent. She is presently being treated for this infection. We assume that the chronicity of the lesion and associated diminution of the inflammation accounted for the lack of contrast enhancement.

CASE EXAMPLE 13-2

Signalment: 13-year-old castrated male shepherd-Akita cross, Caesar
Chief Complaint: Gait disorder
History: This dog, while indoors, suddenly lost its balance and developed a left head tilt and an abnormal gait with his right limbs. The clinical signs had not changed on the third day when he was videoed.
Examination: See **Video 13-32**. Note the quality of the movement of the right limbs with the excessive joint flexion in the hypermetric gait. Note the left head tilt. Not shown on the video were slow postural reactions in the right limbs and an abnormal positional vertical nystagmus.
Anatomic Diagnosis: Right side of the cerebellum
The cerebellar quality ataxia in the right limbs is ipsilateral to the right cerebellar lesion, and the involvement of the right cerebellar peduncles is the cause of the paradoxical left vestibular system dysfunction (left head tilt).
Differential Diagnosis: Vascular compromise, neoplasia, inflammation

VASCULAR COMPROMISE

Injury was not included, as the clinical signs developed suddenly while the dog was indoors. The most presumptive clinical diagnosis is a vascular compromise, causing ischemia or infarction of the cerebellar parenchyma.[6,100] In humans, these vascular compromises

are called *cerebrovascular accidents* (CVA), even though they can also occur in the brainstem and cerebellum. Some authorities refer to these episodes as *strokes*. In the first two editions of this text, vascular compromise in the CNS was considered to be rare in domestic animals. However, we now believe that this event is a more common syndrome based on the advent of MR studies and further pathologic documentation.[6,99] These patients most often exhibit cerebellar-vestibular clinical signs or occasionally clinical signs of a prosencephalic disorder. The cerebellum is the most common site for these strokes to occur in our experience. As a rule, the cerebellar lesions are primarily in the distribution of one of the rostral cerebellar arteries. In one miniature schnauzer with a similar clinical syndrome, a thrombus was found in the rostral cerebellar artery on the side of the cerebellar lesion. In most cases, the cause is unknown. However, hypertension, heart disease, hyperadrenocorticoidism, and hypothyroidism have been seen in some of these patients. MR imaging will show these lesions and define their extent. In particular, fluid-attenuated inversion-recovery (FLAIR) and gradient-echo MR sequences are most useful (Figs. 13-86, 13-87). The prognosis is fair to good, given that many dogs will surprisingly resolve their clinical signs completely, suggesting the lesion is ischemia and not infarction. We have studied a large number of greyhounds with similar clinical signs and MR images that supported ischemia or infarction of the cerebellum. Hypertension was found in many of these patients.

(Continued)

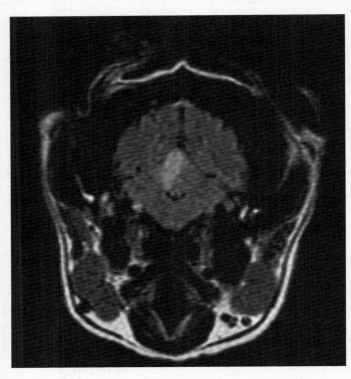

FIGURE 13-86 FLAIR MR image of the brain of a 11.5-year-old castrated male wire fox terrier at the level of the rostral cerebellum and pons. This dog had an acute onset of clinical signs of a left cerebellar disorder. Note the sharply demarcated hyperintensity in the left side of the rostral cerebellum caused by edema associated with a vascular compromise of the left rostral cerebellar artery.

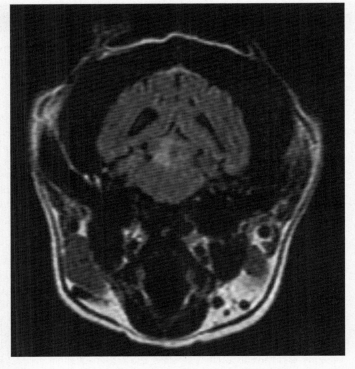

FIGURE 13-87 FLAIR MR image of the brain of the dog in Fig. 13-86 at the level of the caudal mesencephalon, just rostral to the image in Fig. 13-86. Note the same hyperintensity involving a portion of the left caudal colliculus.

Most improved with appropriate medical management and treatment of the hypertension. The cause of the hypertension was not found. Dogs with primary hypothyroidism and severe hyperlipidemia are at risk for developing atherosclerotic lesions or ischemia related to increased blood viscosity.[136]

Caesar, the dog in this case example, had clinical signs of a cardiac disorder and was euthanized. Necropsy showed an infarction of the left side of the cerebellum and endocarditis. The assumption was that a thromboembolism related to the endocarditis compromised the blood supplied by the right rostral cerebellar artery, which caused the cerebellar infarction.

See **Video 13-33**. This video shows Knight, a 3-year-old castrated male Doberman pinscher, that the owner left in her car to go shopping. When she returned to her car, the windows were all steamed up, and she found Knight on the floor thrashing wildly and exhibiting a shaking action of the eyes (a resting abnormal nystagmus). Examination of Knight 36 hours after the onset was difficult to perform and assess accurately because of his severe disorientation and anxiety. He had powerful voluntary movements, which made him lurch to the right side. He exhibited an abnormal positional vertical nystagmus. Knight improved and was able to stand and walk by the third day when this video was made. Study the video. Your anatomic diagnosis should be the right side of the cerebellum. The clinical signs seen in Knight are the same as those observed in Caesar in the previous case example. A presumptive diagnosis was made of vascular compromise of the blood supplied by the right rostral cerebellar artery. Knight continued to improve and by 3 weeks had only a slight hypermetric gait in his right limbs.

Figs. 13-88 through 13-92 illustrates examples of the cerebellar lesions caused by the compromise of its blood supply.

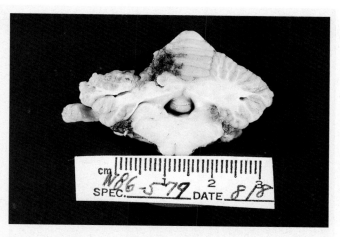

FIGURE 13-89 Higher magnification of the transverse section in Fig. 13-88 through the cerebellum and medulla. Note the sharp demarcation of the right border of the lesion on the median plane of the vermis. This indicates the medial border of the territory of the cerebellum supplied by the left rostral cerebellar artery.

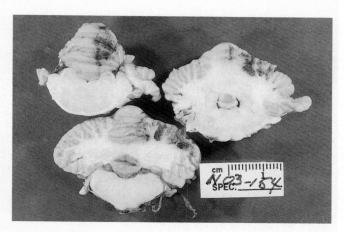

FIGURE 13-90 Transverse sections of the brain of a 10-year-old weimeraner that experienced an acute onset of right cerebellar ataxia and left head tilt similar to the dog described in this case example and the dogs seen in Video 13-32 and Video 13-33. The hemorrhagic infarction and ischemia are limited to the right half of vermis and right cerebellar hemisphere.

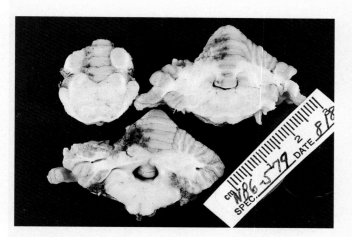

FIGURE 13-88 Transverse sections of the mesencephalon, pons, cerebellum, and medulla of a 12-year-old German shepherd that had an acute onset of left cerebellar ataxia with a right head tilt. These transverse sections show the lesions of a hemorrhagic infarction and ischemia of the left half of the cerebellum. A portion of the malacic cerebellar tissue was lost on removal of the brain at necropsy.

(Continued)

CASE EXAMPLE 13-2—cont'd

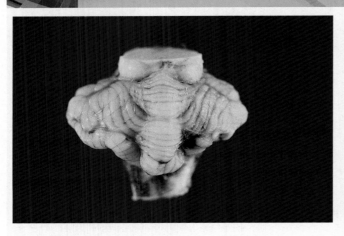

FIGURE 13-91 Dorsal view of the cerebellum from a 9-year-old Samoyed with clinical signs similar to those described for the weimeraner in Fig. 13-90. The clinical signs had not changed for the 4 months prior to euthanasia and necropsy. Note the atrophy of the folia in the right cerebellar hemisphere.

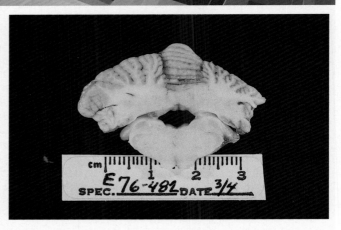

FIGURE 13-92 Transverse section of the cerebellum and medulla of the brain of the dog in Fig. 13-91. Note the folial atrophy in the right vermis and cerebellar hemisphere.

CASE EXAMPLE 13-3

Signalment: 6-year-old spayed female golden retriever, Fawn
Chief Complaint: Abnormal posture and gait
History: Six months before this examination, Fawn fell down a flight of stairs, after which she appeared to be ataxic. The ataxia progressed for 2 months until she was no longer able to stand and walk without assistance. For 4 months, Fawn had to be assisted to walk, as her disorientation progressed.
Examination: See **Video 13-34**. Not shown is an abnormal positional vertical nystagmus and palpation of a hard mass on the caudal right aspect of the calvaria.
Anatomic Diagnosis: Caudal cranial fossa: cerebellum, pons, and medulla

Determining how much of the gait abnormality is the result of dysfunction of the cerebellum and how much is caused by dysfunction of the UMN, GP, and vestibular systems is difficult. All are involved.
Differential Diagnosis: Neoplasm, malformation—cyst, inflammation, abscess

NEOPLASM

The most presumptive clinical diagnosis for these prolonged slowly progressive clinical signs is an extraparenchymal neoplasm. Glioma, ependymoma, and medulloblastoma are less likely to cause such a prolonged course. Meningioma, choroid plexus papilloma, and bone neoplasm are likely considerations for this dog. The fact that a bone mass was palpated in the caudal aspect of the skull is provocative in that it may be the cause of the clinical signs. A malformation with the formation of a dermoid or epidermoid cyst or a subarachnoid cyst is a less common possibility as a cause of these clinical signs. A chronic inflammation is also a consideration. Neosporosis is more likely than a viral, rickettsial, or fungal infection or granulomatous meningoencephalitis. The animal had no history of

a previous or associated otitis media to make an abscess a more serious consideration. MR imaging showed a large bony mass extending from the right temporal muscle through the right parietal and occipital bones into the right side of the cerebellum and occipital lobe compressing the cerebellum and adjacent brainstem (Figs. 13-93 through 13-95). Additionally, significant syringohydromyelia was seen in the cranial cervical spinal cord segments (Figs. 13-96, 13-97), which was

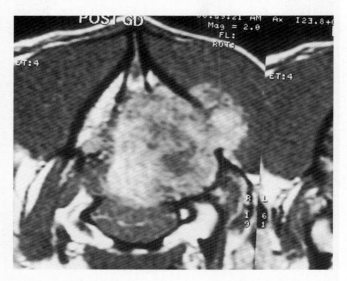

FIGURE 13-93 Axial T1-weighted MR image with contrast of the brain of the 6-year-old golden retriever described in this case example and seen in Video 13-34. Note the contrast-enhanced mass lesion in the right temporal muscle that is continuous with a large mass in the caudal cranial fossa, essentially replacing the cerebellum and compressing the medulla.

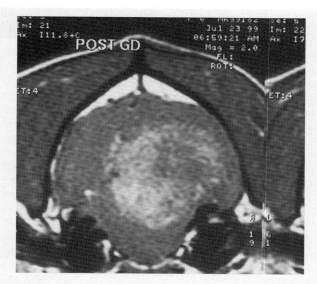

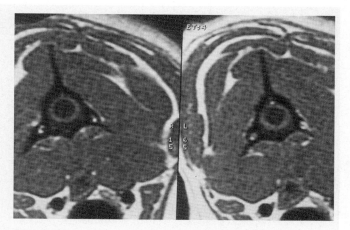

FIGURE 13-96 T1-weighted MR image of the neck of the dog in Figs. 13-93 through 13-95 at the level of the axis. Note the large hypointense cavity in the spinal cord. This image indicates syringohydromyelia.

FIGURE 13-94 Another axial T1-weighted MR image with contrast from the dog in Fig. 13-93 but rostral to it, showing the large contrast-enhanced mass compressing the cerebellum and right occipital lobe.

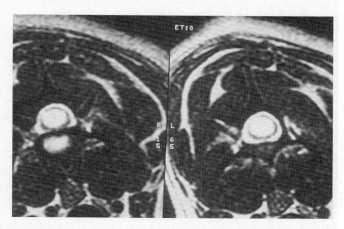

FIGURE 13-97 T2-weighted MR image at the same level of the neck as in Fig. 13-96, showing the hyperintense fluid in the spinal cord cavity.

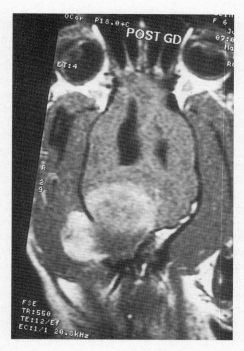

FIGURE 13-95 Dorsal plane T1-weighted MR image of the dog in Figs. 13-93 and 13-94, showing the same contrast-enhancing mass occupying the space normally filled with the cerebellum and right occipital lobe and continuous through the calvaria into the right temporal muscle (left side of figure).

most likely related to the interference with CSF flow pattern at the foramen magnum as a result of the space occupied by the mass lesion in the caudal cranial fossa. The mass lesion had the appearance of a multilobular bone tumor, which is common in the calvarial bones.

The bone mass was surgically removed. The last portion of the video, which shows this dog walking unassisted, was recorded 2 months after the surgery. Microscopic examination of the mass confirmed it to be a multilobular bone tumor.

To review two other dogs and one cat with neoplasms in the caudal cranial fossa and clinical signs that include cerebellar dysfunction, see the following videos. Video 8-1 in Chapter 8 illustrates an example of opisthotonus and extensor rigidity in a dog, and Video 12-7 in Chapter 12, Case Example 12-4, Video 12-19, and Case Example 12-10 highlight examples of dysfunction of the central components of the vestibular system.

CASE EXAMPLE 13-4

Signalment: 1.5-year-old female Parson (Jack) Russell terrier, Misty

Chief Complaint: Abnormal gait and falling

History: The owner purchased Misty when she was 3 months old. At that time, Misty's gait seemed slightly different, which became more obvious over the next few weeks. By 16 months of age, the gait abnormality had progressed to approximately the severity seen on the video. She often falls when excited and has recently fallen down the stairs.

Examination: See **Video 13-35**. Neither abnormal nystagmus nor any head and neck tremor were observed.

Anatomic Diagnosis: Diffuse cerebellum

Differential Diagnosis: Cerebellar cortical abiotrophy, neuronal storage disease, axonopathy (hereditary ataxia), inflammation, neoplasm, malformation—cyst

Cerebellar cortical abiotrophy and neuronal storage disease might explain this anatomic diagnosis, but these abnormalities have not been reported in this breed. Infectious or autoimmune inflammations are strong considerations but are less likely to be confined to the cerebellum and for this long of a period, with the exception of *N. caninum* infection. The young age decreases the likelihood for a cerebellar neoplasm except for the relatively rare medulloblastoma. Dermoid, epidermoid, or subarachnoid cysts are possibilities and require imaging for diagnosis.

AXONOPATHY (HEREDITARY ATAXIA)

Parson (Jack) Russell and Smooth Fox Terriers

Based on the prolonged course of slowly progressive clinical signs of a cerebellovestibular system disorder in this breed, the most presumptive clinical diagnosis is the encephalomyelopathy, described in Parson (Jack) Russell terriers and smooth fox terriers, called hereditary ataxia, a form of spinocerebellar degeneration.[16,18,68] This abnormality is a form of axonopathy with secondary demyelination and astrogliosis that is most prominent in the spinal cord as a bilaterally symmetric lesion, especially in the superficial tracts of the lateral and ventral funiculi. Axonopathy is also extensive with the formation of large spheroids in the trapezoid body but only a mild axonopathy in the cerebellum. The clinical disorder was first described by Bjorck in 25 smooth fox terriers in Sweden in 1957, followed by a description of the lesions in these dogs in 1962.[16,18] In 1973, Hartley and Palmer described a similar syndrome in two Parson (Jack) Russell terriers, a closely related breed.[68] The onset of the clinical signs varies from 2 to 9 months of age and usually starts in the pelvic limbs and progresses to the thoracic limbs. After several months of slow progression, the disease may become static. We have seen dogs 10 to 12 years old with these clinical signs unchanged since 1 to 2 years of age. No antemortem ancillary procedure is available to support this diagnosis except for the brainstem auditory evoked response test (see Chapter 15). In some affected dogs, only the first two wave responses will occur in this test because of the lesion in the trapezoid body. The dysmetric gait disorder with balance loss is typically cerebellovestibular in origin without a head tremor or abnormal nystagmus. The paradox is that the most extensive lesions (excluding the trapezoid body) are in the spinal cord affecting the GP (spinocerebellar), UMN, and vestibulospinal tracts. We assume that additional cerebellar cortical abnormalities exist that are not visible by examination with the light microscope. Bjorck proposed an inheritance of an autosomal recessive gene for the smooth fox terriers. More recently, a polygenic mode of inheritance has been proposed for the Parson (Jack) Russell terriers.[137] These authors also reported observing generalized seizures in approximately one third of their Parson (Jack) Russell terriers. Research on humans has produced a large volume of literature on inherited spinocerebellar ataxia with an established genetic mechanism for many of them.

For another example of this inherited axonopathy, see **Video 13-36**. This video shows Elli, an 8-month-old female Parson (Jack) Russell terrier with a progressive gait disorder since 5 months of age. We thank Dr. Marc Kent at the University of Georgia for the use of this video.

Ibizan Hounds

We have studied a remarkably similar syndrome in Ibizan hounds that is inherited as an autosomal recessive gene.[131] The onset of the gait disorder is approximately the time that these Ibizan hound puppies first begin to walk. Initially, the clinical signs are observed in the pelvic limbs, but the disorder rapidly progresses to the thoracic limbs. The extreme dysmetria causes a bobbing, bouncy, explosive type of ataxia. Trunkal swaying and balance loss is marked. See **Video 13-37** to appreciate the extent of these clinical signs and their cerebellovestibular quality. Three dogs are featured in this video. They are 2-year-old littermates, and their clinical signs have not changed since 1 year of age. All of these dogs lack any patellar reflexes but have normal withdrawal reflexes. Muscle tone is normal to increased, and no muscle atrophy is observed, which suggests that the loss of the patellar reflex involves the sensory portion of the reflex arc. Cranial nerves are normal, and neither abnormal nystagmus nor head and neck tremor is observed. Some of the affected Ibizan hounds have also had generalized seizures. In most affected dogs, the clinical signs progress for 5 to 10 months and become static. Some dogs become recumbent and unable to stand; others remain ambulatory with the type of gait disorder seen on the video. Their lesions are identical to those of the smooth fox terriers and Parson (Jack) Russell terriers and include the unique involvement of the axons in the trapezoid body. In addition, we have observed some mild scattered lesions of axonal and myelin degeneration in spinal nerve roots and specific named peripheral nerves.

CASE EXAMPLE 13-5

Signalment: 7-month-old male Portuguese water dog, George
Chief Complaint: Abnormal gait
History: George was considered to be normal until he was approximately 5 months old when his gait changed. The owners described a high stepping wobbly gait and a swaying of his body. These clinical signs progressed. A littermate exhibited similar clinical signs starting at 4 months of age. He was euthanized at 6 months of age because of the progression of his gait disorder. No necropsy was performed.
Examination: See **Video 13-38**. Three Portuguese water dogs are featured on this video, starting with George. The other two dogs are 6 months old with clinical signs that started at approximately 4 months of age.
Anatomic Diagnosis: Diffuse cerebellum
Differential Diagnosis: Cerebellar cortical abiotrophy, neuronal storage disease, inflammation, neoplasm, malformation—cyst

See the previous discussion for the differential diagnosis of Case Example 13-4. If the littermate had the same disease as George, the possibility of an inherited degenerative disease becomes a strong consideration. At the time of euthanasia and necropsy of George, our presumptive clinical diagnosis was a cerebellar cortical abiotrophy, which had not been reported in this breed at the time of this study in the early 1980s, but there always has to be a first time, and we had this experience in other breeds. Additionally, no reports had been issued of a neuronal storage disease in this breed at the time of this study. No other clinical signs to suggest a diffuse CNS disorder were observed, as occurs in many neuronal storage diseases. The fairly short period of observation might account for the absence of any prosencephalic clinical signs or any diffuse whole-body tremors that are common in neuronal storage diseases.

NEURONAL STORAGE DISEASE

Portuguese Water Dogs

George was euthanized, and necropsy showed a diffuse distribution of neuronal cell bodies with vacuoles distending their cytoplasm. This distribution was especially pronounced in the Purkinje neurons, but no population of neurons was spared (Fig. 13-98). The vacuoles are the result of the accumulation of a substrate because the neuron lacks the necessary degradative lysosomal enzyme to break it down. This feature is classic of a neuronal storage disease. We had not saved fresh-frozen tissue for biochemical examination; thus we were unable to identify the stored substrate in these neurons accurately. In 1987,

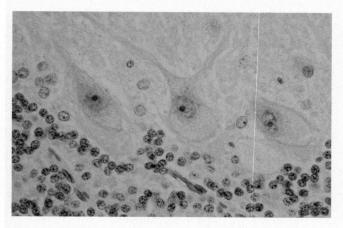

FIGURE 13-98 Microscopic section of a cerebellar folium from the 7-month-old Portuguese water dog described in Video 13-38. Note the swelling of the cytoplasm caused by the accumulation of the GM1 ganglioside substrate.

Dr. Linda Shell studied a Portuguese water dog with this same clinical syndrome that started at 5 months of age. She obtained tissue for biochemical analysis and determined this syndrome to be a GM1 gangliosidosis caused by a deficiency of the degradative enzyme beta galactosidase.[117,122] This neuronal storage disease is presumed to be inherited as an autosomal recessive gene. Enzyme analysis of red blood cells can be used to determine affected and carrier dogs.

American Bulldog

See **Videos 13-39 and 13-40**. These videos show two 4.5-year-old American bulldogs with an onset of a similar gait disorder between 1 and 3 years of age that slowly progressed. At least nine of these American bulldogs have been studied by Drs. Donald Levesque and Jason Evans from breeders in the Las Vegas, Nevada, area.[60,93] We thank Dr. Levesque and Dr. Evans for providing these two videos. After several years of progression, an affected dog may become unable to stand to walk but retain some voluntary movement (nonambulatory tetraparesis and ataxia). Study the videos. The dysmetria and mild balance loss have a cerebellar quality, but excluding involvement of the UMN and GP systems in the brainstem or spinal cord is difficult, especially in the pelvic limbs, which appear to exhibit a mild degree of spastic paresis and GP ataxia. A precise anatomic diagnosis is difficult to make. When a similar clinical syndrome occurs in several animals of a single breed and has a diffuse or multifocal anatomic diagnosis, an inherited degenerative disease needs strong consideration.

Pathologic study of all of the affected American bulldogs that were euthanized revealed a diffuse neuronal storage disease with autoflourescent, periodic acid-Schiff–positive lipopigment inclusions in the cytoplasm of neuronal cell bodies throughout the CNS, including the retinae. Axonal spheroids were abundant, especially in the proprioceptive nuclei in the medulla and in the spinal cord gray matter. Immunocytochemical analysis showed these inclusions to be products of lipid peroxidation that were identified as ceroid lipofuscin on ultrastructural examination. This ceroid lipofuscinosis is a variant form that causes a late onset of a slowly progressive gait disorder that is inherited in the American bulldog as an autosomal recessive gene.[60,93] A genetic test is now available for diagnosis of affected and carrier dogs.

Dachshunds

In 1976, Dr. John Cummings and I (AD) studied a 4-year-old wirehair dachshund that had a progressive gait disorder of all four limbs for over 1 year.[41,135] Our anatomic diagnosis was a cerebellar disorder. At necropsy, microscopic examination of the brain showed an extensive loss of Purkinje neurons, and the remaining few exhibited a swollen cytoplasm containing a lipid material. Similar swollen neurons were present in numerous brainstem nuclei and the spinal cord gray matter. The cerebral cortex was least affected. Histochemical and ultrastructural studies showed the stored lipid material to be a ceroid lipofuscin. A similar neuronal ceroid-lipofuscinosis is described in other older dachshunds without recognized clinical signs of cerebellar ataxia.

Cairn Terrier

See Video 10-47, Case Example 10-23, in Chapter 10. This video shows a 9.5-week-old cairn terrier puppy with clinical signs of a diffuse or multifocal spinal cord disorder, as well as a suggestion of cerebellar involvement. This puppy has globoid cell leukodystrophy, which is an inherited disorder of myelin maintenance. The clinical signs can initially relate to the cerebellar lesion or the thoracolumbar spinal cord lesion and then progress to involve both areas.

REFERENCES

1. Altman J: Postnatal development of the cerebellar cortex in the rat. I. The external germinal layer and the transitional molecular layer, *J Comp Neurol* 145:353, 1972.
2. Altman J: Postnatal development of the cerebellar cortex in the rat. II. Phases in the maturation of the Purkinje cells and of the molecular layer, *J Comp Neurol* 145:399, 1972.
3. Altman J: Postnatal development of the cerebellar cortex in the rat. III. Maturation of the components of the granular layer, *J Comp Neurol* 145:465, 1972.
4. Altman J: Experimental reorganization of the cerebellar cortex. I. Morphological effects of elimination of all microneurons with prolonged x-irradiation started at birth, *J Comp Neurol* 146:355, 1972.
5. Altman J: Experimental reorganization of the cerebellar cortex. II. Effects of elimination of most microneurons with prolonged x-irradiation at 4 days, *J Comp Neurol* 149:123, 1973.
6. Bagley RS, et al: Cerebellar infarction caused by arterial thrombosis in a dog, *J Am Vet Med Assoc* 192:785-787, 1988.
7. Bagley RS, Silver GM, Gavin PR: Cerebellar cystic meningioma in a dog, *J Am Anim Hosp Assoc* 36:413-415, 2000.
8. Baird JD, MacKenzie CD: Cerebellar hypoplasia and degeneration in part Arab horses, *Aust Vet J* 50:25, 1974.
9. Barlow RM: Further observations on bovine familial convulsions and ataxia, *Vet Rec* 105:91, 1979.
10. Barlow RM: Morphogenesis of cerebellar lesions in bovine convulsions and ataxia, *Vet Pathol* 18:151, 1981.
11. Barlow RM, Linklater KA, Young GB: Familial convulsions and ataxia in Angus calves, *Vet Rec* 83:60, 1968.
12. Barone G, Foureman P, de Lahunta A: Adult onset cerebellar cortical abiotrophy and retinal degeneration in a domestic shorthair cat, *J Am Anim Hosp Assoc* 38:51-54, 2002.
13. Bedard P: The nigrostriatal pathway. A correlative study based on neuroanatomical and neurochemical criteria in the cat and monkey, *Exp Neurol* 25:365, 1969.
14. Bildfell RJ, Mitchell SK, de Lahunta A: Cerebellar cortical degeneration in a Labrador retriever, *Can Vet J* 36:570-572, 1995.
15. Bistner S, Rubin LF, Saunders LZ: The ocular lesions of bovine viral diarrhea-mucosal disease, *Vet Pathol* 7:275, 1970.
16. Bjorck G, Dyrendahl S, Olsson SE: Hereditary ataxia in smooth-haired fox terriers, *Vet Rec* 69:871, 1957.
17. Bjorck G, et al: Congenital cerebellar ataxia in the Gotland pony breed, *Zentralbl Veterinaermed* 20:341, 1967.
18. Bjorck G, et al: Hereditary ataxia in fox terriers, *Arch Neuropathol* (Suppl) 1:45, 1962.
19. Borghesani PR, et al: BDNF stimulates migration of cerebellar granule cells, *Development* 129:1435, 2002.
20. Brown TT, et al: Pathogenetic studies of infection of the bovine fetus with bovine viral diarrhea virus. II. Ocular lesions, *Vet Pathol* 12:394, 1975.
21. Brown TT: *Pathogenetic studies of bovine viral diarrhea infection in the bovine fetus* [doctoral thesis], Ithaca, NY, 1973, Cornell University.
22. Brown TT, et al: Pathogenetic studies of infection of the bovine fetus with bovine viral diarrhea virus. I. Cerebellar atrophy, *Vet Pathol* 11:486-505, 1974.
23. Brown TT, et al: Virus-induced congenital anomalies of the bovine fetus. II. Histopathology of cerebellar degeneration (hypoplasia) induced by the virus of bovine viral diarrhea-mucosal disease, *Cornell Vet* 63:561-578, 1973.
24. Cantile C, Arispici M: Necrotizing cerebellitis due to Neospora caninum infection in an old dog, *J Vet Med Series A* 49:47-50, 2002.
25. Carmichael KP, Richey LJ: Cerebellar Purkinje cell degeneration and hepatic microvascular dysplasia in Havana Brown kittens [abstract], *Vet Pathol* 42:689, 2005.
26. Carpenter MB, Donald H: A study of congenital feline cerebellar malformations, *J Comp Neurol* 105:51, 1956.
27. Chambers WW, Spraque JM: Functional localization in the cerebellum. I. Organization in longitudinal corticonuclear zones and their contribution to the control of posture both extrapyramidal and pyramidal, *J Comp Neurol* 103:105, 1955.
28. Chambers WW, Spraque JM: Functional localization in the cerebellum. II. Somatotopic organization in cortex and nuclei, *Arch Neurol Psych* 74:653, 1955.
29. Chan-Palay V, Palay SL, Wu JY: Gamma-aminobutyric acid pathways in the cerebellum studied by retrograde and antegrade transport of glutamic acid decarboxylase antibody after in vivo injections, *Anat Embryol* 157:1, 1979.
30. Cho DY, Leipold HW: Cerebellar cortical atrophy in a Charolais calf, *Vet Pathol* 15:264, 1978.
31. Coates JR, O'Brien DP, Kline KL: Neonatal cerebellar ataxia in Coton de Tulear dogs, *J Vet Intern Med* 16:680-689, 2002.
32. Cordy DR, Snelbaker HA: Cerebellar hypoplasia and degeneration in a family of Airedale dogs, *J Neuropathol Exp Neurol* 11:324, 1952.
33. Cork LC, Troncoso JC, Price DL: Canine inherited ataxia, *Ann Neurol* 9:492, 1981.
34. Courville J, Faraco-Cantin F: On the origin of the climbing fibers of the cerebellum: an experimental study in the cat with an autoradiographic tracing method, *Neurosci* 3:797, 1978.
35. Csiza CK: *Feline panleukopenia virus as an etiological agent of ataxia: pathogenesis and immune carrier state* [doctoral thesis], Ithaca, NY, 1970, Cornell University.
36. Csiza CK, et al: Spontaneous feline ataxia, *Cornell Vet* 62:300, 1972.
37. Csiza CK, et al: Pathogenesis of feline panleukopenia virus in susceptible newborn kittens. I. Clinical signs, hematology, serology, and virology, *Infect Immunol* 3:833, 1971.
38. Csiza CK, et al: Pathogenesis of feline panleukopenia virus in susceptible kittens. II. Pathology and immunofluorescence, *Infect Immunol* 3:838, 1971.
39. Csiza CK, et al: Feline viruses. XIV. Transplacental infections in spontaneous panleukopenia of cats, *Cornell Vet* 61:423-439, 1971.
40. Csiza CK, et al: Respiratory signs and central nervous system lesions in cats infected with panleukopenia virus. A case report, *Cornell Vet* 62:192, 1972.
41. Cummings JF, de Lahunta A: An adult case of canine neuronal ceroid-lipofuscinosis, *Acta Neuropathol* 39:43, 1977.
42. Deforest ME, Eger CE, Basrur PK: Hereditary cerebellar neuronal abiotrophy in a Kerry blue terrier dog, *Can Vet J* 19:198, 1978.
43. de Lahunta A: Cerebellar degeneration. In Andrews EJ, Ward BC, Altman NH, editors: *Spontaneous animal models of human disease*, New York, 1979, Academic Press.
44. de Lahunta A: Comparative cerebellar disease in domestic animals, *Compend Cont Ed* 2:8, 1980.
45. de Lahunta A: Abiotrophy in domestic animals, *Can J Vet Res* 54:65-76, 1990.
46. de Lahunta A, Averill DR Jr: Hereditary cerebellar cortical and extrapyramidal abiotrophy in Kerry blue terriers, *J Am Vet Med Assoc* 168:1119, 1976.
47. de Lahunta A, et al: Hereditary cerebellar cortical abiotrophy in the Gordon setter, *J Am Vet Med Assoc* 177:538, 1980.
48. Del Cerro MP, Snider RS: Studies on the developing cerebellum. II. The ultrastructure of the external granule layer, *J Comp Neurol* 144:131, 1972.

49. Done JT, et al: Bovine virus diarrhea mucosal disease virus: pathogenicity for the fetal calf following maternal infection, *Vet Rec* 106:473, 1980.

50. DeSilva U, et al: The human reelin gene: isolation, sequencing, and mapping on chromosome 7, *Genome Res* 7:157-164, 1997.

51. Dorling PR, Huxtable CR, Vogel P: Lysosomal storage in Swainsona Spp. toxicosis. An induced mannosidosis, *Neuropathol Appl Neurobiol* 4:285, 1978.

52. Dow RW: Partial agenesis of the cerebellum in dogs, *J Comp Neurol* 72:569, 1940.

53. Dungworth DL, Fowler ME: Cerebellar hypoplasia and degeneration in a foal, *Cornell Vet* 55:17, 1966.

54. Eager RP: Efferent corticonuclear pathways in the cerebellum of the cat, *J Comp Neurol* 120:81, 1963.

55. Eccles JC: The development of the cerebellum of vertebrates in relation to the control of movement, *Naturwissenschaften* 56:525, 1969.

56. Eccles JC, Llinas R, Sasaki K: Golgi cell inhibition in the cerebellar cortex, *Nature* 204:1265, 1964.

57. Edmunds L, Crenshaw D, Shelby LA: Micrognathia and cerebellar hypoplasia in an Aberdeen Angus herd, *J Hered* 64:62, 1973.

58. Ekerot CF, Larson B: Correlation between sagittal projection zones of climbing and mossy fiber paths in cat cerebellar anterior lobe, *Brain Res* 64:446, 1973.

59. Emmerson JL, Delez AL: Cerebellar hypoplasia, hypomyelinogenesis and congenital tremors of pigs associated with prenatal hog cholera vaccination in sows, *J Am Vet Med Assoc* 147:47, 1965.

60. Evans J, et al: A variant form of neuronal ceroid lipofuscinosis in American bulldogs, *J Vet Intern Med* 19:44, 2005.

61. Finnie EP, Leaver DD: Cerebellar hypoplasia in calves, *Aust Vet J* 41:287, 1965.

62. Galano HR, et al: Choroid plexus cyst in a dog, *Vet Radiol Ultrasound* 43:349-352, 2002.

63. Gardner C: *Cerebellar degeneration in three pigs*. Presented at the Senior Seminar, Flower Veterinary Library, Ithaca, NY, 1972, NYS College of Veterinary Medicine, Cornell University.

64. Gearhart MA, de Lahunta A, Summers BA: Cerebellar mass in a dog due to granulomatous meningoencephalitis, *J Am Anim Hosp Assoc* 22:683-686, 1986.

65. Gowers WR: A lecture on abiotrophy, *Lancet* 1:1003, 1902.

66. Green HJ: Congenital hydranencephaly and cerebellar hypoplasia in calves, *J Am Vet Med Assoc* 173:1008, 1978.

67. Hartley WJ, et al: Inherited cerebellar degeneration in the rough coated Collie, *Aust Vet Pract* 8:1-7, 1978.

68. Hartley WJ, Palmer AC: Ataxia in Jack Russell terriers, *Acta Neuropathol* 26:71, 1973.

69. Higgins RJ, LeCouteur RA, Kornegay JN: Late onset progressive spinocerebellar degeneration in Brittany spaniels, *Acta Neuropathol* 96:97-101, 1998.

70. Holden M: *Unusual ataxia in three Samoyeds*. Presented at the Senior Seminar, Flower Veterinary Library, Ithaca, NY, 1974, NYS College of Veterinary Medicine, Cornell University.

71. Holliday TA: Clinical signs of acute and chronic experimental lesions of the cerebellum, *Vet Sci Comm* 3:259-278, 1980.

72. Hong SE, et al: Autosomal recessive lissencephaly with cerebellar hypoplasia is associated with human RELN mutations, *Nat Gen* 26:93-96, 2000.

73. Inada A, Mochizuki M, Izumo S: Study of hereditary cerebellar degeneration in cats, *Am J Vet Res* 57:296-301, 1996.

74. Innes JRM, Rowlands WT, Parry HB: An inherited from of cortical cerebellar atrophy in (daft) lambs in Great Britain, *Vet Rec* 61:225, 1949.

75. Innes IMR, Russell DS, Wilsdon AJ: Familial cerebellar hypoplasia and degeneration in Hereford calves, *J Pathol Bacteriol* 50:455, 1940.

76. Innes JRM, MacNaughton WM: Inherited cortical cerebellar atrophy in (daft) lambs in Great Britain, *Cornell Vet* 40:127, 1950.

77. Jackson W, et al: Neospora caninum in an adult dog with progressive cerebellar signs, *Prog Vet Neurol* 6:124, 1995.

78. Johnson KR, Fourt DL, Ross RH: Hereditary congenital ataxia in Holstein-Fresian calves, *J Dairy Sci* 41:1371, 1958.

79. Johnson RH, Margolis G, Kilham L: Identity of feline ataxia virus with feline panleukopenia virus, *Nature* 214:175, 1967.

80. Jolly RD, et al: Mucopolysaccharidosis IIIA (Sanfilippo syndrome) in a New Zealand Huntaway dog with ataxia, *N Z Vet J* 48:144-148, 2000.

81. Kahrs RF, et al. *An epizootiological investigation into bovine viral diarrhea-mucosal disease as the suspected etiological agent of a series of abortions, still-births, early neonatal deaths and congenital cerebellar disease in a New York State dairy herd*. Paper No. 1 Epizootiology Series from Department of Large Animal Medicine Obstetrics and Surgery, NYS Veterinary College, Cornell University, Ithaca NY, 1969.

82. Kahrs RF, Scott FW, de Lahunta A: Congenital cerebellar hypoplasia and ocular defects in calves following bovine viral diarrhea-mucosal disease infection in pregnant cattle, *J Am Vet Med Assoc* 156:1443-1450, 1970.

83. Kahrs RF, Scott FW, de Lahunta A: Bovine viral diarrhea-mucosal disease abortion and congenital cerebellar hypoplasia in a dairy herd, *J Am Vet Med Assoc* 156: 351-357, 1970.

84. Kahrs RF, Scott FW, de Lahunta A: Epidemiological observations on bovine viral diarrhea-mucosal disease, virus-induced congenital cerebellar hypoplasia and ocular defects in calves, *Teratology* 3:181-184, 1970.

85. Kato M, Dobyns WB: Lissencephaly and the molecular basis of neuronal migration, *Human Molec Genet* 12: R89-R96, 2003.

86. Kay WJ, Budzelovich GN: Cerebellar hypoplasia and agenesis in the dog, *J Neuropathol Exp Neurol* 29:156, 1970.

87. Kent ME, Glass E, de Lahunta A: Cerebellar cortical abiotrophy in a beagle, *J Sm Anim Pract* 41:321-323, 2000.

88. Kilham L, Margolis G: Viral etiology of spontaneous ataxia of cats, *Am J Pathol* 48:991, 1966.

89. Kilham L, Margolis G: Cerebellar disease in cats induced by inoculation of rat virus, *Science* 148:244, 1965.

90. Kilham L, Margolis G, Colby ED: Cerebellar ataxia and its congenital transmission in cats by feline panleukopenia virus, *J Am Vet Med Assoc* 158:888, 1971.

91. Kilham L, Margolis G, Colby ED: Congenital infection of cats and ferrets by feline panleukopenia virus manifested by cerebellar hypoplasia, *Lab Invest* 17:465, 1971.

92. Knecht CD, et al: Cerebellar hypoplasia in chow chows, *J Am Anim Hosp Assoc* 15:51, 1979.

93. Koppang N: Canine ceroid-lipofuscinosis—a model for human neuronal ceroid-lipofuscinosis and aging, *Mech Aging Dev* 2:421, 1973.

94. Kornegay JN: Cerebellar vermian hypoplasia in dogs, *Vet Pathol* 23:374-379, 1986.

95. Leiner HC, Leiner AL: *The treasure at the bottom of the brain* (website): www.newhorizons.org/neuro/leiner.htm. Accessed December 2007.

96. MacKillop E, Schatzberg S, de Lahunta A: Intracranial epidermoid cyst and syringohydromyelia in a dog, *Vet Rad Ultrasound* 47:339-344, 2006.

97. Margolis G, Kilham L: In pursuit of an ataxic hamster or virus-induced cerebellar hypoplasia. In Bailey OD, Smith DE, eds: *The central nervous system*, Baltimore, 1968, Williams and Wilkins.

98. Margolis G, Kilham L: Virus-induced cerebellar hypoplasia. In: Infections of the nervous system, *Res Publ ARNMD* 44:113, 1968.

99. Margolis G, Kilham L, Johnson RH: The parvoviruses and replicating cells: insight into the pathogenesis of cerebellar hypoplasia, *Prog Neuropathol* 1:168, 1971.

100. McConnell JF, Garosi L, Platt SR: Magnetic resonance imaging findings of presumed cerebellar cerebrovascular accident in twelve dogs, *Vet Radiol Ultrasound Radiol* 46: 1-10, 2005.

101. Mettler FA, Goss LJ: Canine chorea due to striocerebellar degeneration of unknown etiology, *J Am Vet Med Assoc* 108:377, 1946.

102. Montgomery DL, Storts RW: Hereditary striatonigral and cerebello-olivary degeneration in the Kerry blue terrier, *Proc Am Col Vet Pathol* 31:119, 1980.

103. O'Brien DP, et al: Genetic mapping of canine multiple system degeneration and ectodermal dysplasia loci, *J Hered* 96:727-734, 2005.

104. Oliver JE, Geary JC: Cerebellar anomalies-two cases, *Vet Med Sm An Clin* 60:697, 1965.

105. Orman HK, Grace OD: Hereditary encephalopathy, a hydrocephalus syndrome in newborn calves, *Cornell Vet* 54:229, 1964.

106. O'Sullivan BM, McPhee CP: Cerebellar hypoplasia of genetic origin in calves, *Aust Vet J* 51:468, 1975.

107. Palmer AC: Pathogenesis and pathology of the cerebello-vestibular syndrome, *J Sm Anim Pract* 11:167, 1970.

108. Palmer AC, et al: Cerebellar hypoplasia and degeneration in the young Arab horse: clinical and neuropathological features, *Vet Rec* 93:62, 1973.

109. Palmer AC, Payne JE, Wallace ME: Hereditary quadriplegia and amblyopia in the Irish setter, *J Sm Anim Pract* 14:343, 1973.

110. Percey DH, et al: Lesions in puppies surviving infection with the canine herpesvirus, *Vet Pathol* 8:37, 1971.

111. Phemister RD, Young S: The postnatal development of the canine cerebellar cortex, *J Comp Neurol* 134:243, 1968.

112. Porter MB, et al: Neurologic disease putatively associated with ingestion of Solanum viarum in goats, *J Am Vet Med Assoc* 223:501-504, 2003.

113. Rakic P: Neuron-glia relationship during granule cell migration in developing cerebellar cortex. A Golgi and electromicroscopic study in Macacus rhesus, *J Comp Neurol* 141:283, 1971.

114. Regnier AM, Ducos de Lahitte MJ, Delisle MB: Dandy-Walker syndrome in a kitten, *J Am An Hosp Assoc* 29:514-518, 1993.

115. Riet-Correa F, et al: Intoxication by Solanum fastigiatum var. fastigiatum as a cause of cerebellar degeneration in cattle, *Cornell Vet* 73:240-256, 1983.

116. Satterthwaite WR, Talbott RE, Brookhart JM: Changes in canine postural control after injury to anterior vermal cerebellum, *Brain Res* 164:269, 1979.

117. Saunders GK, et al: GM1 gangliosidosis in Portuguese water dogs: pathologic and biochemical findings, *Vet Pathol* 25:265-269, 1988.

118. Schatzberg SJ, et al: Polymerase chain reaction (PCR) amplification of parvoviral DNA from brains of dogs and cats with cerebellar hypoplasia, *J Vet Intern Med* 17:501-504, 2003.

119. Schmid VS, Lang JL, Wolf M: Dandy-Walker like syndrome in four dogs: cisternography as a diagnostic aid, *J Am An Hosp Assoc* 36:34-41, 1992.

120. Scott FW, et al: Virus induced congenital anomalies of the bovine fetus. I. Cerebellar degeneration (hypoplasia), ocular lesions and fetal mummification following experimental infection with bovine virus diarrhea-mucosal disease virus, *Cornell Vet* 63:536-560, 1973.

121. Shamir M, Perl S, Sharon L: Late onset of cerebellar abiotrophy in a Siamese cat, *J Sm Anim Pract* 40:343-345, 1999.

122. Shell LG, Potthoff A, Carithers R: Neuronal-visceral GM1 gangliosidosis in Portuguese water dogs, *J Vet Intern Med* 3:1-7, 1989.

123. Sievers J, et al: A time course study of the alterations in the development of the hamster cerebellar cortex after destruction of the overlying meningeal cells with 6-hydroxydopamine on the day of birth, *J Neurocytol* 23:117-134, 1994.

124. Smith DE, Downs I: Postnatal development of the granule cell in the kitten cerebellum, *Am J Anat* 151:527, 1978.

125. Speciale J, de Lahunta A: Cerebellar degeneration in a mature Staffordshire terrier, *J Am Anim Hosp Assoc* 39: 459-462, 2003.

126. Sponseller ML: Equine cerebellar hypoplasia and degeneration, *Proc Am Assoc Eq Pract* 13:123, 1967.

127. Sponseller ML: Equine cerebellar hypoplasia and degeneration, *J Am Vet Med Assoc* 152:313, 1968.

128. Steinberg H, Galbreath EJ: Cerebellar medulloblastoma with multiple differentiation in a dog, *Vet Pathol* 35: 543-546, 1998.

129. Steinberg S, et al: Clinical features of inherited cerebellar degeneration in Gordon setters, *J Am Vet Med Assoc* 179:886, 1981.

130. Steinberg S, et al: Cerebellar degeneration in Old English sheepdogs, *J Am Vet Med Assoc* 217:1162-1165, 2000.

131. Summers BA, Cummings JF, de Lahunta A: *Veterinary neuropathology*, St Louis, 1995, Mosby.

132. Tipold A, et al: Presumed immune-mediated cerebellar granuloprival degeneration in the Coton de Tulear breed, *J Neuroimmunol* 110:130-133, 2000.

133. Van Bogaert L, Innes JRM: Cerebellar disorders in lambs, *Arch Pathol* 50:36, 1950.

134. Van der Merwe LL, Lane E: Diagnosis of cerebellar cortical degeneration in a Scottish terrier using magnetic resonance imaging, *J Sm Anim Pract* 42:409-412, 2001.

135. Vandevelde M, Fatzer R: Neuronal ceroid-lipofuscinosis in older Dachshunds, *Vet Pathol* 17:686, 1980.

136. Vitali CL, Olby NJ: Neurologic dysfunction in hypothyroid hyperlipidemic Labrador Retreivers, *J Vet Intern Med* 21:1316-1322, 2007.

137. Wessmann A, et al: Hereditary ataxia in the Jack Russell terrier—clinical and genetic investigations, *J Vet Intern Med* 18:515-521, 2004.

138. White ME, Whitlock RH, de Lahunta A: A cerebellar abiotrophy of calves, *Cornell Vet* 65:476, 1975.

139. White RG, Rowlands WT: An hereditary defect of newly-born lambs, *Vet Rec* 44:491, 1945.

140. Wilson TM, de Lahunta A, Confer L: Cerebellar degeneration in dairy calves: clinical, pathologic and serologic features of an epizootic caused by bovine virus diarrhea virus, *J Am Vet Med Assoc* 183:1076-1080, 1983.

141. Zaki FA, Kay WJ: Carcinoma of the choroid plexus in a dog, *J Am Vet Med Assoc* 164:1195, 1974.

14 VISUAL SYSTEM

EMBRYOLOGY OF THE EYEBALL

HISTOLOGY OF THE PARS OPTICA RETINA

Pigment Epithelium of the Retina
Photosensitive Layer
External Limiting Membrane
External Nuclear Layer
External Plexiform Layer
Internal Nuclear Layer
Internal Plexiform Layer
Ganglion Layer
Nerve Fiber Layer
Internal Limiting Membrane
Area Centralis
Optic Disk

CENTRAL VISUAL PATHWAY

Optic Nerve
Optic Chiasm and Tract
Pathway for Conscious Perception—Visual Cortex
Reflex Pathway

CLINICAL EVALUATION

Clinical Tests
  Menace Response Test
  Pupillary Light Reflex
Clinical Signs

DISEASES OF THE VISUAL SYSTEM

Abnormal Pupils
  CASE EXAMPLE 14-1
  CASE EXAMPLE 14-2
  CASE EXAMPLE 14-3
    Optic Neuritis
    SARDS
  CASE EXAMPLE 14-4
  Microphthalmia
  Optic Nerve Hypoplasia
  Optic Nerve Injury
  Vitamin A Deficiency
Clinical Evaluation of Prosencephalic Disorders
Diseases of the Visual System
  Normal Pupils

CASE EXAMPLE 14-5
  Necrotizing Meningoencephalitis,
  Necrotizing Leukoencephalitis
CASE EXAMPLE 14-6
  Cuterebra Myiasis
CASE EXAMPLE 14-7
  Thiamin Deficiency Encephalopathy
  Amprolium, Mercury, Postanesthetic
    Hypoxia
  Equine Neonatal Encephalopathy
  Osmolar Imbalance
  Nervous Ketosis
CASE EXAMPLE 14-8
  Equine Leukoencephalomalacia
  Cerebrospinal Nematodiasis
  Intracarotid Drug Injection
  Hepatic Encephalopathy
Adult Cheetah
  Leukoencephalopathy
Storage Diseases

◼ EMBRYOLOGY OF THE EYEBALL

The eyeball (bulbus oculi) is derived from neurectoderm (retina), surface ectoderm (lens and cornea), and mesoderm-neural crest (cornea, sclera, and uvea). In the bird, ectodermal neural crest contributes to the cornea, sclera, and uvea.[152] The amount of contribution of neural crest in the mammal remains to be determined.

The neurectodermal contribution to the eyeball is induced in the neural plate stage at its rostral end on the median plane just before closure to form the neural tube. This portion of the neural tube is destined to form the prosencephalon and subsequently the diencephalon. This initially single primordial optic field area (eye field) is influenced by the adjacent head mesenchyme, which includes mesoderm and neural crest cells. This portion of head mesenchyme is rostral to the notochord and is therefore designated prechordal mesenchyme. The morphogenesis of the eye is controlled by the *Pax 6* gene that is expressed by the prechordal mesenchymal and neurectodermal eye fields. Sonic hedgehog is the signaling protein secreted by these cells that has a diverse role in this morphogenesis.[222] This signaling molecule plays a critical role in establishing the bilateral eye fields from the initial single optic field area of neurectoderm. This area first appears as two depressions within the neural tube, the optic pits, in

each half of the initial prosencephalon. They proceed to grow laterally as evaginations from the neural tube known as *optic vesicles* (Fig. 14-1). Evidence in lower vertebrates indicates that the prosencephalic cells that contribute to each optic vesicle come from both sides of the prosencephalon.[99] This arrangement may relate to the subsequent development of optic nerve axon crossing at the optic chiasm. Improper separation of the single optic area into two primordia by the prechordal mesenchyme leads to the development of the cyclopic malformation with a single median-plane eyeball. The *Veratrum* sp. cyclopamine alkaloid ingested by the ewe interferes with the action of the sonic hedgehog molecule which results in the cyclopic malformation. This occurs specifically at 14 days of gestation.[57] See Chapter 3 for a description of this malformation with the brain malformation holoprosencephaly.

The optic vesicles bulge laterally from the prosencephalon and lie adjacent to the surface ectoderm, where their cells proliferate and induce the surface ectoderm to proliferate to form the lens placode. Differential growth in the wall of the optic vesicle results in the invagination of the portion of the optic vesicle adjacent to the lens placode. This infolding and the more rapid growth of the outer wall of the optic vesicle result in the formation of an optic cup. As the optic vesicle cup grows away from the prosencephalon, its connection elongates into the optic stalk, which is the

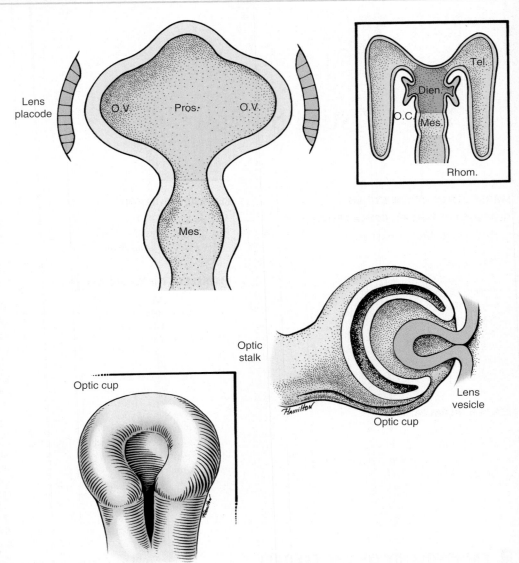

FIGURE 14-1 Development of the eyeball. *Dien.,* Diencephalon; *Mes.,* mesencephalon; *O.C.,* optic cup; *O.V.,* optic vesicle; *Pros.,* prosencephalon; *Rhom.,* rhombencephalon; *Tel.,* telencephalon.

precursor of the pathway of the optic nerve. The optic cup is incomplete ventrally where the optic or choroidal fissure forms. The embryonic hyaloid vasculature enters the developing eye through this fissure. In time, fusion of the edges of this fissure will close the fissure, except for a small notch. The infolding that produces the optic cup also involves the optic stalk, which provides a pathway for the optic nerve axons to enter the brain. The two walls of the optic cup differentiate into the retina.

As the optic vesicle invaginates to form the optic cup, the lens placode that is developing in the surface ectoderm also invaginates to form the lens vesicle, which ultimately separates from the overlying surface ectoderm and remains located at the opening of the optic cup. A fine fibrous connection remains between the inner wall of the optic cup and the posterior surface of the lens vesicle. The anterior cells of the lens vesicle remain cuboidal. The posterior cells elongate to form the primary lens fibers that eventually obliterate the cavity of the lens vesicle. These primary lens fibers lose their nuclei and become the embryonic lens nucleus. The anterior cuboidal cells remain as the lens epithelium. Proliferation and elongation of these cells around the equator

of the lens gives rise to secondary lens fibers. These fibers grow anteriorly between the anterior epithelium and the embryonic nucleus and posteriorly over the embryonic nucleus beneath the lens capsule. Secondary fibers are continually formed at the equator for the life of the animal. The characteristics of these lens fibers impart transparency to the lens. Congenital cataracts develop in the primary lens fibers of the embryonic lens nucleus.[7]

The lens is thought to be partially responsible for the induction of the remaining surface ectodermal cells to form the surface epithelium of the cornea. A rare malformation in cattle is the development of a rudimentary ectopic lens within the cornea. This malformation results from the failure of the lens vesicle to separate from the surface ectoderm that ultimately forms the corneal epithelium.

As these primordial ectodermal structures are forming internal components of the eyeball, a component of mesodermal-neural crest is added to the external surface of the optic stalk and cup. This structure can be considered as an extension of the two supporting layers that are formed around the entire central nervous system, the dense protective dura, and the thinner vascular pia-arachnoid (Fig. 14-2).

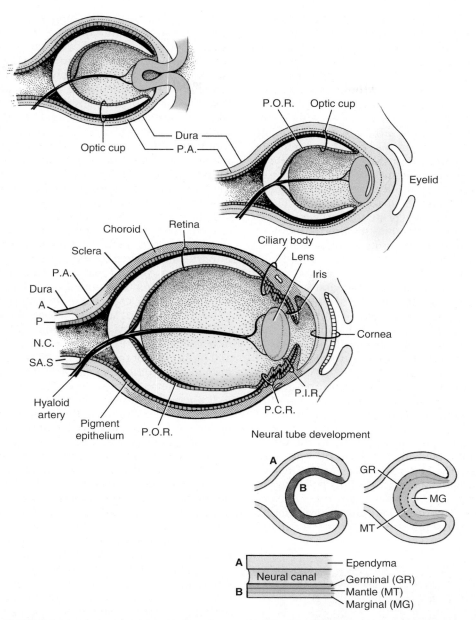

FIGURE 14-2 Development of the eyeball. **A,** Pigment epithelium of the retina; **B,** pars optica retinae (POR). *A,* Arachnoid; *N.C.,* neural canal; *P,* pia mater; *P.A.,* pia arachnoid; *P.C.R.,* pars ciliaris retina; *P.I.R.,* pars iridica retina; *P.O.R.,* pars optica retina; *SA.S,* subarachnoid space.

As the loose mesoderm-neural crest surrounding the brain differentiates into the vascular pia-arachnoid (leptomeninges), this process of differentiation continues along the optic stalk and over the optic cup and lens vesicle. The subarachnoid space found between the pia and the arachnoid over the brain continues along the optic stalk to the posterior surface of the optic cup where it stops. This subarachnoid space is implicated in the spread of disease between the brain and the eyeball. At the optic cup, this space is obliterated, and the mesoderm-neural crest, homologous with the pia-arachnoid, differentiates into the uveal coat of the eyeball (choroid, ciliary body, and iris) and forms the endothelial layer on the posterior (inner) surface of the cornea. This initially loose mesoderm-neural crest completely fills the area between the lens vesicle and the corneal endothelium. A space forms in this tissue, leaving the mesoderm-neural crest anteriorly as the corneal endothelium and posteriorly as the body of the iris and pupillary membrane. This space is the anterior chamber, which fills with aqueous humour. The pupillary membrane is the mesoderm-neural crest located centrally over the lens. Ultimately, it disintegrates to form the pupil. Abnormalities in this disintegration result in a persistent pupillary membrane. This condition is thought to be inherited in Basenji dogs.[139,172] The space formed in the mesoderm-neural crest between the iris and the lens is the posterior chamber, which also fills with aqueous humour. The uvea is the vascular tunic of the eyeball that at the optic stalk is continuous with the pia-arachnoid, the vascular tunic of the central nervous system (CNS). The cells of these layers have some similar histologic characteristics.

The space between the inner wall of the posterior portion of the optic cup and the posterior surface of the lens is the vitreous chamber. The vitreous body that fills this space is derived from secretions from the optic cup, the lens, and the enclosed mesenchyme. Hyaloid blood vessels course in the mesoderm from the base of the brain along the optic stalk in the optic fissure to supply the optic cup, vitreous, and lens. Branches of these blood vessels course through the vitreous to the posterior surface of the lens. These hyaloid vessels normally disappear after birth. Remnants may persist in dogs to around 4 months of age and in cattle until 1 year or more. These reminants are seen emerging from the optic disk that forms at the site of the optic stalk. Abnormal persistence of this hyaloid vasculature to the lens results in the development of cataracts of the posterior lens capsule and an accumulation of blood pigment and fibrovascular tissue posterior to the lens. This lesion is called persistent hyperplastic tunica vasculosa lentis and persistent hyperplastic primary vitreous.[120,159,168] A hereditary basis has been suggested for this disorder in the Doberman pinscher.[194]

As the outer layer of the mesoderm-neural crest surrounding the brain differentiates into the dense pachymeninx (the dura), this process of differentiation continues along the optic stalk and optic cup. Over the optic cup, this layer forms the fibrous tunic of the eyeball, the sclera. It continues anteriorly deep to the surface ectoderm to form the substance of the cornea, the substantia propria. Thus the fibrous tunic of the brain (the dura) and the eyeball (the sclera and corneal substantia propria) have a similar origin that reflects the initial origin of the eyeball from the neural tube.

Differentiation of the optic cup is similar to the differentiation of the neural tube, with two adjacent walls separated by a neural canal (Fig. 14-3; see also Fig. 14-2). The wall of the optic vesicle originally consisted of a single layer of columnar neuroepithelial cells, similar to any other component of the neural tube. These cells were rapidly proliferating neuroepithelial cells. As the lumen of the vesicle is reduced

to a small space by the infolding of the anterior surface, this area forms an outer and inner wall to the optic cup. The differentiation of each of these walls can be compared with that of the neural tube, with the formation of germinal (ventricular zone), mantle, and marginal layers. The entire outer wall of the optic cup, which initially proliferated, later regresses to a single layer of cells. Posterior to where the ciliary body will form and adjacent to the choroid, this optic cup outer wall is the pigment layer of the retina. Anterior to this, it forms the outer layer of the two cell layers that cover the posterior surface of the ciliary body (pars ciliaris retina) and iris (pars iridica retina). Thus this differentiated outer wall of the optic cup is homologous to the ependymal layer of the differentiated neural tube that lines the ventricular system and the central canal and forms the epithelial portion of the choroid plexuses (see Chapter 3). The inner wall of the optic cup, posterior to the level of the ciliary body, differentiates into the multilayered sensory portion of the retina, the pars optica retina. Anterior to this structure, the inner wall of the optic cup differentiates into a single layer of cells that joins with the single layer of cells of the outer wall of the optic cup to form the two-cell layer that covers the posterior surface of the ciliary body (pars ciliaris retina) and the iris (pars iridica retina). Thus these two layers of cells derived from the outer and inner walls of the optic cup are called the *pars ciliaris retina* and *pars iridica retina,* named for the structures that they cover on the posterior surface. The rostral extent of the pars iridica retina determines the margin of the iris, which is the border of the pupil. Beyond this structure, the mesoderm-neural crest of the pupillary membrane degenerates to produce the pupillary space, the pupil. Improper degeneration of this membrane leaves persistent remnants, which may be an inherited abnormality in the Basenji breed.

The outer nonpigmented cells in the pars iridica retina proliferate to form the smooth muscle cells of the dilator muscle of the iris. Thus ectodermal cells are forming smooth muscle at this site.

In the inner wall of the optic cup posterior to the ciliary body, the neuroepithelial cells proliferate as the germinal layer (see Fig. 14-3). With development, this germinal layer differentiates into three layers of neurons. The outer layer of cells closest to the choroid and sclera forms the photoreceptor neurons. These neurons are separated from the pigment epithelium of the retina by the collapsed slitlike lumen of the neural canal and are homologous to the ependymal layer of the nervous system. Two other layers of neurons differentiate in this inner wall of the optic cup. These layers include the layer of bipolar neurons and the ganglion neuron layer. This latter name is another inappropriate use of the term *ganglion,* given that this collection of neuronal cell bodies is within the CNS. Nevertheless, the name has been retained as the acceptable term. The combined layer of bipolar neurons and the ganglion neuronal layer are homologous to the mantle layer of the neural tube. The nerve fiber layer is a layer of axons from the ganglion cell neurons located on the inner surface of this inner wall facing the vitreous. This layer is homologous to the marginal layer on the surface of the neural tube. The axons of these ganglion neurons course to the optic stalk and grow through it to the brain to form the optic nerve. As these axons penetrate the optic stalk, some optic stalk cells degenerate; others differentiate into the glial cells of the optic nerve. The oligodendroglia of the optic stalk myelinate the axons of the ganglion neurons.

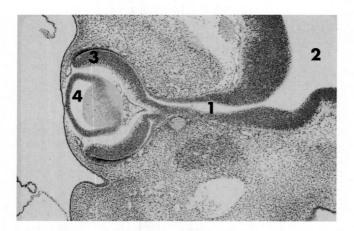

FIGURE 14-3 Microscopic section of the developing eye of a 20-day-old feline embryo. Note the extension of the optic stalk (1) from the diencephalon (2) on the right to the optic cup on the left. All of the cellular proliferation in the optic cup involves the inner layer, where the pars optic retina will form (3). Pigment is evident in the single layer of cells in the outer layer of the optic cup, which is the pigment epithelium of the retina. The optic cup partially surrounds the lens vesicle (4). The anterior epithelium of the lens is in contact with the corneal epithelium. Note the hyaloid blood vessels where the vitreous will form between the optic cup and the posteriors lens.

Myelination occurs in the optic nerve from the brain to the eyeball. This feature is apparent in the white color of the optic disk seen with the ophthalmoscope in the back of the eyeball. The area seen with this instrument is the fundus of the eyeball. No myelination occurs in the nerve fiber layer of the retina.

In dogs and cats at birth, the single layer of ganglion neurons is separated from an outer thick layer of undifferentiated cells that represent the primordia of the photoreceptor neurons and the bipolar neurons.[65,100,187,196] These neuronal cell bodies become separated by the external plexiform layer in the first 7 days of life so that the three definitive layers of retinal neurons are established. In retinal development, an overproduction of neurons occurs, which leads to significant apoptosis to attain the normal population by a few weeks after birth. Their normal development and survival is dependent on these neurons forming synapses on neurons in the brain (i.e., lateral geniculate nucleus, rostral colliculus, pretectal nucleus).[222] Ganglion neurons that do not make appropriate synapses degenerate by apoptosis. In the chicken, up to 20% of the ganglion neuron population degenerates in normal retinal development.[95] In the fetal kitten there are approximately 600,000 ganglion neurons at 47 days of gestation. These neurons progressively decrease to the permanent number of approximately 150,000 by 2 weeks after birth. The histologically mature retina is apparent by 6 weeks of age in the dog, which coincides approximately with the development of visual function. The various media of the eyeball are not transparent until 5 to 6 weeks after birth. The following sequence of development of the eye has been observed in the dog.[6,65]

Gestational day:

Day 15: Optic vesicle and lens placode are well developed.

Day 19: Optic vesicle invaginates to form the optic cup.

Day 25: Lens vesicle is separated from the surface ectoderm. Multicellular inner wall of the optic cup is differentiated into outer nuclear (mantle) and inner marginal zones. The outer wall of the optic cup remains a single layer of cells. Retinal development progresses from central to peripheral in the optic cup inner wall as a *wave* of maturation.

Day 33: Inner neuroblastic (ganglion neuron) layer is separated from outer neuroblastic layer. The optic nerve is formed. Eyelid buds meet and adhere.

Birth: Retina consists of outer neuroblastic layer, inner plexiform layer, ganglion neuron layer, and nerve fiber layer.

Postnatal days:

Days 7-13: The inner and outer nuclear layers of retina are formed.

Day 14: Eyelids separate (9 days in kittens).

Days 16-35: Distinct inner and outer segments of photoreceptor neurons are formed.

Day 21: Optic nerve is myelinated; pupillary light reflex is detectable.

Day 35: Electroretinogram is first detectable.

Day 42: Normal retinal histology is developed.

The tapetum lucidum develops its normal color by 12 to 16 weeks. Before this time, the tapetum lucidum has a blue color when you examine the fundus with an ophthalmoscope.

In contrast to the dog with its short gestational period, the bovine eyeball is fully developed at birth. Studies have shown that the bovine eyeball appears well developed by the end of the second trimester of gestation. The following sequence of development has been observed in the bovine embryo-fetus.[20] Gestational size (mm) and approximate days:

6 mm, 26-30 days: Optic vesicle and lens placode are well developed.

10 mm, 30 days: Optic cup is formed, and lens vesicle is separated from surface ectoderm. The multicellular inner wall of optic cup is differentiated into outer mantle and inner marginal zones.

14-33 mm, 40-50 days: Inner and outer nuclear layers of pars optica retina are separated.

20-40 mm, 40-50 days: Nerve fiber layer is formed. Outer wall of optic cup is transformed from a multicellular layer to a single cell layer.

24 mm, 40 days: Optic nerve is well developed.

40 mm, 50 days: Eyelid buds meet and fuse.

410 mm, 150-180 days: All layers of retina are present.

Birth: Eyelids are separated.

HISTOLOGY OF THE PARS OPTICA RETINA

Ten layers of the pars optica retina are described here, progressing from the outer (scleral) surface to the inner (vitreal) surface. These layers include three groups of neurons, two types of interneurons, astrocytes, and numerous neurotransmitters (Fig. 14-4).[156,186,187]

Pigment Epithelium of the Retina

This epithelium is composed of a single layer of cuboidal cells with their base on a basement membrane apposed to the choroid and their apex facing the photosensitive layer across the potential space of the neural tube (lumen of the optic cup).[159,217] This epithelium is entirely derived from the outer wall of the optic cup. Numerous processes of the apical cell membrane and cytoplasm interdigitate with the processes of the external segments of the photoreceptor rods and cones. In cats, this structure is quite elaborate, with specialized sheetlike projections from the apical surface of the pigment epithelium ensheathing the external segments of the cones and, to a lesser degree, the rods. This close arrangement may facilitate the role of the pigment epithelium in the regeneration of rhodopsin, the visual pigment in the rods, and the removal of degenerate rod membranous lamellae by pigment-cell phagocytosis. Many melanin granules fill the apical cytoplasm of the pigment cells throughout the retina, except over the area occupied by the tapetum lucidum in the adjacent choroid. The presence of these pigment granules partly accounts for the dark color of the non-tapetal portion of the fundus observed with the ophthalmoscope. The tapetum lucidum in the choroid is rendered more visible by the absence of melanin pigment in this pigment epithelium. These pigment cells and the photoreceptor neurons are nourished by the vessels of the choriocapillaris layer of the choroid. This layer is adjacent to the scleral side of the pigment epithelial cells. Exchange of substances between these choroidal vessels and the photoreceptor neurons must pass through the pigment epithelial cells.

Definitive layer   **External (scleral) surface**   **Embryonic derivative**

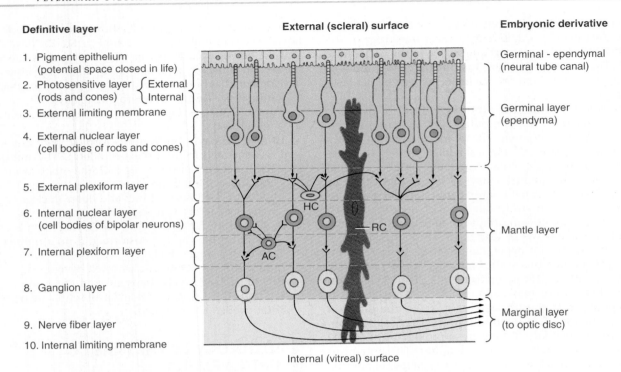

1. Pigment epithelium
   (potential space closed in life)

2. Photosensitive layer ⎰ External
   (rods and cones)   ⎱ Internal

3. External limiting membrane

4. External nuclear layer
   (cell bodies of rods and cones)

5. External plexiform layer

6. Internal nuclear layer
   (cell bodies of bipolar neurons)

7. Internal plexiform layer

8. Ganglion layer

9. Nerve fiber layer

10. Internal limiting membrane

Germinal - ependymal
(neural tube canal)

Germinal layer
(ependyma)

Mantle layer

Marginal layer
(to optic disc)

Internal (vitreal) surface

FIGURE 14-4 Microscopic anatomy of the pars optica retina. *AC,* Amacrine cell (interneuron); *HC,* horizontal cell (interneuron); *RA,* radial astrocyte (Muller neuroglial cell).

Photosensitive Layer

The photosensitive layer,[2] divided into two segments, represents the dendritic zone and cell body of the special somatic afferent neuron, the photoreceptor cell.[210,217] The external and internal segments of the layer are composed of modifications of the cell processes and the bodies of the rod and cone cells. Their nuclei are in the external nuclear layer. The external segment of the photosensitive layer represents the dendritic zones of these neurons. For each neuron (rod and cone), the component in the external segment consists of parallel lamellae within an elongate cell process. These lamellae are orderly stacks of flattened, double-membrane sacs in the form of disks. These membranes are oriented transversely to the axis of the cell process. They are formed at the base of the external segment from the modified cilium located there. These membranes are continually being produced. They migrate distally (away from the vitreous) and are cast off at the outer portion, where they are phagocytized by the pigment epithelial cells.[73,131,220] In the rods, these membranes contain the visual pigment rhodopsin, the photoreceptor substance responsible for light absorption and the initiation of the visual stimulus. A similar substance, iodopsin, is in the cone membranous lamellae. The rod cells are sensitive to low levels of illumination (night vision) and are more abundant in nocturnal animals. Cone cells respond to high levels of illumination (day vision) and are responsible for initiating color vision.

The external segment is connected to the internal segment by a slender stalk containing the modified cilium. The internal segment, called the ellipsoid, is elongated in rods and oval in cones and is composed mostly of endoplasmic reticulum and numerous mitochondria. The ellipsoid is a modification of the cell body of these photoreceptor special somatic afferent neurons.

External Limiting Membrane

The external limiting membrane consists of the junctional complexes between the photoreceptor neurons and the supporting radial astrocytes (the cells of Muller). These latter cells surround and support all the neural elements of the retina between the internal limiting membrane adjacent to the vitreous and the external limiting membrane, which is on the scleral side of the external nuclear layer between the internal segments and the nuclei of the photoreceptor neurons.

External Nuclear Layer

The external nuclear layer is composed of the nuclei of the cell bodies of the photoreceptors, which are special somatic afferent neurons. The cone nuclei are located adjacent to the external limiting membrane. The rod nuclei are smaller than cone nuclei and constitute most of this layer. They extend in several layers toward the vitreal surface of the retina. In the dog retina, the ratio of rod cells to cone cells is estimated to be approximately 18 to 1. The number of cone cells increases toward the central area of the retina. Rod cells predominate in the retinas of all the domestic animals that have been studied and are more common in animals that are active during the night when illumination is limited. Axons of the rod and cone cells course vitreally into the next layer.

External Plexiform Layer

The external plexiform layer[122] is composed of the axons and telodendria of the photoreceptor neurons and the axons and dendritic zones of the bipolar neurons and their synaptic arrangements. Intermingled with these neuronal processes are the processes of horizontal cells. The horizontal cell is an interneuron transmitting between different groups of photoreceptor neurons.

Internal Nuclear Layer

The internal nuclear layer consists primarily of the nuclei in the small cell bodies of bipolar neurons, which are the second neurons in the visual pathway and, similar to the photoreceptor neurons, are restricted to the retina. Bipolar neurons connect photoreceptor neurons with the ganglion neurons in the visual pathway. The dendritic zone of the bipolar neuron is in the external plexiform layer. The axon courses from the external plexiform layer, through the internal nuclear layer, and into the internal plexiform layer, where the telodendron is located. The cell body with its nucleus is situated along the axon in the internal nuclear layer, accounting for its bipolar characteristics. On the scleral surface of this internal nuclear layer are the cell bodies of the horizontal interneurons. On the vitreal surface are the cell bodies of another interneuron, the amacrine cell. This interneuron is in synaptic relationship with the bipolar neurons, ganglion neurons, and other amacrine interneurons. In addition, the nuclei of the radial astrocytes are located in this layer. Whereas many rod cells are in synaptic contact with one bipolar neuron, only one cone cell may be synapsing on a bipolar neuron. Thus convergence of rod cell activity on the bipolar neurons takes place.

Internal Plexiform Layer

The internal plexiform layer[123,124] is composed primarily of the axons and telodendria of the bipolar neurons and the axons and dendritic zones of the ganglion neurons and their synaptic arrangements. In addition, the processes of the amacrine interneurons extend throughout this layer.

Ganglion Layer

This neuronal ganglion layer contains the cell bodies and nuclei of the third neuron in the visual pathway.* These cell bodies and nuclei are large multipolar neurons with a large cell body and nucleus that comprise an incomplete layer one to two cells thick between the internal plexiform layer and the nerve fiber layer. This neuron transmits the visually induced impulse to the brain by way of its axon in the optic nerve. Endoplasmic reticulum, Nissl substance, is evident in the cytoplasm of these neuronal cell bodies. These cell bodies vary in size from 6 to 35 microns in diameter. The smallest cell bodies have axons that project to the rostral colliculus. The larger cell bodies have axons that project mostly to the lateral geniculate nucleus. Functional differences may be found between the medial (nasal) and lateral (temporal) portions of the retina. Mean ganglion neuron size is greater in the lateral retina than in the medial retina, suggesting a greater projection from the lateral retina (medial visual field in space) to the lateral geniculate nucleus of the thalamus for cerebral projection. An increased number of ganglion neurons can be found in the area centralis, where the

smaller cell bodies predominate. Remember that the term for this layer, *ganglion,* is a misnomer because it implies that these neurons are outside the CNS, which is incorrect.

Nerve Fiber Layer

The nerve fiber layer consists of the axons of the ganglion neurons coursing on the vitreal surface of the retina to the optic disk. These axons are unmyelinated until they penetrate the sclera at the optic disk. Their myelination by oligodendrocytes at this point accounts for the white color of the optic disk. The nerve fiber layer is most thick in the vicinity of the optic disk. The separation of scleral collagen fibers at the point where the axons of ganglion neurons penetrate the sclera to form the optic nerve is called the *area cribrosa.* Stellate astrocytes are located in this nerve fiber layer.

Internal Limiting Membrane

The internal limiting membrane is formed by the basal cell membrane of the radial astrocyte and a basement membrane adjacent to the vitreous.

Figs. 14-5 and 14-6 show examples of these layers in a dog and horse eye.

Area Centralis

Humans have a round area for most distinct vision located dorsolateral to the optic disk known as the macula (spot), fovea, or central area. This portion of the retina has the

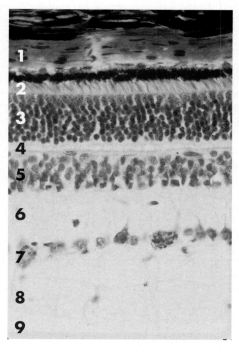

FIGURE 14-5 Microscopic section of the pars optica retina of a dog's eye. The pigment at the top is in the inner (vitreal) portion of the choroid. Beneath this portion, in order, is the tapetum lucidum of the choroid (1), the pigment epithelium of the retina (without pigment), the external segments of the photosensitive layer, (densely stained), the internal segments of the photosensitive layer (2), the external nuclear layer (nuclei of rods and cones) (3), outer plexiform layer (4), inner nuclear layer (primarily nuclei of bipolar cells) (5), inner plexiform layer (6), ganglion cell layer (single layer of large neurons) (7), and nerve fiber layer (8). The vitreous (9) is at the bottom.

*References 79, 87, 196, 198, 202, 203, 208.

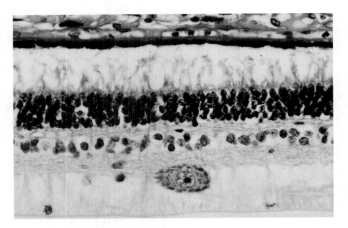

FIGURE 14-6 Microscopic section of the pars optica retina of a horse eye. At the top is a small inner (vitreal) portion of the choroid where no tapetum lucidum is found. The single layer of pigmented cells adjacent to the choroid is the pigment epithelium of the retina. The remaining layers can be identified below as in the previous figure of the dog retina.

highest resolving power necessary for acute vision. In this area, the retina is composed of only cone cells in the photoreceptor layer, and other modifications occur to facilitate its function for visual acuity. For most precise close-up vision such as reading extraocular neuromuscular mechanisms are responsible for the visual field being focused on this central area in each eyeball. Domestic animals have various modifications of this area. In no species of domestic animal is this area readily seen with the ophthalmoscope, except possibly in some cats. In the cat, this area may be identified as a pale streak or oval in the area of the tapetum lucidum dorsolateral to the optic disk in which the blood vessels (arterioles) converge (Fig. 14-7).[209] The area itself is devoid of any large blood vessels. In this area centralis in the cat, an increase in the number of cone cells relative to rod cells can be found in the photosensitive layer, with an overall increase in thickness of the external nuclear layer. The length of the external segments of the photoreceptor cells is increased. The bipolar

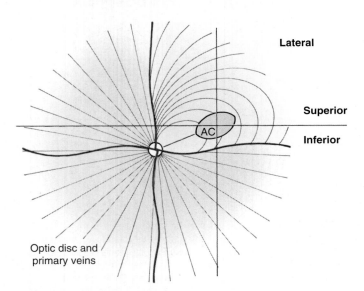

Lateral

Superior

Inferior

AC

Optic disc and primary veins

FIGURE 14-7 Relationship of optic disk and the area centralis (AC) in the retina of a cat.

and ganglion neurons in this area are increased in number as well. The axons in the nerve fiber layer form an arc as they leave the area centralis and course to the optic disk. If the area centralis is defined as a region of the pars optica retina in which ganglion neuron density increases to a peak, then, in all ungulates, this is evident as a streak of high cell density extending horizontally dorsal to the optic disk. This increase in ganglion neurons is maximal near the lateral end of the visual streak, which corresponds approximately to the location of area centralis in cats.

Optic Disk

The optic disk at the origin of the optic nerve varies in shape in the domestic animals, as well as between breeds of dogs, from round to oval to triangular.[15,141,218] It is usually slightly ventrolateral to the posterior pole of the eyeball and varies in its relationship to the level of the tapetum lucidum. In toy breeds, the optic disk may be in the retina entirely inferior to the inferior border of the tapetum lucidum. In medium-size breeds, it is usually halfway over the inferior border of the tapetum lucidum. In large breeds, it may be entirely over the area of the tapetum lucidum. In cats, the optic disk is small, round, and always over the area of the tapetum lucidum. In horses and ruminants, it is just inferior to the inferior border of the tapetum lucidum. The degree of myelination of the optic disk varies between species of domestic animal, with it being the most developed in the dog and least in cattle. The size and arrangement of the blood vessels at the optic disk also vary between species and are the least prominent in the horse and limited to the periphery of the optic disk. Some examples of photographs of the fundus of a normal dog, cat, cow, and horse can be found in Figs. 14-8 through 14-11.

■ CENTRAL VISUAL PATHWAY

Optic Nerve

The growth of the ganglion neuronal axons through the embryonic optic stalk produces the optic nerve.* In reality, the term *optic nerve* is a misnomer, given that a nerve is defined as a bundle of neuronal axons outside the CNS and myelinated by Schwann cells. The optic nerve is, in fact, a tract of the CNS based on its origin within the optic cup, which is an extension of the rostral portion of the neural tube that forms the prosencephalon. The axons in the optic nerve are myelinated by oligodendroglia, and this nerve contains astrocytes. The optic nerve is surrounded by meninges and a subarachnoid space. Extensions of the pia course through the nerve as septa. This structure has clinical importance because the optic nerve is subject to diseases of the CNS and not the peripheral nervous system. When contrast is injected into the cerebellomedullary cistern to produce a myelogram and the head is lowered to direct the contrast into the cranial cavity, an encephalogram is produced. The contrast in the subarachnoid space around the brain surrounds the optic nerve from the middle cranial fossa rostrally to the posterior surface of the eyeball, forming an optic thecogram.

*References 116, 117, 130, 146, 190, 199.

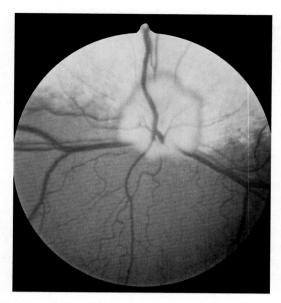

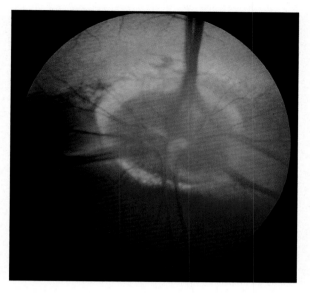

FIGURE 14-8 Fundus of the eye of a medium-sized dog breed. Note the abundant myelination of the optic disk, which is at the inferior border of the choroidal tapetum lucidum. Note the veins located in the center of the optic disk.

FIGURE 14-10 Fundus of a cow eye. Note the optic disk at the inferior border of the choroidal tapetum lucidum with the large tortuous blood vessels and the minimal myelination.

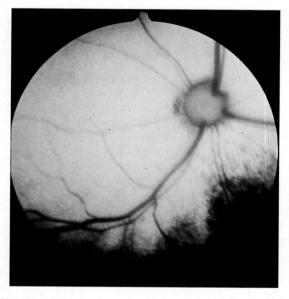

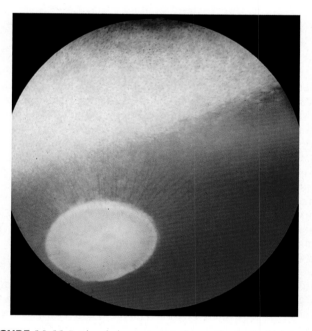

FIGURE 14-9 Fundus of a cat eye with the optic disk positioned over the area of the choroidal tapetum lucidum. Note that the optic disk is small, and all of the blood vessels are at the margin of the optic disk.

FIGURE 14-11 Fundus of a horse eye. Note the prominent optic disk just below the inferior border of the choroidal tapetum lucidum (non–tapetal nigrum area). Note the very small blood vessels only located at the margin of the optic disk.

The optic nerves course caudally in the orbit surrounded by their meninges, extraocular muscles, and periorbita. They enter the skull through the optic canals of the presphenoid bone, which have considerable length in the horse. The optic nerves join at the optic chiasm ventral to the rostral aspect of the hypothalamus and rostral to the hypophysis.

Optic Chiasm and Tract

At the optic chiasm in domestic animals, a majority of the axons in each optic nerve cross to enter the opposite optic tract. These axons are destined to influence the contralateral occipital lobes of the cerebral hemispheres (Fig. 14-12).[31,37,89,188] This arrangement corresponds to the pattern that most sensory modalities that can be localized in space (general proprioception, general somatic afferent) are represented contralaterally in the brain. The factor that determines whether ganglion neuronal axons cross or not in the chiasm is the subject of extensive ongoing investigations. Research has shown that the signal molecule, sonic hedgehog, that is produced in retinal ganglion neurons plays a role in this development.

In fish and birds, all of the optic nerve axons cross in the optic chiasm. In mammals, partial decussation develops in relationship to the development of a binocular field of vision, with frontal positioning of the eyes and the ability to perform coordinated conjugate movements of the

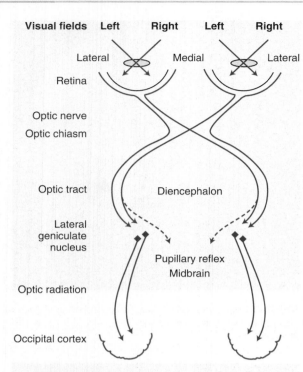

FIGURE 14-12 Central visual pathway for conscious perception.

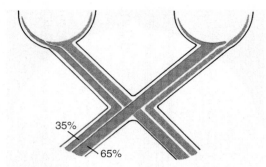

FIGURE 14-13 Origin in retinal ganglion layer of axons in the optic tract of the cat.

eyeballs, including convergence. In primates, in whom this feature is most developed, the degree of decussation is slightly over 50%. Estimates suggest that the degree of decussation in the cat is 65%; in dogs, 75%; and in the horse and farm animals, 80% to 90%. Based on this information, the cat most closely resembles the primate in degree of decussation, frontal positioning of the eyes, and presumably conjugate movements of the eyeballs. As the visual system becomes more complex along with the capability for binocular vision, decussation in the optic chiasm decreases. In avian species, decussation is 100%. The Siamese cat and white Persian tiger have been found to have an increased number of axons that cross in the optic chasm, which is reflected in an altered lamination of the lateral geniculate nucleus. Congenital pendular nystagmus and a convergent strabismus have been considered to be related to this altered visual system architecture in these species.* This feature was described in Chapter 12.

The axons that cross in the optic chiasm come from ganglion neurons in the medial (nasal) aspect of the retina (see Fig. 14-12).[197,200] Axons from ganglion neurons in the lateral (temporal) aspect of the retina remain ipsilateral in their course through the central visual pathway. Neuroanatomic studies in the cat have determined that this division between medial and lateral portions of the retina, based on the axons that cross in the chiasm, is a vertical line approximately through the area centralis. This arrangement was initially determined by cutting one optic tract and studying the retrograde degeneration that occurred in the ganglion neurons of the retina, the axons of which were severed (Fig. 14-13). Studies using horseradish peroxidase injected into the lateral

geniculate nucleus of the thalamus have further confirmed this nasotemporal division of the retina.

The optic tracts course caudodorsolateral over the side of the diencephalon, progressing from ventral to lateral to caudal in relationship to the internal capsule to reach the lateral geniculate nucleus.[19] This nucleus forms a caudodorsolateral protrusion of the thalamus (see Figs. 2-2 through 2-6). Each optic tract contains axons mostly from the medial retina of the contralateral eyeball and the lateral retina of the ipsilateral eyeball. The visual field is defined as the area in space observed by each eyeball when fixed at any one moment. Therefore light from the lateral half of the visual field of each eyeball will stimulate the medial retina, and light from the medial half of the visual field will stimulate the lateral retina. Thus each optic tract contains the axons of neurons in which light generates an impulse from the same half of the visual field of each eyeball. That is, the left optic tract contains the axons of neurons stimulated by light from the right half of the visual field of the left and right eyeballs. Objects in the right visual field of each eyeball are therefore represented in the left central visual pathways.

When the optic tract reaches the level of the lateral geniculate nucleus, two basic courses can be followed: (1) a pathway for conscious perception and (2) a reflex pathway.

Pathway for Conscious Perception— Visual Cortex

Approximately 80% of the optic tract axons in the cat terminate in the lateral geniculate nucleus (see Figs. 2-4 through 2-6). This nucleus contains neuronal cell bodies organized in specific laminae.* A retinotopic anatomic relationship is maintained throughout the central visual pathway. This relationship is reflected in the laminar pattern of the lateral geniculate nucleus. The axons of the neuronal cell bodies in the lateral geniculate nucleus project into the internal capsule and course caudally as the optic radiation in the caudal limb of the internal capsule, which forms the lateral wall of the lateral ventricle (see Figs. 2-5, 2-6). These axons terminate in the cerebral (visual) cortex on the lateral, caudal, and medial aspects of the occipital lobe.[72,150] The gyri that comprise this area include the caudal part of the marginal, ectomarginal (laterally), occipital (caudally), and the splenial (medially) gyri. This pathway from the optic tract to the lateral geniculate nucleus to the optic

*References 4, 22, 32, 77, 78, 94, 114, 176, 182, 183, 200, 204.

*References 53, 75, 76, 82, 83, 93, 113, 173, 175, 201.

radiation of the internal capsule to the visual cortex must be intact for normal conscious visual perception to occur.

Various portions of the visual cortex have connections to the visual cortex of the opposite cerebrum via the corpus callosum, to the motor cortex of both cerebral hemispheres, to the cerebellum by way of the pons, to the rostral colliculus, and to the mesencephalic tegmentum and nuclei of cranial nerves III, IV, and VI directly or indirectly through the rostral colliculus.

Similar to the arrangement in the optic tract, the lateral geniculate nucleus, optic radiation, and visual cortex on one side of the brain contain neurons stimulated by light from objects in the contralateral half of the visual fields of each eyeball. This route is a retinotopic pathway in that specific anatomic portions of the retina are represented in specific anatomic portions of the optic tract, lateral geniculate nucleus, optic radiation, and visual cortex. These retinal areas have a specific representation in the visual field of each eyeball.

In primates, the visual cerebral cortex is divided into functional areas. Area 17 is for vision of stationary objects. Areas 18 and 19 function in panoramic vision for movement, spatial relationship, and depth perception. For normal object vision, interaction is required between the visual cortex and the rostral colliculus. For normal panoramic vision, interaction is required between the visual cortex and the mesencephalic tegmentum. Removal of the rostral colliculus on one side causes hemianopsia in the contralateral visual field for object vision. Bilateral rostral collicular lesions cause blindness for stationary objects. Visual perception of movement and spatial orientation are lost with lesions of the mesencephalic tegmentum. Unilateral lesions of the tegmentum cause a contralateral deficit in addition to causing a severe torsion of the head such that it tilts more than 90 degrees to the side opposite the lesion. Blindfolding corrects this postural dystonia, indicating its visual basis.

In cats, functional differences between the medial (nasal) and lateral (temporal) portions of the retinal ganglion neurons have been found. These neurons in the lateral retina have a greater projection to the thalamus and visual cortex, whereas more of the medial retinal ganglion neurons project to the rostral colliculus. After bilateral removal of the visual cortex of the occipital lobes, some visual orienting responses persist. These cats can detect objects introduced into the lateral visual field of each eye presumably by using their rostral collicular projection, which is more abundant from the medial retina. Total bilateral rostral colliculectomy causes immediate inattention to all visual stimuli and loss of both visual placing and the menace responses. These functions return in a few days to a week. Obviously the cerebral cortex and rostral midbrain have extensive interaction in mediating visually guided behavior. From a clinical perspective, we do not feel confident that we can make an anatomic diagnosis of a rostral collicular lesion.

Reflex Pathway

Two reflex pathways exist for the optic tract axons. One pathway subserves the pupillary light reflex function, and the other pathway involves reflexes concerned with somatic motor responses to retinal activity.

For the pupillary light reflex, approximately 20% of the optic tract axons in the cat pass over the lateral geniculate nucleus to terminate in the mesencephalic pretectal nucleus or the rostral colliculus (see Figs. 2-5 through 2-7). The pretectal nucleus functions in the pupillary light reflex pathway. Optic tract axons terminate in this nucleus. Most of the axons of the neuronal cell bodies in the pretectal nuclei cross in the caudal commissure to synapse in the contralateral general visceral efferent (GVE) parasympathetic oculomotor nucleus. Thus light entering one eye will have its greatest effect on the pupil of that eye because of the crossing of the majority of the axons in the optic chiasm and again at the caudal commissure.

For somatic motor responses to retinal activity, the axons that course into the rostral colliculus form the brachium of the rostral colliculus, which lies between the lateral geniculate nucleus and the rostral colliculus. The rostral colliculus is also a laminated structure, and, in addition to the optic tract axons, it receives axons from the cerebral cortex (especially the visual cortex) and the spinal cord via the spinomesencephalic (spinotectal) tract in the ventral funiculus. Recall from Chapter 3 that the tectum of the mesencephalon is the roof composed of the four colliculi. Tectonuclear axons of cell bodies in the rostral colliculus project to the tegmentum of the midbrain and medulla to influence the nuclei of cranial nerves III, IV, and VI. A tectospinal tract courses caudally from the rostral colliculus, decussates in the midbrain, and continues through the medulla into the ventral funiculus of the cervical spinal cord to contribute to the upper motor neuron that influences the lower motor neurons in the gray matter of the cervical spinal cord.[153] These rostral collicular efferent tracts are important in the activation of muscles concerned with the orientation of the eyes, head, and neck in response to visual input. Think of the muscles that are activated for you to follow the action in a sports event or in your response to a flashbulb. Tectothalamic axons project to the thalamus for feedback to the cerebral cortex, and tectocerebellar axons project to the cerebellum via the rostral cerebellar peduncle. All of these pathways function in the coordination of head, neck, and eyeball movements in response to visual stimuli.

■ CLINICAL EVALUATION

Clinical Tests

Vision can be tested by watching the patient walk in a strange environment or through a maze of obstacles. Owners may be unaware of a loss of vision in their pet if its activity is confined to their home or yard and especially if no stairs are available to negotiate. Owners rarely detect unilateral visual loss. In the neurologic examination, vision is evaluated by the menace response and pupillary light reflexes. [44,46]

Menace Response Test

The menace response test consists of making a menacing gesture with the hand directed at one eye while the other eye is covered and observing closure of the eyelids. You can perform this test as you face your patient or while standing over your patient facing in the same direction. Care must be taken not to touch any of the facial hairs or to create too much air turbulence because a palpebral reflex will be elicited. Cover one eye with your hand that is holding the head and lightly tap the eyelids or the side of the face of the eye being tested so that the patient is aware of the test and to be sure the facial nerve functions normally. The menace response is a learned response that requires the entire peripheral and central components of the visual system pathway and connections from the cerebrum to the brainstem with activation of the facial neurons in the medulla. Being a learned response, it is often absent in young animals. It is, however, usually present in foals and calves by 1 to 2 weeks of age and by 10 to 12 weeks of age in puppies and kittens. In patients with facial nerve paralysis, look for retraction of the eyeball away from the menacing gesture, which will be indicated by a brief protrusion of the third eyelid. Occasionally, this patient will retract its entire head away from the gesture. Based on the observation of numerous kinds of lesions located in the cerebral components of this visual pathway, it has been established that these areas are all necessary for the perception of vision required for this menace response. Experimental studies have defined a role for the rostral colliculus in the normal menace response, but the rarity of lesions localized to one or both rostral colliculi does not permit any similar clinical conclusion.

In all domestic animals, diffuse cerebellar disorders, especially those that involve the interposital and lateral cerebellar nuclei, have often been observed to cause a failure of the menace response to elicit eyelid closure bilaterally. The palpebral reflex is normal, as is their vision, based on eyeball or head retraction. The assumption is either that the pathway that mediates this response passes through the cerebellum to reach the facial neurons (Fig. 14-14) or that the cerebellar lesion causes inhibition of the cerebrocortical neurons involved in this response. An anatomic pathway was described in Chapter 13 on the cerebellum that involves a synapse in the pontine nuclei, a cerebropontocerebellar pathway. Alternatively a pathway may involve the rostral colliculus with or without a pontine relay, a cerebrotectopontocerebellar pathway[115] or cerebrotectocerebellar pathway. See Video 13-22 and Video 13-23 in Chapter 13 for a good example of this feature in Arabian foals with a diffuse cerebellar cortical abiotrophy. In the horse and dog, we have observed a unilateral loss of the menace response in patients with a large unilateral cerebellar lesion on the same side as the menace deficit. This loss may be explained by the crossing that occurs from the cerebrum to the cerebellum at the pontine nucleus (see Fig. 14-14).

Pupillary Light Reflex

The pupillary light reflex was described in Chapter 7. Fig. 7-1 highlights this pathway. The cones are probably the most receptive to this bright light stimulus. Light should be directed toward the lateral (temporal) retina, where the area centralis is located. This procedure tests the visual components of the eyeball and the central visual pathway to the level of the mesencephalic pretectal nuclei at the junction of the thalamus and midbrain. The light reflex pathway continues to the adjacent GVE parasympathetic preganglionic neurons in the rostral portion of the oculomotor nuclei, which mediate the motor response. No involvement of any component of the cerebrum occurs in this reflex. Recall that the direct response to light directed into one eye is greater than the indirect (consensual) response in the other eye because of the majority of optic nerve axons crossing in the optic chiasm and

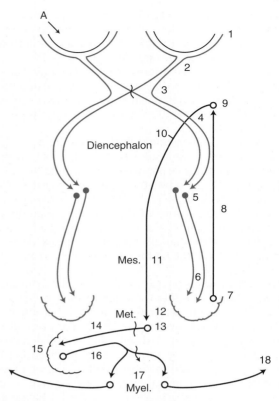

FIGURE 14-14 An anatomic pathway for the menace response. *Mes.,* Mesencephalon; *Met.,* metencephalon; *Myel.,* myelencephalon. ⟨ indicates axons crossing the midline of the brain. A lesion in the left cerebellar hemisphere would prevent a response to a menace directed at the left eye from its left visual field (*A*) because 65% to 90% of the optic nerve axons cross in the optic chiasm.

1. Retina
2. Optic nerve
3. Optic chiasm
4. Optic tract
5. Lateral geniculate nucleus
6. Optic radiation
7. Visual cortex
8. Internal capsule association fiber
9. Motor cortex
10. Internal capsule projection fiber
11. Crus cerebri
12. Longitudinal fibers of the pons
13. Pontine nucleus
14. Transverse fibers of the pons and middle cerebellar peduncle
15. Cerebellar cortex
16. Efferent cerebellar pathway
17. Facial nuclei
18. Facial muscles-orbicularis oculi

the majority of the pretectal nuclear axons crossing through the caudal commissure. This feature is more pronounced in horses and farm animals than in small animals. Lesions in the afferent (visual) portion of this pathway must be severe to cause a loss of this reflex. Remember that the rate of pupil constriction varies among species of domestic animal, being most rapid in cats and slowest in horses. Occasionally, when this reflex is tested, the bright light causes the eyelids to close. This reaction is called the *dazzle reflex,* or squint, and involves optic tract axons that synapse in the rostral colliculus and tectonuclear axons that synapse in the facial nucleus to elicit this motor response. This route is a brainstem pathway similar to the pathway for constriction of the pupils and does not involve the cerebrum.

Clinical Signs

See Table 14-1. Refer to Fig. 7-1 to help you determine what to expect with the following location of lesions. The degree

TABLE 14-1 Clinical Signs of Visual System Lesions

Lesion	OS Menace	Left Eye (OS) Pupil	OD Menace	Right Eye (OD) Pupil
Right optic nerve	Present	Normal size Light in OS; both constrict	Absent	Normal size to partial dilation Light in OD; neither constricts
Right cranial nerve III	Present	Normal size Light in OS; only OS constricts	Present	Complete dilation Light in OD; only OS constricts
Right retrobulbar	Present	Normal size Light in OS; only OS constricts	Absent	Complete dilation Light in OD; neither pupil constricts
Right optic tract	Mostly absent	Normal size Light in OS; both pupils constrict	Mostly present	Normal size Light in OD; both pupils constrict
Right visual cortex	Mostly absent	Normal size Light in OS; both pupils constrict	Mostly present	Normal size Light in OD; both pupils constrict

of visual deficit depends on the location and extent of the lesion in the visual pathway.

Lesions that destroy the retina or optic nerve in one eye cause blindness and a normal to slightly dilated pupil in that eyeball. Pupil size may be normal in the affected eye if enough light enters the normal eyeball to stimulate both oculomotor nuclei. This lesion does not usually cause any disorientation observable in the gait or posture in domestic animals. No head tilt or any neck curvature is observed; in birds, the lesion may cause a head tilt toward the blind eye. No palpebral closure to the menace gesture made toward the affected eye is observed, but the palpebral reflex is normal. Light directed into the affected blind eyeball produces no response in either eyeball. Light directed into the normal eyeball causes both pupils to constrict. In the pupillary light reflex pathway, many of the afferents cross both in the optic chiasm, as well as in the pretectum, to influence both oculomotor nuclei. Observing both eyes simultaneously is often difficult. The best way to observe the pupillary response in both eyes is to swing the light source, which is held close to the eye, continually from one eye to the other and back again. This action is called the *swinging light maneuver*. The speed is determined by how fast you can observe the response in the eye when you swing the light to that eye. As you swing the light from one eye to the other, both pupils constrict when the light is directed into the normal eyeball, However, as the light swings back to the affected eye, that pupil will be dilating back to its original size in room light. If the pupil had not constricted when the light was directed into the normal eye, no change would be seen when the light was moved into the affected eye. If you cover the normal eye with your hand, the pupil in the affected eye will dilate because you have eliminated the only source of light to the oculomotor nuclei.

Bilateral retinal or optic nerve disease that is total causes blindness with both pupils widely dilated and unresponsive to light directed into either eyeball. Sudden acquired retinal degeneration syndrome (SARDS) and optic neuritis are each a common causes of this. Ordinarily, very severe retinal or optic nerve lesions are needed to prevent the pupils from constricting to a bright source of light. In most instances, vision will disappear before the loss of the pupillary light reflex. Therefore an animal may be blind from retinal or optic nerve disease but still have pupils that respond to a bright source of light. However, the pupils may be slightly dilated in the relatively subdued room light. Remember that

the light source used for the pupillary light reflex is very bright, and if any retinal or optic nerve axons are intact, a pupillary light reflex will be observed. Another way to consider this factor is that, as a disease process progressively interferes with retinal or optic nerve function, vision will be lost before the pupillary light reflex. If blindness occurs slowly and the patient is confined to a small environment, the visual deficit may not be noticed. Blind animals may adjust well to their normal surroundings. Owners often describe an acute onset of blindness in their dogs that have either SARDS or optic neuritis, both of which are progressive diseases. These patients have undoubtedly been losing their vision for some time and only when most of these structures have lost their function does the patient appear to be *suddenly* blind.

Unilateral lesions in the optic tract, lateral geniculate nucleus, optic radiation, and visual cortex result in a visual deficit in the contralateral visual field of each eyeball. Because of the degree of decussation in the optic chiasm, the visual deficit can be appreciated only in the contralateral eyeball. This abnormality is called *hemianopsia* because a visual field deficit occurs in 50% of the total visual field. In the dog, this level represents approximately a 25% retinal dysfunction in the ipsilateral eyeball and a 75% retinal dysfunction in the contralateral eyeball. In the dog and cat, the visual deficit is most evident in the failure of the menace response in the contralateral eye. This aspect is very reliable despite the still-intact function of the lateral retinal neurons that do not decussate in the optic chiasm. The visual deficit may be difficult to detect as the patient moves around in its surroundings. Occasionally, an object may be bumped on the side opposite to that of the lesion. However, in many instances, no evidence of a visual deficit is observed. Unilateral blindfolding and maze testing of the patient may be helpful. In the large animals with 80% to 90% of the optic nerve axons crossing in the optic chiasm, a greater tendency exists for the patient to walk into objects on the side of the visual deficit, contralateral to the lesion.

All domestic animals with these unilateral lesions in the central visual pathway exhibit a poor to absent palpebral closure response to menacing gestures to the eyeball that is contralateral to the lesion. If the examiner is careful, this test can be reliably performed without using a transparent barrier between the hand and the eyeball to prevent air currents and direct contact with facial hairs. The dropping of cotton balls, which some recommend instead of the menace test, is unreliable and awkward to perform. In small animals, the eye not being tested must be covered. By menacing the eye from both the medial and lateral visual fields when a lesion exists in the contralateral central visual pathway, you may determine that the deficit is more pronounced when the lateral visual field is tested.

In unilateral lesions of the central visual pathway caudal to the optic chiasm, the pupillary light reflex responses are usually normal. The logical assumption is that a unilateral lesion in the optic tract will cause a decreased pupillary light reflex in the contralateral eyeball because most of the optic nerve axons cross in the optic chiasm and most of the axons of pretectal neurons cross back to the oculomotor nucleus on the side of the eyeball that is stimulated (see Fig. 7-1). In our experience, this difference in the pupillary light reflex response between the two eyeballs with a unilateral optic tract lesion has been difficult to appreciate.

Bilateral lesions in the optic tracts and the lateral geniculate nuclei that involve the pathway to the pretectal nuclei, if complete, will cause blindness with dilated pupils that are unresponsive to light. More often the lesions here are partial, and clinical signs are difficult to determine. Canine distemper virus often produces extensive demyelinating lesions in the optic tracts without obvious clinical deficits of vision or pupillary function.

The central visual pathway from the lateral geniculate nucleus to the visual cortex contains no neurons in the pupillary light reflex pathway, and therefore lesions here cannot interfere with this reflex. Bilateral lesions here can cause complete blindness with normal pupillary light reflexes.

DISEASES OF THE VISUAL SYSTEM

Abnormal Pupils

The following four case examples provide cases of clinical disorders that involve the pupillary light reflex. See Table 7-1 and the description of similar clinical disorders in Chapter 7.

CASE EXAMPLE 14-1

Signalment: 3-year-old male Doberman pinscher
Chief Complaint: Widely dilated left pupil
History: For at least the past 6 days, the left pupil was noticed to be wider than the right pupil.
Examination: This dog's physical and neurologic examinations were normal, except for the cranial nerve examination. Menace responses were normal in both eyes.

In room light, the left pupil was widely dilated. Light directed into the left eyeball constricted only the right pupil. Light directed into the right eyeball constricted only the right pupil. Slight ptosis of the left palpebral fissure and slightly decreased adduction of the left eye on testing normal physiologic nystagmus were observed.
Anatomic Diagnosis: Left oculomotor nucleus or nerve with complete dysfunction of the GVE components and only slight dysfunction of the general somatic efferent (GSE) components
Differential Diagnosis: Retrobulbar abscess or neoplasm, middle cranial fossa neoplasm, neuritis—ganglionitis

No protrusion of the left eyeball was noted, and no resistance was felt or discomfort elicited on applying pressure to the left eyeball through the closed eyelids. We have never seen a neuritis limited to one oculomotor nerve and ciliary ganglion, but this finding has been reported in humans. Our presumptive clinical diagnosis was a neoplasm in the middle cranial fossa compromising the left oculomotor nerve with no clinical signs of brain dysfunction.

No ancillary studies were performed, and 1 week later, this patient was examined again because of progressive depression. This dog was now obtunded and reluctant to stand. If stimulated, he could stand and walk with a normal but slow gait. Postural reactions were slow bilaterally. The cranial nerve examination was unchanged. These observations supported involvement of the ascending reticular activating system (ARAS) in the rostral brainstem. The severity of the obtundation in a dog that could still walk indicated involvement of the ARAS in the diencephalon. At this level, the oculomotor nerve is ventral to the hypothalamus. With the initial clinical signs limited to the left oculomotor nerve, an extraparenchymal (extraaxial, extramedullary)

lesion was presumed, and a mass lesion that compressed this nerve and subsequently the hypothalamus was the presumptive clinical diagnosis. At this age, a germ-cell neoplasm is more common than a pituitary neoplasm or a meningioma. Most pituitary neoplasms grow dorsally into the hypothalamus and do not usually involve the cranial nerves passing through the middle cranial fossa to enter the orbital fissure. They also usually spare the optic nerves and chiasm. This dog was euthanized, and a large germ-cell neoplasm was found at necropsy (Fig. 14-15). In humans, the GVE preganglionic neurons in the oculomotor nerve are on the surface of the nerve where it courses through the middle cranial fossa. Thus these neurons are more at risk for compressive lesions, and pupillary light reflex abnormalities usually precede clinical signs of involvement of the GSE lower motor neurons in this cranial nerve. This neoplasm is readily demonstrated on magnetic resonance (MR) imaging (Fig. 14-16).

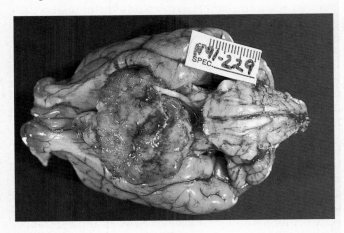

FIGURE 14-15 Ventral surface of the brain of a 4.5-year-old golden retriever with a germ cell neoplasm compressing the rostral brainstem and the cranial nerves coursing through the middle cranial fossa. This lesion is similar to the one seen in this case example at necropsy.

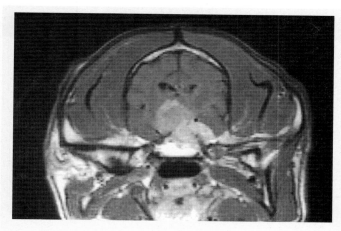

FIGURE 14-16 Axial T1-weighted MR image with contrast of the brain of a 2-year-old mixed-breed dog. Note the hyperintense, contrast-enhanced mass in the middle cranial fossa compressing the rostral brainstem. This lesion is a germ-cell neoplasm.

See **Video 14-1**. This video shows Zeus, a 3-year-old castrated male Doberman pinscher with a history of 7 to 10 days of progressive lethargy and reluctance to perform any activity.

Study the video. Note the obtunded sensorium but the ability to walk without any obvious deficit and the normal hopping responses. The menace responses do not show well on the video but were considered normal. The left pupil is widely dilated. Light directed into the dilated left pupil caused pupillary constriction only in the right pupil. Light directed into the normal-size right pupil caused pupillary constriction only in the right pupil. Both palpebral fissures were narrowed. Poor eye movements were observed on testing normal physiologic nystagmus. The anatomic diagnosis is similar to that in this case example at the time of that dog's second examination. A diencephalic lesion best explains the degree of obtundation caused by an ARAS dysfunction with a normal gait. The most profound cranial nerve deficit is dysfunction of the left oculomotor GVE neurons. The poor eye movement supports mild deficiency of the GSE neurons in cranial nerves III and VI bilaterally. The small palpebral fissures may be caused by the dog's obtunded state or deficiency of oculomotor GSE neurons to the levator palpebrae superioris muscles. A germ-cell neoplasm best explains this anatomic diagnosis at this young age. Zeus was euthanized, and necropsy revealed a large germ-cell neoplasm in the middle cranial fossa (Fig. 14-17).

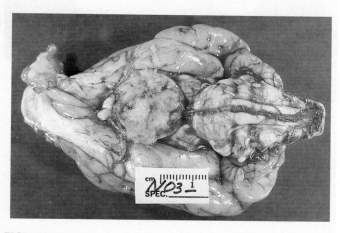

FIGURE 14-17 Ventral surface of the brain of Zeus, the 3-year-old Doberman pinscher seen in Video 14-1. This mass lesion is a germ-cell neoplasm.

CASE EXAMPLE 14-2

Signalment: 5-year-old female miniature poodle
Chief Complaint: Seizures and abnormal behavior
History: Over the past week, this dog had five seizures that were described as generalized. For the past 3 days, she had become more lethargic and occasionally walked in circles or stood in a corner with her head pressed against the wall.
Examination: This dog was responsive but acted very lethargic. She tended to walk in a circle to her right with a normal gait. No paresis or ataxia was noted. Postural reactions were slightly slow in her left limbs. She exhibited no menace response bilaterally. Both pupils were widely dilated. Light directed into the left eye caused no constriction of either pupil. Light directed into the right eye caused no constriction of either pupil until it was directed laterally, and then both pupils constricted.
Anatomic Diagnosis: Intracranial optic nerves, optic chiasm, or both optic tracts with involvement of the adjacent prosencephalon

The seizures require a prosencephalic lesion. See Chapter 18. The cranial nerve examination requires a bilateral retinal, optic nerve, optic chiasm, or both optic tracts lesion with slight sparing in the right retina, right optic nerve, optic chiasm, or left optic tract. The fact that the light caused a bilateral pupil constriction at one site in the right retina indicated that the GVE components of both oculomotor nerves were

normal. A dog with a rostral brainstem lesion will have a normal gait but may exhibit slow postural reactions. In this dog, they were only slow in the left limbs, which implicates involvement of the upper motor neuron (UMN) and general proprioception (GP) systems on the right side of the prosencephalon. In this dog with the lesion in its visual system where it first enters the cranial cavity, a disorder of the diencephalon is presumed. Most dogs that propulsively circle will circle toward their prosencephalic disorder.
Differential Diagnosis: Neoplasia—pituitary tumor, germ-cell tumor, meningioma, sphenoid bone tumor; inflammation—autoimmune optic neuritis (granulomatous meningoencephalitis), canine distemper

The location of the visual system lesion suggests that the lesion is more likely extraparenchymal with invasion or compression (or both) of the diencephalon. Having enough of a diencephalic lesion to cause this degree of lethargy and propulsion is less common for a dog with optic neuritis. Although canine distemper commonly causes demyelinating and inflammatory lesions in the optic nerves and tracts, this degree of visual deficit is unlikely.

Computed tomographic (CT) and MR imaging were not available at the time this dog was studied. She was euthanized, and a macroadenoma of the pituitary gland was diagnosed at necropsy, which extensively compressed and displaced the diencephalon (Fig. 14-18). A rostral

(Continued)

CASE EXAMPLE 14-2—cont'd

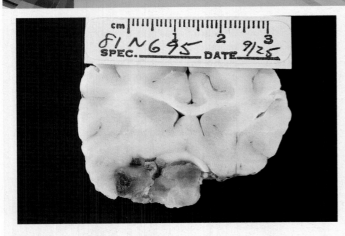

FIGURE 14-18 Transverse section of the preserved brain of the 5-year-old miniature poodle described in this case example. Note the large pituitary macroadenoma elevating and compressing the optic chiasm.

component compressed the intracranial portion of the optic nerves, optic chiasm, and initial portion of the optic tracts. A pituitary macroadenoma is a common tumor in dogs, but compression of the optic nerve or chiasm is less common, given that the gland is just caudal to these structures and usually expands directly dorsally into the hypothalamus. Surgical removal of pituitary neoplasms via a transsphenoidal approach has been described and used for pituitary glands in dogs with pituitary-dependent hyperadrenocorticoidism.[9] Pituitary macroadenomas can be only partially debulked by this procedure. Radiation therapy may result in cessation of growth and some reduction in size of a pituitary macroadenoma.

CASE EXAMPLE 14-3

Signalment: 8-year-old male Welsh corgi cross-breed
Chief Complaint: Blindness
History: The owner reported that this dog suddenly became blind the morning of this examination when he could not find his feed dish.
Examination: This dog was alert and very responsive, craved attention, and walked and played as though he was normal, except he was blind. He would bump into any object that was placed in his pathway, which included the examiner. Postural reactions were normal. Cranial nerve examination was normal except for the eyes. No menace response was elicited bilaterally. Palpebral reflexes were normal. The pupils were moderately dilated in room light. Light directed into the left eye caused both pupils to constrict. Light directed into the right eye caused both pupils to constrict.
Anatomic Diagnosis: Both retinas, both optic nerves, the optic chiasm, or both optic tracts. However, you ask, why do we select this location if the pupillary light reflexes are normal? This question has two answers. Remember: As lesions develop in this portion of the visual system, the vision will be lost before the pupillary light reflex is lost. The latter is the last function to be lost. The pupils are too large in this dog in normal room light, reflecting some degree of loss of the afferent pathway. In addition, your other choice for an anatomic basis for bilateral blindness with normal pupillary responses to light is bilateral cerebral hemispheres, and what prosencephalic lesion will suddenly develop bilaterally and cause blindness with no effect on the dog's sensorium or behavior? The most important clue in this dog is the size of the pupils in room light. The light source that you use

for testing the pupillary light reflex is very intense, and if you do not assess the size of the pupils before you use this bright light, you will miss the fact that the intensity of the room light is insufficient to cause normal constriction.
Differential Diagnosis: Retinal degeneration (sudden acquired retinal degeneration syndrome [SARDS]), inflammation—optic neuritis, other inflammations, neoplasm

OPTIC NEURITIS

SARDS

Neoplasm and inflammation other than an autoimmune optic neuritis are less likely with this degree of visual deficit and no other clinical signs of neurologic disease. Optic neuritis is nonsuppurative and is presumed to be an autoimmune disorder that is often considered to be a focal form of granulomatous meningoencephalitis (GME) (Figs. 14-19, 14-20).[60,149,192] Although minor inflammatory lesions may be scattered in other portions of the brain, they usually do not cause clinical signs. Both optic neuritis and SARDS are progressive disorders. Nonetheless, approximately one half of all cases of either disorder are reported as a sudden onset of blindness. More likely, the owner's *observation* is sudden, but the visual deficit had been progressing without the owner being aware of it, especially with the pet being in its own familiar environment. Clinical blindness occurs when the last of the visual system structure is lost with the disorder. The cause of SARDS is unknown. It begins with a loss of the external segments of the photoreceptor layer, and therefore, at the onset of the blindness, it may not cause any recognizable changes on examination of the fundus with an ophthalmoscope. Thus this abnormality has also been called *silent retinal degeneration*. SARDS is a disease of older dogs that is more common in the medium-size breeds and in dogs that are often obese and may have some association with hyperadrenocorticoidism.

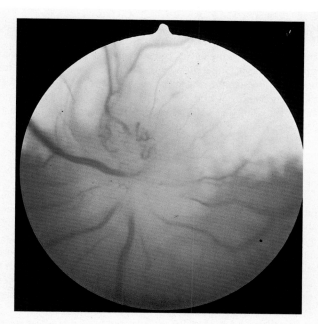

FIGURE 14-21 Photograph of the fundus of a dog with optic neuritis. Note the poor demarcation associated with the edema and discoloration of the optic disk caused by the inflammation in the optic nerve.

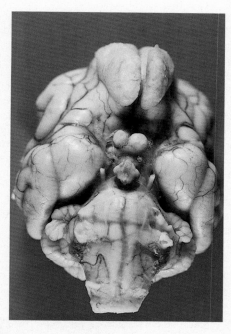

FIGURE 14-19 Ventral surface of the brain of a dog with the form of GME that affects primarily the optic nerves, called optic neuritis. Note the swollen optic nerves and optic chiasm.

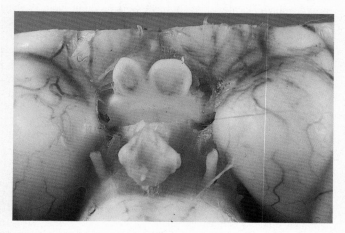

FIGURE 14-20 Higher magnification of the optic nerves and chiasm of the brain in Fig. 14-29 after removing a dorsal plane section of these structures. Note the swelling and discoloration of the optic nerves and optic chiasm caused by the lymphoproliferative inflammation.

An electroretinogram (ERG) determines whether the retina can function and generate impulses when it is exposed to light. In these dogs with retinal degeneration, the readings will be abnormal. In dogs with optic neuritis, the ERG is normal because no lesion exists in the retina other than the optic disk in some dogs. Dogs that have

optic neuritis usually have a swollen and or hemorrhagic optic disk that can be seen with the ophthalmoscope (Fig. 14-21). If the optic neuritis is only in the retrobulbar portion of the optic nerve, the ophthalmoscopic examination will be normal. Remember that the optic nerve is surrounded by cerebrospinal fluid (CSF), and therefore inflammation in this nerve may cause an abnormal CSF evaluation when it is obtained from the cerebellomedullary cistern. The ERG should be performed first because general anesthesia is necessary to obtain the CSF, and the ERG requires only sedation. The dog in this case example had a normal ophthalmoscopic examination, but the ERG showed no retinal activity; thus a diagnosis of SARDS was made. No treatment is available for this disorder, but this patient can remain an acceptable pet as long as the owner protects it from potential injury. This dog needs a seeing eye person for help. Optic neuritis is treated with immunosuppresant drugs.

See **Video 14-2** of Ryan, a 9-year-old castrated male mixed-breed dog, that was suddenly noticed to be blind 2 weeks before this examination. Note the moderately dilated pupils in room light followed by their response to a bright light. This dog has the same anatomic and differential diagnoses as the dog in this case example. The ophthalmoscopic examination was normal. The ERG did not record any retinal activity when Ryan's eyes were exposed to light, indicating a diffuse retinal degeneration and a presumptive clinical diagnosis of SARDS.

See **Video 14-3** of Duffy, an 8-year-old castrated male golden retriever with loss of vision. The owner reported a progressive loss of vision to complete blindness over a period of 3 months. Note the similarity of the ocular examination to that of the miniature poodle in Case Example 14-2. No menace response was observed bilaterally. Both pupils are dilated in room light. Light directed into one eyeball (the right eye in this dog) elicits no response in either eyeball. Light directed into the other eye (the left in this dog) elicits a response in both eyeballs. As the light source swings from the right eye to the left, the dilated left pupil constricts. On swinging the light back to the right eyeball, the right pupil, which had constricted to the light when

(Continued)

it was directed into the left eyeball, is now dilating back to its original size in room light. The remainder of the neurologic examination was normal. The anatomic diagnosis is both retinas, both optic nerves, the optic chiasm, or both optic tracts with slight neuronal sparing in the left retina, left optic nerve, optic chiasm, or right optic tract. No clinical signs on the neurologic examination or any history of clinical signs were observed to implicate a prosencephalic lesion, as occurred in Case Example 14-2. Therefore the differential diagnosis was primarily SARDS or optic neuritis—less likely other inflammations or a neoplasm.

The ophthalmoscopic examination was normal, as was the ERG. See Video 14-3 for CT images after injection of contrast, which showed a hyperdense mass involving the presphenoid bone where the optic canals are located. This bone mass was presumed to be a multilobular bone tumor. It had not displaced the prosencephalon enough to cause any clinical signs. This case emphasizes the value of advanced imaging procedures for all patients with sudden blindness without evidence of ocular disease. If the ERG is normal, the patient should have advanced imaging.

See **Video 14-4** of Renee, an 8-year-old spayed female golden retriever with a 5-day history of progressive loss of vision and loss of any response to her owner. Note the severe degree of obtundation in this dog. However, when she is urged, she can walk without obvious paresis or ataxia, and her postural reactions are normal. She has normal nasal septum nociception. She has bilateral absence of menace responses with dilated pupils that are unresponsive to light. The anatomic diagnosis is intracranial bilateral optic nerves, optic chiasm, optic tracts, and diencephalon. In this dog, in addition to the visual system lesion at this level, is a possible loss of oculomotor GVE lower motor neurons, and the bilateral ptosis may be from slight involvement of the GSE neurons in this nerve, or it may be a result of this dog's obtundation. The profound obtundation in the presence of the ability to walk without obvious paresis or ataxia supports interference with the ascending reticular activating system at the level of the diencephalon. Complete involvement of the optic nerves, optic chiasm, or optic tracts at this level will cause the ocular clinical signs observed in this dog. At this age, an intracranial extraparenchymal neoplasm is the most presumptive clinical diagnosis. CT imaging (see Video 14-4) showed a large contrast-enhancing neoplasm with a broad base on the floor of the cranial cavity at the level of the rostral and middle cranial fossae. A presumptive meningioma was diagnosed.[18] Renee was euthanized, and no necropsy was performed.

Signalment: 3-year-old male collie

Chief Complaint: Seizures

History: This dog had been having seizures approximately once a month since he was 2 years old. The owners described generalized seizures.

Examination: This dog's neurologic examination was normal except for the cranial nerve examination. No menace response was elicited in the left eye. The size of both pupils in room light was normal. Light directed into the left eye caused no response in either eye. Light directed into the right eye caused both pupils to constrict. On swinging the light back to the left eye, the pupil was dilating back to where it started. When the right eye was covered by your hand, the left pupil widely dilated. On removal of your hand the pupil constricted to its original size, which was the same as the right pupil.

Anatomic Diagnosis: Prosencephalon and the left retina or optic nerve

The seizures require a disorder within the prosencephalon. Considering this combination of anatomic diagnoses together is difficult. Possibly, a retrobulbar abscess or neoplasm might extend along the left optic nerve into the cranial cavity and involve the prosencephalon located there, but why were no other clinical signs of progression of the prosencephalic lesion seen over this past year? Remember: With any blindness that involves the retina or optic nerve, an ophthalmoscopic examination is necessary. When this examination was performed in this collie, the right eye was normal, but the left eye showed a large depression at the optic disk. This depression is called a coloboma and is part of an inherited ocular malformation that is common in this breed.[51,219] This dog has been blind in its left eye since birth, a fact that was never recognized by the owner, which is no surprise. Therefore this part of the anatomic diagnosis has nothing to do with the prosencephalic disorder that is causing the seizures. The differential diagnosis for the seizures in this collie are described in Chapter 18. Based on the age of this dog, the history of regularly repeated seizures, and the normal neurologic examination, a presumptive diagnosis of idiopathic epilepsy is most likely.

Microphthalmia

Microphthalmia has been observed in three kittens in one litter of a queen who had been treated throughout gestation with the antifungal agent griseofulvin.[180] Microscopic examination of the orbital tissues revealed remnants of retinal neuroepithelium, indicating that an optic cup had formed in the embryo. No recognizable optic nerves were observed (Figs. 14-22, 14-23). In Chapter 3, a meningoencephalocele was described in kittens and attributed to this same drug. In addition, a cyclopic kitten has also been seen in a litter of a queen receiving this drug during gestation.

Optic Nerve Hypoplasia

Bilateral hypoplasia of the optic nerve has been observed in the cat, dog, and horse, with no other CNS abnormalities.[17,55,69,121,178] The eyes are normal. The degree of hypoplasia

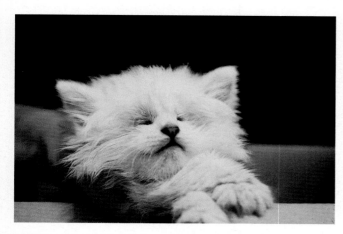

FIGURE 14-22 This kitten is one of the three kittens in the litter of a queen that had been treated for ringworm throughout gestation with oral griseofulvin. No grossly visible eyeballs were observed. On microscopic examination of the orbital tissue, remnants of retinal tissue were recognized, which makes this abnormality bilateral microphthalmia.

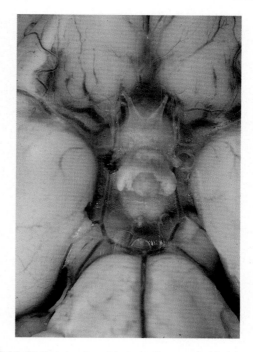

FIGURE 14-24 Ventral surface of the brain of a 4-month-old miniature poodle that was blind since birth with dilated pupils that were unresponsive to a bright light stimulus. Note the empty sleeves of meninges where the optic nerves failed to develop or degenerated perinatally.

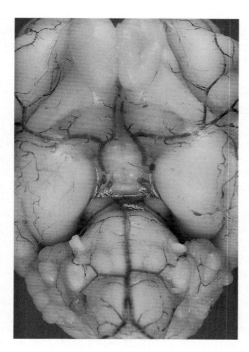

FIGURE 14-23 Ventral surface of the brain of the kitten in Fig. 14-22. Note the absence of any recognizable optic nerves, optic chiasm, or optic tracts.

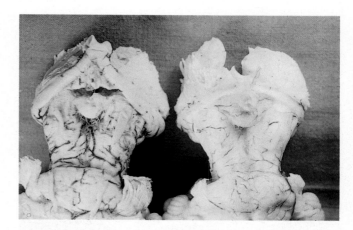

FIGURE 14-25 Ventral surface of the brain of a normal horse on the left and a horse with optic nerve hypoplasia or abiotrophy on the right.

varies from only a meningeal sleeve, where the optic nerves should have been present in the cat and dog, to optic nerves that are approximately one fourth their normal size in the horse (Figs. 14-24, 14-25). Whether this circumstance represents a true hypoplasia or a fetal degenerative disorder such as a retinal abiotrophy is unknown. Optic nerve hypoplasia and atrophy occur in possibly 25% of calves that have the cerebellar hypoplasia and atrophy caused by the in utero infection with the bovine virus diarrhea (BVD) virus (Fig. 14-26).[21]

Optic Nerve Injury

Optic nerve injury may occur with head trauma in any species.[118] Foals are at risk because of the exceptionally long optic canals in this species. Their acute blindness is associated with absent or depressed pupillary light reflexes. The portion of the optic nerve where it courses through the long optic canal is usually affected. If the moving head strikes an object, the head stops, but the eyeballs keep moving, which stretches the optic nerves. Swelling occurs in the nerve from the injury, but the portion within the optic canal is restricted by the bony wall, and the axons are at risk of degenerating from the pressure of the edema (Figs. 14-27, 14-28).

Vitamin A Deficiency

Be aware that, in calves, especially steers, blindness with dilated unresponsive pupils may follow chronic vitamin A deficiency.[3,43,48,193] This type of deficiency occurs on ranges

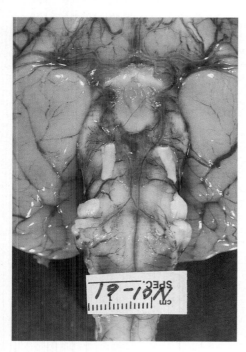

FIGURE 14-26 Ventral surface of the brain of a 2-month-old calf that was blind since birth with dilated unresponsive pupils. In addition, this calf exhibited a severe cerebellar disorder when she walked, which was caused by severe hypoplasia and atrophy of the of cerebellum secondary to in utero infection with the BVD virus. Possibly as many as 25% of calves with the BVD-induced cerebellar lesion also have these visual system lesions.

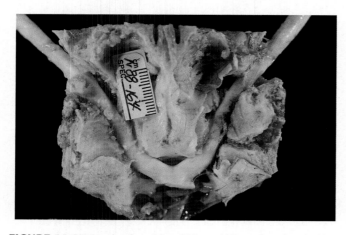

FIGURE 14-27 Dorsal surface of the middle cranial fossa of an 8-month-old colt that was clinically blind after a head injury at pasture. Euthanasia and necropsy were performed 2 months after the presumed injury when the colt's vision did not improve. The optic canals have been opened to show their extensive length and the mild narrowed appearance of the optic nerves.

in the western states when a dry season results in a lack of green feed, which is a source of vitamin A, or in feedlots with the same deficiency. Night blindness results from the loss of rod photoreceptor function because of the inability to produce rhodopsin. However, complete blindness is caused by compression and degeneration of the optic nerves where they course through the optic canals. Stenosis occurs at this location because of a thickening of the dura and a failure of the optic canals to enlarge as the calves grow. These same

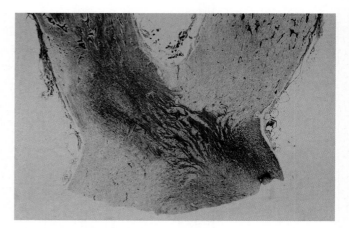

FIGURE 14-28 Microscopic section of the optic erves adjacent to the optic chiasm from the horse in Fig. 14-27, stained for myelin. The absence of myelin is the result of wallerian degeneration caused by the axonal disruption in the portion of the optic nerves within the optic canals and is most severe in the right optic nerve where no pupillary light reflex was observed in the right eye.

animals usually have an elevated CSF pressure caused by the dural fibrosis affecting the arachnoid villi. Optic disk edema may be evident on fundic examination (Box 14-1).

Clinical Evaluation of Prosencephalic Disorders

It is appropriate to pause here and consider how we evaluate the prosencephalon in our neurologic examination because it includes the central visual pathways.[24] In Chapters 8 and 9, the prosencephalic components of the UMN, GP, and general somatic afferent (GSA) systems are described and the clinical signs that would result from their dysfunction. In this chapter, the prosencephalic components of the visual system have been described, as well as the clinical signs that result from their dysfunction. In Chapter 4, the clinical signs of prosencephalic dysfunction are summarized with the discussion of hydrocephalus. You should review this material now. From the perspective of the owner, these circumstances include various forms of seizures, changes in an animal's behavior, and changes in its sensorium. From your perspective in evaluating the neurologic examination, three clinical observations should be made that, if abnormal, may reflect a prosencephalic disorder: (1) postural reactions, (2) nociception, and (3) vision. See Figs. 9-16 and 14-12 for diagrams of the neuronal pathways that provide the anatomic basis for these three clinical observations.

1. With unilateral prosencephalic disorders, the postural reactions will be delayed or absent in the contralateral limbs because of the dysfunction in the prosencephalic components of the UMN and GP systems. This dysfunction is most reliably observed in the hopping response. The gait will be normal. No hemiparesis or ataxia is observed in the gait on a level surface except for a mild deficit in the first 1 to 2 days after a peracute lesion, such as a hemorrhage, infarction, or head injury. After this point, only the postural reaction deficit will be observed. For a clear understanding of the clinical signs, these should be described as a normal gait with abnormal postural reactions. Abnormal postural reactions by

BOX 14-1 Neurophthalmology—Review of Clinical Signs

EXTRAOCULAR

Size of palpebral fissure: Levator palpebrae superioris (III); levator anguli oculi medialis (VII) in the horse and farm animals; orbitalis (sympathetic)

  Narrow: Ptosis-oculomotor nerve paralysis with strabismus and mydriasis

    Sympathetic nerve paralysis—Horner syndrome

    Facial paralysis in the horse and farm animals

  Wide: Facial paralysis in small animals occasionally

Protrusion of third eyelid:

  Sympathetic paralysis—Horner syndrome

    Tetanus when stimulated

    Facial paralysis when menaced

    Severe depression in cats

    Hyperplasia of the gland of the third eyelid

Strabismus:

  Oculomotor nerve paralysis—ventrolateral—constant

  Abducent nerve paralysis—medial—constant

  Trochlear nerve paralysis—dorsal deviation of the medial angle—constant

  Vestibular system dysfunction—ventrolateral in some head positions

Nystagmus:

  Vestibular system dysfunction—jerk to opposite side with peripheral disease

  Congenital blindness—pendular

  Congenital nystagmus—pendular

Hypalgesia-analgesia:

  Cornea: Trigeminal nerve—ophthalmic branch—neurotrophic keratitis

  Eyelids: Trigeminal nerve—ophthalmic and maxillary branches

INTRAOCULAR

Size of pupil

Mydriasis:

  Oculomotor nerve paralysis with ptosis and strabismus

  Retinal or optic nerve disease with blindness

  Glaucoma

  Iris atrophy

Miosis:

  Sympathetic nerve paralysis—Horner syndrome

  Acute prosencephalic disease—release of oculomotor neurons

  Ocular discomfort: Oculopupillary reflex

  Iritis

Blindness:

  Cornea—aqueous—lens—vitreous—retina—optic nerve—central visual pathway

---

themselves should not be called hemiparesis. In addition, calling the condition *hemiparesis* is a misnomer because the deficit also involves dysfunction of the GP system.

2. With unilateral prosencephalic disorders that involve components of the nociceptive pathway, hypalgesia of the contralateral side of the body will be present. These areas include the face, neck, trunk, and limbs, but hypalgesia is best appreciated in the nasal septum mucosa, where testing sensitivity is most reliable.

3. With unilateral prosencephalic disorders of the central visual pathway—optic tract, lateral geniculate nucleus, optic radiation, and visual cortex—a contralateral menace deficit with normal pupillary light reflexes will be observed.

Be aware that all three of these clinical signs can result from a large lesion that affects one entire cerebral hemisphere (telencephalon) or a small lesion on one side of the diencephalon where it can affect the internal capsule or crus cerebri, the adjacent optic tract, and the thalamic relay nucleus for nociception. See Fig. 2-3 and note how close the optic tract fibers are to the projection fibers of the internal capsule that will enter the crus cerebri.

Diseases of the Visual System

Normal Pupils

The following case examples involve unilateral and bilateral prosencephalic disorders that include the central visual pathways without interfering with the pupillary light reflexes.

CASE EXAMPLE 14-5

Signalment: 10-year-old castrated male boxer, Casey

Chief Complaint: Abnormal behavior

History: One month before this examination, Casey was anesthetized for removal of a skin tumor on his tail. After his recovery from anesthesia, he became less responsive and began to walk in circles to his left side. These clinical signs progressed in severity.

Examination: See **Video 14-5**. You cannot appreciate from this video that Casey had a poor menace response in his right eye, and his pupils were normal in size and response to light.

Anatomic Diagnosis: Left prosencephalon

Casey exhibits all three of the prosencephalic clinical signs that can be determined on neurologic examination. He exhibits a normal gait with postural reaction deficits in his right limbs, a right-side nasal septum hypalgesia, and a right-side menace deficit, with normal pupillary size and light reflexes. In addition, Casey is lethargic, is poorly responsive to his environment, paces in a circle to his left side, and will stand with his head in a corner. His occasional tendency to drift to either side suggests the possibility of a slight compromise of the vestibular system, which most likely results from increased intracranial pressure from a prosencephalic mass lesion rather than a separate lesion site. Occasionally, an acute thalamic lesion that affects the medial geniculate nucleus may result in clinical signs of a vestibular system disorder caused by involvement of the conscious projection pathways of that system.

(Continued)

CASE EXAMPLE 14-5—cont'd

Differential Diagnosis: Neoplasm, inflammation

A neoplasm is the presumptive diagnosis for Casey based on the high risk of neoplasia in this breed, his age, and the focal asymmetric nature of his clinical signs. The onset of clinical signs immediately after general anesthesia suggests that the neoplasm was present at that time but was subclinical because of the autoregulation to maintain normal cerebral perfusion in the face of increasing intracranial pressure. The general anesthesia compromised this autoregulation enough to result in postanesthetic clinical signs, which then continued to progress. Some of the gas anesthetics cause vasodilation of the intracranial blood vessels, which can exacerbate the intracranial pressure. A focal form of granulomatous meningoencephalitis, a fungal granuloma, or bacterial abscess are other possibilities but are less likely.

CT and MR imaging were not available at the time Casey was studied. He was euthanized, and necropsy showed a large malignant astrocytoma in the left prosencephalon (Figs. 14-29 through 14-32).

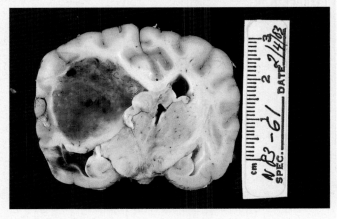

FIGURE 14-31 Transverse section of the preserved brain of the dog in Figs. 14-29 and 14-30 at the level of the caudal thalamus, where the neoplasm obliterates the thalamocortical fibers and origin of the optic radiation.

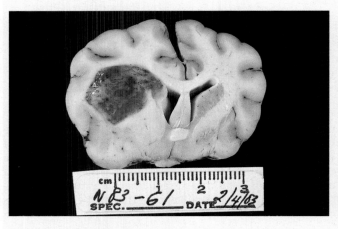

FIGURE 14-29 Transverse section of the preserved brain of the 10-year-old boxer in Video 14-5. This view is the first of four transverse sections to show the anatomic location of a large aggressive malignant astrocytoma. This figure shows the glioma obliterating the left caudate nucleus and internal capsule at the level of the optic nerves and rostral commissure.

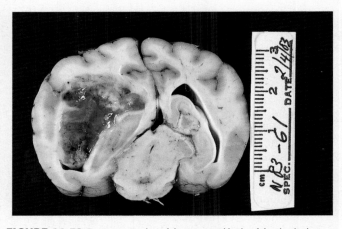

FIGURE 14-32 Transverse section of the preserved brain of the dog in the previous three figures at the level of the temporal and occipital lobes, where the neoplasm obliterates the optic radiation of the internal capsule. Note the compression of the mesencephalon. You should understand how the location of this astrocytoma readily explains the clinical signs observed in this boxer dog.

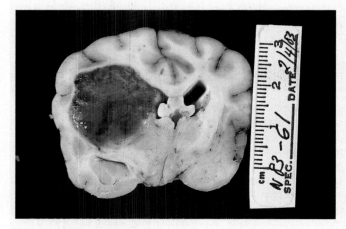

FIGURE 14-30 Transverse section of the preserved brain of the dog in Fig. 14-29 at the level of the midthalamus, where the neoplasm obliterates the internal capsule and thalamocortical fibers.

See **Video 14-6**. This video shows Otter, an 11-year-old male Labrador retriever with a history of generalized seizures over the past 3 months and approximately 3 weeks of a slowly progressive abnormal behavior that included depression and a tendency to walk in circles to his right side. Study the video. Your anatomic diagnosis should be right prosencephalon. In addition, Otter has a mild lameness in his left pelvic limb associated with a palpable mass in his left thigh muscles. The differential diagnosis for his prosencephalic lesion is the same as this case example: neoplasm or focal inflammation. MR imaging (see Video 14-6) showed a contrast-enhancing mass in the dorsolateral aspect of the right thalamus that bulged into the right lateral ventricle. The ring-enhancement feature of the contrast images makes a glioma a strong possibility, but the location also suggests a meningioma or choroid plexus papilloma. Otter was euthanized, and no necropsy was allowed.

See **Video 14-7**. This video shows Peanut, a 9-year-old female toy fox terrier with a history of seizures that were described by the owner as generalized seizures. At least three of these seizures had been observed in the past 2 months. For 1 month, she had been less responsive to the owner and recently started to walk in circles to her left side.

Study the video. Your anatomic diagnosis should be left prosencephalon based on her normal gait and right-side postural reaction deficits, right-side menace deficit, and right-side nasal hypalgesia, as well as her circling to the left side. The differential diagnosis is neoplasm or focal inflammation. A seizure is the most common neurologic reason for owners to seek examination by a veterinarian. All seizures represent a prosencephalic disorder. Seizures are the subject of Chapter 18. Most seizures are caused by idiopathic epilepsy, and the patient has a normal neurologic examination. If a structural basis exists for the seizures, then one or more of the three clinical signs observed on these last three videos may be present. The presence of any one of these three clinical signs excludes the diagnosis of idiopathic epilepsy.

NECROTIZING MENINGOENCEPHALITIS, NECROTIZING LEUKOENCEPHALITIS

Two necrotizing inflammatory disorders of unknown cause are observed worldwide in young adult toy and small-breed dogs. Necrotizing meningoencephalitis most commonly affects pug dogs, and necrotizing leukoencephalitis most commonly affects Yorkshire terriers.[33,195,207] We have seen confirmation of one or the other of these two forms of encephalitis in the Chihuahua, Maltese, Lhasa apso, and shih tzu breeds and have made the presumptive diagnosis in other toy and small-breed dogs. The characteristic description of these diseases emphasizes a meningeal and neocortical location for the necrotizing meningoencephalitis with extension into the corona radiata and a deep cerebral white matter location (i.e., centrum semiovale, internal capsule, thalamocortical fibers) with extension into the adjacent gray matter in the necrotizing leukoencephalitis. Overlap in the topography of these two disorders is often observed. Whether these are two distinct pathogenetic disorders or a continuum from one to the other remains to be determined. We suspect the latter possibility may be more realistic. The character of the lesions observed tends to depend on the severity of the disease and the length of time the patient has been affected before death or euthanasia. The inflammation is nonsuppurative with an extensive accumulation of lymphoplasmacytic cells around blood vessels and throughout the involved parenchyma in both disorders and in the meninges in necrotizing meningoencephalitis. Extensive edema is common in the white matter lesions. Necrosis of white matter is more severe in the chronic cases with cavitation more common in necrotizing leukoencephalitis. In dogs with necrotizing leukoencephalitis that are necropsied early in the course of the disease, evidence can be found for primary demyelination. No infectious agent has been identified that is associated with this inflammation. This search includes polymerase chain reaction studies for viral DNA of herpesvirus, adenovirus, and canine parvovirus in the brain tissue of dogs diagnosed at necropsy.[179] At the present time, both disorders are thought to be autoimmune inflammations and possibly the involved epitope antigenic determinant is different between the two disorders. Molecular mimicry may play a role in the pathogenesis of these two disorders where an infectious virus may share epitopes—antigenic protein characteristics—with a protein expressed by a CNS parenchymal cell such as the oliogodendroglial cell. The immune system, responding to the viral protein, in turn, also attacks the CNS protein, resulting in an autoimmune inflammation and destruction of the CNS tissue. This event has been demonstrated in mice and proposed for the pathogenesis for multiple sclerosis and the polyneuritis of the Landry-Guillain-Barré syndrome in humans.[56] We discussed a consideration of molecular mimicry for the pathogenesis of polyradiculoneuritis (coonhound paralysis) in dogs in Chapter 5. A familial predisposition is suspected for these inflammatory disorders, especially in the pug dogs, where related dogs have been affected. We await the results of investigations to prove this pathogenesis and identify the infectious agents that are involved.

Both disorders occur most commonly in young adult dogs usually younger than 5 years. Generalized seizures are the most common initial clinical sign reflecting the primary involvement of the prosencephalon. Because these dogs have cerebral lesions that tend to predominate in one cerebral hemisphere, they often exhibit one or more of the three clinical signs of prosencephalic disease that you can determine on your neurologic examination. These clinical signs were described and illustrated in Peanut, the fox terrier in Video 14-7. Brainstem and cerebellar lesions can occur in both disorders.

The clinical expression of these two disorders varies in severity. most dogs have an acute onset of generalized seizures, behavioral changes, or both, and some dogs die in 7 to 10 days. Others have a slower onset and progression of clinical signs. Many of these dogs are euthanized because of the frequency and severity of the seizures and the interictal prosencephalic clinical signs. A few dogs will live for weeks to even many months with sporadic seizures and varying degrees of interictal clinical signs. Dogs with brainstem or cerebellar lesions are usually euthanized because of their gait disorder and the lack of any successful therapy. The CSF frequently contains significant elevations of protein and mononuclear cells. MR imaging is the most useful diagnostic procedure. In the classic necrotizing meningoencephalitis that is common in pug dogs, MR imaging will show abnormalities that predominate in the neocortex and corona radiata, especially in one cerebral hemisphere. Whereas, in the classic necrotizing leukoencephalitis that is common in Yorkshire terriers, the MR imaging will show abnormalities predominantly in the deep cerebral white matter and adjacent diencephalon. Lesions may be bilateral but are usually worse in one cerebral hemisphere.

No satisfactory treatment is available for these two disorders. The use of immunosuppressant drugs may slow the progression of the disorder and extend the life of the patient for a few weeks but will not resolve the lesions. Corticosteroids, cyclosporine, and cytarabine (Cytosar), as well as whole-brain radiation, have been used with variable success. Anticonvulsive drugs are necessary in an attempt to control the seizures.

MR imaging of the brain of Peanut, the dog in Video 14-7, revealed a mild enlargement of the white matter in her left cerebrum that was hypointense on T1-weighted images and hyperintense on T2-weighted and fluid-attenuated inversion-recovery (FLAIR) images, and scattered contrast enhancement occurred throughout these same regions. The nature and topography of these changes strongly supported the diagnosis of a necrotizing leukoencephalitis. Figs. 14-33 through 14-37 show examples of these lesions and MR images of affected patients.

(Continued)

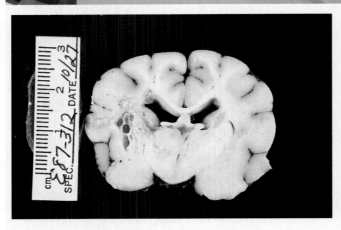

FIGURE 14-33 Transverse section of the preserved brain of a 5-year-old Yorkshire terrier at the level of the rostral diencephalon. This dog exhibited many weeks of primarily a left prosencephalic disorder. Note the cavitating lesion in the deep cerebral white matter, the internal capsule, which is the result of the necrosis associated with the necrotizing leukoencephalitis that is a common disorder in this breed and that is presumed to be a form of autoimmune disease.

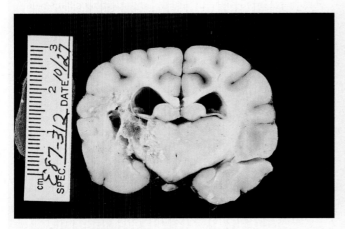

FIGURE 14-34 Transverse section of the brain of the dog in Fig. 14-33 at the level of the midthalamus. Note the cavitating lesions of necrotizing leukoencephalitis centered in the internal capsule and thalamocortical fibers.

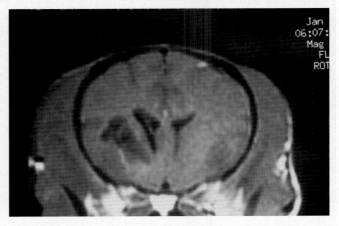

FIGURE 14-35 Axial T1-weighted MR image with contrast of the head of another adult Yorkshire terrier with asymmetric clinical signs of a prosencephalic disorder for many weeks. Note the hypointensity where a cavitating lesion is located similar to those seen in Figs. 14-33 and 14-34.

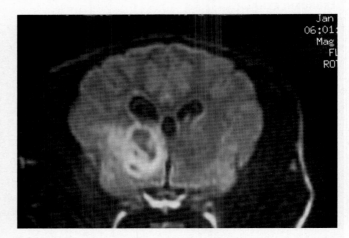

FIGURE 14-36 Axial T1-weighted MR image with contrast of the dog in Fig. 14-35. Note the contrast enhancement and the extension of the lesion into the lateral portion of the rostral diencephalon. The contrast enhancement is caused by the inflammatory portion of this lesion.

FIGURE 14-37 Axial T1-weighted MR image with contrast of the head of a 3-year-old Chihuahua with clinical signs of a chronic disorder primarily of the prosencephalon. Note the hypointensity of the cavitation bordered by contrast enhancement of the inflammation. This abnormality is another example of necrotizing leukoencephalitis in a small-breed dog.

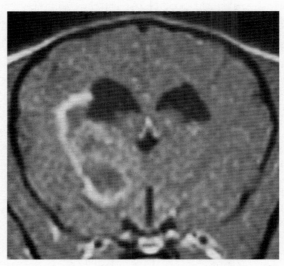

CASE EXAMPLE 14-6

Signalment: 5.5-year-old castrated male domestic shorthair, Geebau

Chief Complaint: Abnormal behavior

History: Geebau was normal when he was put outdoors for the evening on 25 August 1994. The next morning the owner found him on the doorstep acting strange. He seemed afraid, remained crouched, and refused to move or to respond to the attempts by the owner to pet him. The next day, he would walk more, and the owner noted that his left limbs slid out from him on the linoleum-covered kitchen floor.

Examination: See **Video 14-8**, which was made on the third day of his illness. Note that when he looks to the right, his left forepaw turns on to its dorsal surface, but he walks with a normal gait. Note that when he is backed up on his pelvic limbs, the left pelvic limb is slow to move. This sign should be interpreted similar to his hopping deficit.

Anatomic Diagnosis: Right prosencephalon

You should have recognized the postural reaction deficits in his left limbs, his left-side menace deficit with normal pupillary size and light reflexes, and his left-side hypalgesia, especially in his nasal septum. Remember that these clinical signs can reflect a disorder of the entire right cerebral hemisphere or just a small portion of the right side of the diencephalon.

Differential Diagnosis: *Cuterebra spp.* larval myiasis, vascular compromise (*Cuterebra spp.* larval myiasis, hypertension), injury, neoplasm, abscess—granuloma

No external wounds or any bulbar conjunctival hemorrhage was observed to suggest a head injury, but the possibility still exists. A prosencephalic neoplasm, abscess, and granuloma are less likely to cause such an acute onset of clinical signs. Hypertension is associated with vascular compromise in older cats and especially in those with chronic renal disease. At this age and this time of the year, the intracranial myiasis of a *Cuterebra* spp. larva with or without vascular compromise is the most presumptive clinical diagnosis.

CUTEREBRA MYIASIS

In the second edition of this textbook, *feline ischemic encephalopathy* or *feline cerebral infarction* were terms used to describe a vascular disease of unknown origin in cats that caused an acute onset of prosencephalic clinical signs.[45] We now strongly believe that most of these cases were the result of intracranial migration of the larva of a species of *Cuterebra* bot fly.[216] There are thirty-four species of *Cuterebra* in North America. These species use a wild rodent or rabbit in their normal life cycle. The cat is an aberrant host for this parasite, but only cats that have access to the outdoors are affected. This unique feline brain disorder is not found outside of North America where this bot fly is not located. This intracranial disorder is rare in other species. We have seen it in one dog.[136]

In the normal life cycle, the *Cuterebra* bot fly lays its eggs in the early summer on vegetation near the rodent or rabbit burrow. When the rodent or rabbit pass by this vegetation, the warmth of the animal's body causes the egg to hatch into a 1- to 2-mm first instar larva that attaches to the hairs of the animal's coat. The larva moves to a body orifice, usually the mouth, where it enters and penetrates the mucosa. The larva migrates through the connective tissues to a subcutaneous site. At some point, it molts to a second instar larva (5 to 10 mm in length). At the subcutaneous site, the larva molts to a third instar larva and grows to as large as 3 to 4.5 cm. This larva

produces subcutaneous swelling and a breathing hole through the skin. In the fall, this third instar larva extrudes through the skin onto the ground, where it pupates to survive through the winter months. In the spring, the bot fly emerges from the pupa, reproduces, and repeats this life cycle. When the first instar larva attaches to the coat hair of the cat that comes in contact with this infested vegetation, it may enter the oral cavity and migrate through the mucosa to a subcutaneous site, as in the rodent or rabbit. However, the larva may also enter the nasal cavity, where it may cause one or more episodes of sneezing. On a few occasions, we have observed a first instar larva that has been sneezed out of the nasal cavity. The larva moves caudally through the nasal cavity and passes through the cribriform plate of the ethmoid bone to enter the cranial cavity. Within the cranial cavity, the larva may be found in the subarachnoid space or within the brain parenchyma. Rarely do we find it in the spinal cord subarachnoid space. Its intracranial survival is tenuous, given that only remnants of larvae may be found on histologic sections. The presence of a degeneration of only the superficial layers of a large portion of the cerebral cortex or occasionally the surface of the ventricular system suggests that the larva may secrete a toxic substance into the CSF, and degeneration occurs where a sufficient concentration of the toxin contacts the brain surface. This lesion is in addition to large areas of ischemia or infarction secondary to compromise of cerebral arteries, especially the middle cerebral artery. Observing arterial lesions such as vasculitis or thrombosis is uncommon. We suspect that the vascular compromise is usually secondary to a vasospasm that may be the result of hemorrhage in the subarachnoid space caused by the migrating larva or the result of the effects of the presumptive larval toxin. In the normal connective tissue migration to a subcutaneous site, this larval secretion may be used to digest the tissues to facilitate its migration. Focal areas of hemorrhage and necrosis also occur in the CNS parenchyma from the migration of the larva, and these areas may be the primary lesions in some cats. Eosinophils may be seen where the larva has migrated, but they are not common enough in the meninges to be reliable for diagnosis on CSF evaluation. Usually, a differential cell count of a blood sample contains no eosinophilia.[70] Figs. 14-38 through 14-46 illustrate examples of the brain lesions caused by this parasitic migration.

Cuterebra spp. larval myiasis occurs primarily in young adult cats that have access to the outdoors from July through September. Clinical neurologic signs may be preceded by clinical signs of an upper respiratory system disorder. Intracranial signs are usually very acute and are often limited to the disruption caused by the vascular compromise of the middle cerebral artery. Seizures and behavioral changes are most commonly observed by the owners. On the neurologic examination, you will usually appreciate some aspect of the behavior change. The cat may be depressed or lethargic, fearful, or distant, as if in a world of its own and you are not part of it. The cat may continuously walk in a circle. Your *hands-on* examination will usually show one or more of the three clinical signs observed with prosencephalic disorders. Be aware that, if the larva migrates into the intracranial optic nerves or the optic chiasm, bilateral blindness with dilated unresponsive pupils may develop. In many cats, the clinical signs do not progress, and those that are present often improve enough for the cat to be acceptable to the owner as a pet. The persistence of unacceptable behavior or poorly controlled seizures has sometimes led to the decision for euthanasia. In some cats in which parenchymal migration of the larva is more extensive, the clinical signs progress and may involve the brainstem and even the

(Continued)

CASE EXAMPLE 14-6—cont'd

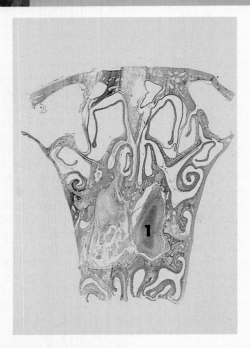

FIGURE 14-38 Microscopic section of the head of a cat at the level of the ethmoid bone cribriform plate and the olfactory bulbs. The normal olfactory bulb is on the right (1). The left olfactory bulb is necrotic where a *Cuterebra spp.* first instar larva migrated from the nasal cavity into the cranial cavity.

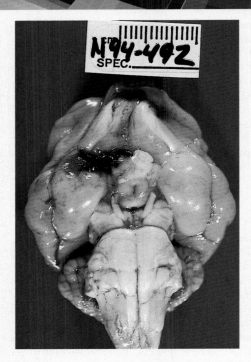

FIGURE 14-40 Ventral surface of the brain of a cat with hemorrhage obscuring the origin of the right middle cerebral artery and containing remnants of a *Cuterebra spp.* larva. Note the swollen optic nerve and optic chiasm. This cat was blind with dilated pupils that were unresponsive to light.

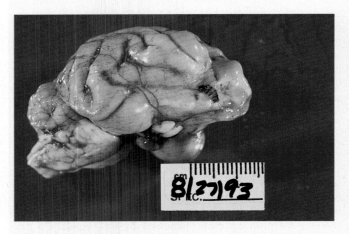

FIGURE 14-39 Lateral view of the brain of a cat with a second instar larva of a *Cuterebra spp.* on the side of the right olfactory peduncle just caudal to a necrotic olfactory bulb.

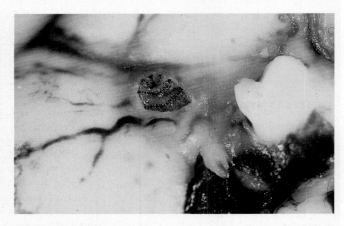

FIGURE 14-41 Ventral surface of the brain of a cat at the level of the optic chiasm. Note the second instar *Cuterebra spp.* larva emerging from or entering into the rostral aspect of the right piriform lobe at the origin of the right middle cerebral artery.

cerebellum. See Video 12-20 in Chapter 12. This diagnosis can be best supported by MR imaging, which may show the area of ischemia or infarction, as well as the track lesion made by the migrating larva and the area of superficial degeneration of the cerebral cortex (Figs. 14-47 through 14-50).

Treatment consists of phenobarbital for seizure control; to attempt to kill the larva and prevent any allergic reaction that might occur, the following combination of drugs has been used without any proof of its efficacy. Administer diphenhydramine intramuscularly at 4 mg/kg 1 to 2 hours before giving ivermectin subcutaneously at

200 to 500 mcg/kg and methylprednisolone succinate intravenously at 30 mg/kg. This treatment is repeated at 24 and 48 hours after the first injection of ivermectin. In addition, the patient should receive orally twice daily for 14 days prednisone at 5 mg/cat and enrofloxacin at 22.7 mg/cat. Ivermectin is not approved for use against *Cuterebra spp.* in cats and therefore requires owner permission.

See **Video 14-9** of Chez, a 2-year-old castrated male domestic shorthair that was found wandering aimlessly along a road. Study the

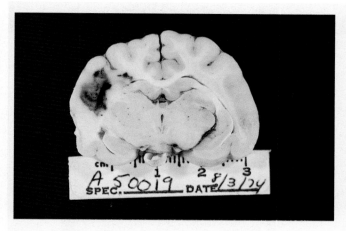

FIGURE 14-42 Transverse section of the brain of a cat with an acute hemorrhagic infarct in the vascular distribution of the left middle cerebral artery.

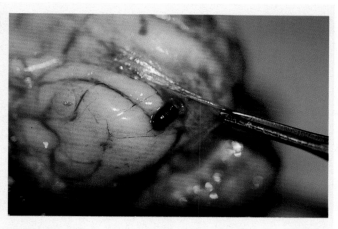

FIGURE 14-45 Dorsal surface of the left cerebral hemisphere with the dura retracted to expose a second instar *Cuterebra spp.* larva.

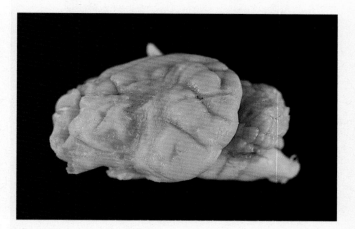

FIGURE 14-43 Lateral view of the brain of an adult cat 2 months after an acute onset of clinical signs of a left prosencephalic disorder. Note the atrophy in the area of the infarct caused by the compromise in the vascular distribution of the left middle cerebral artery.

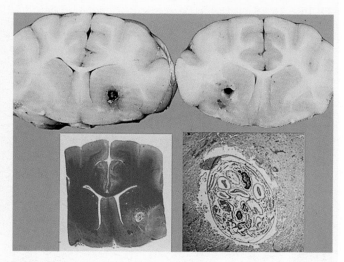

FIGURE 14-46 Four transverse sections of the brain of a cat showing the pathway of migration of a second instar *Cuterebra spp.* larva and the larva itself within the necrotic parenchyma (lower right).

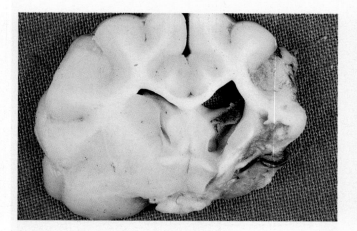

FIGURE 14-44 Transverse section of the brain of the cat in Fig. 14-43. Note the severe atrophy and loss of cerebral parenchyma secondary to the compromise of the left middle cerebral artery many weeks before euthanasia and necropsy. The loss of the left internal capsule at this level would account for a right-side postural reaction deficit with a normal gait, and the loss of the left caudate nucleus may have contributed to the tendency of this cat to walk propulsively in a circle towards its left side.

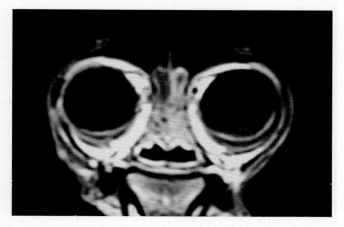

FIGURE 14-47 Figs. 14-47 through 14-50 are T1-weighted MR images with contrast of the head of a 2.5-year-old domestic shorthair with an acute onset of clinical signs of a left prosencephalic disorder presumed to be caused by the intracranial migration of a *Cuterebra spp.* larva. Fig. 14-47 is an axial image at the level of the ethmoid bone cribriform plate and olfactory bulbs. Note the hyperintensity in this area on the cats left side (right side of image).

(Continued)

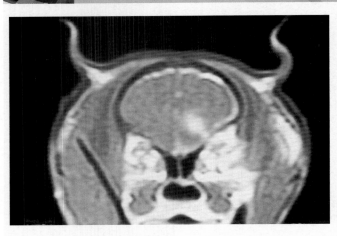

FIGURE 14-48 Axial image of the cat in Fig. 14-47 at the level of the frontal-parietal lobes. Note the focal hyperintensity adjacent to the olfactory peduncle and the diffuse narrow hyperintensity on the surface of the left cerebral hemisphere. The latter represents the superficial degeneration of the neocortex that we believe is related to a toxin secreted from the larva and circulating in the CSF.

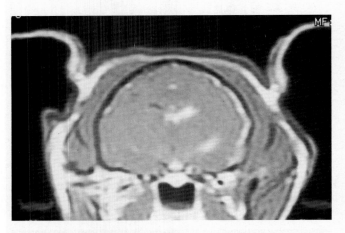

FIGURE 14-49 Axial image of the head of the cat in Figs. 14-47 and 14-48 at the level of the diencephalon. Note the hyperintensity at two sites in the left thalamus and the diffuse surface-related hyperintensity of the cat's left cerebral hemisphere.

video and note the similarity to this case example, except that this cat has no menace response in either eye. Not shown was nasal septum hypalgesia bilaterally. The anatomic diagnosis is bilateral prosencephalon that is worse on the left side. No ancillary studies were performed, and Chez did not receive any antiparasitic therapy. Six days later, he was more alert. Nine days after this point, he began to circle constantly to his right side, and his sensorium varied from lethargy to aggression. He was euthanized, and necropsy showed lesions compatible with a migrating *Cuterebra spp.* larva.

Figs. 14-51 and 14-52 show a 3-year-old cat with a right cerebral abscess from a dog bite in which a tooth penetrated the right parietal bone. Initially, this cat had all three clinical signs of a left prosencephalic lesion. As the lesion enlarged and cerebral herniation compressed the brainstem, the clinical signs progressed and the cat became recumbent.

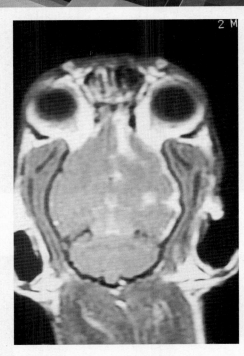

FIGURE 14-50 Dorsal plane MR image of the head of the cat in the previous three figures. Note the tract of hyperintensity from the left olfactory bulb area (right side of figure) into the left thalamus and the superficial hyperintensity on the surface of the left cerebrum. We believe these MR abnormalities are diagnostic for an intracranial migration of a larva of a *Cuterebra spp.*

Meningiomas are common in aging cats, and the majority of cases involve the prosencephalon. Changes in behavior are the most common initial clinical sign of the prosencephalic disorder recognized by the cat's owner. Loss of vision depends on the location of the meningioma. A menace response loss may be an early clinical sign

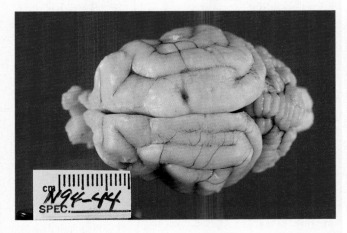

FIGURE 14-51 Dorsal view of the preserved brain of a young adult domestic shorthair with clinical signs of a chronic right prosencephalic disorder. Note the swollen gyri of the right cerebral hemisphere and the focal depression in the right marginal gyrus, which we believe was made by the tooth of a dog. A hole was discovered in the parietal bone at this same site.

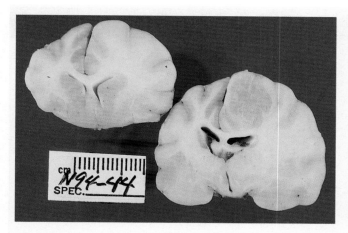

FIGURE 14-52 Transverse section of the brain of the cat in Fig. 14-50. Note the large abscess in the right cerebral hemisphere and the vasogenic edema in the cerebral white matter adjacent to the abscess and rostral to it.

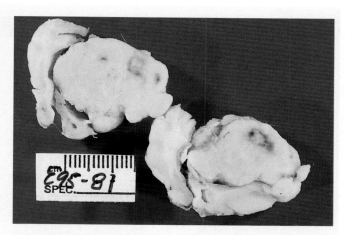

FIGURE 14-54 Transverse section of the cat brain in Fig. 14-53 at the level of the olfactory bulb and frontal lobe.

observed on your neurologic examination if the neoplasm involves the optic tract, lateral geniculate nucleus, optic radiation, or visual cortex. Alternatively, loss of vision may result from vasogenic edema in the cerebral white matter or herniation of the occipital lobes caused by the enlarging neoplasm and the consequent increase in intracranial pressure (Figs. 14-53 through 14-57). The clinical signs of a meningioma compressing an occipital lobe may be mimicked both clinically and on MR imaging by a cryptococcal granuloma.[71]

Figs. 14-58 through 14-64 illustrate examples of horses that exhibited menace deficits as part of their neurologic signs. Figures 14-58 and 14-59 show an abscess caused by *Streptococcus equi* in the left cerebrum of a 2-year-old Standardbred gelding. This gelding consistently had a right-side menace response deficit, but his state of alertness varied, presumably with the waxing and waning of the vasogenic edema associated with this mass lesion. At the time of his euthanasia and necropsy, he was recumbent from the cerebral herniation and the compression of the brainstem.[164] Note the brainstem hemorrhages that resulted from this compression.

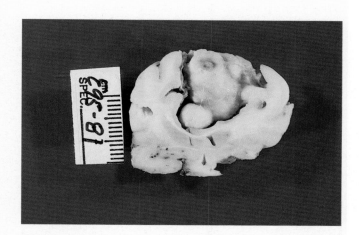

FIGURE 14-55 Transverse section of the cat brain in Fig. 14-53 at the level of the rostral diencephalon.

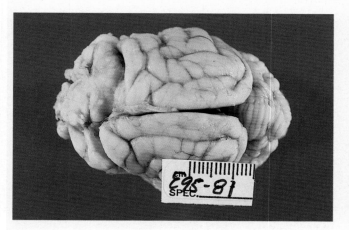

FIGURE 14-53 Dorsal view of the preserved brain of a 9-year-old domestic shorthair with a large meningioma compressing the right frontal lobe.

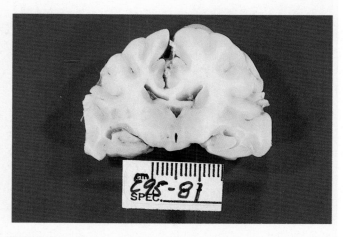

FIGURE 14-56 Transverse section of the cat brain in Fig. 14-53 at the level of the mid-diencephalon just caudal to the meningioma. Note the extensive vasogenic edema in the right cerebral white matter.

(Continued)

CASE EXAMPLE 14-6—cont'd

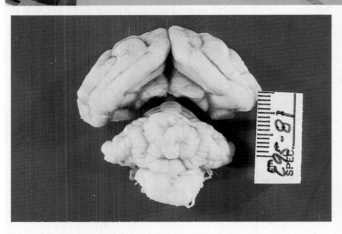

FIGURE 14-57 Caudal view of the cat brain in Fig. 14-53. Note the grooves on the ventromedial aspect of the occipital lobes caused by herniation of the cerebral hemispheres ventral to the tentorium cerebelli as a result of the vasogenic edema. Note the indentation in the caudoventral cerebellar vermis caused by the occipital bone at the foramen magnum when the cerebellum and medulla herniated out of the cranial cavity.

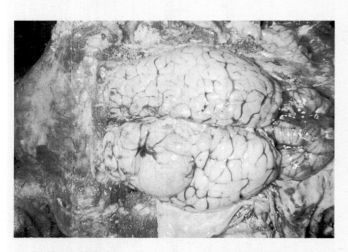

FIGURE 14-58 Dorsal view of an abscess in the left cerebral hemisphere of a 2-year-old Standardbred gelding after removal of the calvaria at necropsy. Rostral is on the left of the figure. This abscess was caused by *S. equi.*

Figs. 14-60 through 14-64 show examples of cholesterinic granulomas of the lateral ventricles that commonly cause lethargy or obtundation and occasionally a loss of vision secondary to cerebral vasogenic edema and occipital lobe herniation. Fig. 14-65 shows a large sarcoma in the right cerebrum of a 15-year-old Quarter horse used for calf roping.[59] The owner who rode this horse first noted that something was wrong when the horse failed to follow the calf when it ran to the horse's left side. This horse lost the calf when the calf ran into the left visual field of the horse. This situation represents a unique way to determine a left-side menace deficit!

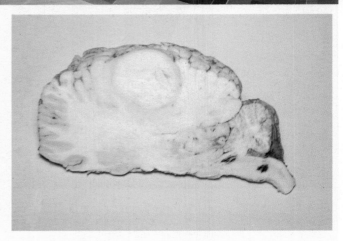

FIGURE 14-59 Lateral view of the preserved brain of the horse in Fig. 14-58 after making a sagittal section through the brain and abscess. Note the portion of the left occipital lobe that has herniated ventral to the tentorium cerebelli and compressed the brainstem and cerebellum. Note the hemorrhages in the pons and medulla secondary to their compression and displacement.

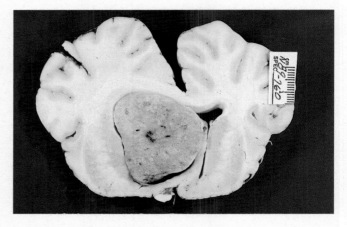

FIGURE 14-60 Transverse section of the preserved brain of a 14-year-old Morgan with a cholesterinic granuloma of the choroid plexus of the left lateral ventricle.

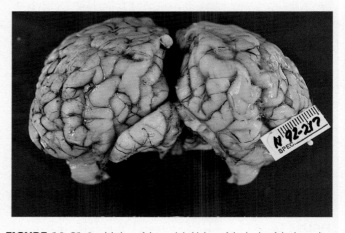

FIGURE 14-61 Caudal view of the occipital lobes of the brain of the horse in Fig. 14-60. Note the groove in the caudal ventromedial portion of the left occipital lobe, where it had herniated ventral to the tentorium cerebelli.

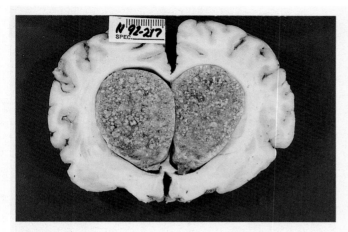

FIGURE 14-62 Transverse section of the preserved brain of an 11-year-old Percheron with bilateral cholesterinic granulomas of the choroid plexuses of the lateral ventricles.

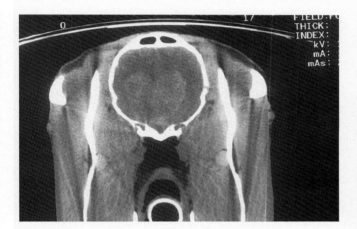

FIGURE 14-63 Axial CT image of the head of a 12-year-old Quarter horse after contrast administration. Note the mildly hyperdense appearance of bilateral cholesterinic granulomas filling the lateral ventricles.

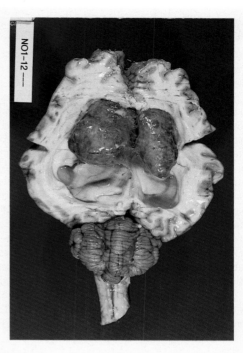

FIGURE 14-64 Dorsal view of the preserved brain of the horse in Fig. 14-63 after removal of the dorsal portion of the cerebrum. Note the bilateral cholesterinic granulomas in the lateral ventricles.

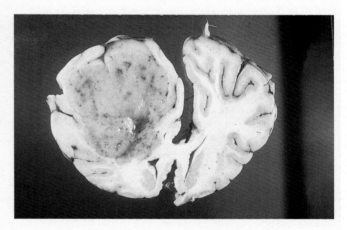

FIGURE 14-65 Rostral surface of a transverse section of the preserved brain of the 15-year-old Quarter horse described in the text, with a large sarcoma in the right cerebral hemisphere. The vasogenic edema caudal to the neoplasm interrupted the optic radiation to cause a left hemianopsia.

CASE EXAMPLE 14-7

Signalment: 6-month-old female Holstein
Chief Complaint: Unable to stand
History: This calf initially became depressed, blind, and mildly ataxic, which rapidly progressed over 24 hours to obtundation, recumbency, and opisthotonus.
Examination: See **Video 14-10**. The heifer in this video had no menace response from either eye, and not shown well on the video were bilateral miotic, almost linear, pupils and a dorsomedial

strabismus bilaterally when the head was held in line with the body. In addition, an occasional abnormal positional nystagmus was seen. We would describe this heifer's sensorium as semicoma (stupor) based on her being unresponsive except for a noxious stimulus.
Anatomic Diagnosis: Diffuse brain
Differential Diagnosis: Encephalopathy caused by thiamin deficiency, sulfur toxicity, lead toxicity, osmolar imbalance—salt or water toxicity, cerebral anoxia

(Continued)

CASE EXAMPLE 14-7—cont'd

All of these disorders cause a similar lesion known as cerebrocortical necrosis or polioencephalomalacia. In lambs, copper deficiency is another cause of this lesion. These two terms describe the lesion and not the cause of the lesion, but most veterinarians relate these terms to thiamin deficiency. An important point to remember is that, even though the majority of cattle that have these clinical signs are the result of a thiamin deficiency, other causes must be considered. The farm history should readily determine whether any possibility exists of cerebral anoxia or a shortage of water, such as from pipes freezing in the winter followed by an excessive consumption of water. The most common source of lead is from licking lead-based paint on the farm buildings or discarded vehicle batteries that are available to the cattle on pasture.[2] The most common source of sulfur is in the water or in feed grown in sulfur-rich soils. The inflammatory diseases were not included in this list because they rarely cause such an acute onset of initial severe prosencephalic clinical signs. This group of inflammatory diseases includes rabies despite its variable clinical signs. Remember that listeriosis is primarily a caudal brainstem disease, and blindness is not seen with this inflammation.

THIAMIN DEFICIENCY ENCEPHALOPATHY

Thiamin deficiency cerebrocortical necrosis (polioencephalomalacia) is the most presumptive clinical diagnosis for this heifer.[133] It is more common in calves than adults. The deficiency of thiamin is related to the amount available to be absorbed from the digestive tract. When the diet is changed abruptly, especially a change that increases the dietary source of carbohydrates, such as the addition of grain, the bacterial population in the rumen may change, resulting in an increase in bacteria that produce thiaminase. The increase in this enzyme causes a decrease in the ruminal thiamin available for absorption. Neurons are dependent on aerobic metabolism for their survival and function, and thiamin acts as a coenzyme in the aerobic energy–producing metabolic cycles. The distribution of lesions caused by thiamin deficiency is similar to that caused by hypoxia. These lesions occur in the populations of neurons that are the most sensitive to anything that interferes with their aerobic metabolism. These areas include the neocortex, lateral geniculate nuclei, and the caudal colliculi (Fig. 14-66). This anatomic location of lesions will not explain the diffuse anatomic diagnosis, largely because, as a metabolic disorder, many populations of neurons exist that are not functioning but have not yet degenerated to the point of being recognized on a microscopic examination of the brain. The earliest recognizable histologic lesions are a cytotoxic edema of cerebrocortical astrocytes and then adjacent neurons. Although ancillary procedures are used to support this diagnosis, including determination of erythrocyte transketolase activity, which is thiamin dependent, these methods are time consuming, not always readily available, and expensive. Time is critical! The earlier the clinical signs of this disorder are recognized, the more effective the treatment with thiamin will be. Cytotoxic edema should be treated intravenously with mannitol, a hypertonic fluid. Remember that other cattle will have been exposed to this same dietary change and are at serious risk for developing the same clinical disorder and should also be treated with thiamin or have thiamin added to their feed, which should have the grain slowly replaced with hay fiber. The description of the clinical signs observed by the owner of this heifer and the ones that you observed on the video are typical for this disorder: an acute onset of depression, mild ataxia, blindness, and occasionally tremors

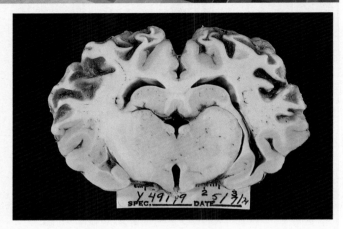

FIGURE 14-66 Transverse section of the preserved brain of a 9-month-old steer that 2 months before euthanasia and necropsy was treated with thiamin for an acute onset of diffuse brain disease that was diagnosed as polioencephalomalacia secondary to a deficiency of thiamin. The steer recovered the ability to walk but remained lethargic and blind. Note the symmetric bilateral atrophy of the neocortex where the polioencephalomalacia occurred, leaving uncovered corona radiata.

followed by rapid progression to recumbency (nonambulatory tetraparesis) with opisthotonus, abnormal positional nystagmus, semicoma (stupor), extremely miotic pupils with dorsal deviation of the medial aspect of both pupils (dorsomedial strabismus), and occasional seizures. As patients respond to treatment, the blindness is usually the last deficit to resolve and the one that occasionally persists.

The heifer in this case example died the day after being video-taped. A diffuse necrotizing polioencephalopathy was diagnosed at necropsy that was assumed to be due to a thiamin deficiency.

Encephalopathy caused by thiamin deficiency occurs in cats and less commonly in dogs.[111,134] It occurs in cats fed a fish diet in which the species of fish contains thiaminase, in cats that are fed a diet with an inadequate level of thiamin, or those fed food that is cooked, which destroys thiamin. Prolonged anorexia may also lead to thiamin deficiency. In cats with marginal levels of thiamin that are stressed with clinical illness, the period of anorexia necessary to produce a deficient state may be shortened. In dogs, this disease is most commonly associated with feeding cooked food. In small animals, the degenerative lesions are more severe in the brainstem nuclei than the neocortex, in contrast to ruminants with thiamin deficiency. Lesions in cats and dogs are especially prominent in the vestibular nuclei, caudal colliculi, oculomotor nuclei, red nuclei, and lateral geniculate nuclei (Fig. 14-67). The initial neurologic signs usually consist of a cerebellovestibular ataxia followed by dilation of the pupils that respond poorly to light. Seizures, head and neck flexion, coma, and death follow. Seizures are sometimes elicited by handling the cat, which induces a severe flexion of the entire neck and trunk. The cat will act as if it were trying to roll itself into a ball. Immediate therapy with thiamin may resolve these clinical signs. Dogs with thiamin deficiency usually show an initial depression and spastic paraparesis and pelvic limb ataxia that progress to vestibular ataxia, circling, and recumbency. Wide head excursions may reflect the bilateral vestibular nuclear lesions. Seizures usually occur after the dog is recumbent.

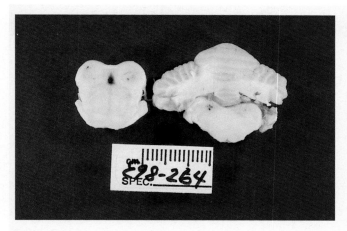

FIGURE 14-67 Transverse sections of the mesencephalon, cerebellum, and medulla of a 1-year-old domestic shorthair with thiamin deficiency. Note the bilateral discolorations of the medullary vestibular nuclei and the mesencephalic caudal colliculi caused by their acute degeneration.

In both species, the menace response may be absent because of the thalamic nuclear or the neocortical lesions. MR imaging may show the bilaterally symmetric brainstem nuclear lesions (Figs. 14-68, 14-69).[68]

See **Video 14-11** of a 6-month-old female Holstein with a history identical to the animal in this case example: an acute onset of depression, blindness, and ataxia that progressed in 24 hours to recumbency and opisthotonus similar to what you observed in Video 14-10. Treatment with thiamin was started shortly after she became recumbent, and this video shows her 4 days later. Note that she is lethargic and blind. Her pupils were small and reactive to light. She exhibits a mild vestibular ataxia.

AMPROLIUM, MERCURY, POSTANESTHETIC HYPOXIA

Be aware that the use of amprolium as a coccidiostat in lambs and calves has caused a cerebrocortical necrosis and clinical signs similar to those that occur with thiamin deficiency.[147]

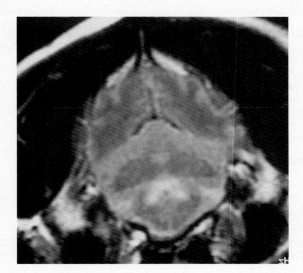

FIGURE 14-68 Axial T1-weighted MR image with contrast of the head of a 7-year-old castrated male mixed-breed dog with thiamin deficiency at the level of the cerebellum and medulla. Note the bilateral hyperintensity of the vestibular nuclei.

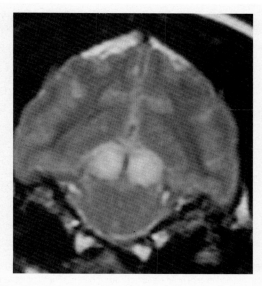

FIGURE 14-69 Axial T1-weighted MR image with contrast of the head of the dog in Fig. 14-68 at the level of the caudal mesencephalon. Note the bilateral hyperintensity in the caudal colliculi. The diagnosis of thiamin deficiency was based on the unique anatomy of the lesions seen in the MR images. The authors thank Dr. Laurent Garosi for the use of these images.

Animals that ingest wheat seed that has been treated with fungicide that contains mercury may develop a chronic degeneration of neuronal populations, especially in the cerebral cortex. Seizures and blindness may result.[112]

Small animals that survive after a period of hypoxia or anoxia during general anesthesia slowly recover from the anesthesia and exhibit varying degrees of diffuse neurologic signs, including blindness with normal pupillary light reflexes.[155] After a variable time period, they often regain their normal sensorium and ability to stand and walk, but they may remain permanently blind. We have seen one dog that regained its vision 6 weeks after one of these hypoxic episodes (Figs. 14-70 through 14-72).

We have observed five adult horses that have been anesthetized for various surgical procedures that from 5 hours to 7 days after recovery from the anesthesia rapidly develop severe prosencephalic clinical signs.[145] These signs include propulsive behavior, blindness, and seizures. Necropsy revealed extensive cerebrocortical necrosis compatible with a period of hypoxia (Fig. 14-73). The hypoxia during anesthesia was documented in two of these horses. In humans, after a global ischemia, a delay in neuronal death of a few hours to days may occur, which is known as a *maturation period*. The reason for this delay is poorly understood but may involve a form of reperfusion injury.

EQUINE NEONATAL ENCEPHALOPATHY

Equine neonatal encephalopathy, a form of maladjustment syndrome, occurs in newborn foals that are normal at birth. From 1 to 14 days postnatally, these foals rapidly develop diffuse neurologic signs but predominantly prosencephalic with lethargy, inability to nurse, blindness, and seizures. Their lesions consist of cerebrocortical necrosis and brainstem nuclear degeneration similar to those observed after hypoxia (Fig. 14-74). The cause of the hypoxia is unknown but may occur before or during birth, and the delay in observation of the clinical signs may reflect the maturation period, as previously described.

(Continued)

CASE EXAMPLE 14-7—cont'd

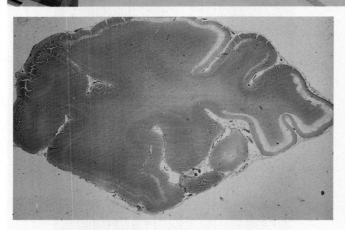

FIGURE 14-70 Microscopic section of the occipital lobe of an adult male boxer dog that had experienced respiratory arrest during general anesthesia. He slowly recovered all of his neurologic function except for vision. After 10 months of blindness, he was euthanized and necropsied. Note the empty space where the cerebrocortical necrosis of the middle portion of the neocortex occurred, which only consists of a few astrocytes.

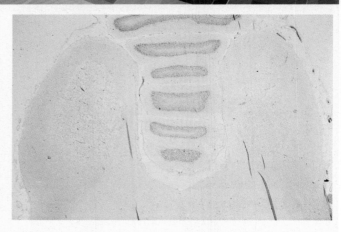

FIGURE 14-72 Microscopic section of the caudal colliculi of the dog in Fig. 14-71. Note the bilateral necrosis similar to that in the neocortex. These neocortical and caudal collicular neurons are especially susceptible to disorders that interfere with aerobic metabolism (i.e., hypoxia, thiamin deficiency).

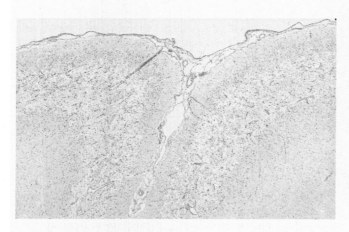

FIGURE 14-71 Higher magnification of a microscopic section of the neocortex of two adjacent occipital lobe gyri from a dog with a history similar to the boxer in Fig. 14-70. Note that the central laminae are most at risk after hypoxia.

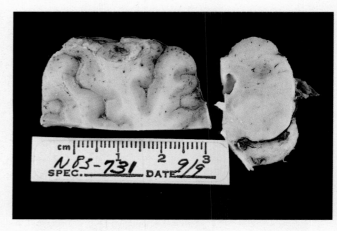

FIGURE 14-73 Transverse sections of a portion of the occipital lobe and the mesencephalon of an adult horse with an acute onset of primarily prosencephalic clinical signs 1 week after recovery from general anesthesia. Note the irregular appearance of the gyri at the top of the section of occipital lobe and the focal discoloration of the center of the rostral portion of the caudal colliculus in the section of mesencephalon. These areas of necrosis are related to the delayed effect of hypoxia that occurred during the general anesthesia.

OSMOLAR IMBALANCE

Osmolar imbalance is usually the result of excessive consumption of salt, causing hypernatremia, followed by excessive water intake or just after excessive water consumption. The administration of inappropriate levels of intravenous saline may be a cause of this polioencephalomalacia lesion in small animals. Salt toxicity is most common in garbage-fed pigs in which the salt content may be excessive. No problem occurs as long as sufficient water is available. Seizures and blindness are common. Be aware that potbellied pigs like potato chips, and without sufficient water, toxicity can result. Correcting the osmolality must be accomplished very slowly to prevent myelinolysis in the brainstem.

NERVOUS KETOSIS

Nervous ketosis is the term used for the occasional occurrence of the encephalopathic form of the metabolic disorder ketosis. The encephalopathy is presumed to be the result of the ketoacidosis and hypoglycemia that interfere with the aerobic metabolism that is critical for normal neuronal function. Nervous ketosis can occur at any time during the first 8 weeks of lactation. These encephalopathic cattle are occasionally blind with normal pupillary size and light responses. They more commonly exhibit bizarre behavior that may include constant licking of one or more sites on their body or inanimate objects in their

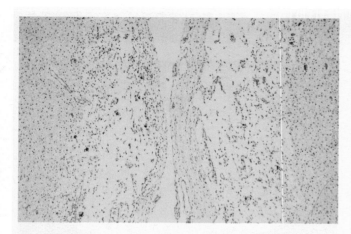

FIGURE 14-74 Microscopic section of two adjacent cerebral gyri from a foal with neonatal encephalopathy. Note the necrosis of the central laminae similar to the dogs in Figs. 14-70 and 14-71, presumably related to a period of hypoxia during birth.

environment, biting and even breaking off the water cups from the water pipes, and propulsively pushing into their stanchion. If these cattle are loose, they may wander aimlessly or head-press against the fence or wall that confines them. They can act obtunded and demented or be very aggressive. The diagnosis is readily made by determining the presence of ketonuria or ketonemia. These clinical signs will usually resolve with appropriate intravenous therapy with dextrose. However, blindness may persist in a severely affected patient as a result of permanent lesions in the visual neocortex.

CASE EXAMPLE 14-8

Signalment: 21-year-old palomino mixed-breed gelding
Chief Complaint: Abnormal behavior and blind
History: This horse lived in a pasture adjacent to the owner's house and was normal until one morning when the owner saw this horse continuously pacing along the inside of the fence and bumping into it at each corner. The horse was hospitalized later that day.
 Examination: Video 14-12 was made on the second day of his hospitalization. The view is from the top of the stall wall looking down into the stall. This horse's sensorium varied from obtundation to almost mania when he would violently force himself into the walls and door of his stall. His pupils were normal in size and in response to light, and no other cranial nerve abnormalities were noted.
Anatomic Diagnosis: Diffuse brain, but primarily bilateral, prosencephalon

Evaluating his gait for degree and quality of paresis and ataxia was difficult, and leading him out of his stall was dangerous. His unsteady appearance indicated some involvement of the brainstem.
Differential Diagnosis: Hepatic encephalopathy; viral encephalitis—eastern equine, rabies, West Nile; leukoencephalomalacia; cholesterinic granuloma; abscess; neoplasm: cerebrospinal nematodiasis

Head injury was excluded because this horse was confined to a small pasture, and no evidence of any gunshot wound was found. This horse is a New York State horse that developed these clinical signs in August when mosquitos are abundant for the viral transmission of either eastern or West Nile encephalitis.

Brain neoplasms are uncommon in horses, except for pituitary adenomas, but the sudden onset of diffuse prosencephalic clinical signs would be unusual for any prosencephalic neoplasm. The most common space-occupying mass lesion in the horse is a cholesterinic granuloma of the choroid plexus of the lateral ventricle.[98] These lesions are thought to result from chronic bleeding from the small blood vessels of the choroid plexus with the precipitation of cholesterol crystals from the degenerate red blood cells and the consequent proliferation of chronic inflammatory cells. These lesions are common in older horses but are usually small and do not cause

any dysfunction. They occasionally become very large in one or both ventricles and cause tentorial herniation of the occipital lobes (see Figs. 14-60 through 14-64). These horses usually exhibit progressive lethargy and occasionally visual deficits. The acute onset of clinical signs as in this horse would not be expected. An abscess caused by *S. equi* or other bacterium is more common in younger horses and usually develops in one cerebral hemisphere; an acute onset of clinical signs would not be expected. The tentorial herniation of the occipital lobes that often occurs with these space-occupying lesions may cause or contribute to the visual system impairment (see Figs. 14-58, 14-59).

EQUINE LEUKOENCEPHALOMALACIA

Equine leukoencephalomalacia is a lesion primarily in the cerebral white matter caused by a mycotoxin ingested with corn or other feed contaminated with the growth of the mold *Fusarium moniliforme*. This mold is a trichothecene toxin known as *fumonisin-1* that affects the brain and liver. This event occurs during warm moist weather conditions and is more common in the Midwestern and Southern United States; it has also occurred in New York State. Many years ago, a localized outbreak in Penn Yan, New York, earned it the name Penn Yan disease. The clinical signs occur abruptly and include lethargy, blindness, ataxia, and dysphagia. The lack of a source of moldy feed made this diagnosis unlikely in this palomino.

CEREBROSPINAL NEMATODIASIS

Cerebrospinal nematodiasis at the present time is most commonly caused by infection with the nematode *Halicephalobus gingivalis* (*Micronema deletrix*). As a rule, this disease causes a fairly acute onset of diffuse CNS clinical signs that progress rapidly. Antemortem diagnosis is difficult to make unless an accompanying subcutaneous infection is present, such as in the prepuce. Lesions can also occur in the kidney and skeletal system. CSF eosinophilia is uncommon. The

(Continued)

widespread use of Ivermectin in horses has essentially eliminated the involvement of the CNS directly with *Strongylus vulgaris* larvae migration or secondary to embolism from verminous lesions in the proximal aorta (Figs. 14-75 through 14-80).

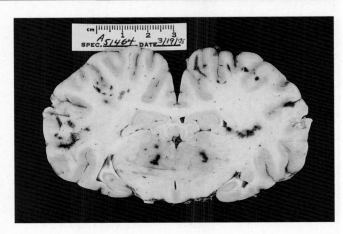

FIGURE 14-77 This transverse section of the brain of the horse in Fig. 14-76 is at the level of the mid-diencephalon, which exhibits numerous infarcts.

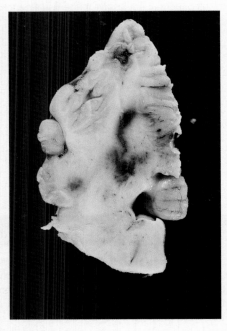

FIGURE 14-75 Transverse section of the preserved cerebellum and medulla from an adult Morgan with an acute onset of predominantly cerebellar vestibular clinical signs. The multiple areas of discoloration represent hemorrhage and necrosis associated with a migrating *S. vulgaris* larva.

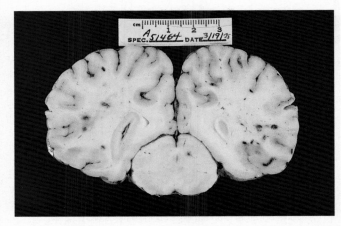

FIGURE 14-78 This transverse section of the brain of the horse in Fig. 14-76 is at the level of the occipital lobes and mesencephalon.

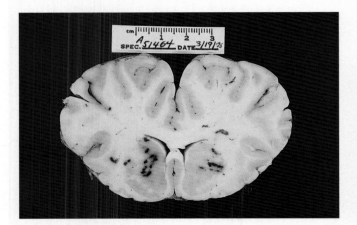

FIGURE 14-76 Figs. 14-76 through 14-79 are transverse sections of the preserved brain of an adult miniature horse with an acute onset of predominantly prosencephalic clinical signs that included head-pressing, blindness, and generalized seizures. The bilateral multiple discolorations are hemorrhagic infarcts associated with fibrin products and *S. vulgaris* larvae that embolized to the brain from a verminous lesion in the wall of the aortic arch and circulation through the brachiocephalic trunk and both internal carotid arteries. Fig. 14-76 is at the level of the frontoparietal lobes of the cerebrum. Note the lesions in both caudate nuclei and internal capsules.

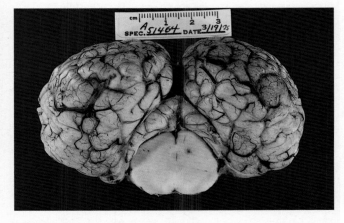

FIGURE 14-79 Caudal view of the occipital lobes and a transverse section of the mesencephalon of the brain of the horse in Fig. 14-76. Note the herniation of the occipital lobes from swelling in the cerebrum. The dark spot to the right of the mesencephalic aqueduct is a transverse section of a *S. vulgaris* larva.

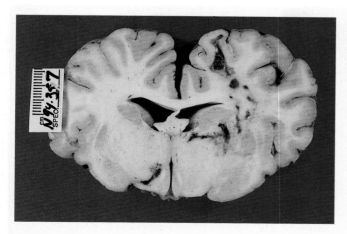

FIGURE 14-80 Transverse section of the preserved brain of an 11-year-old miniature horse at the level of the mid-diencephalon. This horse had an acute onset of predominantly right prosencephalic clinical signs that included a left hemianopsia. The lesions in the right prosencephalon are hemorrhagic infarcts associated with embolic fibrin and *S. vulgaris* larvae from a verminous lesion in the wall of the aortic arch. The embolization circulated through just the right internal carotid artery.

INTRACAROTID DRUG INJECTION

Intracarotid injection of most drugs that are meant to be injected into the venous system will cause ischemic infarction in the prosencephalon on the same side as the injection (Figs. 14-81, 14-82). This location is where the highest concentration of the drug affects the arterial circulation from the side of the cerebral arterial circle supplied by the internal carotid artery that is the branch from the injected common carotid artery. This abnormality will occur in any species but is most common in horses because of their size and the common use of intravenous drugs for therapy.[67] To prevent this event, never attempt a venipuncture with the drug-containing syringe attached. If you have the syringe attached and enter the common carotid artery by mistake, you will not recognize the red color of the arterial blood nor its pulsations. Always insert the needle, observe venous blood, and then attach the syringe.

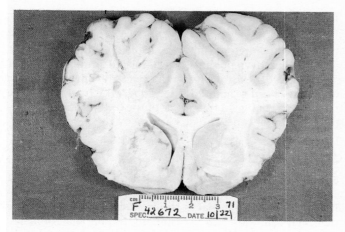

FIGURE 14-81 Transverse section of the preserved brain of a 4-year-old Standardbred with an acute onset of seizures and left prosencephalic clinical signs after an inadvertent injection of a drug into its left common carotid artery. Euthanasia and necropsy occurred 6 weeks later. This transverse section is at the level of the frontal and parietal lobes and exhibits several cavitations caused by the ischemic infarcts related to the vascular compromise associated with the drug in the arterial circulation.

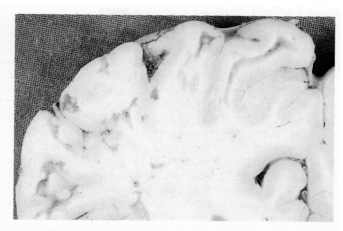

FIGURE 14-82 Transverse section of the same brain as in Fig. 14-81, showing a higher magnification of the cavitations in the left cerebral hemisphere.

Eastern equine, rabies, and West Nile viral encephalitides are all strong possibilities for this diagnosis of the horse in this case example.[47] This horse had received no vaccines for any of these diseases. Of these three viral diseases, eastern equine encephalitis is the most likely to cause such an acute onset of prosencephalic clinical signs.

HEPATIC ENCEPHALOPATHY

Hepatic encephalopathy related to a severe diffuse necrosis of the liver occurs in horses that receive equine plasma or serum products made in horses for a variety of infectious diseases. The most common is tetanus antitoxin. This abnormality was first described by Sir Arnold Theiler in South Africa in 1918 and was called Theiler's disease; it is also called serum hepatitis, despite the lack of inflammation, and a viral cause has been suspected by some for years. However, no virus has been isolated or identified in the liver lesions, nor is the disease transmissible. More likely, hepatic encephalopathy is a peracute hypersensitivity associated with an immune-mediated disorder. It is readily diagnosed by determining elevated serum ammonia levels. It is usually fatal because of the massive destruction of the liver and the difficulty of treating these often maniacal patients. The brain disorder is a metabolic dysfunction unassociated with any neuronal death. Other liver disorders that can lead to hepatic encephalopathy include portosystemic shunts in foals and pyrrolizidine alkaloid hepatopathy from ingesting plants (*Senecio* and *Crotolaria* spp.) that contain this toxin. In addition, a similar metabolic encephalopathy has been seen in unusual cases of colic associated with an overproduction of ammonia by bacteria in the colon and its absorption causing hyperammonemia and an inherited disorder in Morgan foals known as HHH (hyperammonemia, hyperornithinemia, and hyperhomocitrullinuria).

The palomino in this case example had a marked elevation in blood ammonia levels and was euthanized. Necropsy revealed a diffuse liver necrosis and the presence of Alzheimer type II astrocytes in the brain, especially the cerebral cortex. This lesion is the only one seen in the CNS of horses with hepatic encephalopathy and is completely reversible if the metabolic derangement can be corrected. Two months before this illness, this palomino had received tetanus antitoxin, which may have been the source of the presumptive virus or antigenic stimulus that caused the acute liver necrosis.

See Chapter 3 for malformations (hydranencephaly, prosencephalic hypoplasia) and Chapter 4 for cases of obstructive hydrocephalus in which the prosencephalic lesion causes a dysfunction that includes bilateral blindness with normal pupillary function.

Adult Cheetah Leukoencephalopathy

Since the mid-1990s a progressive loss of vision to complete blindness has been recognized in captive adult cheetahs (*Acinonyx jubatus*) in the United States. Dr. Linda Munson at the University of California at Davis has led the study of this disorder.[148] Between 1996 and 2003, 67 of 127 cheetahs that died in the United States had some degree of this leukoencephalopathy, and most had clinical evidence of a loss of vision. Affected cheetahs came from 28 zoological facilities throughout the United States and ranged from 7 to 18 years of age. Sixty were at least 10 years of age. The keepers working with these cheetahs recognized a progressive loss of vision. When blind, subtle changes occured in the behavior of these animals, and they exhibited altered patterns of movement in their enclosures. The cheetah's pupils were normal in size and reacted to bright light. Obviously, completing a neurologic examination on most captive animals is impossible, but these simple observations by the keepers were invaluable. The loss of vision in these cheetahs is caused by a diffuse leukoencephalopathy that affects primarily the cerebral white matter bilaterally. Axonal and myelin degeneration are associated with a profuse astrocytosis with a plethora of bizarre reactive astrocytes. When the lesion is extensive, it can be recognized on examination of preserved transverse sections of the cerebral hemispheres as a gross discoloration of the white matter of the centrum semiovale, internal capsule, and corona radiata (Fig. 14-83). Cavitations occasionally occur. These white matter lesions are observed as hypodense areas on CT images. T1-weighted MR images show a diffuse bilaterally symmetric hypointensity throughout the white matter of both cerebral hemispheres that does enhance after administration of contrast. These same areas are hyperintense on T2-weighted MR images (Figs. 14-84, 14-85). No cause for this lesion has been proven. Extensive efforts to identify an infectious agent have been unrewarding, and the lesion is a degeneration and not an inflammation. A genetic basis could not be established, and the same lesions have been found in three captive Florida panthers. During the period when this disorder was recognized, all of these captive cheetahs were fed a diet from a common

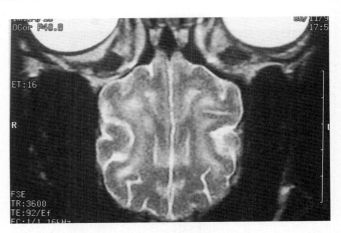

FIGURE 14-84 Dorsal plane T2-weighted MR image of the brain of the cheetah in Fig. 14-83. Note the fairly symmetric hyperintensity of the cerebral white matter including the corona radiata.

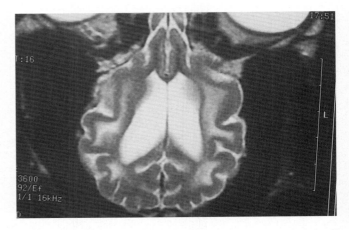

FIGURE 14-85 Dorsal plane T2-weighted MR image of the brain of the cheetah in Figs. 14-83 and 14-84 at the level of the dorsal portion of the lateral ventricles. Note the fairly symmetric hyperintensity of the centrum semiovale and corona radiata.

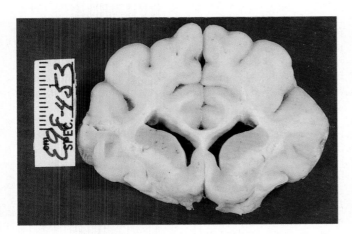

FIGURE 14-83 Transverse section of the preserved brain of a 12-year-old blind cheetah at the level of the parietal lobes just rostral to the diencephalon. Note the bilateral dull tan discoloration of the cerebral white matter. The corpus callosum and the portion of the internal capsule between the caudate nuclei and the lentiform nuclei are more normal in appearance.

vendor. At the present time, the suspicion is that this leukoencephalopathy represents a feed-related intoxication that is directed at the astrocytes in the cerebral white matter. No cases have been diagnosed since 2004, which appears to be related to a change in the source of the feed for captive cheetahs throughout the United States.

Storage Diseases

Storage diseases in the CNS result from a deficiency of a specific degradative lysosomal enzyme causing the accumulation of a substrate that is stored in the cytoplasm of the neuronal cell body and occasionally in glia, macrophages, and the cells of other organs.[9,12,104] An example of this type of storage disease is described in Chapter 13 on the cerebellum with Case Example 13-5. The enzyme deficiency is usually inherited as an autosomal recessive gene. Each storage disease is named for the nature of the stored substrate that accumulates. These metabolic disorders are most common in dogs and cats, and many are models for comparable disorders in humans. Most of these disorders are expressed in neurons by the accumulation of a complex lipid, carbohydrate, or both in the neuronal cytoplasm. One inherited enzymatic deficiency, globoid cell leukodystrophy, affects the myelin in both the central and the peripheral nervous systems, which degenerates and the degraded myelin products accumulate in macrophages (see Case Example 10-23). A partial list of these storage disorders in domestic animals is provided in Table 14-2. The list is partial because these disorders are continually being discovered and described.

The clinical signs are usually observed at a few months of age. The clinical signs are occasionally first observed at a few weeks of age, especially in cats, and a few canine disorders may not be observed until 2 years of age or older. These clinical signs are usually slow to progress and diffuse in origin. Some clinical signs are predominantly prosencephalic; others are mostly cerebellar or more of a diffuse origin. Involvement of the visual cortex results in progressive blindness with normal pupillary light reflexes.

TABLE 14-2 Storage Disorders in Domestic Animals

Disease	Enzyme Deficit (Stored Product)	Species, Breed	Age of Onset of Clinical Signs
Gangliosidosis GM$_1$,[a]			
Type 1	Beta-galactosidase (ganglioside)	Beagle cross	3 mos.
		Portuguese water dog	5 mos.
		Domestic cat	2-3 mos.
		Friesian cattle	1 mo.
Type 2	Beta-galactosidase (ganglioside)	Siamese, Korat, and domestic cat	2-3 mos.
		Suffolk sheep	4 mos.
Gangliosidosis GM$_2$[b]			
Type 1	Hexosaminidase A (ganglioside)	German shorthair pointer	6-9 mos.
		Japanese spaniel	18 mos.
Type 2	Hexosaminidase A,B (ganglioside)	Domestic cat	2 mos.
Type 3	Hexosaminidase A (ganglioside)	Mixed-breed dog	1.5 yrs.
		Yorkshire pig	3 mos.
Unidentified substrate—possible ganglioside—ruminants, grazing species of *Solanum*			
Glucocerebrosidosis[81,129,211,213]	Beta-glucosidase (glucocerebroside)	Sydney silky Abyssinian cat	6-8 mos.
Sphingomyelinosis[13,25,28,215]	Sphingomyelinase (sphingomyelin)	Siamese, Balinese, domestic cat	2-4 mos.
		Poodle	2-4 mos.
Globoid cell leukodystrophy[c]	Galactocerebrosidase (galactocerebroside)	Cairn terrier	2-5 mos.
		West Highland white terrier, beagle, blue tick coonhound	4 mos.
		Miniature poodle	2 yrs.
		Basset hound	1.5-2 yrs.
		Pomeranian	1.5 yrs.
		Domestic cat	5-6 wks.
		Polled Dorset sheep	4-18 mos.
Mucopolysaccharidosis[36,83]	Arylsulfatase B (mucopolysaccharide)	Siamese, domestic cat	4-7 mos.
	Alpha-iduronidase (mucopolysaccharide)	Domestic cat	10 mos.
		Plott hound	3-6 mos.
		Miniature pinscher	6 mos.
		Mixed-breed dog	4-6 mos.
Glycoproteinosis[42,88]	Unknown	Beagle, basset hound, poodle	5 mos.-9 yrs.
Mannosidosis[d]	Alpha-mannosidase (mannoside)	Domestic cat	7 mos.
		Persian cat	2 mos.
		Angus, Murray Grey, Galloway, Holstein cattle; horses and farm animals grazing species of Swainsona[50,93,94]	At birth
	Beta-mannosidase (mannoside)	Nubian goat	Birth-1 yr.
		Salers calf	At birth
Glycogenosis[e]	Alpha-glucosidase (glucoside)	Lapland dog	1.5 yrs.
		English springer spaniel	11 yrs.
		Domestic, Norwegian forest cat	5 mos.
		Corriedale sheep	6 mos.
		Shorthorn, Brahman cattle	3-9 mos.
Fucosidosis[90,206]	Alpha-fucosidase (fucoside)	Springer spaniel	2 yrs.

(Continued)

TABLE 14-2 Storage Disorders in Domestic Animals—cont'd

Disease	Enzyme Deficit (Stored Product)	Species, Breed	Age of Onset of Clinical Signs
Ceroid-lipofuscinosis[f]	Unknown	English setter	1 yr.
		Dachshund	6.5 mos.
		Cocker spaniel	1.5 yrs.
		Chihuahua, saluki	2 yrs.
		Tibetan terrier	3 yrs.
		Australian cattle dog	14 mos.
		Border collie	18-22 mos.
		Blue heeler	1 yr.
		Yugoslavian sheepdog	1 yr.
		American bulldog	1-3 yrs.
		Mixed-breed dog	4 mos.
		Siamese, domestic cat	2-7 yrs.
		South Hampshire sheep	6-18 mos.
		Rambouillet sheep	9-12 mos.
		Devon cattle	14 mos.
		Nubian goat	10 mos.

[a]References 11, 15, 49, 50, 58, 92, 142, 165, 167, 184, 185.
[b]References 34, 35, 41, 127, 128, 160, 166, 169, 174, 189.
[c]References 62-64, 101, 102, 135, 161, 181, 221.
[d]References 1, 14, 23, 26, 40, 52, 54, 82, 86, 91, 96, 97, 103, 106, 107, 109, 110, 132, 137.
[e]References 27, 66, 138, 143, 144, 154, 163, 170, 177, 214.
[f]References 5, 8, 30, 38, 39, 61, 74, 80, 105, 108, 125, 126, 140, 151, 157, 162, 171, 191, 205, 212.

REFERENCES

1. Abbott B: Beta mannosidosis in twelve Salers calves, *J Am Vet Med Assoc* 198:109-113, 1991.
2. Andersen DH, Fisher SK, Steinberg RH: Mammalian cones: disc shedding, phagocytosis and renewal, *Invest Ophthalmol* 17:117, 1978.
3. Anderson WI, et al: The ophthalmic and neuro-ophthalmic effects of vitamin A deficiency in young steers, *Vet Med* 86:1143-1148, 1991.
4. Antonini A, et al: Behavioral and electrophysiological effects of unilateral optic tract section on ordinary and Siamese cats, *J Comp Neurol* 185:183, 1979.
5. Appleby EC, Longstaffe JA, Bell FR: Ceroid lipofuscinosis in two Saluki dogs, *J Comp Pathol* 92:375-380, 1982.
6. Aquirre GD, Rubin LF, Bistner SI: Development of the canine eye, *Am J Vet Res* 33:2399, 1972.
7. Ashton H: Congenital nuclear cataracts in cattle, *Vet Rec* 100:505, 1977.
8. Awano T, et al: A frame shift mutation in canine TPPI (the ortholog of human CLN2 in a juvenile Dachshund with neuronal ceroid lipofuscinosis, *Molec Genet Metabol* 89:254-260, 2006.
9. Axlund TW, et al: Canine hypophysectomy using a paramedian approach, *Vet Surg* 34:179-189, 2005.
10. Baker HJ: Inherited metabolic disorders of the nervous system in dogs and cats. In Kirk RW, editor: *Current veterinary therapy V: small animal practice*, Philadelphia, 1974, Saunders.
11. Baker HJ, et al: Neuronal GM₁ gangliosidosis in a Siamese cat with beta galactosidase deficiency, *Science* 174:838, 1971.
12. Baker HJ, et al: Animal models of human ganglioside storage diseases, *Anim Mod Biomed Res VI Metabolic Dis* 35:1193, 1976.
13. Baker HJ, et al: Sphingomyelin lipidosis in a cat, *Vet Pathol* 24:386-391, 1987.
14. Barlow RM, et al: Mannosidosis in Aberdeen Angus cattle in Britain, *Vet Rec* 109:441, 1981.
15. Barnes I, et al: Hepatic beta galactosidase and feline GM₁ gangliosidosis, *Neuropathol Appl Neurobiol* 7:463, 1981.
16. Barnett KC: Variations of the normal ocular fundus of the dog, *Am Anim Hosp Assoc Proc* 39:1, 1972.
17. Barnett KC, Grimes TD: Bilateral aplasia of the optic nerve in a cat, *Brit J Ophthalmol* 58:663, 1974.
18. Barnett KC, Kelly DF, Singleton WB: Retrobulbar and chiasmal meningioma in a dog, *J Sm Anim Pract* 8:391, 1967.
19. Bishop GM, Clare MC: Organization and distribution of fibers in the optic tract of the cat, *J Comp Neurol* 103:269, 1955.
20. Bistner SI, Rubin LF, Aquirre GD: Development of the bovine eye, *Am J Vet Res* 34:7, 1955.
21. Bistner SI, Rubin LF, Saunders LZ: The ocular lesions of bovine viral diarrhea-mucosal disease, *Pathol Vet* 7:275, 1970.
22. Blake R, Antionetti DN: Abnormal visual resolution in the Siamese cat, *Science* 194:109, 1976.
23. Blakemore W: A case of mannosidosis in the cat: clinical and histopathological findings, *J Sm Anim Pract* 27:447-455, 1986.
24. Braund KG, et al: Central (post-retinal) visual impairment in the dog—a clinical-pathologic study, *J Sm Anim Pract* 18:395, 1977.
25. Bundza A, Lowden JA, Charlton KM: Niemann-Pick disease in a poodle dog, *Vet Pathol* 16:530, 1979.
26. Cavanagh K, Dunston RW, Jones MZ: Plasma alpha and beta mannosidase activities in caprine beta mannosidosis, *Am J Vet Res* 43:1058, 1982.
27. Ceh L, et al: Glycogenoses type III in the dog, *Acta Vet Scand* 17:210, 1976.
28. Chrisp CE, et al: Lipid storage disease in a Siamese cat, *J Am Vet Med Assoc* 156:616, 1970.
29. Christian RG, Tryphonas L: Lead poisoning in cattle: brain lesions and hematologic changes, *Am J Vet Res* 32:203, 1971.

30. Cho D, Leipold H, Rudolph R: Neuronal ceroidosis (ceroid lipofuscinosis) in a blue heeler dog, *Acta Neuropathol* 69:161-164, 1986.

31. Cooper ML, Pettigrew JD: The decussation of the retinothalamic pathway in the cat, with a note on the major meridians of the cat's eye, *J Comp Neurol* 187:285, 1979.

32. Cooper ML, Pettigrew JD: The retinothalamic pathways in Siamese cats, *J Comp Neurol* 187:313, 1979.

33. Cordy DA, Holliday TA: A necrotizing meningoencephalitis of pug dogs, *Vet Pathol* 26:191-194, 1989.

34. Cork LC, Munnell JF, Lorenz MD: The pathology of feline GM_2 gangliosidosis, *Am J Pathol* 90:723-734, 1978.

35. Cork LC, et al: GM_2 ganglioside lysosomal storage disease in cats with beta-hexosaminidase deficiency, *Science* 196:1014-1017, 1977.

36. Cowell KR, et al: Mucopolysaccharidosis in a cat, *J Am Vet Med Assoc* 169:334-339, 1976.

37. Cummings JF, de Lahunta A: An experimental study of the retinal projections in the horse and sheep, *Ann N Y Acad Sci* 167:293, 1969.

38. Cummings JF, de Lahunta A: An adult case of canine neuronal ceroid lipofuscinosis, *Acta Neuropathol* 39:43, 1977.

39. Cummings JF, de Lahunta A, Riis RC: Neuropathological changes in a young adult Tibetan terrier with subclinical neuronal ceroid lipofuscinosis, *Prog Neurol* 1:301-309, 1990.

40. Cummings JF, Wood PA, de Lahunta A: The clinical and pathological heterogeneity of feline alpha mannosidosis, *J Vet Intern Med* 2:164-170, 1988.

41. Cummings JF, et al: GM_2 gangliosidosis in a Japanese spaniel, *Acta Neuropathol* 67:247-253, 1985.

42. Cusick PK, Cameron AM, Parker AJ: Canine neuronal glycoproteinosis: Lafora's disease in the dog, *J Am Anim Hosp Assoc* 12:518-521, 1976.

43. Davis TE: *Bone resorption in hypovitaminosis A* [doctoral thesis], Ithaca, NY, 1968, Cornell University.

44. de Lahunta A: Small animal neuro-ophthalmology, *Vet Clin North Am* 3:491, 1963.

45. de Lahunta A: Feline ischemic encephalopathy—a cerebral infarction syndrome. In Kirk RW, editor: *Current veterinary therapy VI*, Philadelphia, 1977, Saunders.

46. de Lahunta A, Cummings JF: Neuro-ophthalmologic lesions as a cause of visual deficit in dogs and horses, *J Am Vet Med Assoc* 150:994, 1967.

47. Del Piero F, et al: Rabies in horses in New York State: clinical, pathological, immunohistochemical and virological findings, *Eq Infect Dis* 8:291-296, 1999.

48. Divers TJ, et al: Blindness and convulsions associated with vitamin A deficiency in feedlot steers, *J Am Vet Med Assoc* 189:1579-1582, 1986.

49. Donnelly WJC, Kelly M, Sheahan BJ: Leukocyte beta galactosidase activity in the diagnosis of bovine GM_1 gangliosidosis, *Vet Rec* 100:318, 1977.

50. Donnelly WJC, Sheahan BJ, Rogers TA: GM_1 gangliosidosis in Friesian calves, *J Pathol* 111:173, 1973.

51. Donovan EF, Wymann M: Ocular fundus anomaly in a collie, *J Am Vet Med Assoc* 147:1465, 1965.

52. Dorling PR, Huxtable CR, Vogel P: Lysosomal storage in Swainsona spp toxicosis: an induced mannosidosis, *Neuropathol Appl Neurobiol* 4:285, 1978.

53. Elgeti H, Elgeti R, Fleischhauer K: Postnatal growth of the dorsal lateral geniculate nucleus of the cat, *Anat Embryol* 149:1, 1976.

54. Embury DH, Jerrett IV: Mannosidosis in Gallaway calves, *Vet Pathol* 22:548-551, 1985.

55. Ernest JT: Bilateral optic nerve hypoplasia in a pup, *J Am Vet Med Assoc* 168:125, 1976.

56. Evans CF, et al: Viral infection of transgenic mice expressing a viral protein in oligodendrocytes leads to chronic central nervous system autoimmune disease, *J Exp Med* 184:2371-2384, 1996.

57. Evans HE, Ingalls TN, Binns W: Teratogenesis of craniofacial malformations in animals III. Natural and experimental cephalic deformities in sheep, *Arch Environ Health* 13:706, 1966.

58. Farrell DF, et al: Feline GM_1 gangliosidosis: biochemical and ultrastructural comparisons with the disease in man, *J Neuropathol Expt Neurol* 32:1, 1973.

59. Finn JP, Tennant BC: A cerebral and ocular tumor of reticular tissue in a horse, *Vet Pathol* 8:458, 1971.

60. Fischer CA, Jones GT: Optic neuritis in dogs, *J Am Vet Med Assoc* 160:68, 1972.

61. Fiske RA, Storts RW: Neuronal ceroid lipofuscinosis in Nubian goats, *Vet Pathol* 25:171-173, 1988.

62. Fletcher TF, Kurtz HJ, Low DG: Globoid cell leukodystrophy (Krabbe type) in the dog, *J Am Vet Med Assoc* 149:165, 1971.

63. Fletcher TF, Lee DG, Hammer RF: Ultrastructural features of globoid cell leukodystrophy in the dog, *Am J Vet Res* 32:177, 1971.

64. Fletcher TF, Suzuki K, Martin FB: Galactocerebrosidase activity in canine globoid cell leukodystrophy, *Neurology* 27:758, 1977.

65. Fox MW: Postnatal ontogeny of the canine eye, *J Am Vet Med Assoc* 143:968, 1963.

66. Fyfe JC: Familial glycogen storage disease type IV (GSD IV) in Norwegian Forest cats (NWFC), *J Vet Intern Med* 4:12, 1990.

67. Gabel RR, Koestner A: The effects of intracarotid artery injection of drugs in domestic animals, *J Am Vet Med Assoc* 142:1397-1403, 1963.

68. Garosi LS, et al: Thiamin deficiency in a dog: clinical, clinicopathologic and magnetic resonance imaging findings, *J Vet Intern Med* 17:719-723, 2003.

69. Gelatt KN, Leipold HW, Coffman JR: Bilateral optic nerve hypoplasia in a colt, *J Am Vet Med Assoc* 155:627, 1969.

70. Glass E, et al: Clinical and clinicopathologic features in 11 cats with Cuterebra larvae myiasis of the central nervous system, *J Vet Intern Med* 12:365-368, 1998.

71. Glass E, et al: A cryptococcal granuloma in the brain of a cat causing focal signs, *Prog Vet Neurol* 7:141-144, 1996.

72. Glickenstein M, et al: Cortical projections from the dorsal lateral geniculate nucleus of the cat, *J Comp Neurol* 130:55, 1967.

73. Goldman AI, O'Brien PJ: Phagocytosis in the retinal pigment epithelium of the RCS rat, *Science* 201:1023, 1978.

74. Green PD, Little PB: Neuronal ceroid lipofuscin storage in Siamese cats, *Can J Comp Med* 38:207, 1974.

75. Guillery RW: The organization of synaptic interconnections in the laminae of the dorsal lateral geniculate nucleus of the cat, *Z Zellforsch Mikrosk Anat* 96:1, 1969.

76. Guillery RW: The laminar distribution of retinal fibers in the dorsal lateral geniculate nucleus of the cat: a new interpretation, *J Comp Neurol* 139:339, 1970.

77. Guillery RW, Kaas JH: A study of normal and genetically abnormal retinogeniculate projections in the cat, *J Comp Neurol* 143:73, 1971.

78. Guillery RW, Kaas JH: Genetic abnormality of the visual pathways in a "white" tiger, *Science* 180:1287, 1973.

79. Guo X, Sugita S: Topography of ganglion cells in the retina of the horse, *J Vet Med Sci* 62:1145-1150, 2000.

80. Harper PAW, et al: Neurovisceral ceroid lipofuscinosis in blind Devon cattle, *Acta Neuropathol* 75:632-636, 1988.

81. Hartley WJ, Blakemore WF: Neurovisceral glucocerebroside storage (Gaucher's disease) in a dog, *Vet Pathol* 10:191-201, 1973.

82. Hartley WJ, Blakemore WF: Neurovisceral storage and dysmyelinogenesis in neonatal goats, *Acta Neuropathol* 25:325, 1973.

83. Haskins ME, Jezyk PF, Desnick RJ: Animal models of mucopolysaccharidosis. In Desnick RJ, Patterson DF, Scarpello DG, editors: *Animal models of inherited metabolic diseases*, New York, 1982, Alan R Liss.

84. Hayhow WR: Experimental degeneration of optic axons in lateral geniculate body of the cat, *Acta Anat* 37:281, 1958.

85. Hayhow WR: The cytoarchitecture of the lateral geniculate body in the cat in relation to the distribution of crossed and uncrossed optic fibers, *J Comp Neurol* 110:1, 1958.

86. Healy PJ: Beta mannosidase deficiency in Anglo Nubian goats, *Aust Vet J* 57:504, 1981.

87. Hebel R: Distribution of retinal ganglion cells in five mammalian species (pig, sheep, ox, horse, dog), *Anat Embryol* 150:45, 1976.

88. Hegreberg GA, Padget GA: Inherited progressive epilepsy of the dog with comparisons to Lafora's disease of man, *J FASEB* 35:1202-1205, 1976.

89. Herron MA, Martin JE, Joyce JR: Quantitative study of the decussating optic axons in the pony, cow, sheep and pig, *Am J Vet Res* 39:1137, 1978.

90. Herrtage ME: Canine fucosidosis, *Vet Ann* 28:223-227, 1988.

91. Hocking JD, Jolly RD, Batt RD: Deficiency of alpha mannosidase in Angus cattle, *Biochem J* 128:69, 1972.

92. Holmes EW, O'Brien JS: Feline GM$_1$ gangliosidosis: characterization of the residual liver acid beta galactosidase, *Am J Hum Genet* 30:505, 1978.

93. Howard DR, Breazile JE: Optic fiber projections to dorsal lateral geniculate nucleus in the dog, *Am J Vet Res* 34:419, 1973.

94. Hubel DH, Wiesel TN: Aberrant visual projections in the Siamese cat, *J Physiol* 218:33, 1971.

95. Huges WF, McLoon SC: Ganglion cell death during normal retinal development in the chick. Comparisons with cell death induced by early target field destruction, *Exp Neurol* 66:587, 1979.

96. Huxtable CR, Dorling PR, Colegate SM: Mannosidosis induced by Swainsonine—a model to study pathogenetic aspects of neuronal lysosomal storage disease, *Proc Am Coll Vet Pathol* 31:118, 1980.

97. Huxtable CR, Dorling PR, Walkely SU: Onset and regression of neuraxonal lesions in sheep with mannosidosis induced experimentally with Swainsonine, *Acta Neuropathol* 58:27, 1982.

98. Jackson CA, et al: Neurological manifestations of cholesterinic granulomas in three horses, *Vet Rec* 135:228-230, 1994.

99. Jacobsen M, Hirose G: Origin of retina from both sides of the embryonic brain: a contribution to the problem of crossing at the optic chiasm, *Science* 202:637, 1978.

100. Johns PR, Russhof AC, Dubin MW: Postnatal neurogenesis in the kitten retina, *J Comp Neurol* 187:545, 1979.

101. Johnson GR, Oliver JE, Selcer R: Globoid cell leukodystrophy in a Beagle, *J Am Vet Med Assoc* 167:380, 1975.

102. Johnson KH: Globoid cell leukodystrophy in the cat, *J Am Vet Med Assoc* 157:2057, 1970.

103. Jolly RD: Mannosidosis and its control in Angus and Murray Grey cattle, *N Z Vet J* 26:194-198, 1978.

104. Jolly RD, Hartley WJ: Storage diseases of domestic animals, *Aust Vet J* 53:1, 1977.

105. Jolly RD, et al: Ovine ceroid lipofuscinosis: a model of Batten's disease, *Neuropathol Appl Neurobiol* 6:195, 1980.

106. Jolly RD, Thompson KG: The pathology of bovine mannosidosis, *Vet Pathol* 15:141, 1978.

107. Jolly RD, et al: Beta mannosidosis in a Salers calf: a new storage disease of cattle, *N Z Vet J* 38:102-105, 1990.

108. Jolly RD, West DM: Blindness in South Hampshire sheep: a neuronal ceroid lipofuscinosis, *N Z Vet J* 24:123, 1976.

109. Jones LF, Van Kampen KR, Hartley WJ: Comparative pathology of Astragalus (locoweed) and Swainsona poisoning in sheep, *Pathol Vet* 7:116, 1970.

110. Jones MZ, Dawson G: Caprine beta mannosidosis: inherited deficiency of beta-D-mannosidase, *J Biol Chem* 256:5185, 1981.

111. Jubb KV, Saunders LZ, Coates HV: Thiamin deficiency encephalopathy in cats, *J Comp Pathol* 66:217-277, 1956.

112. Kahrs RF: Chronc mercurial poisoning in swine: a case report of an outbreak with some epidemiological characteristics of hog cholera, *Cornell Vet* 58:67, 1968.

113. Kalil R: Development of the dorsal lateral geniculate nucleus in the cat, *J Comp Neurol* 182:265, 1978.

114. Kalil RE, Jhaveri SR, Richards W: Anomalous retinal pathways in the Siamese cat: an inadequate substrate for normal binocular vision, *Science* 174:302, 1971.

115. Kanamura K, Brodal E A: Tectopontine projection in the cat: an experimental anatomical study with comments on pathways for receptive impulses to the cerebellum, *J Comp Neurol* 3:371, 1973.

116. Karamanlidis AN, Magras J: Retinal projections in domestic ungulates. I. The retinal projections in the sheep and the pig, *Brain Res* 44:27, 1972.

117. Karamandilis AN, Magras J: Retinal projections in domestic ungulates. II. The retinal projections in the horse and ox, *Brain Res* 6:209, 1974.

118. Kelly DF, Pinsent PJN: *Optic neuropathy in a horse*, Berlin, 1979, Springer Berlin/Heidelberg.

119. Kelly WR, et al: Canine L fucosidosis: a storage disease of Springer spaniels, *Acta Neuropathol* 60:9-13, 1983.

120. Kern TJ: Persistent hyperplastic primary vitreous and microphthalmia in a dog, *J Am Vet Med Assoc* 178:1169, 1981.

121. Kern TJ, Riis RC: Optic nerve hypoplasia in three miniature poodles, *J Am Vet Med Assoc* 178:49, 1980.

122. Kolb H: The organization of the outer plexiform layer in the retina of the cat: electron microscopic observations, *J Neurocytol* 6:131, 1977.

123. Kolb H: The inner plexiform layer in the retina of the cat: electron microscopic observations, *J Neurocytol* 8:295, 1979.

124. Kolb H, West RW: Synaptic connections of the interplexiform cell in the retina of the cat, *J Neurocytol* 6:155, 1977.

125. Koppang N: Neuronal ceroid lipofuscinosis in English setters: juvenile amaurotic familial idiocy in English setters, *J Sm Anim Pract* 10:639, 1970.

126. Koppang N: Canine ceroid lipofuscinosis: a model for human neuronal ceroid lipofuscinosis and aging, *Mech Aging Develop* 2:421, 1973-1974.

127. Kosanke SD, Pierce KR, Bay WW: Clinical and biochemical abnormalities in porcine GM$_2$ gangliosidosis, *Vet Pathol* 15:685, 1978.

128. Kosanke SD, Pierce KR, Read WW: Morphogenesis of light and electron microscopic lesions in porcine GM$_2$ gangliosidosis, *Vet Pathol* 16:6, 1979.

129. Lange AL, Van den Berg PB, Baker MK: A suspected lysosomal storage disease in Abyssinian cats. Part II. Histopathological and ultrastructural aspects, *J S Afr Vet Med Assoc* 48:201, 1977.

130. Laties AM, Sprague JM: The projection of optic fibers to the visual centers in the cat, *J Comp Neurol* 127:35, 1966.

131. LaVail MM: Rod outer segment disk shedding in rat retina. Relationship to cyclic lighting, *Science* 194:1071, 1976.

132. Leipold HW, et al: Mannosidosis of Angus calves, *J Am Vet Med Assoc* 175:457, 1979.

133. Little PB, Sorenson DK: Bovine polioencephalomalacia, infectious embolic meningoencephalitis and acute lead poisoning in feedlot cattle, *J Am Vet Med Assoc* 155:1892, 1969.

134. Lowe FM, Martin CL, Dunlop RH: Naturally occurring and experimental thiamin deficiency in cats receiving commercial cat food, *Cornell Vet* 11:109-113, 1970.

135. Luttgen PJ, Braund KG, Storts RW: Globoid cell leukodystrophy in a Basset hound, *J Sm Anim Pract* 24: 153-160, 1983.

136. MacDonald JM, de Lahunta A, Georgi J: Cuterebra encephalitis in a dog, *Cornell Vet* 66:372-380, 1976.

137. Maenhout T, et al: Mannosidosis in a litter of Persian cats, *Vet Rec* 122:351-354, 1988.

138. Manktelow CD, Hartley WJ: Generalized glycogen storage disease in sheep, *J Comp Pathol* 85:139-145, 1975.

139. Mason TA: Persistent pupillary membrane in the Basenji, *Aust Vet J* 52:343, 1976.

140. Mayhew I, Jolly R: Ovine ceroid lipofuscinosis, *ACVIM Proc* 11:57-59, 1986.

141. McCormack JE: Variations of the ocular fundus of the bovine species, *Vet Scope* 18:21, 1974.

142. McGrath JT, Kelly AM, Steinberg SA: Cerebral lipidosis in the dog, *J Neuropathol Exp Neurol* 27:141, 1968.

143. McHowell J, Dorling PR, Cook RD: Infantile and late onset form of generalized glycogenosis type II in cattle, *J Pathol* 134:266-277, 1981.

144. McHowell J, Palmer AC: Globoid cell leukodystrophy in two dogs, *J Sm Anim Pract* 12:633, 1971.

145. McKay JS, et al: Postanesthetic cerebral necrosis in five horses, *Vet Rec* 150:70-74, 2002.

146. Meikle TH Jr, Sprague JM: The neural organization of the visual pathways in the cat, *Int Rev Neurobiol* 6:150, 1964.

147. Morgan KT: Amprolium poisoning of preruminant lambs: an ultrastructural study of the cerebral malacia and the nature of the inflammatory response, *J Pathol* 112: 229-236, 1974.

148. Munson L, et al: Leukoencephalopathy in cheetahs (Acinonyx jubatus). In Callanan JJ, Munson L, Stronach N, editors: *Report of workshop on ataxia in cheetah cubs*, Dublin, 1999, University College.

149. Nafe L: Canine optic neuritis, *Compend Cont Ed* 3:978, 1981.

150. Niimi K, Sprague JM: Thalamo-cortical organization of the visual system in the cat, *J Comp Neurol* 138:219, 1970.

151. Nimmo Wilkie JS, Hudson EB: Neuronal and generalized ceroid lipofuscinosis in a Cocker spaniel, *Vet Pathol* 19: 623-628, 1982.

152. Noden DM: Interactions directing the migration and cytodifferentiation of avian neural crest cells. In Garrod DR, editor: *Specificity of embryological interactions*, London, 1978, Chapman and Hill.

153. Nyberg-Hansen R: The location and termination of tectospinal fibers in the cat, *Exp Neurol* 9:212, 1964.

154. O'Sullivan BM: Generalized glycogen storage disease in Brahman cattle, *Aust Vet J* 57:227-229, 1981.

155. Palmer AC: Cardiac arrest and cerebrocortical necrosis, *Vet Rec* 80:390, 1967.

156. Parry HB: Degenerations of the dog retina. I. Structure and development of the retina of the normal dog, *Br J Ophthalmol* 37:385, 1953.

157. Patel V, et al: Alpha-phenylenediamine-mediated peroxidase deficiency in English setters with neuronal ceroid lipofuscinosis, *Lab Invest* 30:366, 1974.

158. Peiffer RL, Gelatt KN, Gwin RM: Persistent primary vitreous and a pigmented cataract in a dog, *J Am Anim Hosp Assoc* 13:478, 1977.

159. Pfeffer BA, Fisher SK: Development of retinal pigment epithelial surface structures ensheathing cone outer segments in the cat, *J Ultra Res* 76:158, 1981.

160. Pierce KR, et al: Porcine cerebrospinal lipodystrophy (GM_2 gangliosidosis), *Am J Pathol* 83:419, 1976.

161. Pritchard DH, Napthine DV, Sinclair A: Globoid cell leukodystrophy in polled Dorset sheep, *Vet Pathol* 17:399, 1980.

162. Rac R, Giesecke PR: Lysosomal storage disease in Chihuahuas, *Aust Vet J* 51:403, 1975.

163. Rafiquzzaman M, et al: Glycogenoses in the dog, *Acta Vet Scand* 17:196, 1976.

164. Raphel CF: Brain abscess in three horses, *J Am Vet Med Assoc* 180:874, 1982.

165. Read DH, et al: Neuronal-visceral GM_1 gangliosidosis in a dog with beta galactosidase deficiency, *Science* 194:442, 1976.

166. Read WK, Bridges CH: Cerebrospinal lipodystrophy in swine. A new disease model in comparative pathology, *Pathol Vet* 5:67, 1969.

167. Read WK, Bridges CH: Neuronal lipodystrophy: occurrence in inbred strain of cattle, *Pathol Vet* 6:235-243, 1969.

168. Rebhun WC: Persistent primary hyperplastic vitreous in a dog, *J Am Vet Med Assoc* 169:620, 1976.

169. Ribelin WE, Kintner LD: Lipodystrophy in the central nervous system in a dog: a disease with similarities to Tay Sachs disease in man, *Cornell Vet* 46:532, 1956.

170. Richards RB, et al: Bovine generalized glycogenosis, *Neuropathol Appl Neurobiol* 3:45, 1977.

171. Riis RC, et al: Tibetan terrier model of canine ceroid lipofuscinosis, *Am J Med Genet* 42:615-621, 1992.

172. Roberts SR, Bistner SI: Persistent pupillary membrane in Basenji dogs, *J Am Vet Med Assoc* 153:533, 1968.

173. Robertson TW, Hickey TL, Guillery RW: Development of the dorsal lateral geniculate nucleus in normal and visually deprived Siamese cats, *J Comp Neurol* 191:573, 1980.

174. Rotmistrovsky RA, et al: GM_2 gangliosidosis in a mixed breed dog, *Prog Vet Neurol* 2:203-208, 1991.

175. Sanderson KJ: The projections of the visual field to the lateral geniculate and medial interlaminar nuclei in the cat, *J Comp Neurol* 143:101, 1971.

176. Sanderson KJ, Guillery RW, Shackelford RM: Congenitally abnormal visual pathways in mink (Mustela vision) with reduced retinal pigment, *J Comp Neurol* 154:225, 1974.

177. Sandstrom B, Westman J, Ockerman PA: Glycogenosis of the central nervous system in the cat, *Acta Neuropathol* 14:194-200, 1969.

178. Saunders LZ: Congenital optic nerve hypoplasia in collie dogs, *Cornell Vet* 42:67, 1952.

179. Schatzberg SJ, et al: Polymerase chain reaction screening for DNA viruses in paraffin embedded brains from dogs with necrotizing meningoencephalitis, necrotizing leukoencephalitis and granulomatous meningoencephalitis, *J Vet Intern Med* 19:553-559, 2005.

180. Scott FW, et al: Teratogenesis in cats associated with griseofulvin therapy, *Teratology* 11:79, 1974.

181. Selcer ES, Selcer RR: Globoid cell leukodystrophy in two West Highland terriers and one Pomeranian, *Compend Cont Ed* 6:621-624, 1984.

182. Shatz CJ: A comparison of visual pathways in eastern and midwestern Siamese cats, *J Comp Neurol* 171:205, 1977.

183. Shatz CJ, Levay S: Siamese cat: altered connections of visual cortex, *Science* 204:328, 1979.

184. Sheahan BJ, Roche E, Donnelly WJC: Studies on skin fibroblasts from calves with GM_1 gangliosidosis, *J Comp Pathol* 87:205, 1977.

185. Shell LG, Potthoff A, Carithers R: Neuronal visceral GM_1 gangliosidosis in Portuguese water dogs, *J Vet Intern Med* 3:1-7, 1989.

186. Shively J, Epling G, Jensen R: Fine structure of the canine eye: retina, *Am J Vet Res* 31:1339, 1970.

187. Shively J, Epling G, Jensen R: Fine structure of the postnatal development of the canine retina, *Am J Vet Res* 32:383, 1971.

188. Silver J, Sidman RL: A mechanism for the guidance and topographic patterning of retinal ganglion cell axons, *J Comp Neurol* 189:101, 1980.

189. Singer HS, Cork LC: Canine GM$_2$ gangliosidosis: morphological and biochemical analysis, *Vet Pathol* 26:114-120, 1989.

190. Singleton MC, Peele TL: Distribution of optic fibers in the cat, *J Comp Neurol* 125:303, 1965.

191. Sisk DB: Clinical and pathological features of ceroid lipofuscinosis in two Australian cattle dogs, *J Am Vet Med Assoc* 197:361-364, 1990.

192. Smith JS, de Lahunta A, Riis RC: Reticulosis of the visual system in a dog, *J Sm Anim Pract* 18:634, 1977.

193. Spratling FR, et al: Experimental hypovitaminosis A in calves: clinical and gross postmortem findings, *Vet Rec* 77:1532-1542, 1965.

194. Stades FC: Persistent hyperplastic tunica vasculosa lentis and persistent hyperplastic primary vitreous (PHTVL/PHPV) in 90 closely related Doberman pinschers. Clinical aspects, *J Am Anim Hosp Assoc* 16:739, 1980.

195. Stalis IH, et al: Necrotizing meningoencephalitis of Maltese dogs, *Vet Pathol* 32:230-235, 1995.

196. Stone J: A quantitative analysis of the distribution of ganglion cells in the cat's retina, *J Comp Neurol* 124:337, 1965.

197. Stone J: The naso-temporal division of the cat's retina, *J Comp Neurol* 126:585, 1966.

198. Stone J: The number and distribution of the ganglion cells in the cat's retina, *J Comp Neurol* 180:753, 1978.

199. Stone J, Campion JE: Estimate of the number of myelinated axons in the cat's optic nerve, *J Comp Neurol* 180:799, 1978.

200. Stone J, Campion JE, Leicester J: The naso-temporal division of retina in the Siamese cat, *J Comp Neurol* 180:783, 1978.

201. Stone J, Hansen SM: The projection of the cat's retina in the lateral geniculate nucleus, *J Comp Neurol* 126:601, 1966.

202. Stone J, Keens J: Distribution of small and medium-sized ganglion cells in the cat's retina, *J Comp Neurol* 192:235, 1980.

203. Stone J, et al: Gradients between nasal and temporal areas of the cat retina in the properties of retinal ganglion cells, *J Comp Neurol* 192:219, 1980.

204. Stone J, Rowe M, Campion JE: Retinal abnormalities in the Siamese cat, *J Comp Neurol* 180:773, 1978.

205. Taylor R, Farrow BRH: Ceroid lipofuscinosis in Border collie dogs, *Acta Neuropathol* 75:627-631, 1988.

206. Taylor R, Farrow BRH, Healy P: Canine fucosidosis: clinical findings, *J Sm Anim Pract* 28:291-300, 1987.

207. Tipold A, Fatzer R, Zurbriggen A: Necrotizing encephalitis in Yorkshire terriers, *J Sm Anim Pract* 34:623-628, 1993.

208. Trousse F, et al: Control of retinal ganglion cell axon growth: a new role for Sonic hedgehog, *Development* 128:3927-3936, 2001.

209. Tucker GS: Light microscopic analysis of the kitten retina: postnatal development in the area centralis, *J Comp Neurol* 180:489, 1978.

210. Tucker GS, et al: Anatomic and physiologic development of the photoreceptor of the kitten, *Exp Brain Res* 37:459, 1979.

211. Van den Berg PB, Baker MK, Lange A: A suspected lysosomal storage disease in Abyssinian cats. Part I: Genetic, clinical and pathological aspects, *J S Afr Vet Med Assoc* 48:195, 1970.

212. Vandevelde M, Fatzer R: Neuronal lipofuscinosis in older Dachshunds, *Vet Pathol* 17:686, 1980.

213. Van de Water NS, Jolly RD, Farrow BRH: Canine Gaucher disease. The enzymic defect, *Aust J Exp Biol Med* 57:551, 1979.

214. Walvoort HC: Canine glycogen storage disease type II: a clinical study of four affected Lapland dogs, *J Am Anim Hosp Assoc* 20:279-286, 1984.

215. Wenger DS, et al: Niemann-Pick disease: a genetic model in Siamese cats, *Science* 208:1471, 1980.

216. Williams KJ, Summers BA, de Lahunta A: Cerebrospinal cuterebriasis in cats and its association with feline ischemic encephalopathy, *Vet Pathol* 35:330-343, 1998.

217. Wouters L, De Moor A: Ultrastructure of the pigment epithelium and the photoreceptors in the retina of the horse, *Am J Vet Res* 40:1066, 1979.

218. Wyman M, Donovan EF: The ocular fundus of the normal dog, *J Am Vet Med Assoc* 147:17, 1965.

219. Yakely WL, et al: Genetic transmission of an ocular fundus anomaly in collies, *J Am Vet Med Assoc* 152:457, 1968.

220. Young RW, Bok D: Participation of the retinal pigment epithelium in the rod outer segment renewal process, *J Cell Biol* 42:392, 1969.

221. Zaki F, Kay WJ: Globoid cell leukodystrophy in a miniature poodle, *J Am Vet Med Assoc* 163:248, 1973.

222. Zhang X-M, Yang X-Z: Regulation of retinal ganglion cell production by sonic hedgehog, *Development* 128:943-957, 2001.

15 AUDITORY SYSTEM: SPECIAL SOMATIC AFFERENT SYSTEM

ANATOMY

Receptor
Cranial Nerve VIII: Vestibulocochlear
  Nerve, Cochlear Division
Brainstem Nuclei and Tracts

Thalamocortical Pathway

DEAFNESS

Conduction Deafness
Sensorineural Deafness

*Congenital Inherited Sensorineural
  Deafness*
Acquired Sensorineural Deafness

ANATOMY

Receptor

The development of the bony and membranous labyrinths of the receptor in the auditory system is described with the development of the vestibular system in Chapter 12. Fig. 12-1 outlines the basic components; Fig. 15-1 shows their relationship to the other components of the ear. The cochlea is the coiled portion of the bony labyrinth in the petrosal portion of the temporal bone that contains perilymph. The degree of coiling varies with the species of animal. There are 3.5 turns in the dog cochlea, compared with 2.5 turns in the human cochlea. The portion of the bone that forms the center, or axis, of the coiled cochlea is the modiolus. It contains the cochlear division of the vestibulocochlear nerve. At the base of the modiolus, the cochlea is continuous with the vestibule, and there is an opening into the tympanic cavity that is called the cochlear window. A shelf of bone projects into the cochlea from the modiolus. This is the spiral lamina, which partially divides the cochlea into two portions and is absent at the apex, or most distal extent of the cochlea (Fig. 15-2).

The cochlear duct is the coiled portion of the membranous labyrinth derived from the embryonic ectodermal otocyst. It is located inside the cochlea and contains endolymph. It is a tubular structure that, in transverse section, is triangular in shape. The apex of the triangle attaches medially to the spiral lamina, and the base of the triangle attaches laterally to the outer wall of the cochlea (see Fig. 15-2). This completes the partitioning of the cochlea into two portions, each filled with a continuous column of perilymph. The two sections are the scala vestibuli and the scala tympani. The scala vestibuli is situated dorsal to the cochlear duct; it communicates proximally with the vestibule and distally at the apex of the cochlear duct, with the scala tympani. The latter occurs because the cochlear duct does not reach the apex of the cochlea, leaving an opening between the two scali that is known as the helicotrema. The scala tympani is situated ventral to the cochlear duct. It communicates distally, at the helicotrema, with the scala vestibuli. Proximally, at the base of the coiled cochlea, the scala tympani terminates at the cochlear window, which is covered by a membrane that retains the perilymph within the bony labyrinth. On the other side of this membrane, at the cochlear window, is the air-filled tympanic cavity of the middle ear in the tympanic bulla. Perilymph fills the scala vestibuli and scala tympani (see Fig. 15-1). A small perilymphatic duct connects the scala tympani with the subarachnoid space medial to the petrosal portion of the temporal bone via the cochlear canaliculus. At the level of the origin of the cochlea from the vestibule, the cochlear duct communicates with the saccule by way of the ductus reuniens. Figs. 15-3 through 15-5 show the microscopic features of this anatomy.

The base of the triangular cochlear duct, when viewed in transverse section, is attached to the outer wall of the bony cochlea and consists of a stria vascularis and a spiral prominence (see Figs. 15-2 and 15-5). A thin layer of tissue called the vestibular membrane forms the dorsal border of the cochlear duct. This membrane is between the perilymph of the scala vestibuli and the endolymph of the cochlear duct. It extends from the stria vascularis dorsolaterally to the spiral lamina medially. The basilar membrane extends between the spiral lamina and the ventrolateral extent of the stria vascularis at the middle of the lateral wall of the cochlea (Fig. 15-6; see also Fig. 15-5). The basilar membrane is a highly organized layer of collagen fibers. The spiral organ (organ of Corti) is the specialized sensory neuroepithelium that is located on this basilar membrane.[31] This spiral organ is composed of hair cells and several types of supporting cells. The hair cells have, on their luminal surfaces, modified microvilli known as stereocilia. The tips of these stereocilia are embedded in a proteinaceous membrane, the tectorial membrane, which covers the hair cells and is attached medially along the apex of the cochlear duct. The hair cells are associated with various types of supporting cells located on the basilar membrane. The dendritic zones of the neurons in the cochlear portion of the eighth cranial nerve are in synaptic relationship with the bases of the hair cells.[29]

Sound waves are transmitted from the air medium of the external ear canal to the solid medium of the tympanum

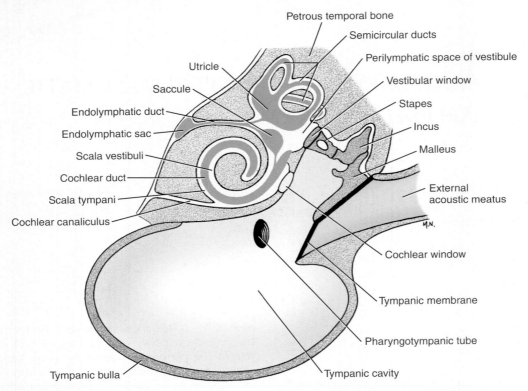

FIGURE 15-1 Schematic section through the inner ear, middle ear, and external ear of a dog. The membranous labyrinth is drawn in blue within the bony labyrinth. *(From Evans HE: Miller's anatomy of the dog, ed 3, Philadelphia, 1993, Saunders.)*

and the chain of three ear ossicles, which extends to the vestibular window, and to the fluid medium of the perilymph in the scala vestibuli. Wave flow through the perilymph in the scala vestibuli is reflected to the basilar membrane by way of the vestibular membrane and the endolymph of the cochlear duct or by continuing through the helicotrema to the perilymph in the scala tympani. Movement of the highly organized basilar membrane causes the hair cells of the overlying spiral organ to move and their stereocilia, embedded in the tectorial membrane, to bend. This action causes an impulse to be generated in the cochlear neurons. The basilar membrane acts as a resonator, and different portions respond maximally to sound waves of specific frequencies. This function may be related to the length of the basilar membrane, which is longest at the base of the cochlear coil and progressively shortens through the coils to the apex. Low frequencies cause maximal vibration of the basilar membrane at the base of the cochlear duct. High frequencies affect the apical portion of the basilar membrane maximally. In dogs, the basilar membrane is sensitive to a frequency range of 2 to 47 Hertz, compared with a range of 1 to 19 Hertz in humans.

Cranial Nerve VIII: Vestibulocochlear Nerve, Cochlear Division

The neurons of the vestibulocochlear nerve are derived from placode ectoderm associated with the otocyst. The dendritic zone of the cochlear division of the eighth cranial nerve is in synaptic relationship with the base of the hair cells in the spiral organ. The axons course medially along the basilar membrane into the modiolus. The cell bodies of these

bipolar neurons are located in the modiolus at the origin of the spiral lamina, where they form the spiral ganglion. The axons course though the center, or axis, of the modiolus to the internal acoustic meatus, where they are joined by the vestibular division of the eighth cranial nerve. Within the vestibulocochlear nerve, the axons of the cochlear division course to the region of the cerebellomedullary angle at the junction of the medulla and the pons, caudal to the transverse fibers of the pons. They terminate in telodendria on cell bodies in the dorsal and ventral cochlear nuclei that are located on the side of the medulla where the nerve enters. These nuclei bulge from the lateral side of the rostral medulla where they appear to be in the vestibulocochlear nerve (see Figs. 2-11, 2-12).

Brainstem Nuclei and Tracts

The axons of the cell bodies in the cochlear nuclei pass into the medulla by one of two pathways: ventrally through the trapezoid body or dorsally over the caudal cerebellar peduncle by way of the acoustic stria (see Figs. 2-12, 2-13). Numerous pathways involving a number of synapses are available in the brainstem to the auditory system for reflex activity and conscious perception (Fig. 15-7).

Reflexes are mediated directly, through the influence of cochlear nuclei neurons on the lower motor neurons (LMNs) in brainstem nuclei; or they are mediated indirectly by transmission through the neurons of the caudal colliculus or other auditory nuclei in the brainstem. Reflex regulation of the sound wave frequency occurs by way of the afferent neurons of the cochlear division of the eighth cranial nerve,

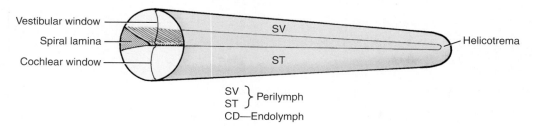

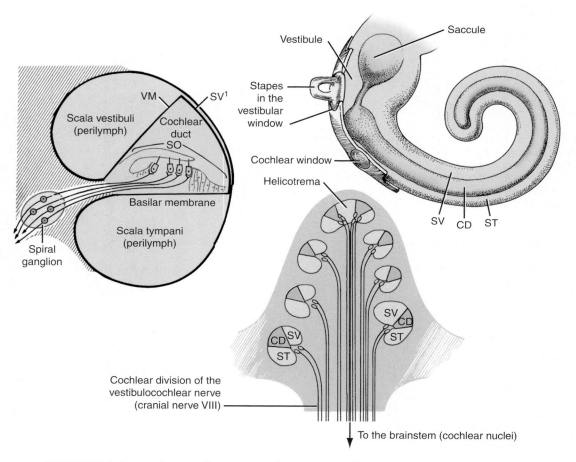

FIGURE 15-2 Receptor of somatic afferent system: auditory system (special somatic afferent). *CD,* Cochlear duct; *SO,* spiral organ; *ST,* scala tympani; *SV,* scala vestibuli; *SV¹,* stria vascularis; *VM,* vestibular membrane.

the cochlear nuclei, and the efferent neurons of the motor nucleus of the trigeminal nerve in the pons that innervate the tensor tympani muscle and the efferent neurons in the facial nucleus in the medulla that innervate the stapedius muscle. These muscles control the degree of mobility of the ear ossicles.

Other neurons that belong to the auditory system and function in both reflex and conscious perception pathways include the dorsal and ventral nuclei of the trapezoid body, the nucleus of the lateral lemniscus, and the caudal colliculus.[12] The neuronal cell bodies of the ventral nucleus of the trapezoid body are scattered without specific arrangement throughout the axons of the trapezoid body. The dorsal nucleus of the trapezoid body forms a distinctly

encapsulated nucleus ventrally in the rostral medulla, dorsal to the trapezoid body and dorsolateral to the pyramid, from the level of the facial nucleus in the medulla to the motor nucleus of the trigeminal nerve in the pons (see Figs. 2-11, 2-12). The lateral lemniscus is composed mostly of ascending axons in the auditory system as they course from the rostral medulla through the pons to the caudal mesencephalon on the lateral surface of the brainstem (see Figs. 2-8 through 2-10).[12] The lateral lemniscus contains axons from the cochlear nuclei or the various nuclei of the trapezoid body on the same side or the opposite side. The lateral lemniscus is formed medial to the middle cerebellar peduncle and is exposed on the lateral surface of the caudal mesencephalon rostral to the transverse fibers of the pons that

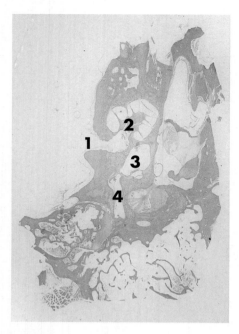

FIGURE 15-3 Microscopic dorsal plane section of dog petrosal and tympanic parts of the right temporal bone. The rostral aspect is at the top, and the medial side is on the left of the figure, where the open space is the internal acoustic meatus (1). From the top to the bottom of the section, you should be able to identify the cochlea coiled around the modiolus (2), the vestibule (3), and one semicircular canal (4) in the petrosal part of the temporal bone.

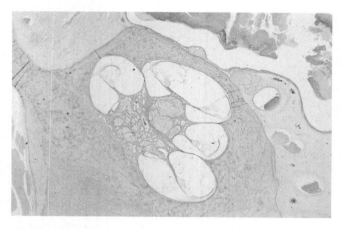

FIGURE 15-4 Higher magnification of the cochlea and cochlear duct coiled around the modiolus of a 1-month-old calf.

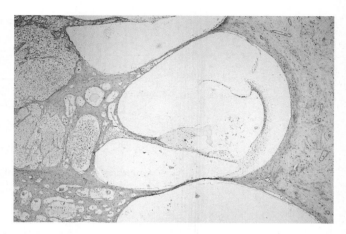

FIGURE 15-5 Higher magnification of one complete transverse section of the cochlea and cochlear duct of the calf in Fig. 15-4. The stria vascularis is on the right, with artifactitious separation from the wall of the cochlea.

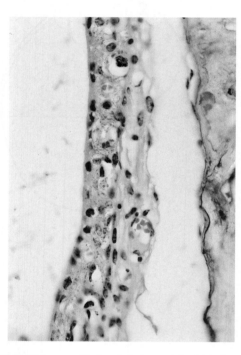

FIGURE 15-6 Higher magnification of a stria vascularis. This is the source of the endolymph, within which it maintains the normal endocochlear potential. Note the scattered melanin granules.

form the middle cerebellar peduncle. Embedded along the ventromedial aspect of this lateral lemniscus is the nucleus of the lateral lemniscus (see Fig. 2-9). The lateral lemniscus terminates at the caudal colliculus.

The caudal colliculus consists of cell bodies of neurons and axonal processes organized in laminae (see Figs. 2-8, 2-9).[23] It functions as a reflex center for the auditory system. Efferent axons project to LMNs in the brainstem by way of the tectonuclear pathway and to LMNs in the cervical spinal cord through the tectospinal pathway in the ventral funiculus. The latter arises from the rostral colliculus. Efferent axons project to the thalamus in the brachium of the caudal colliculus located on the lateral side of the mesencephalon ventral to the rostral colliculus (see Figs. 2-7, 2-8). They terminate in the medial geniculate nucleus (see Figs. 2-5, 2-6).

Thalamocortical Pathway

Axons in the conscious projection pathway arise primarily from cell bodies in the caudal colliculus that project rostrally in the brachium of the caudal colliculus. This brachium is located on the lateral side of the mesencephalon and courses rostrally to the medial geniculate nucleus of the thalamus. This nucleus protrudes from the caudolateral aspect of the thalamus and extends caudally beside the mesencephalon (see Figs. 2-5, 2-6). It is the specific thalamic projection nucleus for the auditory system, and it projects

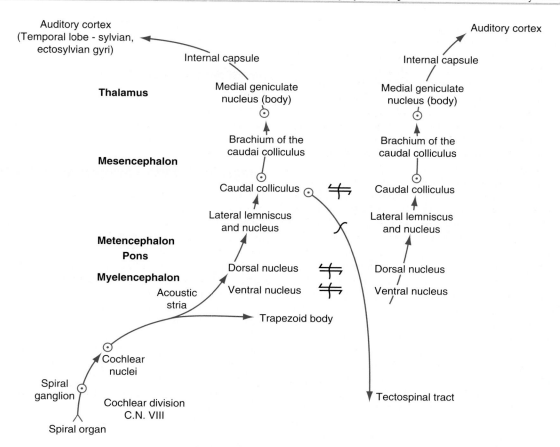

FIGURE 15-7 The auditory pathway.

axons by way of the internal capsule to the neocortex of the temporal lobe. This auditory system cortex is located primarily in the sylvian and ectosylvian gyri. Studies in the dog have localized the auditory conscious projection pathway to the ectosylvian gyrus, where the various frequencies can be arranged from rostral (high frequencies) to caudal (low frequencies).[38-40]

This rostrally projecting auditory pathway is characterized by diffuseness and a bilateral distribution. Despite this, at the cortical level there is predominance of a contralateral representation of each cochlear duct. Thus, impulses stimulated in one cochlear duct are conducted predominantly to the opposite temporal lobe. The crossing occurs at the level of the trapezoid body, between the nuclei of the lateral lemniscus, and at the commissure of the caudal colliculus.

DEAFNESS

By recording brainstem auditory evoked potentials, researchers have found that there is some evidence of perception of sound at 10 to 11 days of age in puppies. In normal dogs it may take as long as 2 weeks for the external acoustic meatus to open completely.[28] Audiometry studies first detect sound perception at 5 days of age in kittens and 14 days in puppies. Normal hearing of environmental sounds in dogs usually develops by 4 to 5 weeks of age. For that reason, as well as the practicality in handling puppies at this age, it is best

to delay electrophysiologic tests for hearing until at least 6 to 8 weeks of age.

Partial bilateral loss of hearing and complete unilateral loss of hearing are difficult to establish on the clinical physical examination of domestic animals. Complete bilateral deafness usually is caused by direct or indirect interference with the function of the receptor organ. For central lesions to produce deafness, there must be extensive damage to both cerebral hemispheres or to the conscious projection pathways on both sides of the brainstem. Such a lesion would most likely produce severe neurologic signs referable to the interference with other systems adjacent to the auditory pathways. Because of the multitude of brainstem pathways available for the auditory system, there is a large margin of safety for this function.

Therefore, when you are presented with a deaf animal, your attention should be directed to diseases that affect the receptor portion of this system. The best clinical test for total deafness is to confront the sleeping patient with a loud noise. Inability to arouse the patient in this manner is the best evidence of total inability to hear. Less obvious degrees of deafness are difficult for you to appreciate clinically, and careful observation by the owner of the patient in its own environment may be the most reliable means of determining any degree of deafness.

Sophisticated procedures have been developed to determine hearing in animals, including the technique of monitoring changes in respiration in response to hearing sounds as well as recording electroencephalographic responses to auditory stimuli.[6,25,41,42] Brainstem responses to far-field auditory stimuli can be recorded percutaneously in the brains of animals.[7] The various wave forms that are observed have been related to specific components of the peripheral and central portions of the auditory system. The most common procedure used by practicing neurologists is the recording of brainstem auditory evoked responses. This technique can be used to determine an auditory defect and to specify the level of the interference with this system between the peripheral receptor and the thalamus. The procedure can be performed in an awake, sedated, or anesthetized patient. It consists of a specialized ear plug that is the source of an auditory stimulus in the form of clicks. The evoked responses are recorded through subcutaneous electrodes inserted over the calvaria. The evoked responses consist of four to six waves seen within 10 ms of the delivery of the clicks. The first wave is generated by the vestibulocochlear nerve. The origin of waves two through five is less precise. Wave two is thought to be from the cochlear nuclei; wave three from the dorsal nucleus of the trapezoid body; wave four from the lateral lemniscus and its nucleus; wave five from the caudal colliculus; and wave six from the medial geniculate nucleus. Normal animals have four to six recognizable wave forms. Animals that are deaf due to lesions that involve the receptor organ show a flat line with no wave forms. Patients with brainstem lesions may show a delay in the appearance of wave forms two through six. This procedure is most valuable in determining unilateral deafness in puppies that are being tested for the inherited forms of receptor organ deafness. It is also useful in determining brain death in patients being maintained on life-support systems. Impedance audiometry, including tympanometry, have been used to evaluate the integrity of the conduction components of hearing in the external and middle ears.[25]

There are two forms of deafness related to the peripheral components of the auditory pathway: conduction deafness and sensorineural deafness.[14,18,35-37,43]

Conduction Deafness

Conduction deafness results from any obstruction to the passage of sound waves from the external environment to the spiral organ. Obstacles include the air pathway in the external acoustic meatus, the tympanum and bony pathway of the ossicles through the middle ear, and the fluid medium of the perilymph in the cochlea. The receptor is still functional and responds to vibrations induced in the petrosal part of the temporal bone with a tuning fork but not to sound waves that are prevented from reaching the receptor organ. Using a tuning fork in animals is unreliable. Congenital absence of an external acoustic meatus is rare. Acquired causes of conduction deafness include inflammatory lesions, which are common in the external acoustic meatus and in the tympanic cavity of the middle ear. Neoplasms can also involve these structures and prevent the passage of sound waves. The cause of the deafness that is associated with aging (presbycusis) is poorly understood except that it most likely results from dysfunction of the peripheral components of the auditory pathway. It may involve arthrosis of the articulations between ear ossicles that prevents their movement (conduction deafness) or a late form of abiotrophy of the hair cells in the spiral organ (sensorineural deafness).

Sensorineural Deafness

Sensorineural deafness involves an abnormality in the receptor organ or in the neurons of the cochlear division of the vestibulocochlear nerve. There are congenital and acquired forms of sensorineural deafness.

Congenital Inherited Sensorineural Deafness

Congenital inherited sensorineural deafness is a common disorder, especially in dogs; numerous breeds are affected.[1,2] Electrophysiologic testing has determined that hearing is usually present in affected dogs in the first few weeks of life but is absent by about 60 days of age. This supports a degenerative pathogenesis, rather than hypoplasia or aplasia. This form of deafness involves the function of the cochlear duct. Two pathogenetic mechanisms have been described using terminology that seems confusing to us. One is related to albinism and involves dysfunction of the stria vascularis (cochleosaccular). The other involves abiotrophy of the hair cells (neuroepithelial). We prefer the use of the terms *albinotic* and *abiotrophic* for these two forms of congenital sensorineural deafness.

Albinotic Form. Albinotic inherited congenital sensorineural deafness is associated with dysfunction of the stria vascularis because of the lack of melanocytes at this location. The production of endolymph and the maintenance of its normal endocochlear potential is a function of the stria vascularis (see Fig. 15-6). The latter involves the transfer of potassium ions into the endolymph. In the absence of melanocytes in the stria vascularis, this function is inhibited. The abnormal endocochlear potential leads to degeneration of the hair cells of the spiral organ and hence to deafness. Thus, this form of deafness occurs in animals that are partially or completely albinotic. The deafness may be unilateral or bilateral. White-coated, blue-eyed cats are notorious for this form of deafness; the incidence is nearly 50%. Dalmatians have a 30% incidence of the albinotic form of deafness, which is inherited as an autosomal dominant gene.[3,17,19,21] Deafness has been recognized in at least 12 different breeds of white-coated cats, in numerous breeds of dogs with predominantly white or merle coat colors, and in white mink.*

Abiotrophic Form. Abiotrophic inherited congenital sensorineural deafness directly affects the hair cells of the spiral organ. The endocochlear potential is normal in these animals. The lesion is usually bilateral and occasionally also affects the hair cells of the vestibular system receptors. The inheritance usually involves an autosomal recessive gene. Although most of these abiotrophies cause deafness at a few weeks of age, occasionally the onset of deafness occurs later in life. In the cavalier King Charles spaniel, deafness may not be apparent until 3 or 4 years of age.[27]

Our understanding of the pathogenesis of congenital deafness is markedly compromised by the difficulty in processing the inner ear after death to obtain histologic sections

---

*References 4, 5, 9-11, 15, 16, 20, 24, 26, 30, 32-34, 44.

as free from artifact as possible. This is due to the difficulty of rapid preservation of the structures in the membranous labyrinth of the inner ear after death and the need to decalcify the petrosal portion of the temporal bone to obtain these sections. Although a list of 69 dog breeds with congenital deafness has been published, in most cases, it is not known whether they have the albinotic or abiotrophic form of deafness or some other pathogenesis, such as a hypoplasia or aplasia.

Acquired Sensorineural Deafness

Acquired sensorineural deafness occurs most commonly secondary to infections that cause inflammation of the middle ear and extend into the structures of the inner ear. The clinical signs of dysfunction of the peripheral components of the vestibular system predominate, and deafness is not recognized clinically unless the lesion is bilateral. See Case Example 12-9. Temporal bone neoplasia is a less common cause of unilateral deafness. Be aware that the small perilymphatic duct provides a direct connection between the cerebrospinal fluid in the subarachnoid space and the perilymph in the scala tympani of the bony labyrinth. Meningitis and otitis interna may occur concomitantly more often than we appreciate. As a rule, the clinical signs of the meningitis mask the clinical signs of the otitis interna. A less common cause of acquired deafness is ototoxicity. The list of drugs and chemicals that are potentially ototoxic is very long.[8,13,22] You should be especially concerned with long-term administration of the aminoglycoside antibiotics. Many ear cleaning agents are ototoxic if they gain access to the middle ear through a ruptured tympanum. Some of the chemotherapeutic agents used in the treatment of neoplasms may be ototoxic, and you must be aware of their published toxic effects. The specific effects of these drugs and chemicals vary according to the dose used, the duration of administration, and the species in which it is used. Some affect the receptors of the auditory system; others affect the vestibular system receptors; or both may be affected.

Age-related deafness is common, especially in older dogs, and is referred to as presbycusis.[27] The causes of this form of deafness are not well understood. Some cases may involve conduction deafness due to arthrosis of the ear ossicles and their consequent immobility. Other cases may be age-related degeneration of the hair cells in the spiral organ. Be aware that this form of deafness may not be recognized by the owner until the dog receives general anesthesia for some minor procedure, such as dentistry or ear cleaning. What role the anesthesia has in precipitating the sudden observation of deafness is not known. Presumably, the patient had already lost most of its hearing before the anesthesia but it had not been appreciated by the owner.

Hearing aids for dogs have been utilized by some clinicians. However, they have little utility in veterinary medicine, from our perspective. The patients do not tolerate the apparatus well and eventually shake it from the ear. On occasion, the patient has consumed the fairly expensive equipment. That said, if an owner wants to explore this option, cooperation with a human medical group is recommended.

REFERENCES

1. Adams EW: Hereditary deafness in a family of foxhounds, *J Am Vet Med Assoc* 128:302, 1956.
2. Altmann F: Histologic picture of inherited nerve deafness in man and animal, *Arch Otolaryngol* 51:852, 1950.
3. Anderson H et al: Genetic hearing impairment in the Dalmatian dog, *Acta Otolaryngol* 232:1, 1968.
4. Bergsma DR, Brown KS: White fur, blue eyes, and deafness in the domestic cat, *J Hered* 61:171, 1971.
5. Bosher SK, Hallpike CS: Observations on the histologic features, development and pathogenesis of the inner ear degeneration of the deaf white cat, *Proc R Soc Biol Series B* 162:147, 1965.
6. Bradford ZJ et al: Measurement of hearing in dogs by respiration audiometry, *Am J Vet Res* 34:1183, 1973.
7. Cazals Y et al: Acoustic responses after total destruction of the cochlear receptor: brainstem and auditory cortex, *Science* 210:83, 1980.
8. Crowell WA, Divers TJ, Byars TD: Neomycin toxicosis in calves, *Am J Vet Res* 42:29, 1981.
9. Faith RE, Woodard JC: Animal models of human disease: Waardenburg's syndrome, *Comp Pathol Bull* 5:3, 1973.
10. Flottrop G, Foss I: Development of hearing in hereditary deaf white mink (Hedlund) and normal mink (Standard) and the subsequent deterioration of the auditory response in Hedlund mink, *Acta Otolaryngol* 87:16, 1979.
11. Foss I, Flottrop G: Measurements of hearing and morphological examination of the inner ear in deaf white mink (Hedlund) and normal mink (Standard), *Proc 7th Int Cong Electron Microsc* 3:761, 1970.
12. Goldberg JM, Moore RY: Ascending projections of the lateral lemniscus in the cat and monkey, *J Comp Neurol* 129:143, 1967.
13. Hawkins JR, Lurie MH: The ototoxicity of dihydrostreptomycin and neomycin in the cat, *Ann Otol Rhinol Laryngol* 62:1128, 1953.
14. Hayes HM et al: Canine congenital deafness: epidemiologic study of 272 cases, *J Am Anim Hosp Assoc* 17:473, 1981.
15. Hilding DA, Siguira A, Nakai Y: Deaf white mink: electron microscopic study of the inner ear, *Ann Otol Rhinol Laryngol* 76:647, 1967.
16. Howe HA: The reaction of the cochlear nerve to destruction of its end organ: a study of deaf albino cats, *J Comp Neurol* 62:72, 1935.
17. Hudson WR, Ruben RJ: Hereditary deafness in the Dalmatian dog, *Arch Otolaryngol* 75:213, 1962.
18. Johnson LG, Hawkins JE: Symposium on basic ear research. II. Strial atrophy in clinical and experimental deafness, *Laryngoscope* 81:1105, 1972.
19. Lurie MH: The membranous labyrinth in the congenitally deaf Collie and Dalmatian dog, *Laryngoscope* 58:279, 1948.
20. Mair IWS: Hereditary deafness in the white cat, *Acta Otolaryngol Supp* 314:5, 1973.
21. Mair IWS: Hereditary deafness in the Dalmatian dog, *Otorhinolaryngology* 212:1, 1976.
22. McGee TM, Olsezewski J: Streptomycin sulfate and dihydrostreptomycin toxicity; behavioral and histopathologic studies, *Arch Otolaryngol* 75:295, 1962.
23. Merzenich MM, Reid MD: Representation of the cochlea within the inferior colliculus of the cat, *Brain Res* 77:397, 1974.
24. Pcyol R, Rebillard M, Rebillard G: Primary neural disorders in the deaf white cat cochlea, *Acta Otol* 85:59, 1977.
25. Penrod JP, Coulter DB: The diagnostic uses of impedance audiometry in the dog, *J Am Anim Hosp Assoc* 16:941, 1980.
26. Platt S et al: Prevalence of unilateral and bilateral deafness in border collies and association with phenotype, *J Vet Intern Med* 20:1355-1362, 2006.

27. Podel M: Advances in assessing canine degenerative hearing loss, *Proc Am Coll Vet Intern Med* 17:291-293, 1999.

28. Pujol R, Marty R: Postnatal maturation in the cochlea of the cat, *J Comp Neurol* 139:115, 1970.

29. Raphael Y, Altschuler RA: Structure and innervation of the cochlea, *Brain Res Bull* 60:397-422, 2003.

30. Rebillard G et al: Histophysiologic relationships in the deaf white cat auditory systems, *Acta Otol* 82:48, 1976.

31. Represa J, Frenz DA, Van De Water TR: Genetic patterning of embryonic ear development, *Acta Otolaryngol* 120:5-10, 2000.

32. Roberts S: Color dilution and hereditary defects in Collie dogs, *Am J Ophthalmol* 63:1762, 1967.

33. Saunders LZ: The histopathology of congenital hereditary deafness in white mink, *Pathol Vet* 2:256, 1965.

34. Sigiura AS, Hilding DA: Cochlear-saccular degeneration in Hedlund white mink, *Acta Otol* 69:126, 1970.

35. Steinberg SA: Inherited deafness in the dog, *Proc Am Coll Vet Intern Med* 16:337-338, 1998.

36. Strain GM: Congenital deafness and its recognition, *Vet Clin North Am Sm Anim Pract* 29:895-907, 1999.

37. Strain GM: Deafness prevalence and pigmentation and gender associations in dog breeds at risk, *Vet J* 167:23-32, 2004.

38. Tunturi AR: Audio frequency localization in the acoustic cortex of the dog, *Am J Physiol* 141:397, 1944.

39. Tunturi AR: The pathway from the medial geniculate body to the ectosylvian auditory cortex in the dog, *J Comp Neurol* 138:131, 1970.

40. Tunturi AR: Classification of neurons in the ectosylvian auditory cortex of the dog, *J Comp Neurol* 142:153, 1971.

41. Whidden SJ, Redding RW: Evaluation of the origins in the brainstem of far field averaged auditory responses in the canine, *Proc Am Coll Vet Intern Med* 7:112, 1979.

42. Whidden SJ, Redding RW, Grover J: Evaluation of the normative far field averaged auditory evoked responses in the canine, *Proc Am Coll Vet Intern Med* 7:112, 1979.

43. Willems PJ: Genetic causes of hearing loss, *N Engl J Med* 342:1101-1109, 2000.

44. Wolff D: Three generations of deaf white cats, *J Hered* 33:39, 1942.

16 VISCERAL AFFERENT SYSTEMS

GENERAL VISCERAL AFFERENT SYSTEM

ANATOMY

Receptor: Peripheral Nerve

Brainstem and Tracts
Functional Concepts
Referred Pain

SPECIAL VISCERAL AFFERENT SYSTEM: TASTE

SPECIAL VISCERAL AFFERENT SYSTEM: OLFACTION

▋ GENERAL VISCERAL AFFERENT SYSTEM

The visceral afferent systems consist of neurons whose dendritic zones are located primarily in the viscera of the body as opposed to the somatic afferent system, which innervates primarily the surface of the body. The general visceral afferent (GVA) system consists of neurons whose cell bodies are located in all of the spinal ganglia and in many of the cranial ganglia. Many of the tissues that are innervated are derived from embryonic splanchnopleura. These GVA neurons are concerned with body temperature, blood pressure, gas concentration and pressure, and movement of viscera. The special visceral afferent (SVA) system consists of neurons restricted in their location to specific cranial nerves that function in taste and smell.

▋ ANATOMY

Receptor: Peripheral Nerve

The receptors of the GVA system are located throughout the viscera of the body, where they are stimulated by a number of different modalities. Stretch, distention, and pressure on or in a viscus are the most common modalities. Some receptors are sensitive to chemical changes in the environment. Free endings and a variety of encapsulated endings are found at the dendritic zones of the neurons in this system.[7,10,17,19] The axons course over the peripheral nerves that are most readily available to the viscus. In the head, they are the facial nerve to the middle ear and blood vessels of the head; the glossopharyngeal nerve to the caudal tongue, pharynx, carotid body, and carotid sinus; and the vagus nerve to the pharynx and larynx. In the thoracic and abdominal cavities, they are the vagus nerve and the peripheral branches of the sympathetic trunk that include the splanchnic nerves in the abdominal cavity. Here in the body cavities, the GVA axons course toward the central nervous system (CNS) in nerves that contain neurons of the parasympathetic and sympathetic portions of the general visceral efferent (GVE) system (Fig. 16-1). GVA axons from peripheral blood vessels course through the peripheral nerves to the segmental spinal nerves.

The cell bodies of these GVA neurons are located in the geniculate ganglion of the facial nerve, the distal ganglia of the glossopharyngeal and vagus nerves, and the spinal ganglia of the involved spinal nerves.[18] Horseradish peroxidase studies of the esophageal innervation of the dog have shown GVA neuronal cell bodies diffusely distributed in the distal ganglia of the glossopharyngeal and vagal nerves and the cervical and thoracic spinal ganglia.

Brainstem and Tracts

The axons continue from the various ganglia into the CNS. Those axons in the facial, glossopharyngeal, and vagal nerves enter the ventrolateral aspect of the medulla and course to a position near the lateral aspect of the fourth ventricle adjacent to the sulcus limitans. There, the axons course rostrally in a column called the *solitary tract* (see Figs. 16-1, 2-14, and 2-15). This tract is surrounded by neurons that form the nucleus of the solitary tract in which the axons in the tract terminate. This solitary tract and its nucleus develop in the alar plate adjacent to the motor column of the GVE system. Therefore, it is found dorsolateral to the parasympathetic nuclei of the facial, glossopharyngeal, and vagal nerves. The solitary tract stands out in myelin-stained sections as a densely cylindric structure surrounded by the unstained cell bodies of the nucleus. It extends from the level of the facial nucleus (GSE) rostrally to caudal to the obex caudally. Caudally, the nucleus gracilis and medial cuneate nucleus are dorsal to the solitary tract and rostrally, the medial vestibular nucleus is dorsal to it.

The nucleus of the solitary tract participates mostly in reflex activity and projects to neuronal cell bodies in the GVE system directly or indirectly by way of interneurons in the reticular formation that participate in the various metabolic centers that regulate visceral functions. These include respiratory and cardiovascular activity, swallowing, and micturition. The area postrema receives afferents from the solitary nucleus and participates with the medullary vomiting center.[12]

The area postrema is located on both sides of the caudal medulla at the level of the obex. It is adjacent to the

441

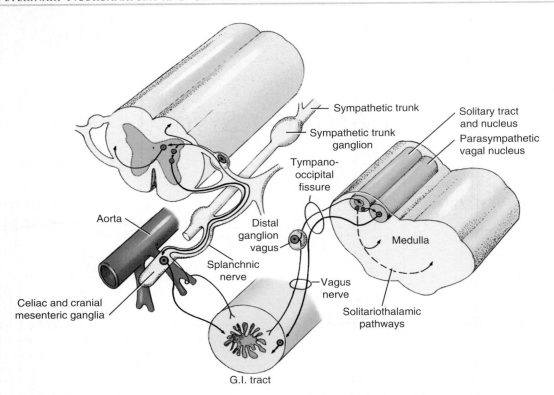

FIGURE 16-1 GVA system. Reversal of the GVE sympathetic pathway (conscious perception) and parasympathetic pathway (reflex function). *G.I.,* Gastrointestinal.

floor of the fourth ventricle, dorsal and slightly lateral to the parasympathetic nucleus of the vagus. It is a unique parenchymal structure that is readily recognized microscopically by its abundance of small capillaries and glial cells adjacent to a flat layer of ependymal cells that line the fourth ventricle. It is easily mistaken for a neuropathologic lesion. The area postrema is one of the circumventricular organs that have in common the absence of a blood-brain barrier and an anatomic position adjacent to the ventricular system. Other circumventricular organs include (1) the subfornical organ on the caudal surface of the columns of the fornix, where they form the rostral borders of the third ventricle; (2) the subcommissural organ that projects ventrally into the rostral mesencephalic aqueduct ventral to the caudal commissure; (3) the pineal gland that projects caudally from the dorsal portion of the third ventricle; and (4) the hypothalamic vascular organ adjacent to the ventral portion of the third ventricle. These sites are thought to be involved in such functions as chemoreception, neurosecretion, and the control of various visceral activities. They play important roles in the communication between the parenchyma and the cerebrospinal fluid and in communication with other organs via blood-borne products.

Some neuronal cell bodies in the nucleus of the solitary tract project axons rostrally in a pathway of conscious perception. These course mostly on the contralateral side of the brainstem in an ill-defined solitariothalamic pathway that closely parallels the medial lemniscus and spinothalamic pathway. These axons terminate at a synapse in the ventral caudal medial nucleus of the thalamus, which, in turn, projects axons via the internal capsule to the sensory neocortex.

Some of the axons of the GVA system receptors in the thoracic and abdominal organs also course centrally over the branches of the thoracic sympathetic trunk and the abdominal splanchnic nerves. Here they are accompanied by the GVE neurons, which are coursing toward the organ innervated (see Fig. 16-1). From the sympathetic trunk, each of these GVA axons courses through a ramus communicans to the segmental spinal nerve, where it enters the dorsal root. The neuronal cell body of the GVA neuron is located in the segmental spinal ganglion. The axon continues over the dorsal root, enters the spinal cord at the dorsolateral sulcus, and continues into the dorsal gray column, where it terminates on a neuronal cell body located there.

For a reflex pathway, a dorsal gray column interneuron passes into the adjacent intermediate gray column in segments T1-L4 to synapse on a preganglionic sympathetic GVE neuron located there. The pathway for conscious perception involves the synapse of a GVA telodendron on a neuronal cell body in the dorsal gray column that projects its axon into the same-side or the opposite-side lateral funiculus and courses cranially along with the axons of the spinothalamic pathway. This is probably a multisynaptic system that follows the same course as that of the spinothalamic system (general somatic afferent; GSA), including the synapse in the ventral caudal lateral thalamic nucleus for projection to the sensory neocortex.

There is some evidence that for the organs of the body cavities, the GVA neurons in the vagus nerve are concerned with reflex activity, and those entering the spinal cord by way of the sympathetic trunk are concerned primarily with the conscious projection of visceral afferent stimuli, the source of "visceral pain."

In addition to these pathways from the dendritic zones in the gastrointestinal organs to the CNS, there are some, possibly many, GVA neurons that reside entirely within the wall of the viscus in an enteric plexus in which intrinsic reflex activity can occur. They are components of what is referred to as the enteric nervous system, which can function autonomously.

Functional Concepts

Most smooth muscle regulation is involuntary and occurs at a reflex level not reaching the level of conscious perception. The enteric plexus and ganglia (enteric nervous system) within the wall of the bowel can function autonomously, independent of their extrinsic innervation and the CNS. Autonomous pacemaker activity has been recognized in selected areas of the bowel. Visceral surfaces are for the most part insensitive to many of the stimuli to which the surface of the body is sensitive. There is no conscious perception of touching, pinching, or cutting of normal viscera. This is exemplified by the surgical rumenotomy or cesarean sections performed in cattle, in which only the body wall and the parietal peritoneum have to be desensitized by local anesthesia. The wall of the rumen or the uterus is incised without anesthesia and without causing any discomfort to the patient.

Conscious perception (nociception) of visceral sensation is usually referred to as visceral pain. It occurs following tension or distention of the wall of the viscus or traction on their mesenteries. Diseased, inflamed visceral surfaces are sensitive to touching and cutting. Loss of blood supply (ischemia) to the wall of a viscus is a cause of visceral nociception.

Visceral nociception is poorly localized to its specific source; it is reflected as a dull, deep, painful sensation in the body cavity. This may reflect the fact that compared with the GSA system, there are fewer GVA neurons, and they are stimulated only occasionally by modalities that are projected to the level of conscious perception. Thus, the cerebrum has little experience in localizing the source of these visceral modalities that come from structures that cannot be visualized. This provides part of the basis for the phenomenon of referred pain, in which a specific area of the body surface is hypersensitive and is considered to be where the visceral afferent stimulus that is perceived as pain is arising.

Referred Pain

In referred pain, the visceral nociception is referred to the surface of the body innervated by GSA neurons whose axons terminate in the same spinal cord segment and on the same neuronal cell bodies as the GVA neurons from a viscus (Fig. 16-2). Thus there is a dermatomal distribution of referred visceral nociception, and the surface of the body can be mapped to represent the areas of pain referral of the various visceral organs. For example, the diaphragm is referred to the shoulder and neck region innervated by GSA neurons in cervical spinal nerves 5, 6, and 7. The stomach is referred to the midthoracic region (T6-T9). The ureter is referred to the area of the scrotum (L3 and L4). Many theories have been proposed to explain this mechanism. The common pool theory proposes that both the GSA and GVA neurons synapse in the dorsal gray column on the

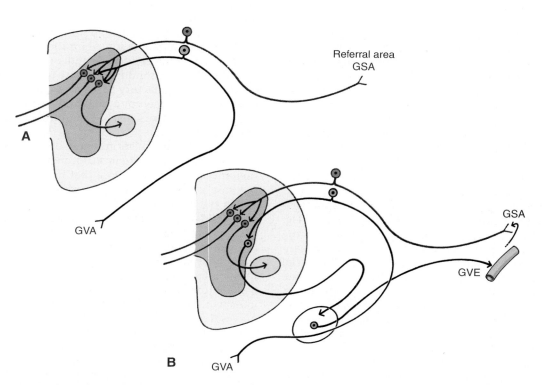

FIGURE 16-2 Anatomy of the dermatomal rule for referred visceral pain. **A,** Theory of a common pool of neurons for GSA and GVA that project to the brain. **B,** Theory of a GVA viscerovisceral reflex arc causing tonic spasm of peripheral blood vessels, which alters tissue metabolism with the accumulation of by-products that stimulate the local GSA receptors.

same neuronal cell bodies that serve as the conscious projection pathway by way of the spinothalamic system. The GSA system is stimulated frequently, whereas the GVA system is stimulated only occasionally. The site of stimulus by the GSA neurons is readily recognized on the surface of the body, and the brain has learned this source of the stimulus. When the same dorsal gray column neurons are stimulated by excessive activity in the GVA neurons, the brain misinterprets the source and refers it to the origin of the GSA neurons on the body surface.

The viscerovisceral reflex arc theory proposes that excessive GVA neuronal stimulation causes a reflex spasm in blood vessels of the peripheral body wall by way of sympathetic GVE neurons located in the same spinal cord segments. Release or accumulation of abnormal substances at the site of the vasospasm then stimulates the dendritic zones of the GSA neurons in that area of GVE distribution. These impulses are then conducted into the segmental dorsal gray column and projected to the somesthetic cortex, which projects the pain to the surface of the body innervated by the GSA neurons. In reality, referred pain is rarely recognized or utilized clinically in veterinary medicine. There is anatomic evidence that supports a much more diffuse location of visceral sensory neurons than was formerly assumed, which may explain this observation. In the dog, there are 22 spinal cord segments that supply GVA innervation to the stomach.

SPECIAL VISCERAL AFFERENT SYSTEM: TASTE

The primary receptors for the sense of taste, the gustatory sense, are responsive to chemical agents introduced into the mouth and are organized in taste buds, which are small structures associated with the various glossal papillae. Taste buds also occur in the soft palate, pharynx, larynx, lips, and cheeks.[5] The taste bud consists of supporting cells and neuroepithelial cells arranged so that the shorter neuroepithelial cells are centrally located. This cell has a hair-like process on the distal extremity that extends into a depression in the center of the taste bud known as the taste pore.[16] Here the hair-like process is sensitive to chemical substances dissolved in the saliva. There is a rapid turnover of neuroepithelial receptor cells in the taste bud.[1] Following denervation, the taste bud degenerates and reforms 1 to 2 days after the reinnervation of the tongue papillae.[3]

These neuroepithelial receptor cells are in synaptic relationship with the dendritic zones of the SVA neurons (Fig. 16-3). The cell bodies of these neurons are located in the geniculate ganglion of the facial nerve and the distal ganglia of the glossopharyngeal and vagal nerves. The facial SVA neurons are distributed to the taste buds of the palate and the rostral two thirds of the tongue by way of branches of the trigeminal nerve.[18,19] The glossopharyngeal SVA neurons innervate taste buds in the caudal third of the tongue and the rostral pharynx. The vagal SVA neurons innervate taste buds in the caudal pharynx and the larynx.[4]

The course and central pathway of reflex activity and conscious perception are the same as those described for the GVA neurons in these three cranial nerves.[2,6,11,13,14] In the cat, taste perception is located primarily in the presylvian gyrus. As an example of these pathways in action, think of how a dog reacts to the prehension of a bitter foodstuff or how you would react. The immediate excessive salivation is the result of reflex activity between these SVA neurons and the parasympathetic nuclei of cranial nerves VII, IX, and X that innervate the salivary glands. The continual chewing motions and other attempts made to eliminate this bitter foodstuff from the animal's mouth result from the animal's conscious perception of the bitter taste of the foodstuff and voluntary upper motor neuron corticonuclear activation of the GSE neurons in the motor nucleus of cranial nerve V in the pons and the hypoglossal nucleus in the medulla.

The perception of taste is a psychologic phenomenon involving the central projection of many afferent systems and the role of the higher centers such as the limbic system, which contributes the factors of memory of past experiences. Although the primary afferent for taste is the chemoreceptor in the taste bud, thermoreceptors and mechanoreceptors in the oral cavity and pharynx and olfactory receptors in the caudal nasal cavity also contribute to the sensation of taste.

SPECIAL VISCERAL AFFERENT SYSTEM: OLFACTION

The telencephalic cortex can be divided on a developmental evolutionary basis into the archipallium, the paleopallium, and the neopallium. The archipallium and paleopallium make up the rhinencephalon or "smell brain." On an anatomic and functional basis, the rhinencephalon consists of an olfactory portion (paleopallium) and a nonolfactory portion or limbic system (archipallium). The limbic system has evolved extensively in the higher species of mammals and in addition to the telencephalic components also involves nuclei and tracts in the brainstem.

The olfactory (paleopallial) portion of the rhinencephalon is the SVA system designed for the conscious perception of smell. The nonolfactory portion, or limbic system, is concerned with the emotional response to afferent stimuli, one of which is the olfactory SVA system. Reflect on your own reaction to the smell of a delightful perfume as compared with a rotten animal carcass. That difference is a function of the limbic system.

The specialized chemoreceptor of the olfactory rhinencephalon is a bipolar neuron located in the olfactory epithelium of the nasal mucosa that lies in the caudal part of the nasal cavity.[8,15] This is primarily the nasal mucosa that covers the ethmoid labyrinth. The cell body and dendritic zone reside in the epithelium. Between six and eight long cilia project from the apex of the olfactory cell and lie in the secretions on the surface of the olfactory epithelium, where they are stimulated by chemical substances dissolved in the secretions. The axon courses caudally from the cell body into the connective tissue of the nasal mucosa and joins with other olfactory axons to form the olfactory nerves (cranial nerve I). They pass through the foramina of the cribriform plate of the ethmoid bone and into the adjacent olfactory bulbs. There are four highly organized layers of neuronal cell bodies and their processes on the surface of the olfactory bulb. Here the olfactory nerve telodendria synapse in glomeruli with the dendritic zones of the brush and mitral cells. Many olfactory neurons converge on a few neurons of the olfactory bulb.

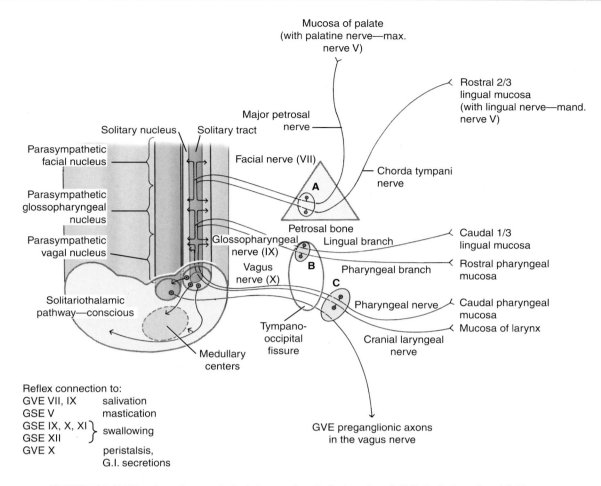

FIGURE 16-3 SVA pathways for taste. **A,** Geniculate ganglion; **B,** distal ganglion of CN IX; **C,** distal ganglion of CN X. *G.I.,* Gastrointestinal.

The axons of the brush and mitral cells of the olfactory bulb project through the olfactory tract on the surface of the olfactory peduncle and the lateral olfactory stria to the pisilateral olfactory cortex that covers the piriform lobe (Fig. 16-4; see also Figs. 2-2 and 2-3). Synapse may occur with neurons in the cortex of the olfactory peduncle (the lateral olfactory gyrus); in the lateral olfactory stria; or in the olfactory tubercle. The last is a nucleus located between the medial and lateral olfactory striae. The majority of the central olfactory projections are ipsilateral and project to the piriform cortex without a relay through a thalamic nucleus. This is the only sensory system that lacks a specific thalamic nucleus for cortical projection.

The functions of the two olfactory bulbs are correlated by axons of the brush neurons in one olfactory bulb that course through the ipsilateral olfactory tract and medial olfactory stria, through the rostral commissure, and then rostrally in the contralateral medial olfactory stria and olfactory tract to the contralateral olfactory bulb (see Fig. 16-4). The olfactory peduncle includes the olfactory tract and the adjacent cortex of the lateral olfactory gyrus ventral to the rostral lateral rhinal sulcus. Commissural axons in the rostral commissure also pass between the cortices of the two piriform lobes.

This is the conscious perception pathway for the olfactory SVA system. The so-called reflex pathway involves projections into the nuclear areas of the limbic system. Axons in the medial olfactory stria enter the septal area (septal nuclei and subcallosal area). Axons in the lateral olfactory stria enter the amygdaloid nucleus and hippocampus.

The development of the olfactory portion of the rhinencephalon (the SVA system) varies extensively among species of mammals. In the dog, the sense of smell is highly developed functionally and anatomically, and the canine species is referred to as a macrosmatic species. Primates are microsmatic, lacking a well-developed olfactory system. This is obvious just by comparing the size of the olfactory bulbs. The olfactory bulb in the human and the nonhuman primate is very small when compared with the olfactory bulb in any domestic animal. It is remarkably large in all species of bears as well as in sea lions and also in opossums. In the last species, the olfactory system is well developed, whereas the remaining telencephalon and its neocortex are poorly developed. See examples of some of these species differences in Fig. 13-12 (dog); Fig. 13-23 (bear); and Fig. 13-31 (gibbon).

Experimental lesions in one olfactory bulb or peduncle produce unilateral anosmia. Bilateral lesions in the olfactory mucosae, bulbs, peduncles, or piriform lobes cause complete anosmia. Lesions in any part of the nonolfactory rhinencephalon, the limbic system, do not interfere with the sense of smell.

Deficiencies in the sense of smell are difficult to verify by clinical testing. The owner's observations of the animal's behavior on sensing the presence of food or game in the

Olfactory rhinencephalon

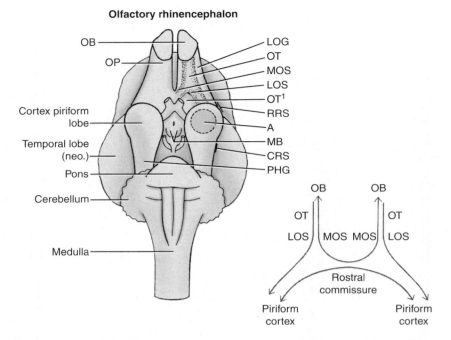

FIGURE 16-4 Anatomy of the SVA olfactory system. *A,* Amygdala; *CRS,* caudal rhinal sulcus; *LOG,* lateral olfactory gyrus; *LOS,* lateral olfactory stria; *MB,* mamillary bodies; *MOS,* medial olfactory stria; *OB,* olfactory bulb; *OP,* olfactory peduncle; *OT,* olfactory tract; *OT¹,* olfactory tubercule; *PHG,* parahippocampal gyrus; *RRS,* rostral rhinal sulcus.

field may be more reliable information. Substances such as cloves, cinnamon, perfume, xylol, and benzol can be used to test olfaction, but you have to be careful about using irritating compounds that stimulate the GSA neurons of the trigeminal nerve that innervate the nasal mucosa. Anosmia is an uncommon clinical complaint. The most common cause is severe rhinitis with involvement of the olfactory nasal mucosa. Head injury may cause a shearing of the olfactory nerves as they pass through the cribriform plate, resulting in anosmia. There is unsubstantiated information that infection by the canine distemper virus may cause anosmia without other clinical signs. Most often, in the few dogs that are seen with anosmia, the cause is never determined and speculations are never proven.

We have performed numerous surgeries in both dogs and cats to remove unilateral neoplasms located in one olfactory bulb or frontal lobe and have excised the olfactory bulb and peduncle unilaterally without apparent clinical consequence for the sensation of smell. In addition, in dogs with relatively large nonresectable neoplasms that involve the cribriform plate and olfactory bulb both unilaterally and bilaterally, we have not appreciated anosmia clinically.

Inappropriate urine spraying and marking in cats is a behavioral disorder that in the past has been treated by olfactory tractotomy.[9] The surgical method resulted in apparently minimal to no adverse side effects in these cats. The close proximity of other neural structures made unwanted behaviors and neurologic deficits a significant postsurgical possibility. Thankfully, this dramatic procedure has fallen out of favor because of the discovery of clumping litter and a much better understanding of these behaviors by veterinary behaviorists. Olfactory tractotomy, from our perspective, should not be considered a therapy until all other avenues of treatment have been ineffective.

REFERENCES

1. Beidler LM, Smallman RL: Renewal of cells within taste buds, *J Cell Biol* 27:263, 1965.
2. Bell FR, Kitchell RL: Taste reception in the goat, sheep and calf, *J Physiol* 183:145, 1966.
3. Cheal M, Oakley B: Regeneration of fungiform taste buds. Temporal and spatial characteristics, *J Comp Neurol* 172:609, 1977.
4. Cottle MK: Degeneration studies of primary afferents of the IXth and Xth cranial nerves in the cat, *J Comp Neurol* 122:329, 1964.
5. Davies RO, Kare MR, Cagan RH: Distribution of taste buds on fungiform and circumvallate papillae of bovine tongue, *Anat Rec* 195:443, 1979.
6. Emmers R: Localization of thalamic projection of afferents from the tongue in the cat, *Anat Rec* 148:67, 1964.
7. Fletcher TF, Bradley WE: Afferent nerve endings in the urinary bladder of the cat, *Am J Anat* 128:147, 1970.
8. Graziadei PPC: The ultrastructure of vertebrate olfactory mucosa. In Friedman I, editor: *The ultrastructure of sensory organs,* Amsterdam, 1973, North Holland Publishing.
9. Hart BL: Olfactory tractotomy for control of objectionable urine spraying and urine marking in cats, *J Am Vet Med Assoc* 179:231-234, 1981.
10. Khurana RK, Petras JM: Anatomic demonstration of the afferent innervation of the dog's stomach: a possible implication for visceral pain in humans, *Neurology* 32:A71, 1982.
11. Kitchell RL: Taste perception and discrimination by the dog, *Adv Vet Sci Comp Med* 22:287, 1978.
12. Morest DK: Experimental study of the projections of the nucleus solitarius and the area postrema in the cat, *J Comp Neurol* 130:277, 1967.
13. Morrison AR, Hand PJ, Ruderman MI: Cortical gustatory and facial somestheic areas of the cat as revealed by an anatomicophysiological technique, *Anat Rec* 172:462, 1972.

14. Morrison AR, Tarnecki R: A new location for the gustatory cortex of the cat, *Anat Rec* 181:431, 1975.

15. Moulton DG, Beidler LM: Structure and function in the peripheral olfactory system, *Physiol Rev* 47:1, 1967.

16. Murray RG: The ultrastructure of taste buds. In Friedmann I, editor: *The ultrastructure of sensory organs*, Amsterdam, 1973, North Holland Publishing.

17. Paintal AS: Vagal sensory receptors and their reflex effects, *Physiol Rev* 53:159, 1973.

18. Rhoton AL Jr: Afferent connections of the facial nerve, *J Comp Neurol* 133:89, 1968.

19. Nemura E, Fletcher TF, Bradley WE: Distribution of lumbar afferent axons in muscle coat of cat urinary bladder, *Am J Anat* 139:389, 1974.

17 NONOLFACTORY RHINENCEPHALON: LIMBIC SYSTEM

ANATOMY
Telencephalon
Diencephalon
Mesencephalon

FUNCTION
Self-Stimulation
Direct Stimulation
Experimental Destruction
Diseases

Frontal Lobotomy
Behavioral Abnormalities
English Springer Spaniel Rage Syndrome

The prosencephalon consists of the telencephalon and the diencephalon. The diencephalon is composed of the thalamus, epithalamus, metathalamus, subthalamus, and hypothalamus, with the third ventricle in the center. The telencephalon is the cerebrum, which consists of two cerebral hemispheres. The cell bodies of the neurons in the cerebrum are located in two general areas. One area is on the external surface of the gyri in the laminations of the cerebral cortex. The other area is deep to the surface in basal nuclei. The caudate nucleus, pallidum, and putamen are basal nuclei that function in the extrapyramidal system. The amygdaloid body and septal nuclei function mainly in the limbic system.

The cerebral cortex covers the external surface of the cerebrum and can be divided into three general regions on the basis of the evolution of each. The paleopallium (pall-cloak) consists of the olfactory bulb, the olfactory peduncle, and the cortex of the piriform lobe. The archipallium is the hippocampus, which is an internal gyrus that is rolled into the lateral ventricle during development. The neopallium is the most recently evolved and makes up the remainder of the cerebrum, which includes all the gyri dorsal to the rhinal sulcus.

Another grouping of brain components is called the rhinencephalon, the "smell brain." It consists of an olfactory component, the paleopallium (see Chapter 16), and a nonolfactory component, which is referred to as the limbic system. In the telencephalon, this includes the archipallium.

The term *limbic system* refers to the anatomic arrangement of the telencephalic neurons and tracts that are components of this system and are arranged primarily as two incomplete ring-like structures on the medial aspect of the cerebral hemisphere at its border with the diencephalon (Fig. 17-1). *Limbus* means edge or border, and these telencephalic structures form the border of the main mass of the cerebral hemisphere. The term has been expanded in usage to include the major nuclei and pathways in the rostral brainstem that are connected with these telencephalic structures anatomically and functionally (Box 17-1).

ANATOMY

Telencephalon

The telencephalic components of the limbic system form two "cortical rings" at the border of the diencephalic-telencephalic junction (see Fig. 17-1). The inner ring consists of the amygdaloid body, the hippocampus, and its fornix. The outer ring consists of the cingulate gyrus and its cingulum and the septal area.

The amygdaloid body, one of the basal nuclei of the telencephalon, is a complex of nuclei located in the piriform lobe deep to the olfactory cortex (Fig. 17-2; see also Fig. 2-3). A projection pathway of the neurons in the amygdaloid nuclei, the stria terminalis, courses in the angle between the thalamus and the caudate nucleus. It forms an incomplete circle shaped like a C that progresses from the amygdaloid body in a caudal, then dorsal, and then rostral and ventral direction to terminate in the septal area and the rostral hypothalamus. A diagonal band courses on the ventral surface of the cerebrum, connecting the amygdaloid body with the septal area.

The hippocampus is a unique gyrus of the cerebrum that in lower mammals is found on the external surface of the cerebrum but in higher mammals has been rolled into the lateral ventricle and is not visible on the external surface. The hippocampus is shaped like a C. The hippocampus extends in a curve, starting from the amygdaloid body ventrally in each piriform lobe and progressing caudally and dorsally and then rostrally over the diencephalon. It forms part of the medial and dorsal wall of the lateral ventricle ventrally, and part of the medial and ventral wall of the lateral ventricle dorsally (see Figs. 2-4 through 2-6). It lies adjacent to the lateral geniculate nucleus from which it is separated by meninges with cerebrospinal fluid. Dorsal to the caudal thalamus, the hippocampus of each cerebral hemisphere meets at the median plane, and a commissure is formed here, the hippocampal commissure. On the ventral surface of the brain, caudal to the piriform lobe, the hippocampus is covered superficially by the parahippocampal gyrus,

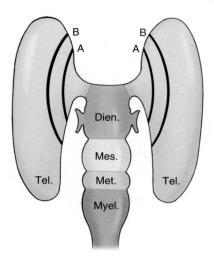

FIGURE 17-1 Schematic diagram of developing brain vesicles, with approximate site of telencephalic components of the limbic system at the "border" of the telencephalic cerebral vesicle. *A,* Inner ring: amygdala, hippocampus; *B,* Outer ring: cingulate gyrus, septal area; *Dien.,* diencephalon; *Mes.,* mesencephalon; *Met.,* metencephalon; *Myel.,* myelencephalon; *Tel.,* telencephalon.

which is bounded laterally by the caudal lateral rhinal sulcus and medially where it joins the hippocampus at the hippocampal sulcus (see Fig. 2-4). The parahippocampal gyrus is continued dorsally, dorsal to the corpus callosum, by the cingulate gyrus (see Figs. 2-4 through 2-6).

Axons course to and from the hippocampus along its lateral side, forming the fimbria and the crus of the fornix.

BOX 17-1 Nonolfactory Rhinencephalon: Limbic System, Summary of Major Structures

I. Telencephalon
  A. Inner cortical ring
    Amygdaloid body
    Hippocampus
      Fimbria-fornix—septal area hypothalamus, mamillary bodies
  B. Outer cortical ring
    Cingulate gyrus and cingulum
    Septal area
    Medial forebrain bundle, hypothalamus
      Brainstem general visceral efferent, lower motor neuron
II. Diencephalon
  A. Thalamus
    Habenular nucleus
      Stria habenularis thalamus
      Habenular intercrural tract
    Rostral thalamic nucleus
  B. Hypothalamus
    Mamillary bodies
      Mamillothalamic tract
      Mamillotegmental tract—reticular formation
III. Mesencephalon
  A. Intercrural nucleus—reticular formation

The two crura meet rostral to the hippocampal commissure and continue rostrally as the body of the fornix (see Figs. 17-2, 2-2, and 2-3). After coursing rostrally a short distance, the body of the fornix bends ventrally and dorsal to the rostral commissure. Two distinct cylindric columns emerge from the body on each side. Each column of the fornix splits at the rostral commissure. On each side, a small bundle of axons courses rostrally into the septal area, and a larger portion of the column courses caudal to the rostral commissure and ventrally through the hypothalamus beside the third ventricle to terminate in the mamillary body (see Figs. 2-3 and 2-4). The body of the fornix and the proximal portion of each column are attached dorsally to the corpus callosum by the septum pellucidum. The caudal portion of this septum is not visible unless the lateral ventricle is enlarged and the septum appears as a thin sheet between the body of the fornix and the corpus callosum. Rostrally, this septum contains neuronal cell bodies of the septal nucleus. The leptomeninges extend rostrally between the diencephalon and the hippocampi and body of the fornix to the level of the interventricular foramen. The columns of the fornix that course caudal to the rostral commissure form the rostral border of this foramen on each side. The caudal border of this foramen is the portion of choroid plexus that is continuous from the third ventricle to the lateral ventricle. Here, the rostral extent of the leptomeninges between the diencephalon and telencephalon is associated with this choroid plexus.

The cingulate gyrus consists of cerebral cortex and its corona radiata, the cingulum. It is located dorsal to the corpus callosum and is continuous caudally with the parahippocampal gyrus and rostrally with the septal area (see Figs. 2-2 through 2-6). The cingulum is a long association tract consisting of longitudinal axons in the white matter (corona radiata) of the cingulate gyrus (see Fig. 17-2). These axons course from the parahippocampal gyrus, located caudally, to the septal area and frontal lobe gyri located rostrally.

The septal area consists of the subcallosal area, which is the cerebral cortex ventral to the genu of the corpus callosum and the septal nuclei. The septal nuclei are a collection of neuronal cell bodies in the rostral septum pellucidum that bulges into the medial side of the lateral ventricle. This is dorsal and just rostral to the bend in the body of the fornix, where it forms the columns of the fornix. The septal area connects with the hippocampus by way of the adjacent columns of the fornix; with the amygdaloid body through the diagonal band and stria terminalis; and with the habenular nucleus via the stria habenularis thalamus (see Fig. 2-3). The medial forebrain bundle courses caudally from the septal area into the hypothalamus. By way of this pathway, limbic system efferents can influence the hypothalamic centers that control the activity of the general visceral efferent (GVE) system. The function of the limbic system involves visceral motor activation. Hypothalamic nuclei serve in the upper motor neuron system that regulates the GVE system. These hypothalamic nuclei receive numerous limbic system efferents.

Diencephalon

In the thalamus, the habenular nucleus and the rostral thalamic nucleus function mainly in the limbic system

I. Telencephalon

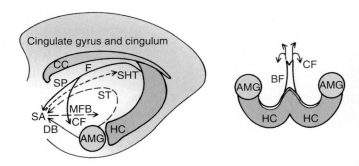

II. Diencephalon: thalamus—hypothalamus

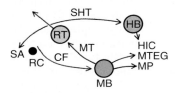

III. Mesencephalon

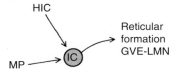

FIGURE 17-2 Anatomy of the limbic system. Telencephalon inner ring: *AMG,* amygdaloid nucleus; *F,* fornix; *HC,* hippocampus. Telencephalon outer ring: *Cingulate gyrus and cingulum; CC,* corpus callosum; *MFB,* median forebrain bundle; *SA,* septal area; *SHT,* stria habenularis thalamus; *SP,* septum pellucidum; *ST,* stria terminalis. *BF,* Body of fornix; *CF,* column of fornix; *DB,* diagonal band; *GVE-LMN,* general visceral efferent-lower motor neuron; *HB,* habenular nucleus; *HIC,* habenulointercrural tract; *IC,* intercrural nucleus; *MB,* mamillary body; *MP,* mamillary peduncle; *MT,* mamillothalamic tract; *MTEG,* mamillotegmental tract; *RC,* rostral commissure; *RT,* rostral thalamic nucleus.

(see Fig. 17-2).[4] The habenular nucleus is part of the epithalamus, located dorsally, adjacent to the third ventricle and rostral to the pineal body (see Fig. 2-4). It connects with the telencephalic septal area by way of the stria habenularis thalamus, which is a column of axons located in the dorsal thalamus adjacent to the dorsal component of the third ventricle. The choroid plexus of the third ventricle attaches to this stria on both sides. The habenular nucleus connects with the intercrural nucleus of the mesencephalon via the habenulointercrural tract. A short habenular commissure connects the two adjacent habenular nuclei. The rostral thalamic nucleus receives afferents from the mamillary body of the hypothalamus through the mamillothalamic tract (see Figs. 2-3 and 2-4). The rostral thalamic nucleus projects predominantly to the cingulate gyrus and adjacent neopallium.

The limbic system component of the hypothalamus is the mamillary body. The paired mamillary bodies are located adjacent to the ventral midline in the most caudal part of the hypothalamus. They protrude from the ventral surface of the hypothalamus just caudal to the infundibulum of the hypothalamus (see Fig. 2-4). They connect with the hippocampus by way of the columns of the fornix and with the rostral thalamic nucleus via the mamillothalamic tract. The paired columns of the fornix and mamillothalamic tracts pass through the hypothalamus adjacent to the ventral portion of the third ventricle. In addition to

these pathways, the mamillary bodies connect with the mesencephalic tegmentum and the visceral motor nuclei in the medulla through the mamillotegmental tract. The mamillary peduncle connects caudally with the mesencephalic intercrural nucleus (see Fig. 17-2).

Mesencephalon

The intercrural nucleus is the only limbic system nucleus in the mesencephalon. It is located ventrally, adjacent to the intercrural fossa and between the two crus cerebri on the ventral surface of the mesencephalon (see Figs. 2-7 and 2-8). It connects with the habenular nucleus by way of the habenulointercrural tract; with the mamillary bodies via the mamillary peduncle; and with the reticular formation in the brainstem which, in turn, influences the visceral motor nuclei, the general visceral efferent lower motor neuron in the medulla.

█ FUNCTION

The limbic system receives and associates impulses from the olfactory (special visceral afferent); optic (special somatic afferent); auditory (special somatic afferent); exteroceptive (general somatic afferent); and interoceptive (general visceral afferent) sensory systems. It projects predominantly to the hypothalamus and caudal brainstem, influencing primarily the visceral motor neurons.

The limbic system is involved mostly with emotional and behavioral patterns.[23,24] Emotion involves visceral reaction, which is controlled largely by the autonomic nervous system. This system is regulated centrally by the hypothalamus, which accounts for the multitude of connections between the limbic system and the hypothalamus. The limbic system is considered to function in humans as the higher center controlling the psychic and motor aspects of behavior. It is the portion of the brain involved in basic human drives—sexual activity, emotional experiences, memories, fears, and pleasures.

Dr. James Papez, Professor of Neurology at Cornell University, suggested in 1937 that the part of the rhinencephalon now classified as the limbic system was concerned with activity other than the perception of smell.[26] Following his observations of the distribution of the rabies lesions in these rhinencephalic structures in dogs and the bizarre behavior exhibited by rabid animals, he attributed to these structures a role in the control of normal behavior.

Since then, many different experimental procedures and clinical observations have substantiated this role of the limbic system in the control of an animal's behavior. These observations have included the effect of direct stimulation of rhinencephalic structures, the effect of ablation of portions of these structures, and the clinical syndromes produced by diseases causing lesions in these structures. The specific results have varied, even with the use of similar procedures, because of the difficulty in the exact placement of stimulating electrodes and the variable spread of excitation to adjacent structures, coupled with the fact that adjacent nuclei may have diametrically opposed functions. Surgical ablations that were repeated often lacked specificity. Nevertheless, the general conclusion drawn from all of these observations is that the alteration of the animal's behavior suggests that a basic drive has been satisfied or that the condition of an unsatisfied basic drive has been created. Some examples of these observations follow.

Self-Stimulation

Self-stimulation experiments were designed in which electrodes were implanted in various specific areas of the limbic system, and stimulation occurred when the experimental animal stepped on a lever or bar in the floor of its cage.[8,25,30] The response observed was presumed to be pleasurable when it was sought and continually repeated by the animal, to the exclusion of feeding. A painful experience was assumed to have occurred when the stimulation was actively avoided. Such self-stimulation of the intercrural nucleus, septal area, and rostral hypothalamus in cats and rats was sought so actively that the animals continually pressed the bar and did not eat. These areas have been called pleasure centers.[25] Similar stimulation of the lateral hypothalamus and selected mesencephalic areas resulted in complete avoidance of the source of the stimulus. These areas were referred to as pain centers.

Direct Stimulation

Direct stimulation of the feline cingulate gyrus, amygdaloid body, or hippocampus results in the production of a complex partial seizure, also known as a psychomotor seizure.[10,12,20,21]

This form of seizure is characterized by marked abnormal behavior preceding the tonic-clonic somatic motor phase of the seizure. Expression of arousal, fear or rage, or both are observed. Direct stimulation of the temporal lobe in humans under local anesthesia has caused individuals to completely recall a past experience and express the full emotional impact of that event. Upon cessation of the stimulus, the person does not remember recalling the event.

Experimental Destruction

Ablation experiments have resulted in variable responses, all of which show an alteration in the animal's behavior.[10,29] In cats, amygdalectomy results in unfriendliness and fear or even a rage response. The latter involves a complete sympathetic response, with a tendency to attack animate and inanimate objects.

Hypersexuality in males and hyperphagia also have been observed. All of these behaviors represent unsatisfied basic drives that the animal is attempting to remedy. Amygdalectomy has caused aggressive monkeys to be tame, nonaggressive and sometimes hypersexual and to show no emotional response when confronted by objects or events that formerly elicited an emotional response. Lesions in the temporal lobe in humans often cause psychomotor seizures. Removal of the temporal lobe may stop the seizures but seriously blunts the emotional responses of the individual, and the memory of past events is often lost. As a form of therapy, bilateral lesions have been produced in the amygdaloid body in dogs that showed variable degrees of aggression and viciousness. This procedure has seemed to be helpful only in alleviating the aggressive behavior in nervous, fearful biting dogs. Destruction of the amygdaloid body or hippocampus in cats, by applying aluminum oxide cream directly to the area, resulted in psychomotor seizures.

Diseases

Diseases that cause lesions in the temporal lobe in humans often are the source of psychomotor seizures. Neonatal or childhood trauma and infectious diseases that cause encephalitis of this area such as the measles virus may cause damage to the temporal lobe. The temporal lobe is closely associated with the amygdaloid body and hippocampus. Their functions overlap, and the lesions described as occurring in the temporal lobe usually involve the hippocampus as well. Psychomotor seizures in humans are characterized by loss of contact with the external environment, by hallucinations of visual events, or by visceral sensations (tastes and smells) that are pleasing or distasteful. They are accompanied by visceral motor activity, such as pupillary dilation, salivation, mastication, and fecal and urinary excretions, and by somatic motor activity consisting of wildly running around as though searching for something, along with an excessive expression of emotion. They usually culminate in a generalized seizure characterized by falling on one side, opisthotonus, and tonic (rigid extension) and clonic (rapidly alternating contraction and relaxation of a muscle) activity of the limbs, alternating with paddling or running movements of the limbs. Complete recovery follows. The duration may range from 1 to 3 or from 10 to 15 minutes.

Complex partial seizures (psychomotor seizures) have been observed in dogs that have lesions in the piriform lobe or hippocampus. When agenized flour was used in dog foods, it caused necrosis in these areas bilaterally and produced this kind of seizure.[23,27] Similar necrosis resulting from ischemia of unknown origin, seizure-induced excitotoxic degeneration, and inflammations caused occasionally by the canine distemper virus produce this same abnormal behavior. In dogs, a complex partial seizure may be referred to as a "running fit" because before the dog falls on its side and exhibits tonic-clonic motor activity of its limbs and opisthotonus, it may have a period of uncontrolled, wild running around in its environment, combined with barking and growling and complete lack of awareness of anyone or anything in its environment. Occasionally, the psychic stage of the seizure is manifested in what might be called a hallucination. The dog may stand in a corner, barking and growling, with dilated pupils and erect hair along its back as if it were going to attack an object, although nothing is there. Extreme fear may be manifested. This dog is usually unresponsive to the owner during these episodes. A common cause in dogs of seizures that are accompanied by psychic stages with bizarre and abnormal behavior is lead poisoning. There have been no adequate studies of the distribution of the lesions to determine whether the limbic system structures are more seriously affected in these dogs.

Frontal Lobotomy

Frontal lobe structures are closely connected with the limbic system and hypothalamus and are involved in the status of an animal's behavior. Frontal lobotomies have been performed in humans and in animals to alleviate violent, aggressive behaviors that are destructive in nature. In lobotomized humans, extensive changes in personality and loss of intellect accompany the alleviation of the aggressive behavior, so the procedure is infrequently used. The results in dogs have been variable.[1-3,22]

In one study, frontal lobotomies were performed on two groups of aggressive animals.[1] One group consisted of malamutes used as sled dogs that had marked aggression toward each other. The other group of dogs and cats consisted of house pets that had histories of aggressive behavior toward humans. The lobotomies performed on the malamutes with intraspecies aggression were more successful than those performed on the animals aggressive toward humans. In most instances, the lobotomized malamutes were able to return to the sled-dog team and to function without attacking the other dogs on the team. However, this surgical procedure is not without serious sequelae and should be performed only as a last resort. Electroconvulsive shock therapy has been used alone or together with lobotomies on dogs with aggressive behavior.

Behavioral Abnormalities

Behavioral abnormalities are common in domestic animals.[5-7,9,11,13-19] The abnormalities can be defined as changes in an animal's normal habits, personality, attitude, and reaction to its environment and in its general sensorium. Some of the clinical signs that make up this abnormal behavior include depression (dullness), lethargy, obtundation, and stupor (semicoma). Dementia; failure to recognize owners, familiar environments, and objects; and the inability to learn are referred to collectively as cognitive disorders. Other clinical signs include destructive behaviors, propulsive pacing or circling, hypersexuality, polydipsia, polyphagia, pica, and anorexia.

Normal behavior requires a complex integrated involvement of the entire nervous system but predominantly the prosencephalon. Some of these behavioral abnormalities are caused by structural lesions in the prosencephalon, such as neoplasia, ischemia, inflammation, or inherited degeneration that involves some component of the limbic system. Some abnormal behaviors are psychologic disturbances in which there are no recognized structural or metabolic disturbances of brain function. Some of them may be explained as abnormalities in neurotransmitter levels or interactions. Other abnormal behaviors represent inappropriate behavior for the environment in which the animal is expected to live. The latter include aggression or destruction, which are normal animal behaviors but may be inappropriate in its environment, where it is inconvenient or dangerous to the owner or others in that environment.

Almost any disturbance of the prosencephalon will cause one or more of these clinical signs that are considered to be abnormal behavior. A few signs are more specifically related to individual clinical signs, such as polydipsia with pituitary-hypothalamic neoplasia. Encephalitis, neoplasia, intoxications, malformations, injuries, ischemia and infarction, and metabolic disorders must be considered in the differential diagnosis of a prosencephalic disorder that causes abnormal behavior.

A structural brain lesion is supported as the cause if neurologic deficits other than the abnormal behavior are determined during the neurologic examination, especially if the deficits are asymmetric. If the neurologic examination is normal and ancillary blood and urine studies do not support a metabolic disorder, a psychologic disturbance or inappropriate behavior must be considered. For these latter disorders, all ancillary procedures, such as blood chemistry, evaluation of the cerebrospinal fluid, and advanced imaging (computed tomography and magnetic resonance imaging), will be normal.

The evaluation of animals for the cause of their psychologic disturbance or inappropriate behavior requires detailed analysis of their environments, training, and all their experiences since birth. Frequently, environmental alterations or the lack of training or inappropriate training are identified and, with correction, the problem can be rectified. Obviously, this requires extensive cooperation on the part of the owners. There are numerous publications that deal with the recognition, diagnosis, and control of these kinds of behavioral abnormalities. Animal behavior is now recognized as a specialty in veterinary medicine, and these specialists should be consulted in some of the complex clinical situations.

English Springer Spaniel Rage Syndrome

An episodic behavioral abnormality has been recognized in the English springer spaniel.[28] This disorder occurs in dogs that are normally well-behaved, well-adapted house pets. It consists of an episodic sudden change in behavior that lasts a few seconds to a few minutes, with the dog returning to normal immediately after the episode. The first clinical signs may be a sudden snapping and a marked bilateral mydriasis, with a glazed appearance to the eyes. This often follows a mild provocation such as approaching or attempting to pet the animal. A few fine tremors may occur in the pelvic limbs. The dog will often wag its tail, growl, and attack and bite animate or occasionally inanimate objects. This aggression is often directed at just one member of the family with whom it lives. The affected dog is completely unresponsive to its normal environment, including the owner. At times, the dog may crouch under a table or desk and not allow anyone near it. Be acutely aware that these dogs are not predictable, so appropriate action must be considered, especially in families with children.

The episodes may occur sporadically, weeks apart at first, but often increase in frequency to many times a day. In the majority of dogs, the clinical signs begin at around 18 months of age, but the range of onset varies from about 3 months to 4 years. The disorder occurs predominantly in males.

In these dogs, all ancillary studies are normal. In the few dogs in which magnetic resonance images have been obtained, no abnormalities have been observed. Electroencephalography has not been found to show evidence of a consistently abnormal tracing. The use of high levels of progestins and vigorous training programs may help to control the disease, but neither will completely eliminate all aggressive behavior. No light microscopic lesions have been found in necropsy studies of euthanized dogs.

This disorder resembles a complex partial seizure that involves the limbic system, in that it is an episodic disturbance of brain function that resolves spontaneously and recurs at varying intervals. However, it is completely unresponsive to anticonvulsant therapy. The lack of any electroencephalographic abnormality and the lack of response to anticonvulsant therapy suggest that this is a behavioral disorder. It is hoped that neurochemical studies will reveal the basis for this behavioral disorder and that genetic studies will define the presumed inherited basis. An inherited idiopathic epilepsy has also been diagnosed in this breed and should not be confused with this behavioral disorder.

REFERENCES

1. Allen BD, Cummings JF, de Lahunta A: The effects of prefrontal lobotomy on aggressive behavior in dogs, *Cornell Vet* 64:201, 1974.
2. Andersson B: A case of nervous distemper treated with prefrontal lobectomy, *Nord Vet Med* 8:17, 1956.
3. Andersson B, Olsson K: Effects of bilateral amygdaloid lesions in nervous dogs, *J Sm Anim Pract* 6:301, 1965.
4. Bandler R, Flynn JP: Neural pathways from thalamus associated with regulation of aggressive behavior, *Science* 183:96, 1974.
5. Beaver BL: Mental lapse aggression syndrome, *J Am Anim Hosp Assoc* 16:937, 1980.
6. Beaver BL: *Veterinary aspects of feline behavior*, St Louis, 1980, Mosby.
7. Beaver B: *Canine social behavior: canine behavior, a guide for veterinarians*, Philadelphia, 1999, Saunders.
8. Bruner A: Self-stimulation in the rabbit: an anatomical map of stimulation effects, *J Comp Neurol* 11:615, 1967.
9. Caldwell DS, Little PB: Aggression in dogs and associated neuropathology, *Can Vet J* 21:152, 1980.
10. Egger MD, Flynn JP: Further studies on the effects of amygdaloid stimulation and ablation on hypothalamically elicited attack behavior in cats. In Adey WR, Tokizane T, editors: *Progress in brain research: structure and function of the limbic system*, New York, 1967, Elsevier.
11. Fox MW: *Abnormal behavior in animals*, Philadelphia, 1968, Saunders.
12. Gol A: Relief of pain by electrical stimulation of the septal area, *J Neurol Sci* 5:115, 1967.
13. Hart BL: Objectionable urine spraying and marking in cats: evaluation of progestin treatment on gonadectomized males and females, *J Am Vet Med Assoc* 177:529, 1980.
14. Hart BL: Progestin therapy for aggressive behavior in male dogs, *J Am Vet Med Assoc* 178:1070, 1981.
15. Hart BL: Olfactory tractotomy for control of objectionable urine spraying and urine marking in cats, *J Am Vet Med Assoc* 179:231, 1981.
16. Hart BL: *Behavior of domestic animals*, New York, 1985, WH Freeman.
17. Hart BL, Ladewig J: Effects of medial preoptic-anterior hypothalamic lesions on development of sociosexual behavior in dogs, *J Comp Physiol* 93:566, 1979.
18. Houpt KA: Aggression in dogs, *Compend Cont Ed* 123:123, 1979.
19. Houpt KA: Equine behavior, *Eq Pract* 1:20, 1979.
20. Hunsberger RW, Bucher VM: Affective behavior produced by electrical stimulation in the forebrain and brainstem of the cat. In Adey WR, Tokizane T, editors: *Progress in brain research: structure and function of the limbic system*, New York, 1967, Elsevier.
21. Kling A, Coustan D: Electrical stimulation of the amygdala and hypothalamus in the kitten, *Exp Neurol* 10:81, 1964.
22. Kramer W, Beigers JD: Frontale leucotomie bij de hond, *Tijdschre Diergeneesk* 83:589, 1958.
23. Mellanby E: Diet and canine hysteria, experimental production by treated flour, *Br Med J* 2:288, 1947.
24. Olds J: The limbic system and behavioral reinforcement. In Adey WR, Tokizan T, editors: *Progress in brain research: structure and function of the limbic system*, New York, 1967, Elsevier.
25. Olds J: Pleasure centers in the brain, *Sci Am* 195:105, 1956.
26. Papez J: A proposed mechanism of emotion, *Arch Neurol Psychiatry* 38:725, 1937.
27. Parry HB: Canine hysteria in relation to diet, *Vet Rec* 60:389, 1948.
28. Reisner I, Houpt KA, Shofer FS: National survey of owner-directed aggression in English springer spaniels, *J Am Vet Med Assoc* 227:1594-1603, 2005.
29. Summers TB, Kaelber WW: Amygdalectomy: effect in cats and a survey of its present status, *Am J Physiol* 203:1117, 1962.
30. Wilkinson HA, Peele TL: Intracranial self-stimulation in cats, *J Comp Neurol* 121:425, 1963.

18

SEIZURE DISORDERS: NARCOLEPSY

DEFINITION

TERMINOLOGY

CLASSIFICATION

PATHOGENESIS
Neuronal Environmental Alterations
Intracranial Disorders
Extracranial Disorders
Idiopathic Epilepsy

EXAMINATION
Chief Complaint
Signalment
    Age
    Breed
    Sex
    Use
History
    Description
    Onset and Course

Environment
Diet
Medical History

PHYSICAL EXAMINATION
Neurologic Examination
Ancillary Examination
    Complete Blood Count
        and Differential Cell Count
    Blood Chemistry
    Cerebrospinal Fluid
    Imaging
Examination Summary

CASE EXAMPLES
    CASE EXAMPLE 18-1
    CASE EXAMPLE 18-2
    CASE EXAMPLE 18-3
    CASE EXAMPLE 18-4

GENERALIZED AND PARTIAL SEIZURES

INCIDENCE

TREATMENT
Maintenance Anticonvulsant Therapy
    Phenobarbital
    Potassium Bromide
    Alternative Anticonvulsants
Anticonvulsant Therapy for Cluster Seizures
    and Status Epilepticus
    Diazepam
Vagal Stimulation
Surgery

NARCOLEPSY AND CATAPLEXY
Diagnosis
Cataplectic Diagnostic Tests and Therapy
Treatment
Narcolepsy and Cataplexy

SLEEP-ASSOCIATED MOVEMENT DISORDER

DEFINITION

 See **Video 18-1** to introduce yourself to the subject of seizure disorders and so you can better appreciate the following discussion. This video shows Victory Forth, a 9-year-old female quarter horse, that has had a series of generalized seizures for the first few weeks after her last three foalings. Two seizures are shown on the video between which she was normal for approximately 1 hour.

Remember that *a neuron is an excitable tissue constantly held in check.* When this constant inhibition is interrupted, a seizure may be the result! Neurons communicate with each other via excitatory and inhibitory connections. Normal neuronal activity represents a balance of these excitatory and inhibitory influences. When imbalance results in excessive excitation, abnormal neuronal activity occurs and is manifested as a seizure. A seizure represents the uncontrolled synchronous discharge of neurons that is initiated in the prosencephalon. It is usually a brief episode as the brain usually rapidly corrects the imbalance in these neuronal influences. A seizure is the most common clinical complaint that involves the nervous system that a practicing veterinarian will encounter.

The terms *seizure, convulsion, epilepsy,* and *fit* are synonyms for a brain disorder expressed as a paroxysmal

transitory disturbance of brain function that has a sudden onset, ceases spontaneously, has a tendency to recur, and originates in the prosencephalon. The term *epilepsy* is usually used for seizures that are recurrent. Those of unknown cause are called *idiopathic epilepsy.* The initial seizure focus may involve only a small number of highly unstable neurons that spontaneously discharge. This first episode may induce surrounding neurons to discharge, resulting in a progressive spread, or generalization, of the seizure. The pathogenesis of seizures has been and still is currently the subject of extensive investigation.*

TERMINOLOGY

The period of the seizure is known as the *ictus,* or the attack. The manifestation of the seizure is variable. Any unusual involuntary phenomenon that is episodic and recurrent in nature should be evaluated as a seizure disorder. Such phenomena include loss or derangement of consciousness, excessive or decreased voluntary muscle tone or movement, visceral muscle activity, and altered behavior.

Postictal depression refers to the period of recovery after a seizure when the patient may wander around in a state of confusion, may propulsively walk in circles or bump into objects because of its central blindness, or may sleep for a prolonged period or exhibit hyperphagia. This phase has the appearance of a patient whose neurons are exhausted

*References 10, 17, 19, 28, 58, 59, 67, 70, 80, 93, 98, 99.

from the excessive activity of the seizure. The length and form of postictal depression are variable. No correlation exists between the severity and length of the seizure and the severity, duration, or nature of the postictal phase. A short partial seizure may be followed by a longer, more complex postictus than a generalized seizure. As a rule, the postictal phase lasts less than an hour, but much longer periods of up to 1 to 2 days are possible. In horses, the postictal phase may last for 3 to 4 days.

The interictal period is the period between seizures after the patient has recovered from the postictal period. This phase is when the neurologic examination should be performed.

An isolated seizure is a seizure that occurs only once in a 24-hour period. Cluster seizures are when two or more seizures occur in 24 hours separated by normal interictal periods. Status epilepticus is when the seizure state is continual for more than 5 minutes or when a series of seizures occur without full recovery of consciousness between the seizures for 30 minutes.[5,93] The seizure is continually repeated with no interictal period. Cluster seizures and status epilepticus are medical emergencies.

Descriptions of seizures usually include the terms *aura* and *prodrome*. The prodrome or prodromal period precedes the seizure and consists of a change in the sensorium of the patient that is exhibited in its behavior. The aura is defined as the initial focal motor or sensory signs that may precede a generalized seizure by a few seconds. If the aura is observed, it may suggest the site of the seizure focus. We do not regularly use these terms because they are often difficult to recognize in our patients. However, some owners will report recognizing a change in their pet's behavior, a prodrome or aura, that is predictive of a seizure.

CLASSIFICATION

The classification of seizures in animals is controversial and cannot be directly correlated with that used in humans.[80] We believe the following discussion best serves the experience we have had with seizures in domestic animals, which are most common in the canine species. Seizures can be classified as focal, partial, or general; those that begin as partial seizures may subsequently generalize.

A **focal seizure** is a nonclinical spontaneous discharge of a small group of prosencephalic neurons without any spread. It can be observed only on an electroencephalogram (EEG) and should not be confused with a partial seizure, which is a clinical entity. Focal seizures are sometimes present in the interictal period of dogs diagnosed as idiopathic epileptics. Notably, some clinicians use the terms *focal* and *partial* as synonyms, which is technically incorrect.

A **partial seizure** is a focal seizure that has a limited spread and is observed clinically. The nature of the clinical signs will reflect the area of the prosencephalon where the seizure focus is located and consists of varying degrees of abnormal motor and sensory behavior with or without loss of consciousness. Lateralizing clinical signs often indicate which side of the prosencephalon is affected. Most partial seizures occur in animals that have a structural lesion in the prosencephalon. Occasionally, partial seizures are idiopathic. Two categories are described for partial seizures.

1. A **simple partial seizure** reflects primarily abnormal motor neuron discharge with no disturbance of the patient's sensorium. Episodic tremors, head turning, limb flexion, facial muscle twitches, head and neck sporadic myoclonus, sialosis, and mydriasis are examples. In Chapter 8, see Videos 8-29 through 8-31 for examples of sporadic myoclonus, which is a form of simple partial seizure. Some of these simple partial seizures may also be difficult to differentiate from a movement disorder, which we describe in Chapter 8. A simple partial seizure that involves only the limbs or face on one side of the body is considered as a lateralizing clinical sign and indicates that the seizure focus or lesion is in the opposite cerebral hemisphere. For most simple partial seizures, the seizure focus is thought to be in the motor area of the cerebral hemisphere. In humans, a simple partial (focal motor) seizure that consists of an initial tonic contraction followed by clonic contractions of one hand that spreads to the rest of that forelimb, the ipsilateral face, and pelvic limb is called a *Jacksonian seizure*. This type of seizure indicates a focus in the contralateral motor cortex.

2. A **complex partial seizure** includes some disturbance of the patient's sensorium, which is expressed as a behavioral abnormality.[33] Some examples are episodes of staring into space, maniacal running, tail chasing, flank attacking, fly or light biting, abnormal aggression or rage, and just brief episodes of loss of consciousness. These complex partial seizures are often called psychomotor seizures because of the behavioral component. The presence of abnormal behavior in the seizure suggests that the seizure focus includes involvement of the limbic system. A complex partial seizure may terminate in a generalized seizure.

A **generalized seizure** is the most common form that occurs in domestic animals and affects the brain diffusely. This form of seizure has been called a *grand mal seizure*. The *petit mal seizures* that are described in humans consist of brief lapses in the conscious state with a specific EEG pattern. These types of seizures have not been recognized in domestic animals. A generalized seizure is the form of seizure seen in the 9-year-old Quarter horse in the introductory video (Video 18-1) for this chapter. The initial seizure focus may be in one cerebral hemisphere that immediately spreads to the thalamus, which diffusely activates the entire cerebrum through its neurons that function in the diffuse cortical projection system, or the seizure may originate in this thalamic system. The result is a loss of the conscious state by the patient, a tonic contraction of most of the antigravity skeletal muscles, recumbency followed by periods of tonic muscle activity, and clonic muscle activity, which causes running-like movements of the limbs. Jaw clinching or chewing movements may occur along with sialosis, dilated pupils, hair erection, and sometimes urinary and fecal excretions. Apnea may occur during a tonic phase of the seizure. This form of seizure usually lasts from 30 seconds to 3 minutes, followed by a variable period of postictal clinical signs and then complete recovery.

PATHOGENESIS

To understand the basis for seizures, consider that neurons have what we call a *seizure threshold*. This neuronal threshold is determined by their environment, which is genetically determined. Seizures result when this neuronal environment is disturbed and the threshold is lowered. Most commonly, the seizure originates in disturbed prosencephalic neurons. Consider this neuronal threshold in the following simple graph diagram.

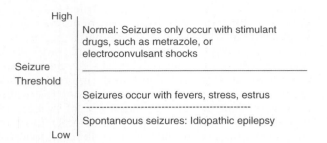

What comprises this neuronal environment? This concept is obviously very complex, but at the least it includes (1) the structure of the dendritic zones and all their synapses, as well as those on the neuronal cell body; (2) the neuronal lipoprotein cell membrane, including the plethora of ion channels that are influenced by the neurotransmitters and the enzymes involved with their activity, such as sodium-potassium-adenosine triphosphatase; (3) the ionic environment of the neurons that includes the availability of sodium, chloride, calcium, and potassium; and (4) the concentration of neurotransmitters that includes those concerned with excitation—glutamate, aspartate, and acetylcholine—and those concerned with inhibition—gamma aminobutyric acid, glycine, taurine, and norepinephrine. In addition, this neuronal environment includes the adjacent neurons and the astrocytes, which also have synapses with neurons and other astrocytes. Astrocytes regulate the transfer of metabolites and ions through the blood vessel walls and have a role in metabolizing many of the neurotransmitters.[73] Fig. 18-1 will help you appreciate the anatomic background of this neuronal environment. Alteration of any one or more of these components may lower the neuronal threshold enough to precipitate a seizure. These alterations comprise the differential diagnosis for seizures.

Neuronal Environmental Alterations

Neuronal environmental alterations in the prosencephalon that precipitate seizures include intracranial (structural), extracranial (metabolic, toxic), and idiopathic disorders. Many of these disorders have already been described in this text. Remember that seizures are the result of uncontrolled discharge of living neurons in the prosencephalon. When necrosis occurs as part of a lesion, the live neurons associated with the disease process are the source of what we observe as seizure activity.

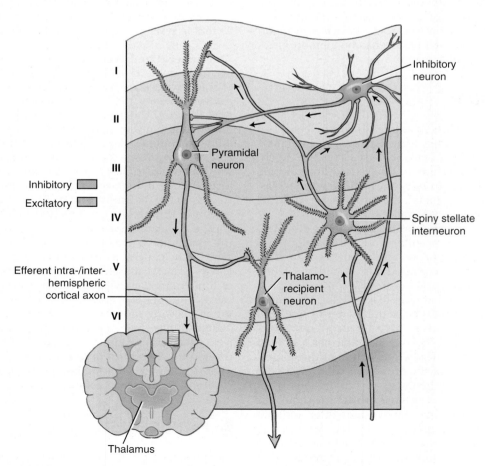

FIGURE 18-1 Neocortex showing some of the cellular components of the neuronal environment where seizures are initiated. *(From: March PA: Seizures: Classification, etiologies, and pathophysiology,* Clin Tech Sm Anim Pract *13:119–131, 1998.)*

Intracranial Disorders

Intracranial in this discussion refers to structural disorders.[101] A thorough neurologic examination will often reveal one or more neurologic deficits in the interictal examination, which indicates a structural lesion.

1. **Malformation.** Many of the malformations described in Chapter 3 that involved the prosencephalon are possible causes of seizures. Obstructive hydrocephalus is the most common. Lissencephaly is another cause, with the onset of seizures at a few years of age. Hydranencephaly is rare in dogs, but we have seen a miniature poodle with unilateral hydranencephaly that began to have seizures at a few months of age. Abnormalities in neuronal migration that cause various cerebrocortical dysplasias are relatively subtle malformations that are more difficult to identify. Considerable interest exists in these cortical dysplasias being a cause of seizures in some dogs diagnosed with idiopathic epilepsy.

2. **Injury.** Brain injury may cause seizures at the time of the injury, or the seizures may be delayed for a few weeks to months after the injury occurred and the tissues have healed. The astrocytic proliferation, neuronal reorganization, and the formation of new synapses that are all part of the healing process in the brain may serve as a seizure focus when this healing occurs in the prosencephalon. These seizures occur only if the patient has had significant intracranial disturbance at the time of the injury with the occurrence of clinical neurologic signs.

3. **Neoplasia.** In our experience, neoplasms are the most common structural cause of seizures, as well as the most common lesion to cause seizures initially and no other clinical neurologic deficit.[16,100,102] Never exclude a brain neoplasm or other structural lesion because the interictal neurologic examination is normal. Lesions can occur in large areas of cerebrum that we cannot recognize on the clinical neurologic examination. For example, we often see large neoplasms of the olfactory bulbs and frontal lobes in dogs; these neoplasms cause seizures without any apparent neurologic abnormalities on our neurologic examination. Primary prosencephalic neoplasms (neurectodermal) are much more common than metastatic neoplasms, and they are more common in dogs and cats than other species of domestic animals. In cats, meningiomas are the most common brain neoplasm. However, in our experience, brain neoplasms in cats, especially meningiomas, do not seem to cause seizures as frequently as they do in dogs.

4. **Inflammation.** Encephalitis that involves the prosencephalon commonly causes seizures. The specific cause of the inflammation is irrelevant to the basis for the seizures but includes viral, bacterial, protozoal, rickettsial, and fungal agents. The relative incidence of these depends on your geographic location. In dogs, the inflammations also include those that may be autoimmune disorders: granulomatous meningoencephalitis, necrotizing meningoencephalitis (common in pug dogs), and necrotizing leukoencephalitis (common in Yorkshire terriers).

5. **Degeneration.** A wide variety of disorders cause various forms of neuronal degeneration in the prosencephalon.[51] *Vascular compromise, cerebrovascular accident,* and *stroke* are all terms related to varying degrees of ischemia or infarction of the brain that, when they occur in the prosencephalon, are possible causes of a seizure. These lesions include those associated with *Cuterebra* spp. myiasis in cats, hypertensive vasculopathy most commonly associated with chronic renal disease, or hyperthyroidism in cats and chronic hypothyroidism in dogs associated with the rare occurrence of cholesterol plaque formation in the walls of cerebral blood vessels. The neonatal encephalopathy of foals is another example.[79] Other degenerations include thiamin deficiency encephalopathy in cats and ruminants, osmolar disorders related to excessive salt or water ingestion, and lead intoxication, as well as other toxicities that include organophosphates, chlorinated hydrocarbons, the artificial sweetener xylitol, caffeine in chocolate, and ethylene glycol.[48,131] Metabolic disorders such as the inherited storage diseases and mitochondrial encephalopathies often cause seizures, as does heat stroke.[21]

Extracranial Disorders

Extracranial causes of seizures are disorders that affect primarily other body systems that, in turn, affect the metabolism of neurons in the central nervous system (CNS). The interictal neurologic examination is usually normal in these patients. However, the physical examination may reflect a systemic abnormality that is related to the cause of the seizures. Some overlap exists with the intracranial group because some of these disorders cause degenerative lesions in the prosencephalon. This group emphasizes what needs to be considered when you study the history, do your physical examination, and order ancillary studies.

1. **Hypoglycemia.** Hypoglycemia from any origin is a common cause of seizures.[69] The most common cause is a functional neoplasm of the beta cell in the pancreatic islet that produces insulin.[14,23,25,106] The common but inappropriate term for this neoplasm is *insulinoma*, which, by its derivation, means a swelling of insulin. My younger colleague, Eric Glass, would say, "Go figure!" Hypoglycemia occurs in dogs older than 4 years. Seizures often occur soon after feeding, which is related to the stimulus of feeding on the release of excessive amounts of insulin in these patients. Although seizures are the most common clinical sign observed with this neoplasm, the episodes associated with a sudden drop in blood glucose occasionally consist of altered behavior or neuromuscular paresis, or both, with or without a mild ataxia. Other causes of hypoglycemia include other neoplasms that produce paraneoplastic hypoglycemia, a functional form observed in hunting dogs associated with vigorous exercise, an unexplained form seen in young 6- to 12-week-old toy breed puppies, a glucose-6-phosphatase deficiency in puppies that is similar to von Gierke disease in children, and any puppy stressed by cold, starvation, gastrointestinal, or other systemic disease and pre- or postpartum hypoglycemia. Clinicians should be aware that a blood sample held overnight before submission to a laboratory for analysis will often be low in blood glucose. If hypoglycemia is a concern, the analysis should be performed as soon as the blood is obtained from the patient. If a functional pancreatic islet cell neoplasm is suspected, be sure to save enough blood for determination of insulin levels before administering intravenous dextrose.

2. **Hepatic encephalopathy.** Hepatic encephalopathy occurs in small animals most commonly associated with congenital portosystemic shunts.[13,27,37] This metabolic

disorder is related to the increased levels of ammonia and other metabolites that the liver fails to remove from the blood adequately, and therefore these substances circulate to the brain. This metabolic encephalopathy can also result from any severe acquired liver disorder. In horses, it is most commonly associated with an acute, presumably autoimmune, necrosis of the liver, known as Theiler disease. See Case Example 14-8 and Video 14-12 in Chapter 14 for an example of this disorder causing behavioral abnormalities and blindness. Seizures may also occur in this disease. Other causes of hyperammonemia in horses are discussed with this case example. Xylitol, an artificial sweetener found in many gum products, has recently been associated with hepatic necrosis and seizures in one dog late in the disease process. Xylitol is a common food additive, and its toxic effects bear close watching.

3. **Electrolyte abnormalities.** The encephalopathy associated with severe osmolar disorders may cause seizures along with other clinical signs of prosencephalic or diffuse brain dysfunction. The most common of these disorders is the salt poisoning that occurs in garbage-fed pigs that have a restricted source of water. We also see this hypernatremia in dogs that spend a day at the beach ingesting salt water. Hypernatremia may occur in dogs with hypothalamic lesions that cause dysfunction of the osmolar receptors located in the hypothalamus that results in adipsia. Encephalopathy may occur in animals that after a period of water deprivation suddenly engorge on water and create a hypoosmolar condition. This circumstance may occur in farm animals if the water pipes freeze for a period. Periparturient hypocalcemia in dogs may cause seizures.[4,114] Hypocalcemia is also a rare occurrence in vigorously exercised hunting dogs and in dogs with chronic renal disease.[72] Severe parathyroiditis may be a cause of hypocalcemia.[117] Seizures may occur in cattle that are hypomagnesemic (grass tetany). Hyperkalemia from adrenocortical insufficiency (Addison disease) or sudden withdrawal of corticosteroid therapy after prolonged use may cause seizures.

4. **Uremia.** Chronic uremia is a rare cause of renal encephalopathy, with seizures as one of the possible clinical signs observed. The cause is poorly understood but has been blamed on the associated acidosis, hypoglycemia, or hypocalcemia. It occurs more commonly in young dogs with congenital renal disease. Chronic renal failure, especially in cats, may also cause hypertension and a vasculopathy that results in an ischemic encephalopathy with seizures.

5. **Hypoxia.** The most common cause of a global hypoxia or anoxia is that related to anesthesia-induced cardiovascular dysfunction. This diffuse encephalopathy was discussed in Chapter 14 as a cause of cortical blindness. Seizures also may occur with this lesion. Hypoxia is thought to be a component of the neonatal encephalopathy that occurs in foals.[103] Acquired cardiovascular disorders that interrupt cerebral blood flow may also be a source of this global hypoxia.

6. **Hyperlipidemia.** Dogs with hyperlipidemia from a dysfunction of lipid metabolism may have seizures.[115] This abnormality is most common in the miniature schnauzer, with an onset of seizures between 2 and 7 years of age.

7. **Hyperthermia.** Heat stroke occurs when the hypothalamic thermal regulatory center can no longer maintain body temperature when an animal is confined in a poorly ventilated space with a high environmental temperature.[21] One of the clinical signs may be seizures. Be aware that the seizure itself can elevate body temperature.

8. **Intestinal parasitism.** Puppies that are heavily infested with intestinal parasites may have seizures that disappear when the parasites are removed. The basis for this is poorly understood but hypocalcemia, hypoglycemia, or some toxin have been considered but not proven.

Idiopathic Epilepsy

Idiopathic epilepsy, the most common cause of seizures in dogs,* is a syndrome characterized by repeated episodes of seizures for which no known demonstrable clinical or pathologic cause has been found. It is a diagnosis based on exclusion of all known causes of seizures. The interictal physical and neurologic examinations are normal, as are the blood studies, cerebrospinal fluid (CSF) evaluation, and imaging studies that rule out the intracranial and extracranial disorders that can cause seizures. Some of these patients may show an abnormality in their EEG readings during the interictal period, but this does not have diagnostic value. Much to the dismay of the owner of a patient with seizures, no conclusive diagnostic test is available for this disorder. In patients with idiopathic epilepsy, the alteration of the neuronal environment in the prosencephalon that lowers their threshold for seizures cannot be recognized by any laboratory procedure or microscopic examination of the brain. The development of this seizure threshold is likely genetically determined. The assumption is that dogs with idiopathic epilepsy have a lowered threshold as a result of a genetic alteration that may be inherited. Pedigree analysis and breeding studies have determined an inherited epilepsy in a large number of breeds that include the following: German shepherd (Alsatian),[39] Belgian Turvuren,[126] keeshond, beagle,[35] English springer spaniel,[107] dachshund, vizsla,[108] Bernese mountain dog,[66] Irish wolf hound,[24] Finnish spitz,[127] golden retriever,[122] standard poodle,[75] and Labrador retriever.[15] The incidence is high in many other breeds that may yet be proven to be inherited, and idiopathic epilepsy also occurs in mixed-breed dogs. Where data is sufficient, it supports an autosomal recessive or polygenic recessive inheritance.

In idiopathic epilepsy, the seizures are usually generalized, but a variety of partial forms do occur. The onset of seizures is usually between 6 months and 6 years of age, but both younger and older onsets have been recognized. Owners may recognize a prodrome that is some subtle change in the behavior of their dog just before the seizure. The seizure usually lasts from 30 seconds to 3 minutes. If the seizure is a partial seizure, the form it takes is consistent and does not usually vary in an individual dog. Large breeds such as the German shepherd, Saint Bernard, and Irish setter often have very severe generalized seizures that may occur in clusters. Miniature and toy poodles may exhibit a mild form of generalized seizure but without loss of consciousness. They act disoriented and exhibit some loss of balance as they develop spasticity of their neck, trunk, and limbs and uncontrolled diffuse trembling but still try to move close to their owners. Their seizure may last up to 30 minutes. We often see simple partial seizures in Labrador retrievers that we diagnose as idiopathic epilepsy. Idiopathic partial seizures are recognized in Finnish spitz dogs with normal magnetic resonance (MR) imaging[127] and are

---

*References 6, 20, 36, 38, 44, 47, 60, 76, 125.

documented in the standard poodle as an autosomal recessive inherited disorder.[75] Most dogs with idiopathic epilepsy are depressed and occasionally blind in the immediate postictal period, which usually lasts for less than an hour. The interval between seizures varies from one or a few weeks to months. The frequency of the seizures may increase as the dog ages, and the dog may occasionally develop status epilepticus during which death can occur. In many of these dogs, the seizures can be controlled to an acceptable level for the owner with the use of anticonvulsant therapy.

Idiopathic epilepsy is a diagnosis of exclusion in which MR imaging plays a significant role in demonstrating the lack of structural lesions in the prosencephalon. However, dogs with presumptive idiopathic epilepsy occasionally have lesions on MR imaging that are likely the effect rather than the cause of the repetitive seizures. These dogs may have bilaterally symmetric to asymmetric lesions in the piriform lobe, the adjacent hippocampal portion of the temporal lobe, or both.[3,40,83] Similar lesions have been reported in the frontal and parietal lobes and less commonly in the cingulate gyrus and the thalamus. The lesions are typically hypointense on T1-weighted images, hyperintense on T2-weighted and fluid-attenuated inversion-recovery (FLAIR) images, and may or may not have scant contrast enhancement. The margins are not well demarcated, and they lack any mass effect. These lesions are usually transient and not visible on repeat imaging once seizure control is achieved. On microscopic examination, these lesions consist of edema, vascular proliferation, neuronal loss, reactive astrogliosis, and occasionally necrosis. Similar findings are reported in humans and are presumed to be related to the excitotoxic effect of accumulated glutamic acid.

Idiopathic epilepsy occurs in cats but is much less common.[12,67,70] It is uncommon in farm animals[2] and the horse, except for the Arabian foals; an idiopathic seizure disorder occurs in Arabian foals.[1] The onset is 3 to 9 months of age, and after a period of weeks the seizures may spontaneously cease. A familial basis is suspected. A form of idiopathic epilepsy has been observed in horses that may be related to the estrus period when the estrogen levels are increased. The horse in the introductory Video 18-1 for this chapter had seizures that occurred only in the first few weeks after foaling. A postpartum hormonal irregularity was presumed to be responsible, given that no lesions were found in the brain after euthanasia and necropsy when the horse was 10 years old. Occasionally, one or more seizures may occur in a patient over a few days with no identifiable cause and then cease spontaneously, which can occur at any age in dogs but more commonly occurs in puppies.

Terminology with seizures can be confusing. One term that will occasionally be seen in the literature is *symptomatic epilepsy,* which refers to recurrent seizures that have an intracranial or extracranial cause. *Primary epilepsy* is idiopathic epilepsy. *Secondary epilepsy* refers to recurrent seizures caused by a structural prosencephalic lesion, and *reactive epilepsy* refers to seizures caused by a metabolic disorder. We do not use these terms.

▌ EXAMINATION

The following discussion is an example of a dog presented with the chief complaint of a possible seizure. This description demonstrates what the veterinarian should

be considering and the historical information that needs to be obtained in attempting to diagnose the cause of the seizure.

Chief Complaint

Seizure

Signalment

Age

Less than 1 year—canine distemper encephalitis, lead poisoning, hepatic encephalopathy from a portosystemic shunt, hydrocephalus, hypoglycemia of toy-breed puppies, puppies with severe intestinal parasitism, occasionally idiopathic epilepsy

1 to 5 years—idiopathic epilepsy

Over 5 years—prosencephalic neoplasia, hypoglycemia from a beta-cell neoplasm of the pancreas, occasionally idiopathic epilepsy

Breed

Hypoglycemia of toy-breed puppies, hydrocephalus in toy and brachycephalic breeds, portosystemic shunt in Yorkshire terriers, neoplasm in boxers, idiopathic epilepsy in German shepherds and other breeds at risk (see earlier discussion), leukodystrophy in cairn and West Highland white terriers, neuronal storage disease in specific breeds (see Table 14-2), lissencephaly in the Lhasa apso, hyperlipidemia in miniature schnauzers, necrotizing meningoencephalitis in pug dogs, necrotizing leukoencephalitis in Yorkshire terriers

Sex

Mammary gland adenocarcinomas may metastasize to the brain. Seizure threshold may be lowered during estrus.

Use

Hypoglycemia in hunting dogs

History

Description

Obtain a complete description of the episode that is being considered as a seizure to be sure that the event is a seizure. Seizures rarely occur when you can see them, and if the description is questionable, have the owner video the episode for you to study. The motor activity in a simple partial seizure may be lateralizing and indicate the site of the seizure focus (i.e., frontoparietal lobes of one cerebral hemisphere). Most generalized seizures from many causes are symmetric and not lateralizing. These causes include toxins and idiopathic epilepsy. Bizarre behavioral abnormalities sometimes precede seizure generalization with lead intoxication. Seizures in cats with marked flexion of the neck and trunk occur with thiamin deficiency. Idiopathic epileptics usually have short generalized seizures.

Onset and Course

An explosive onset of cluster seizures or status epilepticus can occur with neoplasms, intoxications, or occasionally idiopathic epilepsy. A progressive course with increasing frequency and duration of seizures occurs with inflammations or neoplasms. Regular intervals are more common in idiopathic epilepsy. Hypoglycemic seizures often occur just before or shortly after feeding. Seizures often follow a high-protein meal in hepatic encephalopathy.

Environment

Littermates may also be affected with infectious diseases such as canine distemper. Multiple animals may be affected by a common toxin. Sources of lead include paint, linoleum, tarpaper, wall board, and roofing materials. Other intoxicants to consider are metaldehyde in snail bait, hexachlorophene soap, ethylene glycol antifreeze, chlorinated hydrocarbon and organophosphate insecticides, fluoroacetate (1080) rodenticide, fungicides with mercury, arsenicals in insecticides, and phenol and cresol germicides. We studied one young basset hound with seizures secondary to the ingestion of cement that contained ethylene glycol antifreeze, which prevents the cement from freezing during construction in cold weather.

Diet

An all-fish diet that contains thiaminase may precipitate thiamin deficiency, especially in cats. Cooking the food will deplete the thiamin and lead to a deficiency in small animals.

Medical History

Seizures may follow the recovery from significant intracranial injuries by weeks to months. A febrile illness associated with the systemic clinical signs of canine distemper infection may precede the seizures from the subsequent encephalitis. A difficult parturition may cause cerebral hypoxia or brain injury. A delay of weeks may occur between smoke inhalation or radiation therapy overdose and the onset of encephalopathy with seizures. A previous diagnosis of neoplasia in another body system may herald a brain metastasis. The owner's recognition of other neurologic dysfunction in the patient suggests a structural lesion. Evidence of a behavior change, polyuria, polydipsia, or a voracious indiscriminate appetite suggests possible hypothalamic involvement by a pituitary neoplasm. Clinical signs of hyperadrenocorticoidism may accompany a functional pituitary adenoma. A recent change in behavior often accompanies a frontal lobe neoplasm. Episodic behavioral alterations occur in the young dog with hepatic encephalopathy.

▎ PHYSICAL EXAMINATION

Extracranial causes of a seizure may reflect abnormal function of another organ system, which may be evident in your physical examination of these systems, as well as in the ancillary procedures. These organs include the liver, pancreas, kidney, and cardiorespiratory organs. Systemic disease may accompany the encephalitis caused by infectious agents.

Neurologic Examination

Abnormal = Structural brain disease
Normal = Structural brain disease in a quiet area
              Metabolic disorder—intoxication
              Idiopathic epilepsy

To be reliable, the examination must be performed in the interictal period. Abnormalities in the interictal neurologic examination suggest intracranial structural brain disease. Focal clinical signs suggest a neoplasm, vascular compromise, previous injury, or focal infection (granuloma, abscess). See Chapter 14 for the discussion of prosencephalic disorders and the three clinical signs that can be recognized in your neurologic examination indicating a prosencephalic dysfunction. Recognition of any one of these in an otherwise normal patient is critical for the diagnosis of a structural lesion that is the cause of the seizures. See Video 14-6 and Video 14-7 that follow Case Example 14-5 in Chapter 14, in which seizures were the chief complaint. Patients with frontal lobe lesions may circle toward the side of the structural lesion (the adversive syndrome). This is a common clinical sign that helps locate the side of a prosencephalic disorder. Multifocal clinical signs suggest an inflammation or multiple neoplasms. Clinical signs of diffuse prosencephalic or brain dysfunction may occur with inflammations, degenerative diseases, or a metabolic disorder that is neuronal or extracranial in origin.

In the absence of interictal neurologic signs, the cause of the seizures can still be intracranial, as well as extracranial, in origin or idiopathic. Remember that large areas of prosencephalon may have a lesion causing neuronal dysfunction, but this dysfunction may not be reflected in the animal's behavior or on its neurologic examination. We refer to these areas as "quiet areas" because we cannot test them for dysfunction in our neurologic examination. Most extracranial disorders do not cause interictal neurologic signs (i.e., hypoglycemia, hepatic encephalopathy, cardiac arrhythmias). The interictal neurologic examination is always normal in dogs with idiopathic epilepsy.

Further study to determine the cause of the seizure requires ancillary examinations.

Ancillary Examination

Complete Blood Count and Differential Cell Count

Nucleated red blood cells, basophilic stippling, and a low packed cell volume may be present in lead poisoning. A microcytic anemia may occur with a portosystemic shunt. The complete blood count (CBC) is usually normal in viral encephalitis. Leucocytosis and neutrophilia may be present with suppurative meningoencephalitis. Leucocytosis may occur with portosystemic shunts. Polycythemia with a packed cell volume greater than 70 cells/mm^3 may cause enough viscosity to result in a seizure.

Blood Chemistry

The blood urea nitrogen (BUN) may be increased in chronic renal disease or decreased with portosystemic shunts. Most animals with hepatic encephalopathy will be hyperammonemic and show variable evidence of liver dysfunction on serum studies. Hypoglycemia or abnormal glucose-to-insulin ratios may be diagnostic for a pancreatic beta-cell neoplasm or other disease process. Electrolyte abnormalities may be recognized. Bile acid evaluation will be abnormal with diffuse liver disorders such as the portosystemic shunt. Hyperlipidemia may relate to seizure genesis.

Cerebrospinal Fluid

The CSF is normal in all idiopathic epileptics and may be normal in many of the structural brain disorders. We do not routinely measure the CSF pressure and avoid obtaining CSF if we suspect that intracranial pressure may be markedly elevated. Whenever possible, we rely on the results of the MR imaging to dictate whether the CSF is obtained for evaluation.

Imaging

By far the most reliable imaging for the recognition of prosencephalic disorders that cause seizures is MR imaging. Radiographs rarely show a structural lesion unless it involves the calvaria directly or indirectly. Meningiomas adjacent to the calvaria may cause a thickening of the bone. Computed tomographic (CT) imaging, using a soft tissue window, will reveal many prosencephalic lesions, but their characteristics to allow differentiation and further treatment options are much less useful when compared with MR imaging. Rectal scintigraphy may confirm a portosystemic shunt.

Examination Summary

The extent of the examination for the cause of the seizure disorder depends on the number of seizures, the age of the patient at the time of the examination, the priority of the disorders in your differential diagnosis, and the cost of the ancillary procedures. All patients require a physical and neurologic examination. For a young dog with a single seizure and normal neurologic examination, this may be sufficient. In an older dog with a single seizure and normal neurologic examination, a CBC, differential cell count, and a complete blood chemistry panel should comprise the minimal database. Recurrent seizures with or without interictal neurologic signs require this minimal database, as well as consideration of a serum lead level and serum antibody levels for infectious diseases plus imaging studies, preferably MR imaging, if the owner can afford the expense. CSF evaluation is dependent on whether imaging studies are performed and your consideration of its value in determining the clinical diagnosis.

█ CASE EXAMPLES

The following case examples exemplify the four major conclusions from the neurologic examination of a patient with the chief complaint of seizures.

CASE EXAMPLE 18-1

Signalment: 6-year-old female Boston terrier

History: Seven weeks before this examination, she had her first episode of generalized seizures, which occurred as a cluster over 2 hours. Clusters of seizures recurred at 10 days and 2 days before this examination, as well as in the hour before this examination. The owners described her as being normal between these clusters of seizures.

Examination: On the initial examination when she was presented to the hospital, she was depressed and blind, with normal pupil size and response to light. She drifted to either side as she walked and had slow postural reactions in all four limbs.

Anatomic Diagnosis: Diffuse brain but primarily the prosencephalon bilaterally

Because of the history of a seizure just before hospitalization and this examination, the concern was that these clinical signs represented the postictal effects of that seizure, and the examination should be repeated if and when she reached an interictal stage.

Second Examination: This examination was performed 24 hours after the initial examination. She was alert, responsive, and visual, and she had a normal gait. Hopping was consistently slow in the right limbs. Hypalgesia was found on the right side of the nasal septum.

Anatomic Diagnosis: Left prosencephalon, possibly the left frontoparietal lobe region that spared the left central visual pathway

Differential Diagnosis: Structural disease: neoplasm, necrotizing meningoencephalitis or leukoencephalitis, granulomatous meningoencephalitis, abscess, vascular compromise

Progressive seizures in a brachycephalic breed at this age suggest a neoplasm. Necrotizing encephalitides are uncommon in this breed. A focal form of the lymphoproliferative granulomatous meningoencephalitis is a possibility. A bacterial or fungal abscess or granuloma is uncommon. Be aware of brain infections with *Coccidioides immitis* in the southwestern states. Vascular compromise is unlikely to only cause a seizure at the onset and then cause progressive seizures.

Imaging procedures are necessary to define the clinical diagnosis further. Advanced imaging was not available at the time of this study. CSF contained 2 white blood cells (WBCs)/mm³ (normal <5) and 39 mg/dl of protein (normal <25), which supported a structural disorder and suggested that a neoplasm was more likely than an inflammatory process.

The patient was euthanized, and necropsy revealed a well-defined astrocytoma in the left side of the diencephalon at its junction with the telencephalon (Fig. 18-2).

For two video examples of dogs with a history of seizures and clinical signs of a unilateral prosencephalic disorder, see Chapter 14, Case Example 14-5, Videos 14-6 and 14-7.

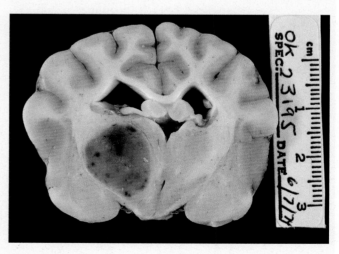

FIGURE 18-2 Transverse section of the preserved brain from the 6-year-old Boston terrier in this case example. Note the astrocytoma in the left side of the diencephalon.

CASE EXAMPLE 18-2

Signalment: 7-year-old female German shepherd

History: This female had her first generalized seizure 6 months before this examination. Seizures recurred at variable intervals that became weekly this past month. A cluster of seizures occurred 1 week before this examination. The owner described that, for the past week, this dog acted different. The dog seemed less interested in the owner, sometimes paced around the house, and occasionally howled for no obvious reason.

Examination: Her physical and neurologic examinations were normal.

Anatomic Diagnosis: Prosencephalon

Differential Diagnosis:

1. A structural lesion in a *quiet area* of the prosencephalon. See the list for Case Example 18-1.
2. A metabolic disorder or toxicity. See the list of extracranial disorders that may cause seizures.
3. Idiopathic epilepsy. Although this breed is at risk for idiopathic epilepsy, it is less likely with an onset at this age.

This history of progressive seizures and the more recent change in behavior supports a structural lesion, especially a neoplasm, but metabolic and toxic causes must still be considered. The discussion of possible structural lesions in Case Example 18-1 is applicable to this patient. We have never seen the necrotizing encephalitides in a large-breed dog.

The CBC, differential cell count, blood chemistry panel, and urinalysis were all normal. The CSF contained 2 WBCs/mm³ and 119 mg/dl of protein, which supported a structural brain lesion and more likely a neoplasm than an inflammatory disease. Skull radiographs were normal. Advanced imaging was not available when this dog was studied. Scintigraphy showed increased uptake of radioisotope in the area of the left olfactory bulb.

This dog was euthanized, and necropsy revealed a large extraparenchymal mass adjacent to the left olfactory bulb and peduncle, which were displaced along with the left frontal lobe. The mass was a fibroblastic meningioma (Figs. 18-3 through 18-5).

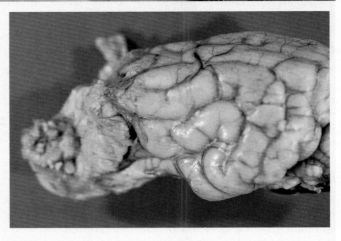

FIGURE 18-4 Lateral view of the preserved brain from the dog in Fig. 18-3. Note the meningioma compressing the left frontal lobe, olfactory bulb, and olfactory peduncle.

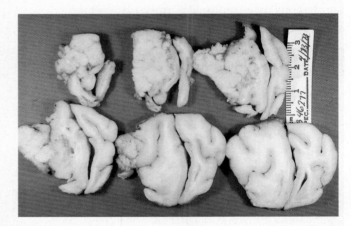

FIGURE 18-5 Transverse sections of the rostral portion of the brain in Fig. 18-4. The extraparenchymal mass on the left side is a fibroblastic meningioma.

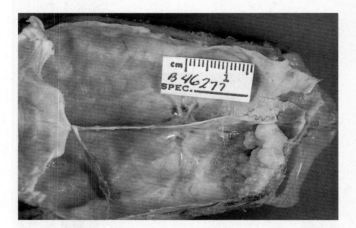

FIGURE 18-3 Ventral surface of the preserved calvaria with the dura attached from the 7-year-old German shepherd in this case example. The rostral edge of the tentorium cerebelli is at the left, and the falx cerebri is in the center. The protruding attached irregular tissue on the surface of the left side of the rostral calvarial dura is a meningioma.

CASE EXAMPLE 18-3

Signalment: 12-year-old male miniature poodle

History: Generalized seizures began 6 weeks before this examination. Each seizure was followed by 90 minutes of lethargy and mild ataxia. Seizures had been increasing in frequency and often occurred in the early evening when the owner returned from work and the dog became very excited. Recently the dog had exhibited episodes of fatigue or ataxia associated with moderate exercise.

Examination: The physical and neurologic examinations were both normal.

Anatomic Diagnosis: Prosencephalon

Differential Diagnosis:

1. Structural lesion in a *quiet area* of the prosencephalon. See the list for Case Example 18-1.
2. Metabolic disease or toxicity. See the list of extracranial disorders that will cause seizures.
3. Idiopathic epilepsy would be very unlikely with onset at 12 years of age.

The CBC, differential cell count, and urinalysis were normal. The blood chemistry panel showed significantly low blood glucose level of 30 mg/dl (normal is 60 to 100). A radioimmunoassay for serum insulin showed a significant elevation above normal levels. Ultrasound examination revealed a small pancreatic mass, which was presumed to be a beta-cell islet neoplasm. It was reasonable to assume that these findings explained the cause of the seizures and the other neurologic signs observed by the owner of this dog. Therefore performing advanced imaging, which would have required general anesthesia, was considered unnecessary.

Because of the frequency that this neoplasm has for metastasis to adjacent lymph nodes and the liver, this dog was euthanized, and the diagnosis was confirmed at necropsy. Many of these patients can be managed with frequent feeding, corticosteroids, and diazoxide therapy.[106] Other drugs sometimes used for this disease include octreotide and somatostatin. Medical or surgical therapy (or both) may successfully control the seizures for approximately 4 to 12 months.

CASE EXAMPLE 18-4

Signalment: 2-year-old male German shepherd

History: The first generalized seizure occurred 7 months before this examination. After the third seizure, which occurred 1 month after the first one, this dog had a physical and neurologic examination, both of which were normal. The CBC, differential cell count, blood chemistry panel, and urinalysis at that time were all normal. The dog was started on anticonvulsant therapy with phenobarbital. Despite this therapy, the seizures continued and became more frequent. A cluster of seizures occurred 3 weeks before this examination, as well as the day of the examination.

Examination: See **Video 18-2** of this dog on admission to the hospital. Reread the description of a generalized seizure and appreciate that this abnormality is what you are observing here. This dog is having serial seizures without recovery between them, and he is therefore in status epilepticus. On the video, the dog is given diazepam intravenously in an attempt to stop the seizures. The following day, this dog was interictal, and a physical and neurologic examination at that time was normal.

Anatomic Diagnosis: Prosencephalon

Differential Diagnosis:

1. Structural lesion in a *quiet area* of the prosencephalon. See the list for Case Example 18-1.

2. Metabolic disease or toxicity. See the list of extracranial disorders that will cause seizures.
3. Idiopathic epilepsy. The age of onset, progressive course, and the breed make this diagnosis the most presumptive at this point in the clinical study. The seizures that occur in this disorder in the large breeds of dogs, especially in German shepherds, can be very difficult to control with anticonvulsant therapy.

The CBC, differential cell count, blood chemistry panel, and urinalysis were all normal in this patient. CSF was normal. Advanced imaging was not available when this dog was studied, but brain scintigraphy was normal. The presumptive clinical diagnosis was idiopathic epilepsy.

This dog's serum level of phenobarbital was considered to be inadequate to control the seizures. The decision was made to increase the dose of phenobarbital and monitor his clinical response in relationship to his serum levels. If this therapy proved to be ineffective, then the addition of potassium bromide would be considered before adding or changing to other anticonvulsant therapies.

GENERALIZED AND PARTIAL SEIZURES

The following videos are examples of generalized and partial seizures resulting from a variety of causes.

Video 18-3. This video shows Corky, a 7-year-old castrated male miniature schnauzer that was diagnosed with idiopathic epilepsy at 3 years of age. Anticonvulsant therapy partially controlled the seizures until the day before this video was made and status epilepticus occurred. The only value in doing a neurologic examination during a brief interval between a series of seizures or in the postictal period

is to look for any obvious asymmetry in the three clinical signs of prosencephalic disease. The presence of any asymmetry would support a structural lesion. No such asymmetry was found in this dog, and a presumptive diagnosis was made of idiopathic epilepsy in which anticonvulsant control was lost. An MR imaging study should be recommended for this dog to support this presumed diagnosis further, and serum levels of the anticonvulsants used should be obtained.

Video 18-4. This video shows a 4-month-old spayed female beagle dog with canine distemper encephalitis in status epilepticus having a series of generalized seizures. Note the postictal obtundation, blindness, and propulsive circling. These postictal neurologic signs are not useful by themselves in making a more precise anatomic diagnosis.

Video 18-5. This video shows a 6-month-old spayed female vizsla with canine distemper encephalitis in status epilepticus having a series of generalized seizures. The chewing motions and sialosis make the dog appear as if it had eaten an irritating substance. This sign is the basis for the term *chewing gum fits,* which has no diagnostic significance other than being a component of a generalized seizure.

Video 18-6. This video shows a 9-year-old spayed female boxer with a 3-week history of progressive generalized seizures that was presented to the hospital in status epilepticus. This dog was euthanized, and necropsy revealed diencephalic glioma.

Video 18-7. This video shows a 2-month-old female mixed-breed pig in status epilepticus caused by salt intoxication. It is typical for these pigs with this osmotic encephalopathy to back up during their seizures. No explanation for this unique behavior is known.

Video 18-8. This video shows a 6-week-old male Arabian that was found in its stall having a generalized seizure. Epistaxis was present, and a small area of hemorrhage near its left ear was noted. The foal was hospitalized later that day when the video was made. The initial portion of the video shows the foal in a postictal state. It is lethargic, mildly ataxic and paretic, and blind, with normal pupil size and light response. The last portion of the video shows the foal recumbent at the end of another generalized seizure. Diazepam was given intravenously to stop the seizures. As the foal recovered from its postictal state, the menace response returned in the left eye before the right eye. This finding suggested that a more significant lesion may have been present in the left cerebral hemisphere. The interictal neurologic examination was normal, as were all the ancillary studies that were performed. No advanced imaging was performed. Idiopathic epilepsy is seen in young Arabian foals 3 to 9 months old. In this foal, the young age, the associated hemorrhage, and the delay in the return of the menace response in the right eye suggested that these seizures were secondary to intracranial injury, possibly by the foal's mare that was in the stall with this foal.

Video 18-9. This video shows an adult lion in status epilepticus in the Serengeti National Park in Tanzania. This lion has canine distemper encephalitis from exposure to unvaccinated dogs. Unfortunately, many lions died from this viral infection during the 1990s.

Video 18-10. This video shows BJ, a male Indian rhinoceros at the Metro Zoo in Miami, Florida. He is having a generalized seizure in his moat where he was kept at the zoo. He was treated with large doses of phenobarbital and potassium bromide, which kept the seizure frequency and duration at an acceptable level for 5 years before he was euthanized. Necropsy showed mild inflammatory lesions in the brain suggestive of the remains of a nonsuppurative inflammation of unknown cause. We thank Dr. Chriss Miller of the Metro Zoo for this video.

Video 18-11. This video shows Kiki, a 15-month-old Shiba Inu that has exhibited episodes of sporadic myoclonus in the form of facial twitches for the past week that are now almost continuous. The neurologic examination revealed a depressed sensorium but a normal gait and postural reactions. The video shows a decreased menace response in the left eye and decreased nociception in the left nasal cavity. Pupil size and light responses were normal. This abnormality is an example of a simple partial seizure. The anatomic diagnosis was right prosencephalon. MR imaging showed scattered contrast enhancement and hyperintensity on T2-weighted images in the area of the right frontal and parietal lobes. Kiki was euthanized, and necropsy revealed a nonsuppurative encephalitis of unknown cause, located primarily in the frontoparietal lobes.

Video 18-12. This video shows a 20-year-old palomino Saddle horse that has been exhibiting brief twitches of the right side of its body for the past 7 days with an increasing frequency. At the start of the video, before an episode, the menace response is normal bilaterally. Note that, during the seizure, the muscle contractions occur only on the right side of the body. You cannot see the left side well in this video, but the contractions are not present there. Note that the postictal examination shows a loss of the menace response on the right side. Within 15 minutes, this menace response returned. This postictal abnormality supports a structural lesion in the left prosencephalon, as does the simple partial seizure, which is caused by a seizure focus with limited spread in the left motor area of the prosencephalon. Radiographs showed a bony proliferation on the inner surface of the left calvaria, presumably the result of some previous traumatic event. This bony proliferation was removed surgically, but the horse developed severe postoperative cerebral edema and was euthanized. At necropsy, an extensive depression was found in the left cerebral hemisphere where the bone protrusion penetrated the brain. This depression was located on the dorsolateral aspect at approximately the middle of the left cerebral hemisphere. Microscopic examination revealed extensive neuronal degeneration and astrogliosis at this site.

Video 18-13. This video shows Oscar, a 5-year-old castrated male domestic shorthair with the episodes that you see on this video for the past 18 months. They only occur when he is scratched over the lumbar and sacral area. This seizure is a simple partial seizure that is often known as feline hyperesthesia syndrome, which we believe was first described by Dr. Jean Holzworth from the Angell Memorial Animal Hospital. Feline hyperesthesia syndrome is quite common in cats and can be prevented in many cats by not stimulating this area. The use of phenobarbital, prednisone, or both together has produced variable results. An unusual myopathy of unknown cause has been diagnosed in the lumbar muscles in some of these cats.[81] This myopathy may be the cause of the lumbar area hypersensitivity. The excessive sensory stimulation of the prosencephalon may be the basis for the initiation of these partial seizures in cats with an especially low seizure threshold. This relationship needs further study.

Video 18-14. This video shows Walter, a 5-year-old castrated male domestic shorthair with severe simple partial seizures that partially generalize when his lumbosacral area is stimulated. This abnormality is a severe form of feline hyperesthesia syndrome. Note the urination that occurs during the episode. Walter's hypersensitivity was so severe that performing all of the neurologic examination on him was difficult.

Video 18-15. This video shows Chelsae, a 6-year-old spayed female Bernese mountain dog with episodes as seen on the video that had been occurring at varying intervals over a 1-year period. She was examined at a veterinary hospital and diagnosed with dyschezia. Extensive diagnostic procedures and treatments had been performed on Chelsae for a presumptive gastrointestinal system disorder with no cause found and no response to the various therapies, which included a lumbosacral laminectomy. We believe these are complex partial seizures, psychomotor seizures, and what appears to be dyschezia is the excretory component of the seizure. Note the vague, disoriented expression in the dog's head after some of the spinning episodes.

 Video 18-16. This video shows Claire, a 4-year-old Labrador retriever with presumably complex partial seizures that can be described as *fly-biting* episodes. These episodes had been occurring sporadically for approximately 6 months. Differentiating these kinds of episodes from the obsessive-compulsive syndrome is often difficult. In these situations, we usually recommend a trial therapy with the anticonvulsant drug phenobarbital, and if this therapy produces no effect, we try therapy with a behavioral drug such as clomiprazine.

 Video 18-17. This video shows a 1-year-old pit bull terrier that has exhibited the episodes that are seen on the video for approximately 3 months. Anticonvulsant therapy was ineffective.

Are these *bug-searching* episodes a complex partial seizure, or is this an example of the obsessive-compulsive syndrome? The owner elected euthanasia, and necropsy showed no lesions, which does not answer the question.

 Video 18-18. This video shows Rascal, an 11-month-old castrated male Pekinese, that has exhibited these *flank-attacking* episodes that are seen on this video for the past 5 months. He is lame in his right pelvic limb, but his neurologic examination was normal, as was his CBC, differential cell count, blood chemistry panel, and urinalysis. No advanced imaging was performed. We believe this disorder is a complex partial seizure. This belief is supported by a study of tail-attacking dogs that had focal seizure activity in their interictal EEGs.[31]

 Video 18-19. This video shows Bubbles, a 2.5-year-old spayed female Dalmatian, that has exhibited the episodes that are seen on the video for the past month. We interpreted this *foot-attacking-the-dog* episode as a complex partial seizure. A few months later, this dog developed generalized seizures and was euthanized. No necropsy was performed.

See Videos 8-29, 8-30, and 8-31 in Chapter 8 for two dogs and one cat with sporadic myoclonus, which is a form of simple partial seizure.

INCIDENCE

Seizures are the most common neurologic disorder that you will encounter in small-animal practice. Various reports cite an incidence in up to 5% of all dogs, and the majority of these will be idiopathic epileptics. For comparison, approximately 5% of all humans will have at least one seizure in their lifetime. In approximately 30% of human patients with seizures, a neurologic or systemic disorder will be identified, and 70% will be idiopathic.

Between 2% and 5% of all children with fevers will have seizures in the United States.

TREATMENT

The treatment of seizures should be directed toward the primary disease that is causing the seizures when it is recognized and if it is a treatable disorder. Surgical removal of structural prosencephalic lesions is now a common procedure in small-animal practice. The seizures themselves should be controlled as much as possible with current pharmacologic anticonvulsant therapy. A dog that is presented for a single seizure and that has normal physical, neurologic, and routine ancillary examinations need not be treated. No one knows for any individual patient if an acceptable number of seizures exists for any given time period that will not be life threatening at any time. We believe that dogs that have a second seizure are at risk for an increasing frequency or duration of seizures, and anticonvulsant therapy should be considered. You cannot accurately predict if and when seizures will cluster or become continuous (status epilepticus), which is life threatening. Seizure control is paramount because the seizure itself can cause brain lesions resulting from the hypoxia associated with the apnea that occurs during a prolonged seizure and the accumulation of excessive amounts of glutamic acid, which causes an excitotoxic degeneration of neurons.[3,40,73] In addition, the hyperthermia secondary to the prolonged or recurring seizures can cause disseminated intravascular coagulation and death.

Experimentally, spontaneous seizures can be induced by the *kindling phenomenon,* which involves frequent repeated experimental stimulations to cerebral neurons.[38,128] This event sets up an electrical circuitry that can ultimately initiate a seizure spontaneously. No evidence has been found to date that a greater tendency exists for more seizures to occur after one clinical seizure because of this kindling phenomenon, but it may play a role as seizures are repeated. The kindling phenomenon has been used to test the efficacy of anticonvulsant drugs in dogs.

The two most common anticonvulsants presently in use are phenobarbital and potassium bromide. Most clinicians initiate treatment with phenobarbital, but either drug may be used as the initial therapy with the addition or replacement by the other if control is unsatisfactory. Serum levels of the anticonvulsant drug should be determined before changing the dose or changing the drug in use. Patients must be carefully observed for side effects, and drug adjustments must be made in accordance with the pharmacodynamics of the drug and the clinical situation for the patient. Both phenobarbital and potassium bromide are inexpensive and relatively safe for the patient. Although complete elimination of the seizures is the most desirable result, it is often difficult to achieve. The seizures that occur in approximately 25% to 30% of all dogs diagnosed with idiopathic epilepsy are poorly controlled using phenobarbital, potassium bromide, or both at acceptable serum levels. The treatment goal should be to reduce the incidence and severity of the seizures to a level that is acceptable to the owner and least disruptive to the patient while avoiding significant drug-induced side effects. Without an owner's cooperation, effective seizure control will not be obtained. This control is a daily treatment that cannot be interrupted because interruption itself may precipitate a seizure. The owner must appreciate the importance of this daily routine.

Occasionally, relapses occur even in well-controlled patients. The exacerbation of a seizure disorder after successful management does not necessarily indicate the presence of a progressive structural lesion, but it may simply require more vigorous therapy. Similarly, seizures that change in pattern do not necessarily imply the presence of a structural lesion. In many instances, no correlation exists between the severity and duration of the seizure and the underlying disease. Some dogs with idiopathic epilepsy have more serious seizures than dogs with large intracranial neoplasms. The prognosis in serious seizure disorders, including status epilepticus, is not necessarily grave if no indication of structural brain disease is found during the examination of the patient. Except in status epilepticus, dogs usually do not die from a seizure.

Numerous excellent resources describe in detail the pharmacology and dose levels of these anticonvulsant drugs and the newer drugs that are being investigated.[31,32,109,111] The following section provides a brief description of the drugs presently available.

Maintenance Anticonvulsant Therapy

Phenobarbital

Phenobarbital is considered the standard anticonvulsant therapy in all domestic animals. Its action is to raise the threshold of neurons to the initiation of a seizure. It is rapidly effective in producing this effect. Most clinicians initiate oral therapy with 2.5 to 3.0 mg/kg of body weight twice daily. Owners should be made aware that many patients will be depressed by this dose but will recover their normal sensorium in 1 to 4 weeks without reducing the dose of the drug. Overdose causes persistent sedation. The half-life of phenobarbital is 1 to 3 days, and a steady-state serum level takes 7 to 15 days to achieve. Therefore determining the serum levels is unreliable until at least 1 week after the initiation of therapy. Effective serum levels vary for each patient but are thought to be between 15 and 45 mcg/ml. A loading dose of phenobarbital may be used when more prompt seizure control is necessary. With this therapy, the patient receives a total loading dose of 16 mg/kg over 16-24 hours. This level is usually accomplished by giving 4 mg/kg intravenously, intramuscularly or orally every 4 to 6 hours. Serum levels can be checked at the end of giving this medication. If the patient becomes too sedate, the loading protocol is discontinued and maintenance therapy is initiated. If the decision is made to stop using this drug for any reason, never stop it suddenly; otherwise, serious seizures may result. Slowly withdraw the drug over several weeks by decreasing the dose used. Chronic use of high levels of the drug may cause polydipsia and polyphagia with weight gain and sedation to the point of causing mild paresis and ataxia. Blood dyscrasia and a superficial necrotizing dermatitis are rare. Phenobarbital is excreted through the liver and commonly elevates the serum levels of alkaline phosphatase. Hepatopathy is an uncommon side effect, but you should monitor the patient's liver function with blood chemistry panels every few months to evaluate other liver enzymes.[22] Bile acid testing is a better way to evaluate liver function. Phenobarbital may also alter the results of thyroid function tests, which can be confused with hypothyroidism.[29] Phenobarbital is the preferred anticonvulsant in cats.

Potassium Bromide

Potassium bromide is a halide salt most commonly used as an add-on anticonvulsant drug to phenobarbital when the latter is ineffective or not as effective as desired.[112,113] It also may permit you to decrease the dose level of the phenobarbital. Potassium bromide may also be used initially as the sole anticonvulsant drug. Its action is similar to phenobarbital in that it raises the threshold of neurons to seizure initiation. Potassium bromide is excreted through the kidneys and is therefore useful in dogs with liver disease, but the drug needs to be decreased in dose in dogs with any renal disease. Potassium bromide is dissolved in double distilled water to form a solution of 200 or 250 mg/ml. The oral dose is 30 to 40 mg/kg of body weight once daily if used with phenobarbital and 30 to 80 mg/kg of body weight if used alone. A loading dose of bromide may be used when faster seizure control is necessary. With this therapy, the patient receives a total loading dose of 400 to 600 mg/kg over 1 to 2 days. This level is usually accomplished by giving 100 to 150 mg/kg orally twice a day for 2 days. If the patient becomes too sedate, the loading dose is discontinued and maintenance therapy is initiated. The bromide ion is handled the same as the chloride ion, and high-chloride diets will increase the elimination of bromide and lower the blood levels, which requires an increase in the dose used. The elimination half-life is 24 to 36 days in dogs, and 80 to 120 days are needed to reach a steady state in the blood. Determination of serum levels for maintenance dose can be performed after 3 to 4 months. The serum level therapeutic range is 1 to 2.5 mg/ml when the drug is used with phenobarbital and 1 to 3 mg/ml when it is the sole anticonvulsant drug. The side effects are similar to those observed with phenobarbital (i.e., sedation, polydipsia, polyphagia, mild paresis and ataxia in the pelvic limbs). Rarely, aggressive behavior has been related to the use of this drug. The long half-life of this drug has the advantage of allowing you to stop treatment with this drug all at once, permitting the blood level to decrease slowly on its own. It has the disadvantage that if side effects are observed and the drug is stopped, some time will be required before the clinical signs will resolve. If absolutely necessary, intravenous sodium chloride fluid supplementation can be administered to reduce the serum levels of bromide rapidly. The threat of bronchial asthma and pancreatitis in cats along with less efficacy has reduced the use of potassium bromide in this species.

Alternative Anticonvulsants

Alternative anticonvulsant drugs that are used in humans are still unapproved and under clinical investigation in dogs. These drugs are generally more expensive than those mentioned previously, which may be prohibitive in large-breed dogs. They have been used as add-on drugs to standard anticonvulsant therapy or as the sole drug used. When used as an add-on drug, reducing the dose of the initial drug used may be possible. This group of drugs includes zonisamide, felbamate, gabapentin, and levetiracetam. Most of these drugs act on neurons to raise their threshold to the initiation of seizures. At the present time, zonisamide and felbamate appear to be the most helpful in dogs that have seizures that cannot be satisfactorily controlled with phenobarbital and potassium bromide. In recent studies, when used as an add-on drug to phenobarbital or as the sole drug, either drug showed greater than 50% improvement in the control of the seizures. However, these drugs are very expensive.

Zonisamide. Zonisamide (Zonegran) is a sulfonamide-based anticonvulsant. It has a half-life of 15 to 20 hours and is metabolized for excretion by hepatic microsomal enzymes. As a sole therapy, the recommended oral dose is 5 to 8 mg/kg of body weight twice daily. If zonisamide is administered as an add-on drug to dogs on phenobarbital, use an oral dose of 10 mg/kg of body weight twice daily. Serum levels can be determined after 1 week of therapy, with the therapeutic range being 10 to 40 mcg/ml. The increased dose is necessary because the phenobarbital will already have stimulated the activity of hepatic microsomal enzymes for its metabolism. Zonisamide has a high margin of safety in dogs. Occasionally, the drug may cause mild sedation, ataxia, and vomiting.

Felbamate. Felbamate (Felbatol) is a dicarbamate anticonvulsant drug with a half-life of 4 to 8 hours in dogs. The majority of the drug is excreted unchanged through the kidneys, with the remainder being metabolized in hepatocytes. The recommended initial oral dose is 15 mg/kg of body weight three times daily. If the initial dose is ineffective, it can be increased in increments of 15-20 mg/kg of body weight every 2 weeks. This drug has a wide margin of safety in dogs, and sedation is not observed. The toxic dose in dogs is 300 mg/kg of body weight. Evaluation of serum levels of this drug is seldom performed because of the expense, wide therapeutic range, and low toxicity. Felbamate is effective both as an add-on drug and as the sole therapy. Liver function should be periodically evaluated for potential hepatotoxicity.

Gabapentin. Gabapentin (Neurontin) is a structural analog of gamma aminobutyric acid, but its mechanism of action is poorly understood. It has a half-life of 3 to 4 hours in dogs. Gabapentin is excreted primarily through the kidneys, with a portion metabolized and excreted by the hepatocytes. The recommended oral dose is 10 mg/kg of body weight three times daily. Side effects are uncommon except for occasional sedation. Serum level evaluations are not usually performed in dogs. The need for at least three-times-daily therapy makes the drug less desirable.

Levetiracetam. Levetiracetam is a pyrrolidine acetamide that has a half-life of 3 to 4 hours, with most of the drug being excreted through the kidneys. It is used as an add-on drug in both dogs and cats. The recommended initial oral dose is 10-20 mg/kg of body weight three times daily. The dose can be increased in increments of 20 mg/kg of body weight to achieve efficacy. Toxicity studies in dogs indicate it to be a very safe drug. Levetiracetam is well tolerated in cats and appears to be useful as an add-on drug to phenobarbital in this species.

Anticonvulsant Therapy for Cluster Seizures and Status Epilepticus

Both cluster seizures (two or more in less than 24 hours) and status epilepticus (continuous seizures for greater than 5 minutes or recurrent seizures with incomplete recovery between seizures for 30 minutes) are medical emergencies. The hypoxia, hyperthermia, altered blood pressure, and accumulation of glutamic acid may cause irreversible brain lesions. Seizure control is critical and must be accomplished as soon as possible.[97]

Diazepam

Diazepam (Valium), a benzodiazepine, is most useful for stopping the seizures in dogs with cluster seizures or status epilepticus.[5] It is ineffective as an oral maintenance therapy in dogs. Diazepam is usually the first treatment administered to stop these life-threatening seizures. The drug is administered intravenously in 0.5 to 0.1 mg/kg of body weight every 15 minutes until the seizures stop. In violent patients, it may be used intramuscularly. If the diazepam is effective, it may be added to the intravenous fluid line at 0.5 to 2.0 mg/kg of body weight/hour in 5% dextrose or 0.9% saline. If three or four doses are ineffective, an alternative intravenous drug should be used such as intravenous phenobarbital or pentobarbital. Use 2 to 6 mg/kg of body weight of phenobarbital or 2 to 15 mg/kg body weight of pentobarbital to effect. Propofol may be used intravenously as a bolus dose at 1 to 6 mg/kg of body weight to effect. Propofol can also be used in a constant flow infusion.

Diazepam may be administered per rectum at 2 mg/kg of parenteral solution (5 mg/cc).[110] This drug is especially useful for owners who live some distance from a veterinary emergency hospital and who also may recognize a change in their pet's behavior just before a seizure. Prompt initiation of this therapy may abort the seizure or reduce its severity. Rectal administration of diazepam may be repeated up to three times in 24 hours.

The following discussion provides a guideline that is useful for veterinarians and their technicians to facilitate the rapid administration of diazepam (Valium) in a crisis situation:

Small-size dogs (<10 kg): 5 mg, 1 cc intravenously
Medium-size dogs (10 to 25 kg): 10 mg, 2 cc intravenously
Large-size dogs (25-40 kg): 15 mg, 3 cc intravenously
Extra large–size dogs (40-60 kg): 20 mg, 4 cc intravenously
Cats: 2.5 to 5 mg, 0.5 to 1 cc intravenously

Vagal Stimulation

In humans who are refractory to anticonvulsant therapy, vagal stimulation may be an alternative consideration.[94,121] A pacemaker-like device is implanted subcutaneously that, when activated, will stimulate the vagus nerve in the neck. The basis for the anticonvulsant effect is thought to involve the large number of general visceral afferent neurons in the vagus nerve and their synapses in the solitary nucleus. The solitary nucleus has numerous subcortical and cortical connections that, when stimulated, might interrupt the seizure activity. One study of the use of this therapy in dogs suggests that vagal stimulation may be an effective alternative in selected patients and is worth further investigation.[94]

A practical procedure that involves stimulation of afferent neurons to interrupt seizure activity is eyeball compression.[121] This procedure has practical value when you encounter a patient that is in status epilepticus and its thrashing interferes with introducing an intravenous catheter. If you apply firm pressure on both eyeballs through the closed eyelids, the seizure activity may stop and allow you to administer intravenous anticonvulsant drugs such as diazepam. The neuroanatomic basis for this event is not well understood but is assumed to be initiated through the general somatic afferents in the ophthalmic nerve from the trigeminal nerve. Whether this action, in turn, involves the spinal nucleus of the trigeminal nerve or the solitary nucleus with their cerebral connections is unknown. A decrease in the heart rate occurs, which supports involvement of the vagal general visceral efferent neurons.

Surgery

A final alternative in uncontrolled human patients may be to section the corpus callosum to interrupt the spread of the seizure activity. The surgical procedure has been successfully performed in dogs, but whether it is useful in a patient with uncontrolled seizures remains to be seen.[8,9] Determination of seizure foci and surgical removal of these foci have not yet been adequately explored in veterinary patients to our knowledge.[105]

◼ NARCOLEPSY AND CATAPLEXY

Narcolepsy is an incurable disorder of the normal sleep mechanism in which genetic and acquired disorders have been discovered to explain the pathogenesis. This disorder is still being extensively investigated for a better understanding of its pathogenesis and therapy.[74] In general, sleep has two major components, slow-wave sleep and paradoxical or rapid eye movement (REM) sleep.[62,77,89] In the normal sleep cycle, the initial sleep is always the slow-wave sleep. During the sleep cycle, the individual goes in and out of paradoxical sleep. These two phases of sleep are named for their EEG patterns. In the awake state, the EEG pattern consists of low-amplitude fast waves. In slow-wave sleep, the pattern changes to one of high-amplitude slow waves. In paradoxical sleep, the EEG pattern resembles that of the awake state. However, the individual is physiologically asleep, which is the basis for the name *paradoxical sleep*. During slow-wave sleep, normal resting muscle tone exists. In paradoxical sleep, complete atonia of all skeletal muscles occurs, except those necessary for respiration. This state causes a flaccid paralysis. Sporadically, the extraocular muscles break through this lower motor neuron (LMN) inhibition and contract, causing eye movements, which is the basis for also naming paradoxical sleep *rapid eye movement* sleep. This portion of the sleep cycle is when we dream. Sorry, but you cannot run during your dream. Despite how active we may be in our dream, our muscles are completely atonic. Occasionally, other muscle groups break through this inhibition and contract. This breaking through is what we observe in our small animals when, during their sleep, they exhibit facial muscle twitches or sporadic movements of their digits. During slow-wave sleep, a decrease occurs in the heart and respiratory rates. In paradoxical sleep, respirations are shallow, more rapid, and irregular. Normally in small animals, slow-wave sleep occurs in 10- to 15-minute intervals, with approximately 5 minutes of paradoxical sleep.[46,54]

Narcolepsy is a syndrome that, in humans, has four recognizable components: (1) excessive sleepiness, (2) cataplexy, (3) hypnagogic hallucinations, and (4) sleep paralysis. Cataplexy is the spontaneous collapse that occurs from the complete atonia of the skeletal muscles. This collapse is the most common clinical sign observed in animals with the narcoleptic syndrome. In a laboratory environment, excessive sleepiness can be observed in these patients.[62] Only human patients can appreciate the hypnagogic hallucinations and the sleep paralysis. The narcoleptic syndrome is a manifestation of the abrupt occurrence of paradoxical sleep without a preceding period of slow-wave sleep. It is the result of a dysfunctional paradoxical sleep center that is suddenly freed from the normal inhibitory mechanisms. This state results in one or more of the four clinical signs that comprise this syndrome. Narcolepsy and cataplexy refer to the same disorder, with cataplexy being the clinical sign of this syndrome that is easiest for us to observe in our domestic animal patients.[63,64]

The maintenance of the awake state, as well as sleep, is a function of the reticular formation. Understanding the clinical signs of cataplexy requires an understanding of the anatomy and physiology involved with paradoxical sleep.[49,74] The anatomic components that regulate sleep are poorly defined but are thought to be primarily located in the brainstem reticular formation, especially in the pons and medulla, but these are diffusely connected rostrally with the prosencephalon and caudally with the spinal cord. These components involve a large number of neurotransmitters, the knowledge of which is important in understanding cataplexy and its treatment. The neurons in the pons and rostral medulla involved with paradoxical sleep use both monoaminergic and cholinergic mechanisms.[30,41,42] Two of these nuclei are the locus ceruleus and the dorsal raphe nucleus. The locus ceruleus is in the central gray substance adjacent to the rostral portion of the fourth ventricle (see Fig. 2-9). These locus ceruleus neurons release norepinephrine, which is inhibitory to the pontomedullary nuclei that are responsible for the diffuse inhibition of the general somatic efferent (GSE) LMN that causes the flaccid paralysis observed in cataplexy.[130] A closely related group of neurons called *dorsal raphe neurons* release serotonin, which contributes to this inhibition.[56] Paradoxical sleep occurs when the activity of these inhibitory nuclei is decreased.[130]

The following list describes some of the anatomic components that regulate sleep and in particular paradoxical sleep along with the neurotransmitters that have been recognized (Fig. 18-6).

1. Light stimulates retinal neurons.
2. Optic nerve axons activate neurons in the suprachiasmatic nucleus in the rostral ventral hypothalamus.
3. Axons from the suprachiasmatic neurons terminate in a ventrolateral nucleus in the hypothalamus.
4. These latter hypothalamic neurons project diffusely in the prosencephalon and brainstem and release the neuropeptide hypocretin (orexin), a facilitory neurotransmitter involved with appetite control and neuromodulation of sleep.
5. Neurons in the locus ceruleus and dorsal raphe nucleus have receptors for hypocretin and are activated by its release from the hypothalamic neurons.
6. Locus ceruleus neurons release norepinephrine, and dorsal raphe neurons release serotonin, both of which are inhibitory at their termination in the pontine reticular formation nucleus, the neurons of which are involved in the pathway for inhibiting GSE-LMNs.
7. The neurons in this pontine reticular formation center release acetylcholine at their termination in the medullary reticular formation center that projects to the spinal cord and brainstem to inhibit the GSE-LMNs.

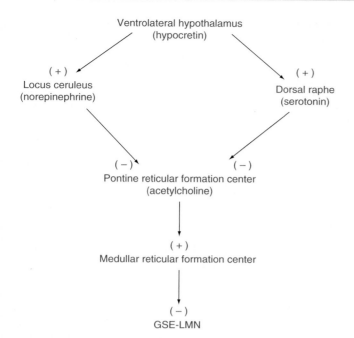

Ventrolateral hypothalamus
(hypocretin)

(+)
Locus ceruleus
(norepinephrine)

(+)
Dorsal raphe
(serotonin)

(−)   (−)
Pontine reticular formation center
(acetylcholine)

(+)
Medullar reticular formation center

(−)
GSE-LMN

FIGURE 18-6 Diagram of neural control of paraoxical sleep.

The critical point, or *switch,* in this mechanism is the level of activity of the inhibitory neurons in the locus ceruleus and dorsal raphe nucleus. When these neurons are inactive, the pontomedullary centers are released from inhibition, and the atonia of paradoxical sleep occurs. A decrease in hypocretin activity may be one possible source that deactivates the inhibitory neurons in the locus ceruleus and dorsal raphe nucleus to permit paradoxical sleep during slow-wave sleep. At the same time that this GSE-LMN inhibition occurs, a release occurs from inhibition of the thalamic neurons that normally activate the cerebral cortex, which results in the low-amplitude fast waves observed in the EEG during paradoxical sleep.

Another way to look at this complex mechanism is to consider the clinical sign of cataplexy and then consider where the dysfunction may occur to cause the abrupt activation of paradoxical sleep in the awake patient.

1. The clinical sign of cataplexy is caused by the diffuse inhibition of spinal cord GSE-LMNs. This diffuse inhibition is the atonia of paradoxical sleep.
2. This inhibition is a function of a group of neurons in the reticular formation of the medulla. We are not aware of the specific neurotransmitter released by these medullary neurons.
3. This medullary center is activated by a group of neurons in the pontine reticular formation that release acetylcholine. Thus this release is a cholinergic action.
4. This pontine center is normally inhibited by neurons in the locus ceruleus that release norepinephrine and neurons in the dorsal raphe nucleus that release serotonin. Thus this release provides a monoaminergic action.
5. The neurons in the locus ceruleus and the dorsal raphe nucleus have receptors for hypocretin, which is a facilitory neuropeptide neurotransmitter released by a group of neurons in the ventrolateral nucleus of the hypothalamus. The activity of the neurons in the locus ceruleus and dorsal raphe nucleus is necessary for the inhibition

of the pontine center to prevent the activation of the medullary center and the consequent inhibition of the GSE-LMNs.

Only in the last few years has the role of hypocretin in sleep been discovered, which has enhanced our understanding of the pathogenesis of cataplexy.[84,87,119] Hypocretin has numerous functions but plays a major role in appetite control and as a neuromodulator of sleep. In the latter role, hypocretin is involved in maintaining the awake state and suppressing entry into paradoxical sleep. In domestic animals, cataplexy is most commonly a genetic disorder, with the onset of clinical signs from birth to a few weeks or months of age. A less common acquired form usually occurs in older dogs and horses. An inherited basis has been determined for Doberman pinschers, Labrador retrievers, and dachshunds.[88] The inherited gene is known as the *canarc gene,* which is on chromosome 12. This gene codes for a hypocretin receptor that is found on neurons in the locus ceruleus and dorsal raphe nucleus. Although hypocretin levels in the CSF are normal in these dogs, the inherited receptor abnormality prevents the binding necessary to activate the neurons in the locus ceruleus and dorsal raphe nucleus. The gene mutation that results in cataplexy is inherited as an autosomal recessive gene. Some question still exists as to whether the immune system also plays a role along with this genetic mutation, but this area needs further study.[17] A genetic basis is assumed for the miniature poodle, the miniature horse,[76] and Shetland ponies, but the mode of inheritance has not been established. A 1924 report of feinting in Suffolk draft horse foals reads like a description of narcolepsy, with an inherited pathogenesis.[118] The mutation may also be spontaneous, given that this syndrome occurs abruptly in young dogs of many breeds, as well as mixed breeds. Sporadic cases occur in farm animals.[104,123] See Videos 18-33 and 18-34.

In the acquired form of narcolepsy that is usually seen in older dogs, a depletion of hypocretin in the CSF has been recognized, which suggests dysfunction of the neurons in the ventral lateral nucleus of the hypothalamus. In humans with acquired narcolepsy and a depletion of hypocretin in the CSF, necropsy studies have shown a degeneration and loss of neuronal cell bodies in this hypothalamic nucleus. The cause is unknown, but an autoimmune inflammation has been proposed. Intense effort is presently underway to find a way to supply a synthetic hypocretin in these patients artificially. In the list of videos of narcolepsy, see Video 18-24. This video shows a weimaraner with severe narcolepsy associated with a depletion of hypocretin in his CSF.[116] A catheter was placed in the cervical spinal cord subarachnoid space and was attached to an implanted source of synthetic hypocretin. This measure was not effective in this dog but shows the value of the canine patient in the development of new therapeutic measures for humans. CSF hypocretin levels have not been studied in adult horses with narcolepsy.

Paradoxical sleep is influenced by cholinergic mechanisms.[30,68] Physostigmine and arecoline facilitate it, and atropine and scopolamine depress it. The monoamines norepinephrine and serotonin depress paradoxical sleep. Normal paradoxical sleep requires a critical balance of serotonergic, adrenergic, and cholinergic activity in the pons and medulla. An increase in cholinergic mechanisms (pontine reticular formation center) or a decrease in monoaminergic mechanisms (locus ceruleus and dorsal raphe nucleus) in the brainstem will result in cataplexy. Thus cataplexy can be explained by brainstem cholinergic hypersensitivity, by monoaminergic hypoactivity, or by a combination of both circumstances.[82]

Biochemical studies on the brains and CSF of affected Doberman pinschers support a defect in the release of the three catecholamines—serotonin, dopamine, and norepinephrine. These dogs also have a higher concentration of cholinergic receptors in brainstem nuclei than control dogs, which supports a higher sensitivity of the cholinergic system in dogs with narcolepsy. Studies in narcoleptic dogs have shown that blocking the alpha$_1$-adrenergic receptor with the antagonist prazosin will exacerbate the cataplexy.[86] Cataplexy is inhibited by the administration of alpha$_1$-adrenergic agonists or alpha$_2$-adrenergic antagonists. Studies on dopaminergic receptors have shown overactivity of the D$_2$-dopamine receptor in narcoleptic dogs.[95] Blocking this receptor with the antagonist raclopride decreases the incidence of cataplexy. Much of this research on narcolepsy in dogs has been done at two sleep disorder laboratories in California. One is at Stanford University,[77,85,90] and the other is at the University of California at Los Angeles.[120] At these facilities for dogs with inherited narcolepsy, researchers have determined that the onset of the clinical signs is approximately 2 to 4 months of age, with intensification of clinical signs to approximately 1 year of age. This phase is followed by a very slow decrease in clinical signs until approximately 4 to 5 years, when the clinical signs may nearly disappear. However, the incidence and severity of the clinical signs vary considerably between dogs, the basis for which remains to be explained. Dogs with the acquired form of narcolepsy can show clinical signs at any age and usually exhibit these sign for the remainder of their lives.

Obviously, the regulation of paradoxical sleep is dependent on the precise interaction of a large number of neurotransmitters. On rare occasions, this balance can be upset and result in cataplexy. In a few dachshunds, a breed at risk for narcolepsy, we have observed cataplexy after general anesthesia for surgery to treat thoracolumbar protruded or extruded intervertebral disks. For approximately 1 week postoperatively, these dogs exhibited cataplexy every time they started to eat, and then it resolved. Emotion inducing events or feeding are recognized as stimulants for cataplexy in patients with the narcoleptic syndrome. These dogs had never shown any cataplectic events before the general anesthesia, according to their owners. We assume that these dogs have a canarc gene mutation that results in cataplexy only when their CNS is exposed to a general anesthetic. We studied a young cat that the Society for the Prevention of Cruelty to Animals (SPCA) found collapsed beside the road (see Video 18-28). When she was hospitalized, we observed the cataplexy that can be seen on this video. Her neurologic examination was normal. After approximately 10 days, the cataplectic episodes slowly resolved completely. Narcolepsy is uncommon in cats. We assumed that this cat may have experienced minor brainstem trauma that temporarily affected the brainstem to cause cataplexy. Cataplexy is rarely observed in domestic animals that show clinical signs of a pontomedullary lesion. An interesting observation is that you can induce cataplexy in the newborn foal or calf by holding it up and compressing its thorax. The newborn will suddenly become limp (atonic) and collapse as you hold it suspended and recover when you place it back on the ground surface. This reaction varies in degree and usually disappears after 1 to 2 days. This response may be a normal physiologic response of the fetus to the compression that occurs during birth to prevent the newborn from resisting the pressure and thus facilitate the birth.

The adult horse presents a unique problem in trying to differentiate hypersomnia caused by sleep deprivation from narcolepsy.[34,57,92,124] Horses may stand during slow-wave sleep but are more often recumbent in a sternal position. They must be recumbent for paradoxical sleep to occur and are usually in lateral recumbency. The entire sleep cycle is approximately 15 minutes, with a mean duration of 6.4 minutes of slow-wave sleep and 4.2 minutes of paradoxical sleep. These cycles occupy approximately 4 hours of each day. Sleep deprivation occurs primarily in two situations. One circumstance is when a horse has a disorder that causes severe discomfort when it lies down or stands up, and therefore to prevent this event from occurring, the horse remains standing and is deprived of its paradoxical sleep. The second circumstance involves environmental insecurity, such as moving to a new barn or moving from a box stall to a slip stall. If the horse is not comfortable with its environment, it refuses to lie down, and paradoxical sleep does not occur. Of all the domestic animals, the horse appears to exhibit the clinical signs of excessive sleepiness along with its cataplexy. While standing, the head and neck will slowly drop toward the ground surface followed by a buckling of the thoracic limbs. The horse usually catches itself before collapsing, but it will occasionally fall on the thoracic limbs before standing again, and then the event is often repeated. Sleep deprivation is considered to be much more common than narcolepsy. The only practical way to differentiate these disorders is to examine the patient carefully for any physical reason to prevent the horse from lying down and to evaluate its environment to determine if some aspect exists that might contribute to the insecurity of the horse such that it refuses to lie down. Most likely, the poor response of adult horses to drug therapy for narcolepsy is because most of them do not have this disorder but are instead sleep deprived. Reports of this presumed narcolepsy involve many breeds, with a median age of 10 years. The episodes tend to increase slowly in frequency and severity and on rare occasions have occurred while being ridden. An inherited form of narcolepsy does occur in Shetland ponies, the American miniature horse, and probably the Suffolk draft horse (1924), but there are no reports of the efficacy of drug therapy.[78,118]

Diagnosis

The clinical sign of cataplexy is unique and should not be confused with a seizure disorder or the exercise-induced neuromuscular paresis that accompanies several disorders of this system that were described in Chapter 5.* Cataplexy causes atonia. Seizure disorders produce uncontrolled muscle contractions. The neuromuscular disorders do not cause such an abrupt onset of the collapse or the sudden recovery from the collapse. An acute cardiac disorder such as a block of the conduction system may cause syncope, which mimics cataplexy, with the sudden onset of the collapse episode and its immediate recovery.[18,43,50] See **Video 18-20** of a

---

*References 10, 11, 26, 45, 65, 71, 91.

9-year-old Australian kelpie that has sporadic episodes of such a heart block. We thank Dr. Brian Farrow at the University of Sydney in Australia for this video.

A diagnostic problem occurs when the cataplexy is partial or the episodes are uncommon and never observed during your examination and you are dependent on the owner's description. Having the owner video an event for your study is helpful, but doing so may be difficult if the events are quite rare. You should consider trying to provoke a cataplectic episode using your knowledge of the neurotransmitters involved and provocative drugs. We have found physostigmine useful in provoking an attack. An intravenous dose of 0.05 to 0.1 mg/kg of body weight should not induce cataplexy in a normal dog but may provoke an episode in the patient that is at risk for such an episode. As a rule, a dog that exhibits cataplectic episodes almost continuously is not a diagnostic problem. However, if you feel the need for assurance, administer imipramine (Tofranil) intravenously at 0.5 mg/kg of body weight, which will temporarily stop the event in a cataplectic patient. This drug is an antidepressant that inhibits the reuptake of norepinephrine and has anticholinergic actions. Intravenous atropine sulfate at 0.1 mg /kg of body weight may also interrupt the episodes. A food-elicited cataplexy test may be useful in making a diagnosis or in monitoring a dog's response to therapy. Ten very small portions of food are placed in a row approximately 3 feet apart, and then the dog is timed on how much time passes before the dog collapses as it consumes the food. This test is best performed in the patient's home environment. Normal dogs will consume all 10 portions in less than 45 seconds. Narcoleptic dogs take 2 minutes or more. Food and excitement are events that often stimulate the onset of a cataplectic episode.

Cataplectic Diagnostic Tests and Therapy

Provocative test—Physostigmine
　　　　　　Food
Preventative test—Imipramine
　　　　　　Atropine
Therapy—Imipramine
　　　Methylphenidate
　　　Selegeline
　　　Yohimbine

Treatment

No single effective drug is available to treat narcolepsy, and research is ongoing for improved methods of treatment that prevent side effects.[7,17,52,96] If the cataplectic episodes are infrequent, the best course of action is to live with the disorder and avoid subjecting the patient to treatment. For patients in which the episodes are frequent enough to interfere with their quality of life, most veterinarians use the same drugs that are used for humans with this disorder. For treatment of acquired narcolepsy in which CSF hypocretin is deficient, a goal is to develop a systemic hypocretin replacement.[61,116] This task has yet to be accomplished clinically. See **Video 18-24**. Imipramine (Tofranil) and desipramine are used primarily for the cataplexy because of their anticholinergic properties, as well as their interference with the reuptake of norepinephrine. For imipramine, an oral dose of 0.5 mg/kg of body weight three times daily is recommended. Methylphenidate (Ritalin) is a stimulant that is used primarily for the excessive sleepi-

ness (an oral dose of 0.25 mg/kg of body weight twice or three times daily). Selegeline (Anapryl) is a monoamine oxidase inhibitor that results in an increase in the concentration of norepinephrine in the CNS. It may be used at an oral dose of 2 mg/kg of body weight once daily and is purported to improve both cataplexy, as well as excessive sleepiness. Yohimbine is an alpha$_2$-adrenergic antagonist that increases the release of norepinephrine and may be helpful in these cases. Modafanil (Provigil) and sodium oxybate (Xyrem) are two drugs presently used in humans for which no reports have been published of their efficacy in domestic animals. Various drug combinations have been tried, such as imipramine and methylphenidate. Tolerance may be a problem that can be decreased by alternating the drugs used. We have much to learn about successful treatment but have had a few dogs that responded and eventually have been taken off the drugs.

Narcolepsy and Cataplexy

The following videos are examples of this syndrome in several domestic animals.

Video 18-21. This video shows Ginger, a 6-month-old female cockapoo with an onset of the episodes that you see on the video at approximately 4 months of age. These events are episodes of cataplexy that had progressed in frequency. Ginger was the first dog with narcolepsy to be diagnosed at Cornell University. Her episodes correlate well with the description that attacks of cataplexy are often similar to turning a light bulb on and then off, which clearly distinguishes this event from the exercised-induced episodes of paresis in dogs with myasthenia gravis. In myasthenia gravis, the patient does not immediately completely collapse or immediately return to normal but requires a variable period of exercise before the progressive collapse and a rest phase for recovery. Neither of these events occurs in the cataplectic patient. An EEG of Ginger showed that these collapsing episodes were associated with periods of low-amplitude fast waves typical of paradoxical sleep along with an absence of muscle contractions on an electromyogram. Ginger was donated to Dr. William Dement at the Stanford University Sleep Disorder Center, where she appeared on the television show "60 Minutes."

Video 18-22. This video shows Dozer, a 6-month-old male Doberman pinscher exhibiting episodes of cataplexy that have been present for approximately 2 months. Three of the five dogs in his litter had similar clinical signs. Remember that narcolepsy is inherited in this breed as an autosomal recessive disorder that involves a mutation of the canarc gene.

Video 18-23. This video shows Chloe, a 4-year-old female dachshund with a sudden onset of collapsing episodes 4 days before this video was made. The attending clinician gave Chloe Tensilon intravenously as a test for myasthenia gravis, which, not surprisingly, had no effect. This test was unnecessary because dogs with myasthenia gravis never suddenly collapse from a normal gait and then just as suddenly stand and walk off. Chloe was treated with oral imipramine, and the episodes slowly decreased in frequency and after 4 to 5 weeks stopped completely. An autosomal recessive inheritance has been determined for dachshunds.

Video 18-24. This video shows Blue, a 2-year-old castrated male weimaraner with a sudden onset of collapsing episodes approximately 1 month before making this video. These episodes were especially apparent when he was fed. Note the almost continuous clinical signs of narcolepsy, which significantly interfere with his quality of life and his ability to interact with the owner's three children. CSF hypocretin levels were very low. Dr. Emmanuel Mignot of the Stanford University Sleep Disorder Center arranged to have an intrathecal catheter placed in the dog's cervical spinal cord subarachnoid space and a pump implanted subcutaneously in his neck to provide a continuous source of synthetic hypocretin. Blue did not respond well to the hypocretin replacement in the CSF and was placed on oral imipramine and yohimbine, which markedly reduced the incidence and severity of the episodes. These drugs were used alternately at 6-week intervals to decrease the chance of tolerance. The owner frequently took Blue to the local schools in the Syracuse, New York area to make the students aware of this sleep disorder that affects approximately 5 in 10,000 humans.[116]

 Video 18-25. This video shows Sheba, an 8-month-old female pit bull terrier with an acute onset of collapse 2 weeks before this video was made. She would have 15 to 20 episodes in a 30- to 45-minute period. She transiently recovered immediately after atropine was administered intravenously. She slowly recovered on oral imipramine.

Video 18-26. This video shows Sammy, a 2-year-old male toy poodle that exhibited the clinical signs of narcolepsy only when the owners started to use him for breeding. The excitement of breeding elicited attacks of cataplexy as seen on this video. This type of excitement is also one of the stimulating events recognized in humans! With the assumed inheritance of this disorder in this breed, Sammy was apparently trying to make more dogs like himself!

Video 18-27. This video shows Carlos, a 10-year-old male mixed-breed dog that was kept as a guard dog at a local junkyard. The owner's complaint was that when Carlos recently attempted to prevent a person from entering the junkyard at off-hours, he would bark vigorously and then collapse. He was hospitalized, and the first portion of the video shows only brief episodes of partial paresis as he is run around on a leash. Each day that he stayed at the hospital, his episodes worsened. The last portion of the video was made after 6 days of hospitalization, and the episodes are nearly continuous. He is then given intravenous imipramine, and you can see the immediate result. His clinical signs were controlled enough with oral imipramine therapy that he was able to resume his occupation as a junkyard guard dog.

Video 18-28. This video shows a young adult female domestic shorthair found by the local SPCA collapsed beside the road. When she was hospitalized, we observed cataplexy that was almost continuous, as can be seen on this video. The neurologic examination was normal. After approximately 10 days, the cataplectic episodes slowly resolved completely. Narcolepsy is uncommon in cats. Our presumption was that this cat may have experienced mild intracranial trauma, which temporarily affected the brainstem, causing narcolepsy. We have seen other animals with structural lesions in the brainstem with clinical signs that included cataplexy, although this observation is rare.

Video 18-29. This video shows a 1-month-old male American miniature horse that, for the past 2 weeks, had exhibited episodes of collapse, especially when he nursed his dam. The owner suspected that the milk was toxic and was about to wean the foal when he was hospitalized for examination. This abnormality is a presumptive inherited form of narcolepsy. He was donated to the animal laboratory at the Stanford University Sleep Disorder Center.

 Video 18-30. This video shows a 6-day-old male American miniature horse that had a normal birth. He was able to stand and nursed three times the first day. At 36 hours, he acted lethargic and stopped nursing and was referred to Cornell at 5 days of age as a septic *dummy* foal. On examination, he was recumbent and initially appeared obtunded. However, when he was pinched with forceps, he immediately aroused and stood up. He would walk a few steps before he stopped, slowly dropped his head and neck, and collapsed into a recumbent posture. When picked up and held suspended, he lost all muscle tone and exhibited total-body flaccidity. This abnormality is severe narcolepsy presumably from a genetic pathogenesis. As he grew, the cataplectic episodes became less frequent but did not disappear.

Video 18-31. This video shows a 7-year-old Westphalian gelding that exhibits episodes of paradoxical sleep when in his stall at night. He had been having these episodes for approximately 2 weeks when this video was made. What you see on this video is characteristic of what is usually known as the adult form of equine narcolepsy. Because this term implies a disorder of the sleep mechanism in the brainstem, the preferred term for this state is paradoxical sleep until you can determine if this is sleep deprivation from refusal to lie down as a result of a lesion causing discomfort or from an environmental change that causes the patient to refuse to lie down. No reliable diagnostic procedure is available that will differentiate narcolepsy from sleep deprivation caused by a change in the environment of the horse. Drug therapy has not been reliable either. Sleep deprivation is a common problem in horses, and a basis for this tendency should be carefully investigated for patients such as this one. Correction of the horse's environment may alleviate the clinical signs.

 Video 18-32. This video shows a 16-year-old Appaloosa gelding that has exhibited the episodes that you observe on this video for the past 3 years. This episode is paradoxical sleep, and with no basis for sleep deprivation, it was considered to be the disease narcolepsy. The assumption is that this abnormality is an acquired form of narcolepsy, but no studies have been conducted on hypocretin levels in the CSF of horses. Histologic studies of the brain have revealed no significant lesions.

Video 18-33. This video shows a 2-week-old alpaca cria that was born 3 weeks premature at 316 days of gestation (normal range is from 335 to 360 days). The cataplexy associated with nursing is spectacular. When this cria was 3 weeks old, the episodes spontaneously stopped. This point in time would be equivalent to the normal age at birth for this species and suggests that the preterm fetus is at risk for cataplexy, which may play a role in the normal process of birth. We thank Dr. Brian Farrow of the University of Sydney for this video.

Video 18-34. This video shows Zorro, a 5-day-old mixed-breed lamb that has exhibited the clinical signs that you see on this video since birth. The gestation period was normal, and although the frequency of the collapses decreased as the lamb grew, they did not disappear. Zorro was donated to the Sleep Disorder Center at the University of California at Los Angeles.[129]

SLEEP-ASSOCIATED MOVEMENT DISORDER

Owners will occasionally describe seizure-like activity in their dog or cat that occurs only when the animal is asleep, or the owner will describe the activity as a violent dream.[53] The assumption is that these uncontrolled movements represent paradoxical sleep during which you normally expect sporadic eye movements, which is the basis for this phase of sleep being called REM sleep. This phase of the sleep cycle is when the normally sleeping dog or cat exhibits facial muscle twitching or digital muscle contractions. In these patients, a GSE-LMN break from inhibition occurs that is massive and causes violent thrashing of the limbs. A cat has been described that threw itself off of a bureau where it normally slept.[55] A large dog may damage adjacent furniture or the wall in the room where it is confined (see Video 18-36). These animals can be immediately aroused and the movements stop. Anticonvulsant therapy is ineffective because these events are not seizures; they represent a disorder of the paradoxical phase of sleep that occurs at its normal time in the sleep cycle. Some anecdotal data suggest that treatment with clonazepam may reduce the severity of these uncontrolled movements. The following two videos are examples of this disorder.

 Video 18-35. This video shows Mully, a 4-year-old spayed female domestic shorthair that exhibits this uncontrolled movement during her sleep cycle. These patients always enter sleep in the slow-wave phase, and the movements follow when they enter the paradoxical phase of sleep.

Video 18-36. This video shows an 8-year-old spayed female Belgian Tervuren with sleep-associated uncontrolled movements that, over a period of 2.5 years, had slowly progressed in severity. The owner described that this dog had kicked holes in the dry wall where it slept. She had been treated for much of this time with phenobarbital with no effect. Her neurologic examination was normal.

REFERENCES

1. Aleman M, et al: Juvenile idiopathic epilepsy in Egyptian Arabian foals: 22 cases (1985-2005), *J Vet Intern Med* 20: 1443-1449, 2006.
2. Alkeson FW, Ibensen A, Eldridge E: Inheritance of an epileptic type character in Brown Swiss cattle, *J Hered* 35:45, 1944.
3. Andersson B, Olson SE: Epilepsy in a dog with extensive bilateral damage to the hippocampus, *Acta Vet Scand* 1:98, 1959.
4. Austad R, Bjerkas E: Eclampsia in the bitch, *J Sm Anim Pract* 17:793, 1976.
5. Averill DA Jr: Treatment of status epilepticus in dogs with diazepam sodium, *J Am Vet Med Assoc* 156:432, 1970.
6. Averill DA, Jr: Idiopathic epilepsy. In Andrews EJ, Ward BC, Altman HH, editors: *Spontaneous animal models of human disease. II*, New York, 1979, Academic Press.
7. Babcock DA, et al: Effects of imipramine, chlorimipramine and fluoxetine on cataplexy in dogs, *Pharmacol Biochem Behav* 5:599, 1976.
8. Bagley RS, et al: Clinical effects of longitudinal division of the corpus callosum in normal dogs, *Vet Surg* 24:122-127, 1995.
9. Bagley RS, Harrington ML, Moore MP: Surgical treatments for seizure. Adaptability for dogs, *Vet Clin North Am Sm Anim Pract* 26:827-842, 1996.
10. Baker TL, et al: Canine model of narcolepsy: genetic and developmental determinants, *Exp Neurol* 75:729-742, 1982.
11. Baker TL, et al: Diagnosis and treatment of narcolepsy in animals. In Kirk RW, editor: *Current veterinary therapy: small animal practice*, Philadelphia, 1983, Saunders.
12. Barnes HL, et al: Clinical signs, underlying cause, and outcome in cats with seizures: 17 cases (1997-2002), *J Am Vet Med Assoc* 225:1723-1726, 2004.
13. Barrett RE, et al: Five cases of congenital portacaval shunt in the dog, *J Sm Anim Pract* 17:71, 1976.
14. Beck AM, Krook L: Canine insuloma. Two surgical cases with relapses, *Cornell Vet* 55:330, 1965.
15. Berent M, et al: A cross-sectional study of epilepsy in Danish Labrador retrievers: prevalence and selected risk factors, *J Vet Intern Med* 16:262-268, 2002.
16. Berryman FY, de Lahunta A: Astrocytoma in a dog with convulsions, *Cornell Vet* 65:212, 1975.
17. Boehmer LN, et al: Treatment with immunosuppressive and anti-inflammatory agents delays onset of canine genetic narcolepsy and reduces symptom severity, *Exp Neurol* 188:292-299, 2004.
18. Branch CE, Beckett SD, Robertson BT: Spontaneous syncopal attacks in dogs: a method of documentation, *J Am Anim Hosp Assoc* 13:673, 1977.
19. Breazile JE: Convulsive disorders in dogs. In Kirk WR, editor: *Current veterinary therapy: small animal practice IV*, Philadelphia, 1971, Saunders.
20. Brietschweidt EB, Breazile JE, Broadhurst JJ: Clinical and electroencephalographic findings associated with ten cases of suspected limbic epilepsy in the dog, *J Am Anim Hosp Assoc* 15:37, 1979.
21. Bruchim Y, et al: Heat stroke in dogs: a retrospective study of 54 cases (1999-2004) and analysis of risk factors for death, *J Vet Intern Med* 20:39-46, 2006.
22. Bunch SE, Baldwin BH, Hornbuckle WE: Compromised hepatic function in dogs treated with anticonvulsant drugs, *J Am Vet Med Assoc* 184:444-448, 1984.
23. Capen CC, Martin SL: Hyperinsulinism in dogs with neoplasia of the pancreatic islets, *Pathol Vet* 6:309, 1969.
24. Casal ML, et al: Epilepsy in Irish wolfhounds, *J Vet Intern Med* 20:131-135, 2006.
25. Caywood DD, et al: Pancreatic islet cell adenocarcinoma: clinical and diagnostic features of six cases, *J Am Vet Med Assoc* 174:714, 1979.
26. Coleman ES: Canine narcolepsy and the role of the nervous system, *Comp Cont Ed Pract Vet* 21:641-649, 1999.
27. Cornelius LM, et al: Anomalous portosystemic anastomoses associated with chronic hepatic insufficiency in six young dogs, *J Am Vet Med Assoc* 167:220, 1975.
28. Cunningham CG: Canine seizure disorders, *J Am Vet Med Assoc* 158:589, 1971.
29. Daminet S, et al: Short-term influence of prednisone and phenobarbital on thyroid function in euthyroid dogs, *Can Vet J* 40:411-415, 1999.
30. Delashaw JB, et al: Cholinergic mechanisms and cataplexy in dogs, *Exp Neurol* 66:745, 1979.
31. Dewey CW: Anticonvulsant therapy in dogs and cats, *Vet Clin North Am Sm Anim Pract* 36:1107-1127, 2006.
32. Dewey CW, et al: Alternative anticonvulsant drugs for dogs with seizure disorders, *Vet Med* 99:786-793, 2004.
33. Dodman NH, et al: Behavioral changes associated with suspected complex partial seizures in bull terriers, *J Am Vet Med Assoc* 208:688-691, 1996.
34. Dreifuss FE, Flynn DV: Narcolepsy in a horse, *J Am Vet Med Assoc* 184:131-132, 1984.
35. Edmonds HL, et al: Spontaneous convulsions in beagle dogs, *Fed Proc* 38:2424, 1979.
36. Ellenberger C, et al: Inhibitory and excitatory neurotransmitters in the cerebrospinal fluid of epileptic dogs, *Am J Vet Res* 65:1108-1113, 2004.

37. Ewing GO, Suter PF, Bailey CS: Hepatic insufficiency associated with congenital anomalies of the portal vein in dogs, *J Am Vet Med Assoc* 10:463, 1974.

38. Fabisiak JP: *The role of cerebral free amino acids and taurine in the kindling models of epilepsy* [master's thesis], Ithaca, NY, 1980, Cornell University.

39. Falco MJ, Barker J, Wallace ME: The genetics of epilepsy in the British Alsatian, *J Sm Anim Pract* 15:685, 1974.

40. Fatzer R, et al: Necrosis of hippocampus and piriform lobe in 38 domestic cats with seizures: a retrospective study on clinical and pathologic findings, *J Vet Intern Med* 14:100-104, 2000.

41. Faull KF, et al: Monoamine metabolite concentration in the cerebrospinal fluid of normal and narcoleptic dogs, *Brain Res* 243:137-143, 1982.

42. Faull KF, et al: Biogenic amine concentrations in the brains of normal and narcoleptic canines, *Sleep* 9:107-110, 1986.

43. Fisher EW: Fainting in boxers—the possibility of vaso-vagal syncope (Adams-Stokes attacks), *J Sm Anim Pract* 12:347, 1971.

44. Foutz AS, et al: Genetic factors in canine epilepsy, *Sleep* 1:413, 1979.

45. Foutz AS, Mitler MM, Dement WC: Narcolepsy, *Vet Clin North Am Sm Anim Pract* 10:65, 1980.

46. Fox MW, Stanton G: A developmental study of sleep and wakefulness in the dog, *J Sm Anim Pract* 8:605, 1967.

47. Gastaut H, et al: Anatomical and clinical study of 19 epileptic dogs. In Baldwin M, Bailey P, editors: *Temporal lobe epilepsy*, Springfield, IL, 1958, Charles C Thomas.

48. Grauer GF, Thrall MA: Ethylene glycol (antifreeze) poisoning in the dog and cat, *J Am Anim Hosp Assoc* 18:492, 1982.

49. Guilleminault C, Heinzer R, Mignot E: Investigations into the neurological basis of narcolepsy, *Neurology* 50:S8-S15, 1998.

50. Hamlin RL, Smetzer DL, Breznock E: Sinoatrial syncope in miniature schnauzers, *J Am Vet Med Assoc* 161:1022, 1972.

51. Hegreberg GA, Edmonds HL Jr: Familial progressive myoclonic epilepsy (Lafora's disease). In Andrews EJ, Ward BC, Altman HH, editors: *Spontaneous animal models of human disease. II*, New York, 1976, Academic Press.

52. Hendricks JC, Hughes C: Treatment of cataplexy in a dog with narcolepsy, *J Am Vet Med Assoc* 194:791-792, 1989.

53. Hendricks JC, et al: Movement disorders during sleep in cats and dogs, *J Am Vet Med Assoc* 194:686-689, 1989.

54. Hendricks JC, Morrison AR: Normal and abnormal sleep in mammals, *J Am Vet Med Assoc* 178:121, 1981.

55. Hendricks JC, et al: A disorder of rapid eye movement sleep in a cat, *J Am Vet Med Assoc* 178:55, 1981.

56. Henley K, Morrison AR: A reevaluation of the effects of lesions of the pontine tegmentum and locus coeruleus on phenomena of paradoxical sleep in the cat, *Acta Neurobiol Exp* 34:215, 1974.

57. Hines MT, Schott HC, Byrne BA: Adult-onset narcolepsy in the horse, *Am Assoc Eq Pract Proc* 38:289-296, 1992.

58. Holiday TA: Epilepsy in cats, *Mod Vet Pract* 51:14, 1970.

59. Holiday TA: Seizure disorders, *Vet Clin North Am* 10:3, 1980.

60. Holiday TA, Cunningham JG, Gutnich MJ: Comparative clinical and electroencephalographic studies on canine epilepsy, *Epilepsia* 11:281, 1970.

61. John J, Wu M-F, Siegel JM: Systemic administration of hypocretin-1 reduces cataplexy and normalizes sleep and waking durations in narcoleptic dogs, *Sleep Res Online* 3:23-28, 2000.

62. Jouvet M: The states of sleep, *Sci Am* 216:62, 1967.

63. Kaitin KI, Kilduff TS, Dement WC: Sleep fragmentation in canine narcolepsy, *Sleep* 9:116-119, 1986.

64. Kaitin KI, Kilduff TS, Dement WC: Evidence for excessive sleepiness in canine narcoleptics, *Electroencephalogr Clin Neurophysiol* 64:447-454, 1986.

65. Katherman AE: A comparative review of canine and human narcolepsy, *Comp Cont Ed* 2:818, 1980.

66. Kathmann I, et al: Clinical and genetic investigations of idiopathic epilepsy in the Bernese mountain dog, *J Sm Anim Pract* 40:319-325, 1999.

67. Kay WJ: Epilepsy in cats, *J Am Anim Hosp Assoc* 11:77, 1975.

68. Kilduff TS, et al: Muscarinic cholinergic receptors and the canine model of narcolepsy, *Sleep* 9:102-106, 1986.

69. Kirk RW: Hypoglycemia. In Kirk RW, editor: *Current veterinary therapy III*, Philadelphia, 1968, Saunders.

70. Kline KL: Feline epilepsy, *Clin Tech Sm Anim Pract* 13:152-158, 1998.

71. Knecht CD, et al: Narcolepsy in a dog and cat, *JAVMA* 162:1052, 1973.

72. Kornegay JN, et al: Idiopathic hypocalcemia in four dogs, *J Am Anim Hosp Assoc* 16:723, 1980.

73. Kurosinski P, Gotz J: Glial cells under physiologic and pathologic conditions, *Arch Neurol* 59:1524-1528, 2002.

74. Larkin KT: The neurobiology of the narcoleptic syndrome, *Inter J Neurosci* 25:1-17, 1984.

75. Licht BG, et al: Clincial characteristics and mode of inheritance of familial focal seizures in standard poodles, *J Am Vet Med Assoc* 231:1520-1528, 2007.

76. Lohi H, et al: Expanded repeat in canine epilepsy, *Science* 307:81, 2005.

77. Lucas EA, et al: Sleep cycle organization in narcoleptic and normal dogs, *Physiol Behav* 23:737, 1979.

78. Lunn DP, Cuddon PA, Shaftoe S: Familial occurrence of narcolepsy in miniature horses, *Eq Vet J* 25:483-487, 1993.

79. Mahaffey LW, Rossdale PD: Convulsive syndrome in newborn foals, *Vet Rec* 69:1277, 1957.

80. March PA: Seizures: classification, etiologies, and pathophysiology, *Clin Tech Sm Anim Pract* 13:119-131, 1998.

81. March PA, Fischer JR, Potthoff A: Electromyographic and histologic abnormalities in epaxial muscles of cats with feline hyperesthesia syndrome, *ACVIM Proc* 13:238, 1999.

82. Mefford IN, et al: Narcolepsy: biogenic amine deficits in an animal model, *Science* 220:629-632, 1983.

83. Mellema LM, et al: Reversible magnetic resonance imaging abnormalities in dogs with seizures, *Vet Radiol Ultrasound* 40:588-595, 1999.

84. Mieda M, Yanagisawa M: Sleep, feeding and neuropeptides: roles of orexins and orexin receptors, *Curr Opin Neurobiol* 12:339-345, 2002.

85. Mignot E, Dement WC: Narcolepsy in animals and man, *Eq Vet J* 25:476-477, 1993.

86. Mignot E, et al: Effects of alpha adrenoceptors blockade with prazosin in canine narcolepsy, *Brain Res* 444:184-188, 1988.

87. Mignot E, et al: The role of cerebrospinal fluid hypocretin measurement in the diagnosis of narcolepsy and other hypersomnias, *Arch Neurol* 59:1553-1562, 2002.

88. Mignot E, et al: Genetic linkage of autosomal recessive canine narcolepsy with a immunoglobulin heavy-chain switch-like segment, *Proc Natl Acad Sci* 88:3475-3478, 1991.

89. Mitler MM, Dement WC: Sleep studies on canine narcolepsy: pattern and cycle comparisons between affected and normal dogs, *Electroencephalogr Clin Neurophysiol* 43:691, 1977.

90. Mitler MM, Foutz A: The diagnosis and treatment of narcolepsy in animals. In Kirk RW, editor: *Current veterinary therapy VII. Small animal practice*, Philadelphia, 1980, Saunders.

91. Mitler MM, Stowe O, Dement WC: Narcolepsy in seven dogs, *J Am Vet Med Assoc* 168:1036, 1976.

92. Moore LA, Johnson PJ: Narcolepsy in horses, *Comp Cont Ed Pract Vet* 22:86-89, 2002.

93. Munana KR: Causes of and diagnostic approach to seizures, *ACVIM Proc* 22:355-357, 2004.

94. Munana KR, et al: Use of vagal nerve stimulation as a treatment for refractory epilepsy in dogs, *J Am Vet Med Assoc* 221: 977-983, 2002.

95. Nashino S, et al: Dopamine D2 mechanisms in canine narcolepsy, *J Neurosci* 11:2666-2671, 1991.

96. Nashino S, Mignot E: Pharmacological aspects of human and canine narcolepsy, *Prog Neurobiol* 52:27-78, 1997.

97. O'Brien DP: Status epilepticus, *ACVIM Proc* 16:275-277, 1998.

98. Oliver JE Jr: Seizure disorders in companion animals, *Compend Cont Ed* 2:77, 1980.

99. Oliver JE Jr, Hoerlein BF: Convulsive disorders of dogs, *J Am Vet Med Assoc* 146:1126, 1965.

100. Palmer AC: Clinical signs associated with intracranial tumors in dogs, *Res Vet Sci* 2:326, 1961.

101. Palmer AC: Pathological changes in the brain associated with fits in dogs, *Vet Rec* 90:167, 1972.

102. Palmer AC, Malinowski W, Barnett KC: Clinical signs including papilloedema associated with brain tumours in twenty-one dogs, *J Sm Anim Pract* 15:359, 1975.

103. Palmer AC, Rossdale PD: Neuropathology of the convulsive foal syndrome, *J Reprod Fertil Suppl* 23:691, 1975.

104. Palmer AC, Smith GF, Turner SJ: Cataplexy in a Guernsey bull, *Vet Rec* 106:421, 1980.

105. Parker AJ, Cunningham JG: Successful surgical removal of an epileptogenic focus in a dog, *J Sm Anim Pract* 12:513, 1971.

106. Parker AJ, O'Brien D, Musselman EE: Diazoxide treatment of metastatic insulinoma in a dog, *J Am Anim Hosp Assoc* 18:315, 1982.

107. Patterson EE, et al: Clinical description and mode of inheritance of idiopathic epilepsy in English springer spaniels, *J Am Vet Med Assoc* 226:54-58, 2005.

108. Patterson EE, et al: Clinical characteristics and inheritance of idiopathic epilepsy in Vizslas, *J Vet Intern Med* 17: 319-325, 2003.

109. Podel M: Antiepileptic drug therapy, *Clin Tech Sm Anim Pract* 13:185-192, 1998.

110. Podel M: High dose benzodiazepine per rectum to treat cluster seizures in dogs, *ACVIM Proc* 16:278-280, 1998.

111. Podel M: Strategies of antiepileptic drug therapy, *ACVIM Proc* 19:430-432, 2001.

112. Podel M, Fenner WR: Bromide therapy in refractory canine idiopathic epilepsy, *J Vet Intern Med* 7:318-327, 1993.

113. Podel M, Fenner WR: Use of bromide as an antiepileptic drug in dogs, *Comp Cont Ed Pract Vet* 16:767-774, 1994.

114. Resnick S: Hypocalcemia and tetany in the dog, *Vet Med Sm Anim Clin* 67:637, 1972.

115. Rogers WA, Donovan EF, Kociba GJ: Idiopathic hyper-lipoproteinemia in dogs, *J Am Vet Med Assoc* 166:1087, 1975.

116. Schatzberg SJ, et al: The effect of hypocretin replacement therapy in a 3-year-old Weimaraner with narcolepsy, *J Vet Intern Med* 18:586-588, 2004.

117. Sheading RG, et al: Primary hypoparathyroidism in the dog, *J Am Vet Med Assoc* 176:439, 1980.

118. Sheather AL: Fainting in foals, *J Comp Pathol Ther* 37:106, 1924.

119. Siegel JM: Narcolepsy: a key role for hypocretins (orexins), *Cell* 98:409-412, 1999.

120. Siegel JM, et al: Neuronal degeneration in canine narcolepsy, *J Neurosci* 19:248-257, 1999.

121. Speciale J, Stahlbrodt JE: Use of ocular compression to induce vagal stimulation and aid in controlling seizures in seven dogs, *J Am Vet Med Assoc* 214:663-665, 1999.

122. Srenk P, et al: Genetische grundlagen der idiopathischen epilepsie beim golden retriever, *Tierarztl Prax* 22:574-578, 1994.

123. Strain GM, Olcott BM, Archer RM: Narcolepsy in a Brahman bull, *J Am Vet Med Assoc* 185:538-541, 1984.

124. Sweeney CR, et al: Narcolepsy in a horse, *J Am Vet Med Assoc* 185:126-128, 1983.

125. Thomas WB: Idiopathic epilepsy in dogs, *Vet Clin North Am Sm Anim Pract* 30:183-206, 2000.

126. Van der Velden NA: Fits in Tervuren shepherd dogs. A presumed hereditary trait, *J Sm Anim Pract* 9:63, 1968.

127. Viitmaa R, et al: Magnetic resonance imaging findings in Finnish Spitz dogs with focal epilepsy, *J Vet Intern Med* 20:305-310, 2006.

128. Wauguer A, Ashton D, Melis W: Behavioral analysis of amygdaloid kindling in beagle dogs and the effects of clonazepam, diazepam, phenobarbital, diphenylhydantoin and flunarizine on seizure manifestation, *Exp Neurol* 64:579, 1979.

129. White EC, de Lahunta A: Narcolepsy in a lamb, *Vet Rec* 149:156-157, 2001.

130. Wu M-F, et al: Locus coeruleus neurons: cessation of activity during cataplexy, *Neuroscience* 91:1389-1399, 1999.

131. Zook BC, Carpenter JL, Leeds EB: Lead poisoning in dogs, *J Am Vet Med Assoc* 155:1329, 1969.

19 DIENCEPHALON

DIENCEPHALON

THALAMUS

Anatomy
Function
    Direct Cortical Projection
      System
    Diffuse Cortical Projection
      System
    Thalamic Reticular System
    Ascending Reticular Activating
      System
    Summary of Thalamic Function

Clinical Signs
Clinical Evaluation of the Obtunded
   to Comatose Patient
    Neurologic Examination

HYPOTHALAMUS

Anatomy
    Hypothalamic Nuclei
    Afferent Hypothalamic Tracts
    Efferent Hypothalamic Tracts
Function

Clinical Syndromes
    Abnormal Behavior
    Abnormal Sensorium
    Abnormal Water Consumption
    Abnormal Appetite
    Abnormal Temperature Regulation
    Abnormal Carbohydrate Metabolism
    Abnormal Heart Rate
    Narcolepsy
    Hemi-Neglect, Hemi-Inattention

To understand the anatomic terminology used in this chapter, the following description is based on terms described in the *Nomina Anatomica Veterinaria,* fifth edition. The prosencephalon is the forebrain that consists of the telencephalon and diencephalon. The telencephalon is the endbrain, the principal components of which are the neopallium, rhinencephalon, and corpus striatum (basal nuclei) of the cerebrum, which consists of two cerebral hemispheres. The diencephalon is the intermediate brain that consists of the thalamencephalon, hypothalamus, and subthalamus. The thalamencephalon includes the thalamus, metathalamus, and epithalamus (Box 19-1).

Box 19-1 Components of Prosencephalon

Prosencephalon
  Telencephalon: Cerebrum
    Neopallium
    Rhinencephalon
    Corpus striatum

Diencephalon
  Thalamencephalon
    Thalamus
    Metathalamus (geniculate nuclei)
    Epithalamus
  Hypothalamus
  Subthalamus

DIENCEPHALON

The components of the diencephalon are distributed symmetrically on both sides of the third ventricle. The hypothalamus consists of specific nuclei that are located lateral and ventral to the ventral portion of the third ventricle, ventral to the interthalamic adhesion (Fig. 19-1). The subthalamus is between the thalamus and substantia nigra of the mesencephalon. It is composed of the subthalamic body and zona incerta. The thalamus is composed of a plethora of nuclei that make up the major part of the diencephalon located dorsal to the ventral portion of the third ventricle and medial to the internal capsule. The metathalamus consists of the medial and lateral geniculate nuclei. The epithalamus includes the habenular nuclei and their connections and the pineal gland. For teaching purposes, this text considers the metathalamic nuclei to be part of the thalamus. This chapter describes the major components of the thalamus and hypothalamus. The epithalamus was previously considered with the limbic system and the subthalamus with the extrapyramidal system.

THALAMUS

Anatomy

The thalamus is related to the hypothalamus ventrally and to the internal capsule laterally (see Fig. 19-1; see also Figs. 2-3 through 2-5).[7,29-32,35] Leptomeninges (pia and arachnoid trabeculations) and cerebrospinal fluid (CSF) cover most of its dorsal surface. It is composed of numerous nuclei partly separated by medullary laminae and arranged in a bilaterally symmetric pattern on either side of the third ventricle. The internal medullary lamina divides each side of the thalamus into medial and lateral halves, and it splits rostrally to enclose a rostral portion, which includes the rostral thalamic nucleus (Fig. 19-2). A dorsal plane through the lateral half separates the thalamus into dorsal

Median section

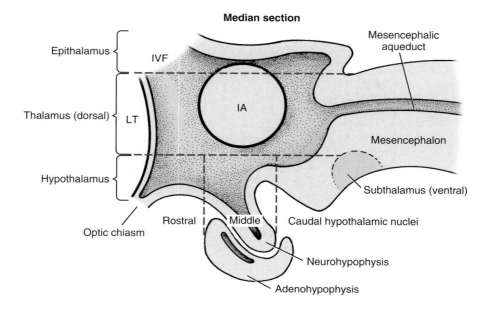

Transverse section through optic tract and internal capsule

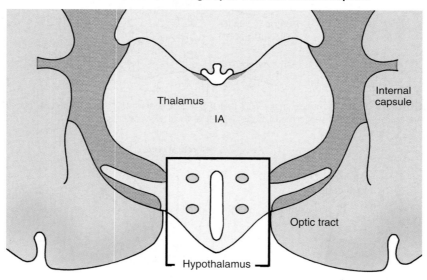

FIGURE 19-1 Divisions of the diencephalon. *IA,* Interthalamic adhesion; *IVF,* interventricular foramen; *LT,* lamina terminalis.

and ventral tiers of nuclei, and two transverse planes through the ventral tier further define these nuclei from rostral to caudal. The thin external medullary lamina forms the external boundary of the lateral half of the thalamus and is separated from the internal capsule by a narrow nuclear area, the thalamic reticular nucleus. These divisions result in the following groups of nuclei with a listing of their specific nuclei.

1. Rostral thalamic group: rostral thalamic nucleus (limbic system)
2. Medial thalamic group: medial dorsal nucleus
3. Lateral thalamic group:
   Dorsal tier:
       Dorsolateral nucleus
       Caudolateral nucleus
   Ventral tier:
       Ventral rostral nucleus (extrapyramidal)
       Ventral lateral nucleus (cerebellum)

Ventral caudal group:
    Ventral caudal medial nucleus (cranial nerves)
    Ventral caudal lateral nucleus (spinal nerves)
4. Caudal thalamic group (metathalamus)
    Medial geniculate nucleus (auditory, vestibular)
    Lateral geniculate nucleus (vision)
5. Intralaminar-midline thalamic group:
    Central medial nucleus
    Paraventricular nucleus
6. Thalamic reticular nucleus (ascending reticular activating system [ARAS])

Function

On a functional basis, the thalamic nuclei can be grouped into three major systems: (1) the direct cortical projection system, (2) the diffuse cortical projection system, and (3) the thalamic reticular system (Fig. 19-3).

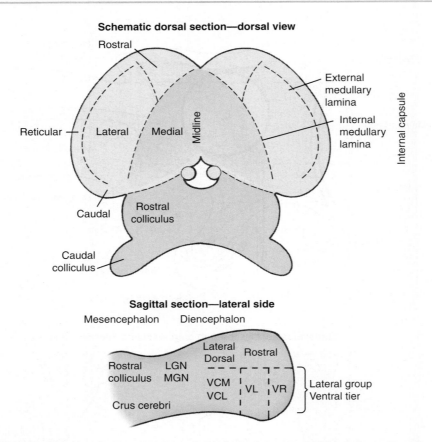

FIGURE 19-2 Thalamic nuclear groups. *LGN,* Lateral geniculate nucleus; *MGN,* medial geniculate nucleus; *VCL,* ventral caudal lateral; *VCM,* ventral caudal medial; *VL,* ventral lateral; *VR,* ventral rostral.

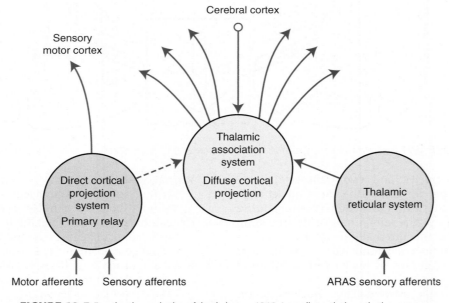

FIGURE 19-3 Functional organization of the thalamus. *ARAS,* Ascending reticular activating system.

Direct Cortical Projection System

The direct cortical projection system is the primary relay system that has been described throughout this text in relation to the conscious perception pathways for sensory systems and the thalamic relay for motor systems.

For the sensory systems, a thalamic relay occurs in the conscious perception pathway of all sensory systems except olfaction. The thalamic nuclei concerned with this relay are located in the ventral tier of the lateral half of the thalamus and in the caudal thalamic group. These thalamic nuclei are listed here with the specific sensory pathways afferent to the thalamic nucleus and the general area of the cerebrum to which each nucleus projects.

1. The **ventral caudal lateral nucleus** receives afferents from spinothalamic tracts (general somatic afferent [GSA], general visceral afferent [GVA]) and the medial lemniscus (general proprioceptive [GP]) and projects efferents to the somesthetic cortex for neck, trunk, and limbs.

2. The **ventral caudal medial nucleus** receives afferents from the quintothalamic tract (GSA, GP) and solitariothalamic tract (GVA, special visceral afferent [SVA]) and projects efferents to the somesthetic cortex for the head region.

3. The **lateral geniculate nucleus** receives afferents from the optic tract and projects efferents to the visual cortex of the occipital lobe.[11]

4. The **medial geniculate nucleus** receives afferents from the brachium of the caudal colliculus (special somatic afferent [SSA]—auditory and special proprioception [SP]) and projects efferents to the temporal lobe.

For the motor systems, a thalamic relay occurs for the extrapyramidal system and the cerebellum in their circuitry to the telencephalon.

1. The **ventral rostral nucleus** receives afferents from the pallidum and red nucleus and projects efferents to the motor cortex of the frontoparietal lobe.

2. The **ventral lateral nucleus** receives afferents from the cerebellar nuclei via the rostral cerebellar peduncle and the red nucleus and projects efferents to the motor cortex of the frontoparietal lobes.

All of these primary relay nuclei also project to other thalamic nuclei.

Diffuse Cortical Projection System

The diffuse cortical projection system is the thalamic association system that receives axons only from other diencephalic nuclei and telencephalic sources. These sources include the primary relay thalamic nuclei and the thalamic reticular system nuclei, the hypothalamus, the cingulate gyrus, the frontal cortex, and the striatum. No afferents are received from the primary afferent pathways in the brainstem. These diffuse cortical projection nuclei project diffusely to all parts of the telencephalon (see Fig. 19-3).

Thalamic nuclei that comprise this system include nuclei in the rostral thalamic group, the medial group, and the dorsal tier of the lateral group.

Thalamic Reticular System

The thalamic reticular system is the most rostral component of the ARAS, which receives afferents from more caudal brainstem levels of the reticular formation and collaterals of all the conscious perception pathways for sensory systems. Efferents from this system project to the thalamic nuclei of the diffuse cortical projection system (thalamic association system), which, in turn, projects diffusely to the telencephalic cerebral cortex (see Fig. 19-3). Thalamic nuclei that comprise this system include nuclei in the intralaminar (midline) group and the thalamic reticular nucleus.

Experimental evidence for the efferent pathways and functions of these various thalamic systems comes from the following studies.[26,28]

1. If the cortex of the telencephalon is removed, retrograde degeneration occurs only in specific thalamic nuclei that project to the cerebral cortex. This group includes the nuclei of the direct cortical projection system and the diffuse cortical projection system but not the nuclei of the thalamic reticular system.

2. Mild electrical stimulation of specific nuclei in the direct cortical projection system produces activity only in the specific areas of the cerebral cortex where the nuclei project. Stimulation of any of the nuclei in the thalamic reticular system produces slow, spreading diffuse activity of the entire cerebral cortex. This activity is mediated by the nuclei of the diffuse cortical projection system.

Ascending Reticular Activating System

The reticular formation is defined in Chapter 8, and the ascending component, the ARAS, is introduced at that time. The ARAS is part of the reticular formation, which, you may recall, consists of a network of neurons in the central portion or core of the brainstem from the medulla through the pons and midbrain and into the diencephalon.[21] The ARAS receives afferents from all the conscious projection pathways of the sensory systems, which includes interoception, exteroception, and proprioception. As these conscious projection pathways (spinal and cranial) course rostrally through the brainstem to the primary relay nuclei in the thalamus, collateral axons are given off into the reticular formation (Fig. 19-4). Most of these collaterals synapse in the reticular formation. Neurons of the reticular formation that project rostrally (the ARAS) continue the impulse flow rostrally in a multisynaptic pattern to one of two areas in the diencephalon, either the thalamic reticular system or the hyposubthalamic reticular system. A few collaterals project rostrally as part of the ARAS without synaptic interruption to terminate on one of these two diencephalic areas. The diencephalic portion of the ARAS stimulates the entire cerebral cortex diffusely. The thalamic reticular system affects the cerebral cortex by way of the diffuse telencephalic connections of the thalamic association system.

The ARAS functions to arouse the cerebral cortex, to awaken the brain to a conscious level, and to prepare the cortex to receive the rostrally projecting impulses from any sensory modality. It is responsible for maintaining the state of wakefulness. Decreased activity of the ARAS is associated with sleep. Sleep is a highly complex mechanism that is mediated through centers near the midline of the pons and medulla. These centers influence the activity of the ARAS. Stimulation of dorsal roots, somesthetic tracts, or any part of the ARAS of the sleeping animal arouses it to the awake state. This activity can be observed in the animal and on its electroencephalogram. The activity does not occur with stimulation of a primary relay nucleus in the thalamus. In this case, only the specific projection area of the cerebral cortex shows activity. Conversely, lesions that destroy the ARAS cause a comatose state.

The ARAS is considered to be the seat of consciousness. Both central nervous system (CNS) depressants and stimulants function on the ARAS. The ARAS may be responsible for the ability to focus attention on particular sources of stimuli with the rejection of others. Thus it monitors the myriad of stimuli that project rostrally to thalamic levels, accepting what is needed for conscious perception and rejecting what is irrelevant.

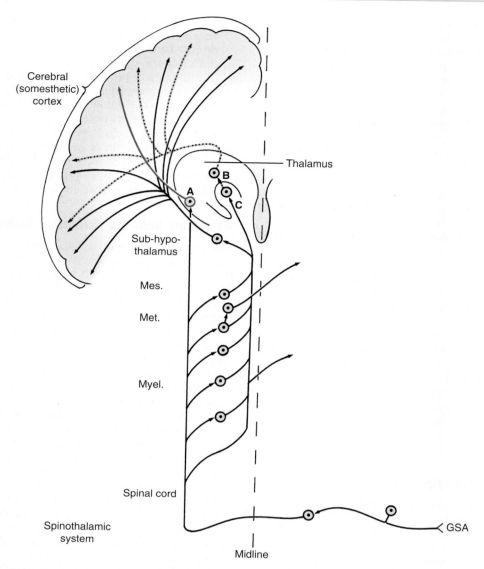

FIGURE 19-4 Ascending reticular activating system. **A,** Direct cortical projection system; **B,** thalamic association system—diffuse cortical projection system; **C,** thalamic reticular system. *GSA,* General somatic afferent; *Mes.,* mesencephalon; *Met.,* metencephalon; *Myel.,* myelencephalon.

Summary of Thalamic Function

1. The thalamus is the chief sensory integrating system of the neuraxis. It functions in the integration and relay of all types of sensory and motor pathways between the caudal brainstem and the cerebrum.
2. The thalamus may serve as the site of conscious perception of some sensory modalities. This activity is most evident after a lesion destroys the somesthetic cortex and the perception of some modalities is preserved. See Video 3-1 in Chapter 3, which shows a newborn Guernsey calf that has no cerebral hemispheres but still appears to have some intact nociception but not vision.
3. The thalamus functions in the ARAS as part of the mechanism for maintaining consciousness, for producing a state of attention, or for producing sleep.

Clinical Signs

Focal thalamic lesions in domestic animals are uncommon and often difficult to localize based on the physical neurologic examination. Involvement of the direct cortical projection nuclei, their projections, or both will produce variable degrees of deficits in their specific systems that may be recognizable on your physical neurologic examination. These nuclei include:

Lateral geniculate nucleus: contralateral loss of vision, hemianopsia

Medial geniculate nucleus: possible vestibular ataxia

Ventral caudal lateral nucleus: contralateral hypalgesia of the neck, trunk, and limbs and contralateral loss of proprioception in the limbs (slow postural reactions)

Ventral caudal medial nucleus: contralateral hypalgesia of the head

Ventral lateral nucleus: possible hypermetric ataxia

Ventral rostral nucleus: possible contralateral slow postural reactions from loss of upper motor neuron (UMN) circuitry

Lesions in the limbic system nuclei or tracts result in behavioral changes such as pacing, circling, aggression, unresponsiveness to owner, and loss of trained habits. Lesions in the thalamic reticular system nuclei result in disturbances of consciousness. In increasing order of severity, disturbances of consciousness progress from depression to lethargy to obtundation to semicoma (stupor) to coma. When determining this level of severity, use your best judgment as to how your patient responds to its environment and your vocal and physical stimulation. This response decreases from depression when it is mild to obtundation when it is quite severe. In semicoma, the patient is generally unresponsive to environmental stimuli, except for a noxious stimulus. A comatose patient will not respond to any stimuli, including those that are noxious, such as rigorous squeezing of the base of the digits with forceps or an electric prod in large animals. Rostral thalamic lesions may cause leaning, propulsive circling, or ocular or head and neck deviation (pleurothotonus), usually toward the side of the lesion. This abnormality is termed adversive syndrome. Animals with thalamic lesions occasionally act as if they were experiencing discomfort and exhibit the clinical signs of pain the "thalamic pain syndrome." See Video 9-4 in Chapter 9. Seizures can result from intrinsic environmental disorders that affect thalamic nuclei.

Clinical Evaluation of the Obtunded to Comatose Patient

A decrease in the level of consciousness can occur from either a diffuse brain lesion or widespread multifocal lesions of both cerebral hemispheres or a focal lesion affecting the ARAS of the brainstem. Except for traumatic lesions with bilateral cerebral edema and the various diseases that produce a polioencephalomalacia in animals, acute organic diseases that destroy both cerebral hemispheres are uncommon. In both bilateral traumatic cerebral edema and polioencephalomalacia, although the primary lesions are cerebral in location, the brainstem will be affected by the brain edema or the metabolic encephalopathy to contribute to the decreased level of consciousness. In our experience, a lesion confined to the cerebral cortex will not likely produce coma. A good example of this circumstance is congenital hydranencephaly of calves, a disorder in which the entire neopallium is replaced by a thin membrane of pial and glial cells. These calves vary from lethargic to obtunded but are still able to stand and walk but are blind. See Chapter 3 for this description and illustrations. Most coma results from brainstem lesions.

Peracute coma is most commonly caused by extensive brainstem lesions associated with intracranial injury, vascular compromise, intoxications, or a metabolic disorder. As a rule, these patients are recumbent with sporadic or no limb movements. The metabolic disorders and intoxications usually spare cranial nerve functions, except for vision. Intracranial injury can produce semicoma (stupor) from diffuse bilateral cerebral edema or from contusion and hemorrhage in the midbrain and pons of the brainstem. See Figures 7-30 and 7-31 in Chapter 7. If the semicomatose patient with an intracranial injury has evidence of voluntary limb movements, normal physiologic nystagmus, no cranial nerve deficits, and pupils that may be asymmetric or miotic but will still respond to a bright light, then the semicoma is probably the result of a prosencephalic dysfunction that may be limited to the cerebrum. The prognosis is guarded but more favorable than a patient who is semicomatose with clinical evidence of a more caudal brainstem lesion that is interfering with the function of the ARAS in the reticular formation.

Lesions confined to the prosencephalon that are not peracute will cause severe obtundation but do not interfere with the gait. See Video 14-4 in Chapter 14. Semicoma and coma are not expected with lesions confined to the prosencephalon. Similar lesions in the brainstem caudal to the diencephalon will cause varying degrees of spastic paresis and ataxia. Most brainstem lesions that are severe enough to cause coma will affect the ARAS at a level of the brainstem that also causes a nonambulatory tetraparesis or tetraplegia (i.e., the mesencephalon and pons).

Progressive space-occupying lesions of the cerebrum will cause herniation and compression of the brainstem. These lesions include neoplasms, hemorrhage and edema, infarcts, and abscesses and other inflammations. Initial clinical signs will be referable to the cerebrum. As the space-occupying lesion enlarges, clinical signs referable to the brainstem caudal to the diencephalon and to the cerebellum will occur that include varying degrees of loss of consciousness, with coma preceding death. Metabolic encephalopathy and most intoxications cause diffuse clinical signs. Remember that a prolonged postictal depression to stupor can follow a seizure.

Neurologic Examination

The following list includes some features of the neurologic examination that are helpful in localizing the cause of the loss of consciousness and in following the response to therapy or lack thereof.

1. **State of consciousness.** Carefully document your impression of the degree of loss of consciousness, especially whether any response to a noxious stimulus is observed. In increasing order of severity, the terms that we use are depression, lethargy, obtundation, semicoma (stupor), and coma.

2. **Posture and voluntary movement.** In the recumbent patient, be sure to determine whether any voluntary limb movement is seen that is not just reflex induced. Decerebrate rigidity occurs with midbrain lesions and is characterized by recumbency accompanied by rigid extension of all the limbs and opisthotonus. Opisthotonus with extensor rigidity of the thoracic limbs and the pelvic limbs flexed at the hips with the other joints extended suggests a lesion involving the rostral cerebellum and is termed decerebellate rigidity.

3. **Vision.** Most prosencephalic lesions that are involved with semicoma or coma will disrupt the central visual pathway and cause a loss of the menace response with normal pupillary size and light response. The return of the menace response is a clinical indication of improvement.

4. **Pupils.** The size of the pupils and their response to light is a reliable way to assess the degree of a brainstem lesion (see Chapter 7). As a rule, the pupillary light reflex is spared in metabolic or toxic disorders. Dilated pupils with a loss of the pupillary light reflex is a strong indication of a primary diencephalic or mesencephalic structural lesion or edema secondary to an enlarging prosencephalic or adjacent brainstem lesion. Loss of the pupillary light reflex suggests a poor prognosis. Pupils that are initially small or normal and reactive to light that progressively dilate and become unresponsive to light are an indication that the disorder is progressing. Remember that acute prosencephalic lesions may cause bilateral miosis from release of oculomotor general visceral efferent (GVE) neurons from inhibitory UMNs located in the prosencephalon. Your observation of pupils that are initially dilated and that return to normal is a good indication of improvement. Space-occupying lesions in the cerebrum that cause herniation and progressive compression of the midbrain will initially cause miosis from UMN release, but this herniation and compression will be followed by progressive dilation of the pupils as the oculomotor GVE neurons become dysfunctional. This dilation will usually be ipsilateral to a space-occupying lesion in one cerebral hemisphere. In a recumbent comatose patient, reactive pupils suggest a metabolic or toxic disorder. Dilated unresponsive pupils suggest a structural disorder.

5. **Physiologic nystagmus.** Physiologic nystagmus requires an intact pathway between the vestibular portion of cranial nerve VIII and the GSE neurons in nuclei of cranial nerves VI, IV, and III. This pathway involves axons of neurons in the vestibular nuclei that course rostrally in the medial longitudinal fasciculus (MLF). Brainstem lesions that disrupt the MLF will prevent the nystagmus that can normally be generated by moving the head in a dorsal plane from side to side. Remember that this physiologic nystagmus will also be absent if bilateral lesions are present in the inner ears. In patients with clinical signs of brainstem dysfunction, the absence of this physiologic nystagmus response is an indication of a poor prognosis. Even severe metabolic disorders may interrupt this response. Physiologic nystagmus is absent in a patient that has no brainstem function and is being maintained on life support systems.

6. **Respiration.** Irregularities of respiration may occur with serious brainstem lesions. Cheyne-Stokes respirations may occur with severe bilateral cerebral disease, diencephalic disease, or both. This abnormal breathing pattern is characterized by gradually increasing and decreasing tidal volume interspersed with periods of apnea and is an indication of increasing intracranial pressure. Mesencephalic lesions may cause a regular sustained hyperventilation known as central neurogenic hyperventilation. More caudal brainstem lesions produce bizarre abnormal breathing patterns, often known as ataxic breathing, which usually precedes cardiac arrest. Obviously, traumatic lesions that injure the thorax may also produce abnormalities in respiration.

Box 19-2 lists some of the extracranial metabolic disorders that, when severe, may result in coma. Box 19-3 is a list of intoxications that, when severe, may also cause coma.

BOX 19-2 Metabolic Disorders That May Produce Coma

Pancreatic disease:
   Beta-cell neoplasia: hypoglycemia
   Diabetes mellitus: hyperglycemia and ketoacidosis
Liver disease: hyperammonemia, hypoglycemia
Renal disease: uremia, acidosis, hypocalcemia
Myocardial disease: ischemic hypoxia
Pulmonary disease: hypoxia, acidosis
Adrenal disease: hypoadrenocortical crisis, hyperkalemia
Anemia: carbon monoxide poisoning, hemorrhage
Osmotic abnormalities:
   Water intoxication—hypoosmolar state
   Salt poisoning—hyperosmolar state, hypernatremia
Nutritional deficiency: thiamin deficiency
Acidosis, if severe
Heat stroke: hyperthermia

BOX 19-3 Poisons That May Produce Coma

Amphetamine sulfate
Arsenic
Barbiturates
Benzene hexachloride, benzene
Carbon tetrachloride
Cyanide
Dinitrophenol
Ethylene glycol
Hexachlorophene
Kerosene
Lead salts
Nitrobenzene
Turpentine
Xylitol
Zinc phosphide

HYPOTHALAMUS

Anatomy

Hypothalamic Nuclei

The hypothalamus is that part of the diencephalon that forms the ventral and lateral walls of the ventral portion of the third ventricle. The hypothalamic nuclei are ventral to the interthalamic adhesion. The hypothalamus extends from the lamina terminalis and optic chiasm rostrally through the mamillary bodies caudally (see Figs. 19-1, 2-3, and 2-4). The ventral surface of the hypothalamus, between these areas, is the tuber cinereum. A ventral extension of the tuber cinereum is the infundibulum or pituitary stalk. Distally, the infundibulum expands to form the neurohypophysis, the neural lobe of the hypophysis (pituitary gland).

The hypothalamus may be divided transversely from rostral to caudal into three regions of nuclei.

1. **Rostral region—the chiasmatic group:** supraoptic nucleus, suprachiasmatic nucleus, paraventricular nucleus, rostral hypothalamic nucleus, preoptic nuclei, and rostral periventricular nucleus
2. **Intermediate region—tuberal group:** dorsomedial and ventromedial nuclei, infundibular nucleus and lateral hypothalamic area
3. **Caudal region—mamillary group:** premamillary nucleus, dorsal, and dorsocaudal hypothalamic areas; lateral and perifornical hypothalamic nuclei; caudal periventricular nucleus; mamillary nuclei

Afferent Hypothalamic Tracts

Telencephalon. Afferents tracts from the rhinencephalon include the columns of the fornix from the hippocampus to the mamillary bodies, the medial forebrain bundle from the septal area, and the stria terminalis from the amygdaloid body. Pallidohypothalamic axons are extrapyramidal projections from the pallidum (globus pallidus).

Diencephalon. Numerous axons enter the hypothalamus from various thalamic nuclei.

Mesencephalon. The mamillary peduncle consists of collateral axons from brainstem GVA and SVA pathways involved in sensory modalities from visceral organs. The dorsal longitudinal fasciculus located in the periventricular central gray substance consists of collateral axons from the axons in the solitary tract, which contains the central projections of GVA and SVA neurons that innervate visceral organs.

Efferent Hypothalamic Tracts

The mamillothalamic tract projects from the mamillary nuclei to the rostral thalamic nucleus. The mamillotegmental tract projects primarily to the mesencephalic reticular formation to synapse on UMNs that, in turn, will influence the brainstem and spinal cord GVE-lower motor neuron (LMN) systems.[10] Periventricular fibers and the dorsal longitudinal fasciculus consist of axons that also project to brainstem and spinal cord GVE-LMN nuclei. The hypothalamo-hypophyseal tracts, which course into the hypophysis (pituitary gland), comprise two systems. The hypothalamo-neurohypophyseal system terminates on blood vessels in the neurohypophysis, and the hypothalamo-adenohypophyseal system terminates on blood vessels in the tuber cinereum and infundibulum. Both systems consist of axons that provide a pathway for neurosecretory substances produced by neuronal cell bodies in the hypothalamus to access blood vessels where these products are released.[38] Neurosecretory products from the supraoptic and paraventricular nuclei (oxytocin, vasopressin—antidiuretic hormone) course through the supraopticohypophyseal and paraventriculohypophyseal tracts to the neurohypophysis in which they are released into the capillary bed and circulate to the effector organ to exert their activity.[4] The neurosecretory products involved with adenohypophyseal regulation are releasing factors that are produced in a variety of hypothalamic nuclei. They pass through the axons of the tuberohypophyseal tract and are released terminally into the capillary plexus in the tuber cinereum and infundibulum, where they circulate by way of the hypophyseal

BOX 19-4 Hypothalamo-Hypophyseal Tracts

HYPOTHALAMO-NEUROHYPOPHYSEAL SYSTEM

Supraoptic, paraventricular nuclei
   Oxytocin, vasopressin—antidiuretic hormone
Supraopticohypophyseal tract
Paraventricular-hypophyseal tract
Tuber cinereum—infundibulum
Capillaries of systemic circulation
Target organ

HYPOTHALAMO-ADENOHYPOPHYSEAL SYSTEM

Hypothalamic nuclei
   Releasing factors
Tuberohypophyseal tract
Tuber cinereum—infundibulum
Capillaries of hypothalamo-hypophyseal portal system
   Sinusoids of pars distalis of adenohypophysis
Target cells of pars distalis
   Trophic hormones to systemic circulation
Target organs

portal system vessels located there to the sinusoids of the adenohypophysis to influence the endocrine activity of the cells in the pars distalis. These neurosecretory products are the adenohypophyseal-releasing factors that are produced in hypothalamic nuclei. These pars distalis cells are their target organ (Box 19-4).

Function

The hypothalamus serves as a higher center for regulation of visceral motor activity. Its nuclei act as the UMN for visceral function. Therefore they are considered to be the UMN for the autonomic nervous system. Stimulation of the rostral hypothalamus elicits parasympathetic activity, whereas stimulation of the caudal hypothalamus elicits sympathetic activity throughout the body. The hypothalamus functions without voluntary control. The neocortex does not order hypothalamic activity. Nevertheless, the hypothalamus is subject to its influence. As an example, consider the gastrointestinal signs that accompany fear, pain, and various emotional states. Visceral motor activity associated with the function of the olfactory and limbic systems is mediated through the hypothalamus. In addition, the hypothalamus regulates the activity of a large portion of the body's endocrine system by way of the neurosecretory-releasing factors that influence the adenohypophysis. The hypophysis is considered to be the master gland of the body, and it is regulated by the hypothalamus. Recall from Chapter 18 the role of the hypothalamus in the synthesis of hypocretin and its involvement in the regulation of sleep.

Clinical Syndromes

Numerous clinical syndromes have been related to lesions that disturb the hypothalamus and related structures.[27]

Abnormal Behavior

The hypothalamus has components, such as the mamillary nuclei, that function with the limbic system. Selective ventral hypothalamic lesions in cats produce rage. Cattle with a pituitary gland abscess are usually lethargic and often hold their head and neck extended as if *star gazing*.

Abnormal Sensorium

Hypothalamic lesions that interfere with its role in the ARAS may result in varying degrees of loss of the conscious state. Most of these lesions are space-occupying lesions, and separating the contributions of the hypothalamus and the thalamus to the loss of ARAS function is difficult. Magnetic resonance imaging will determine the extent and the nature of these lesions and direct the course of therapy. In our experience, profound obtundation approaching semicoma in a patient that is still able to stand and walk usually reflects a diencephalic lesion.

Abnormal Water Consumption

Polydipsia is a clinical sign of diabetes insipidus and hyperadrenocorticoidism. Diabetes insipidus is the loss of control of water excretion caused by the failure of production or transport and release of antidiuretic hormone (ADH) into the blood stream.[6,17,20] Normal ADH function requires a normal pathway from the rostral group of hypothalamic nuclei into the infundibulum of the pituitary gland. Without this hormone, the failure to resorb water from the renal tubules causes polyuria and polydipsia. The urine specific gravity is constantly low (1.002 to 1.005) and does not concentrate when water consumption is stopped but does show some response of the kidney to the intramuscular injection of extracts containing ADH. In one study of 26 dogs with neoplasms of the adenohypophysis, 92% had the clinical diagnosis of diabetes insipidus from direct pressure of the neoplasm on the infundibulum and rostral group of hypothalamic nuclei.[9]

Hyperadrenocorticoidism often accompanies functional neoplasms of the adenohypophysis that produce adrenocorticotrophic hormone or a similar-acting polypeptide hormone. This syndrome has been reported with chromophobe adenomas and pars intermedia neoplasms of the canine pituitary gland.[5,8,9] If the hypothalamus is compromised by the neoplasm, various clinical signs of hypothalamic dysfunction may accompany the clinical signs of hyperactivity of the adrenal cortex. Clinical signs of hyperadrenocorticoidism include:

1. Polyuria, polydipsia, and polyphagia
2. Bilateral symmetric alopecia with sparing of the head and distal extremities, thin skin, patchy hyperpigmentation, comedones, keratin plugs, petechiae or ecchymoses, and calcinosis cutis
3. Pendular hypotonic abdomen
4. Enlarged liver
5. Lameness (osteoporosis), paresis, and skeletal muscle atrophy
6. Atrophic testicles or prolonged anestrus
7. Temporal muscle atrophy
8. Rarely, clinical myotonia (see Chapter 8)

The diagnosis can be supported by ancillary laboratory procedures.

Adipsia may result from hypothalamic lesions that interfere with the osmoreceptor activity of neurons involved with the control of water consumption (thirst).[1] We have seen adipsia and secondary hypernatremia in a young dog with a diencephalic dysplasia that affected primarily the hypothalamus.[3] The osmolar level of both the urine and plasma was elevated. Obtundation, adipsia, anorexia, dehydration, and hypothermia were associated with a severe hypernatremia and a hyperosmolar state in an 8-year-old cat with a B-cell lymphoma in its diencephalon.[25]

Abnormal Appetite

Abnormalities of appetite are expressed as hyperphagia and obesity or anorexia and cachexia.[14,15] A satiety center resides in the ventromedial hypothalamic nucleus of the intermediate region. The neuropeptide hypocretin may be involved in this activity. If this nucleus is destroyed bilaterally, hyperphagia and obesity result, which may be accompanied by a savage behavior. In the lateral hypothalamic area, a feeding center is responsible for the stimulation of appetite. Lesions in this center cause anorexia, resulting in cachexia and eventual death. The amygdaloid body is also involved in appetite control.[14] The adiposogenital syndrome (Fröhlich syndrome) results from hypothalamic lesions that involve the satiety center and the tuberohypophyseal system. The latter system is necessary for adenohypophyseal stimulation of gonadal function. These patients become obese, and their genitalia atrophy.[33,34]

Abnormal Temperature Regulation

Abnormal temperature control may cause hyperthermia, hypothermia, or poikilothermia.[14,18] A heat-loss center is located in the rostral hypothalamus, which normally responds to elevated body temperature by initiating sweating, increased respirations, peripheral vasodilation, and panting. A heat-conservation center is located in the caudal and lateral areas of the hypothalamus that responds to depressed body temperature by initiating piloerection, shivering, peripheral vasoconstriction, and an increased basal metabolic rate. The increased basal metabolic rate results in increased feeding activity. Lesions that disrupt these centers inhibit their normal regulatory function. Loss of function of the heat-loss center results in hyperthermia, and loss of function of the heat-conservation center results in hypothermia. Hyperhydrosis (excessive sweating) may accompany hyperthermia. Cattle with a pituitary abscess that compresses the hypothalamus often are hypothermic. Bilateral destruction of the hypothalamotegmental tracts that function in the conservation and dissipation of body heat may produce poikilothermia. Intracranial injuries that affect the hypothalamus may be a cause of poikilothermia.

Abnormal Carbohydrate Metabolism

The hypothalamus is involved with the regulation of the blood sugar level of the body. The exact mechanism of this control is poorly understood. Lesions that involve the nuclei in the ventral wall of the third ventricle have been associated with hyperglycemia, glucosuria, and abnormal glucose tolerance curves.[16,19] A unique syndrome occurs in aging horses that represents a dysfunction of the pars intermedia that is related to degeneration of its dopaminergic innervation.* Apparently a pathologic continuum exists in these affected horses that ranges from pars intermedia hypertrophy, to hyperplasia, to functional adenoma. Whatever the structural abnormality may be, the enlarged dysfunctional pars intermedia results in an increased uncontrolled secretion of beta-endorphin, alpha-melanotropin, and adrenocorticotrophic hormone. Because of the increased activity of the adrenal cortex, causing an excess of circulating glucocorticoids, this disorder has been called Cushing disease. The clinical signs relate to the excessive circulating glucocorticoids and the physical compression of the neurohypophysis and hypothalamus. These signs include polydipsia, polyuria, hyperglycemia and glucosuria that are unresponsive to insulin, and muscle atrophy. A common clinical sign that is often the first to be observed is the failure to shed the winter hair coat through the warm summer months of the year (hirsutism).[13] Hyperthermia and hyperhydrosis have also been reported with these neoplasms and occasionally diabetes insipidus and hyperphagia. Laminitis may be a sequela of the abnormal carbohydrate metabolism. The cause of the dopaminergic neuronal degeneration is unknown. Treatment with pergolide, a dopaminergic agonist, is recommended, but clinical trials to determine its efficacy are still in progress.

Abnormal Heart Rate

Alterations of cardiac function have been observed in cattle with a pituitary abscess that involves the hypothalamus. Interference with the role of the hypothalamus in control of the autonomic nervous system may result in a marked slowing of the heart (bradycardia).

Narcolepsy

Selective loss of function of ventral hypothalamic neurons that normally produce hypocretin may result in the acquired form of narcolepsy. Lesions have been recognized in these hypothalamic nuclei in humans. This circumstance has not yet been reported in dogs.

Despite all these possible clinical signs related to pituitary-hypothalamic dysfunction, a surprising statistic is how many dogs with very large neoplasms compressing the pituitary gland and hypothalamus show only lethargy or obtundation and sometimes generalized seizures.

Hemi-Neglect, Hemi-Inattention

Unilateral lesions of the diencephalon may cause a behavior abnormality known as the hemi-neglect or hemi-inattention syndrome. The characteristic feature of this syndrome is the patient's lack of response to any environmental stimulus on one side of its body. The failure to respond to visual stimuli may reflect hemianopsia as a result of interference with the optic tract or lateral geniculate nucleus on one side. The reluctance or refusal to eat or drink when food or water are provided from one side may also reflect the hemianopsia or the asymmetric involvement of other diencephalic nuclei responsible for cortical awareness.

*References 2, 12, 13, 19, 22, 23, 24, 36, 37.

REFERENCES

1. Anderson B: Thirst and brain control of water balance, *Am Sci* 59:408, 1971.
2. Backstrom G: Hirsutism associated with pituitary tumors in horses, *Nord Vet Med* 15:778, 1963.
3. Bagley RS, et al: Hypernatremia, adipsia, and diabetes insipidus in a dog with a hypothalamic dysplasia, *J Am Anim Hosp Assoc* 29:267-271, 1993.
4. Bisset GW, Clark BJ, Errington ML: The hypothalamic neurosecretory pathways for the release of oxytocin and vasopressin in the cat, *J Physiol* 217:111, 1971.
5. Brandt AJ: Uber hypophysenadenom bei hund and pferd, *Skand Vet Tidskr* 30:875, 1940.
6. Breitschwerdt EB, Root CR: Inappropriate secretion of antidiuretic hormone in a dog, *J Am Vet Med Assoc* 175:181, 1979.
7. Cabral RJ, Johnson JI: The organization of mechanoreceptive projections in the ventrobasal thalamus of sheep, *J Comp Neurol* 141:17, 1971.
8. Capen CC, Koestner A: Functional chromophobe adenoma of the canine adenohypophysis. An ultrastructural evaluation of neoplasms of pituitary corticotrophs, *Pathol Vet* 4:326, 1967.
9. Capen CC, Martin SL, Koestner A: Neoplasms in the hypophysis of the dogs, *Pathol Vet* 4:301, 1967.
10. Cheatham ML, Matzke H: Descending hypothalamic medullary pathways in the cat, *J Comp Neurol* 127:369, 1966.
11. Cummings JF, de Lahunta A: An experimental study of the retinal projections in the horse and sheep, *Ann N Y Acad Sci* 167:293, 1969.
12. Dybdal NO, et al: Diagnostic testing for pituitary pars intermedia dysfunction in horses, *J Am Vet Med Assoc* 204:627-632, 1994.
13. Eriksson KS, Dyrendahl S, Grunfelt D: A case of hirsutism in connection with hypophyseal tumor in a horse, *Nord Vet Med* 8:807, 1956.
14. Fonberg E: The effect of hypothalamic and amygdalar lesions on alimentary behavior and thermoregulation, *J Physiol* 63:249, 1971.
15. Keesey RE, Pawley TL: Hypothalamic regulation of body weight, *Am Sci* 63:558, 1975.
16. King JM, Kavanaugh JF, Bentinck-Smith J: Diabetes mellitus with pituitary neoplasm in a horse and dog, *Cornell Vet* 52:133, 1962.
17. Koestner A, Capen CC: Ultrastructural evaluation of the canine hypothalamic-neurohypophyseal system in diabetes insipidus associated with pituitary neoplasms, *Pathol Vet* 4:513, 1967.
18. Krum SH, Osborne CA: Heat stroke in the dog. A polysystemic disorder, *J Am Vet Med Assoc* 170:531, 1977.
19. Loeb WF, Capen CC, Johnson LE: Adenomas of the pars intermedia associated with hyperglycemia and glycosuria in two horses, *Cornell Vet* 56:623, 1966.
20. Madewell BR, et al: Clinicopathologic aspects of diabetes insipidus in the dog, *J Am Anim Hosp Assoc* 11:497, 1975.
21. Magoun HW: The ascending reticular activating system, *Res Publ Assoc Res Nerv Ment Dis* 30:480, 1952.
22. McFarlan D, et al: The role of dopaminergic neurodegeneration in equine pituitary pars intermedia dysfunction (Equine Cushing's syndrome), *Am Assoc Eq Pract Proc* 49: 2003.
23. McFarlane D, et al: Nitration and increased alpha-synuclein expression associated with dopaminergic neurodegeneration in equine pituitary pars intermedia dysfunction, *J Neuroendocrinol* 17:73-80, 2005.
24. Moore JN, et al: A case of pituitary adrenocorticotropin-dependent Cushing's syndrome in the horse, *Endocrinology* 104:576-582, 1979.
25. Morrison JA, Fales WA: Hypernatremia associated with intracranial B-cell lymphoma in a cat, *Vet Clin Pathol* 35: 362-365, 2006.

26. Murray M: Degeneration of some intralaminar thalamic nuclei after cortical removals in the cat, *J Comp Neurol* 127:341, 1966.

27. Nelson RW, et al: Diencephalic syndrome secondary to intracranial astrocytoma in a dog, *J Am Vet Med Assoc* 179:1004, 1981.

28. Peacock JH, Combs CM: Retrograde cell degeneration in adult cat after hemidecortication, *J Comp Neurol* 125:329, 1965.

29. Rioch DM: Studies on the diencephalon of carnivores. I. Nuclear configuration of the thalamus, epithalamus and hypothalamus of the dog and cat, *J Comp Neurol* 49:1, 1929.

30. Rioch DM: Studies on the diencephalon of the carnivore. II. Nuclear configuration and fiber connections of subthalamus and midbrain of the dog and cat, *J Comp Neurol* 49:121, 1929.

31. Rioch DM: Studies on the diencephalon of the carnivore. III. Certain myelinated fiber connections of the diencephalon of the dog and cat, *J Comp Neurol* 53:319, 1931.

32. Rose JE: The thalamus of the sheep: cellular and fibrous structure and comparison with pig, rabbit and cat, *J Comp Neurol* 77:469, 1942.

33. Saunders LZ, Rickard CG: Craniopharyngioma in a dog with apparent adiposogenital syndrome and diabetes insipidus, *Cornell Vet* 42:490, 1952.

34. Saunders LZ, Stephenson HC, McEntee K: Diabetes insipidus and adiposogenital syndrome in a dog due to an infundibuloma, *Cornell Vet* 41:445, 1951.

35. Sychowa B: The morphology and topography of the thalamic nuclei of the dog, *Acta Biol Exp* 21:101, 1961.

36. Urman HK, Ozcan HCV, Tekeli S: Pituitary neoplasms in two horses, *Zentrabl Veterinaermed* 19:257, 1963.

37. Van der Kolk JH, et al: Equine pituitary neoplasia: a clinical report of 21 cases (1990-1992), *Vet Rec* 133:594-597, 1993.

38. Zambrano D, de Robertis E: Ultrastructure of the hypothalamic neurosecretory system of the dog, *Z Zellforsch Mikrosk Anat* 81:264, 1967.

20 THE NEUROLOGIC EXAMINATION

**NEUROLOGIC EXAMINATION—
OVERVIEW**

Signalment
History

PHYSICAL EXAMINATION

**NEUROLOGIC EXAMINATION—
SPECIFICS**

Sensorium—Mental Attitude
Gait and Posture
Postural Reactions
Muscle Tone and Size and Spinal Nerve
  Reflexes

Cranial Nerves
Vision—Menace, Pupils
Palpebral Fissure and Third Eyelid
Strabismus
Nystagmus
Facial and Trigeminal Neurons
Cranial Nerves IX, X, and XII

**SUMMARY OF CLINICAL SIGNS
AT SPECIFIC CNS LOCATIONS**

Spinal Cord
  *Lumbosacral: Fourth Lumbar Through
    Caudal Segments*

*Thoracolumbar: Third Thoracic Through
  Third Lumbar Spinal Cord Segments
Caudocervical: Sixth Cervical Through
  Second Thoracic Spinal Cord Segments
Craniocervical: First Cervical Through
  Fifth Cervical Spinal Cord Segments*
Medulla and Pons
Cerebellum
Mesencephalon
Diencephalon
Telencephalon

CONCLUSION

NEUROLOGIC EXAMINATION— OVERVIEW

This chapter provides a complete description of the neurologic examination in one place. It is located near the end of this textbook because it represents the culmination of your understanding of the neuroanatomy of your patients. Most of this information has been described at some point in the various chapters that precede this one. The emphasis of this description is based on what can be performed in a cooperative dog. Features of the examination that apply specifically to the horse or food animal will be noted. Our opinion is that if you learn to perform this examination well on a cooperative dog systematically, you can adapt it to any other species. You would be amazed at how much you can determine in a confined wild animal such as a cheetah by just studying the animal through the barrier that confines it.

Examination of a patient with signs of a neurologic disorder should include a review of the history, a complete physical examination, a neurologic examination, and appropriate ancillary procedures. The purpose of the neurologic examination is to determine the neurologic abnormalities and, based on that, the location of the lesion or lesions responsible for causing these abnormalities. The location is the anatomic diagnosis. The continual use of a routine systematic procedure will provide you with the experience and confidence to make an accurate anatomic diagnosis.

The differential diagnosis must be based on the anatomic diagnosis, and the order of significance of these disorders will depend on your evaluation of the signalment and history. Be sure to consider all five major kinds of lesions in your

differential diagnosis or a list of these with which you are comfortable. Our list is described in Chapter 1 and includes malformation, injury, inflammation, neoplasia, and degeneration (MIIND). Your experience with the anatomic diagnosis together with the signalment and history will often lead to a presumptive clinical diagnosis. Further examination of the patient with ancillary procedures must depend on your differential diagnosis and what you consider to be the most likely clinical diagnosis. Many factors will be considered in this selection, including the cost to the patient's owner.

Be sure to record carefully all your observations from the neurologic examination, and never rely on your memory. Many forms are available for recording your observations. Some of these forms list in detail every possible response that is present or absent, with numbers to estimate the level of response. The considerable variation between individual patients of the same species makes the recording of the degree of a response less reliable and often misleading. We prefer a less time-consuming form that is easier to follow and adaptable to all species (Fig. 20-1).

Signalment

The signalment of the patient provides the examiner with the age, sex, breed, and use of the patient. When considered together with the chief complaint, this information may help direct the line of questioning as you take the history. For example, canine patients younger than 1 year that are presented for seizures are more likely to have an inflammatory lesion than a neoplasm, and lead poisoning is more common in dogs younger than 1 year. Toy breeds with functional hypoglycemia

Neurologic Examination

Patient Identification

Signalment: _____

History: _____

_____

_____

Mental status: _____

Gait and posture: _____

Cranial Nerves

II. Menace   OS   OD   VII.

II-III. Pupils—Size   VIII. Cochlear

    Light in OS = OS   OD   Vestibular

    Light in OD = OD   OS   Head tilt

  III. Strabismus   Nystagmus

  V. Motor

    Sensory   IX, X. Gag

  VI. Strabismus   XII.

Muscle tone

Muscle atrophy

Spinal nerve reflexes: Postural reactions:

  Patellar   L   R   Hopping   LF   RF

  Flexor   LF   RF   LH   RH

        LH   RH   Paw/hoof replacement   LF   RF

                           LH   RH

  Perineal

  Nociception   Other:

Anatomic diagnosis:

Differential diagnosis:

FIGURE 20-1 Neurologic examination form.

usually have seizures when they are younger than 6 months. Hypoglycemic seizures caused by a functional neoplasm of the pancreatic islet beta cells are rarely seen before 4 years of age. Neoplasms of the nervous system usually occur in the older patient, except for lymphosarcoma, which can occur at any age, and a spinal cord nephroblastoma, which occurs in young dogs. Exceptions are common. Intervertebral disk extrusion-protrusion is a concern in the chondrodystrophic breeds any-time after 1 year of age, whereas in the nonchondrodystrophic breeds, it is rarely a concern before 5 years of age.

The sex of the patient is an important consideration when the differential diagnosis includes brain neoplasms, given that mammary gland adenocarcinomas of the female patient rank high among the more common neoplasms that metasta-size to the brain. Estrus may also lower the seizure threshold in animals that have or are at risk for idiopathic epilepsy.

Many disorders of the nervous system are restricted to one or more specific breeds. You must consider these breed-related disorders in your differential diagnosis. This prac-tice is especially true for the inherited degenerative diseases such as the storage diseases, abiotrophies, and movement disorders. Many neurology texts provide a list of these breed-related disorders, and their recognition is a continual process. These disorders can be readily searched for each breed on the Internet.

History

The line of questioning followed in taking the history of the patient depends on the chief complaint. In all cases, this review should include a summary of any medical and surgi-cal history unrelated in time to the present complaint.

If the chief complaint is an injury, the questioning will focus on the authenticity of the trauma, when the clinical signs first appeared, and how they have changed to the present time. By 24 to 48 hours after an injury, the clinical signs usually remain static or improve. Progressive neurologic signs are not usually the result of a single episode of trauma. Be aware that own-ers will often blame the neurologic signs on an injury from a fall when the fall was actually caused by the initial neurologic signs that were not recognized by the owner. This scenario is especially common when a dog falls down a set of stairs.

When a patient is brought in with the complaint of seizures, you need to obtain as thorough a description of the *seizure* event as possible to be certain of its authenticity and to determine the kind (classification) of seizure. The majority of seizures seen in domestic animals are generalized seizures. This type of seizure is the one that most commonly occurs in idiopathic epilepsy, most intoxications, and many prosence-phalic structural disorders. Complex partial seizures (psycho-motor) are more common in lead poisoning and diseases that affect the limbic system. Descriptions of these seizures often include episodic activities of the patient that the owner will describe as bizarre behavior or hysteria. Simple partial seizures may occur with or without confusion but with no loss of consciousness. The episodic activity is limited to groups of skeletal muscles such as the facial muscles or the muscles of one or both limbs on one side. Distinguishing between a simple partial seizure and a movement disorder may be dif-ficult. The latter is described in Chapter 8. It is very useful to have the owner provide a video of the episodic event for you to study, given that these seizures rarely occur in your hos-pital. A thorough description or a video evaluation of a dog

that is exhibiting episodes of collapsing will help distinguish among a seizure, cataplexy, movement disorder, syncope, or neuromuscular disorder. Episodic behavioral disorders are also best evaluated on videos.

Be sure to evaluate the history of each neurologic clinical sign that the owner observed to determine its validity, its progres-sion, and whether these clinical signs represent a lesion that is focal or disseminated through the nervous system. For exam-ple, a patient that initially exhibited a spastic paresis and ataxia of the pelvic limbs that progressed and then developed a head tremor, head tilt, and abnormal nystagmus requires lesions in more than one location to explain these clinical signs (i.e., a lesion in the thoracolumbar spinal cord segments and a lesion in the cerebellomedullary region). Such a multifocal distribu-tion of lesions is characteristic for an inflammatory lesion, such as the encephalomyelitis caused by the canine distemper virus in dogs, toxoplasmosis or cryptococcosis in dogs and cats, or *Sarcocystis neurona* in horses. The clinical signs of inflammatory disease usually progress more rapidly than those from an inher-ited degenerative disorder. Careful questioning may determine that what an owner thought was a sudden onset was, in fact, a progressive disorder. "My 6-year-old male German shepherd fell down the stairs this morning and injured himself. Oh yes, I did notice him stumble once yesterday." As a rule, clinical signs that are precipitous at onset and not progressive after 1 to 2 days are caused by an injury or vascular compromise. The outdoor dog that is found in the morning unable to use its pel-vic limbs is a candidate for an extrinsic spinal cord injury, isch-emic or hemorrhagic myelopathy caused by fibrocartilaginous emboli or an acute intervertebral disk extrusion. Be aware that neoplasms occasionally cause an acute onset of clinical signs that are followed by progression.

As a rule, malformative or inflammatory diseases that occur in utero will cause clinical signs that are observed at birth and are nonprogressive. These signs are readily observed in foals and the newborns of farm animals that are born *on the trot*. In small animals, these clinical signs may not be obvi-ous until the puppy or kitten starts to stand and tries to walk. A good example of this circumstance is the kitten in which the feline panleukopenia virus destroyed its cerebellum in the perinatal period. The cerebellar ataxia may not be appar-ent until 3 to 4 weeks of age. As the kitten develops normally in its second month of life and becomes more active, the cerebellar ataxia may appear to be worse, but the disease is not progressive. Most puppies with inherited cerebellar cor-tical abiotrophy develop normally for a few weeks and then begin to exhibit progressive cerebellar ataxia. Be aware that the onset of clinical signs of a cerebellar disorder at 10 to 12 weeks of age might just as well be the onset of progres-sive canine distemper encephalomyelitis. In a cairn or West Highland white terrier, this sign might signal the onset of clinical signs of inherited globoid cell leukodystrophy.

If intoxication is suspected, a thorough search should be carried out to find a possible source of the toxic agent. Sources of lead include lead-based paints, linoleum, tarpaper, welding equipment, and batteries. Cattle that lick old vehicle batteries are at risk for lead poisoning. Cats seem to enjoy licking antifreeze, which is a source of ethylene glycol. Be aware of the various houseplants that can be toxic if eaten by small animals and pasture plants that large animals consume. Consumption of rotting garbage, compost piles, and animal carcasses left in the woods may also be the basis for the cause of neurologic signs.

Be sure to ask about the patient's behavior in its home environment. The owner will be aware of subtle changes that you cannot appreciate in your hands-on examination.

Inquire about the health of other animals in the same environment. Canine distemper often affects more than one puppy in a litter, as do many of the inherited degenerative disorders. Equine herpesvirus may affect multiple animals on a property. A brain abscess caused by *Streptococcus equi* may occur in a horse that is associated with other horses that are exhibiting signs of a strangles infection caused by the same bacterium.

Always determine the vaccination history of your patient because many of these vaccines involve infectious agents that affect the nervous system (i.e., canine distemper, eastern equine encephalitis, rabies).

The following additional questions should be asked as part of the historical examination:

What diet do you feed? Raw or homemade diets may affect the nervous system.

Is your pet on any medications? Surprisingly, many owners forget to tell you that their pet is on metronidazole, which, at high doses or for prolonged usage, can cause profound neurologic clinical signs.

Is your pet confined indoors, or does it have access to the outdoors? Exposure to the outside environment is necessary for the development of *Cuterebra* spp. myiasis and ischemic encephalopathy.

Has your pet traveled anywhere recently? Certain geographic locations may have endemic diseases such as coccidioidomycosis in the southwest United States and tick paralysis in the middle eastern coastal states.

Does your pet exhibit any polyuria, polydipsia, or polyphagia? These clinical signs may reflect dysfunction of the diencephalon.

Has your pet exhibited any coughing, sneezing, vomiting, or diarrhea on a regular basis? Diseases such as myasthenia gravis can result in regurgitation and secondary aspiration pneumonia with a resultant cough.

PHYSICAL EXAMINATION

All patients presented with neurologic clinical signs must have a thorough general physical examination first. Some inflammatory diseases of the nervous system also affect other body systems. Seizures may occur in patients with extensive liver or kidney disease or in patients that have an islet beta-cell neoplasm of the pancreas. Primary disease of other body systems may cause episodes of paresis or complete collapse. Examples include hypoglycemia, cardiorespiratory disorders, and hypoadrenocorticoidism. Musculoskeletal disorders are often confused with neurologic disease, especially in horses. A rectal examination should be performed in all horses that exhibit any clinical signs of spinal cord disease and in large dogs that exhibit clinical signs of involvement of the lumbosacral intumescence or its spinal nerves.

NEUROLOGIC EXAMINATION— SPECIFICS

The neurologic examination can be divided into five parts:
1. Sensorium—mental attitude
2. Gait and posture
3. Postural reactions
4. Muscle tone, size, and spinal nerve reflexes
5. Cranial nerves

The order in which parts are performed is usually determined by the degree of patient cooperation and your preference. We usually perform the examination in the order listed. If the patient is resting comfortably in its cage, performing the cranial nerve examination first may be preferable. If the patient is excited or apprehensive, performing the cranial nerve examination may be more convenient after the patient has been handled for the examination of its gait, postural reactions, and spinal nerve reflexes.

Remember that, as described in Chapter 5, spinal nerve reflexes require only the specific peripheral nerves that innervate the area being tested and the spinal cord segments with which they connect. Postural reactions depend on the same components as the spinal nerve reflexes plus the cranial projecting pathways in the spinal cord white matter to the brainstem, cerebellum, and frontoparietal portion of the cerebral hemisphere and the caudal-projecting upper motor neuron (UMN) pathways that return from the cerebrum and brainstem and comprise tracts in the white matter of the spinal cord that terminate in the cervical and lumbosacral intumescences. These postural reactions test the integrity of nearly the entire peripheral and central nervous systems. By themselves, the postural reactions are relatively less reliable for lesion location.

Sensorium—Mental Attitude

An assessment should be made and recorded of the patient's sensorium, its mental attitude, and response to the immediate environment and attitude to being handled by you. The owner is the best judge of subtle changes in the patient's behavior in its normal environment. Be sure to explore this issue when you obtain the history. Considerable patient variation exists in how alert and responsive the patient may be in the examination room of a veterinary hospital. Do not mistake a very laidback behavior for depression. Descriptive terms for this portion of your examination include alert and responsive, depressed, lethargic, obtunded, semicoma (stupor), and coma. These states are described with the discussion of the ascending reticular activating system (ARAS) in Chapter 19. Other descriptions include acting vague, disoriented, hyperactive, propulsive, and aggressive.

As a rule, alterations in the patient's normal sensorium reflect disturbances in the ARAS and limbic system components of the cerebrum or rostral brainstem. Be sure to evaluate the sensorium of a recumbent patient thoroughly. Recumbency from diffuse neuromuscular disease or focal cervical spinal cord disease will not alter the patient's sensorium. A horse that is recumbent as a result of botulism may appear to be severely depressed or lethargic because it has no voluntary movement to show a response. The quality of the tetraparesis or tetraplegia with a cervical spinal cord lesion is the same as that caused by a mid- to caudal brainstem lesion, but the latter circumstance will often alter the patient's level of response to its environment. Be aware that horses that suddenly become recumbent from an aortic thromboembolism or spinal cord ischemia and hemorrhage from an equine herpesvirus infection may act delirious as they struggle to stand. Horses that become acutely recumbent from a pontomedullary lesion that involves the vestibular system may be extremely disoriented and thrash wildly and appear maniacal as they try to recover their balance. The behavior is often remarkably altered in horses that have acute encephalitis from infection with the rabies, eastern equine encephalomyelitis, or West Nile viruses, as well as from hepatic encephalopathy. In human neurology, the Glasgow scale is used to report the patient's sensorium objectively. Scales of this nature are presently being modified and evaluated for animals but are not routinely used in veterinary medicine at this time.

Gait and Posture

Examination of the gait should be performed in a place where the patient can be walked with a leash or shank and where the surface is not slippery. Most hospital floors have a very slippery surface, which facilitates cleaning but is poor for evaluating a gait disorder and can be dangerous if the patient slips and falls, especially horses and cattle. A washable carpet is very useful for small animals. A rubberized floor is ideal for large animals. Be careful if you walk horses or cattle on a macadam surface because it is slippery. If you are constructing a small animal hospital, we recommend that you consider having a covered area with a specialized surface used in playgrounds that is relatively soft, provides excellent traction for the patient, and is easily cleaned. The material is Vitriturf and is available from Hanover Specialties, Inc., Hauppauge, New York. Whatever facility you adopt for this gait evaluation in patients with neurologic disorders will also be useful for orthopedic examinations.

Observe the patient while it is standing for a head tilt, lowered position of the neck, trembling, degree of tarsal extension, and its tail position. You should evaluate the gait both as you lead the patient and as an assistant leads the patient. Most deficits are best seen during a slow walk and as it turns. Walk the animal back and forth in a straight line and in circles in each direction. Observe the patient from all directions. In our opinion, most abnormalities are best seen from a side view. Trotting a horse is occasionally helpful. If it is difficult to determine an abnormality, evaluate the patient on a slope or turn the patient loose in a confined area such as a paddock or riding ring. Be aware of breed characteristics that influence the posture and gait. The overflexed tarsus in German shepherds and the excess flexion action in the thoracic limbs of the Paso Fino and Tennessee walking horse are examples.

Is your patient unwilling or unable to move normally? When you see a gait disorder, this question is the first one that you need to answer. This circumstance is especially true when the patient is short strided or does not support weight well on one or more limbs. A loss of support from a femoral or radial nerve disorder will mimic a severe painful disorder causing a reluctance to bear weight.

Pattern recognition is critical in evaluating gait disorders. With experience, clinicians recognize specific patterns in abnormal gaits that suggest an anatomic diagnosis. We can describe these patterns, but observing them on videos is the best way to learn them. These patterns have five components consisting of two qualities of paresis and three qualities of ataxia.

Paresis is defined as "weakness" in the dictionary, but in clinical neurology, it is defined as "a deficiency in the generation of the gait or the ability to support weight." This definition includes the two qualities of paresis, which are lower motor neuron (neuromuscular) and upper motor neuron.

Lower motor neuron (LMN) paresis reflects degrees of difficulty in supporting weight and varies from a short stride that is easily mistaken for a musculoskeletal lameness to complete inability to support weight, causing collapse of the limb whenever weight is placed on it. Animals with LMN disorders affecting both pelvic limbs will occasionally use them simultaneously. This action is described as *bunny hopping*. Be aware that bunny hopping can also be seen in orthopedic disorders, as well as spinal cord dysplasias. UMN paresis causes a delay in the onset of protraction, which is the swing phase of the gait. The stride will usually be longer than normal. Stiffness and spasticity may be apparent in the stride. You may hear the hoof slap the ground in horses that are spastic. Most of the UMN pathways necessary for gait generation are anatomically adjacent to the pathways of the general proprioceptive (GP) sensory system, and lesions usually affect both simultaneously. Therefore the gait that reflects UMN paresis also reflects ataxia caused by dysfunction in the GP system. It is unnecessary to recognize the separate clinical signs of dysfunction of these two systems. Therefore we recognize a pattern that reflects the combined dysfunction of UMN paresis and GP ataxia. To observe and compare these two forms of paresis, see Videos 5-14 and 10-36.

Ataxia is a synonym for incoordination, and we recognize three qualities of ataxia: (1) GP, (2) vestibular (special proprioception [SP]), and (3) cerebellar. GP ataxia reflects the lack of information reaching the central nervous system (CNS) that informs the CNS of where the neck, trunk, and limbs are in space and the state of muscle contraction at any time. Without this GP information, the onset of protraction of a limb may be delayed, and the stride may be lengthened. During protraction, the limb may swing to the side (abduct) or swing under the body (adduct), overflex during protraction, scuff or drag one or more digits, and in the support phase, stand on the dorsal aspect of one or more digits. Remember that these clinical signs overlap with those caused by dysfunction of the UMN. The gait pattern of a patient with a focal cervical spinal cord lesion between the C1 and C5 segments reflects dysfunction of the UMN and GP systems and is observed as spastic tetraparesis and ataxia. This cervical spinal cord pattern is often recognized by the overextension of the thoracic limbs creating an overreaching or floating action. This clinical sign can be augmented by holding the head and neck extended as the patient is led, especially in horses. This unique form of hypermetria must not be confused with cerebellar ataxia in which the limb is overflexed on protraction. At no time do we try to differentiate between conscious (cerebral) and unconscious (cerebellar) GP pathways! No examination will clearly differentiate these two pathways from each other or from the UMN pathways. No pure conscious proprioceptive deficit exists. This term should be dropped from the clinician's vocabulary. See Video 10-36 for this combination of UMN and GP clinical signs. Vestibular ataxia reflects the loss of orientation of the head with the eyes, neck, trunk, and limbs, which results in a loss of balance. Lesions in this system cause the patient to lean, drift, or fall to one side. However, the patient's strength and awareness of where its limbs are in space are normal with lesions confined to this system. This ataxia is usually accompanied by a head tilt and sometimes abnormal nystagmus. We will occasionally blindfold our patients with bandage material in small animals or a towel in horses and cattle to exacerbate vestibular ataxia. See Video 12-1. Cerebellar ataxia most commonly causes hypermetric ataxia characterized by sudden bursts of motor activity with a marked overflexion of the limbs on protraction. Vestibular system components exist in the cerebellum that, if dysfunctional, may cause loss of balance, head tilt, and abnormal nystagmus. Cerebellar ataxia in horses produces more hypertonia than hypermetria when compared with other species of domestic animal. See Videos 13-9 and 13-21.

Many clinicians use a grading system for the clinical signs observed in the gait caused by spinal cord lesions. These systems facilitate determination of a prognosis and provide a basis for monitoring their response to therapy. The grading systems used are different for small animals and large animals. In small animals, the system is designed primarily for lesions that involve the spinal cord segments between T3 and L3 and is a measure of the degree of pelvic limb strength (UMN) and coordination (GP) that is present. In large animals, the system is designed primarily for lesions between the C1 and C5 spinal cord segments and is a measure of the degree of gait deficit.

Small animals:

Grade 5: Normal strength and coordination

Grade 4: Readily stands and walks with minimal paraparesis and ataxia

Grade 3: Able to stand to walk unassisted but with difficulty; often stumbles and falls but can walk; mild to moderate paraparesis and ataxia

Grade 2: Unable to stand unassisted; when assisted, able to move the pelvic limbs but constantly stumbles and often falls; moderate to severe paraparesis and ataxia

Grade 1: Unable to stand unassisted; when assisted, only slight pelvic limb movements; severe paraparesis and ataxia

Grade 0: Unable to stand unassisted; when assisted, complete absence of any pelvic limb movements, paraplegia

Horses:

Grade 0: Normal strength and coordination

Grade 1: Normal gait when walking straight; slight deficit on walking in tight circles or on walking with the head and neck extended or when pulled by the tail (swaying)

Grade 2: Mild spastic tetraparesis and ataxia at all times and especially during the manipulations described for grade 1

Grade 3: Marked spastic tetraparesis and ataxia with a tendency to buckle and fall on vigorous circling, backing, or swaying

Grade 4: Spontaneous stumbling, tripping, and falling

Grade 5: Recumbent; unable to stand

As you observe the gait of your patient, look carefully for any evidence of a head tilt (vestibular system), head and neck deviation or tendency to walk in circles (prosencephalon), neck flexion (neuromuscular), and tail movement.

Postural Reactions

The degree of functional limb deficit will determine the need for postural reaction testing. In a patient that is recumbent with tetraplegia or is paraplegic, you need not perform postural reactions in the affected limbs. However, in the paraplegic patient, you must test the thoracic limb postural reactions so as to prevent overlooking a focal cranial thoracic lesion or a multifocal disorder.

In small animals, we evaluate muscle size and tone just before our evaluation of the postural reactions. Be sure to talk to your patient continually, and use its name to gain its cooperation. Stand over the patient with both of you facing in the same direction. Simultaneously palpate the muscles of the neck and both thoracic limbs from proximal to distal for any evidence of atrophy. Flex and extend each limb for range of motion and to determine the degree of muscle tone. A short stride or stiffness in the gait may be caused by a joint disorder, limiting the range of motion. When you place the limb back on the ground surface, turn the paw over so that its dorsal surface bears the weight of the limb to determine how rapidly the paw is replaced. Most normal small animals immediately return the paw to its normal position. This response is known as the paw or hoof replacement reaction that requires many peripheral and central components to be normal. This test is not just for conscious perception of GP and should not be called the CP test. This term is a misnomer that we are well aware will be difficult to eliminate from the clinical language of veterinarians, even boarded veterinary neurologists. Moving on, palpate the thoracolumbar epaxial muscles and then the muscles of both pelvic limbs followed by flexing and extending those limbs and checking for paw or hoof replacement. Check for the degree of tail tone, and while extending the tail, evaluate the anal tone. In horses and farm animals, make the same evaluation for muscle atrophy. Some equine clinicians will place the hoof on its dorsal surface or place one limb in front of the other or laterally to the side and assess its rate of replacement.

Hopping responses, in our opinion, are the most reliable of the postural reactions that we test. While still straddling the patient, move back to the thoracic limbs, and while elevating the abdomen with one hand, pick up the thoracic limb on the opposite side with your other hand. With all the weight supported on the other thoracic limb, hop the patient laterally on that thoracic limb. Go as far as you can without moving your pelvic limbs. Then switch hands and hop the patient back on the other thoracic limb. Repeat this test many times until you are sure the thoracic limbs are normal or abnormal. As you stand over your patient and look down the lateral aspect of the limb that is being hopped, the limb should move as soon as you move the shoulder region laterally over the paw or hoof. Any delay in this response is abnormal. The hopping movements should be smooth and fairly rapid and not irregular or excessive. The paw or hoof should never drag or land on its dorsal surface. Carefully compare one thoracic limb with the other. To test the hopping responses in the pelvic limbs, stand beside the patient, and place your forelimb that is closest to the patient's head between its thoracic limbs with your hand on its sternum. Lift up on the thorax just enough to take the weight off of the thoracic limbs. With the other hand, pick up the pelvic limb on the side where you are standing and push the patient toward the pelvic limb that is bearing the weight. This action will force the patient to hop on that pelvic limb in a direction away from you. After a few hops, switch sides, and hop the patient back on the other pelvic limb. Keep repeating this test until you have determined that the response is normal or abnormal. The responses should be brisk and smooth but will not be quite as rapid as in the thoracic limbs. While you are hopping the patient, you will also be aware of the degree of tone in the limb that is bearing all the weight. In large dogs or small farm animals that are too heavy to lift for this testing, the same observations can be made while the patient is walked on one side (hemiwalking). Hemiwalking is performed by standing on one side of the patient. Grasp each limb on that side and lift the limbs off the ground surface and push the patient toward its opposite side. The patient will hop with both limbs on that side. Switch sides and repeat the hemiwalking performance on the opposite limbs. Be sure to compare one thoracic limb with the other and one pelvic limb with the opposite pelvic limb.

These hopping response evaluations can be performed on foals and calves and other farm animals that are not too large. Some clinicians will try to evaluate hopping in the adult horse by picking up one limb and using their shoulder to push the horse toward the opposite side, forcing it to hop on that limb. We find this method difficult to evaluate reliably, and the danger of self-injury for questionable value is not worth the effort.

In small animals in which the hopping responses are equivocal or difficult to interpret, testing the placing responses may be useful. Pick up the patient and bring its thoracic limbs to the edge of a shelf, table, or chair so that the dorsal surface of the paw contacts the front surface of the object. The normal patient will immediately place its paws on the horizontal surface of the object. Test both thoracic limbs while holding the patient from both sides. For some unknown reason, occasionally the normal patient will not respond on the side on which it is being held. Blocking the vision of the patient while conducting this test may also be useful. Do this by extending its head and neck so that it cannot see the protruding surface of the shelf, table, or chair. Whether the lack of vision or the position of the head and neck helps exacerbate the placing deficits is unclear.

In cooperative patients in which you are not sure of the thoracic limb function, you can wheelbarrow the patient while holding its head and neck in extension. With one of your forelimbs, elevate the abdomen of your patient, and with the other hand, hold the head and neck in extension and force the patient to walk forward. With this posture, vision is compromised, and the need for GP is increased. In large animals, elevate the head and neck as much as you can and still be able to lead them. With mild cervical spinal cord or brainstem lesions, this test may cause some patients to scuff the dorsal surface of its paws or overreach on protraction.

In large animals in which these postural reactions cannot be performed, we rely on other maneuvers that require more neurologic function of the UMN and GP systems to be normal. These maneuvers may elicit abnormalities that are not seen on observing the patient walking in a straight line. They include the head elevation described previously plus circling, backing, and swaying. Circling is the most useful of these maneuvers. Walk the patient in a tight circle for 8 to 10 times in each direction. The leader should be standing in the center of the circle as this test is conducted. The normal patient will step around briskly with relatively short strides and will not pivot on one hoof or step on itself. Patients with lesions that affect the UMN and GP systems, at most any level of the CNS, will appear awkward as they circle. The patient's movements may be irregular, and the patient will often pivot on the inside limb, which is held

in place and not protracted. The outside pelvic limb may flex and abduct excessively as it is protracted. This action is known as *circumduction*. The excessive flexion on protraction appears occasionally like a stringhalt action. The outside thoracic limb may overextend and cross over the standing limb. During this circling, the abnormal patient may step on itself. Be careful when you circle a patient with a severe deficit because you may cause it to fall. Backing up may be useful in a cooperative patient. Look for the tendency to be reluctant to back with one or both limbs. They may drag the limb or just collapse on one or both pelvic limbs and sit in a dog-like fashion. Sway the standing and walking patient by pulling its tail toward you and then releasing it. The degree of resistance may help you assess the patient's strength, and releasing the tail may alter its balance and precipitate a brief ataxia. Some clinicians will place one limb cranial to the other or as much on the opposite side of the other limb as possible and determine how rapidly it is replaced. A delayed replacement suggests a neurologic deficit similar to paw replacement in small animals. In small animals with suspected spinal cord disease, palpation of the vertebral column may elicit an area of discomfort. In large animals, firm hand compression of the vertebral column that induces some extension may reveal a degree of paresis if the patient tends to collapse from this vertebral extension.

When the clinical signs are subtle, you might want to walk, circle, back up, and sway the equine patient on a gentle slope. Walking the horse back and forth over a road curb may also be helpful. When turned loose in a paddock, a horse with mild UMN and GP dysfunction may exhibit clinical signs only when it has to change directions at the fence corner. If you are suspicious of a subtle dysfunction of the vestibular system, blindfolding the patient may exacerbate the vestibular system signs; this measure has no effect on horses with spinal cord disease. Use a towel and tuck it under the halter where it can be readily grasped and removed. Never tie the blindfold onto the halter!

Remember that patients with LMN disease that still have some voluntary movements will hop or circle rapidly if their weight is supported because their GP is unaffected. This observation may help distinguish between subtle UMN and LMN paresis. When we are presented with a patient that we suspect has LMN paresis, we will hop the patient with and without supporting all the weight on the affected limb or limbs. As already stated, the patient with LMN paresis should know exactly where the limb is located during these postural reactions.

When presented with a recumbent patient, you should pick it up and hold it in a standing position. Get help if the patient is too large for you to handle alone. Use a sling in horses and large farm animals. By holding them in this position and lifting them up and down, you can readily determine the quality of the muscle tone, whether they are hypotonic-flaccid from LMN disease, or hypertonic from spasticity of UMN disease. You can determine whether any voluntary movements are present in the limbs, and while supporting the patient, you can determine the presence and quality of the hopping responses. Muscle tone in recumbent adult horses and cattle is difficult to evaluate, especially in the recumbent limbs.

One might conclude that these postural reactions are relatively nonspecific. This conclusion is absolutely correct. Why then are they useful? First, testing postural reactions acts as a screen for detecting abnormalities in the nervous system. Abnormal responses will be the first clinical sign of any progressive lesion in any part of the central or peripheral nervous system that is involved in limb movement. One or more of these postural reactions may be abnormal before any detectable abnormality in the gait is observed. Second, their importance in localizing lesions is dependent on the results of the rest of the neurologic examination. If the gait is normal in the environment of your examination and one or more of the postural reactions are abnormal in the limbs on one side of the body, a contralateral prosencephalic lesion is strongly suggested. This test is the most useful of the three clinical tests that we use for prosencephalic disorders. If you have a patient with clinical signs of a unilateral vestibular system disorder with a normal gait but the postural reactions are abnormal, then the lesion is in the central components of the vestibular system.

Remember to use terminology that all clinicians can understand. Lesions that affect the UMN pathways also affect the GP pathways; thus when you describe a gait abnormality as paraparesis, also include pelvic limb ataxia. Using hemiparesis and ataxia is preferable when this is visible in the gait. If the gait is normal and the postural reactions are abnormal on one side, describe it that way, and do not refer to this abnormality as hemiparesis. Be sure your reader clearly can understand what you have observed.

Muscle Tone and Size and Spinal Nerve Reflexes

In small animals, examination of these features is performed in the recumbent patient that is gently restrained by an assistant. You can conduct this test unassisted in a cooperative patient by gently kneeling on the patient's neck to hold it in lateral recumbency. For cats, toy breeds, and puppies, you might want to sit on the floor with your back against a wall and your knees held together and flexed. Place the patient with its back resting against your thighs. This position is also useful for the cranial nerve examination.

Flex and extend the limbs on the nonrecumbent side to assess muscle tone, and palpate the muscles again for any indication of atrophy. For the patellar reflex, hold the pelvic limb in partial flexion, and, with the limb as relaxed as possible, lightly strike the patellar ligament with a human pediatric patellar hammer or any blunt instrument. The response is a brisk extension of the stifle. This response can be graded as 2 for normal, 1 for depressed, and 0 for absent; grade 3 is hyperactive, and grade 4 is clonic. A clonic reflex is one that, after the response to a single stimulus, the stifle rapidly relaxes and extends for a brief period, creating a tremor. Grades 3 and 4 occur with UMN lesions. This reflex is the most reliable tendon reflex and determines the integrity of the femoral nerve and the L4, L5, and L6 spinal cord segments. See Chapter 5 for a detailed explanation of spinal nerve reflexes. Always check the patellar reflexes in both limbs while in both recumbencies because, in normal dogs, it will occasionally be absent in one position and not the other. We have no explanation for this phenomenon. Also recall that, in dogs 10 years of age or older, one or both patellar reflexes may be absent with no other neurologic signs present. The presence of normal tone and the lack of any atrophy suggests that the basis for this sign is on the sensory side of the reflex arc, which may involve age-related

sensory neuropathy. However, this suggestion has not been proven. In recumbent horses and cattle, strike the intermediate patellar ligament with the side of your hand.

Other tendon or muscle reflexes elicited by striking the tendon (gastrocnemius muscle—tibial nerve) or muscle (cranial tibial muscle—peroneal nerve) are of limited use because they are not present in all normal small animals. We do not consistently perform these reflexes. Be sure to test the patellar reflexes before the withdrawal reflexes because the latter require a noxious stimulus that may upset your patient.

The withdrawal-flexor reflex is evaluated in both pelvic limbs. This reflex requires an adequate noxious stimulus that differs between species and between individual patients. A pin may be adequate in the standing horse and many cats but not in many dogs. We prefer using tissue forceps because the degree of compression can be adjusted to the individual patient. Compress the skin at the base of the third phalanx of a digit with enough pressure to elicit the reflex and usually a slight conscious response in a normal patient. By increasing the compression of the digit, the stimulus becomes sufficiently noxious to elicit nociception. Your digital pressure is sometimes sufficient, but a pair of tissue forceps is usually more reliable. In horses and farm animals, compress the skin of the coronary band or at the base of the digital pads. Remember that this noxious stimulus tests both the spinal nerve reflex and the pathways in the CNS for nociception. You can have a reflex loss without loss of nociception; therefore you must use care in the amount of pressure that you apply to avoid excessive discomfort to the patient and injury to you by the patient. This withdrawal reflex is a more complex reflex. The sensory neurons tested depend on the digit being tested or the autonomous or cutaneous zone that you select for this noxious stimulus. The motor response involves primarily the sciatic nerve in the pelvic limb, with caudal thigh muscular branches responsible for stifle flexion, the peroneal branch for tarsal flexion, and the tibial nerve branch for digital flexion. Be aware that the flexion of the hip is the responsibility of motor neurons in the femoral nerve and the ventral branches of all the lumbar spinal nerves that innervate the psoas major muscle. An animal with a complete dysfunction of its sciatic nerve can still flex the hip when the medial side of the crusor metatarsus is stimulated. The latter receives sensory innervation from the saphenous nerve branch of the femoral nerve. The spinal cord segments associated with the sciatic nerve are L6, L7, and S1 in small animals and L6, S1, and S2 in horses and farm animals. Remember that these reflexes will still be intact with a transverse lesion cranial to the L4 spinal cord segment, but nociception will be lost in the pelvic limbs. Lesions of peripheral nerves cause both reflex loss and hypalgesia or analgesia. Lesions of the spinal cord tracts cause hypalgesia or analgesia but will spare the reflexes in the limbs caudal to the lesion. As you perform this reflex and observe flexion of the limb that is stimulated, watch the opposite pelvic limb. In some animals with severe UMN dysfunction, you may observe extension of the opposite limb. This reaction is called *cross-extension* and is a clinical sign of release from inhibition and is an abnormal response. Be cautious about your interpretation of spinal nerve reflexes in the recumbent horse or ox. These responses are often absent in the recumbent limb, which has been compressed by the weight of the body in this recumbent position. Nociception may appear to be absent until you use a vigorous stimulus such as an electric cattle prod. In the dog with severe diffuse LMN paralysis caused by polyradiculoneuritis, the only evidence of nociception will be movements of the jaw as the dog attempts to vocalize and movements of the eyes. The same effect occurs in horses and cattle with botulism.

In the thoracic limb, only the withdrawal reflex is reliable. The biceps (musculocutaneous nerve) and triceps (radial nerve) tendon reflexes are not consistently elicited in normal animals. For the biceps reflex, place your finger on the distal portion of the muscle at the elbow, and lightly strike your finger with the hammer and feel the muscle contract or observe a brief elbow flexion. Striking the triceps tendon may elicit a brief elbow extension. Striking the extensor carpi radialis muscle (radial nerve) may elicit a brief carpal extension. Because of the numerous muscles and nerves involved with the withdrawal response from a noxious stimulus of a thoracic limb digit, this evaluation method is a crude test for the entire brachial plexus and the cervical intumescence. The sensory nerve or nerves tested depend on the autonomous or cutaneous zones selected. In small animals, compression of the second or third digits stimulates the sensory components of the radial nerve dorsally and the median and ulnar nerves on the palmar surface. The motor neurons involved are in the axillary nerve (shoulder flexion), musculocutaneous nerve (elbow flexion), and the median and ulnar nerves (carpal and digital flexion).

With your patient still being restrained in lateral recumbency, evaluate the tail and anal tone, and gently pinch the skin of the perineum and observe for a tightening of the anus. This response is the perineal reflex (pudendal nerve, sacral spinal nerves, and sacral spinal cord segments). This reflex is often accompanied by tail flexion (caudal nerves and segments).

Be aware that, in some patients with severe UMN dysfunction, this stimulus may elicit a *mass reflex,* which includes flexion of the pelvic limbs along with the anal closure and tail flexion and occasionally urination.

When this testing is completed, return your patient to a standing position, and perform the cutaneous trunci reflex evaluation. See Fig. 5-9 in Chapter 5. Using your tissue forceps and starting at the level of the sacrum, pinch the skin on the dorsal midline or on either side of the trunk and look for a reflex contraction of the cutaneous trunci muscle. In normal animals, this response will usually be bilateral. Progress cranially with your midline stimulus until a response is elicited or until you determine that it is absent. Some variation exists on where you will first elicit a muscle contraction in normal animals. In most dogs, this contraction will occur by approximately the mid-lumbar level. Sometimes the contraction cannot be elicited in some normal dogs and cats. The forceps compression stimulates the sensory nerves in the dorsal branches of the spinal nerves that innervate the area of skin stimulated. Because of the short caudal distribution of these dorsal branches, each spinal nerve innervates the skin for a distance of approximately two vertebrae caudal to the intervertebral foramen where the spinal nerve emerged from the vertebral canal. The general somatic afferent (GSA) neurons that are stimulated synapse in the respective dorsal gray column on long interneurons, the axons of which enter the adjacent fasciculus proprius bilaterally with a predominance on the contralateral side. Here, these axons course cranially to the C8 and T1 spinal cord segments to terminate in the ventral gray columns by synapsing on the general somatic efferent (GSE) neurons that innervate the cutaneous trunci via the brachial plexus and the lateral

thoracic nerve. Recall that this reflex is absent in injuries that cause an avulsion of the roots of the brachial plexus. In these patients, this reflex will be present only on the side opposite to the injury. This reflex may help locate a transverse thoracolumbar spinal cord lesion where it will be absent when the stimulus is applied caudal to a line that is approximately two vertebrae caudal to the lesion.

At this point in your neurologic examination, if any indication exists of a possible spinal cord dysfunction, carefully palpate the vertebral column for any location of discomfort.

In standing horses and cattle that are able to walk, most spinal nerve reflexes in the limbs will be intact, and no reliable way exists to test if they are depressed or hyperactive.

Cutaneous muscle reflexes can be readily determined by pinching the skin of the neck where the cutaneous colli muscle is innervated by the facial nerve and the skin of the trunk where the cutaneous muscles are innervated by the lateral thoracic nerve. Cutaneous stimulation in the neck of horses induces contraction of the cutaneous colli, as well as ear muscles, resulting in a movement of the ear on the side stimulated. Horses are the species that are most responsive to minimal cutaneous stimulation. In many instances, a pin or the point of a pen or pencil is sufficient to get a response. More vigorous stimulation may be necessary in cattle and other farm animals. Always check the tail and anal tone and perineal reflex by standing beside the pelvic limb and reaching across the area of the hip to elevate the tail and feel the anus. The normal horse anus is very tight compared with many small animals. Be sure to observe and palpate the muscles of the neck, trunk, and limbs on both sides to detect any atrophy that may be present.

Cranial Nerves

The cranial nerve examination should be performed when the patient is the most relaxed. In most cooperative patients, this examination is performed after the examination of the gait and spinal nerve reflexes. With very young animals, the examination is often performed before you handle them at all. When examining a young farm animal, especially a pig that is ambulatory, perform as much of the cranial nerve examination as you can without any restraint. The less restraint you use, the better your examination will be. As soon as you try to restrain young farm animals, the ensuing struggle will make the cranial nerve evaluation very difficult. Puppies and kittens may be wrapped in a towel and placed between your thighs when you sit on the floor with your back against the wall and your knees flexed. This same floor position can be used for toy breeds. For all other small animals and young farm animals, we examine the cranial nerves while standing over the standing patient, similar to when we performed the postural reactions. For horses and cattle and adult Camelidae, stand in front of their heads, with an assistant holding the lead. The cranial nerve examination can be performed by the numbers I through XII or by regions. We prefer the latter method, starting with the eyes, where either part or all of cranial nerves II through VIII are evaluated.

Vision—Menace, Pupils

We always start with the menace response. Cover one eye with your hand. In small patients, use the hand that is holding the head to cover one eye and menace the opposite eye. This reaction is a learned response that may not be developed until 10 or 12 weeks in puppies and kittens and 7 to 10 days in foals and young farm animal species. Before this age, you may be able to assess vision by determining their ability to follow objects moving in their environment. The menace response requires normally functioning eyes, the optic nerves (cranial nerve II), and the central visual pathway to the visual cortex in the occipital lobe, along with an efferent pathway that includes the facial neurons. The majority of this central visual pathway caudal to the optic chiasm is contralateral to the eye being menaced. Some normal patients need a mild stimulus to get a response. We usually tap their orbital or frontal bone region with our hand to arouse their attention and to observe for an intact palpebral reflex to be sure the facial nerve is functioning. In the normal menace response, the menacing gesture elicits eyelid closure. Eyelid closure is dependent on normal facial nerve innervation of the orbicularis oculi. Be careful to avoid touching any part of the face, especially the hair of the eyelids or the long vibrissae (whiskers), and to avoid creating a sudden air movement that might stimulate the skin of the face. This action creates a cranial nerve V-VII reflex. If the menace response is absent, we immediately touch the eyelid to be sure the facial nerve innervation is intact to cause its closure. If facial paralysis is present, then we look for eyeball retraction and third eyelid elevation or head retraction movements to determine if vision is present. Setting up a maze of objects in the patient's environment is sometimes necessary to determine if the animal can see and avoid these objects when walking around them.

Immediately after the menace test, the pupil size and response to light should be evaluated. Most patients have a dark-colored iris, which makes seeing the border of the pupil difficult without some light assistance. Cats with a yellow iris are an exception. You need a bright source of light such as that you get from a new penlight. Initially, hold the light on the midline over the nose just close enough so that you can see the pupillary margins and determine their size and if any anisocoria is present. Then bring the light source as close as possible to one eye without touching the patient's face. If no response occurs, move the light so that it shines on all aspects of the ocular fundus. Quickly swing the light into the opposite eye and observe what happens to that pupil. Then quickly return the light source to the original eye. Keep repeating this swinging light action until you are comfortable with your findings, and record them accurately. To prevent confusion, record what happens in each eye when the light is directed into one eye, and perform this maneuver for both eyes. See how this pupillary light reflex is recorded on the neurologic examination form in this chapter. In the normal patient, the pupil will rapidly constrict when the light is directed into it (the direct response), and the opposite pupil will also constrict without moving the light (the indirect or consensual response). Because of the major axonal crossing that occurs at the optic chiasm and at the level of the pretectal nuclei, light directed into one eye will cause a stimulus that will reach both oculomotor nuclei. The details of this anatomy are described in Chapters 7 and 14. When you swing the light to the opposite eye, the pupil had already constricted from the light directed into the first eye, and it stays constricted. As you repeatedly swing the light back and

forth between the eyes, the pupils remain constricted in the normal animal. The pupillary light responses are the same in horses and farm animals, but the response is slower, especially in adult horses. The process we have described here is the way in which we observe the direct and indirect (consensual) pupillary light responses, but avoid using these terms, which can be confusing to students and clinicians alike. We will sometimes evaluate pupil size in a darkened room to help determine the origin of anisocoria.

Test yourself on the anatomic diagnosis of the following examples of eye examinations. See Chapter 14 for similar case studies and further discussion of the involved anatomy and differential diagnoses. (OS is oculus sinister and refers to the left eye. OD is oculus dextra and refers to the right eye. OU is oculi uterque and refers to both eyes.)

1. A patient has no menace response in OS with a normal palpebral reflex. No anisocoria is observed. Light directed into OS causes no response OU. Light directed into OD causes a normal response OU. As you swing the light from OD where the pupil is constricted back to OS, the OS pupil that was constricted from the stimulation of OD is now dilating back to its original size. This asymmetry is repeated as you swing the light back and forth between the two eyes. When you cover OD with your hand, the OS pupil fully dilates.

Anatomic diagnosis: In OS or the left optic nerve.

In most cases with this anatomic diagnosis, room light entering the normal eye is sufficient to keep the pupil in the affected eye constricted. Occasionally the pupil on the affected side will be slightly larger than the pupil in the unaffected side in room light.

2. A patient has normal menace responses. Anisocoria is present with the pupil in OD widely dilated. Light directed into OD causes the pupil to constrict only in OS. Light directed into OS causes only the OS pupil to constrict.

Anatomic diagnosis: Right oculomotor nerve general visceral efferent (GVE) component, ciliary ganglion, ciliary nerves.

Be aware that this reaction may be the first clinical sign of an extramedullary mass lesion ventral to the diencephalon compressing the oculomotor nerve and causing a loss of function of the GVE preganglionic neurons, which may precede the loss of function in the GSE neurons. This disparity between the altered pupil size without ptosis or strabismus is useful in making an anatomic diagnosis of the different components of the oculomotor nerve.

3. A patient has no menace response OD with a normal palpebral reflex. Anisocoria is present with the OD pupil widely dilated. Light directed into OD causes no response OU. Light directed into OS causes only the OS pupil to constrict.

Anatomic diagnosis: Right optic nerve and the GVE neurons of the right oculomotor nerve, ciliary ganglion, ciliary nerves.

A retrobulbar neoplasm or abscess might produce this result.

4. A patient acts blind and has no menace response OU with normal palpebral reflexes. In room light, the pupils are mildly dilated. Light directed into OS causes the pupils to constrict OU. Light directed into OD causes the pupils to constrict OU. This dog's sensorium is normal.

Anatomic diagnosis: Both eyeballs, optic nerves, optic chiasm, or optic tracts.

Patients with lesions in the retina (retinal degeneration, sudden acquired retinal degeneration) or optic nerves (optic neuritis) OU often lose their vision and are clinically blind but still have light-responsive pupils when a bright light is directed into the eyes. However, room light is insufficient to cause normal constriction, and the pupils will appear mildly dilated. This response can be explained by the disease process sparing the retinal neurons involved with these light responses or, more likely, with progressive loss of function of retinal neurons, the threshold for loss of vision is lower than that for pupillary constriction to light. In other words, the pupillary light reflex neurons are the last to lose function when lesions disrupt the retina or optic nerve.

Anisocoria may result from many intraocular disorders. Iris atrophy is fairly common in older dogs and creates dilated unresponsive pupils with no interference with vision. Be sure to evaluate the iris thoroughly with your bright light source. Neurologic causes of anisocoria include disturbances to cranial nerves II and III and the sympathetic ocular innervation. Examination of the patient in a darkened room may help determine the cause of anisocoria in your patient.

Palpebral Fissure and Third Eyelid

Observe the size of the palpebral fissures and their symmetry. In small animals, the fissure will be smaller with oculomotor nerve dysfunction (loss of function of the levator palpebrae superioris muscle causing ptosis), sympathetic innervation dysfunction (loss of the orbitalis smooth muscle function in the orbit), and secondary to atrophy of the muscles of mastication from dysfunction of the mandibular nerve from the trigeminal nerve or chronic myositis. In the horse and farm animals, a narrow palpebral fissure occurs with facial nerve dysfunction (loss of function of the levator anguli oculi medialis muscle).

An elevated third eyelid will be apparent with sympathetic denervation, as well as secondary to atrophy of the muscles of mastication. The third eyelid elevates in tetanus secondary to the tetanus of the extraocular muscles that results in retraction of the eyeball and in animals with a facial paralysis when they are menaced.

Strabismus

Strabismus is an abnormal position of the eyeball. While examining the eyes, you can appreciate whether they are normally positioned in the orbits. Normal ocular position is dependent on the innervation of the extraocular muscles by cranial nerves III, IV, and VI and the normal function of the vestibular system. Repeatedly move the head in a horizontal (dorsal) plane from one side to the other. Watch the excursions of the eyeballs. The degree of adduction (medial rectus, cranial nerve III) should be the same as the abduction (lateral rectus, cranial nerve VI), which is normal physiologic nystagmus and requires a normal vestibular system. Remember that, in some cats, you will only see this response at the end of the head movement. A ventrolateral strabismus occurs with oculomotor nerve dysfunction, a medial strabismus with abducent nerve dysfunction, and an ocular extorsion with trochlear nerve dysfunction. The last of these abnormalities causes the dorsal aspect of the pupil to rotate laterally in cats and the medial aspect of the pupil to rotate dorsally in horses and farm animals. In dogs, in which the pupil is round, a fundic examination will show a lateral deviation of the retinal vein that emerges from the superior edge of the optic disk and normally courses in a superior direction. A vestibular strabismus is usually ventrolateral and is present only in some positions of the head. Testing physiologic nystagmus will confirm the normal ability to adduct the eye, which is a function of the oculomotor nerve.

Nystagmus

Nystagmus is an involuntary oscillation of the eyeball. In normal animals, a jerk nystagmus occurs when the head is moved rapidly. This normal physiologic nystagmus was observed when the eyes were examined for the function of cranial nerves III and VI. Abnormal nystagmus occurs with dysfunction of the vestibular system. In severe cases, it is continual and is observed when the head is resting in its normal posture, as well as in any change of the head position. This disorder is a resting or spontaneous nystagmus. In less severe and chronic disorders, the abnormal nystagmus may be seen only when the head is held in different positions. This disorder is called a positional nystagmus. While you are holding the head in its normal resting position, look at the eyes for any resting nystagmus. To facilitate this, use one hand to pull the facial muscles caudally enough so that the retraction of the eyelids will expose the limbus of the eye to better observe it for any abnormal nystagmus. Move the head laterally to one side, hold it there, and observe for any development of a positional nystagmus. Repeat this maneuver on holding the head directed to the opposite side. Then hold the head and neck in extension and observe for any positional nystagmus. If you are suspicious of subtle vestibular system dysfunction and you have not observed any abnormal nystagmus with the head held in a laterally flexed or dorsally extended position, place the patient on its back. Extend the patient's head and neck, and look for any positional nystagmus. Be sure to record the direction of the abnormal nystagmus, as well as the plane of rotation. The direction is defined as the direction of the quick phase of the jerk nystagmus. The plane of rotation may be horizontal, rotatory, or vertical. As a rule, a consistently vertical nystagmus with no rotatory component indicates involvement of the central components of the vestibular system. Look for possible change in this direction with different positions of the head. Recall that with peripheral vestibular system disorders, the nystagmus is always directed away from the side of the lesion and is in either a horizontal plane or is rotatory. If the direction of the nystagmus changes with different head positions, then a disorder of the central components of the vestibular system is present. When you have the head and neck in extension, look at the position of the eyeballs, without retracting the eyelids, to observe in small animals that both eyeballs have also elevated and are still centered in the palpebral fissure and no sclera is exposed dorsal to the limbus. Sclera that is exposed dorsally indicates inadequate elevation of the eyeball and either an oculomotor nerve dysfunction or a vestibular system dysfunction; the latter disorder is a vestibular strabismus. With vestibular strabismus, this eyeball deviation is present only in some head positions, and the eyeball adducts normally when physiologic nystagmus is examined. In normal horses and farm animals, the eyeballs do not elevate completely when the head and neck are extended so that normally some sclera is exposed dorsal to the eyeballs on this maneuver and it is the same degree for both eyeballs.

Facial and Trigeminal Neurons

Up to this point in your cranial nerve examination, all of your evaluations have been directed at the eyes and orbital structures. Some of these evaluations have involved part of the innervation that is dependent on normal facial and trigeminal nerve function. At this point, we reevaluate all of the facial and trigeminal nerve functions that are practical. For the facial nerve, repeat the palpebral reflex (cranial nerves V and VII) by touching both corners of the eyelids for each eye. The sensory nerves are branches of both the ophthalmic and maxillary nerves from the trigeminal nerve and the closure of the fissure is a function of the palpebral branch of the facial nerve. Observe the symmetry of the face. In facial nerve paralysis, the ear will be drooped in all horses and the farm animals that have normally erect ears. The erect ears of all cats, some breeds of dogs, and those dogs that have had ear crop surgery will not droop with facial paralysis because of the rigidity of the auricular cartilage. You will feel atonia when you palpate the ear, and the ear will not move when the skin of the ear canal is stimulated with your forceps or by blowing in the ear. In horses, you will observe a marked deviation of the nose and upper lip directed toward the normally innervated side. This deviation will also be present in all the farm animals, except for the ox, in which the large planum nasolabiale prevents this deviation. In all domestic animals, you may be able to palpate the loss of tone in the lips, and, in many of them, you may observe a droop of the lips. In small animals, elevate the head and observe the lips at the angle of the mouth. More lip mucosa may be exposed on the denervated side, and the animal may tend to drool on that side. In sheep, goats, and the Camelidae, you may see a deviation of the philtrum toward the normal side. Be aware that a deviated philtrum in a dog is most likely the result of tetany of the facial muscles on the side to which the philtrum is directed. Facial paralysis does not cause a deviation of the philtrum in dogs and cats. This hemifacial tetanus can be confirmed with the aid of anesthesia, as described in Chapter 6. In older literature, this observation is known as hemifacial spasm, which is a misnomer. For the trigeminal nerve, palpate the muscles of mastication for any denervation atrophy caused by dysfunction of the mandibular nerve from the trigeminal nerve. The only evidence of unilateral loss of function of the mandibular nerve from the trigeminal nerve will be unilateral atrophy of the muscles of mastication. Be sure to palpate for this atrophy because you will not see it in breeds with a thick hair coat, such as an Old English sheepdog. No clinical evidence of any loss of jaw function will be observed; they can still bite vigorously. A dropped jaw that the patient cannot move

requires dysfunction of both mandibular nerves from the trigeminal nerves. The observation of a dropped jaw is sometimes aided by holding only the upper jaw and associated lips elevated and observing the gap created by the inability to elevate the lower jaw to close the mouth. Place the blunt end of your tissue forceps against the nasal septum. The normal patient will immediately move its head away from the stimulus. This action tests two anatomic pathways. One is the integrity of the ipsilateral branch of the ophthalmic nerve from the trigeminal nerve that innervates the mucosa of the nasal septum. The other is the nociceptive pathway that projects predominantly to the opposite side of the rostral brainstem and the somesthetic cortex of the opposite cerebral hemisphere. Recall that this evaluation is one of the three clinical examinations that we routinely use for prosencephalic dysfunction. We do not routinely check the autonomous zones of the other two branches of the trigeminal nerve.

Cranial Nerves IX, X, and XII

Cranial nerves IX, X, and XII are examined together with the so-called gag reflex. This examination is performed rapidly because the patient usually objects to the manipulation that is necessary, especially cats. Grasp the upper jaw with one hand and pull down on the lower jaw with the other hand to open the mouth. The resistance felt is the result of the function of the muscles that close the mouth that are innervated by the mandibular nerves from the trigeminal nerves. Quickly look at the surface of the tongue for its size and any movement that is present. Push the tongue with your finger and observe for any movement. This maneuver evaluates the hypoglossal nerve (cranial nerve XII) function. Then insert your finger through the oral cavity into the oropharynx and laryngopharynx. Feel for the muscle tone and evaluate the patient's sensory response to this maneuver. This response is the gag reflex. Muscle tone and the gag reflex are predominantly functions of the pharyngeal branches of the glossopharyngeal (IX) and vagal (X) nerves. This assessment of the gag reflex is difficult to evaluate and is usually quite subjective. A more reliable indication of dysphagia usually comes in the form of a complaint by the owner as they watch their animal eating and drinking. In the horse and farm animals, this examination is limited to an assessment of the size and strength of the tongue (cranial nerve XII). Carefully reach into the mouth from the side and grasp and extract the tongue. Evaluate the patient's resistance to this and the size of the tongue. It is much more difficult to do this in cattle than the other species. In horses, do not be too vigorous or you may injure the tongue. These functions can be assessed by watching the patient prehend and swallow food.

We do not routinely test for olfaction or hearing because they are difficult to evaluate objectively, especially when they are incomplete. The owner's observation of their animal's behavior is more reliable for disorders of these functions. Brainstem auditory-evoked potential (BAER) testing is the most reliable way to evaluate hearing function, especially with unilateral disorders. Tests for olfaction have been described.

Order of the Cranial Nerve Examination

Menace response:
  Cranial nerve II—central visual pathway to the occipital lobe; cranial nerve VII—for closure of the palpebral fissure
Pupil size and light response:
  Cranial nerve II—rostral brainstem; cranial nerve III (GVE)—ciliary ganglion; ciliary nerves for pupil constriction—direct and indirect
Eye position:
  Strabismus: cranial nerve III (GSE)—ventrolateral; cranial nerve IV—extorsion; cranial nerve VI—medial; cranial nerve VIII (vestibular)—ventrolateral
Eye movements:
  Normal physiologic (vestibuloocular) nystagmus: cranial nerve VIII (vestibular)—brainstem—MLF; cranial nerve VI for abduction and cranial nerve III (GSE) for adduction
  Abnormal nystagmus: cranial nerve VIII (vestibular) and central vestibular components

Palpebral fissure size:
  Cranial nerve III (GSE), cranial nerve VII (horse and farm animals), sympathetic nerves, cranial nerve V—atrophy of masticatory muscles
Third eyelid:
  Sympathetic nerves: cranial nerve V—atrophy of muscles of mastication, tetanus; facial paralysis when menaced
Cranial nerve VII:
  Facial muscles: position, tone and movement of eyelids, ears, lips and nose; menace response (II-VII); palpebral reflex (V-VII)
Cranial nerve V:
  Muscles of mastication: jaw function, atrophy
  Sensory: palpebral reflex (V-VII); nasal septum for nociception; autonomous zones of three branches
Cranial nerves V, IX, X, and XII:
  Gag reflex: jaw tone (V), tongue size and movement (XII), gagging, and swallowing (IX, X)

GSE, General somatic efferent; *GVE,* general visceral efferent; *MLF,* medial longitudinal fasciculus.

 ## SUMMARY OF CLINICAL SIGNS AT SPECIFIC CNS LOCATIONS

Spinal Cord

Lumbosacral: Fourth Lumbar Through Caudal Segments

Complete dysfunction from the L4 to the last caudal segment
  Flaccid paraplegia: no weight support and no voluntary movement of the pelvic limbs, except for slight hip flexion, and no tail movement
  No pelvic limb postural reactions
  Normal thoracic limbs
  Neurogenic atrophy in nonacute cases
  Atonia: pelvic limbs, anus, and tail; dilated anus
  Areflexia: patellar, flexor, and perineal reflexes
  Analgesia: pelvic limbs, anus, perineum, tail, and penis
Partial dysfunction of gray and white matter from the L4 to the last caudal segment
  Flaccid paraparesis and ataxia of the pelvic limbs
  Postural reactions in the pelvic limbs attempted but abnormal
  Normal thoracic limbs
  Mild neurogenic atrophy in nonacute cases
  Hypotonia or normal tone in the pelvic limbs, anus, and tail
  Hyporeflexia or areflexia of patellar, flexor, and perineal reflexes
  Hypalgesia or normal nociception in pelvic limbs, perineum, and tail

Thoracolumbar: Third Thoracic Through Third Lumbar Spinal Cord Segments

Complete dysfunction at a focal site between the T3 and L3 spinal cord segments

  Spastic paraplegia with reflex support if held up in a standing position but no voluntary pelvic limb or tail movement
  No pelvic limb postural reactions
  Normal thoracic limbs; with peracute transverse lesions, the thoracic limbs hypertonic and held in extension when in lateral recumbency (the Schiff-Sherrington syndrome); with cranial thoracic spinal cord lesions, difficulty standing up on thoracic limbs from a recumbent position, loss of trunk support when the patient is suspended by the base of the tail and made to walk on its thoracic limbs; and trunk swaying abnormally to either side
  No neurogenic atrophy
  Hypertonia (spasticity) or normal tone in the pelvic limbs
  Hyperactive or normal reflexes: patellar (+3, +2) and flexor
  Occasionally repeated flexor responses to one stimulus, crossed extensor reflexes, or both
  Analgesia caudal to the level of the lesion by approximately two spinal cord segments
  Absent cutaneous trunci reflex caudal to the level of the lesion by approximately two spinal cord segments
  Unilateral lesions cause ipsilateral paralysis and contralateral hypalgesia and decreased cutaneous trunci reflex
Partial dysfunction of gray and white matter at a focal site between the T3 and L3 spinal cord segments
  Spastic paraparesis and pelvic limb ataxia
  Postural reactions attempted but abnormal in the pelvic limbs
  Normal thoracic limbs
  No neurogenic atrophy
  Hypertonia (spasticity) or normal tone in the pelvic limbs
  Hyperactive or normal reflexes in the pelvic limbs: patellar reflexes (+3, +2); normal or hyperactive flexor reflexes with occasional cross extension

Hypalgesia or normal nociception caudal to the level of the lesion—possible decreased cutaneous trunci relflex

Unilateral lesions cause ipsilateral limb movement and spinal reflex clinical signs, contralateral hypalgssia, and decreased cutaneous trunci reflex

Note: Lesions that only affect the white matter from the L4 to the L6 or L7 spinal cord segments may produce similar clinical signs.

Caudocervical: Sixth Cervical Through Second Thoracic Spinal Cord Segments

Complete dysfunction of these segments possibly causing death from the loss of respiratory function

Partial dysfunction of gray and white matter from the C6 to the T2 spinal cord segments

Tetraparesis and ataxia of all four limbs or nonambulatory tetraparesis or tetraplegia; thoracic limb deficits possibly worse resulting from their loss of ability to support weight; short strides in the thoracic limbs with long, ataxic strides in the pelvic limbs—a *two-engine* gait; postural reactions attempted if not tetraplegic and are abnormal in all four limbs; thoracic limb responses possibly worse

Thoracic limb neurogenic atrophy with nonacute lesions

Hypotonia or normal tone in the thoracic limbs and hypertonia or normal tone in the pelvic limbs

Hyporeflexia or areflexia in the thoracic limbs and hyperactive or normal reflexes in the pelvic limbs; crossed extension possibly occurring in the pelvic limbs; lesions confined to the white matter at this location having normal to hyperactive thoracic limb reflexes

Hypalgesia or normal nociception in all four limbs or only hypalgesia in the thoracic limbs

Miosis, ptosis, protruded third eyelid, and enophthalmos with lesions from T1 to T3

Unilateral lesions causing ipsilateral clinical signs

Craniocervical: First Cervical Through Fifth Cervical Spinal Cord Segments

Complete dysfunction at a focal site between these segments causing death from the loss of respiratory function

Partial dysfunction of gray and white matter at a focal site between the C1 and C5 spinal cord segments

Spastic tetraparesis and ataxia of all four limbs or nonambulatory spastic tetraparesis or spastic tetraplegia; recumbent patients when held up exhibiting hypertonia and supporting their weight by hyperactive extensor muscle tone in all limbs, which differentiates them from patients that are tetraplegic from diffuse neuromuscular disorders that have a flaccid tetraparesis or tetraplegia and are atonic in all their neck, trunk, and limb muscles

Postural reactions abnormal in all four limbs, if they are performed at all

No neurogenic muscle atrophy

Hyperactive or normal reflexes in all four limbs; crossed extension possibly occurring with the flexor reflexes

Hypalgesia possibly caudal to the level of the focal lesion but is rarely determined

Unilateral lesions causing ipsilateral clinical signs

Medulla and Pons

Spastic tetraparesis and ataxia of all four limbs or nonambulatory spastic tetraparesis or spastic tetraplegia

Unilateral lesions causing ipsilateral clinical signs

Depression, irregular respirations, hypalgesia of trunk and limbs

Central vestibular signs; facial hypalgesia or analgesia (cranial nerve V); inability to close mouth, atrophy of masticatory muscles (cranial nerve V); facial paresis or paralysis (cranial nerve VII); medial strabismus (cranial nerve VI); dysphagia (cranial nerves IX, X, and XI); tongue paresis, atrophy (cranial nerve XII)

Cerebellum

Spasticity, hypermetric ataxia with support preserved, balance loss, abnormal nystagmus, head and neck tremor and menace deficit; unilateral lesions causing ipsilateral clinical signs except for the paradoxical vestibular syndrome; severe rostral lesions causing opisthotonus and extensor rigidity of all four limbs with flexed hips (decerebellate rigidity)

Mesencephalon

Opisthotonus with extensor rigidity of all four limbs (decerebrate rigidity)

Mild spastic tetraparesis and ataxia of all four limbs; unilateral lesions possibly causing mild spastic hemiparesis and ataxia ipsilateral or contralateral to the lesion

Depression to coma; hypalgesia of head, neck, trunk, and limbs; extorsion strabismus (cranial nerve IV); ventrolateral strabismus and ptosis (cranial nerve III—GSE); mydriasis (cranial nerve III—GVE); head and neck deviated to one side (pleurothotonus); propulsive pacing or circling

Diencephalon

Normal gait with nonperacute bilateral lesions but slow postural reactions bilaterally; blind with dilated unresponsive pupils (optic chiasm, optic tracts)

Total-body hypalgesia (thalamic direct cortical projection nuclei); unilateral lesions causing contralateral postural reaction deficits, hypalgesia, and menace deficit with normal pupillary light responses; depression to coma (ARAS); propulsive circling usually toward the lesion, abnormal behavior; seizures; clinical signs of dysfunction of the hypothalamo-hypophyseal system; alterations in thermoregulation, appetite, and thirst

Occasionally, vestibular signs with acute thalamic lesions

Telencephalon

Seizures; abnormal behavior; propulsive activity; abnormal head and neck postures; movement disorders; depression to semicoma; normal gait in nonperacute disorders but slow postural reactions bilaterally; blind with normal pupillary light responses; bilateral hypalgesia of entire body; unilateral lesions causing contralateral postural reaction deficits, vision loss, and hypalgesia; occasionally, slight facial, tongue, and pharyngeal paresis (cranial nerve UMN) (Table 20-1).

TABLE 20-1 Relationship of Clinical Signs to Anatomic Site of Central Nervous System Lesion

Clinical Sign	Functional System	Anatomic Location
Inability to prehend	Masticatory and tongue muscles	Cranial nerves V, XII, pons, and medulla
Dysphagia	Tongue, palatal, pharyngeal esophageal muscles	Cranial nerves IX, X, XI, XII, medulla
Drooling	Facial paralysis	Cranial nerve VII, middle ear, medulla
	Dysphagia	Cranial nerves IX, X, XI, XII, medulla
Head tilt, balance loss, abnormal nystagmus	Vestibular system	Inner ear, pons, medulla, cerebellum; rarely thalamus
Rolling	Vestibular system	Pons, medulla, cerebellum
Strabismus	Extraocular muscles	Cranial nerves III, IV, VI, midbrain, medulla
	Vestibular system	Inner ear, pons, medulla, cerebellum
Circling (with balance loss)	Vestibular system	Inner ear, pons, medulla, cerebellum; rarely thalamus
Circling (propulsive)	Basal nuclei, limbic system	Prosencephalon (midbrain)
Lateral head and eye, deviation, pacing, head pressing	Basal nuclei, limbic system	Prosencephalon (midbrain)
Opisthotonus	UMN	Midbrain, rostral cerebellum
Bradycardia, hypothermia, hyperthermia	UMN for autonomic GVE system	Hypothalamus
Polydipsia, polyuria	Endocrine system	Hypothalamus, hypophysis
Irregular, ataxic respirations	UMN for respiratory muscle LMN control	Pons, medulla

GVE, General visceral efferent; *LMN*, lower motor neuron; *UMN*, upper motor neuron.

CONCLUSION

The neurologic examination provides you with the anatomic diagnosis. The differential diagnosis depends entirely on the anatomic diagnosis. The disorders considered must be able to cause dysfunction of the components of your anatomic diagnosis. The ancillary studies to be considered will depend on the priority order that you have established for the disorders in your differential diagnosis based on the signalment and history of the disorder in your patient.

21 CASE DESCRIPTIONS

This chapter was written for the second edition of this textbook, and despite the change for this third edition to a case-based format throughout the book, we decided to retain most of this chapter in its original form and have added a few new *bonus* cases. Consider this chapter a test of what you have learned from the preceding chapters. The format is the same as that used for the case examples throughout the book. You must appreciate that magnetic resonance (MR) and computed tomographic (CT) imaging were not available when many of the patients in the original case descriptions were studied.

CASE EXAMPLE 21-1

Signalment: 4-year-old female Great Dane mixed breed

Chief Complaint: Abnormal gait

History: Starting 5 months before this examination, this dog had episodes of coughing and gasping. Repeated examinations during this time did not result in a definitive diagnosis. The owner commented that the dog's eyes looked different during this time period. One month before this examination, the referring veterinarian noted anisocoria with a smaller left pupil. Approximately 10 days before this examination, the dog began to stumble with the pelvic limbs and developed a left head tilt.

Examination: The dog was alert and responsive but acted disoriented. Her head was tilted to the left. She was reluctant to stand but could do so unassisted and then leaned against the wall on her left side. When excited, she nearly fell over toward her left side. The gait was normal except for the balance problem.

Postural reactions were difficult to test because of the patient's disorientation and her frantic struggling when picked up to perform these tests. However, hopping in the left pelvic limb was definitely slow.

Hypertonia was marked in the thoracic limbs and mild in the pelvic limbs. No muscle atrophy was observed. Patellar reflexes were hyperactive (+3) bilaterally. Biceps and triceps reflexes were present. Flexor reflexes and the perineal reflex were all normal, as was nociception.

On cranial nerve examination, menace responses were normal, but the left pupil was smaller than the right pupil in room light and during the normal pupillary light reflexes. A smaller left palpebral fissure and a slight protrusion of the left third eyelid were observed. The head was tilted to the left (left ear more ventral). On holding the head and neck in extension, the left eyeball did not elevate normally in the palpebral fissure and when held in this position, a rotatory nystagmus occurred directed to the right side. Physiologic nystagmus was normal. Moderate muscle atrophy was observed on the left side of the tongue. The gag reflex was normal.

Anatomic Diagnosis: These clinical signs indicate a caudal brainstem lesion on the left side involving predominantly the region of the medulla. The clinical signs of a vestibular system disorder were severe (head tilt, body leaning significantly to the left, strabismus, and abnormal nystagmus). The degree of severity suggested a disorder of the central components of the vestibular system. This evidence was supported by the abnormal postural reactions in the left pelvic limb and the dysfunction of the left hypoglossal neurons. These dysfunctions cannot occur with middle- and inner-ear disorders that often cause clinical signs of vestibular system dysfunction. The clinical signs of Horner syndrome (miosis, protruded third eyelid, and smaller palpebral fissure) were the result of a loss of sympathetic innervation of orbital structures. Horner syndrome can occur with middle-ear disease. It is unlikely for it to be caused by a lesion affecting the upper motor neuron (UMN) tracts that course through the medulla that control the sympathetic lower motor neuron (LMN) without a significant left-side hemiparesis and ataxia. Be aware that Horner syndrome may be caused by a LMN involvement anywhere from the T1-T3 spinal nerve ventral roots to the orbital smooth muscle, and it may be a separate neurologic problem. The history of coughing and gagging suggested paresis of the pharyngeal muscles and might occur with dysfunction of the pharyngeal branches of cranial nerves IX and X on one side or their origin in nucleus ambiguus in the medulla. Dysphagia would not accompany an otitis media.

Differential Diagnosis: Neoplasm; inflammation—abscess, granulomatous meningoencephalitis; epidermoid-dermoid cyst

If the earliest observations of gagging, coughing, and anisocoria were reliable, they suggest involvement of the nerves responsible for these clinical signs long before any clinical signs of vestibular system or brainstem dysfunction. Clinical signs of brainstem dysfunction occurred later in the progression of the disease process and would be best explained by an extramedullary or possibly extracranial mass lesion involving the pharyngeal branches of cranial nerves IX and X and the sympathetic trunk or the cranial cervical ganglion, which then expanded into the cranial cavity and compressed the left side of the medulla. The failure to observe any facial paresis indicated that the lesion should be caudal to the internal acoustic meatus. In the medulla, the vestibular nuclei extend further caudal than the facial nucleus, where they might be affected by a compressing mass at that level.

Inflammations in the medulla of the dog do not commonly cause such specific cranial nerve deficits. An abscess at this level would most likely result from the intracranial extension of a suppurative otitis media-interna, and the history and clinical signs did not support the diagnosis of an otitis. In addition, you would expect this lesion to also cause a facial paralysis. The focal form of granulomatous meningoencephalitis (GME) often occurs in the caudal brainstem, cerebellum, or both. This lesion would not readily explain the initial clinical signs of partial dysphagia or the anisocoria. These clinical signs are best explained by an extracranial lesion in the vicinity of the tympanooccipital fissure. The caudal fossa is a site where congenital epidermoid or dermoid cysts are most common, but they would not be expected to cause the asymmetric cranial nerve clinical signs observed in this dog. Degenerative disorders were not considered because of the anatomic diagnosis.

Ancillary Studies: Cerebellomedullary cerebrospinal fluid (CSF) contained no leucocytes and 71 mg/dl of protein (normal <25). The protein level suggested some noninflammatory disruption of the blood-brain barrier in the central nervous system (CNS). Skull and neck radiographs were normal. A slight uptake of radioisotope occurred on the left side of the caudal cranial fossa on scintigraphy. These ancillary studies were compatible with our presumptive diagnosis of an extramedullary neoplasm.

Outcome: After administering anesthesia for the ancillary studies, the clinical signs of vestibular system dysfunction were remarkably exacerbated. The dog was recumbent and continually attempted to roll to its left side, which indicated more severe disturbance of the vestibular system in the medulla. This medullary location was further supported by the deficient hopping responses in the left limbs when the dog was held up. The prognosis was poor without surgical intervention and very guarded with it; thus the decision was made for euthanasia.

Necropsy revealed marked enlargement of the vagosympathetic trunk in the cranial cervical region. This enlargement included the distal ganglion of the vagus nerve and the cranial cervical ganglion (Fig. 21-1). This nerve enlargement extended into the cranial cavity through the tympanooccipital fissure and jugular foramen. Within the cranial cavity, this mass measured 14 mm in diameter and compressed the medulla caudal to the trapezoid body and cranial nerves VII and VIII (Figs. 21-2, 21-3). The intracranial portion of the hypoglossal and accessory nerves were distended with neoplasm. Cranial nerves IX and X were directly involved with the neoplasm. On microscopic examination, the

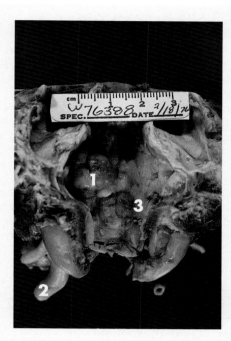

FIGURE 21-2 Dorsal view of the caudal cranial fossa of the skull in Fig. 21-1. The neoplasm (1) on the left is continuous through the jugular foramen and tympanooccipital fissure with the enlarged vagosympathetic trunk (2) and associated ganglia seen in Fig. 21-1. Note the normal jugular foramen (3) with branches of cranial nerves IX, X, and XI in it.

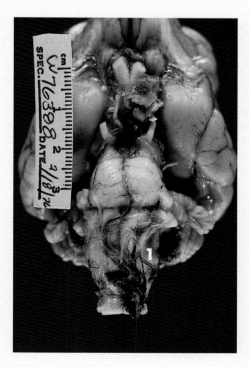

FIGURE 21-3 Ventral surface of the preserved brain of the Great Dane mixed breed in this case example. Note the depression on the left side of the medulla (1) just caudal to the vestibulocochlear nerve and trapezoid body caused by the neoplasm seen in Fig. 21-2.

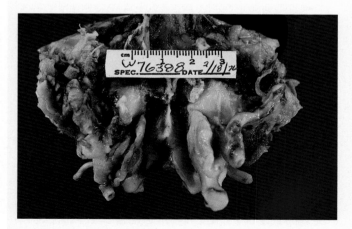

FIGURE 21-1 Ventral surface of the preserved caudal skull of the Great Dane mixed breed in this case example. The tympanic bullae (1) have been exposed. Note the enlarged left vagosympathetic trunk (2) and the associated ganglia (3) caused by the proliferation of a malignant nerve sheath neoplasm.

(Continued)

CASE EXAMPLE 21-1—cont'd

neoplasm was diagnosed as a malignant nerve sheath neoplasm. This neoplasm more commonly affects the trigeminal nerve in our experience and results in unilateral atrophy of the muscles of mastication.

The course of the clinical signs, with the sympathetic and pharyngeal nerves being the first presumed to be involved, is highly suggestive that the neoplasm began outside the cranial cavity in the region of the tympanooccipital fissure. This suggestion is further supported by the late onset of the vestibular system dysfunction. No indication was found as to when the hypoglossal involvement began because this information would have required direct visualization of the hemiatrophy of the tongue. The involvement of the intracranial portion of the accessory nerve, the extracranial portion of the vagus nerve, or both may also have

caused a left laryngeal hemiparesis, which might have contributed to the coughing seen initially.

Remember that Horner syndrome can be caused by lesions in a wide range of anatomic locations. The presence of other clinical signs of neurologic dysfunction usually determines the site of the lesion in the sympathetic system. Dogs with persistent choking, gagging, or coughing for which no explanation can be found in the pharynx should be evaluated for a possible partial paralysis of the pharyngeal muscles. If paralysis is suspected, remember to palpate the area of the tympanooccipital fissure through the dorsolateral wall of the laryngopharynx via the mouth. The mass in this dog may have been palpated antemortem if paralysis had been suspected. CT or MR imaging would facilitate detection of this mass lesion but would not likely have altered the long-term outcome.

CASE EXAMPLE 21-2

Signalment: 11-year-old female collie

Chief Complaint: Inability to use the pelvic limbs

History: Ten days before the examination, this dog became lame in the left thoracic limb. One week later, she began to drag the left pelvic limb, and within 3 days, she became recumbent in the pelvic limbs and unable to stand up with either pelvic limb.

Examination: This collie had been recumbent for the entire day before this examination. She lay in lateral recumbency and was unable to assume a sternal position. When held up and supported by the trunk and tail, she walked on the thoracic limbs with short stiff strides. She was paraplegic (grade 0) and dragged the motionless stiff pelvic limbs. The trunk had to be supported, otherwise she would sway to the side and fall. No postural reactions were observed in the pelvic limbs. The right thoracic limb was stiff but hopped normally. The left thoracic limb hopped slowly with a mild delay in the onset of protraction. Both pelvic limbs and the right thoracic limb were hypertonic. The left thoracic limb was hypotonic, and most of its muscles were mildly atrophied. Both patellar reflexes were brisk (+3). The flexor reflexes were normal in all four limbs. Nociception was depressed in the pelvic limbs (hypalgesia) but normal in the thoracic limbs. Testing for nociception along the trunk revealed a suspicious line in the cranial thoracic region with hypalgesia caudal to it. On cranial nerve examination, the only abnormalities involved the left orbit, where slight miosis, protrusion of the third eyelid, and a smaller palpebral fissure were seen.

Anatomic Diagnosis: Cranial thoracic spinal cord lesion that is functionally transverse at T3 and extends cranially on the left side into the cervical intumescence. The nearly transverse lesion at T3 is the cause of the paraplegia and the loss of trunk strength (UMN paresis), causing it to sway unless supported. Partial involvement of the left side of the T2 and T1 spinal cord segments or ventral roots along with the T3 lesion is the cause of the left-side Horner syndrome. Partial involvement of the left side of the T1 and C8 spinal cord segments or ventral roots is the cause of the mild left thoracic limb deficit and muscle atrophy.

Differential Diagnosis: Neoplasm—nerve sheath, meningioma, metastatic, glioma; intervertebral disk extrusion-protrusion; inflammation

The localizing clinical signs, their asymmetry, and the progressive course are all supportive of a presumptive diagnosis of an extramedullary neoplasm compressing the spinal cord. Extramedullary

neoplasms are more common than intramedullary neoplasms and are more likely to cause asymmetric clinical signs as observed here.

Nerve sheath neoplasms commonly affect spinal nerves and occasionally the sympathetic trunk and often extend into the vertebral canal and compress the spinal cord. If the sympathetic trunk were involved with a nerve sheath tumor at the level of the cervicothoracic ganglion, Horner syndrome would have preceded the clinical signs of spinal cord involvement. A vertebral body or epidural metastasis at this site might also explain the clinical signs. Extramedullary neoplasms may grow slowly to substantial size and slowly compress the spinal cord without causing any clinical signs. The amount of compression that can occur is quite extraordinary, as long as the process is very slow. However, a critical point apparently exists in the ability of the CNS autoregulation that maintains normal spinal cord perfusion to function, and when this limit is surpassed, ischemia occurs with an abrupt onset of clinical signs that rapidly progress. Anesthesia for ancillary studies of these patients may precipitate the loss of autoregulation and result in the presence of more severe clinical signs after recovery from the anesthesia.

Intervertebral disk extrusion-protrusion is uncommon in the cranial thoracic vertebral column and would be less likely to cause the asymmetric thoracic limb clinical signs. Of the various inflammations that affect the spinal cord, focal granulomatous meningomyelitis, or a focal fungal myelitis would be the most likely candidates. Most viral or rickettsial infections cause multifocal or diffuse lesions. Vascular compromise such as fibrocartilaginous embolic myelopathy (FCEM) was not considered because of the progressive nature of the clinical signs.

Ancillary Procedures: Radiographs were normal. A lumbar myelogram showed the contrast to stop abruptly at the caudal aspect of the body of T2, where a small amount of contrast escaped from the subarachnoid space, and the vertebral canal to appear dorsally adjacent to the spine of T3 and ventrally along the ventral aspect of the vertebral body of T2. The lumbar CSF contained no leucocytes and 31 mg/dl of protein (normal <25). These findings were considered to be supportive of the presumptive diagnosis of an extramedullary neoplasm and compressive myelopathy.

Outcome: Exploratory surgery was recommended. However, based on the age of the dog and the severity of the clinical signs, the owner elected euthanasia.

At necropsy, a large firm nodular mass was found in the thorax on the surface of the left longus colli muscle involving the cranial aspect of the thoracic sympathetic trunk and left cervicothoracic ganglion. The mass extended dorsally between the first two ribs and entered the vertebral canal through the intervertebral foramen between the first and second thoracic vertebrae. It compressed the left first thoracic spinal nerve and expanded into the epidural space where it compressed the spinal cord to the right side (Fig. 21-4). The second and especially the third spinal cord segments were the most compressed. The third thoracic spinal cord segment was compressed to less than one half of its normal width. On microscopic examination this neoplasm was diagnosed as a malignant nerve sheath neoplasm.

This case emphasizes the importance of doing a complete neurologic examination regardless of the chief complaint. Recognition of Horner syndrome was especially of value in localizing the level of the lesion in the spinal cord of this dog. This syndrome probably occurred before the gait deficit if it can be assumed that the sympathetic trunk and cervicothoracic ganglion were affected by the neoplasm initially before the neoplasm extended into the vertebral canal. Most extramedullary spinal cord neoplasms are good candidates for surgical removal. However, recurrence is common for this nerve sheath neoplasm, given that removing all the neoplastic cells is impossible. Surgery or radiation therapy would not likely have significantly altered the long-term outcome in this dog given the location of the lesion in

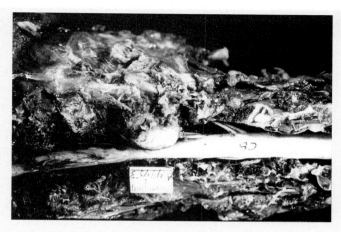

FIGURE 21-4 Necropsy dissection of the collie in this case example to show the malignant nerve sheath neoplasm in the epidural space compressing the left first thoracic spinal nerve roots and the second and third thoracic spinal cord segments.

the thoracic sympathetic trunk and the relatively aggressive nature of this particular neoplasm. These types of neoplasms are readily identified by CT or MR imaging. See Video 7-2 and Case Example 7-1 for a similar disorder.

CASE EXAMPLE 21-3

Signalment: 8-year-old male coonhound mixed breed
Chief Complaint: Unable to stand up
History: Approximately 4 weeks before the examination, this dog was noticed to be slow on treeing a raccoon. This slow reaction occurred 1 month after the dog had been bitten by a raccoon. The dog continued to slow down when hunting and then exhibited a persistent abnormal gait that progressively worsened. Six days before the examination, the dog became recumbent and was unable to stand up without assistance.

Examination: See Video 8-1. This dog was considered to be mildly depressed. He was unable to stand unassisted. When held up, he veered off to the right side and made slow walking attempts with stiff awkward movements as he leaned to the right side. The limbs were markedly hypertonic (spastic), and his ability to support weight was unimpaired. However, he acted very disoriented. The head was tilted to the right, and the neck was curved, with the concavity on the right side (pleurothotonus). He would occasionally exhibit an opisthotonic head and neck posture with the thoracic limbs extended and the pelvic limbs extended but usually flexed at the hips. The trunk often weaved from side to side, and a mild head tremor was evident.

The dog had to be held up to test the postural reactions. The hopping responses were slow in all four limbs but were slower in the left limbs. He fell when hemiwalking was attempted with the left limbs. Paw replacement was absent with the left paws.

He preferred to lie in left lateral recumbency. All the limbs were hypertonic, but hypertonia was worse in the left limbs when he was

placed in right lateral recumbency. No muscle atrophy was observed. Patellar reflexes were brisk (+3). All flexor reflexes were normal, as was the perineal reflex. Nociception was normal.

On cranial nerve examination, the only abnormalities were referable to the vestibular system. A right head tilt was seen. On neck extension, a rotatory right positional nystagmus was observed, and the right eyeball did not elevate fully in the palpebral fissure. No strabismus was seen in other head positions, and physiologic nystagmus was normal.

Anatomic Diagnosis: Caudal cranial fossa—cerebellum, pons, and medulla

Despite the breed and use of this dog and the observed exposure to raccoon bites, these clinical signs are the antithesis of the clinical signs of polyradiculoneuritis of coonhound paralysis, which are diffuse neuromuscular signs. The vestibular system dysfunction was severe with the head tilt, the leaning to one side, the abnormal nystagmus, and the strabismus. The spastic tetraparesis and general proprioceptive (GP) ataxia and decerebellate posture clearly indicate that the clinical signs of vestibular system dysfunction are caused by involvement of its central components. Note that the direction of the abnormal nystagmus also supports a central lesion in this system. The decerebellate posture implicates dysfunction of the rostral portion of the cerebellum. The spastic tetraparesis and GP ataxia support involvement of the pontomedullary UMN and GP systems, with the left side more affected. At this level, the UMN system is primarily ipsilateral to the limbs it controls. The portion of the GP system

(Continued)

CASE EXAMPLE 21-3—cont'd

primarily involved here on the left side would be the spinocerebellar tracts, which are also primarily conducting sensory information from the ipsilateral left limbs. The loss of the left medial lemniscus may contribute to the right limb deficits. The predominance of right-sided central vestibular system clinical signs may reflect an asymmetric bilateral caudal cranial fossa lesion or a multifocal lesion, or these may be paradoxical vestibular clinical signs from a left-side lesion involving the left cerebellar peduncles.

Differential Diagnosis: Neoplasm, focal inflammation, epidermoid or dermoid cyst

The 1 month of slowly progressive clinical signs with a rapid deterioration in the last week supports a presumptive diagnosis of an extramedullary neoplasm such as a meningioma, choroid plexus papilloma, multilobular bone tumor, or some form of sarcoma. These extramedullary neoplasms at this location commonly cause a slow progression of clinical signs. An intramedullary neurectodermal tumor is a strong consideration but only slightly less likely as a result of the prolonged progressive history. Any possibility of a progressive caudal cranial fossa masslike lesion must include an abscess from an intracranial extension of an otitis media-interna. Focal GME occasionally occurs in the cerebellar white matter with involvement of the adjacent pons and medulla. A fungal granuloma can occur at this level of the CNS. The protozoal infections must be considered. Toxoplasmosis is not common and is usually multifocal, but it might cause a large granuloma at this level. *Neospora caninum* is noted for causing an extensive chronic inflammation in adult dogs that can be remarkably limited to the cerebellum. The viral and rickettsial infections are less likely to produce such severe focal caudal cranial fossa clinical signs. Although epidermoid and dermoid cysts are most common in the caudal cranial fossa, the age of this patient and the severity of the clinical signs make this consideration less likely. The progressive course of this disorder eliminates any consideration of a vascular compromise despite the risk of a cerebellar infarction in older dogs. The clinical signs were too focal, asymmetric, and severe to give any consideration for an inherited degenerative disorder.

Ancillary Studies: Radiographs revealed an oval, hyperdense lesion that engulfed the tentorium cerebelli (Fig. 21-5). A meningioma or sarcoma was suspected to be the cause of this hyperdense mass lesion. Cisternal CSF on day 2 of hospitalization contained 14 mononuclear cells/mm³ (normal <5) and 98 mg/dl of protein (normal <25). A second cisternal CSF obtained on day 4 of hospitalization contained 40 white blood cells (WBCs)/mm³, most of which were mononuclear cells, and 176 mg/dl protein. The CSF opening pressure was 265 mm water (normal <180). These ancillary results were compatible with an extramedullary neoplasm involving the tentorium cerebelli, causing compression of the cerebellum and caudal brainstem. Be aware that obtaining CSF from a dog with an intracranial space-occupying lesion has the risk of possible brain herniation secondary to increased intracranial pressure. Today, a delay in obtaining CSF until after advanced imaging has determined the nature of the brain lesion is usually standard procedure.

Outcome: On the second day of hospitalization, all the clinical signs were slightly worse. In addition, the left pupil was slightly dilated but still responsive to light. Occasionally, dysfunction of the cerebellar nuclei will cause an anisocoria and may therefore be the result of the cerebellar compression in this dog or the result of a direct compression of the left side of the mesencephalon, with partial dysfunction of the parasympathetic general visceral efferent neurons of the oculomotor nerve. On day 4 of hospitalization, the patient's clinical signs of decerebellation were worse, and he made fewer attempts to stand. Surgery to remove the neoplasm was recommended, but the owners declined and elected euthanasia.

Necropsy confirmed the presence of a large very firm nodular mass that enveloped the tentorium cerebelli (Fig. 21-6) and primarily projected ventrally where it severely compressed the rostral and central portions of the cerebellum (Figs. 21-7, 21-8). At the most compressed level of the cerebellum, it only measured 7 mm in height. The caudal cerebellar vermis projected caudally into the foramen magnum. The entire pons and medulla were compressed by the adjacent cerebellar compression. Dorsal to the tentorium cerebelli, the neoplasm compressed the medial portions of both occipital lobes. On microscopic examination, the neoplasm was diagnosed as an osteogenic sarcoma.

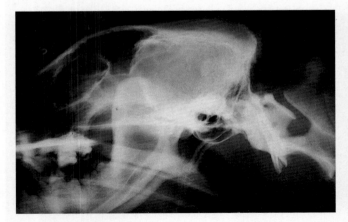

FIGURE 21-5 Lateral radiograph of the head of the coonhound mixed breed in this case example. Note the radiodensity at the site of the tentorium cerebelli.

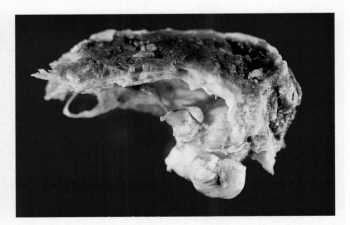

FIGURE 21-6 Lateral view of the preserved calvaria from the skull of the dog in Fig. 21-5, showing an osteogenic sarcoma involving the tentorium cerebelli.

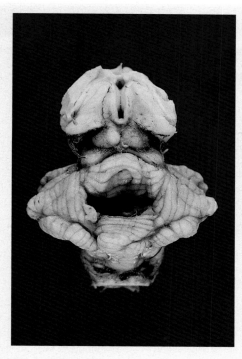

FIGURE 21-7 Dorsal view of the preserved brainstem and cerebellum of the dog in Figs. 21-5 and 21-6. Note the deep depression in the center of the cerebellum where the tentorial neoplasm was removed with the calvaria.

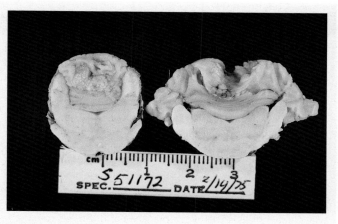

FIGURE 21-8 Transverse sections of the preserved caudal brainstem and cerebellum of the dog in Figs. 21-5, 21-6, and 21-7, showing the depression in the cerebellum and compression of the pons and medulla caused by the tentorial osteogenic sarcoma.

CASE EXAMPLE 21-4

Signalment: 3-year-old female setter mixed breed

Chief Complaint: Abnormal pelvic limb function

History: Five days before examination, this dog ran off from its home. She was found 4 days later lying alongside the road and unable to stand up and exhibiting extreme discomfort. She tried to bite anyone who attempted to move her.

Examination: She was alert and responsive and stood up on her thoracic limbs but refused any attempts to stand on her pelvic limbs. When assisted to a standing position, she walked normally on the thoracic limbs, supported her trunk well, and supported her weight on her right pelvic limb, which she moved slowly but without any obvious neurologic deficit. The dog was reluctant to stand on her left pelvic limb but was able to bear weight if positioned carefully. She often stood on the dorsal surface of her left paw and could move the limb only by mild hip flexion.

Muscle tone, spinal nerve reflexes, and nociception were all normal in the right pelvic limb. The left pelvic limb was mildly hypotonic. The patellar reflex was normal. No flexor reflex was observed when a noxious stimulus was applied to digits 3, 4, and 5, and nociception was absent from these digits. Analgesia was observed from all aspects of the paw except for the medial side. A noxious stimulus to the skin on the medial aspect of the limb at any level resulted in slight hip flexion and intact nociception but no flexion of the stifle, tarsus, or digits. Cutaneous analgesia was observed in the caudal thigh, as well as all of the crus, tarsus, and paw, except for the medial side of the entire left limb. The tail was atonic, areflexic, and analgesic. The anus was hypotonic and partially dilated. A slight anal closure response to stimulation of the perineum was seen on the right side but none from the left side. Nociception was intact on the right side of the perineum but the left side was analgesic. The bladder was distended and required manual evacuation. In addition to these neurologic deficits was swelling at the base of the tail, and crepitus was palpated. The normal space between the right greater trochanter and the right tuber ischium was enlarged.

Anatomic Diagnosis: Left sciatic nerve or L6, L7, and S1 spinal nerve ventral branches, spinal nerves, spinal nerve roots, or spinal cord segments; branches of the left sacral plexus, sacral spinal nerves, spinal nerve roots and spinal cord segments; bilateral pelvic nerve and caudal spinal nerve branches, spinal nerve roots, and spinal cord segments

The femoral nerve and its L4 and L5 spinal cord and spinal nerve components were normal based on the normal patellar reflexes and normal nociception from the medial side of the paw and crus via the saphenous nerve branch of the femoral nerve. The normal cutaneous sensation over the cranial thigh resulted from the unaffected lateral cutaneous femoral nerve (L3 and L4) and over the proximal medial thigh from the intact genitofemoral nerve (L3 and L4). The normal hip flexion resulted from the intact innervation of the psoas major muscle from the ventral branches of most of the lumbar spinal nerves. The bladder paralysis requires a bilateral loss of the pelvic nerve innervation (S1, S2, and S3) The loss of the left perineal reflex,

(Continued)

CASE EXAMPLE 21-4—cont'd

nociception, and anal tone requires dysfunction of the left pudendal nerve or its sacral plexus and nerve origin on the left side. The tail deficit requires a bilateral loss of caudal spinal cord segment or spinal nerve innervation.

Differential Diagnosis: The nature of the onset of the clinical signs is unknown because of the lack of observation of the dog during that time period. Finding the dog beside the road in significant discomfort with palpable skeletal abnormalities in the area of the pelvis is strongly presumptive of a traumatic event of external origin. Most likely this dog was struck by a vehicle, and the clinical signs are the result of injury, primarily of the peripheral nerve components of the structures listed in the anatomic diagnosis. The sciatic nerve or its spinal nerve branches of origin are commonly injured by fractures of the ilium or ischium or sacroiliac luxations because of their close anatomic relationship. Sacrocaudal nerves are commonly injured by sacrocaudal vertebral fractures. Pelvic nerve dysfunction can result from hemorrhage in the connective tissues of the pelvic cavity.

Ancillary Studies: Radiographs revealed a right coxofemoral joint luxation with a craniodorsal dislocation of the right femur, a fracture of the sacrum at the left sacroiliac joint with subluxation, and a fracture of the sacrocaudal articulation with complete ventral displacement of the caudal vertebral portion (Figs. 21-9, 21-10). The ventral branches

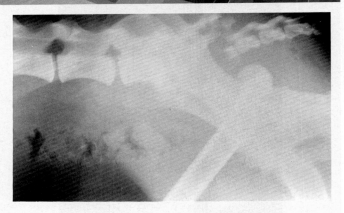

FIGURE 21-10 Lateral radiograph of the pelvis of the dog in Fig. 21-9, showing the sacrocaudal fracture and the luxated right femur. Note the asymmetry of the ilia caused by the subluxation of the left sacroiliac joint.

of the L6 and L7 spinal nerves that contribute to the formation of the sciatic nerve course caudally on the ventral surface of the sacroiliac joint to be joined by the ventral branches of the first and second sacral spinal nerves to form the sciatic nerve at the level of the greater ischiatic notch of the ilium. The skeletal lesions seen here correlate well with the anatomic diagnosis and the clinical signs observed in this dog. Remember that your neurologic examination determines a functional abnormality in the nervous system and not the structural basis for it. Therefore be cautious about your prognosis, especially with injuries such as this one.

Outcome: The right coxofemoral luxation was manually replaced under general anesthesia. Within a few days, this dog recovered its sensation in the distribution of the left sciatic nerve, but motor function remained absent. The right pelvic limb was normal in all functional respects. Within the following 10 days, the dog began to stand and make slow attempts at walking with the left pelvic limb. She supported her weight well (normal femoral nerve) and would advance the left pelvic limb by hip flexion (normal iliopsoas muscle and lumbar spinal nerves). However, she walked with the tarsus overflexed and the stifle extended and often placed the paw on its dorsal surface on the ground. The tarsus was lax from loss of muscle tone. These clinical signs were caused by the persistent sciatic nerve paralysis. Incontinence persisted from the pelvic nerve injury, and the tail remained paralyzed and analgesic. After 1 more month with no further improvement, the owners requested euthanasia for their dog.

At necropsy the skeletal lesions were observed that were diagnosed on the radiographs. The caudal spinal nerves were torn and fibrosed at the sacrocaudal fracture. The left L7 spinal nerve ventral branch was discolored and entirely embedded in fibrous tissue ventromedial to the left sacroiliac joint subluxation. A portion of the left L6 spinal nerve ventral branch was involved in the same fibrous adhesion. The ventral branches of the sacral spinal nerves were embedded in old hemorrhage and fibrous tissue. No spinal cord lesions were observed.

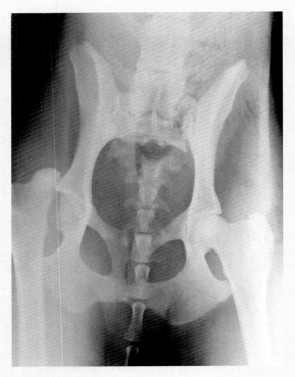

FIGURE 21-9 Ventrodorsal radiograph of the pelvis of the setter mixed breed in this case example. Note the luxated right coxofemoral joint (left side of photograph) and the fractured sacrum at the left sacroiliac joint.

CASE EXAMPLE 21-5

Signalment: 8-year-old female terrier mixed breed
Chief Complaint: Head tilt
History: Six weeks before examination, this dog rapidly developed a mild right head tilt. The degree of head tilt slowly worsened, and for the past 10 days, she tended to move to her right as she walked.
Examination: The patient was alert and responsive. Her head was held markedly tilted to her right side. Her gait was normal except for a tendency to drift to the right side.

Hopping responses were slow in the right limbs. Muscle size and tone and all spinal nerve reflexes were normal. Nociception was normal. Cranial nerve examination revealed anisocoria caused by a slightly enlarged right pupil. Menace responses and pupillary light reflexes were normal, except that the right pupil never would constrict as much as the left pupil. The right eyeball was frequently held in a ventrolateral position but did not persist in all head positions. On testing physiologic nystagmus by moving the head back and forth, both eyeballs adducted and abducted fully. No spontaneous resting nystagmus was observed, but a positional rotatory left-to-vertical nystagmus developed when the head was held flexed to the left side.
Anatomic Diagnosis: Two considerations: (1) focal right side caudal cranial fossa lesion—pons, medulla, cerebellum and (2) focal right middle- and inner-ear plus left prosencephalon
1. Most lesions at the level of the pons and medulla that affect their UMN and GP systems cause an observable ipsilateral hemiparesis and ataxia, but occasionally a very mild dysfunction of these two systems is reflected only in the ipsilateral postural reactions. The clinical signs of vestibular system dysfunction are caused by dysfunction of its central components in the pons, medulla, and cerebellum. The position of the eyeball was interpreted as a vestibular strabismus. The anisocoria may reflect some involvement of the cerebellar nuclei. This anatomic diagnosis is the most likely, but you should at least consider the possibility of the following second choice.
2. The normal gait, except for a mild vestibular ataxia, with abnormal right-side postural reactions may be caused by a left-side prosencephalic lesion involving the UMN and GP systems at that level. If this lesion is present, then the vestibular system clinical signs may all be caused by a dysfunction of the portion of the vestibular system located in the right inner ear. The partly dilated pupil is not accounted for in this anatomic diagnosis unless the left prosencephalic lesion is occupying space and has caused a herniation of the left occipital lobe with compression of the adjacent rostral mesencephalon.

Differential Diagnosis for Anatomic Diagnosis 1:
Neoplasm; focal inflammation—granulomatous meningoencephalitis, abscess, viral, protozoal, fungal, rickettsial; epidermoid or dermoid cyst
Differential Diagnosis for Anatomic Diagnosis 2:
Prosencephalon—neoplasm, focal inflammation; vestibular nerve: otitis media-interna, neoplasm

Neoplasms include meningioma, neurectodermal tumors, or a metastatic neoplasm. An abscess is more of a consideration for the caudal cranial fossa lesion because of the adjacent temporal bone and possible middle- and inner-ear infection. Focal GME can occur in the white matter of either location. Viral, protozoal, fungal, and rickettsial lesions are more often multifocal. A cyst would be unlikely at this age.
Ancillary Studies: Radiographs of the skull that included the tympanic bullae were normal. Cisternal CSF contained 103 WBCs/mm³ (normal <5) that were all mononuclear cells and 286 mg/dl of protein/dl (normal <25).
Outcome: These ancillary studies, without advanced imaging, support a diagnosis of a focal GME. This disease may be controlled for a period with immunosuppressant drug therapy or therapeutic radiation, but the long-term prognosis is very guarded. The owners elected euthanasia.

Necropsy revealed, on transverse sections of the preserved brain, a large red-brown firm lesion centered in the right cerebellar peduncles with extension into the right side of the medulla oblongata and cerebellar medulla (Fig. 21-11). On microscopic examination, this lesion was diagnosed as a focal GME. Smaller lesions were found in the left septal nuclei, caudate nucleus, rostral commissure, column of the fornix, adjacent rostral diencephalon, the right parahippocampal gyrus, and hippocampus. These smaller lesions were clinically quiet. Surprisingly, with the size of this cerebellomedullary lesion, the clinical signs were so mild, and this observation emphasizes the value of carefully evaluating the postural reactions especially the hopping responses.

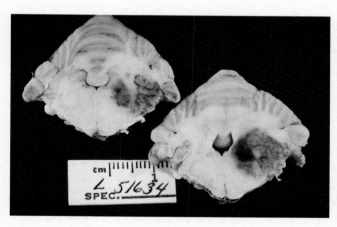

FIGURE 21-11 Transverse sections of the preserved cerebellum and medulla of the terrier mixed breed in this case example. The focal area of discoloration centered in the right cerebellar peduncles is caused by a focal GME.

CASE EXAMPLE 21-6

Signalment: 10-month-old female Arabian horse
Chief Complaint: Abnormal gait
History: At 3 to 4 weeks of age, this filly was noticed to stumble occasionally and even fall when running free in a paddock. The pelvic limbs were noticed to splay out occasionally. No history was elicited of any difficulty following when this filly was foaled. The gait abnormality slowly worsened and was more noticeable in the pelvic limbs.

Examination: The filly was alert and responsive and had normal cranial nerves. Her gait was remarkably abnormal in all four limbs, with a symmetric abnormality. The clinical signs seemed mildly worse in the pelvic limbs. She walked with a base-wide posture in the pelvic limbs with a prolonged stride, causing her to sway from one side to the other. The hooves were occasionally dragged on their dorsal surface at the onset of protraction. On turns, the

(Continued)

CASE EXAMPLE 21-6—cont'd

hindquarters swayed to the side, and the outside pelvic limb often abducted excessively during protraction. When walking, the thoracic limbs were stiff and overreached with the limbs in extension. The dorsal surface of the hooves was occasionally scuffed at the onset of protraction. When she was turned loose in a paddock, her gait abnormality was exaggerated when she made abrupt turns. See Video 11-3 for a yearling Arabian horse with a similar history and clinical signs.

Turning the filly in a tight circle exaggerated the gait abnormality. The pelvic limb on the outside of the circle overflexed or abducted excessively during protraction. The pelvic limb on the inside of the circle was occasionally slow to protract and remained in one position on the ground, causing the filly to pivot on it as she turned. When the limb did protract, it sometimes stepped on the opposite hoof. The thoracic limbs were occasionally slow to protract, stepped on each other, or the outside limb would cross over the opposite limb in an overreaching motion. Swaying the filly as she walked by pulling on her tail caused her to stumble. During this procedure, resistance was less than normal. Compression of the midline of her trunk caused her to sink and almost collapse.

Muscle tone and size were normal, as were the cutaneous and perineal reflexes. Nociception was normal. The cervical vertebrae were normal on palpation, and their manipulation caused no discomfort.

Anatomic Diagnosis: Focal or diffuse spinal cord lesion between the C1 and C5 segments

The clinical signs are typically those that occur with a dysfunction of the UMN and GP systems to all four limbs. The gait represents the combined dysfunction of these two systems. Distinguishing between the deficits of the two systems is impossible and is unnecessary to make the anatomic diagnosis.

Differential Diagnosis: Equine degenerative myeloencephalopathy, occipitoatlantoaxial malformation, cervical vertebral malformation-malarticulation, diskospondylitis, equine protozoal myelitis, equine herpesvirus-1 vasculitis and myelopathy

The age of onset, the slowly progressive symmetric clinical signs, and the normal atlantooccipital joint on palpation are most compatible with the diagnosis of degenerative myeloencephalopathy. The Arabian breed has two presumably inherited CNS disorders that affect the gait at this age. One is a cerebellar cortical abiotrophy that was described in Chapter 13 and does not satisfy the anatomic diagnosis for this Arabian filly (see Video 13-21). The other disorder of the Arabian breed is the skeletal malformation known as occipitoatlantoaxial malformation (OAAM). This abnormality might cause the clinical signs seen on the neurologic examination of this filly, but the skeletal malformation, which can be palpated, was not present. OAAM may cause a unique extended head and neck posture, which was not present in this filly (see Video 11-2). An acquired cervical vertebral malformation-malarticulation is a reasonable consideration, although the age of onset in this breed makes this less likely. A radiographic study is necessary to support this diagnosis. A diskospondylitis is most common at a few weeks of age, and in the setting of clinical signs of spinal cord dysfunction, their progression is fairly rapid and associated with cervical discomfort and often systemic signs of a bacterial infection. Only the age of onset in this Arabian filly is suggestive of

this diagnosis. Equine protozoal myelitis is uncommon at this age of onset, 3 to 4 weeks, and would not be expected to progress so slowly for such an extended time period. Equine herpesvirus-1 vasculitis and myelopathy would also be unlikely at this age and would cause a sudden onset of clinical signs that would not progress for more than 2 to 3 days at the most.

Ancillary Studies: Radiographs of the cervical vertebrae, including a cisternal myelogram with flexed and extended views, were normal. Lumbar and cisternal CSF specimens were normal. A presumptive clinical diagnosis of degenerative myeloencephalopathy was made.

Outcome: Although the clinical signs usually become static in horses with degenerative myeloencephalopathy, they do not resolve even with rigorous vitamin E therapy. This abnormality is an axonopathy, and the patient cannot grow new axons in the CNS! Because this filly was unable to be used for riding, the owners elected euthanasia.

Necropsy confirmed the diagnosis of a diffuse degenerative myeloencephalopathy. The lesions of axonopathy and secondary demyelination and astrogliosis are most pronounced in the spinal cord, with a bilateral symmetric distribution. Although multiple tracts are affected, a predilection exists for the tracts on the superficial surface of the dorsolateral and ventral funiculi (Fig. 21-12). Spheroids are common in the nucleus of the dorsal spinocerebellar tracts in the thoracic and cranial lumbar spinal cord segments and in the medullary proprioceptive nuclei at the level of the obex. A deficiency of vitamin E is considered to play a primary role in the pathogenesis of this disorder. See Chapter 11 for an extensive description of this equine disorder.

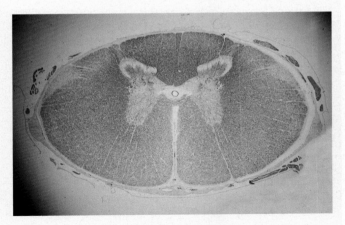

FIGURE 21-12 Microscopic transverse section of the T15 spinal cord segment of the Arabian horse in this case example, stained for myelin. Note the symmetric pale areas on each side of the spinal cord caused by secondary demyelination that are most pronounced in the dorsolateral and ventral funiculi adjacent to the surface of the spinal cord. This lesion, which occurs diffusely at all levels of the spinal cord, is characteristic of the degenerative myelopathy associated with a vitamin E deficiency in young horses. The demyelination is secondary to a primary axonopathy.

CASE EXAMPLE 21-7

Signalment: 7-year-old female domestic shorthair

Chief Complaint: Seizures and behavioral change

History: This cat lived in upstate New York and had access to the outdoor environment. She was found one August morning very depressed and had been confined to the house that evening. She would not respond to the owners and exhibited episodes of "jerky movements" of her face and left thoracic limb. The following day, she was examined by the referring veterinarian, who observed two of these episodes and described the cat as turning its head with jerky, shaking movements to her left side, and extending her left thoracic limb caudally along her trunk in a series of clonic movements. Similar clonic movements occurred in the left pelvic limb. These movements were accompanied by facial muscle twitching, excessive salivation, and pupillary dilation. Each episode lasted approximately 1 minute, after which the cat exhibited a normal gait, but her depression continued, and she expressed considerable resentment on being handled. These episodes were considered to be simple partial seizures and she was treated with phenobarbital and thiamin. No seizures were observed during 2 more days of hospitalization, and she was discharged. Two weeks later, she was returned to this veterinarian for euthanasia because of her persistent aggressive behavior that made her unmanageable and no longer compatible as a pet. The owner allowed the cat to be donated to us for clinical study, euthanasia, and necropsy.

Examination: This cat was alert and responsive and seemed to be well oriented to her environment. She resented any prolonged handling and would growl and strike without provocation. Her gait was normal, but her hopping responses were slow in her left limbs. When she was walked backwards on her pelvic limbs, the left pelvic limb was slower to protract than the right pelvic limb. On being wheelbarrowed with her head and neck extended, her left thoracic limb was slow to protract, and the paw was occasionally dragged on its dorsal surface. Muscle tone and size were normal, as were the patellar and withdrawal spinal nerve reflexes. Nociception from the digits was normal. Cranial nerve examination revealed a persistent poor menace response in the left eye with normal palpebral reflexes. The pupils were normal in size and symmetric in room light and responded well to a bright light. No other cranial nerve abnormalities were observed.

Anatomic Diagnosis: Right prosencephalon

The left-side simple partial seizures suggest a seizure focus in the area of the right frontoparietal motor cortex. The normal gait and left-side postural reaction deficits indicate a dysfunction of the right-side prosencephalic components of the UMN and GP systems. The menace deficit in the left eye with normal pupillary function indicates a lesion affecting the right-side central visual pathway in the prosencephalon.

Differential Diagnosis: *Cuterebra spp.* myiasis, injury, neoplasm, inflammation, thiamin deficiency

The sudden onset of unilateral prosencephalic signs that did not progress to the more caudal brainstem strongly suggests an external injury or a vascular compromise. External injury is unlikely to have occurred because this cat was indoors when the clinical signs began. With the date of onset of clinical signs being mid-August, a vascular compromise related to the intracranial migration of a larva of a species of *Cuterebra* is the most presumptive clinical diagnosis. Many of these cats have areas of ischemia or infarction in the distribution of the blood supplied by the middle cerebral artery. Such a compromise

of the right middle cerebral artery would result in the clinical signs observed in this cat. The most common neoplasm that affects the cat brain is a meningioma. Owners commonly observe changes in the behavior of their cat and occasionally seizures when a meningioma is present. The clinical signs observed on examination of this cat are typical of a meningioma affecting one cerebral hemisphere. The abruptness of the onset of clinical signs would be unusual for a meningioma, and the majority of meningiomas occur in cats over 9 years old. Nevertheless, this diagnosis justifies recommending advanced imaging for the correct diagnosis. The majority of cerebral meningiomas can be surgically removed with satisfactory recovery for many months to years. Intracranial lymphoma rarely produces such focal clinical signs or such an abrupt onset. The most common CNS inflammation in cats is that caused by the virus that causes feline infectious peritonitis. The onset of clinical signs is very slow and insidious and usually reflects dysfunction in the caudal brainstem and spinal cord and rarely one cerebral hemisphere. A cerebral abscess is rare in cats and usually requires a penetrating injury such as a dog bite. A *Toxoplasma gondii* or fungal granuloma in one cerebral hemisphere are considerations but are quite rare. Seizures are the most common clinical sign of thiamin deficiency, but these seizures are usually generalized, and interictal clinical signs of a unilateral prosencephalic disorder would not be present. The interictal asymmetric clinical signs make toxicities and inherited degenerative disorders unlikely considerations.

Ancillary Studies: Radiographs of the skull were normal. Meningiomas that grow in contact with the calvaria sometimes cause a sclerosis of the adjacent bone. Cisternal CSF contained 9 WBCs/mm^3 (normal <5) and 18 mg/dl protein (normal <20). No eosinophiles were observed. A presumptive clinical diagnosis of *Cuterebra spp.* myiasis was made and the owners elected euthanasia for their cat.

Outcome: Necropsy revealed a slight yellow discoloration and softening on the surface of the right cerebral hemisphere near where the right middle cerebral artery courses over the cerebral gyri and included the piriform lobe. No parasitic larva was seen on the surface of the brain or in the area of the cribriform plates of the ethmoid bones. On the transverse sections of the preserved brain, a few areas of softening in the right cerebral hemisphere and both piriform lobes were seen. Microscopic examination revealed extensive ischemic-type degeneration in the neocortex and to a lesser degree in the white matter of the associated corona radiata and the centrum semiovale, predominantly in the lateral portions of the frontoparietal lobes of the right cerebral hemisphere. In less-affected areas of the right cerebral hemisphere was a superficial degeneration of the neocortex. A few scattered lymphocytic perivascular cuffs were seen in the parenchyma and meninges. Ischemic-type neuronal cell body degeneration was observed in the hippocampus and piriform lobes that may have been caused by excitotoxicity associated with the seizures. Despite the inability to find a larva of a *Cuterebra* species, these lesions are typical of those seen in cat brains in which the larva is found. Fig. 21-13 shows a brain from a cat with similar clinical signs and anatomic diagnosis that was euthanized 2 months after the onset of the clinical signs. Note the atrophy in the distribution of the right middle cerebral artery from the infarction that had occurred 2 months before euthanasia. With MR imaging, we can now often recognize a tract lesion extending from one olfactory bulb where the larva enters the cranial cavity through various components of the prosencephalon (Figs. 21-14, 21-15).

(Continued)

CASE EXAMPLE 21-7—cont'd

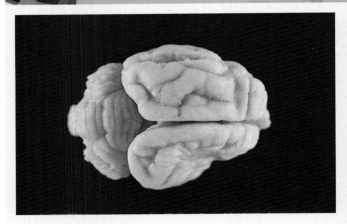

FIGURE 21-13 Dorsal view of the preserved brain of an adult domestic shorthair, showing atrophy of the right cerebral hemisphere in the distribution of the right middle cerebral artery. *Cuterebra* spp. myiasis was the presumptive cause. An acute onset of prosencephalic clinical signs similar to those in this case example had occurred 2 months before this necropsy.

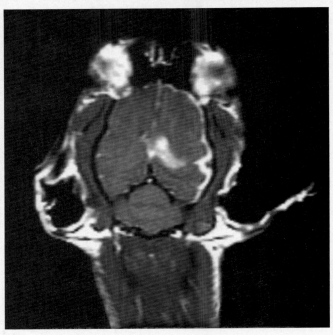

FIGURE 21-15 Dorsal plane T1-weighted MR image with contrast of the head of the cat in Fig. 21-14 but at a more dorsal level through both cerebral hemispheres. Note the hyperintensity of the track lesion in the left cerebral hemisphere, as well as the superficial neocortex of the left cerebral hemisphere.

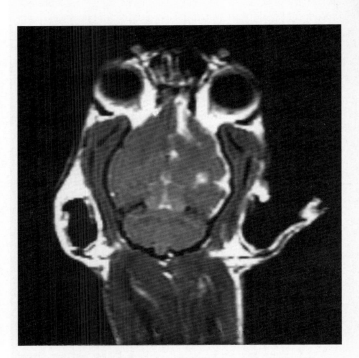

FIGURE 21-14 Dorsal plane T1-weighted MR image with contrast of the head of an adult cat with an acute onset of left prosencephalic clinical signs. Note the hyperintensity in the area of the left olfactory bulb and frontal lobe (right side of image) caused by the necrosis associated with a *Cuterebra* spp. larva that entered the brain through the ethmoidal cribriform plate. Note the thin layer of hyperintensity in the left neocortex, which is caused by the cerebrocortical degeneration of superficial laminae thought to be the result of a toxin released by the larva into the CSF.

CASE EXAMPLE 21-8

Signalment: 8-month-old female cairn terrier

Chief Complaint: Depression and abnormal behavior

History: At 6 months of age, this dog was presented to a veterinarian for lethargy, polyuria, polydipsia, and carrying her tail between her pelvic limbs. A granular yellow discharge was noted at her vulva. She was treated for cystitis, and these signs resolved after 4 days of hospitalization. Her vaccination status was up to date at that time.

At 8 months of age, she was reexamined for 24 hours of depression, circling, standing with her head pressed against a wall, and abnormal use of her pelvic limbs. The owner recalled that other brief periods were observed when her pet stood quietly staring off into space and seemed oblivious of her environment. Ancillary studies at that hospital admission revealed a leucocytosis (23,800/mm^3) and neutrophilia (19,278/mm^3). The total plasma protein was 4.5 g/dl (normal 6.0-7.8). The blood urea nitrogen level was 9 mg/dl (normal 10-20), serum alanine aminotransferase was 192 IU (normal <50), and serum alkaline phosphatase was 263 IU (normal <30). After 24 hours of hospitalization and treatment with intravenous fluids, antibiotics, and corticosteroids, the dog's behavior returned to normal. After discharge from the hospital and before referral to Cornell University, subsequent episodes of depression were treated successfully with removal of the dog's food.

Examination: This dog was small for this breed at this age. Her physical and neurologic examinations were normal.

Anatomic Diagnosis: Diffuse prosencephalon

Although the neurologic examination was normal, the history of this patient involved primarily an abnormal sensorium and changes in behavior that strongly suggested an episodic prosencephalic disorder affecting the ascending reticular activating system (ARAS) and limbic system. The history of an occasional associated gait abnormality indicated a more diffuse CNS disorder affecting the caudal brainstem and/or spinal cord during some of these episodes.

Differential Diagnosis: Metabolic encephalopathy—hepatic, hypoglycemic, renal

These episodic clinical signs are typical of metabolic encephalopathy. Major structural lesions such as malformations, injuries, inflammations, vascular compromise, or neoplasia rarely produce such extensive prosencephalic clinical signs other than seizures that are episodic and followed by a rapid and complete spontaneous recovery when food is withheld. Intoxications such as lead poisoning may initially cause seizures with normal interictal periods but in time cause lesions such as cerebrocortical degeneration and persistent interictal neurologic signs referable to the prosencephalic lesions.

The most common metabolic encephalopathy in dogs and cats that have episodic bizarre changes in behavior and sometimes seizures is hepatic in origin. Severe diffuse liver dysfunction will cause these clinical signs at any age. However, in the young animal, a portosystemic shunt is the most common cause. Portosystemic shunts also occur in foals and young farm animals but are much less common in these species. These shunts cause the portal system blood to bypass the liver and expose the brain to excessive levels of ammonia and other metabolites that are not metabolized by the liver and may interfere with neuronal function in the CNS. Hypoglycemic encephalopathy more commonly causes seizures but may occasionally cause periods in which the sensorium is abnormal but rarely causes the bizarre behavior changes that occur with hepatic encephalopathy. Hypoglycemic encephalopathy in the young toy-breed dog may reflect an aberration of glycogenolysis. In dogs that are 4 years or older, the cause of hypoglycemia is usually a functional neoplasm of the pancreatic islet beta cells that produce an excessive amount of insulin. Renal encephalopathy is uncommon and at this age might be caused by a renal hypoplasia.

Ancillary Studies: The laboratory studies performed by the referring veterinarian indicate liver dysfunction. These studies were repeated at Cornell with similar results. In addition, serum ammonia levels were significantly elevated. A urinalysis determined the presence of biurate crystals in the urine. In retrospect, the crystals found at the vulva of this dog when she was brought in at 6 months of age were most likely biurate crystals, which can occasionally cause a urethral obstruction. At the present time, the most reliable diagnostic test for diffuse hepatic dysfunction is the determination of pre- and postprandial serum bile acid levels. Further confirmation of a portosystemic shunt can be obtained with ultrasound evaluation of the liver and its vasculature. Rectal scintigraphy is another procedure that requires only sedation and can confirm this diagnosis but cannot differentiate an intrahepatic shunt from an extrahepatic shunt. Ultrasound can often accomplish this differentiation, but for the most reliable anatomic demonstration of the vascular abnormality, an intravenous contrast portogram is necessary. This procedure was performed in this patient via cannulation of a jejunal vein exposed by a celiotomy. See Fig. 21-16 and note the small liver shadow and the majority of the contrast entering a looping vessel caudal to the liver that connects to the caudal vena cava. This shunt is an extrahepatic portocaval shunt. A small amount of contrast has entered the liver vasculature.

Outcome: The ancillary studies confirmed the diagnosis of hepatic encephalopathy secondary to a portocaval shunt. Surgical ligation was performed along with a change of diet to one with a low-protein and high-carbohydrate content. The antibiotic, neomycin, was administered orally to decrease the intestinal bacterial population that convert protein to ammonia. No further clinical signs occurred for the 3 years of follow-up after this therapy. Be aware that hyperammonemia and encephalopathy can also occur with inherited urea cycle enzyme deficiencies. See Case Example 14-4 for an example of hepatic encephalopathy in an adult horse.

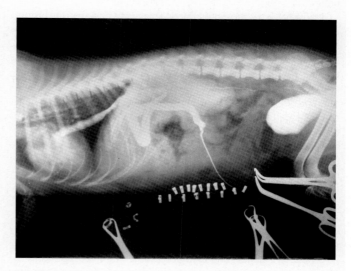

FIGURE 21-16 Lateral radiograph of a contrast portogram of the cairn terrier in this case example. The cannula is in a jejunal vein. Note that the bolus of contrast that enters the portal vein shunts through a looping vessel into the caudal vena cava. Only a very small amount of contrast enters the liver portal system. Note also the relatively small liver size.

CASE EXAMPLE 21-9

Signalment: 8-year-old castrated male West Highland white terrier

Chief Complaint: Dragging the left pelvic limb

History: Four weeks before examination, this dog was reluctant to climb stairs. Three weeks before examination, he began to intermittently drag his left pelvic limb when walking. At that time, the dog was diagnosed with Lyme disease and treated with doxycycline. The clinical signs worsened until presentation when the patient was constantly dragging the left pelvic limb on the dorsal surface of the paw.

Examination: The patient was alert and responsive. His gait was normal, except for the left pelvic limb in which protraction of that limb was delayed. He often dragged or placed the left pelvic limb on the dorsal surface of the paw. Postural reactions were dramatically slow or absent in the left pelvic limb. A slight delay in hopping in the right pelvic limb was observed. The left pelvic limb was hypertonic. The patellar reflex in the left pelvic limb was clonic (+4), and it was brisk (+3) in the right pelvic limb. Flexor reflexes were normal in both pelvic limbs, as was nociception. The cutaneous trunci response was less frequent when the skin of the right side of the trunk was stimulated caudal to the midthoracic region when compared with the stimulation of the left side. Skin stimulation cranial to the midthoracic region resulted in normal cutaneous trunci responses bilaterally. The cranial nerve examination was normal. No significant discomfort was elicited on palpation of the neck and trunk.

Anatomic Diagnosis: Focal left-side partial spinal cord lesion between the T3 and L3 segments. The abnormal cutaneous trunci reflex indicates that the lesion is in the midthoracic spinal cord segments. This clinical observation of a cutaneous trunci reflex deficit contralateral to the side of the unilateral spinal cord lesion supports that the major fasciculus proprius components of this reflex are contralateral to the side stimulated similar to the pathway for nociception. Thus, for example, a hemisection of the spinal cord at T8 would be expected to cause an ipsilateral pelvic limb spastic monoplegia and a contralateral hypalgesia and decreased cutaneous trunci reflex caudal to the T10 or T11 vertebrae.

Differential Diagnosis: Neoplasm, intervertebral disk extrusion-protrusion, inflammation, diskospondylitis, FCEM

Neoplasia is the most presumptive diagnosis based on the history of progressive clinical signs and their asymmetry. Intervertebral disk extrusion-protrusion can occasionally result in asymmetric clinical signs but usually not to the degree of asymmetry that is present in this patient. In addition, intervertebral disk extrusions-protrusions are uncommon in the midthoracic region, and hyperesthesia is often present on palpation of the affected vertebrae. Inflammation can be focal and asymmetric, especially GME. Infectious causes of myelitis can produce asymmetric lesions and clinical signs but are more common in younger animals in our experience. Diskospondylitis is a less common cause of such asymmetric clinical signs and often causes significant discomfort. FCEM can be a cause of such asymmetric clinical signs but is *not* a progressive disorder.

Ancillary Procedures: Radiographs of the thorax and thoracolumbar vertebrae were normal. A complete blood count (CBC), blood chemistry panel, and serologic test for canine distemper virus, *N. caninum, T. gondii,* and *Cryptococcus neoformans* were normal. MR imaging revealed a strongly enhancing mass lesion on the left side of the vertebral canal of the T8 and T9 vertebrae. This lesion was best observed on the sagittal sections in the T1-weighted MR images after gadolinium administration (Figs. 21-17, 21-18). The mass appeared to be intradural and extramedullary. These findings

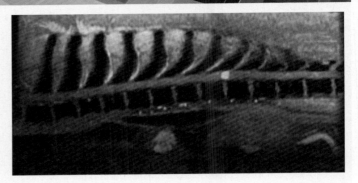

FIGURE 21-17 Sagittal T1-weighted MR image with contrast of the thoracic vertebral region of the West Highland white terrier in this case example. Note the hyperintensity from contrast enhancement of a mass lesion dorsal to the normal-appearing intervertebral disk between the T8 and the T9 vertebral bodies.

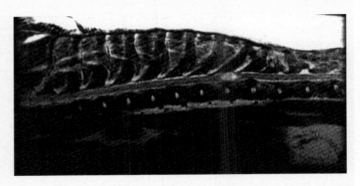

FIGURE 21-18 Sagittal T2-weighted MR image of the dog in Fig. 21-17. Note the moderate hyperintensity of the mass lesion that was contrast enhanced in Fig. 21-17. Note the marked hyperintensity curved around the caudal border of the mass, which is obstructed CSF, indicating that the mass is in the subarachnoid space and is therefore intradural and extramedullary. The mass was removed surgically and was diagnosed as a meningioma.

were most supportive of an extramedullary neoplasm, which resulted in a compressive myelopathy. The two most common neoplasms in this location are a meningioma and a nerve sheath neoplasm. The older age of the patient and the level of the spinal cord cranial to T10 would be unusual for a nephroblastoma.

Outcome: A hemilaminectomy was performed on the left side of the T8 and T9 vertebrae.

The meninges were incised, and a gray mass was exposed compressing the spinal cord to the right side. The mass was relatively well encapsulated and easily pealed away from the spinal cord parenchyma. Postoperatively, the patient was dramatically improved within 24 hours of surgery. Two days later, at the time of discharge, the dog's gait was normal.

Microscopic examination of the surgical specimen diagnosed a meningioma. In our experience, dogs with spinal cord meningiomas do quite well after surgery, with many living for 2 to 5 years without recurrence of clinical signs. Postoperative radiation therapy will usually lengthen this time before recurrence of this type of neoplasm.

CASE EXAMPLE 21-10

Signalment: 7.5-year-old spayed female boxer

Chief Complaint: Neck discomfort and abnormal use of her limbs on her right side

History: Approximately 10 months before examination, this patient began to exhibit discomfort in her neck region. She was treated with corticosteroids and glucosamine. The clinical signs improved, but as the dose of the corticosteroids was progressively decreased and stopped, the neck discomfort recurred. Six months before the examination, the patient again exhibited neck discomfort and was again treated with corticosteroids, which resulted in complete recovery until the dose of the corticosteroids was decreased. One month before the examination, she began to stumble on the right thoracic limb. The clinical signs progressed to involve both right limbs.

Examination: The patient was alert and responsive. Her gait was abnormal in the right thoracic and pelvic limbs. The right pelvic limb delayed on protraction and was often dragged on its dorsal surface. The stride in the right thoracic limb was prolonged. She would often stand with the right pelvic limb paw resting on its dorsal surface. While standing, the right thoracic limb would occasionally buckle. When walking, the protraction phase in the right thoracic limb was prolonged, creating an overreaching or floating effect. Both hopping and paw replacement reactions were delayed in both right limbs. Hemiwalking with the right limbs resulted in the dog falling on its right side. The right limbs were hypertonic. The right patellar reflex was exaggerated (+3). Flexor reflexes and nociception were normal. The patient exhibited discomfort with any manipulation of her neck region. Cranial nerve examination revealed an equivocal left head tilt but no abnormal nystagmus.

Anatomic Diagnosis: Focal lesion on the right side of the first or second cervical spinal cord segments or both

The gait and postural reaction deficits can be explained by dysfunction of the UMN and GP systems on the right side of the pons, medulla, or C1-C5 spinal cord segments. The equivocal left head tilt may reflect dysfunction of the spinovestibular pathways from the first two cervical spinal cord segments or dysfunction of the vestibular nuclei in the caudal brainstem. Possibly multifocal lesions are present in this dog, with at least one right C1-C5 spinal cord segment lesion plus another lesion in the pons, medulla, or cerebellum or even an unrelated lesion in the left inner ear. The equivocal nature of the clinical signs of a vestibular system involvement suggests that the lesion is in the cranial cervical spinal cord and not the brainstem.

Differential Diagnosis: Neoplasm, intervertebral disk extrusion-protrusion, inflammation, FCEM, congenital vertebral malformation, acquired vertebral malformation-malarticulation

Based on the age and breed involved and the slowly progressive nature and asymmetry of the clinical signs, an extramedullary neoplasm is the most presumptive clinical diagnosis. Intervertebral extrusion-protrusion is uncommon in this breed and even if the intervertebral disk lesion were at the articulation between the second and third cervical vertebrae, it would not likely cause the equivocal clinical signs of vestibular system dysfunction. A focal lesion of granulomatous meningomyelitis is a possibility for this anatomic diagnosis. Most infectious diseases are multifocal or diffuse disorders, but a fungal or protozoal granuloma occasionally causes focal clinical signs. FCEM is a nonprogressive disorder and does not usually cause vertebral column discomfort. Atlantoaxial subluxation is a disorder of young small breed dogs, which is not compatible with this patient. Vertebral malformation-malarticulation does not occur at this level, nor does it cause such asymmetric signs.

Ancillary Studies: The CBC, blood chemistry panel, and serologic test for the canine distemper virus, *N. caninum, T. gondii,* and *C. neoformans* were all normal. Thoracic and cervical vertebral radiographs were normal. MR imaging revealed a large well-defined mass within the first cervical vertebral foramen. The mass appeared to be intradural and extramedullary and significantly displaced the first cervical spinal cord segment ventrally and to the left, with compression of the right side more than the left. The mass was strongly enhanced on the T1-weighted images after the administration of gadolinium. The cranial portion of the mass was located at the level of the cerebellomedullary cistern. Figs. 21-19 and 21-20 show the sagittal

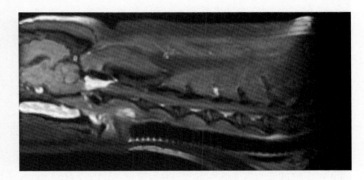

FIGURE 21-19 Sagittal T1-weighted MR image with contrast of the head and neck of the boxer in this case example. Note the marked hyperintensity from contrast enhancement of the mass filling most of the vertebral foramen of the atlas with its greatest height cranially.

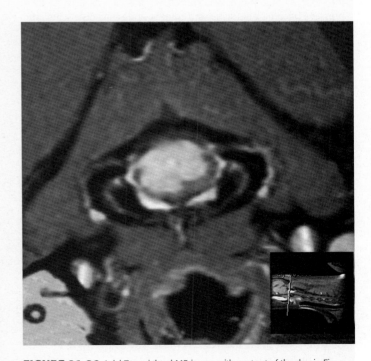

FIGURE 21-20 Axial T1-weighted MR image with contrast of the dog in Fig. 21-19 at the level of the atlantooccipital joint. Note the marked hyperintensity of the contrast-enhanced mass lesion occupying most of the vertebral foramen of the atlas with the spinal cord severely compressed and displaced ventrally and to the left side (right side of image). At necropsy, this mass was diagnosed as a meningioma.

(Continued)

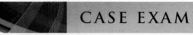

CASE EXAMPLE 21-10—cont'd

and axial (transverse) images of this lesion. The location and MR imaging characteristics of this lesion are most presumptive for a diagnosis of a meningioma.

Outcome: Surgery was recommended for this patient, but the owners elected euthanasia. At necropsy, a firm beige mass was found when the meninges were incised at the level of the C1 and C2 spinal cord segments. The mass was intradural and extramedullary on the right side and severely compressed the spinal

cord segments to the left, leaving only a thin rim of compressed parenchyma. The cause of the slight left head tilt is most likely caused by the interruption in the spinovestibular axons in the compressed parenchyma but may possibly reflect associated vasogenic edema in the adjacent medulla affecting the vestibular nuclei.

In our experience, this location is the most common site for meningiomas that affect the spinal cord.

CASE EXAMPLE 21-11

Signalment: 8-year-old castrated male domestic shorthair

Chief Complaint: Not behaving normally

History: Six months before examination, the owner noted that his cat was becoming lethargic. A few weeks later, the cat stopped eating and would wander into a corner of a room and get stuck there or stand with his head pressed against the wall of a room. Three weeks before examination, the patient was examined at a referral center, where his condition was diagnosed as hepatic encephalopathy, and he was treated with supportive therapy that included prednisone. The basis for this diagnosis was not revealed. Before treatment, the examiner noted that this cat was blind with bilaterally dilated pupils in room light that would not respond to a bright light. The clinical signs rapidly improved when the prednisone therapy was started. As the dose of prednisone was decreased, the clinical signs of head pressing, becoming stuck in room corners, and acting distant recurred. CT imaging was performed at this referral center that revealed a small mass at the level of the pituitary gland.

Examination: The patient was obtunded and poorly responsive. He would walk into a corner of the examination room and just stand there, or he would walk up to the examination room wall and press his head against it. When placed in the middle of the room, he would propulsively circle in either direction. Loud noises and objects thrown near him did not alter his propulsive circling. His gait was normal, as were his postural reactions. Muscle tone and spinal nerve reflexes were all normal. The cranial nerve examination was normal except for mildly dilated pupils in room light that still responded to a bright light source. The menace response was normal in each eye. No hypalgesia of the nasal septum or any surface of the body was noted.

Anatomic Diagnosis: Bilateral prosencephalon with the lesion most likely in the diencephalon affecting the components of the visual system, the ARAS, and the limbic system. The propulsive activity often reflects a dysfunction of the frontal lobes or rostral thalamus, and the degree of mental dysfunction suggests a diencephalic lesion. The history of blindness with dilated unresponsive pupils in each eye indicates involvement of the intracranial optic nerves, the optic chiasm, or both optic tracts. This anatomic location was supported by the CT imaging at the referral center that showed a mass at the level of the pituitary gland.

Differential Diagnosis: Neoplasm, granuloma

Based on the signalment and the referral center CT study, the most presumptive diagnosis is a macroadenoma of the pituitary gland.

Other possible neoplasms located at this site include a meningioma, lymphoma, glioma, and germ-cell neoplasm. Granulomas include those caused by fungal agents such as *C. neoformans* and the protozoan *T. gondii*.

Ancillary Studies: A CBC; chemistry panel; serologic test for feline leukemia virus, feline infectious peritonitis virus, *T. gondii*, and *C. neoformans*; and thoracic radiographs were all normal. CSF was not obtained for evaluation because of the risk of brain herniation associated with the presence of a space-occupying lesion and the possibility of increased intracranial pressure. MR imaging when the patient first was examined revealed a multilobular, strongly enhancing extraparenchymal mass at the level of the middle cranial fossa that measured approximately 1 cm high and 0.75 cm wide. The mass compressed and displaced the diencephalon dorsally. The mass was hyperintense on both the T2-weighted images and the T1-weighted images before the administration of gadolinium. These findings support the presence of blood products, calcification, fat, or melanin-containing substances within the lesion. Moderate perilesional edema was observed. The history of improvement associated with prednisone therapy was most likely caused by the reduction of this perilesional edema.

Outcome: Given the location and size of the lesion, radiation therapy was recommended. The patient received 18 fractions to 45 Gy over a period of 3 weeks. The patient was also maintained on a low dose of prednisone and reevaluated periodically for the next 18 months. Over this period, the patient was considered normal by the owner and examining veterinarian and in the opinion of the owner had an excellent quality of life. After 18 months, this cat suddenly developed an altered mentation and began to circle propulsively to the right side. MR imaging at the time of this recurrence of clinical signs revealed that the mass had grown to 1.4 cm high and 1.2 cm wide (Figs. 21-21, 21-22). Because of the recurrence of these clinical signs and the size of the mass lesion, the owner elected euthanasia. A necropsy diagnosed the mass to be a pituitary macroadenoma. In our experience, radiation therapy has been quite effective at prolonging the life of patients with pituitary macroadenomas in small animals, which is most likely the result of the reduction in the rate of growth of these neoplasms, as well as potentially by slightly reducing the size of the neoplasm. This case is a good example of a severe diencephalic lesion with profound disturbance of the patient's sensorium and behavior but no alteration of its gait. Surprisingly, the postural reactions and nociception remained normal.

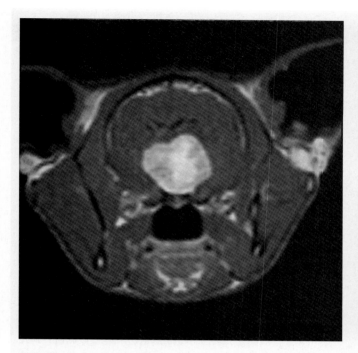

FIGURE 21-21 Axial T1-weighted MR image with contrast of the head of the cat in this case example at the level of the rostral diencephalon. Note the markedly hyperintense contrast enhancement of a large mass with sharp borders that obliterates the rostral diencephalon.

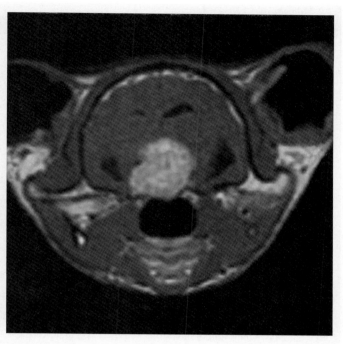

FIGURE 21-22 Axial T1-weighted MR image with contrast of the cat in Fig. 21-21 at the level of the caudal diencephalon. At necropsy, this mass was diagnosed as a pituitary macroadenoma.

CASE EXAMPLE 21-12

Signalment: 2.5-year-old female Australian cattle dog, Kate

Chief Complaint: Recumbent and unable to stand

History: Complex partial seizures occurred when Kate was 7 months old. These seizures were successfully controlled with phenobarbital. When Kate was 20 months old, the owner noticed that this dog's gait appeared to be too stiff, especially in the thoracic limbs, and her activity decreased. This stiffness slowly progressed in the thoracic limbs and began to involve the pelvic limbs. By 24 months of age, Kate became recumbent and unable to stand unassisted. At that time, the thoracic limbs were held in constant rigid extension. Two other littermates were unaffected.

Examination: See **Video 21-1**. Kate was alert and responsive and laid in lateral recumbency with rigidly extended, tetanic, thoracic limbs. Some slight voluntary movement was present in the pelvic limbs, trunk, and neck, but she was unable to get into sternal position. When held up in a standing position, she would try to walk with the hypertonic pelvic limbs but was only able to move them slightly, and no movement was observed in the thoracic limbs. The tetanic thoracic limbs resisted manual flexion, and these efforts caused considerable discomfort. Noxious stimuli were perceived throughout the thoracic limbs and elicited struggling with no withdrawal reflex. Mild to moderate diffuse atrophy of the muscles of both thoracic limbs was noted. The pelvic limbs were extremely hypertonic, but we could flex these manually. Patellar reflexes were depressed. Withdrawal reflexes were normal, as was nociception in the pelvic limbs.

The cranial nerve examination was normal, except that normal physiologic nystagmus was difficult to elicit, and abnormal nystagmus occurred when the head was positioned in lateral flexion to either side or in extension. The direction of the nystagmus was variable.

Anatomic Diagnosis: Cervical and lumbosacral intumescences (C6-T2 and L4-S1 spinal cord segments); pons, medulla, and cerebellum; prosencephalon

The rigid degree of hypertonia was defined as tetanus based on the severity and resistance to manual flexion as opposed to the hypertonia that occurs with lesions that disrupt the inhibitory UMN system. Therefore the thoracic limb tetanus was thought to be the result of loss of function of the inhibitory interneurons (Renshaw cells) in the ventral gray columns in the cervical intumescence with relative sparing of most of the alpha motor neurons. The muscle atrophy suggested disuse or denervation from partial loss of alpha motor neurons. The same pathogenesis might explain the pelvic limb dysfunction but with a less extensive lesion. Involvement of the UMN and GP pathways in the spinal cord white matter could not be ruled out because it might be masked by the gray matter lesions, especially in the thoracic limbs. The abnormal positional nystagmus with variable direction and poor physiologic nystagmus implicated the vestibular system in the pons, medulla, or cerebellum. The extent of the spinal cord lesions masked any evidence of a balance loss or dysmetria from the lesions involving the structures in the caudal cranial fossa. The history of seizures suggested a prosencephalic component.

(Continued)

CASE EXAMPLE 21-12—cont'd

Differential Diagnosis: A multifocal anatomic diagnosis suggests inflammatory, degenerative, or, less commonly, neoplastic diseases. The inflammatory diseases include those caused by the canine distemper virus; protozoal, fungal and rickettsial agents; and meningoencephalitis of unknown origin, such as GME. Degenerative disorders in the context of this case include the inherited neuronal storage diseases and metabolic disorders. Tetanic thoracic limbs represent a unique clinical sign, which is unreported except in the focal form of the disease tetanus. The history of seizures that occurred prior to other neurological signs, the slow progressive course, and the clinical signs of vestibular system dysfunction would not be expected in the disease tetanus. We have never observed thoracic limb tetanus in any of the inflammatory diseases, and it had not been reported in any of the neuronal storage diseases or metabolic CNS disorders at the time this dog was studied.

Ancillary Studies: CBC and serum chemistry studies were normal. Cisternal CSF evaluation was normal. Electromyographic study of the thoracic limb muscles revealed continuous muscle fasciculations in the proximal limb muscles and denervation potentials in numerous thoracic limb muscles. The latter finding supported the involvement of the general somatic efferent neurons in the cervical intumescence in the lesion.

Outcome: A clinical diagnosis of a novel degenerative disorder was the presumptive diagnosis. The owner elected euthanasia, and a necropsy study was permitted.

Necropsy revealed no gross lesions on the surface of the CNS tissues. Transverse sections of the preserved CNS tissues showed grossly visible discrete bilateral symmetric malacic (soft), depressed, tan foci in numerous gray matter areas. This area included spinal cord segments C5-T1 and L4-S2 centered in the ventral gray columns, the vestibular and lateral cuneate nuclei in the medulla, the caudal colliculi, and the interposital nuclei of the cerebellum. The gray matter appeared liquefied in these affected areas (Figs. 21-23, 21-24). On microscopic examination, the central portions of all of these gross lesions were nearly empty spaces consisting of a loose meshwork of blood vessels and slender processes of astrocytes, axons, and scattered neuronal cell bodies of large motor neurons. The neuronal cell bodies appeared to be suspended in this loose meshwork

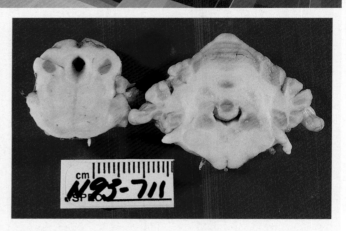

FIGURE 21-24 Transverse sections of the preserved mesencephalon, medulla, and cerebellum of the brain of the dog in this case example. Note the bilateral symmetric tan discolorations where necrosis has occurred in the caudal colliculi, vestibular, and interposital nuclei.

(Figs. 21-25, 21-26). Reactive astrocytes, many of which were vacuolated, populated the borders of these rarefied spaces (Fig. 21-27), and macrophages infiltrated the perivascular spaces and lesion borders. The nuclear lesions in the brain were similar to those in the spinal cord gray matter on microscopic examination (Figs. 21-28, 21-29). Where the lesion was most pronounced in the cervical intumescence, vacuolated myelin sheaths created a cribriform appearance in the adjacent funiculi. Loss of small gamma motor neurons and interneurons was profound, and some of the spared large motor neurons were vacuolated. The extent of the degenerative changes in the reactive astrocytes suggested that a biochemical derangement of these glial cells may have played a significant role in the pathogenesis of this novel CNS degenerative disorder. No microscopic lesions were identified in the prosencephalon. Therefore the assumption was that a functional disorder was responsible for the seizures.

In this novel encephalomyelopathy, vacuolar degeneration was recognized in astrocytes, neurons, and myelin sheaths. Although bilaterally symmetric gray matter vacuolar degeneration in the CNS has

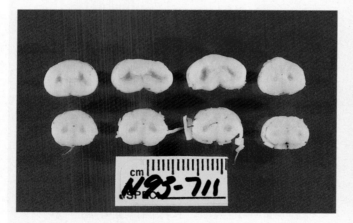

FIGURE 21-23 Transverse sections of the spinal cord of the dog in this case example. The top row includes sections from the C6-T1 segments. The bottom row includes sections from the L4-S1 segments. Note the bilateral symmetric tan discolorations primarily in the gray matter where necrosis has occurred.

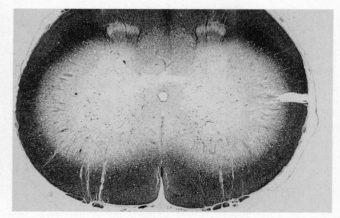

FIGURE 21-25 Low-power magnification of a microscopic section of the C8 spinal cord segment of the dog in this case example stained with Luxol fast blue (myelin) and cresyl echt violet (Nissl substance–neuronal RNA). Note the extent of the necrosis in the gray matter and adjacent white matter.

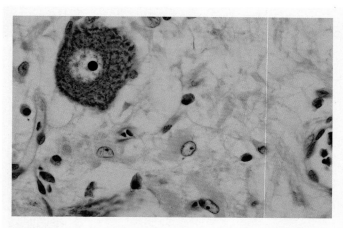

FIGURE 21-26 Higher magnification of the ventral gray column in the C8 spinal cord section in Fig. 21-25. Note the normal large motor neuron surrounded by a loose network of reactive astrocyte processes and capillaries. Most small neurons and myelin have degenerated.

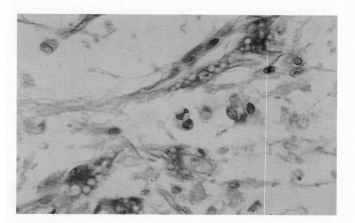

FIGURE 21-27 Higher magnification of the ventral gray column in the C8 spinal cord segment of the dog in this case example, stained histochemically for glial fibrillary astrocyte protein in the intermediate fibers of reactive astrocytes. Note the extensive vacuolation of these reactive astrocytes.

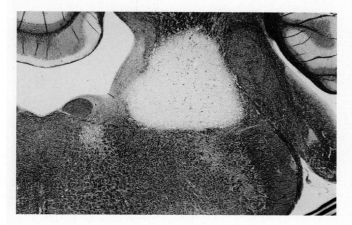

FIGURE 21-28 Low-power magnification of a section of medulla from the brain of the dog in this case example stained with Luxol fast blue and cresyl echt violet. Note the well-defined necrosis of the vestibular nuclei. Compare this figure with the gross lesion in Fig. 21-24.

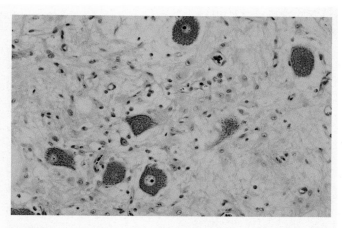

FIGURE 21-29 Higher magnification of the vestibular nucleus in Fig. 21-28, showing normal neuronal cell bodies within the necrotic lesion.

been described in a variety of conditions affecting domestic animals and humans, the encephalomyelopathy in these Australian cattle dogs differs from these previously reported entities. Some resemblance to the human disorder subacute necrotizing encephalopathy, now known as Leigh syndrome, can be found.[1]

Kate was one of three affected dogs that were studied from three litters in one small kennel of Australian cattle dogs in which tight line breeding was employed. None of the parents were affected. Inheritance of a simple autosomal recessive gene with complete penetrance was proposed as the cause of this novel degenerative disorder.

See **Video 21-2**. This video shows Midgit, a 1.5-year-old female Australian cattle dog from the same kennel as Kate. Complex partial seizures occurred when Midgit was 1 year old and were controlled with phenobarbital. Shortly after the onset of seizures, she developed stiffness in her thoracic limbs and had difficulty walking. These clinical signs of motor dysfunction slowly progressed and by a few months later, she was recumbent. Midgit's clinical signs, anatomic, differential, and necropsy diagnoses were the same as Kate in this case example.

See **Video 21-3**. This video shows Kara, a 21-month-old female Australian cattle dog that was studied by Dr. Ken Harkin at Kansas State University for a history of seizures and a progressive gait abnormality of the thoracic limbs.[3] We thank Dr. Harkin for the use of this video. The seizures began at 8 months of age and were controlled with phenobarbital. The gait abnormality began 2 months before this examination, with left thoracic limb lameness. This abnormality slowly progressed to the right thoracic limb, and a right head tilt was seen, as well as an abnormal nystagmus. In the video, note that Kara's thoracic limb gait is similar to a dog that has the disease tetanus but is still able to walk (see Videos 8-14 and 8-15 for a comparison). However, Kara exhibits a mild right head tilt and a truncal ataxia, and she readily looses her balance and falls. She has an abnormal positional nystagmus, and her normal physiologic nystagmus was considered difficult to elicit. Note the severity of the thoracic limb rigidity in lateral recumbency but the ability of the examiner to readily flex the limbs. The muscles in both thoracic limbs were atrophied. These clinical signs are similar to those exhibited by Kate and Midgit but to a lesser degree. Therefore the anatomic and differential diagnoses are the same, and Kara was presumed to have the same novel degenerative disorder. To further support this presumption, MR imaging of the brain was performed, which revealed well-defined bilateral symmetric gray matter lesions in the brainstem and cerebellum identical to those found at necropsy in Kate and Midgit (Fig. 21-30). Kara's clinical signs continued to

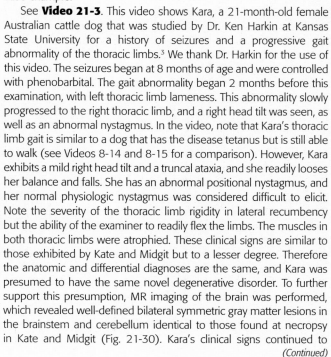

(Continued)

CASE EXAMPLE 21-12—cont'd

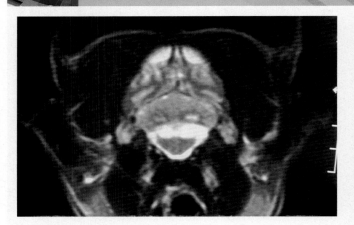

FIGURE 21-30 T2-weighted MR image of the medulla and cerebellum of Kara, the 21-month-old Australian cattle dog seen in Video 21-3. Note the bilateral symmetric hyperintensity of the vestibular nuclei in the medulla and the interposital nuclei in the cerebellum. This MR abnormality reflects the fluid accumulated in the necrotic lesions.

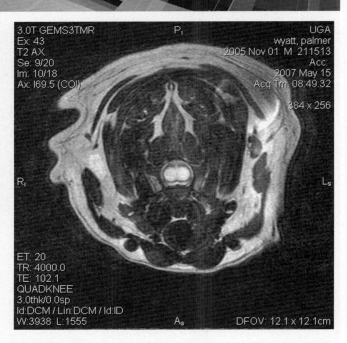

FIGURE 21-31 T2-weighted MR image of the C8 spinal cord segment of the shih tzu with the diffuse neuromuscular disorder. Note the bilateral symmetric hyperintensity of the gray matter and adjacent white matter. Compare this with the lesion seen in Fig. 21-25.

progress; she was euthanized, and necropsy was performed. On gross and microscopic examination, a polioencephalomyelopathy was recognized that was similar to that observed in the previously mentioned two Australian cattle dogs. Bilateral symmetric lesions were present in the C4-T1 spinal cord segments; the interposital and lateral nuclei of the cerebellum; the vestibular nuclei, spinal nucleus of the trigeminal nerve, and lateral reticular nuclei in the medulla and pons; the dorsal nuclei of the trapezoid body in the pons; and the caudal colliculi in the mesencephalon and nuclei in the ventral thalamus.

Recently, an 18-month-old castrated male shih tzu was examined by Dr. Marc Kent at the University of Georgia for a progressive gait disorder primarily in the thoracic limbs. At 7 months of age, the gait in the right thoracic limb was noticed to be abnormal. This abnormality slowly progressed to involve both thoracic limbs by 13 months of age, when the clinical signs progressed rapidly. Examination at 18 months of age revealed clinical signs of a severe neuromuscular disorder in the thoracic limbs and very mild clinical signs of a UMN and GP disorder in the pelvic limbs. The anatomic diagnosis was a lesion involving the C6-T2 spinal cord segments. Thoracic limb electromyography and biopsy of the triceps brachii revealed evidence of denervation. MR imaging of the brain and spinal cord revealed extensive bilateral symmetric lesions similar to those observed in the MR images of the brain of Kara, the Australian cattle dog studied at Kansas State University that was still ambulatory (Figs. 21-31, 21-32). These brain and spinal cord MR image lesions closely correlated with the necropsy lesions of the three Australian cattle dogs previously described. This shih tzu was euthanized, and a necropsy study revealed a polioencephalomyelopathy similar to that observed in the Australian cattle dogs (Figs. 21-33, 21-34). The presumption was that this shih tzu had a more severe loss of the large alpha motor neurons in the cervical intumescence to account for the thoracic limb neuromuscular clinical signs. The involvement of the adjacent white matter in this intumescence would account for the mild pelvic limb clinical signs.

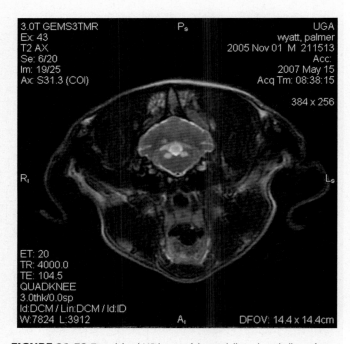

FIGURE 21-32 T2-weighted MR image of the medulla and cerebellum of the brain of the shih tzu, exhibiting bilateral symmetric hyperintense lesions in the vestibular nuclei of the medulla and the interposital nuclei of the cerebellum. Compare this with the lesions seen in Figs. 21-24 and 21-28.

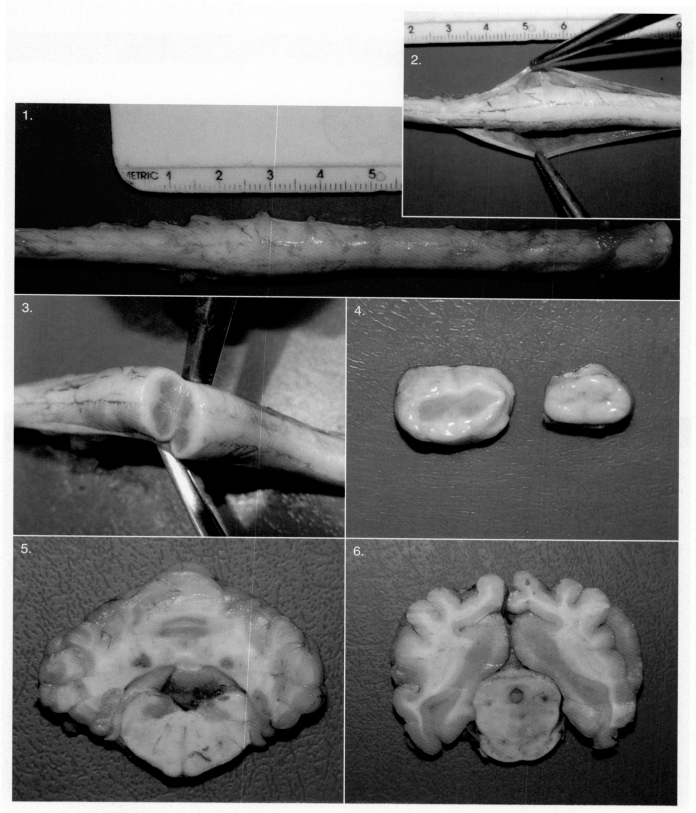

FIGURE 21-33 Gross lesions observed at the necropsy of the shih tzu with the lesions revealed by the MR images in Figs. 21-31 and 21-32. *1* through *4* are photos of the spinal cord lesion prior to preservation. *1,* Mild enlargement of the cervical intumescence that was soft on palpation. *2,* Same as *1* with the dura reflected. *3* and *4* are transverse sections of the cervical intumescence. Note the bilateral symmetrical discoloration primarily in the gray matter that was soft on palpation. *5* and *6* are transverse sections of the preserved brain. *5,* Transverse section of the cerebellum and medulla. Note the bilateral symmetrical gray discoloration of the vestibular and interposital nuclei. *6,* Transverse section of the mesencephalon. Note the discolorations in the caudal colliculi.

(Continued)

CASE EXAMPLE 21-12—cont'd

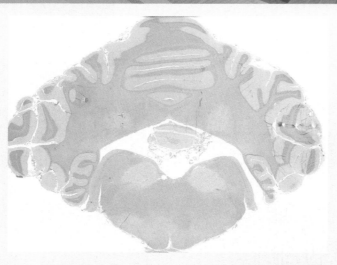

FIGURE 21-34 Low-power magnification of a section of the medulla and cerebellum seen in Fig. 21-33, stained with hematoxylin and eosin. Note the well-defined areas of necrosis in the vestibular nuclei of the medulla and the interposital nuclei of the cerebellum.

CASE EXAMPLE 21-13

Signalment: 10-month-old female Alaskan husky

Chief Complaint: Seizures, abnormal behavior and gait

History: An acute onset of seizures occurred 10 days before examination. After the seizures, this dog was recumbent, obtunded, and blind. By the time of hospitalization and examination, the dog had improved to the extent of being able to stand and walk.

Examination: See **Video 21-4A**. Note the obtundation, propulsive movements, tetraparesis and ataxia, lack of postural reactions, blindness, and facial and oropharyngeal hypalgesia. The ataxia includes GP, vestibular, and cerebellar components. Pupil size and light responses were normal in each eye. Not shown was her difficulty in food prehension.

Anatomic Diagnosis: Diffuse brain

The propulsive activity, degree of obtundation, blindness, and history of seizures reflect a prosencephalic lesion. The tetraparesis and ataxia are caused by a lesion in the caudal brainstem and cerebellum. The hypalgesia and dysphagia may be caused by a rostral brainstem (diencephalon) or caudal brainstem (pons, medulla) lesion.

Differential Diagnosis: Inflammatory and degenerative diseases are the two major disease categories for consideration to cause this progressive diffuse disorder. The diffuse nature of the clinical signs, the acute onset, the age of the patient, and the improvement without therapy make neoplasia less likely. Inflammatory diseases include viral (canine distemper), protozoal, fungal, and rickettsial diseases, as well as meningoencephalitis of unknown origin, such as GME. All of these diagnoses are less likely to cause such profound clinical signs and then improve spontaneously. At the time of this study, no neuronal storage disease or metabolic encephalopathy had been described in the Alaskan husky breed, but the diffuse nature of the intracranial clinical signs and the progressive course are features expected with these diffuse degenerative disorders. A metabolic disorder would best explain the improvement that was observed.

Ancillary Study: CBC and serum chemistry results were normal, as were serum pyruvate and lactate levels. Cisternal CSF evaluation was normal for the number of leucocytes, as well as for the levels of protein, pyruvate, and lactate.

A presumptive clinical diagnosis was made of a metabolic degenerative disorder.

Outcome: Over the next few weeks, this Alaskan husky slowly improved, which can be seen in **Video 21-4B**. She is more alert but still acts confused. Her gait is nearly normal, but postural reactions are very slow. She has no menace response but will follow a rolling object. Her facial hypalgesia is improved, but she still has some problem with prehension. Most of these remaining clinical signs reflect prosencephalic dysfunction. After a few weeks, she relapsed with severe clinical signs that included recumbency and obtundation. She was euthanized, and necropsy was performed.

Necropsy showed no gross lesions on the external surface of the brain or spinal cord. Transverse sections of the preserved CNS tissues revealed distinct bilaterally symmetric malacic (soft) gray discolorations and cavitations. This gross lesion was most pronounced in the lateral aspect of the thalamus on both sides where cavitation was evident (Fig. 21-35). These cavities were obliquely oriented from dorsolateral to ventromedial. This lesion was continuous caudally through the brainstem where cavitations were less evident, but the ventromedial portions of the bilateral soft discolorations met on the median plane, forming a V-like appearance in the center of the brainstem. The extent of the lesion decreased in the more caudal brainstem. On microscopic examination, these gross lesions represented varying degrees of necrotizing lesions that consisted of active and inactive areas distributed in the following two patterns: (1) a bilateral symmetric pattern in basal nuclei in the cerebrum

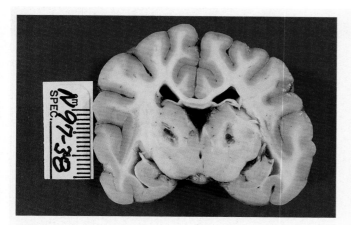

FIGURE 21-35 Transverse section of the preserved prosencephalon of an Alaskan husky with subacute necrotizing encephalopathy. Note the bilateral symmetric cavitations in the midlateral thalamus.

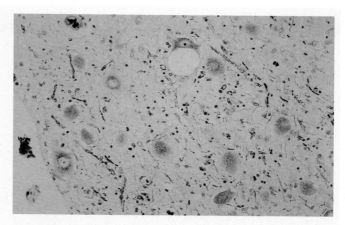

FIGURE 21-37 Higher magnification of the lesion in Fig. 21-36. Note the normal neurons surrounded by a loose network of reactive astrocytes and capillaries within the necrotic lesion.

and the entire central portion of the brainstem, with the most extensive lesions in the thalamus (Figs. 21-36, 21-37), and (2) a multifocal pattern at the base of cerebrocortical sulci mostly in the parietal and temporal lobes and the cerebellar cortex in the ventral vermis. The lesion affected primarily gray matter. All of these brain lesions exhibited neuronal depletion but with variable neuronal sparing within areas of necrosis, prominence of small blood vessels, spongiosis, and gliosis. Active lesions contained normal neurons interspersed with ischemic neurons, glial necrosis, spongiosis, cavitation, and occasionally secondary accumulations of inflammatory cells. Inactive lesions exhibited sclerosis with abundant reactive astrocytes and macrophages surrounding cavitations.

Necrotizing lesions were observed in the dorsolateral caudate nuclei, dorsal putamen, dorsal claustrum, midlateral thalamus, mesencephalic tegmentum, caudal colliculi, reticular formation of the pons and medulla, cerebral cortex at the base of sulci in the parietal and temporal lobes, and ventral cerebellar vermis. This distribution is important when evaluating MR imaging studies (Figs. 21-38 through 21-42). The pathologic diagnosis was a unique encephalopathy with a topography suggestive of a metabolic disorder. These lesions closely resemble those of the human disorder subacute necrotizing encephalomyelopathy, now known as Leigh syndrome.

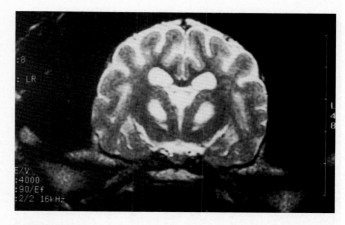

FIGURE 21-38 T2-weighted MR image of the brain of an Alaskan husky with subacute necrotizing encephalopathy. Note the hyperintensity of the bilateral symmetric lesions in the midthalamus. Compare with Fig. 21-35.

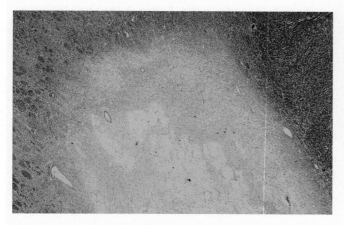

FIGURE 21-36 Low-power magnification of a microscopic section of one of the gross lesions seen in Fig. 21-35, stained with Luxol fast blue (myelin) and cresyl echt violet (neuronal RNA). Note the sharp demarcation of the necrotic lesion.

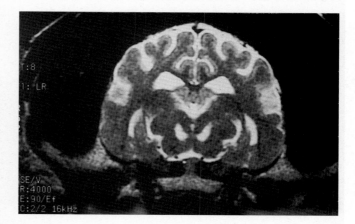

FIGURE 21-39 T2-weighted MR image of the brain the Alaskan husky in Fig. 21-38. Note the bilateral symmetric hyperintensity of the lesions in the mesencephalic tegmentum.

Subacute necrotizing encephalomyelopathy occurs in juvenile individuals and consists of episodic neurologic signs and cumulative neurologic deterioration. Recognized biochemical defects have been heterogenous, but most involve pathways of oxidative metabolism.

(Continued)

CASE EXAMPLE 21-13—cont'd

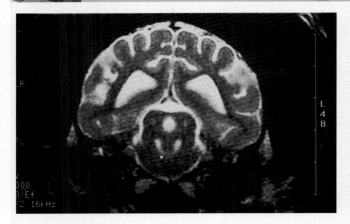

FIGURE 21-40 T2-weighted MR image of the brain of the Alaskan husky in Figs. 21-38 and 21-39. Note the bilateral symmetric hyperintensity of the lesions in the mesencephalic tegmentum and caudal colliculi.

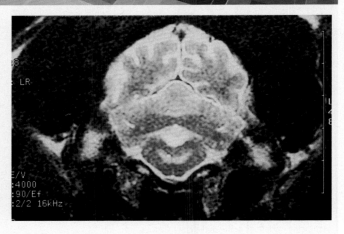

FIGURE 21-42 T2-weighted MR image of the brain of the Alaskan husky in Figs. 21-38 through 21-41. Note the confluent hyperintensity of the lesion in the reticular formation of the medulla.

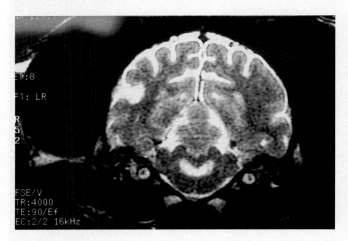

FIGURE 21-41 T2-weighted MR image of the brain of the Alaskan husky in Figs. 21-38 through 21-40. Note the confluent symmetric hyperintensity of the lesion in the reticular formation of the pons.

See **Video 21-5A** showing the first of three sequences of the clinical course of this subacute necrotizing encephalopathy in a 2.5-year-old female Alaskan husky named Yette. This dog had an acute onset of cluster seizures, which were controlled, but she remained tetraplegic and in lateral recumbency. Video 21-5A shows

Yette 3 days later when she was still recumbent and obtunded and exhibited a spastic tetraplegia. She was hypertonic and had brisk patellar reflexes and normal withdrawal reflexes with depressed nociception. No menace response in each eye or any evidence of vision was observed, but the pupil size and light responses were normal in each eye. These clinical signs represent diffuse brain dysfunction. She continued to improve, and **Video 21-5B** shows her approximately 1 week after Video 21-5A. She was able to stand and walk but exhibited a hypermetric ataxia in her propulsive walking. MR imaging was performed at that time and revealed bilateral symmetric lesions in the brainstem typical for that described for the Alaskan husky's degenerative encephalopathy. These images can be seen on **Video 21-5C**. Yette's improvement continued, and **Video 21-5D** shows her approximately 2 weeks after Video 21-5B. At this time, she had no observable clinical signs. Shortly after, diffuse clinical signs recurred, and she was euthanized. A necropsy confirmed this unique subacute necrotizing encephalopathy that has been described here in these Alaskan huskies.

At least 12 cases of this encephalopathy have been confirmed at necropsy from kennels widely distributed throughout the United States. Some of these cases have involved littermates. The assumption is that this abnormality is an inherited metabolic encephalopathy of juvenile and occasionally young adult Alaskan huskies, but the mode of inheritance has not been determined.[2,4]

REFERENCES

1. Brenner O, et al: Hereditary polioencephalomyelopathy of the Australian cattle dog, *Acta Pathol* 94:54-66, 1997.
2. Brenner O, et al: Alaskan husky encephalopathy—a canine neurodegenerative disorder resembling subacute necrotizing encephalomyelopathy (Leigh syndrome), *Acta Neuropathol* 100:50-62, 2000.
3. Harkin KR, et al: Magnetic resonance imaging of a dog with hereditary polioencephalomyelopathy, *J Am Vet Med Assoc* 214:1342-1344, 1999.
4. Wakshlag JJ, et al: Subacute necrotizing encephalopathy in an Alaskan husky, *J Small Anim Pract* 40:585-589, 1999.

Page numbers followed by *f,* indicate figures; *t,* tables; *b,* boxes.

A

Abducent nerve
  anatomy of, 135
  lesions of, 137
  strabismus, direction following
    paralysis, 138*f*
Abiotrophy, 100–101, 407*f*
Abscess, 162
  cholesterinic granuloma in Morgan,
    418*f*
  prevalence of, 423
  Streptococcus equi, cause of, 418*f,*
    417
Absorption of CSF, 59–60
Accessory nerve, 152*f,* 153, 188–189
Acetylcholine, 89–90
  release of, 78–79
Acetylcholinesterase, 78–79
Acquired action-related repetitive
  myoclonus, 215
Acquired idiopathic laryngeal
  paralysis, 159–160
Acquired myotonia, 209
Acquired obstructive hydrocephalus,
  69–70
  in golden retriever
    at columns of fornix, 69*f*
    dilated left lateral ventricle, 69*f*
    at rostral diencephalon, 69*f*
Acquired vertebral malformation-
  malarticulation, 269*f,* 290
Action-related repetitive myoclonus,
  214–215
  acquired, 215
  congenital, 214–215
Acute caudal myopathy, 113–114
Acute polyradiculoneuritis (PRN), 90–91
Acute prosencephalic disease, 187–188
Adenohypophysis, 479, 483
Adipsia, 484
Adrenergic system, 168–169
Adult cheetah leukoencephalopathy,
  426, 426*f*
Adversive syndrome, 72
Afferent neuron, 2
Afghan hound myelinolysis, 264,
  264*f,* 266*f*
Akabane virus, 44, 44*f,* 45*f,* 68*f*
Alar layer, 27, 27*f*
Alpha-2 adrenoreceptors, 185–186

American brown bear
  brain of, 357*f,* 358*f*
  cerebellum of, 358*f*
American Eskimo dog, malignant
  nerve sheath neoplasm in, 142*f*
Ampulla, 320
Amygdaloid body, 448
Anatomic diagnosis, 1
Anencephaly, 39
Anesthesia
  hypoxia, delayed effects of, 422*f*
  hypoxia/anoxia from, 421, 422*f*
  respiratory arrest during, 422*f*
Anisocoria, 182
Anticholinesterase, overdose of, 94
Anticonvulsant therapy
  for cluster seizures and status
    epilepticus, 467
  felbamate for, 467
  gabapentin for, 467
  levetiracetam as, 467
  phenobarbital for, 466
  potassium bromide for, 466
  zonisamide for, 467
Anus, examination in large
  animal, 287
Aortic thromboembolism, 115–116
Apnea, 455
Appetite, abnormal, 484
Arachnoid membrane
  characteristics of, 55–56
  view of, 55*f,* 56*f*
Archicerebellum, 349–352
Archipallium, 36, 448
Area centralis, 395–396, 396*f*
Area postrema, 441
Arnold Chiari malformation, 46–47
  Type I, 47
Arrhinencephaly, 42
Arthrogryposis, 101
Ascending reticular activating system,
  479–480, 480*f*
Aspergillus, 154–156
Association axon, 36–37
Astrocyte, 24–25, 379*f*
Astrocytoma, 410*f*
Ataxia, 228, 254–261, 264–265,
  271–278
  neurologic examination and,
    491–492
  vestibular, 324

Athetosis, 217
Atlantoaxial subluxation, 268–269, 269*f*
Atlas, 290*f*
  disarticulation of, 291*f*
  ossification of, 268, 268*f*
Atonia, 470–471
Atrophy
  of equine gluteal muscles, 164*f*
  of equine tongue, 164*f*
  head and pelvic muscles in horse,
    163–166
Atropine sulfate, 471
Auditory pathway, 437*f*
Auditory system
  anatomy of, 433–437
  inner ear, 319
  receptor of, 435*f*
Autoimmune myositis, 96
Autonomic nervous system
  anatomy of, 168
Autonomous zone, 231
  pelvic limb, cutaneous innervation
    of, 231*f*
  thoracic limb, cutaneous
    innervation of, 232*f*
Autosomal recessive polymyopathy,
  type II deficiency, 98–99
Avulsion
  of brachial plexus, 104–105, 105*f*
  of dorsal root, 105*f*
Awake state, 468, 469
Axis, 290*f*
  disarticulation of, 291*f*
  ossification of, 268, 268*f*
Axon, 2, 2*f*
  axonal buds and, 88
  growth of, 27–28
  processes of, 36–37
  projection, development of, 36
Axonal bud, 88
Axonal neuropathy, inherited
  giant, 125
Axonopathy (hereditary ataxia)
  Ibizan hound, 384
  Parson (Jack) Russell terriers, 384
Axoplasma calcium, 78–79

B

Backing, 286
Backing up, 493

Balance. *See* Vestibular system
Ballism, 217
Basal ganglia, 36
Basal layer, 27, 27f
Basal nuclei, 195–196, 198f
Basset hound, intramedullary mass
    lesion in, 67f
Beagle
    as cyclop, 43f
    developmental obstructive
        hydrocephalus in, 39, 71f, 76f
    malignant nerve sheath neoplasm
        in, 103f, 104f, 140f
Bear
    brain of, 357f, 358f
    cerebellum of, 358f
Behavior, abnormal
    hypothalamic lesions causing, 484
    seizure causing, 452–453
Benign idiopathic peripheral
    vestibular disease
    in canine, 328–329
    in feline, 335
    in horse, 341
Bicep reflex, 84f, 85–86
Bilateral nonsuppurative trigeminal
    neuritis, 142–144
Bilateral optic tract lesion, 402
Bilateral otitis media, 149f
Bilateral retinal lesion, 401
Bladder
    external sphincter of, 186
    lower motor neuron, 187
    manual evacuation of, 187
    neuroanatomy of function, 184f
    upper motor neuron, 187
Blindness
    in calf, 408f
    in colt, 408f
    in kitten, 407f
    in miniature poodle, 407f
    night blindness, 407–408
    prosencephalic hypoplasia and, 39
    vitamin A deficiency and,
        406–407
Blood, CSF collection, 65
Blood-brain barrier, 60
Blood-CSF barrier, 60
Bluetongue virus, 43
    in Hereford calf, 44f
Bony labyrinth, 435f
    fluid-filled portions of, 320
    formation of, 319
Botulism, 92
Bovine viral diarrhea virus, 44
Bovine virus diarrhea (BVD), 371
Brachial plexus neuritis, 104
Brachial plexus root avulsion,
    104–105, 105f
Brain
    of American brown bear, 357f, 358f
    of dog, 236f, 353f, 354f, 358f
    extrapyramidal pathways of, 200f
    of gibbon, 359f
    hemorrhage from trauma, 183f
    of horse, 407f
    hydrocephalus of, 37, 48
    lesion causing behavioral
        abnormalities, 452

Brain *(Continued)*
    malformations of, 37–48
    right cerebral hemisphere, 197f
    of sea lion, 235f, 358f
    transverse plane proton density
        MR images of, 7f
    transverse sections of, 6, 6f
    vesicles, development of, 25f
Brain parenchyma, 60
Brainstem
    abducent level through medulla,
        137f
    cerebellum and, 352
    cranial nerve nuclei, organization
        of, 135f
    dorsal and lateral views of, 6f
    dorsal view of, 224f
    dorsolateral view of, 352f
    hypoglossal level through
        medulla, 137f
    neuronal cell bodies in, 323
    nuclei and tracts, 434–436
    oculomotor nuclei level through
        mesencephalon, 136f
    spinal tract formation, 234–235
    trochlear level through
        mesencephalon, 136f
Brainstem auditory-evoked potential
    (BAER) testing, 498
Brainstem center
    for defecation, 187–188
    for micturition, 186
Brown Swiss myelopathy, 312
Brucella canis, 256
Bug-searching episode, 465
Bünger band, 88
Bunny-hop movement, 49–50
    lower motor neuron disease and,
        86–87
    in Manx cats, 51
    testing responses of, 87, 491
    in weimaraners, 51–52
    See also Hopping
Burmese cat
    craniofacial malformation in, 40
    meningoencephalocele with facial
        duplication, 41f
    meningoencephalocele with
        philtrum/whisker pad
        duplication, 41f

C

Calf
    cerebellar folium of, 354f
    with cerebellar hypoplasia, 68f
    cerebellar malformation in, 372f,
        373f
    complex malformations of, 46–47
    congenital tetany in, 211f
    diastematomyelia in lumbosacral
        spinal cord, 49f
    diplomyelia in lumbar spine, 49f
    hepatic encephalomyelopathy in,
        311–312
    otitis media
        bilateral, 149f
        facial paralysis from, 148f
    otitis media-interna in, 343–344

Calf *(Continued)*
    poliomyelomalacia in, 118
    postoperative poliomyelomalacia
        in, 117
    segmental hypoplasia in, 49f
    vitamin A deficiency in, 70
Caloric nystagmus, 326
Calvaria
    cerebral meninges/arachnoid villi, 57f
    fracture of, 59f
    lipomeningocele, Holstein cow
        with, 41f
Calvarial ossification, 48
Camelid spinal cord disease, 306–308
Campylobacter jejuni, 91
Canarc gene, 469
Canine
    ventricular system of, 57f
    See also Dog
Canine laryngeal paralysis
    acquired, 159–160
    inherited, 159
Canine meningeal polyarteritis,
    281–282, 281f
Canine sensory neuropathy, 232
Caprine arthritis encephalitis (CAE),
    161
    cervical spinal cord of
        dorsal view, 309f
        halved section of, 309f
        macrophages, 310f
        transverse section of, 309f
    diagnosis of, 310
    lesion from, 311f
    prevention of, 310
    in Toggenburg goat, 309–310
Carbohydrate metabolism, abnormal,
    484–485
Carcinoma, in choroid plexus, 37
Cat
    cerebellar abiotrophy in, 370
    cerebellar folium of, 354f
    cerebellar malformation in
        congenital, 369
        feline panleucopenia virus,
            369–370, 369f, 370f
    cervical spinal cord of, 201f
    cuterebra larval myiasis in,
        337–338, 338f
    Cuterebra species larva migration in,
        67–68, 68f
    feline infectious peritonitis (PIF), 69
    feline ischemic encephalopathy,
        67–68, 68f
    Horner syndrome, facial paralysis
        from, 148f
    Horner syndrome in, 174f
    infectious peritonitis viral
        meningoencephalomyelitis in,
        339, 339f, 340f
    lymphoma in, 107f, 260f
    meningioma in, 59f
    meningoencephalitis in, 70f
    mesencephalic aqueduct obstruction
        in, 70f
    neoplasm in, 337, 337f
    otitis media-interna in, 335–336
    paraplegia in, 115–118
    spinal cord of, 252f

Cat *(Continued)*
  trigeminal neuritis in, 144*f*
  tympanic bulla in, 330*f*, 331*f*
  vertebrae versus sacral segments, 63*t*
  vestibular system disorders in, 335
  See also Manx cat
Cataplexy
  clinical signs of, 469–472
  diagnosis of, 470–471
  diagnostic tests and therapy for, 471
  examples of, 471–472
  overview of, 468–472
Catarrhal fever, malignant, 162–163
Cattle. *See* Calf; Cow; Holstein cow
Cauda equina, 111*f*
  in German Shepherd, 112–113
  neuritis of, 111–112
Caudal cerebellar vermis, 48*f*
Caudal cervical dysfunction, 500
Caudal cervical lesion, 247
Caudal colliculus, 436–438
Caudal cranial fossa, 47
Caudal diencephalon, 34*f*
Caudal diskospondylitis, 289–315
Caudal lumbar sympathetic
  GVE-LMN, 185–186
Caudal mesencephalon, 34*f*
Caudate nucleus, 195
Caudoventral cerebellar vermis, 47
Cavalier King Charles spaniel
  movement disorder in, 217–218
  occipital bone malformation
    syndrome in, 60*f*
Cell body, 2
  telencephalic neuronal, location
    of, 36
Cell differentiation, 24–27
Centaurea repens, 205–206
Centaurea solstitalis, 205–206
Central chromatolysis, 89
Central nervous system (CNS)
  layers of, 55–56
  neoplasia of, 2
  protection by CSF, 60–61
  storage disease in, 426
  upper motor neuron (UMN) in, 192
Central vestibular system disease,
  325, 327
Central visual pathway
  for conscious perception, 398–399,
    398*f*
  optic chiasm and tract, 397–398
  optic nerve, 396–397
Cerebellar abiotrophy
  in Arabian horses, 370–371
  in cats, 370
  in cow, 375
  in dogs, 363–369
    beagles and samoyed, 369–370
    Gordon setter, 367–368, 368*f*, 385
    Kerry blue terrier, 363–367, 364*f*,
      365*f*, 366*f*, 367*f*
    Old English sheepdog, 368
    Scottish terrier, 368–369
  in pig, 376
Cerebellar afferent, 355–356
  general proprioception and, 355
  special proprioception and, 355
Cerebellar ataxia, 375–376, 491–492

Cerebellar cortex, 352–356
Cerebellar cortical abiotrophy, 370–371
Cerebellar dysfunction, 228
Cerebellar efferents, 356–357
Cerebellar folium
  in calf, 354*f*
  in cat, 354*f*
Cerebellar herniation, 47
Cerebellar hypoplasia
  in calf, 68*f*
  in wire fox terrier, 46*f*
Cerebellar malformation, 46
  in cats, 369–370, 369*f*, 370*f*
  in cow, 372*f*, 373*f*
  in cows, 371–373
  in dogs, 360–369
    Irish setter, 362*f*, 363*f*
    Labrador retriever, 361*f*
    wire fox terrier, 362*f*
Cerebellar nuclei, 356–357
Cerebellar projection, 224*f*
Cerebellar transmission
  from thoracic limbs and cervical
    region, 222–225
  from trunk and pelvic limb, 222
Cerebellar-vestibular disorder,
  376–377, 376*f*, 377*f*
Cerebellomedullary cistern, CSF
  collection, 61–63, 62*f*
Cerebellum
  of American brown bear, 358*f*
  anatomy of, 349–356
  degeneration of, 377
  development of, 348–349, 349*f*
  disease of
    clinical signs of, 359–360
    in dogs, 360–369
    malformation-abiotrophy, 360–376
  dorsocaudal view of, 353*f*
  dorsolateral view of, 351*f*
  dysfunction of, 500
  of foal, 350*f*
  formation of, 32
  functional cerebellar disorder,
    373–375, 374*f*, 375*f*
  function of, 357–359
  of great horned owl, 357*f*
  inflammation of, 376–377
  injury to, 377
  lesions of, 381*f*, 382*f*
  motor function control, role in, 356*f*
  neoplasm in, 377
  neuronal cell bodies in, 324
  Parelaphostrongylus tenuis in sheep,
    308*f*
  of puppy, 350*f*
  regions of, 357
  of sea lion, 359*f*
  ventral surface of, 351*f*
  zones of, 357
Cerebral abscess
  in cat, 416*f*, 417*f*
  cause of, 416
Cerebral aplasia, 360–369
Cerebral cortex
  extrapyramidal neurons in, 195
  histology of, 194–195, 194*f*
  regions of, 36, 448
  topography of, 193*f*

Cerebral hemisphere, right, 197*f*
Cerebral projection, 227*f*
Cerebrocortical necrosis, 420
  amprolium, use of, 421
  mercury, use of, 421
  postanesthetic hypoxia, 421
Cerebropontocerebellar pathway,
  355–356
Cerebrospinal fluid (CSF)
  absorption, site of, 59–60
  absorption of, 59–60
  characteristics of, 54
  circulation of, 56
  clinical application of, 61
  collection of, 61–63
    from cerebellomedullary cistern, 62*f*
    from lumbosacral, 63–65
    from lumbosacral spinal cord, 64*f*
  compression of flow space, 58
  in equine protozoal myelitis,
    300–301
  evaluation of, 65
  function of, 60–61
  hydranencephaly and, 67–68
  hydrocephalus and, 67
  obstruction of flow, 47–48
  pressure, measurement of, 61–62
  production of, 54–55
  prosencephalic hypoplasia and, 39
Cerebrospinal nematodiasis, 423–425
Cerebrovascular accidents (CVA),
  379–381
Cerebrum
  formation of, 35–37
  pathways for voluntary movement,
    203*f*
  See also Telencephalon
Cervical intumescence
  components of, 85
  segmental innervation from, 85*f*
Cervical scoliosis, 306*f*
  in 19-month old Arabian, 306*f*
  Dutch Warmblood with, 305*f*
  prevalence of, 305–306
Cervical spinal cord
  disease of, 267*f*
    hypervitaminosis A, 267
    progressive compressive cervical
      myelopathy, 267–268
    tetraplegia, 266–271
  in human, cat and horse, 201*f*
  lesions of, 229
  transverse sections of, 248*f*
Cervical spinal cord
  syringohydromyelia, 48*f*
Cervical vertebrae
  eighth, 276*f*, 277*f*
  fifth, 270*f*, 271*f*
  fourth, 270*f*, 292*f*, 306*f*
  seventh, 269*f*, 270*f*, 271*f*, 279*f*, 294*f*
  sixth, 270*f*, 271*f*
  third, 279*f*, 292*f*, 306*f*
  See also Spinal cord segments
Cervical vertebral malformation-
  malarticulation, 289–294
Cervicospinocerebellar pathway,
  224–225
Cervicospinovestibular pathway, 225
Channelopathy, Ions, 217–218

Charolais leukodystrophy, 312
Chewing gum fits, 464
Chiasmatic group, 483
Chihuahua, molera in, 48
Cholesterinic granuloma, 418*f*
  bilateral, Percheron horse with, 38*f*
  diagnosis of, 37
  in Morgan horse, 418*f*
  in Percheron, 419*f*
  prevalence of, 423
  in Quarter horse, 419*f*
  unilateral, Morgan horse with, 38*f*
Cholesterol crystals, 37
Cholinergic system, 168–169
Chondrosarcoma, 181–182
Chorea, 217
Choroid plexus
  cerebrospinal fluid and, 54
  cholesterol crystals in, 37
  development of, 35*f*
  transverse sections of, 55*f*
  See also Cholesterinic granuloma
Choroid plexus of the fourth
    ventricle, 30
  development of, 32*f*
Chronic neuritis, 104
Circling, 286, 493
Circumduction, 493
Cisternal myelogram
  of extradural mass lesion, 66*f*
  of intradural-extramedullary
    lesion, 67*f*
Clonic reflex, 494
Clostridium botulinum, 92
Clostridium tetani, 209
Cluster seizure, 455, 467
Cochlea, 320, 436*f*
Cochlear duct, 433, 436*f*
Cochlear window, 320
Coma
  clinical evaluation for, 481–482
  metabolic conditions causing, 482
  neurologic examination for, 481–482
  peracute, 481
  poisons causing, 482
Comatose patient, clinical evaluation
    of, 481–482
Commissural axon
  groups of, 37
  processes of, 36–37
Compensatory hydrocephalus
  CSF collection in, 67–68
  examples of
    in calf, 68*f*
    in cat, 68*f*
    in steer, 68*f*
Complex partial seizure, 451–452,
    455
Complex regional pain syndrome, 190
Compressive myelopathy, 290*f*, 294*f*
Conduction deafness, 438
Congenital action-related repetitive
    myoclonus, 214–215
Congenital idiopathic megaesophagus,
    153–154
Congenital inherited sensorineural
    deafness
  abiotrophic form of, 438–439
  albinotic form of, 438

Congenital myotonia, inherited,
    207–209, 208*f*
Congenital nystagmus, 345–346, 345*f*
Congenital occiptoatlantoaxial
    malformation, 289–290
Congenital peripheral vestibular
    system disease, 336
Congenital tetany, inherited, 211*f*
Consciousness
  decreased level of, 481
  state of, 481
Conscious pathway, 223*f*
Conscious perception
  central visual pathway for, 398–399,
    398*f*
  GSA pathway for, 230*f*, 233–234,
    236
  for olfaction, 445
Conscious proprioception, 221
Constant repetitive myoclonus,
    213–214
Coordination, loss of, 324
Copper deficiency-enzootic ataxia,
    310
Corpus callosum, 37
Corpus striatum, 195
Cortical projection system
  diffuse, 479
  direct, 478–479
Cow
  Brown Swiss myelopathy in, 312
  cerebellar abiotrophy in, 375
  cerebellar malformation, 371–373
  dystocia injury, femoral nerve,
    126–127
  encephalitis, facial paralysis from,
    146*f*
  focal tetany in, 212
  fracture at T4 in, 312
  functional cerebellar disorder in,
    373–375
  Horner syndrome in, 175*f*
  hypokalemic myopathy in, 78
  listeriosis in, 161–162, 343–344
  listeriosis with tongue paralysis in,
    161*f*
  lumbosacral discospondylitis
    in, 313
  paraparesis in, 123–124, 126–127
  recumbency in, 98, 98*f*
  risus sardonicus, tetanus causing,
    210*f*
  sciatic nerve paralysis in, 124*f*
  sympathetic GVE-LMN innervation,
    loss of, 175–176
  tetanus, risus sardonicus from, 210*f*
  tibial nerve paralysis in, 124*f*
  See also Calf
Cranial cervical dysfunction, 500
Cranial cervical lesion, 247–248
Cranial mediastinal, lesions of, 159
Cranial nerve
  functional organization of, 31*f*
  GSA system and, 234–236
  location of, 30
  lymphoma in, 141
  malignant nerve sheath neoplasm
    in, 139–140
  neurologic examination of, 246

Cranial nerve examination
  order of, 499
  performance of, 495
Cranial nerve general proprioception,
    227–228
Cranial nerve III, 32–33
  abnormalities of, 136–137
  anatomy of, 134–135
  function of, 135–139
  neoplasm, clinical signs of, 139
Cranial nerve IV, 32–33
  abnormalities of, 136–137
  anatomy of, 135
  function of, 135–139
  neoplasm, clinical signs of, 139
Cranial nerve IX, 30, 31*f*
  anatomy of, 152–153
  evaluation of, 498–499
Cranial nerve V, 31–32, 32*f*
  anatomy of, 139
  function, loss of, 139
Cranial nerve VI, 30, 31*f*
  abnormalities of, 136–137
  anatomy of, 135
  function of, 135–139
  neoplasm, clinical signs of,
    139
Cranial nerve VII, 30, 31*f*
  anatomy of, 144–145
  lesions of, 145–147
Cranial nerve VIII, 30, 31*f*, 321–322,
    434*f*
Cranial nerve X, 30, 31*f*
  anatomy of, 152–153
  evaluation of, 498
Cranial nerve XI, 30, 31*f*
  anatomy of, 152–153
Cranial nerve XII, 30, 31*f*
  anatomy of, 160
  diseases of, 160–161
  evaluation of, 498
  lesions of, 160
Cranial placodes, 30
Cranial spinocerebellar tract, 224
Cranial thoracic fracture, 288–289
Craniosacral system, 168–169
Cranioschisis, 39–40
Cranium bifidum, 39–40
Crista ampullaris, 320–321
Cuneocerebellar tract, 222–225
Cupula, 320–321
Cutaneous area, 231
Cutaneous reflex, 287
Cutaneous sympathetic innervation,
    dysfunction of, 190
Cutaneous trunci reflex, 495
  usefulness of, 86
  view of, 86*f*
Cuterebra larval myiasis
  in cat, 337–338, 338*f*, 414*f*, 415*f*,
    416*f*, 512*f*
  cause of, 413–418
Cuterebra species larva migration,
    67–68, 68*f*
Cyclop
  beagle as, 43*f*
  kitten as, 43*f*
  lamb as, 42*f*
Cytoarchitectonics, 194, 194*f*

D

Dachshund
  diffuse myelomalacia in, 119, 119*f*
  tetraplegia in, 118–119
Dancing Doberman disease, 125
Dazzle reflex, 400
Deafness, 437–439
Decerebellate rigidity, 204–205, 205*f*
Decerebrate rigidity, 204–205
Defecation, 187–188
Degeneration, 2
Degenerative joint disease, 270–271, 293*f*, 294*f*
  in horse, 293–294, 293*f*, 294*f*
Degenerative joint disease (DJD), 263–264
Degenerative myeloencephalopathy, 294–296, 295*f*, 296*f*, 510*f*
Degenerative myelopathy, 261–263, 261*f*, 262*f*
Dendritic zone, 2, 2*f*
Denervation
  effects of, 89
  of muscles, 88
  sweating and, 176
Dermatomal mapping, 231
Dermatomyositis, 96
Developmental obstructive
  hydrocephalus beagle with, 39, 71*f*, 76*f*
  characteristics of, 70–71
  diagnosis of, 74–75
  differential diagnosis of, 74
  Labrador retriever with, 74*f*
  miniature horse with, 74*f*
  prosencephalic signs of, 72–74
  signalment, history and clinical signs of, 72–74
  signs in dogs, 72
  treatment of, 75–76
Diabetes insipidus, 484
Diagnosis, accuracy of, 1–2
Diastematomyelia, 48–49, 49*f*
Diazepam, 467
Dicephalus
  cerebral hemisphere of calf, view of, 42*f*
  characteristics of, 41–42
  Holstein calf with, 41*f*
Diencephalon, 23, 25*f*
  afferent hypothalamic tract, 483
  anatomy of, 449–450, 450*f*
  cerebral hemisphere, view of, 42*f*
  choroid plexus and ventricular system, development of, 35*f*
  components of, 196–198, 196*f*, 448, 476
  divisions of, 476–477, 477*f*
  dysfunction of, 500
  extrapyramidal nuclei of, 198*f*
  neural tube development in, 33–35
  prosencephalic hypoplasia, calf with, 39*f*
  rostral and caudal, transverse view of, 34*f*
  See also Interbrain
Differential diagnosis, 1

Diffuse cortical projection system, 479
Diffuse glial neoplasm, 279*f*
Diffuse lower motor neuron disease, 161
Diffuse metabolic encephalopathy, 205, 205*f*
Diffuse myelomalacia, 119–120, 119*f*
Digestion chamber, 88
Diplomyelia, 48–49
  in lumbar spine of calf, 49*f*
Diprosopus
  characteristics of, 41–42
  Holstein calf with, 41*f*
Direct cortical projection system, 478–479
Direct stimulation, 451
Discospondylitis, 113, 123–124, 256, 297–301
  in horse, 296–297
Doberman pinscher
  with extradural mass lesion, 66*f*
  germ cell neoplasm in, 402, 403*f*
  infraspinatus contracture in, 108
  inherited neuromyopathy-dancing in, 125
  intervertebral disk extrusion in, 127
  paraparesis in, 127
  plantigrade posture in, 129*f*
Dog, 66*f*
  beagle, 76*f*
    as cyclop, 43*f*
    developmental obstructive hydrocephalus in, 71*f*, 76*f*
    malignant nerve sheath neoplasm in, 140*f*
  benign idiopathic canine peripheral vestibular disease in, 328–329
  boxer
    otitis media, facial paralysis from, 146*f*
    trigeminal neuritis in, 143*f*
  brain of, 236*f*, 353*f*, 354*f*, 358*f*
  caudal cerebellar vermis, 48*f*
  cerebellar abiotrophy in, 363–369
    beagles and samoyed, 369
    Gordon setter, 367–368, 368*f*, 385
    Kerry blue terrier, 363–367, 364*f*, 365*f*, 366*f*, 367*f*
    Old English sheepdog, 368
    Scottish terrier, 368
  cerebellar malformation in, 361–362
    Irish setter, 362*f*, 363*f*
    Labrador retriever, 361*f*
    wire fox terrier, 362*f*
  cervical spinal cord syringohydromyelia, 48*f*
  developmental obstructive hydrocephalus in, 39, 73*f*, 74*f*
  ear, anatomy of, 434*f*
  English Springer spaniel rage syndrome, 452–453
  episodic falling in, 212
  extradural mass lesion in, 66*f*
  facial tetanus in, 151*f*
  fibrocartilaginous embolic myelopathy in, 110, 110*f*

Dog *(Continued)*
  golden retriever, 383*f*
    acquired obstructive hydrocephalus in, 69*f*
    neoplasm in, 333, 382–383, 382*f*
    neosporosis in, 378–379, 378*f*
  Horner syndrome in, 174–175, 174*f*
  infraspinatus contracture in, 108–109, 108*f*
  inherited congenital myotonia in, 207–209
  intramedullary mass lesion in, 67*f*
  ischemic encephalopathy in, 334
  Labrador retriever
    with intradural-extramedullary lesion, 67*f*
    leukodystrophy in, 335
    nephroblastoma in, 254*f*
  laryngeal paralysis in
    acquired, 159–160
    inherited, 159
  lumbosacral myeloschisis/rachischisis in, 50*f*
  malignant nerve sheath neoplasm in, 141*f*, 142*f*
  molera in, 48
  monoplegia in, 254*f*
  neoplasm in, 331–332, 332*f*
  nephroblastoma in, 255*f*
  normal CT image of, 330*f*
  occipital bone malformation syndrome in, 60*f*
  otitis media-interna in, 329–331
  paraparesis in Leonberger, 124–125
  pelvic limb monoplegia in, 120–123
  syringohydromyelia in, 47–48
  tetanus, risus sardonicus from
    in Airedale terrier, 210*f*
    in Brittany spaniel, 210*f*
    in coonhound, 210*f*
  tetraplegia in dachshund, 118–120
  tick paralysis in, 95
  trigeminal neuritis
    in boxer, 143*f*
    in English setter, 143*f*
  vertebrae versus sacral segments, 63*t*
  vestibular system disorders in, 328–342
  See also Canine
Dorsal funiculus, 225
Dorsal raphe neuron, 468
Dorsal raphe nucleus, 468
Dorsal root
  avulsion of, 105*f*
  formation of, 29*f*
Dorsal spinocerebellar tract, 222
Dorsal subluxation, 269*f*
Dummy lamb, 43
Dural metaplasia-ossification, 265*f*
Dural ossification, 265
Dura mater
  characteristics of, 55–56
  view of, 55*f*
Dying-back neuropathy, 156–158
Dynamic stenosis, 291–292
Dysautonomia, 189–190, 190*f*
Dysmetria, 359
Dysphagia, 153

Dystocia injury, femoral nerve, 126–127
Dystonia, 217
Dystonia of antigravity extensor muscles. *See* Tetany
Dystrophinopathy, 99–100

E

Ear ossicles, 319–320
Ectoderm, 23, 24*f*
Electrodiagnostic technique, 89–90
Electrolyte abnormality, 458
Elso heel, 212
Embryo, spinal cord segments and vertebral column, 79–80
Encephalitis
    clinical signs of, 161
    facial paralysis from, 146*f*
    paresis/paralysis from, 143
Encephalomyelopathy, 384
Endolymph, 320
Endopenduncular nucleus, 196–198, 196*f*
English Springer spaniel rage syndrome, 452–453
Ependyma, 37, 69
Epilepsy, 207, 454
Episodic falling, 212
Episodic repetitive myoclonus, 216–217
Epithalamus, 449–450
    components of, 476
    transverse view of, 34*f*
Equine degenerative myeloencephalopathy, 294–296, 295*f*, 296*f*
Equine grass sickness, 176
Equine herpesvirus 1, 164
Equine herpesvirus-1 myelopathy, 302–304, 302*f*, 303*f*
Equine laryngeal hemiparesis-hemiplegia, 156–158
    endoscopic view of, 159*f*
    grades of, 158
    severe denervation atrophy from, 158*f*
Equine leukoencephalomalacia, 423
Equine motor neuron disease, acquired, 101–102, 101*f*, 102*f*
Equine neonatal encephalopathy, 421, 423*f*
Equine protozoal encephalomyelitis, 164, 297–298, 298*f*, 341–342
    S. neuroma, infection from, 342*f*
Equine protozoal myelitis, 107, 111–112, 295–296, 300*f*, 304
Escherichia coli, 256
Esophagus
    dysfunction of, 153–154
    GVE/GVA innervation of, 154*f*
Exencephaly
    characteristics of, 40–41
    Pomeranian puppies with, 41*f*
Exercise-induced collapse, 100
Exercise-induced fatigue, 100
Experimental destruction, 451
Extensor carpi radialis reflex, 85–86
External ear, 434*f*

External ear canal, 319–320
External germinal layer, 348
External limiting membrane, 394
External sphincter, 186
Exteroceptor, 221
Extracranial disorder, 457–458
Extradural lesion
    in Doberman pinscher, 66*f*
    examples of, 66
Extraocular muscle, functional anatomy of, 138*f*
Extrapyramidal nuclear lesion, 205–206
Extrapyramidal nuclei
    of diencephalon, 196–198, 198*f*
    of telencephalon, 197*f*
Extrapyramidal system, 195–200
    components of, 192, 196*f*
Eye
    parasympathetic GVE-LMN innervation of, 169
    sympathetic GVE-LMN innervation of, 173–182
    third eyelid, protrusion of, 183–184
    See also Pupil; Vision
Eyeball
    development of, 390*f*, 391*f*, 392*f*
    embryology of, 389–393
    gestation in dog, 393
    strabismus of, 497

F

Facial hypalgesia/analgesia, 238
Facial nerve
    evaluation of, 498
    parasympathetic nucleus of, 188–189
Facial nerve tetanus, 150–151
    in cocker spaniel, 151*f*
    in mixed breed dog, 151*f*
    prognosis for, 139
Facial neuron
    anatomy of, 144–145
    lesions of, 145–147
Facial paralysis
    from encephalitis, 146*f*
    from Horner syndrome, 148*f*
    lesions causing, 147
    from otitis media
        in boxer, 146*f*
        in Holstein calf, 148*f*
        in horse, 146*f*
Fainting disease, 207
Falx cerebri, 57*f*
Familial reflex myoclonus, 212
Fasciculus cuneatus, 225
Fasciculus gracilis, 225
Fasciculus proprius, 86
Feedback circuit, 199
Felbamate, 467
Feline hyperesthesia syndrome, 454
Feline infectious peritonitis (PIF), 69
Feline infectious peritonitis viral meningoencephalomyelitis, 339, 339*f*, 340*f*
    decerebellate posture, 339*f*

Feline ischemic encephalopathy, 67–68, 68*f*
Feline laryngeal paralysis, 160
Feline panleukopenia virus, 44, 369–370, 369*f*
Fibrillation, 89–90
Fibroblastic meningioma, 462*f*
Fibrocartilaginous embolic myelopathy (FCEM), 110, 110*f*, 250–251, 304, 315, 315*f*, 316*f*
Fibrocartilaginous embolus, 278*f*, 279*f*
Fibrosis, caudomedial thigh muscle, 128, 128*f*
Fibrous band, 128, 128*f*
Flaccid tetraplegia, 87
Flank-attacking episode, 465
Flexor reflex, 84, 84*f*, 85*f*
    anatomy of, 231
    evaluation of, 287
    pelvic limb, 231*f*, 232
    requirements of, 230–231
    testing for, 233
    thoracic limb, 232, 232*f*
Flexor-withdrawal reflex, 85
Floating, 359
Floor plate, 27, 27*f*
Fluid-attenuated inversion recovery (FLAIR), 379–381, 380*f*
Fly-biting episode, 465
Focal lesion, 228, 509*f*
Focal seizure, 455
Focal tetany, 212–213
Fontanelle, 48
Foot-attacking-the-dog episode, 465
Fracture
    L1 in pig, 315–316
    in setter mixed dog, 508*f*
    T17 in foal, 305
    T4 in cow, 312
Frequency, 433–434
Frontal lobotomy, 452
Functional cerebellar disorder, 373–375, 374*f*, 375*f*
Fundus
    of cat eye, 397*f*
    of cow eye, 397*f*
    of dog, 405*f*
    of dog eye, 397*f*
    of horse eye, 397*f*
Fusarium moniliformis, 161

G

Gabapentin, 467
Gait
    abnormalities of
        in Labrador retriever, 99–102
        large animal, 285
        small animal, 243–244
    cerebellum role in, 357
    grading system for, 492
    neurologic examination of, 491–492
    two-engine, 274
Gait generation, 202–204
Gamma efferent neuron, 202
Gamma trail neuron, 202
Ganglion, 392–393

Ganglion layer, 395
Gastrocnemius reflex, 84
Generalized autoimmune myositis, 82–83
Generalized polymyositis, 83
Generalized seizure, 455, 462f
General proprioception
    abnormal gait, 243–244
    cerebellar afferents and, 355
    cranial nerve, 227
    dorsal spinocerebellar tract, 222
    lesions of
        clinical signs of, 228–229
        postural reactions, 229
        testing for, 221
    pathways
        for cerebellar transmission, 222
        to cerebellum-spinocerebellar, 223f
        for conscious perception, 225–227
        for reflex activity, 222, 223f
        at second cervical spinal cord segment, 223f
        in sensory system, 222
        to somesthetic cortex, 225–227, 226f
    prosencephalic anatomic pathways for, 239f
    spinal cord anatomic pathways for, 240f
    spinal nerve, 222–227
    ventral spinocerebellar tract, 222–225
General proprioception ataxia, 228
General proprioception system, 3t, 4
    disease of, 229
    dysfunction, signs of, 228
General somatic afferent (GSA), 135f
General somatic afferent (GSA)-lower motor neurons (LMN). See GSE-LMN
General somatic afferent (GSA) neuron, 2, 2f
General somatic afferent (GSA) system, 3, 229–239
    canine sensory neuropathy, 232
    cranial nerve and, 234–236
    disease of, 237–239
    facial hypalgesia/analgesia, 238
    lesions of, 236–237
    nociceptive pathway, 233–234
    pain syndrome, 238–239
    pathways, 233–235
        for conscious perception, 236–237
        trigeminal nerve, 235f
    pathways for, 233–235
    prosencephalic anatomic pathways for, 239f
    reflex pathway, 235–236
    sensory ganglioradiculitis, 237–238
    spinal cord anatomic pathways for, 240f
    spinal nerve, 229–234
General somatic efferent (GSE), 3t
General somatic efferent (GSE) neuron, 2f
General somatic efferent (GSE) system, 4
General visceral afferent (GVA) neuron
    dendritic zones of, 186

General visceral afferent (GVA) system, 3t, 3–4, 442f
    brainstem and tracts of, 441–443
    components of, 441
    functional concepts of, 443
    receptor of, 441
General visceral efferent (GVE), 135f
General visceral efferent (GVE) neuron
    development of, 29f
General visceral efferent (GVE) system, 3t, 4
    anatomy of, 168–169
    components of, 168–169
German shepherd
    abnormal gait in, 97–98
    cauda equina syndrome in, 112–113
    inherited giant axonal neuropathy in, 125
    intervertebral disk protrusion in, 113
    nephroblastoma in, 255f
    pelvic limb dysfunction in, 128–129
    sacrocaudal dysfunction in, 112–114
    tetraparesis in, 97–98
Germ cell neoplasm
    in cranial nerves, 139
    in Doberman pinscher, 402, 403f
    in golden retriever, 402f
    in middle cranial fossa, 172f
    in mixed breed dog, 403f
    prevalence of, 402
Giant axonal neuropathy, inherited, 125
Gibbon, brain of, 359f
Glial cell, 24–25
Glial neoplasm, diffuse, 279f
Glossopharyngeal nerve, 152f, 153
    parasympathetic nucleus of, 189
Goat
    caprine arthritis encephalitis virus, 309–310
    inherited congenital myotonia in, 207
    listeriosis in, 144f
    spastic hemiparesis and ataxia in, 311f
    stiffness in kid, 129–130
    sympathetic GVE-LMN innervation, loss of, 175–176
    vestibular system disorders in, 344
    Vitamin E deficiency myopathy, 130
Golden retriever
    acquired obstructive hydrocephalus in
        at columns of fornix, 69f
        dilated left lateral ventricle, 69f
        at rostral diencephalon, 69f
    neoplasm in, 382–383, 382f, 383f
Golgi tendon organs, 202
Gradient-echo MR, 379–381
Grand mal seizure, 455
Granule neuron, 194–195
Granulomatous meningocephalitis, 333
    in dog, 405f
Granuloprival hypoplasia, 369–370
Grass sickness, equine, 176
Gray column, 27, 27f
Gray matter, 25–26
Great horned owl, cerebellum of, 357f
Griseofulvin, effects of, 39–40

GSE-LMN
    neuromuscular disease of, 90–130
    role in cranial nerves, 134
GSE neuron, 78
Guttural pouch
    dissection of, 157f
    fungal infection of, 154–156
    normal mucosa of, 158f
    view of, 155f, 156f
Guttural pouch mycosis, 154–156

H

Habenular nucleus, 449–450
Hair cell, 320
Hairy shaker, 214
Halicephalobus gingivalis, 423–424
Head, 320
    static position of, 321
Head bobber, 216
Head elevation, 286
Head rebound phenomenon, 360
Heart rate, abnormal, 485
Hemianopsia, 401
Hemifacial spasm, 150–151
Hemi-inattention, 485
Hemi-neglect, 485
Hemiparesis, 271–279
    spastic, 311f
Hemiplegia, 277–279
Hemiwalking, 492–493
Hemorrhage
    diffuse subarachnoid, 281f, 282f
    trauma to brain, 183f
Hepatic encephalomyelopathy
    in calf, 311–312
Hepatic encephalopathy, 425
    in Cairn terrier, 513f
    seizure, as cause of, 459–460
Hereditary ataxia, 384
Hereditary spinal muscular atrophy, 101
Herniation
    caudal cerebellar vermis/cervical spinal cord syringohydromyelia, 48f
    cause of, 47
    subfalcine, 58–59
Herpesvirus 1, equine, 164
Herpesvirus-1 myelopathy, equine, 302–304, 302f
Hippocampus, 36, 448–449
Histophilus somnus, 161
Holoprosencephaly-arrhinencephaly
    Morgan brain with, 43f
    occurrence of, 42
Holstein cow
    bone and neural tube malformation, 46–47
    calvarial lipomeningocele, 41f
    cerebellar malformation in, 372f
    as dicephalic, 41f
    dystocia injury, femoral nerve, 126–127
    encephalitis, facial paralysis from, 146f
    listeriosis with tongue paralysis in, 161f

Holstein cow *(Continued)*
  with malformed tail, spina bifida,
    meningomyelocele, 46*f*
  otitis media
    bilateral, 149*f*
    facial paralysis from, 148*f*
  paraparesis in, 126–127
  sciatic nerve paralysis in, 124*f*
  tibial nerve paralysis in, 124*f*
Hoof replacement test, 492
Hopping
  large animals, testing in, 245
  pelvic limb, testing for, 245
  postural reaction testing, 492–493
  small animals, testing response
    in, 245
  thoracic limb, testing for, 245
  See also Bunny-hop movement
Horner syndrome
  in cat
    with facial paralysis, 148*f*
    with right thyroid
      adenocarcinoma, 174*f*
    from withdrawing blood, 174*f*
  characteristics of, 142–143
  clinical signs of, 174–175
  in cow, 175*f*
  diagnosis of, 179*f*
  in dog, 143*f*, 174–175, 174*f*
  in horse, 176, 176*f*
  lesions, summary of, 178*t*
  sweating and, 176, 178–179
  sympathetic paralysis, 287–288
  third eyelid, protrusion of, 177–178
Horse, 59*f*, 290*f*
  cauda equina in, 111*f*, 111–112
  cerebellar abiotrophy in, 370–371
  cervical scoliosis in, 305, 305*f*, 306*f*
  cervical spinal cord of, 201*f*
  cervical vertebral malformation-
    malarticulation, 289–294
  cholesterinic granuloma in, 423
  CSF collection
    from cerebellomedullary cistern, 62*f*
    from lumbosacral spinal cord,
      63, 64*f*
  degenerative joint disease, 293*f*, 294*f*
  degenerative joint disease in,
    293–294
  degenerative myeloencephalopathy
    in, 294–296, 295*f*, 296*f*
  developmental obstructive
    hydrocephalus in, 71*f*, 72*f*, 74*f*
  diskospondylitis in, 296–297
  facial paralysis from surgery, 147*f*
  grading system for, 289
  Horner syndrome in, 176*f*, 176
  larynx
    cranial-to-caudal view of, 158*f*
    dorsal view of, 158*f*
  lavender Arabian foal syndrome
    in, 212
  lymphoma in, 106*f*, 107*f*
  muscle atrophy in, 163–166
  NMD monoparesis in, 106–108
  otitis media
    bone lesion and, 148–149
    facial paralysis from, 146*f*
  otitis media-interna in, 340

Horse *(Continued)*
  palpation of spinal cord segments, 65
  paraparesis in, 126
  postoperative poliomyelomalacia in,
    117, 117*f*
  protozoal myelitis in, 295–296
  S. neuroma, infection from, 342*f*
  sacrocaudal dysfunction in, 111–112
  spinal cord segments, C3, C4 and
    C5, 306*f*
  stenosis in, 290–291
  stylohyoidosteopathy in, 150*f*
  sweating in, 177, 177*f*, 178*f*
  temporohyoid osteopathy in,
    340–341
  tetanus in, 210
  vertebrae versus sacral segments,
    63*t*
  vertebral malformation-
    malarticulation
    acquired, 290
    congenital, 289–290
  vestibular system disorders in,
    340–341
Human, cervical spinal cord of, 201*f*
Huntington chorea, 217
Hydranencephaly
  cause of, 43–45
  CSF collection in, 67–68
  in DSH kitten, 44
  in Hereford calf, 44–45
  unilateral, in miniature poodle,
    44–45, 44*f*, 45*f*
Hydrocephalus
  cause of, 37–38
  compensatory, 67–68
  types of, 67
Hydromyelia, 47–48
Hypercapnia, 58
Hyperexplexia, 212
Hyperlipidemia, 151–152, 458
Hyperreflexia, 204
Hyperthermia, 458
Hypertonicity, 212
Hypertrophic neuropathy
  affecting tibial nerve, 125*f*
  inherited, 125*f*
Hypertrophy, muscle, 207*f*
Hypervitaminosis A, 267
Hypocretin
  decrease in activity of, 469
  role of, 469
Hypoglossal axon, 355–356
Hypoglossal neuron
  anatomy of, 160
  atrophy from meningioma, 160*f*
  diseases of, 160–166
  lesions of, 160
Hypoglossal nucleus, 165*f*, 166*f*
Hypoglycemia, 458–459
Hypokalemic myopathy
  in cattle, 98
  tetraparesis, as rare cause of, 97–98
Hypothalamic nuclei, 482
Hypothalamic tract
  afferent, 483
  efferent, 483
Hypothalamo-adenohypophyseal
  system, 483

Hypothalamo-neurohypophyseal
  system, 483
Hypothalamus
  anatomy of, 482–483
  clinical syndromes of, 483–485
  function of, 483
  lesions, abnormalities caused by, 484
  limbic system component of,
    449–450
  nuclei of, 23
  parts of, 33–35
  transverse view of, 34*f*
Hypothyroidism, 151–152, 159–160
Hypoxia
  anesthesia and, 421
  seizure, as cause of, 458

I

Ictus, 454
Idiopathic epilepsy, 454, 458–459
Idiopathic facial neuropathy, 151–152
Ilium
  fracture of, 122*f*
  mass in, 122*f*
Imipramine, 471
Immunosuppressant, 94–95
Incontinence
  neurogenic sphincter, 188
  urinary, 187
Infarction, 248–249
Inflammation
  seizure, as cause of, 457
  types of, 1
Infraspinatus contracture, 108*f*,
  108–109
Inherited congenital myotonia,
  207–209
Inherited congenital tetany, 211*f*
Inherited encephalomyelopathy-
  polyneuropathy, 273–274
Inherited giant axonal neuropathy,
  125
Inherited hypertrophic neuropathy,
  125, 125*f*
Inherited neuromyopathy-dancing
  Doberman, 125
Inhibition, release from, 204–205
Injury
  cause of, 1
  CSF collection causing, 62
  L7 fracture, 113
  lameness in horse, 107–108
  laryngeal paralysis from, 160
  to pelvic limb, 84
  seizure, as cause of, 457
Inner ear, 319, 320*f*, 434*f*
Innervation
  of bladder, 187
  of esophagus, 154*f*
  of pelvic limb muscles, 84*f*
  sympathetic GVE-LMN, 173*f*,
    173–182
  of thoracic limb muscles, 85
Inspiratory dyspnea, 153
Intention tremor, 359–360
Interbrain
  neural tube development in, 33–35
  See also Diencephalon

Intercranial vasodilation, 58
Internal limiting membrane, 395
Interphase, 24
Intervertebral disk extrusion, 127
Intervertebral disk extrusion-
    protrusion, 257–260, 258f, 259f
    clinical sign of, 259
    diagnosis of, 259
Intervertebral disk protrusion, 113
Intestinal parasitism, seizures
    and, 458
Intracarotid drug injection, 425
Intracranial disorder, 457
Intracranial pressure, 60–61
Intradiscal osteomyelitis, 256
Intradural-extramedullary lesion
    examples of, 66
    in Labrador retriever, 67f
Intramedullary lesion
    in basset hound, 67f
    examples of, 67
Intumescence, cervical and
    lumbosacral, 84f
Iohexol, 65
Ion channelopathy, 217–218
Ipsilateral hemiparesis, 203–204,
    203f
Ipsilateral hemiplegia, 203–204,
    203f
Ischemic encephalopathy, 334
Ischemic infarct, 303f, 304f
Ischemic infarction, 425f
Ischemic poliomyelomalacia, 116f,
    116–117

J

Jacksonian seizure, 454
Jerk nystagmus, 136–137, 215,
    320–321, 497–498
Jugular compression, 58

K

Keratitis sicca, 189
Kindling phenomenon, 465–468
Kinocilium, 320
Knuckling over, 228
Kyphosis, vertebral malformation
    with, 315

L

Labrador retriever
    with abnormal gait and prehension,
        99–102
    cerebellar malformation in, 361f
    developmental obstructive
        hydrocephalus in, 74f
    exercise-induced collapse in, 100
    exercise-induced fatigue in, 100
    with intradural-extramedullary
        lesion, 67f
    leukodystrophy in, 335
    malignant nerve sheath neoplasm
        in, 104f
    monoparesis in, 103–105
    nephroblastoma in, 254f
    with tetraparesis, 98–99

Lamb
    caudal diskospondylitis in, 297–315
    cranial thoracic fracture in, 297–315
    cyclopic newborn, 42f
    "dummy lamb," 43
    listeriosis in, 297–311
    obstructive hydrocephalus in, 70f
Lameness
    in Brittany spaniel, 108–109
    in Doberman pinscher, 108f
    in horse, 106–108
Landry-Guillain-Barre disease, 91
Laryngeal adduction reflex, 288
Laryngeal paralysis, 153
    in canine
        acquired, 159–160
        inherited, 159
    in felines, 160
    progressive, 159
    See also Equine laryngeal
        hemiparesis-hemiplegia
Larynx
    cranial-to-caudal view of, 158f
    dorsal view of, 158f, 273f
Lateral cervical nucleus, 226
Lateral geniculate nucleus, 398–399,
    402, 479
Lateral lemniscus, 435–436
Lavender Arabian foal syndrome, 212
Lead poisoning, 159
Lens, 390
Lentiform nucleus, 195–196
Leonberger, paresis in, 124–125
Leonberger inherited neuropathy, 124
Leptomeninges, 30, 54
Lesion
    from CAE, 311f
    of caudal cervical region, 247
    of cervical spinal cord, 229
    classification of, 66
    of cranial cervical region, 247–248
    focal, 228
    intracranial space, compromising of,
        58–59
    of lumbosacral region, 247
    in pons and medulla, 229
    prosencephalic, 229
    of thoracolumbar region, 247
    unconsciousness, as cause of, 481
Leukodystrophy, 335
Leukoencephalitis, necrotizing,
    399–415
    in chihuahua, 412f
    in Yorkshire terrier, 412f
Leukoencephalomalacia, equine, 423
Leukoencephalopathy, adult cheetah,
    426, 426f
Levetiracetam, 467
Lhasa apso, lissencephaly in, 45f, 46
Limber tail syndrome, 113–114
Limbic system
    anatomy of, 450f
    diencephalic components of,
        449–450
    frontal lobotomy, 452
    function of, 450–453
    mesencephalic components of, 450
    telencephalic components of,
        448–450, 449f

Lipomeningocele, 41
Lissencephaly
    characteristics of, 45–46
    in Lhasa apso dog, 45f
    in wire fox terrier, 46f
Listeria monocytogenes, 160–162
Listeriosis, 129–130
    in cow, 161–162, 343–344
    in goat, 144f
    in lamb, 297–311
    tongue paresis in cow with, 161f
Llama, vertebrae versus sacral
    segments, 63t
Lobotomy, frontal, 452
Locomotion, 202
Locus ceruleus, 468
Lower motor neuron, 89f
    Wallerian degeneration of, 89f
Lower motor neuron (LMN)
    bladder, 187
Lower motor neuron (LMN) disease
    characteristics of, 86–90
    diffuse, 161
    of GSE, 90–130
    tetraparesis-ataxia, pelvic limb,
        274–276
    See also Neuromuscular disease
        (NMD); General visceral efferent
        system
Lower motor neuron (LMN)
    paresis, 491
Lumbar myelogram
    of extradural mass lesion, 66f
Lumbosacral discospondylitis, 313
Lumbosacral dysfunction, 499
Lumbosacral intumescence, 84f
Lumbosacral lesion, 247
Lumbosacral myeloschisis, 50f
Lumbosacral spinal cord
    CSF collection from, 63–65
        standing horse, 64f
    diastematomyelial in calf, 49f
    segmental hypoplasia in
        calf, 49f
    segments versus vertebrae, 63t
Lumbosacral stenosis, 112–113
Lumbosacral syndrome, 112–113
Lymphoma, 106–107
    in cat, 260f
    in cattle, 123
    in Clydesdale, 107f
    in cranial nerves, 141
    in horse, 107f
    in spinal cord, 260–261
    of trigeminal nerve, 142f

M

Macula
    characteristics of, 321–322
    view of, 321f
Maladjustment syndrome, 421–422
Malformation, 1
    Arnold Chiari, 46–47
    Arnold Chiari, type I, 47
    cerebellar, 46
    complex, of calf, 46–47
    of occipital bone, 47–48
    pathogenesis of, 52

Malformation (*Continued*)
  seizure, as cause of, 457
  of Simmenthal calf spinal cord, 50, 50*f*
  of spinal cord, 48–50
Malformation, in brain, 37–52
Malignant catarrhal fever, 162–163
Malignant nerve sheath neoplasm, 103–104
  in beagle, 103*f*, 104*f*
  in Labrador retriever, 104*f*
Mamillary group, 483
Mantle layer, 25–26
Manx cat
  malformations of, 40
  meningomyelocele in, 51, 51*f*
  sacrocaudal spina bifida in, 51
Masticatory myositis, 95–96
Medial cuneate nucleus, 225
Medial geniculate nucleus, 477
Medial lemniscus, 225, 229
Medulla oblongata
  dysfunction of, 500
  formation of, 30
  lesions of, 229
  parasympathetic GVE in, 188–189, 188*f*
  pathways for voluntary movement, 203*f*
  schematic drawing of, 152*f*
  transverse sections of, 140*f*
  See also Myelencephalon
Medulla spinalis. *See* Spinal cord
Megaesophagus, 153
Membranous ampulla, 320
Membranous labyrinth, 435*f*
  fluid-filled compartments of, 320
  formation of, 319
  special proprioception and, 322*f*
Menace deficit, 418–419, 418*f*
Menace response test, 399–400, 400*f*, 495–496
Meningeal fibrosis, C2-C3, 271
Meningeal polyarteritis, canine, 281–282, 281*f*
Meninges
  anatomy of, 55–56
  ultrastructure of, 56*f*
  ventricular system, relationship to, 55–56
Meningioma
  atrophy from, 160*f*
  in boxer, 515*f*
  in cranial nerves, 139
  development of, 37
  in German Shepherd, 462*f*
  prevalence of, 416–417
  in shorthair cat, 59*f*
  in West Highland terrier, 514*f*
Meningocele, 39–40
Meningoencephalitis
  necrotizing, 411
  in Siamese cat, 70*f*
Meningoencephalocele
  Burmese kitten with, 41*f*
  cause and characteristics of, 39–40
  newborn Holstein calf with, 40*f*
  newborn kitten with, 40*f*
  stillborn Belgian foal with, 40*f*
Meningoencephalomyelitis, 339

Meningomyelocele, 46*f*, 51, 51*f*
Mental attitude, neurologic examination and, 490–491
Mesencephalic aqueduct, 23
  CSF flow and, 69
  obstructive hydrocephalus of, 70*f*
Mesencephalon, 23, 25*f*
  afferent hypothalamic tract, 483
  anatomy of, 450, 450*f*
  cranial nerves in, 32–33
  development of, 33*f*
  dysfunction of, 500
  extrapyramidal nuclear areas of, 198–199
  extrapyramidal nuclei of, 199*f*
  rostral, transverse view of, 34*f*
  See also midbrain
Metabolic neuropathy, 124–125
Metastatic melanoma, 304–305
Metastatic neoplasia, 2
Metathalamus, 476
Metencephalon, 25*f*, 31–32, 32*f*
Metronidazole toxicity, 334
Microphthalmia, 406, 407*f*
Micturition
  centers for, 186
  control of, 184–187
  neuroanatomy of bladder function, 184*f*
  urination, 186–187
  See also Urine
Midbrain
  cranial nerves in, 32
  extrapyramidal pathways of, 198–199
  pathways for voluntary movement, 203*f*
  See also Mesencephalon
Mid-diencephalon, 34*f*
Middle ear, 319–320, 434*f*
MIIND system, 1
Miotic pupil, 182
Mitosis, 24, 26*f*
Modified cilium, 320
Modified microvilli, 320
Molera, 48
Monoparesis
  in horse, 92
  in Labrador retriever, 103
Monoplegia, 253–254
  pelvic limb in dog, 120–123
  in Saint Bernard, 254*f*
Mossy fiber, 353–354
Motor (efferent) system, 1–2, 3*t*, 479
Motor ataxia, 228
Motor end plate, 78, 79*f*
  neuromuscular junction of, 80*f*
Motor nerve conduction, 90
Motor neuron, 79*f*
  function of, 78
Motor neuron disease
  congenital, 100–101
  equine, acquired, 101–102, 101*f*
Motor unit, 78
Movement disorder, 205
  definition of, 217
  pathogenesis of, 217
Multiple cartilaginous exostosis, 256
Muscle
  atrophy of, 286–287
  contraction, strength of, 78

Muscle (*Continued*)
  denervation of, 88
  hereditary spinal muscular atrophy, 101
  hypertrophy of, 207*f*, 208*f*
  innervation of, 84*f*
  neurologic examination for tone and size, 494–495
  uncontrolled involuntary contractions of, 206–218, 206*b*
Muscle atrophy, 163–166
Muscle fasciculation, 89–90
Muscular dystrophy with dystrophinopathy, 99–100
Myasthenia gravis, 87–88
  diagnosis of, 93–94
  facial and laryngeal paresis from, 161
  forms of, 93
  treatment of, 94–95
Mycotoxicosis, 215
Mydriatic pupil, 182
Myelencephalon, 25*f*
Myeloarchitectonics, 194, 194*f*
Myelography
  cisternal
    extradural mass lesion, 66*f*
    intradural-extramedullary lesion, 67*f*
    intramedullary mass lesion, 67*f*
  lumbar
    extradural mass lesion, 66*f*
  patterns of, 66*f*
  performance of, 65–67
Myelopathy
  Brown Swiss cattle, 312
  compressive, 290*f*, 294*f*
Myeloschisis, 50–51
Myoclonus, 212
  resting, 217
  sporadic, 213
  types of, 213
  See also Repetitive myoclonus
Myokymia, 216–217
Myopathy-rhabdomyolysis, 130
Myositis, 90, 95, 144
Myotonia, 90
  acquired, 209
  inherited congenital, 207–209
  types of, 206

N

Narcolepsy
  acquired form of, 469
  examples of, 471–472
  hypothalamic lesions causing, 485
  overview of, 468–472
  treatment for, 471
Neck discomfort, 280–282
  evaluation of, 288
  See also Degenerative joint disease
Necrotizing encephalopathy, 523*f*
Necrotizing leukoencephalitis, 411–413
  in chihuahua, 412*f*
  in Yorkshire terrier, 412*f*
Necrotizing meningoencephalitis, 411–413
Needle
  for CSF collection
    dog and cat, 61
    horse, 63*t*

Neocortex, 195, 456*f*
Neopallium, 36, 448
Neoplasia, 2
   CSF flow and, 69
   as metastatic, 2
   seizure, as cause of, 457
Neoplasm, 113
   in cat, 337, 337*f*
   in cerebellum, 377
   in Chesapeake Bay retriever,
      331–332, 332*f*
   in cranial nerves, 139
   diffuse glial, 279*f*
   in golden retriever, 333, 382–384,
      382*f*, 383*f*
Neoplasm-melanoma, at T17, 304–305
Neospora hughesi
   equine degenerative
      myeloencephalopathy, as cause
      of, 297–298
   life cycle of, 298
Neosporosis, 114–115, 378–379, 378*f*
Nephroblastoma, 254–256, 254*f*
   in children, 255–256
   diffuse epithelial cells of, 255*f*
   in German Shepherd, 255*f*
   transverse sections of, 255*f*
Nerve. *See* Cranial nerve
Nerve fiber layer, 395
Nerve sheath neoplasm, malignant,
   103–104, 139–141, 140*f*
   in American Eskimo dog, 142*f*
   in beagle, 103*f*, 104*f*
   in Beagle, 140*f*
   in Great Dane, 503*f*, 505*f*
   in Labrador retriever, 104*f*
   in West Highland terrier, 141*f*
Nervous ketosis, 422–423
Nervous system
   composition of, 2
   functional systems of, 3, 3*t*
   malformations of, 1
   metastatic neoplasia of, 2
   neural tube, 23–27
   tetanus, 209
Neural crest
   characteristics of, 28–30
   general visceral efferent neuron,
      development of, 29*f*
   spinal ganglia development from, 28*f*
Neural crest cell, 23
Neural plate, 23
Neural tube
   cell differentiation in, 24–27
   development of, 23–27
   functional organization of, 26*f*
   malformation in Holstein calf, 46–47
   transverse sections of, 24*f*
Neurectoderm, 23, 24*f*
Neuritis
   brachial plexus, 104
   chronic, 104
   idiopathic facial neuropathy,
      151–152
Neurobiotaxis, 30
Neuroblast, 24–25
Neuroepithelial cell
   differentiation of, 26*f*
Neuroepithelium
   composition of, 321

Neurogenic atrophy, 286–287
Neurogenic sphincter incontinence,
   188
Neuroglia, 24–25
Neurologic examination
   components of
      in large animal, 285
      small animal, 243–244
   cranial nerve, 246
   form for, 488*f*
   gait abnormalities, 491–492
      large animal, 285
      small animal, 243–244
   history if patient, 489–490
   muscle tone and size, 494–495
   overview of, 487–490
   parts of, 490–499
   physical examination and, 490
   postural reaction testing, 492–494
      large animal, 286
      small animal, 243–244
   Schiff-Sherrington syndrome,
      248–250
   signalment of patient, 487–489
   spinal cord disease, signs of, 246*f*
   spinal cord lesions
      caudal cervical region, 247
      cranial cervical region, 247–248
      lumbosacral region, 247
      signs related to, 246–250
      thoracolumbar region, 247
   spinal nerve reflex, 494–495
   spinal reflexes, 245–246
   spinal shock, 248–250
   unconsciousness, determining cause
      of, 481–482
Neuroma, 88
Neuromuscular disease
   of GSE-LMN, 90–130
   tetraparesis
      in German Shepherd, 97–98
      in Labrador retriever, 98–99
   tetraplegia in red bone coonhound,
      90–97
Neuromuscular disease (NMD)
   characteristics of, 86–90
   electrodiagnostic techniques of,
      89–90
   See also Lower motor neuron (LMN)
      disease
Neuromuscular junction (ending), 78
Neuromuscular spindle (NMS), 2, 2*f*
   anatomy and function of, 201*f*
   role of, 200–201
Neuromuscular strabismus
   clinical signs of, 137
Neuron
   definition of, 2
   as immature, 24–25
Neuronal abiotrophy, 101
Neuronal degeneration, 457
Neuronal environment
   alterations of, 456–457
   components of, 456, 456*f*
Neuronal storage disease
   in American bulldog, 385
   in Cairn terrier, 385
   in Dachshund, 385
   in Portuguese water dog, 385
Neuropathy, 125

Neurophthalmology, 409*b*
Neuropore, 23, 24*f*
Neurotrophic keratitis, 237
Night blindness, 393
Nigropallidal encephalomalacia,
   205–206, 206*f*
NMD tetraplegia, 97–98
Nociception, 221–222
   definition of, 236
   neurologic examination of, 494–495
   testing for, 236
Nociceptive pathway, 233–234, 287
Nonolfactory rhinencephalon
   anatomy of
      diencephalon, 449–450
      mesencephalon, 450
      telencephalon, 448–449
   function of, 450–453
   structures of, 449*b*
Nonsuppurative inflammation, 1
Norepinephrine, 168–169
Normotensive communicating
   compensatory hydrocephalus, 67–68
Notochord, 23, 24*f*
Nuclear layer
   external, 394
   internal, 395
Nucleus accumbens, 195
Nucleus ambiguus
   lesions of, 153
   location of, 152
   schematic drawing of, 152*f*
Nucleus gracilis, 225
Nucleus Z, 226–227
Nystagmus, 345*f*
   abnormal, 325–326
   caloric, 326
   congenital, 345–346
   consciousness, determining level of,
      482
   cranial nerve examination for,
      497–498
   definition of, 136–137
   normal, 325
   postrotatory, 326

O

Obstructive hydrocephalus
   acquired, 69–70
   characteristics of, 69–72
   in lamb, 70*f*
Obtunded patient, clinical evaluation
   of, 481–482
Occipital bone malformation, 47–48,
   59*f*
   in Cavalier King Charles Spaniel,
      60*f*
   CSF blockage from, 70
Occiptoatlantoaxial malformation
   (OAAM)
   in Arabian foal, 291*f*
   congenital, 289–290
Oculi uterque (OU), 170
Oculomotor nerve, lesion of, 171
Oculomotor neurons
   anatomy of, 134–135
   lesions of, 139
   strabismus, direction following
      paralysis, 138*f*

Oculus dextra (OD), 170
Oculus sinister (OS), 170
Olfaction, 444–446
Olfactory bulb, function of, 445
Olfactory system, 36
Oligodendrocyte, 24–25
Olivary nucleus, 200
Opisthotonus, 204–205
Opsoclonus, 215
Optic chiasm, 397–398
Optic cup, 391
Optic disk, 396, 396f
Optic nerve
  central visual pathway and, 396–397
  of horse, 408f
  hypoplasia of, 403, 407f
  injury to, 407
  lesions of, 168, 170–171
Optic nerve disease, 401
Optic neuritis, 401, 404
  in dog, 405f
Optic stalk, 33–35
Optic tract
  bilateral lesions of, 402
  central visual pathway and, 398
  unilateral lesion of, 171
Optic vesicle, 389
Organophosphate, 310
Organophosphate anthelmintic
  haloxone, 159
Organophosphate toxicity, 310–311
Orthostatic postural myoclonus, 216
Osmolar imbalance, 422
Ossification, 268
Osteogenic sarcoma, 506f, 507f
Otitis media
  bone lesion in horse, 148–149
  diagnosis of, 148
  facial paralysis
    in boxer, 146f
    in Holstein calf, 148f
    in horse, 146f
    lesions causing, 147–148
  facial tetanus from, 151f
Otitis media-interna
  in calf, 343
  in cat, 148f, 335–336
  in dog, 329–331
  in horse, 340
  in pig, 149f, 330f
  treatment of, 148–149
Otolith (statoconia), 321
Ototoxicity, 329
Overreaching, 359
Owl, cerebellum of, 357f
Ox
  palpation of spinal cord
    segments, 65
  vertebrae versus sacral segments, 63t

P

Pachymeninx. *See* Dura mater, 55–56
Pain
  anatomy of, 443f
  referred, 443–444
  testing for, 236–237
  use of word, 221–222
  visceral, 442

Pain syndrome, 238–239
Paleocerebellum, 357
Paleopallium, 36, 448
Palpebral fissure, size of, 497
Papilloma, 37
Paradoxical sleep
  components that regulate, 468
  influences of, 469–470
  occurrence of, 468
  regulation of, 470
Paradoxical vestibular system
  disease, 327–328
Paralysis
  characteristics of, 86
  from Encephalitis, 143
  sciatic nerve in Holstein calf, 124f
  tibial nerve in Holstein cow, 124f
Paraparesis, 254–261, 264–265
  in cattle, 123–124
  in Doberman pinscher, 127
  in English Springer spaniel, 114–115
  in Holstein cow, 126–127
  in horse, 126
  in Leonberger, 124–125
Paraplegia, 250–253
  in cat, 115–118
  in Great Dane, 109–110
  in small animal, 250–253
Parasitism, seizures and, 458
Parasympathetic GVE, 188–189, 188f
Parasympathetic nucleus
  of facial nerve, 188–189
  of glossopharyngeal nerve, 189
  of vagus nerve, 189
Parasympathetic system, 168–169
Parelaphostrongylus tenuis, 306f
  clinical signs of, 307
  infection from, 307
  life cycle of, 305–306, 307
  sheep
    cerebellum of, 308f
    thoracic spinal cord of, 308f
Parenchyma
  cerebrospinal fluid and, 60–61
  extracellular fluid compartments
    of, 60
  neoplasm growth in, 69
Paresis
  definition of, 491
  from Encephalitis, 143
  upper motor neuron disease
    and, 204
Paroxysmal dystonic choreoathetosis,
  217–218
Pars ciliaris retina, 392
Pars intermedia, dysfunction of,
  484–485
Pars iridica retina, 392
Pars optica retina
  anatomy of, 394f
  area centralis of, 395–396
  of dog eye, 395f
  external nuclear layer of, 394
  external plexiform layer of,
    394–395
  ganglion layer of, 395
  histology of, 393–396
  of horse eye, 396f
  internal nuclear layer, 395

Pars optica retina *(Continued)*
  internal plexiform layer, 395
  limiting membrane of
    external, 394
    internal, 395
  nerve fiber layer of, 395
  optic disk, 396
  photosensitive layer of, 394
  pigment epithelium of, 393–394
Partial seizure, 455, 462f
Patellar reflex, 82f, 82–84
  evaluation of, 287
  neurologic examination of, 494
Pattern recognition, 491
Paw/hoof replacement test, 87, 492
Pelvic limb
  autonomous zones of, 231f
  dysfunction in German shepherd,
    128–129
  flexor reflex, as part of, 232–233
  fracture of, 121f
  hopping, testing for, 245
  injury to, 197–198
Pelvic limb ataxia, 299f, 300f
Pelvic limb spinal reflex, 83
Penicillium, 215
Peracute coma, 481
Peracute thoracolumbar spinal cord
  lesion, severe, 249
Perilymph, 320
Perineal reflex, 84, 495
Perineum, examination in large
  animal, 287
Peripheral nerve, 441
Peripheral nervous system
  lower motor neuron in, 77
  neuron, maturity of, 27
Peripheral vestibular system
  bilateral dysfunction of, 327
  disease of, 336–337
  disorders of, 325
Petit mal seizure, 455
Pharyngeal paresis, 153
Phenobarbital, 466
Photosensitive layer, 394
Physiologic nystagmus, 482
Physostigmine, 471
Pia mater, 56, 56f
Pig
  cerebellar abiotrophy in, 376
  fibrocartilaginous embolic
    myelopathy in, 315, 315f, 316f
  fracture at L1 in, 315–316
  otitis media-interna in, 149f,
    330f
  poliomyelomalacia in, 118
  stifle arthritis in, 315–316
  vertebral malformation with
    kyphosis, 315–316
Pithing, 62–63
Pituitary macroadenoma, 404f, 517f
Placing response, 493
Plantigrade posture, 128–129
  caudal view of, 129
  in Doberman pinscher, 129
  lateral view of, 129
Plexiform layer
  external, 394–395
  internal, 395

Pleximeter, 83
Polioencephalomalacia, 182–183, 205, 205f, 420
Poliomyelomalacia
in calf, 117, 118
ischemic, 116, 116f
in pig, 117–118, 118f
postoperative in horse, 117, 117f
Polydipsia, 484
Polymicrogyria, 44–45
Polymyositis, 95–96
Polyneuritis equi, 106, 111–112, 114–115
Polyradiculoneuritis, 97–98
characteristics of, 90–92
dorsal and ventral root in dog, 91
facial paresis from, 161
recovery rate from, 91
treatment of, 92
Pons, 32
dysfunction of, 500
lesions in, 229
pathways for voluntary movement, 203f
transverse sections of, 145f
Pontine nucleus, 355–356
Positional nystagmus, 497–498
Postganglionic neuron, 29–30, 180
Postictal depression, 454–455
Postrotatory nystagmus, 326
Postural reactions
backing, 286
circling, 286
in large animal, 286, 493
head elevation, 286
in small animal, 1, 492
swaying, 286
Postural repetitive myoclonus, 215–216
Posture
abnormalities of, 324
decerebellate in cat, 339f
Potassium bromide, 466
Preganglionic neuron, 180
Preganglionic neuronal cell body, 169, 173, 184–186
Presumptive autoimmune myositis, 96
Primordial ganglion, 24f
Prodromal period, 455
Progressive compressive cervical myelopathy, 267–268
Projection axon
development of, 36
processes of, 36–37
Proprioception system, 3t, 4
Proprioceptor, 221
Propulsive activity, 205
Prosencephalic disorder, 398
Prosencephalic hypoplasia, 39, 39f
Prosencephalic lesion, 229
Prosencephalon, 23, 25f
behavioral abnormalities, 452
clinical signs of disorders of, 161
duplication of, 41
extrapyramidal pathways of, 198f
seizure initiation in, 454
See also Lesion; Seizure; Thalamus

Protostrongylid nematode, 306f
Protozoal encephalomyelitis, equine, 164, 297–298, 298f, 341–343
S. neuroma, infection from, 342f
Protozoal myelitis, equine, 107, 295–296, 300f
Protozoal radiculitis, 114, 114f
Psychomotor seizure, 451
Pupil
in acute brain disease, 182–183
anatomy of, 169–170
consciousness, determining level of, 482
control of, 169–173, 170f
enlargement from trauma, 183f
lesions of, 170–173
menace response test for, 495–496
See also Eye; Vision
Pupillary light reflex, 400
Purkinje neuron, 3
cerebellar cortex and, 357
view of, 355f
Pyramidal neuron, 194–195
Pyramidal system
axon organization, 193
cell bodies of
characteristics of, 193
location of, 192–193
components of, 192
development of, 192
disturbances in, 193

Q

Queckenstedt maneuver, 58

R

Rabies, 162
Rabies myelitis, 313
Rachischisis
in puppy, 50f
spina bifida versus, 50–52
Radiculitis, 114, 114f
Rapid eye movement sleep, 468
Receptor
anatomy of, 433–434
for auditory system, 319
classification and location of, 221
for vestibular system, 319–321
Recumbency
in cattle, 98, 98f
in Red bone coonhound, 90
tetraparesis, progressing from, 101
Red nucleus, 198–199
Referred pain
anatomy of, 443–444, 443f
Reflex, 224
Reflex activity, 222, 223f, 227
Reflex general somatic afferent pathway, 230–231, 235–236
Reflex pathway, 399, 442
Reflex sympathetic dystrophy, 190
Regurgitation, 153–154
Release from inhibition, 204
Repetitive myoclonus, 213
acquired action-related, 215
action-related, 214–215
congenital action-related, 215

Repetitive myoclonus (Continued)
constant, 213–214
episodic, 216–217
postural, 215–216
Respiration
consciousness, determining level of, 482
Resting myoclonus, 217
Resting nystagmus, 497–498
Reticular formation, 199
Reticulocerebellar axon, 355–356
Retina, 393
Retrobulbar lesion, right, 171
Retrovirus, type C, 161
Rhinencephalon
components of, 448
development of, 445
Rhombencephalon, 23, 25f, 199
Rhombic lip, 348
Right oculomotor nerve, lesion of, 171
Right optic nerve, lesion of, 170–171
Right retrobulbar lesion, 171
Risus sardonicus, tetanus causing
in Airedale terrier, 210f
in Brittany spaniel, 210f
in coonhound, 210f
in Jersey cow, 210f
Roaring, 158
Roof plate, 32f
Rostral commissure, 37
Rostral mesencephalon, 34f
Rottweiler
inherited disorders of, 274
inherited encephalomyelopathy-polyneuropathy in, 243, 273f
Rubrobulbar axon, 199
Ruminant
camelid spinal cord disease, 306
vestibular system disorders in, 343
See also Goat
Russian knapweed, 205–206

S

Sacral GSE-LMN, 186
Sacral parasympathetic GVE-LMN, 184–185
Sacrocaudal dysfunction
in German Shepherd, 112–114
in horse, 111–112
Sacrocaudal spina bifida, 51
Sarcocystis neurona, 108, 144f, 160–161
equine degenerative myeloencephalopathy, as cause of, 297–298
life cycle of, 298
Sarcolemma, 78
Sarcoma
in cerebrum of horse, 419f
left side menace deficit and, 417–418
osteogenic, 506f, 507f
Sarcoplasmic trough, 78
Schiff-Sherrington syndrome, 248–250, 249f
Schirmer tear test, 189
Schwann cell
Bünger band, formation of, 88
neoplasm in, 139–141

Sciatic nerve paralysis, 124
Scoliosis, 47–48
    See also Cervical scoliosis
Scottie cramps, 217–218
Sea lion
    brain of, 235*f*, 358*f*
    brainstem of, 358*f*
    cerebellum of, 359*f*
Segmental innervation
    of pelvic limb muscles, 84
    of thoracic limb muscles, 85
Seizure
    in Boston terrier, 461, 461*f*
    classification of, 455
    definition of, 454
    examination for
        ancillary, 460–461
        histology of patient, 459–460
        neurologic, 460
        physical, 460–461
    extracranial disorder as cause of,
        457–458
    incidence of, 465
    intracranial disorder as cause of, 457
    pathogenesis of, 455–459
    period of, 455–459
    psychomotor, 451
    surgery for, 468
    treatment for, 465–468
Seizure threshold, 455–456
Self-stimulation, 451
Semicircular canal, 320
Semicircular duct, 320
Sensorineural deafness
    acquired, 439
    congenital inherited, 438–439
Sensorium
    abnormalities in, 484
    neurologic examination and,
        490–491
Sensory (afferent) system, 3*t*, 3–4
    thalamic relay for, 478–479
Sensory ataxia, 228
Sensory ganglioradiculitis, 237–238
Sensory nerve conduction velocity,
    90
Sensory neuron, 2
Sensory system, 77
Severe peracute thoracolumbar spinal
    cord lesion, 249
Sex-linked recessive muscular
    dystrophy, 99–100
Sheep
    cerebellar ataxia in, 375–376
    inherited congenital myotonia in,
        207
    Parelaphostrongylus tenuis in, 308*f*
    stiff lamb disease in, 130
    sympathetic GVE-LMN innervation,
        loss of, 175–176
Shivers, 217
Siamese cat
    meningoencephalitis in, 70*f*
    mesencephalic aqueduct obstruction
        in, 70*f*
Silent retinal degeneration, 404–405
Simple partial seizure, 455
Skeletal muscle (SM), 2*f*, 206
Skull, disarticulation of, 291*f*

Sleep-associated movement
    disorder, 473
Sleep cycle
    components that regulate, 468
    disorders of, 468
    hypocretin, role of, 469
Smell, deficiency in, 445
Soft tissue mass, 122*f*
Sole plate, 78
Solitary tract, 441
Somatic afferent system, 3, 3*t*, 435*f*
Somesthetic cortex
    description and location of, 225
    general proprioception pathways to,
        225–227, 226*f*
Sound wave transmission, 433–434
Spastic hemiparesis, 311*f*
Spasticity, 204
Spastic paraparesis, 299*f*, 300*f*
Spastic paresis, 212–213
Spastic syndrome, 213
Spastic tetraplegia, 87
Special proprioception system, 3*t*, 4,
    322*f*
    cerebellar afferents and, 355
Special somatic afferent (SSA) system,
    3, 3*t*
    visual and auditory, 355
Special visceral afferent, 3*t*, 4
Special visceral afferent system
    for olfaction, 444–446, 446*f*
    for taste, 444, 445*f*
Spina bifida
    in Holstein calf, 46*f*
    rachischisis versus, 50–51
Spinal cord
    arterial vasculature of, 243–244
    of cat, 252*f*
    degeneration of, 240*f*
    development and functional
        organization of, 27–30, 27*f*
    disease of
        Camelid, 306
        in horse, 289
        neurologic signs, 246–250, 246*f*
        Schiff-Sherrington syndrome,
            248–250, 249*f*
        spinal shock, 248–250
    duplication of, 48–49, 49*f*
    dysfunction
        cause of, 243–244
        clinical signs of, 499–500
    lesions of, 178–179, 188
        caudal cervical region, 247, 288
        cranial cervical region, 247–248,
            288–289
        fibrocartilaginous embolic
            myelopathy, 250–251
        lumbosacral region, 247, 288
        thoracolumbar region, 247, 249,
            288
    lymphoma in, 260–261
    malformations of, 48–50
    palpation of segments
        in horse, 63–65
        in ox, 65
    pathways for, 239
Simmenthal calf, malformation in,
    50, 50*f*

Spinal cord (*Continued*)
    spinal dysraphism in weimaraner,
        51–52
    syringohydromyelia in, 49*f*
    topography of, 78
    vestibular nerve and, 322–323
    See also Neurologic examination
Spinal cord reflex, 230*f*
Spinal cord segments
    anatomy of, 79
    C3, C4, C5 in horse, 306*f*
    from C5 to T2, 276*f*
    from C6 to C8, 277*f*
    from C6 to T1 in cat, 276*f*
    C8 and T1, tranverse section of, 276*f*
    cervical, thoracic, and lumbar, view
        of, 303*f*
    growth of, 80–81
    lesions of, 165*f*
    vertebral bodies, relationship to,
        81
    See also Cervical vertebrae; Thoracic
        vertebrae
Spinal dysraphism, 51–52
Spinal ganglion (SG), 2*f*, 28–29, 28*f*
Spinal muscular atrophy, hereditary,
    101
Spinal nerve
    distribution of, 79–80
    evaluation of, 286–287
    GSE-LMN, 78
    inflammed extradural, 111*f*
Spinal nerve general proprioception,
    222–227
Spinal nerve general somatic afferent
    system, 229–234
Spinal nerve reflex
    components of, 82
    evaluation of, 286–288
    functioning of, 83
    neurologic examination of, 494–495
    topographical anatomy of, 83
    types of, 82
Spinal shock, 248–250
Spinocerebellar tract
    cranial, 224
    dorsal, 222
    ventral, 222
Spinothalmic system, 234
Spondylosis deformans, 264–265
Spongioblast, 24–25
Spontaneous nystagmus, 497–498
Sporadic myoclonus, 213, 455
Stair test, 359–360
Stapes, 320
Staphylococcus aureus, 256
Startle disease, 212
Static equilibrium, 321
Static stenosis
    indication of, 291–292
    in Thoroughbred, 291*f*
Statoconia (otolith), 321
Status epilepticus, 455, 467
Stellated neuron, 194–195
Stenosis
    dynamic, 291–292
    in horse, 290–291
    in small animal, 269–270
    static, 291–292

Stereocilia, 286
Stiff lamb disease, 130
Stiff man syndrome, 215
Stifle arthritis, 313–316
Stimulation
  self versus direct, 451
  vagal, 467–468
Storage disease
  cause of, 426–427
  clinical signs of, 427
  in domestic animals, 427–428*t*
Strabismus
  cranial nerve examination for, 497
  neuromuscular, 137
  vestibular system disorders and, 326
Streptococcus equi, 159
Streptococcus species, 256
Strongylus vulgaris, 424*f*, 425*f*
Stylohyoidosteopathy
  diagnosis of, 149–150
  in horse, 150*f*
Subarachnoid cyst, 56
Subarachnoid diverticulum, 56, 263
Subarachnoid hemorrhage, 281*f*, 282*f*
Subarachnoid space, 55–56
Subfalcine herniation, 58–59
Substantia nigra, 198–199
Subthalamic nucleus, 33–35, 196*f*
Subthalamus, 33–35, 196–198
Sudden acquired retinal degeneration
  (SARD), 401, 404–406
Sunset eyes, 72
Suppurative inflammation, 1
Swaying, 286
Sweating
  Horner syndrome and, 176, 178–179
  in horse, 177–178, 177*f*, 178*f*
Swimmer syndrome, 115
Swinging light maneuver, 401
Sympathetic GVE-LMN innervation
  clinical signs of loss, 175–176
  of eye, 173–182
  loss in vasoconstrictor smooth
    muscle, 175*f*
Sympathetic paralysis, 287–288
Sympathetic system, 168–169
Sympathetic trunk, 29–30
Synapse, 2
Syncope, 470–471
Syringohydromyelia
  cause and characteristics of, 47–48
  developmental obstructive
    hydrocephalus causing, 72
  transverse view of, 49*f*
Syringomyelia, 47
Syrinx, 56

T

Tail, examination in large animal, 287
Taste, 444
Telencephalic aplasia, 39
Telencephalic commissural pathway,
  development of, 38*f*
Telencephalic neuronal cell body,
  location of, 36
Telencephalon, 25*f*
  afferent hypothalamic tract, 483
  anatomy of, 448–449, 449*f*, 450*f*

Telencephalon (*Continued*)
  basal nuclei of, 198*f*
  choroid plexus and ventricular
    system, development of, 35*f*
  development of, 36*f*
  dysfunction of, 500
  extrapyramidal nuclei of, 197*f*
  formation of, 35–37
  neuronal cell bodies in, 194–200
  neuronal processes in, 37*f*
  See also Cerebrum
Telodendron, 2*f*, 2–3
Temperature regulation, abnormal, 484
Temporal lobe, lesions of, 451–452
Temporohyoid osteopathy, 340–341
Tendon-muscle reflex, 85
Tetanus
  in Brittany spaniel, 210*f*
  definition of, 209
  opisthotonus and extensor rigidity
    form, 209
  risus sardonicus from
    in Airedale terrier, 210*f*
    in Brittany spaniel, 210*f*
    in coonhound, 210*f*
    in Jersey cow, 210*f*
  signs and cause of, 209
Tetany, 217
  clinical signs of, 211–213
  inherited congenital, in Hereford
    calf, 107*f*
  in King Charles spaniels, 212
Tetraparesis, 271–276
  case study
    in German Shepherd, 97–98
    in Labrador retriever, 98–99
  hypokalemic myopathy as cause of,
    97–98
  recumbency, progressing to, 101
Tetraparesis-ataxia
  pelvic limb, case example, 280
  thoracic limb, case example, 279
Tetraplegia
  in dachshund, 118–119
  in small animal, 266, 267
    atlantoaxial subluxation,
      268–269, 269*f*
    degenerative joint disease,
      270–271
    vertebral malformation-
      malarticulation, 268–271
Thalamencephalon, 33–35
Thalamic association system, 479
Thalamic relay, 478
Thalamic reticular system, 479
Thalamocortical pathway, 436–437
Thalamus
  anatomy of, 476–477
  functional organization of, 478*f*
  function of, 480–481
  lesions, clinical signs of, 480–481
  nuclear groups, 478*f*
  nuclei of, 23, 196–198
  transverse view of, 34*f*
Thiamin deficiency encephalopathy,
  182–183, 420–421
  in domestic shorthair, 421*f*
  in mixed breed dog, 421*f*
  in steer, 420*f*

Third eyelid, protrusion of, 183–184,
  497
Thoracic autonomic nerves, 180*f*
Thoracic limb
  autonomous zones of, 232*f*
  flexor reflex, as part of, 232
  hopping, testing for, 245
  postural reaction testing, 492–494
Thoracic limb reflex, 85–86
Thoracic vertebrae
  first, 275*f*, 276*f*
  fourth, 281*f*
  See also Spinal cord segments
Thoracolumbar dysfunction, 499–500
Thoracolumbar lesion, 247, 249
Thoracolumbar system, 168–169
Thorax, radiodense mass in, 181*f*
Three-strikes rule, 62–63
Thromboembolism, aortic, 115–116
Thrombotic meningoencephalitis, 162
  cause of, 344
Thrombus, 303*f*
Tibial nerve
  hypertrophic neuropathy affecting,
    125*f*
  paralysis in cow, 124*f*
  paresis, diabetes-related neuropathy,
    124–125
Tick paralysis, 95, 161
Titubation, 359–360
Tonic neck test, 229
Tonsillar herniation, 58–59
Toxicity
  organophosphate anthelmintic
    haloxone causing, 159
Transtentorial herniation
  in Morgan horse, 59*f*
Tremor. *See* Myoclonus
Tricep reflex, 61, 84
Trigeminal nerve
  evaluation of, 498
  GSA pathway for, 235*f*
  GSA system and, 234
  lymphoma in, 142*f*
  of sea lion, 234, 235*f*
  spinal tract formation, 234
Trigeminal neuritis
  boxer with, 143*f*
  in cat, 144*f*
  effects of, 142–144
  in English setter, 143*f*
  keratitis sicca development, 189
Trigeminal neuron
  anatomy of, 139
  function, loss of, 139
  malignant nerve sheath neoplasm,
    139–141
    in beagle, 140*f*
    in West Highland terrier, 141*f*
Trigeminal neuropathy, 142–144
Trigeminal proprioceptive pathway,
  228*f*
Trochlear nerve
  anatomy of, 135
  lesions of, 138
  strabismus, direction following
    paralysis, 138*f*
Tuberal group, 483
Two-engine gait, 274

Tympanic bulla, 330f, 331f
Tyrosine, 29–30

U

Unilateral optic tract lesion, 171
Unilateral peripheral vestibular
　disease, 324–327
Unilateral retinal lesion, 401
Upper motor neuron (UMN)
　abnormal gait, 243–284
　bladder of, 187
　cerebellum, projection of
　　information, 355–356
　contralateral motor function,
　　control of, 356f
　disease, clinical signs of, 204–206
　dysfunction, signs of, 228
　function of, 200–204
　lesions of, 221
　paresis of, 86
　pathways for voluntary movement,
　　203f
　prosencephalic anatomic pathways
　　for, 239f
　spinal cord anatomic pathways for,
　　240f
　tetraparesis-ataxia, thoracic limb,
　　274–276
Uremia, 458
Urinary incontinence, 187
Urine, 186
Utriculus, 321

V

Vagal stimulation, 467–468
Vagus nerve, 152f, 153, 189
Vascular compromise, 379–382
Vasculitis, 303f
Ventral caudal lateral nucleus,
　479
Ventral caudal medial nucleus, 479
Ventral caudal thalamic nucleus,
　225
Ventral lateral nucleus, 479
Ventral root (VR), 2f
Ventral rostral nucleus, 479
Ventral spinocerebellar tract, 222

Ventral tegmental decussation,
　356–357
Ventricular system
　of canine, 57f
　development of, 35f
　meninges and subarachnoid space,
　　55f
Venturi effect, 47–48
Veratrum californicum, 42
Vertebral column
　development in embryo, 79–80
　growth of, 80–81
　malformations of, 48–50
　spinal cord segments, relationship
　　to, 81f
Vertebral malformation, 297–315
Vertebral malformation-
　malarticulation, 268–269
　acquired, 290
　C5 in Doberman pinscher, 270f
　C7 with narrow cranial orifice,
　　269f, 270f
　congenital, 289–290
　dorsal subluxation, 269f
Vessel wall degeneration, 303f
Vestibular, 320
Vestibular ataxia, 324, 491–492
Vestibular cerebellum, 349–352
Vestibular ganglion, 321–322
Vestibular nuclei, 322–324
Vestibular receptor, 322f
Vestibular strabismus, 139
Vestibular system
　anatomy and physiology of, 319–324
　anatomy of, 321f, 322f
　disease of
　　in cats, 335–336
　　clinical signs of, 324–328
　　in dogs, 328–346
　　in horse, 340–341
　　in ruminants, 343
　　disorders of central components of,
　　　325
　nuclei and tracts, 323f
　postural reaction testing, 326–327
　role of, 319
Vestibule, large, 320
Vestibulocochlear nerve, 321–322, 434
Viral myelitis, 304

Visceral afferent system, 3t, 3–4
Visceral pain, 442, 443f
Vision
　clinical tests for, 399–400
　consciousness, determining level of,
　　481
　deficit, signs of, 171t
　lesions restricting, 170
　menace response test for, 399–400,
　　402–403
　See also Eye; Pupil
Visual cortex, 399
Visual system
　disease of
　　abnormal pupil, 402–403
　　normal pupil, 408–409
　lesions of, 400–402, 401t
Vitamin A
　blindness and, 407–408
　deficiency in calf, 70
Vitamin E
　deficiency myopathy, 130
　equine degenerative
　　myeloencephalopathy,
　　294–295
　equine motor neuron disease and,
　　102

W

Wallerian degeneration
　characteristics of, 88–89
　of lower motor neuron, 89
Water consumption, abnormal, 484
Wheelbarrowing, 493
White shaker syndrome, 215
Wilm tumor, 255–256
Withdrawal-flexor reflex, 494–495
Withdrawal reflex, 83–84
Wobbler syndrome, 269, 290

Y

Yellow star thistle, 205–206

Z

Zona incerta, 196–198, 196f
Zonisamide, 467